BLACKWELL'S NURSING
DICTIONARY

BLACKWELL'S NURSING DICTIONARY

Editors

Dawn Freshwater

Institute of Health and Community Studies,
Bournemouth University, Bournemouth, UK
and Edith Cowan University, Perth

and

Sian E. Maslin-Prothero

University of Southampton, School of Nursing
and Midwifery, Southampton, UK

Blackwell
Publishing

© 1994 Blackwell Science, 2005 by
Blackwell Publishing Ltd

Editorial offices:
Blackwell Publishing Ltd, 9600 Garsington Road, Oxford OX4 2DQ, UK
Tel: +44 (0)1865 776868
Blackwell Publishing Asia Pty Ltd, 550 Swanston Street, Carlton, Victoria 3053, Australia
Tel: +61 (0)3 8359 1011

First published 1994
Reprinted 1997, 1998, 2001, 2002
Second edition published 2005

This second edition is a comprehensive revision of the first edition of *Blackwell's Dictionary of
Nursing*, first published in 1994. The first edition was updated and adapted from *Duncan's
Dictionary for Nurses* by Helen A. Duncan, published by Springer Publishing Co. Inc., New York,
in 1989. Permission for this adaption is acknowledged.

Library of Congress Cataloging-in-Publication Data is available

ISBN 1-4051-0534-8

A catalogue record for this title is available from the British Library

Set in 8 on 9pt Times
by Kolam Informations Services Pvt. Ltd, Pondicherry, India
Printed and bound in Great Britain
by CPI Bath

The publisher's policy is to use permanent paper from mills that operate a sustainable forestry
policy, and which has been manufactured from pulp processed using acid-free and elementary
chlorine-free practices. Furthermore, the publisher ensures that the text paper and cover board used
have met acceptable environmental accreditation standards.

For further information on Blackwell Publishing, visit our website:
www.blackwellnursing.com

CONTENTS

FOREWORD

It gives me great pleasure to introduce this edition of Blackwell's Nursing Dictionary. Those contributing to this edition have produced an excellent textbook, one that will be an invaluable resource and practical guide for both students of nursing and more experienced nurses in clinical practice, research, policy and higher education.

The resources included in this edition cover an impressive range of useful information on professional practice. It includes normal definitions and measures, details of professional organisations and journals, continuing professional development, the Code of Professional Practice, the quality assurance framework for higher education and a guide to understanding and implementing clinical research in practice. The dictionary will, without doubt, add to our understanding of a range of professional issues in clinical practice across all areas of nursing.

The volume of information needed by nurses is increasing all the time, and more and more patients will turn to nurses for health-related information, trusting in them for appropriate help and support. There is a growing desire among patients and the public to take more control of their own health, and to have high quality personalised care, including better access to information and wider choice about their care and treatment. Most patients would like to be more involved in their care and provided with more information about their treatment, tests and investigations.

While much has been achieved, we still need to shift the culture of the NHS from one of dependency to one of increased independence and self care. The language we use – and the way we use it – is an important factor in shifting the balance of power in our relationships with patients and carers.

We need to ensure that patients and carers experience effective communication that is sensitive to their individual needs and preferences, and that it promotes high quality care for the patient.

This highlights the importance of using straightforward language, keeping information up to date and factual, and avoiding jargon and abbreviations in our day-to-day contact with patients and carers. We need to communicate technical and evidence-based information in a way that matches the patient's level of understanding, checking that information given is understood and the meaning is the same for all involved. This will involve developing new relationships with patients, where we see information from the patient's perspective, where information is reviewed by patients, carers and nurses to ensure it is accessible to them and applicable to their needs. We need to look at how we use information and develop a greater awareness of the use of language and its influence on our relationships with patients. Used effectively, it can be a key factor in establishing trusting relationships between patients and nurses.

The contributors have put together an excellent resource and a valuable tool for all areas of nursing. The real challenge lies in how we use this knowledge to build our relationships with patients and carers – so that they are fully engaged in their own care, the way it is planned and delivered, and personalised to their individual needs and choices.

Sarah Mullally
Chief Nursing Officer
Department of Health
England

LIST OF CONTRIBUTORS

Professor Dawn Freshwater PhD BA (Hons) RGN RNT FRCN DipPsych
Professor of Mental Health and Primary Care, IHCS, Bournemouth
University, UK, and Edith Cowan University, Perth, Australia
Dawn is Professor of Mental Health and Primary Care at IHCS Bournemouth University and is leading the development of an Academic Research Centre in Practice with North and Southwest Dorset NHS Trusts. Having completed her nurse training in 1983 she worked in both acute and community settings before undertaking her first degree at the Institute of Advanced Nurse Education, Royal College of Nursing, later completing her PhD at University of Nottingham. The focus of her work has been on critical reflexivity, practice-based research, and therapeutic practice, and she has successfully managed a number of funded research projects in these areas. It was for this work that she was awarded the Sigma Theta Tau Honor Society distinguished nurse researcher award (2000) and a Fellowship of the Royal College of Nursing (2002). She is widely published in her field, with her books being translated into other languages. She sits on a number of editorial boards and committees, including the International Association for Human Caring and the Florence Nightingale Foundation.

Garfield J. Griffiths BEd (Hons) DipN RN ONC RCNT
Senior Lecturer, University of the West of England, Bristol, UK
Garfield Griffiths qualified as a general nurse in South Wales (1970), he practised as a staff nurse on a male mixed speciality ward and went on to specialize in orthopaedics at The Royal National Orthopaedic Hospital, London. In 1973 he took up his first charge nurses post at The Prince of Wales Hospital, Wales. Three years later he became a clinical teacher to the orthopaedic course in that hospital. During this time he studied for the RCN Clinical Teachers Certificate and the London University Diploma in Nursing. His current post is senior lecturer at The University of the West of England, where he has held the roles of award route leader for the Diploma in Professional Studies Award and field leader for the post-qualifying modules.

Dr Sian E. Maslin-Prothero RN RM DipN CertEd MSc PhD
Senior Lecturer at the School of Nursing and Midwifery,
University of Southampton, UK
Sian has worked in academic, education, clinical nursing, and midwifery in a variety of settings in both the United Kingdom and overseas. She has a Master of Science degree from the University of Bristol and a Doctor of Philosophy from the University of Nottingham. Her research interests include policy and practice in the NHS, and the recruitment of women to breast cancer clinical trials, user and carer involvement in health and social care. Sian believes in helping individuals to fulfil their potential by fostering skills and strategies that encourage them to be creative, critical thinkers who can respond to the dynamic health-care environment and the requirements of users.

Abigail Masterson MN BSc RGN PGCEA
Abi has run her own consultancy company since January 1998. Prior to this she held clinical, education, and research posts in organizations including St. Bartholomew's Hospital, the Royal College of Nursing, and the Department of Social Medicine and School for Policy Studies at the University of Bristol. She works with many local and national and international healthcare organizations to develop policies, review services, and carry out research into new roles and service developments across the healthcare professions. Abi has both a Bachelors and Masters degree in nursing, and has a varied list of publications, particularly in new role development, competence assessment, and health policy.

Les Storey FRCN RGN MSc PGDipHE
Principal Lecturer, Faculty of Health, University of
Central Lancashire, UK
Les qualified in 1970 and spent over 14 years in operating theatres before moving into the fields of education and research. Since 1989 he has been involved nationally and internationally in the development and implementation of competency-based approaches within nursing and healthcare. He has been involved in managing a number of research and development projects, has published widely and presented papers at a number of international and national conferences. In 2000 he was conferred as a Fellow of the Royal College of Nursing for his work on competency-based education, and in 2001 was awarded the Edith Cavell scholarship by the Florence Nightingale Foundation.

ACKNOWLEDGEMENTS

When we agreed to undertake this project neither of us realized the amount of effort and concentration that would be required, not only of us, but also of the individuals who had agreed to provide their time and intellect. We would like to thank those people who have supported us in the development and completion of what we believe is a dictionary that is nursing focused, drawing on the dynamic and contemporary health-care context that we now enjoy. In particular, we would like to acknowledge Professor Veronica Bishop, Alison Twycross, Theo Stickley, Abi Masterson, Linda Antoniw Sarah Fisher, Julia Wynn, Tom Tait, Mary Foss, Liz Walsh, and Elizabeth Rosser. We would also like to thank Beth Knight and the staff at Blackwell Publishing for their encouragement and advice.

D.F.
S.M-P.

The publishers would like to thank *Nursing Times* for permission to reproduce the handwashing diagram on page 55, reprinted from the sixth edition of *The Royal Marsden Hospital Manual of Clinical Nursing Procedures*, edited by Lisa Dougherty and Sara Lister and published in 2004 by Blackwell Publishing Ltd; and the Royal Marsden Hospital for permission to reproduce the figures from the same source on pages 494 and 596. Other illustrations in the Dictionary are taken from the following, all published by Blackwell Publishing, who would like to acknowledge their endebtedness to these authors:

Barrett, J. (1983) *Accident and Emergency Nursing*.
Bray, J.J. Cragg, P.A. Macknight, A.D.C. Mills, R.G. and Taylor, D.W. (1989) *Lecture Notes on Human Physiology* Second Edition.
Gibson, J. (1981) *Modern Physiology and Anatomy for Nurses* Second Edition.
Hickman, M. (1985) *Midwifery* Second Edition.
Middleton, D. (1986) *Nursing 2*.
Moffat, D.B. (1987) *Lecture Notes on Anatomy*.

Appendix 4 is reproduced by permission of the Nursing and Midwifery Council, and Appendix 9 by permission of The Quality Assurance Agency for Higher Education.

PRONUNCIATION

The system of pronunciation used has deliberately been kept simple. Words that the nurse might have difficulty pronouncing are broken down into their component syllables and respelled phonetically. The accented syllables are indicated by a slanting mark at their terminations (').

Vowels
Vowels may be pronounced long or short. When short, they are unmarked and are pronounced as follows:

a as in fat or father

e as in bed

i as in fit

o as in for or hot

oo as in tool

u as in but

When long, they are given a long mark and are pronounced as follows:

ā as in tame

ē as in he

ī as in time

ō as in over

ū as in use

Other long vowels are:

ah as in spa

ai as in air

aw as in saw

Words that end with *y* are usually pronounced as though they ended with a short *i*, as, for example, chemistry (kem'-is-tri).

Consonants
Consonants ordinarily take the common English language pronunciation. When this is not the case, the word is respelled phonetically, for example:

c may be pronounced as *s* or *k* as in cicatrix (sik'-a-triks)

ch may be pronounced as *k* as in psychosis (sī-kō'-sis)

g may be pronounced as *j* as in pharyngeal (far-in'-jē-al)

ph is usually pronounced as *f* as in physical (fiz'-i-kal)

psy is pronounced as *sī* as in psyche (sī'-kē)

-sion may be pronounced *shun* as in compassion (kom-pa'shun) or *zhun* as in explosion (eks-plō'zhun)

-tion is usually pronounced *shun*.

ABBREVIATIONS

AA	Alcoholics Anonymous
ABC	airway, breathing, and circulation
Abd	abdomen
ABE	acute bacterial endocarditis
ABGs	arterial blood gases
ACE	angiotensin-converting enzyme
ACTH	adrenocorticotrophic hormone
ADH	antidiuretic hormone
ADHD	attention deficit hyperactivity disorder
ADL	activities of daily living
ADP	adenosine diphosphate
AF	atrial fibrillation
AFP	alpha-fetoprotein
AHF	antihaemophilic factor
AI	(1) aortic insufficiency; (2) artificial insemination
AID	artificial insemination using donor semen
AIDS	acquired immune deficiency syndrome
AIH	artificial insemination using husband's semen
ALG	antilymphocyte globulin
ALS	(1) advanced life support; (2) amyotrophic lateral sclerosis; (3) antilymphocyte serum
AMP	adenosine monophosphate
ANF	antinuclear factor
ANOVA	analysis of variance
anti-HBc	antibody against hepatitis B core antigen
anti-HBe	antibody against hepatitis B e antigen
anti-HBs	antibody against hepatitis B surface antigen
APCL	accreditation (assessment) of prior certificated learning
APEL	accreditation (assessment) of prior experiential learning
APL	accreditation (assessment) of prior learning
APT	alum-precipitated diphtheria toxoid
ARC	AIDS-related complex
ASD	atrial septal defect
ASO	antistreptolysin O
ATP	adenosine triphosphate

ATS	antitetanus serum
ATT	antitetanus toxoid
A-V	atrioventricular
BA	Bachelor of Arts
BACP	British Association of Counselling and Psychotherapy
BAI	Beck anxiety inventory
BAOT	British Association of Occupational Therapists
BBB	blood−brain barrier
BCC	basal cell carcinoma
BCG	bacillus Calmette−Guérin
bd	*bis die* (used in prescriptions, meaning twice daily)
BDI	Beck depression inventory
BEd	Bachelor of Education
BHS	Beck hopelessness scale
BIT	binary digit
BLS	basic life support
BMA	British Medical Association
BMI	body mass index
BMR	basal metabolic rate
BN	Bachelor of Nursing
BNF	British National Formulary
BP	blood pressure
BSc	Bachelor of Science
BSE	bovine spongiform encephalopathy
CAL	computer-assisted learning
CAPD	continuous ambulatory peritoneal dialysis
CARATS	Counselling, Assessment, Referral, Advice, and Throughcare Scheme
CAT	computerized axial tomography
CATS	Credit Accumulation Transfer System
CBT	cognitive behavioural therapy
CCETSW	Central Council for the Education and Training in Social Work
CCF	congestive cardiac failure
CCU	(1) coronary care unit; (2) cardiac care unit
CD	controlled drug
CDC	Centers for Disease Control (USA)
CD-ROM	compact disc read-only memory
CF	cystic fibrosis
CHAI	Commission for Health-care Audit and Inspection
CHC	Community Health Council
CHD	coronary heart disease
CHF	congestive heart failure
CHI	Commission for Health Improvement
CINAHL	Cumulative Index to Nursing and Allied Health Literature
CJD	Creutzfeldt−Jakob disease
CMHT	community mental health team

CMV	cytomegalovirus
CNO	Chief Nursing Officer
CNS	(1) central nervous system; (2) clinical nurse specialist
COAD	chronic obstructive airways disease
COPD	chronic obstructive pulmonary disease
COSHH	Control of Substances Hazardous to Health
CPA	Care Programme Approach
CPAP	continuous positive airways pressure
CPD	continuing professional development
CPK	creatinine phosphokinase
CPN	community psychiatric nurse
CPPIH	Commission for Patient and Public Involvement in Health
CPR	cardiopulmonary resuscitation
CPU	central processing unit
CRP	C-reactive protein
CSF	cerebrospinal fluid
CSP	Chartered Society of Physiotherapists
CSSD	Central Sterile Supplies Department
CSSU	Central Sterile Supply Unit
CT	computed tomography
CV	curriculum vitae
CVA	cerebrovascular accident
CVP	central venous pressure
CVS	(1) cardiovascular system; (2) chorionic villus sampling
CXR	chest x-ray
D and C	dilatation and curettage
DASE	Denver Articulation Screening Examination
DBT	dialectical behavioural therapy
DC	direct current
DDA	Disability Discrimination Act
DES	diethylstilboestrol
DI	donor insemination
DIC	disseminated intravascular coagulation
DipHE	Diploma in Higher Education
DipEd	Diploma in Education
DipN	Diploma in Nursing
DipNEd	Diploma in Nursing Education
DLCC	Disabled Living Centres Council
DN	district nurse
DNA	deoxyribonucleic acid
DOA	death on arrival
DOH	Department of Health
DPhil	Doctor of Philosophy
DPT	diphtheria−pertussis−tetanus (vaccine)
DQ	developmental quotient

DRC	Disability Rights Commission
DSM IV	*Diagnostic and Statistical Manual of Mental Disorders*, 4th edition
DSPD	dangerous and severe personality disorder
DTP	diphtheria–tetanus–pertussis (vaccine)
DTs	delerium tremens
DVT	deep vein thrombosis
EBL	enquiry-based learning
EBM	evidence-based medicine
EBP	evidence-based practice
EC	European Community
ECG	electrocardiogram
ECT	electroconvulsive therapy
ECV	external cephalic version
EDD	expected date of delivery
EDTA	ethylenediamine-tetra-acetic acid
EEG	electroencephalogram
EKG	electrocardiogram
ELISA	enzyme-linked immunosorbent assay
EMG	electromyogram
ENT	ear, nose and throat
ERG	electroretinogram
ERPC	evacuation of retained products of conception
ESR	erythrocyte sedimentation rate
EU	European Union
EUA	examination under anaesthetic
FBC	full blood count
FBS	fasting blood sugar
FEV	forced expiratory volume
FPCert	Family Planning Certificate
FRC	functional residual capacity
FRCGP	Fellow of the Royal College of General Practitioners
FRCN	Fellow of the Royal College of Nursing
FRCOG	Fellow of the Royal College of Obstetricians and Gynaecologists
FRCP	Fellow of the Royal College of Physicians
FRCPath	Fellow of the Royal College of Pathologists
FRCPE	Fellow of the Royal College of Physicians of Edinburgh
FRCPI	Fellow of the Royal College of Ireland
FRCPsych	Fellow of the Royal College of Psychologists
FRCR	Fellow of the Royal College of Radiologists
FRCS	Fellow of the Royal College of Surgeons
FRCSE	Fellow of the Royal College of Surgeons of Edinburgh
FRCSI	Fellow of the Royal College of Surgeons of Ireland
FSH	follicle-stimulating hormone
FVC	forced vital capacity
GABA	gamma-aminobutyric acid

GFR	glomerular filtration rate
GGTP	gamma-glutamyl transpeptidase
GH	growth hormone
GHIH	growth hormone inhibiting hormone
GHRH	growth hormone releasing hormone
GI	gastrointestinal
GIFT	gamete intrafallopian transfer
GM	genetically modified
GMC	General Medical Council
GP	general practitioner
GSCC	General Social Care Council
GTN	glyceryl trinitrate
GUM	genitourinary medicine
GVHD	graft-versus-host disease
HAZ	Health Action Zone
Hb	haemoglobin
HBcAg	hepatitis B core antigen
HBeAg	hepatitis B e antigen
HBIG	hepatitis B immunoglobulin
HBsAg	hepatitis B surface antigen
HBV	hepatitis B virus
HC	head circumference
HCA	health-care assistant
hCG	human chorionic gonadotrophin
HCO	health-care officer
HCV	hepatitis C virus
HDL	high-density lipoprotein
HDU	high dependency unit
HEI	higher education institutions
HGC	Human Genetics Commission
Hib vaccine	*Haemophilus influenzae* type B vaccine
HImP	Health Improvement Programme
HIV	human immunodeficiency virus
HMSO	Her Majesty's Stationery Office
HoNOS	Health of the Nation Outcome Scale
HPC	Health Professions Council
HPV	human papilloma virus
HRT	hormone replacement therapy
HSV	herpes simplex virus
HTLV	human T-cell leukaemia–lymphoma virus
HV	health visitor
HVCert	Health Visitor's Certificate
HTML	hypertext markup language
IBD	inflammatory bowel disease
IBS	irritable bowel syndrome

ICAS	Independent Complaints Advocacy Service
ICD	International Classification of Diseases
ICN	International Council of Nurses
ICPs	integrated care pathways
ICU	Intensive Care Unit
IDDM	insulin dependent diabetes mellitus
IM&T	information management and technology
IPPB	intermittent positive pressure breathing
IPPV	intermittent positive pressure ventilation
IPV	inactivated poliovirus vaccine
IQ	intelligence quotient
IRP	Independent Reconfiguration Panel
IT	information technology
ITU	intensive therapy unit
IU	International Unit
IUCD	intrauterine contraceptive device
IUD	intrauterine device
IV	intravenous
IVF	*in vitro* fertilization
IVI	intravenous infusion
IVP	intravenous pyelogram
IVT	intravenous therapy
LDH	lactic acid dehydrogenase
LDP	Local Delivery Plan
LFT	liver function test
LH	luteinizing hormone
LHRH	luteinizing hormone releasing hormone
LMP	last menstrual period
LREC	Local Research Ethics Committee
LRT	lower respiratory tract
LSD	lysergic acid diethylamide
LSP	Local Strategic Partnership
LVF	left ventricular failure
MA	Master of Arts
MAO	monoamine oxidase
MBA	Master of Business Administration
MCH	mean cell haemoglobin
MCV	mean cell volume
MD	Doctor of Medicine
MDMA	methylenedioxymethamphetamine
ME	myalgic encephalomyelitis
MEd	Master of Education
MI	myocardial infarction
MIND	National Association for Mental Health
MMR	measles, mumps, and rubella vaccine

MPhil	Master of Philosophy
MRC	Medical Research Council
MREC	Multi Research Ethics Committee
MRI	magnetic resonance imaging
MRSA	methicillin-resistant *Staphylococcus aureus*
MRV	minute respiratory volume
MS	multiple sclerosis
MSc	Master of Science
MSU	midstream specimen of urine
NA	Nomina Anatomica
NatPaCT	National Primary and Care Trust Development
NBM	nil (nothing) by mouth
NCSC	National Care Standards Commission
NCVQ	National Council for Vocational Qualifications
NDU	Nursing Development Unit
NEC	necrotizing enterocolitis
NeLH	National Electronic Library for Health
NG	nasogastric
NHS	National Health Service
NHSCRD	National Health Service Centre for Reviews and Dissemination
NICE	National Institute for Clinical Excellence
NICU	neonatal intensive care unit
NIDDM	non-insulin-dependent diabetes mellitus
NIPPV	non-invasive positive pressure ventilation
NMC	Nursing and Midwifery Council
NMR	nuclear magnetic resonance
NPN	non-protein nitrogen
NREM	non-rapid eye movements
NRR	National Research Register
NSAIDs	non-steroidal anti-inflammatory drugs
NSFs	National Service Frameworks
NTO	National Training Organisation
NVQ	National Vocational Qualification
ONS	Office of National Statistics
OPCS	Office of Population Censuses and Surveys
OR	odds ratio
OTC	over the counter
PAF	performance assessment framework
PALS	Patient Advice and Liaison Service
PBL	problem-based learning
p.c.	after meals
PCA	patient-controlled analgesia
PCG	Primary Care Group
PCO_2	partial pressure of carbon dioxide
PCR	practitioner-centred research

PCT	Primary Care Trust
PD	personality disorder
PEEP	positive end expiratory pressure
PFI	Private Finance Initiative
PPD	Purified Protein Derivative
PREP	Post-Registration Education and Practice
p.r.n.	whenever necessary
PROMIS	problem-oriented medical information
PSI	psycho-social intervention
PTSD	post-traumatic stress disorder
PUO	pyrexia of undetermined origin
PV	polycythaemia vera
PVC	premature ventricular contraction
QAA	Quality Assessment Agency for Higher Education
QCA	Qualifications and Curriculum Authority
QUALYs	quality adjusted life years
RAE	Research Assessment Exercise
RCTs	randomized controlled trials
REM	rapid eye movements
RNA	ribonucleic acid
SAD	seasonal affective disorder
SARS	severe acute respiratory syndrome
SCBU	special care baby unit
SCID	severe combined immunodeficiency disease
SCM	State Certified Midwife
SCOTEC	Scottish Technical Education Council
SD	standard deviation
SE	standard error
SHO	senior house officer
SIDS	sudden infant death syndrome
SNOMED	Systemized Nomenclature of Medicine
SPSS	Statistical Package for Social Sciences
SQA	Scottish Qualifications Authority
SRN	State Registered Nurse
stat	statim
STD	sexually transmitted disease
STI	sexually transmitted infection
SVQ	Scottish Vocational Qualification
SVT	supraventricular tachycardia
TABS	temperature, airway, beathing, sugar
TB	tuberculosis (tubercle bacillus)
tds	three times daily
TEDs	thrombo embolic deterrent (stockings)
TENS	transcutaneous electrical nerve stimulation
TIA	transient ischaemic attack

TOP	termination of pregnancy
TOPV	trivalent oral poliovirus vaccine
TPI	*Treponema pallidum* immobilization (test)
TPN	total parenteral nutrition
TPR	temperature, pulse, respiration
TQM	total quality management
TRIC	trachoma and inclusion conjuctivitis
TSH	thyroid-stimulating hormone
TURP	transurethral resection of tumour
TV	tidal volume
UKCC	United Kingdom Central Council for Nursing, Midwifery and Health Visiting
ung	*unguent* (ointment)
UNICEF	United Nations International Children's Fund
UTI	urinary tract infection
UVA	ultraviolet light A
UVB	ultraviolet light B
VC	vital capacity
vCJD	variant Creutzfeldt-Jakob disease
VDU	visual display unit
VF	ventricular fibrillation
VSD	ventricular septal defect
VSO	Voluntary Service Overseas
VT	ventricular tachycardia
WBC	white blood cells/count
WDC	Workforce Development Confederation
WHO	World Health Organization
WTE	Whole Time Equivalent
www	world wide web
ZIFT	zygote intrafallopian transfer

A

Ar: Chemical symbol for argon.

a-; an-: Prefixes denoting absence, separation, away, away from, without, not, less, lacking, lack of; a — when used before a consonant; an — when before a vowel.

AA: Abbreviation for Alcoholics Anonymous (*q.v.*).

ab-: Prefix denoting absent, away from, off, negative, separation, departure from, outside, deviating from.

abacterial (ā-bak-tē'-ri-al): Without bacteria; free from bacteria. A. MENINGITIS aseptic meningitis, see under MENINGITIS.

abaragnosis (a-bar-og-nō'-sis): Lack or loss of the conscious perception of weight, or of the ability to estimate weight.

abarthrosis (ab ar-thrō'-sis): Diarthrosis (*q.v.*).

abarticulation (ab'-ar-tik-ū-lā'-shun): 1. The dislocation of a joint. 2. A synovial or freely movable joint; *e.g.*, the hip. See DIARTHROSIS.

abasia (a-bā'-zi-a): Inability to walk, or unsteadiness of gait, due to motor incoordination. ASTASIA A. see under ASTASIA. — abasic, abatic, adj.

abatement (a-bāt'-ment): A decrease or lessening of a symptom or of pain. — abate, v.

Abbott-Miller tube: A long double-lumen intestinal tube with an inflatable balloon attached to the distal end; used in certain diagnostic tests, to treat an obstruction in the small intestine, and to relieve distension of the intestine.

ABC: In emergency medicine, refers to Airway, Breathing, and Circulation in regard to priority of care.

Abd: Abbreviation for abdomen (*q.v.*).

abdomen (ab'-do-men): The belly. The largest body cavity; lies between the thorax, from which it is separated by the diaphragm, and the pelvis; is enclosed by a wall made up of muscles, the vertebral column and the two ilia; contains the stomach, small and large intestine, liver, gallbadder, pancreas, spleen, the descending aorta and inferior vena cava, and (behind the peritoneum) the kidneys and ureters. It is lined with a serous membrane, the peritoneum, which is also reflected over most of the organs as a cover. ACUTE A. term for a pathological condition within the belly that requires immediate surgery; PENDULOUS A. that which occurs when the anterior wall relaxes and the abdomen sags or hangs down; SCAPHOID A. an A. in which the anterior wall 'caves in'. — abdominal, adj. See REGION, ABDOMINAL.

abdomin-, abdomino-: Combining forms denoting the abdomen.

abdominal (ab-dom'-i-nal): Relating to the abdomen. A. AORTA the part of the descending aorta that passes down through the abdomen; A. BREATHING breathing in which the abdominal muscles and diaphragm are active; the abdomen moves outward during inspiration and inward during expiration. Also called *diaphragmatic breathing*. A. CAVITY the space in the trunk of the body between the diaphragm and the pelvic floor; contains the abdominal organs; A. DELIVERY delivery of an infant through an abdominal incision; A. DROPSYS ascites (*q.v.*); A. FISTULA an artifical opening from an abdominal organ to the surface, *e.g.*, a colostomy; A. GESTATION see ECTOPIC G.; under ECTOPIC; A. HERNIA a hernia of a loop of intestine through the muscles of the abdominal wall; A. HYSTERECTOMY removal of the uterus through an abdominal incision; A. PARACENTESIS removal of fluid from the abdominal cavity by means of a trocar; also called *abdominocentesis* and *abdominal tap*; A. PREGNANCY ectopic pregnancy, see under ECTOPIC; A. REGIONS see under REGION; A. SECTION an incision into the abdominal wall for surgical purposes.

abdominal thrust: An emergency procedure used when a patient's airway is obstructed; may be executed with the patient prone or standing; consists of giving several quick upwards thrusts against the patient's abdomen between the xiphoid (*q.v.*) process and the umbilicus (*q.v.*). If the patient is standing, the rescuer stands behind the patient, grasps one fist in the other and gives the thrust; if the patient is prone, the rescuer may be either beside or astride the patient and makes the thrust with one hand on the heel of the other. Four thrusts are given in fairly rapid succession. See also HEIMLICH MANOEUVRE.

1

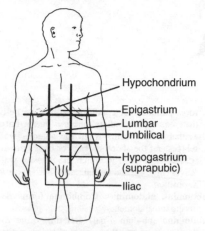

Hypochondrium
Epigastrium
Lumbar
Umbilical
Hypogastrium
(suprapubic)
Iliac

The noughts and crosses grid divides the abdomen into nine regions.

abdominoanterior (ab-dom'-i-nō-an-tē'-ri-or): Relating to a position with the abdomen forward; usually referring to the position of the fetus *in utero*.

abdominocentesis (ab-dom'-i-nō-sen-tē'-sis): Surgical puncture of the abdominal wall for the aspiration of fluid from the abdominal cavity; see PARACENTESIS.

abdominocyesis (ab-dom'-i-nō-sī-ē'-sis): Ectopic pregnancy; see under ECTOPIC.

abdominohysterectomy (ab-dom'-i-nō-his-ter-ek'-to-mi): Operation for the removal of the uterus through an incision in the abdominal wall.

abdominopelvic (ab-dom-i-nō-pel'-vik): Relating to the abdomen and pelvis or pelvic cavity.

abdominoperineal (ab-dom'-i-nō-per-in-ē'-al): Relating to the abdomen and perineum. A. RESECTION OF THE RECTUM an operation in which the proximal end of the bowel is brought out on to the abdominal wall as a permanent colostomy, and the rectum is removed via the perineum.

abdominoposterior (ab-dom'-i-nō-pos-tē'-ri-or): Relating to a position with the abdomen turned backward; usually referring to the position of the fetus *in utero*.

abdominoscopy (ab-dom-i-nos'-ko-pi): Examination or inspection of the abdomen and/or its viscera, either with or without the use of an endoscope.

abdominothoracic (ab-dom'-i-nō-tho-ras'-ik): Pertaining to the abdomen and thorax.

abduct (ab-dukt'): To draw away from the median line of the body or from an adjoining part. Abduce. Opp. to adduct.

abduction (ab-duk'-shun): 1. The drawing away of a part from the midline of the body or of one part from an adjoining part, or the result of such action. Opp. of adduction. 2. The act of turning outward. 3. A position away from the midline. 4. The result of movement away from the midline. 5. In ophthalmology, rotation of the eye outwardly.

abductor (ab-duk'-tor): A muscle that draws a part away from the median line of the body; or a nerve supplying such a muscle. Opp. to adductor.

ABE: Abbreviation for acute bacterial endocarditis; see under ENDOCARDITIS.

aberrant (ab-er'-ant): Deviating or wandering from the normal or expected in some way, as in structure, shape, or course. — aberrancy, n.

aberration (ab-e-rā'-shun): A deviation from normal. MENTAL A. a mild mental abnormality; OPTICAL A. any imperfection in the refraction of a lens of the eye; SPHERICAL A. imperfect focus of light rays by a lens.

abetalipoproteinaemia (a-bē'-ta-lip'-ō-prō-tē-in-ē'-mi-a): A rare hereditary disorder characterized by almost complete lack of lipoprotein in the blood and malabsorption of fat, and later, by retinitis, ataxia, and muscular atrophy; usually manifested early in infancy.

abeyance (a-bā'-ans): 1. Cessation of a function or an activity. 2. A state of suspended or temporary abolition of function.

ABGs: Abbreviation for arterial blood gases; see under ARTERIAL.

ablactation (ab-lak-tā'-shun): 1. Cessation of the flow of milk. 2. Weaning an infant.

ablate (a-blāt'): To excise or amputate a body part completely.

ablatio (ab-lā'-shē-ō): Ablation; detachment. A. PLACENTAE premature detachment of the placenta. A. RETINAE detachment of the retina.

ablation (ab-lā'-shun): Removal; detachment. In surgery, the removal or amputation of a part of the body. — ablative, adj.

ablepharia (a-blef-ai'-ri-a): Congenital absence of the eyelids; may be total or partial. — ablepharous, adj.

ablepsia (ab-lep'-si-a): Blindness.

abluent (ab'-lū-ent): 1. Having a detergent or cleansing action. 2. A cleansing agent such as soap.

ablution (ab-lū'-shun): 1. Washing or cleansing, especially of the body. 2. The pouring of water over the body or part of it as a therapeutic measure.

ablutomania (ab-lū´ -tō-mān´ -i-a): Abnormal interest in washing, bathing, or cleansing oneself.

abnormal (ab-nor´ -mal): Not normal; irregular; different from the usual. — abnormality, n. A. PSYCHOLOGY the study that deals with maladaptive behaviour and deviations in mental functioning, including neuroses and psychoses, whether they occur in people of subnormal, normal, or superior intellect.

ABO: Abbreviation for the international (Landsteiner) classification of human blood types. Blood is typed according to compatibility of the ABO factors in transfusion as A, B, AB, and O. ABO INCOMPATIBILITY a condition usually caused by the mother having O type blood (which has naturally occurring anti-A and anti-B antibodies) and the fetus having either A or B blood; symptoms in infants include those seen in mild anaemia, hyperbilirubinaemia, hepatosplenomegaly, spherocytosis, reticulocytosis. See BLOOD GROUPS.

aboral (ab-aw´ -ral): Away from or opposite to the mouth.

abort (a-bort´): 1. To terminate before full development. 2. To check a disease process in its early stages. 3. To terminate a pregnancy before the fetus is viable.

abortion (a-bor´ -shun): 1. Abrupt termination of a process. 2. Expulsion from the uterus of products of conception before the fetus is viable,

i.e., before the end of the 24th week of pregnancy, the fetus not being born alive. ACCIDENTAL A. one due to an accident; ARTIFICIAL A. one brought on intentionally; COMPLETE A. one in which the entire contents of the uterus are expelled; CRIMINAL A. the illegal intentional evacuation of the uterus; FAILED A. a rare occurrence when a pregnancy persists after incomplete loss of the products of conception; HABITUAL A. repeated successive abortions; preferable term is recurrent abortion; INCOMPLETE A. one in which part of the fetus or placenta is retained within the uterus; INDUCED A., INTENTIONAL A. produced by mechanical or medical means; INEVITABLE A. one that has advanced to a stage where termination of the pregnancy cannot be prevented; MISSED A. one in which early signs and symptoms of pregnancy disappear and the fetus dies but is not expelled for some time, see CARNEOUS MOLE under MOLE; SEPTIC A. one associated with acute infection of the endometrium and myometrium and high fever; evacuation of the uterus is the usual life-saving procedure; SPONTANEOUS A. unexpected expulsion of the products of conception before the 24th week of gestation; THERAPEUTIC A. intentional termination of a pregnancy that is a threat to the mother's life or because there is a substantial risk that the child will be born suffering from such mental and/or physical abnormalities as to be seriously handicapped; has been made legal if carried out in accordance with the

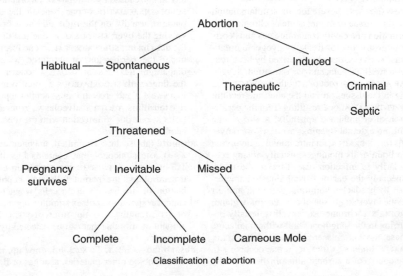

Classification of abortion

provisions laid down in the Abortion Act of 1967, amended 1990; THREATENED A. one with slight blood loss vaginally while the cervix remains undilated; TUBAL A. tubal pregnancy in which the conceptus dies and is expelled from the fimbriated end of the uterine tube.

abrachia (a-brā´-ki-a): Congenital armlessness.

abrachiocephalia (a-brā´-ki-ō-ke, se-fā´-li-a): A malformed fetus that has neither head nor arms.

abrade (a-brād´): To rub, scrape away, wear away, or roughen the skin or a mucous membrane.

abrasion (a-brā´-zhun): Superficial wound to the skin or mucous membrane caused by rubbing, scraping, or erosion; excoriation. — abrade, v.; abrasive, adj.; abrasive, n.

abrasive (a-brā´-siv): 1. Causing abrasion. 2. An agent that erodes, scrapes off, or rubs off the surface or layer of a substance.

abreaction (ab-rē-ak´-shun): In psychoanalysis, a therapeutic reaction resulting from recall of a repressed idea or a traumatic experience or memory; may come about from gaining insight by talking to the analyst or under the influence of light anaesthesia. See NARCOANALYSIS. Also called *catharsis*.

abruptio (ab-rup´-shē-ō): A tearing away; separation. A. PLACENTAE a relatively rare occurrence usually happening prior to the third stage of labour in which there is separation of the placenta accompanied by vaginal bleeding in amounts depending on the degree of separation that occurs.

abscess (ab´-ses): Severe localized inflammation within a tissue or organ, acute or chronic, with formation of a cavity containing pus and debris from destruction of tissue by pyogenic organisms. ACUTE A. one characterized by heat, redness, swelling, pain, and pus formation; ALVEOLAR A. one at the root of a tooth; ANORECTAL A. one in the tissues around the anus and rectum; APPENDICEAL A. one resulting from the perforation of an inflamed appendix; BLIND A. one with no external opening; BONE A. osteomyelitis (*q.v.*); BRAIN A. an intracranial A. involving the brain or its meninges; usually arising secondarily to infection elsewhere in the body, especially the ear or frontal sinus; characterized by headache, vomiting, delirium; BREAST A. one involving tissue of the mammary gland; BRODIE'S A. chronic osteomyelitis, usually occurring in the long bones and without an acute phase; most often seen in young adults; CEREBRAL A. brain A.; CHRONIC A. one occurring in the course of a chronic inflammation; usually

tuberculous; slow-growing with pus formation but slight or no inflammation; COLD A. chronic A.; DRY A. one that dries up without breaking and draining; EPIDURAL A. one outside the dura but inside the cranium or spinal canal; HEPATIC A. one in the liver; HOT A. acute A.; LUNG A. pulmonary A.; LYMPHATIC A. one forming in a lymph node; MAMMARY A. breast A.; METASTATIC A. a secondary A. forming at a distance from the source of infection; PELVIC A. arising in the pelvic peritoneum, often involving the rectouterine pouch; PERINEPHRIC A. one in the kidney cortex or in the tissues surrounding the kidney; PERIDONTAL A. one arising in the periodontium; PERIPROCTIC A. one arising in the tissues around the rectum and anus; PERITONEAL A. one within the peritoneal cavity, frequently following peritonitis; PERITONSILLAR A. one that forms behind the tonsil as an extension of an infection of the tonsil; also called *quinsy*; PRIMARY A. one forming at the site of infection; PSOAS A. one in the psoas muscle, often resulting from tuberculosis of the lower lumbar vertebrae; PULMONARY A. nontuberculous A. of the lung with necrosis of tissue resulting in cavitation; RETROCAECAL A. one posterior to the caecum, often resulting from a ruptured postcaecal appendix; RETROPHARYNGEAL A. one involving the lymph nodes of the lateral and posterior walls of the pharynx; SECONDARY A. an embolic A. STERILE A. one that contains no culturable material; STITCH A. one that forms at the site of a suture; STREPTOCOCCAL A. one caused by a streptococcal organism; SUBDIAPHRAGMATIC A. one beneath the diaphragm, usually on the right side near or involving the liver; SUBDURAL A. one just under the dura mater; SUBPERIOSTEAL A. one forming under the periosteum; SUBPHRENIC A. subdiaphragmatic A.; SUBUNGUAL A. one under the fingernail; SUDORIPAROUS A. one forming in a sweat gland; TONSILLAR A. acute suppurative tonsillitis; TOOTH A. alveolar A.; TUBERCULOUS A. one due to infection with the tubercle bacillus.

absolute (ab´-so-lut): Unlimited, unconditional. A. ALCOHOL alcohol that contains less than 1% of water. A. REFRACTORY PERIOD in electrocardiology, the period following depolarization of the heart muscle cells when they cannot respond to another stimulus regardless of its strength; A. THRESHOLD the smallest amount of stimulus that can be detected by an organism.

absorb (ab-sorb´): 1. To suck up, draw up, take in, or imbibe other material, as a gas or fluid.

2. To take in, through the skin, as medicinal agents or certain rays. **3.** The incorporation by body cells or tissues of substances from the blood or lymph.

absorbable (ab-sorb'-a-bl): Capable of being absorbed.

absorbefacient (ab-sor-be-fā'-shent): Causing absorption; an agent or medication that promotes or causes absorption.

absorbent (ab-sor'-bent): **1.** Having the capability to absorb. **2.** Any agent or substance that has the capability to absorb.

absorption (ab-sorp'-shun): **1.** The assimilation, incorporation, or taking up of one substance by another, *e.g.*, liquids by solids, or gases by liquids or solids. **2.** The passage of water and/or a dissolved substance through a body surface or membrane into the body fluids, tissues, or cells. **3.** The taking up of heat by the body. **4.** In nutrition, the taking up by the mucous membrane of the digestive tract of certain nutrients resulting from digestion, *i.e.*, water, glucose, alcohol, and certain drugs are taken up by the stomach, as well as calcium if protein and vitamin D are also present; water, electrolytes, carbohydrate, amino acids from proteins, fats, iron and calcium — if vitamin D and protein are also present — are taken up by the small intestine; water and electrolytes are taken up by the large intestine while faeces are being held awaiting evacuation. **5.** In pharmacology, the process by which a drug is taken into the bloodstream; the speed and degree to which this is accomplished vary greatly and have a determining influence on the effect of a dose of a particular drug.

abstinence (ab'-stin-ens): Voluntarily denying oneself some experience or substance that has provided gratification in the past, often something to which one has become habituated or addicted; especially certain drugs, food, alcohol, sexual intercourse.

abstract (ab'-strakt): In pharmacology, a preparation made from the soluble principle of a drug, or its fluidextract (*q.v.*), evaporated to twice the original strength of the drug. **A. THINKING** the use of concepts and ideas independent of concrete objects.

abstraction (ab-strak'-shun): **1.** The withdrawal of one or more constituents of a compound or mixture. **2.** The mental process of formulating abstract ideas. **3.** A state of inattention resembling absent-mindedness.

abtortion (ab-tor'-shun): The outward turning of both eyes simultaneously.

abuse (a-būz'): **1.** To put to a bad or improper use. **2.** To treat without compassion and usually in a hurtful manner. See also CHILD ABUSE, ELDER ABUSE, SEXUAL ABUSE.

abused child: A child who has suffered repeated physical or psychological injury, sexual abuse, negligence, or maltreatment, usually inflicted by a parent or parent surrogate. The abuse may consist of fractures; burns; bruises; verbal or sexual abuse; failure to provide adequate food, housing, medical care, or emotional support. See ABUSE.

acampsia (a-kamp'-si-a): Loss or lack of flexibility or movement of a joint; see ANKYLOSIS.

acanth-, acantho-: Combining forms denoting spine, sharp, thorn, spinous.

acanthaesthesia (a kan-thes-thē'-zi-a): The abnormal sensation of being pricked with a sharp point or with needles.

acanthocyte (a-kan'-thō-sīt): A misshapen erythrocyte with many protoplasmic projections, giving it a horny appearance; may be hereditary; seen in such conditions as abetalipoproteinaemia, severe rheumatic disease, gastric carcinoma, bleeding gastric ulcer.

acanthocytosis (a-kan'-thō-sī-to'-sis): The presence of acanthocytes in the blood; a characteristic of congenital abetalipoproteinaemia.

acanthokeratodermia (a-kan'-thō-ker-a-tō-der'-mi-a): Thickening of the horny layer of the skin, particularly that of the hands and feet.

acapnia (a-kap'-ni-a): A condition of diminished carbon dioxide content of the blood; sometimes used when hypocapnia (*q.v.*) is meant. — acapnial, adj.

acardia (a-kar'-di-a): Congenital absence of the heart.

acardiotrophia (a-kar'-di-o-trō'-fi-a): Atrophy of the heart.

acarid (ak'-a-rid): A mite, tick, or other member of the order Acarina.

acarodermatitis (ak'-ar-ō-der'-ma-tī'-tis): Inflammation of the skin, with urticaria and pruritus, caused by the bite of mites, often due to handling mite-infested plants.

acatalasia (a-kat-ā-lā'-zi-a): Absence of the enzyme catalase in the body cells, a rare congenital condition that predisposes the individual to recurrent infections of the gingiva and associated structures in the mouth.

acatalepsy, acatalepsia (a-kat'-a-lep-si,-si-a): **1.** Lack of understanding or comprehension; dementia; impairment of the mental processes. **2.** A state of uncertainty of diagnosis.

acatamathesia (a-kat'-a-ma-thē'-zi-a): Lack or loss of ability to understand or comprehend, particularly speech; usually due to a central nervous system lesion.

acataphasia (a-kat-a-fā′-zi-a): Lack of power to express connected thought or to formulate sentences correctly; due to a brain lesion.

acataposis (a-kat-a-pō′-sis): Difficulty in swallowing; dysphagia (*q.v.*).

acceleration (ak-sel-er-ā′-shun): 1. Increased speed or velocity of action, motion, or rate. 2. Change in velocity. 3. Advancement beyond normal in either physical or intellectual growth. 4. An increase in the rate of a chemical reaction.

acceleration-deceleration injury: One that occurs when the brain is thrown forward against the skull and then back against the opposite side of the skull; the injury at the first site is called 'coup' and that at the second site 'contrecoup'.

accelerator (ak-sel′-er-āt-or): 1. An agent, machine, or device that speeds up something, as a function or process. 2. A nerve or muscle that speeds up the performance of a bodily function.

accessory (ak-ses′-or-i): Supplementary; complementary; concomitant. A. NERVES the 11th pair of cranial nerves.

Access to Health Record Act (1990): Act giving patients statutory rights to see what has been written about them in their medical records since 1 November 1991.

accident (ak′-si-dent): A sudden, unforseen event that produces unintended injury, death, or property damage. CEREBROVASCULAR A. one that occurs within the cerebrum, *e.g.*, cerebral haemorrhage; abbreviation CVA; A. FORM a data sheet used to record an accident or incident to any individual on the premises; data are collated centrally within the hospital and used to rectify health and safety issues. ACCIDENT-PRONE said of one who appears to be more susceptible to accidents than the average person; ACCIDENT-REPETITIVENESS having repeated accidents due to inexperience, age, or maladjustment to the environment; to be differentiated from accident-proneness.

acclimatization (a-klī′-ma-tī′-zā′-shun): 1. The process of becoming accustomed to a new environment, especially to change in temperature and altitude. 2. Structural and physiological changes, such as ventricular enlargement and pulmonary hypertension, which occur in people born and living in high altitudes but which do not interfere with normal activities as long as the person remains in the high altitude.

accommodation (a-kom-mo-dā′-shun): Adjustment or adaptation of an organ or a part to changing circumstances, particularly the automatic adjustment of the lens of the eye so that a distinct image is always obtained, regardless of the nearness or distance of the object being viewed.

accountability (a-kown-ta-bil′-i-ti): In nursing, the obligation of answering for the results or outcomes of one's actions, as differentiated from responsibility which refers to what one *ought* to do. See PRIMARY CARE NURSE under NURSE.

accreditation (a-kred-i-tā′-shun): In healthcare, a voluntary procedure of peer evaluation whereby an educational or healthcare facility and its programme are regularly appraised and recognized as meeting the preset criteria of one or more accrediting agencies. The process involves setting standards, periodic inspections to determine whether the standards have been met, and official approval by the accrediting agency. A. OF PRIOR CERTIFICATED LEARNING a process, through which previously certificated learning is considered and, as appropriate, recognized for academic purposes; this recognition may give the learning a credit value in a credit-based structure and allow it to be counted towards the completion of a programme of study and the award(s) or qualifications associated with it. A. OF PRIOR EXPERIENTIAL LEARNING a process through which learning achieved outside the education or training systems is assessed and, as appropriate, recognized for academic purposes; this recognition may give the learning a credit value in a credit-based structure and allow it to be counted towards the completion of a programme of study and the award(s) or qualifications associated with it. CREDIT ACCUMULATION TRANSFER SCHEME, Appendix 8; A. OF PRIOR LEARNING a process for accessing and, as appropriate, recognizing experiential or certificated prior learning for academic purposes; this recognition may give the learning a credit value in a credit-based structure and allow it to be counted towards the completion of a programme of study and the award(s) or qualifications associated with it, see also A. of prior experiential learning, CREDIT ACCUMULATION TRANSFER SCHEME, Appendix 8.

ACE: Abbreviation for angiotensin-converting enzyme, see under ANGIOTENSIN.

acentric (a-sen′-trik): 1. Not centrally located. 2. Having no centre.

acephalia, acephaly (a-ke-f, se-fā′-li-a, a-kef′, sef′-a-li): A congenital anomaly with absence of the head. — acephalic, adj.

acerbity (a-sur′-bi-ti): Acidity combined with astringency.

acetabular (as-e-tab′-ū-lar): Relating to the acetabulum (*q.v.*). A. LIP a fibrocartilaginous ring that surrounds the acetabulum.

acetabuloplasty (as′-e-tab′-ū-lō-plas-ti): An operation to improve the shape and depth of the acetabulum, sometimes necessary to correct congenital dislocation of the hip, or to relieve osteoarthritis (*q.v.*).

acetabulum (as-et-ab′-ū-lum): A cup-like socket on the external aspect of the innominate bone, into which the head of the femur fits to form the hip joint. — acetabula, pl.; acetabular, adj.

acetate (as′-e-tāt): Any salt of acetic acid.

acetic (a-se′-tik): 1. Relating to acetic acid or vinegar. 2. Sour.

acetic acid The acid present in vinegar. Has several uses in medicine; *e.g.*, in weak solutions as an antidote for alkaline poisons.

acetoacetic acid (as-e′-to-as-e′-tik): One of the ketonic bodies formed in the body during the metabolism of fats. In some metabolic disturbances, *e.g.*, acidosis or diabetes mellitus, it is present in the blood in excessive amounts and appears in the urine; the excess in the blood may produce coma. Also called *diacetic acid*.

acetone (as′-i-tōn): An acrid, colourless, volatile, inflammable liquid with a sweetish odour; found in minute amounts in normal urine and in larger amounts in diabetic urine; used commercially as a solvent. A. BODIES intermediate products in metabolism of fats that become greatly increased in the blood in diabetes mellitus, starvation, pregnancy, after anaesthesia, and other conditions of disturbed metabolism. Also called *ketone bodies*; A. BREATH breath with a fruity odour; usually refers to that of diabetic patients in a state of ketoacidosis. (*q.v.*).

acetonuria (as-i-tō-nū′-ri-a): Excess acetone bodies in the urine that give it a peculiar, sweet smell. Occurs in diabetes, carcinoma, fevers and some digestive disorders. Now usually called *ketonuria*. — acetonuric, adj.

acetylcholine (as′-i-til-kō′-lin): A chemical substance normally present in various body tissues and organs; has several important physiological actions; is released from parasympathetic and voluntary nerve endings to activate muscle, secretory glands and nerve cells. Important in the transmission of nerve impulses across the synapse between one nerve fibre and another. The fibres that release this chemical are described as cholinergic.

acetylcholinesterase (as′-i-til-kō-lin-es′-ter-ās): An enzyme found in red blood cells, nervous tissue, and muscle; it is a catalyst in the hydrolysis of acetylcholine to choline and acetic acid.

acetylsalicylic acid (a-se′-til-sal-i-sil′-ik): An odourless white crystalline powder, soluble in water; readily absorbed from mucous membranes, commonly used in medicine to reduce fever, relieve pain, and as an antirheumatic agent. Aspirin.

achalasia (ak-a-lā′-zi-a): Failure to relax; often referring to sphincter muscles. CARDIAC A. failure of the cardiac sphincter and lower part of the oesophagus to relax to permit food to pass into the stomach, resulting in dilatation of the oesophagus.

ache (āk): A dull, continuous pain as differentiated from one that is sudden, spasmodic or intermittent; may be described according to severity, ranging from dull to severe, or according to location; *e.g.*, headache.

achievement (a-chēv′-ment): Accomplishment. A. AGE a figure obtained by testing; expresses the level of an individual's educational achievement as compared to that of the average individual of the same chronological age; A. QUOTIENT the ratio of a person's achieved educational age to his mental age; A. TEST a standardized test used to measure a person's skill or knowledge in one or more fields of work or study.

Achilles (a-kil′-ēz): Mythical Greek warrior whose entire body was considered invulnerable to injury except the heel by which his mother held him when she immersed him in the river Styx. A. BURSA the bursa between the tendon of Achilles and the calcaneus; A. BURSITIS inflammation of the bursa between the tendon of Achilles and the posterior surface of the calcaneus; A. REFLEX the knee-jerk R., see also under REFLEX; A. TENDON the powerful tendon that attaches the gastrocnemius and soleus muscles to the posterior surface of the calcaneus.

achlorhydria (a-klor-hī′-dri-a): The absence of free hydrochloric acid in the gastric juice. Occurs in pernicious anaemia, iron-deficiency anaemia, gastric cancer, gastritis, pellagra, and sprue. — achlorhydric, adj.

acholia (a-kō-li-a): 1. Lack or absence of bile. 2. Any condition that interferes with the flow of bile into the small intestine.

acholuria (a-ko-lū'-ri-a): Absence of bile pigments from the urine. See JAUNDICE. — acholuric, adj.

achondroplasia (a-kon-drō-plā'-zi-a): congenital, often familial, condition involving disordered chondrification and ossification at the ends of long bones, resulting in dwarfism; the arms and legs are short but the head and body are normal size; the intellect is not usually impaired. — achondroplastic, adj.

achro-: A combining form denoting colourless.

achromasia (a-krō-mā'-zi-a): 1. Lack of normal skin pigmentation. 2. Absence of normal staining reaction in cells or tissue. 3. Lack of pigmentation of the iris.

achromatic (a-krō-mat'-ik): 1. Free from colour. 2. Lacking normal pigment. 3. Not readily coloured by staining agents.

achromatism (a-krō'-ma-tizm): Colour blindness.

achromatopsia (a-krō-ma-top'-si-a): Complete colour blindness. Very rare.

achylia (a-kī'li-a): Absence of chyle (*q.v.*). — achylic, adj.

achylous (a-kī'-lus): 1. Lacking gastric and other digestive juices. 2. Deficiency or lack of chyle.

aciclovir (ā-s-īk'-lō-vēr): An antiviral drug that inhibits DNA synthesis in cells infected by herpes viruses. Administered topically or by intravenous infusion. May also be used prophylactically for patients who are immunocompromised.

acid (as'-id): Any of a group of compounds which, in solution, has a pH of less than 7, turns blue litmus paper red, furnishes hydrogen ions when combined with a metal, and combines with a base to form a salt and water; may also be corrosive. In popular usage any substance with a sour, sharp, or biting taste.

acidaemia (as-i-dē'-mi-a): Abnormal acidity of the blood, with a below normal pH. Cf. acidosis.

acid–base: 1. ACID–BASE BALANCE a normal equilibrium or ratio between the acid and base elements of blood and body fluids. It is influenced by the level of hydrogen ion concentration in the blood. When the blood is in acid–base balance, the pH of the serum remains at 7.35 to 7.45, which is maintained by the regulating systems of the kidney, lungs, skin, adrenal gland and pituitary, and by the buffer system of the blood. 2. ACID–BASE IMBALANCE the condition resulting from loss of the normal balance between the acidity and alkalinity of the blood and body fluids; it occurs in metabolic disturbances that accompany starvation, gastrointestinal diseases, diabetes mellitus, respiratory and renal diseases, toxaemias; correction involves the buffer system of the blood and respiratory and renal regulatory actions.

acid-fast: A bacteriological term describing a bacterium that stains with a basic dye and resists discoloration when treated with an acidic solution, *e.g., Mycobacterium tuberculosis.*

acid intoxication: Severe acidosis causing a toxic condition of the body. May be due to accumulation of acid products resulting from faulty or incomplete oxidation of fats, or by acids introduced into the body from without.

acidosis (as-i-dō'-sis): A disturbance in the acid–base balance in the body, with a depletion of the alkali reserve, accumulation of acid, and lowering of the blood serum pH to below 7.35. May be secondary to some other condition; seen in diabetes mellitus, epilepsy, starvation, cyclic vomiting, diarrhoea, and toxaemias. Acidaemia. COMPENSATED A. results from changes in pulmonary or renal function that restore the normal pH of the blood; DIABETIC A. produced by the accumulation of ketones (*q.v.*) in the blood of patients with uncontrolled diabetes; marked by a sweet fruity breath odour; LACTIC ACID A. an accumulation of lactic acid in the tissues; may occur in circulatory failure, hypotension, malignancies, leukaemia, or lymphoma; when severe it may be life-threatening; METABOLIC A. an increase in the pH of the blood, which may be the result of ingestion of acids, retention of acid products of metabolism, excessive loss of bicarbonate from the body, or excessive elimination of carbon dioxide from the lungs through hyperventilation; MIXED A., A. having a mixed cause, such as when shock and ventilatory failure occur simultaneously, producing both metabolic and respiratory A.; RENAL TUBULAR A. a syndrome characterized by inability to secrete acid urine, by low serum carbonate levels, and by high chloride levels; may occur in osteomalacia or nephrosclerosis; RESPIRATORY A., A. associated with a decrease in the exhalation of carbon dioxide and a consequent increase in the pCO_2 of the bloodstream; occurs in asthma, emphysema, pneumonia, and some other conditions that interfere with normal breathing.

acidotic (as-i-dot'-ik): Relating to or suffering from acidosis.

acid phosphatase (fos'-fa-tās): An enzyme found in many tissues and fluids of the body, including the liver, spleen, pancreas, kidney, blood plasma, red blood cells, seminal fluid. In cancer of the prostate gland the serum A.P. is elevated.

acid rain: Rain, snow, or fog that is polluted by acid in the atmosphere and damages the environment. Two common air pollutants acidify rain: sulphur dioxide and nitrogen oxide. When these substances are released into the atmosphere, they can be carried over long distances by prevailing winds before returning to Earth as acidic rain, snow, fog, or dust. When the environment cannot neutralize the acid being deposited, damage occurs.

acini (as′-in-ī): Minute saccules or alveoli lined or filled with secreting cells, found in various glands and organs; they cluster around a narrow lumen like grapes on a stem; several A. combine to form a lobule. Term commonly applied to the saclike termini of the small tubular passages in the lungs; sometimes used as a synonym for alveoli. — acinus, sing.; acinous, acinar, adj.

acne (ak′-nē): A self-limiting inflammatory condition of the sebaceous glands, common in both sexes during adolescence. A. CONGLO-BATA severe, long-lasting A., occurring mostly in males during late adolescence; characterized by burrowing abscesses and cysts, draining sinus tracts, severe scarring; systemic signs include elevated temperature, malaise, and arthralgia; lesions often form on the lower back, buttocks, and thighs as well as on the face; A. MILIARIS a form in which many small white milia appear on the face; A. PAPULOSA a form characterized by inflammatory papular lesions; A. RHINOPHYMA a form of A. rosacea affecting chiefly the nose; often called *whisky-nose;* A. ROSACEA a pronounced erythema of the brow, cheeks and nose, resulting from dilatation of subcutaneous capillary vessels; seen mostly in adults and is aggravated by hot drinks, alcoholic drinks, and rich or fried food; A. VULGARIS the most common form, which occurs chiefly in adolescents; comedones which develop into papules, and pustules appear on the face, neck and upper part of the trunk.

acousma (a-kooz′-ma): An auditory hallucination in which one hears such nonverbal sounds as buzzing, ringing, hissing.

acoustic (a-koos′-tik): Relating to (1) the sense or organs of hearing, or (2) the science of sound. A. NERVE the eighth cranial nerve, composed of the cochlear nerve, which is concerned with hearing, and the vestibular nerve,

which is concerned with balance and equilibrium; also called *vestibulocochlear nerve* A. NEUROMA, see under NEUROMA.

acoustics (a-koos′-tiks): The branch of physics that deals with sound and sound waves, their production, transmission, and reception, and with the phenomena of hearing and the perception of sounds.

acquired (a-kw-ird′): Not inherited; resulting from learning, experience, or other influences originating outside the organism after birth. A. IMMUNITY any type of immunity that is not inherited. See IMMUNITY. A. REFLEX, same as conditioned reflex, see under REFLEX.

acquired immunodeficiency syndrome (AIDS): A serious worldwide communicable disease in which the body's cellular immune system is suppressed, leaving it defenceless against invasion by bacteria, viruses, fungi, and parasites. First recognized in the US in the early 1980s. The causative virus, Human Immunodeficiency Virus (HIV), is transmitted by sexual contact, unsterilized needles and syringes used by drug users, and contaminated blood and blood products. In addition, HIV-positive women may transmit the virus to unborn fetuses or in breast milk. The incubation period varies from several months to five or more years. Symptoms include fever, enlarged lymph glands, anorexia, severe weight loss, and diarrhoea.

acr-, acro: Combining forms denoting: 1. An extremity of the body. 2. A tip end. 3. Extreme.

acral (ak′-ral): 1. Relating to an apex. 2. Pertaining to or affecting the peripheral parts of body, *e.g.,* the ears, fingers, toes.

acraturesis (a-krat-ū-rē′-sis): Inability to urinate normally, due to atony of the urinary bladder or obstruction in the urethra; may result in incontinence or slow dribbling of urine.

acroasphyxia (ak′-rō-as-fik′-si-a): Episodes of cyanosis, pallor, and red or blue mottling of the skin of the extremities, due to interference with the circulation; may follow exposure to cold or an emotional disturbance; associated with Raynaud's disease (*q.v.*) See also ACRO-CYANOSIS.

acrocentric (ak-rō-sen′-trik): Usually refers to a chromosome in which the centrosome is located close to one end rather than being in the centre.

acrocephalosyndactyly (ak′-rō-sef′-a-lō-sin-dak′-ti-li): A congenital condition characterized by acrocephaly, unnatural facies, webbing of the fingers and toes, obesity, underdeveloped genitalia, and, sometimes, mental handicap. Also called *acrocephalosyndactylism* and *Apert's syndrome*.

acrocephaly (ak-rō-sef′-a-li): A congenital malformation whereby the top of the head is more or less pointed, due to premature closure of the coronal, sagittal, and lambdoid sutures. Also called *acrocephalia* and *oxycephaly*. — acrocephalic, acrocephalous, adj.

acrocyanosis (ak′-rō-sī-a-nō′-sis): Cyanosis of the extremities. Often associated with chilblains when the skin may be bluish or reddish and mottled; usually due to a vasomotor disturbance. In infants, the extremities are blue and cold while the cheeks and trunk are pink; usually due to faulty cardiopulmonary function; tends to clear with warmth. See also ACROASPHYXIA. — acrocyanotic, adj.

acrohyperhidrosis (ak′-rō-hī-per-hī-drō′-sis): Excessive sweating of the hands or feet, or both.

acromania (ak-rō-mā′-ni-a): A severe form of mania characterized by excessive motor activity and sometimes by muteness.

acromegaly (ak-rō-meg′-a-li): A fairly common chronic metabolic disorder, characterized by enlargement of the bones of the hands, face, and feet, and of the viscera. Occurs in adult life and is due to prolonged overproduction of growth-stimulating hormone by the pituitary gland. — acromegalic, adj.

acronyx (ak′-rō-niks): An ingrowing nail.

acropachyderma (ak′-rō-pak-i-der′-ma): A condition marked by thickening of the skin, especially that of the face, scalp and extremities, along with clubbing of the fingers and other skeletal deformities usually associated with acromegaly; due to hypopituitarism (*q.v.*).

acroparaesthesia (ak′-rō-par-es-thē′-zi-a): A condition characterized by attacks of tingling, numbness, or stiffness of one or more of the extremities, particularly the hands and feet, often following sleep; occurs in women more often than men; additional symptoms include pain, pallor, cyanosis.

acrophobia (ak-rō-fō′-bi-a): Morbid fear of being at a height.

acrosclerosis (ak′-rō-sklē-rō′-sis): Hardening and thickening of the skin of the extremities, usually symmetrical, affecting chiefly the distal parts of the extremities as well as the neck and face, the nose especially; combined with features of Raynaud's disease (*q.v.*); occurs most often in women.

acrotic (a-krot′-ik): 1. Relating to the surface, especially to the glands of the skin. 2. Relating to a weak or absent pulse.

acrylic (a-kril′-ik): Relating to a type of cement used for anchoring prosthetic devices or metallic implants to the skeleton. A. RESIN any of a group of several thermoplastic substances derived from acrylic acid; has many commercial uses including the manufacture of prosthetic devices such as contact lenses.

ACTH: Abbreviation for adrenocorticotrophic hormone (*q.v.*).

actin (ak′-tin): A protein in the filaments of muscle fibres which, along with myosin particles, acts to cause contraction and relaxation of muscles.

acting out: 1. Coping with one's feelings and expressing them in action rather than words. In psychiatry, the expression of anxiety or emotional conflict in undesirable, possibly dangerous, behaviour, *e.g.*, stealing or arson. 2. Dramatization or play therapy, in which individuals are encouraged to express their emotional conflicts freely as part of a therapeutic regimen.

actinodermatitis (ak′-ti-nō-der-ma-tī′-tis): Inflammation of the skin resulting from exposure to the sun, ultraviolet light, or x-rays.

action (ak′-shun): The performance of an activity or function by any part of the body or by the whole body. ANTAGONISTIC A. (1) in physiology, the action of a muscle or group of muscles that limits the action of an opposing muscle or muscles; (2) in pharmacology, a drug action that opposes the effect of another drug; BUFFER A. the prevention, by certain chemical substances, of change in a body system or function, as in pH or blood pressure. COMPULSIVE A. one performed independently of one's will or conscious motivation; CUMULATIVE A. sudden increase in intensity of the action of a drug following repeated doses; REFLEX A. an involuntary A. in response to a sensory stimulus; SYNERGISTIC A. (1) the working together of two or more muscles to accomplish what one muscle could not do alone, or (2) the A. of one drug in increasing the effect of another drug.

action potential: The complete cycle of changes in the self-propagating electric impulses set up in the cell membrane of a nerve or muscle cell, or other excitable tissue, in response to a stimulus during which depolarization and repolarization of the nerve or muscle fibre takes place.

action research: A research methodology that pursues action (or change) and research (or understanding) at the same time, achieved by using a cyclic or spiral process that alternates between action and critical reflection, and in the later cycles continuously refines methods, data, and interpretation in the light of understanding developed in the earlier cycles. An emergent process that takes shape as understanding increases and an iterative process that moves towards a better understanding of what happens. In most forms also participative and qualitative.

activation (ak-ti-va′-shun): The process of rendering active or activating, as the action of a pre-enzyme on an enzyme. In nuclear physics, the process of bombarding a material with nuclear particles to make it radioactive.

activator (ak′-ti-vā-tor): A substance that renders something else active or one that converts an inactive substance into an active one.

active (ak′-tiv): Energetic; working; moving; functioning or capable of functioning. Not passive. A. IMMUNITY that acquired naturally by having the disease or artificially by vaccination; A. MOVEMENTS those consciously produced by the individual; A. PRINCIPLE the constituent of a compound or drug that gives it its chief value or characteristic; A. TRANSPORT in physiology, the energy-expending process of moving a substance across a membrane between two areas of differing concentration; A. TREATMENT vigorous medical or surgical treatment, with the objective of curing the illness, not just allaying the symptoms.

activism (ak′-ti-vizm): In healthcare, refers to practice that emphasizes direct action in seeking cures rather than employing palliative treatment for illness. THERAPEUTIC A. the extent to which a physician will intervene to attempt a cure.

activities of daily living: The activities performed by an individual for himself in the course of a normal day, e.g., eating, dressing, toileting, bathing, exercising, etc.

activity (ak-tiv′-i-ti): The quality or state of being active; alertness. A. THERAPY the therapeutic use of a variety of activities, e.g., physical, social, diversional; A. THEORY a theory of ageing that holds that the more older people continue to engage in the activities they enjoyed earlier in life, the better off they will be both physically and mentally.

Act of Parliament (pah′-la-ment): Law written by a parliament. In the UK, the House of Commons and House of Lords will debate proposals for new laws (Bills, q.v.); if both Houses vote for the proposals then the Bill is ready to become an Act. It can only be

described as an Act when it has received Royal Assent.

actomyosin (ak-tō-mī′-ō-sin): A complex network of actin and myosin in the muscle fibrils which contract when stimulated and thus are responsible for the contraction and relaxation of muscles.

acuity (a-kū-i-ti): Sharpness, clearness, keenness, distinctness. AUDITORY A. ability to hear clearly and distinctly. Tests include the use of tuning fork, whispered voice and audiometer. In infants, simple sounds, e.g., bells, rattles, cup and spoon are utilized; VISUAL A. extent of visual perception; dependent on the clarity of retinal focus, integrity of nervous elements and cerebral interpretation of the stimulus. Usually tested by Snellen's letters. See SNELLEN'S TEST TYPE.

acupoint (ak′-ū-poynt): Specific sensitive points on the surface of the body which are precisely described in the Chinese explanation of the theoretical foundation for acupuncture, acupressure, and moxibustion as being located on 'conduits of energy'. Stimulation at these points may affect the function or sensitivity of a specific area or body part. Also called *acupuncture points*.

acupressure (ak′-ū-presh-ur): An ancient Chinese healing method used to cure many common ailments. Pressure is applied to certain points throughout the body to relieve pain and promote good health.

acupuncture (ak′-ū-pungk-chur): A system for treating illness through the insertion of fine needles into the body, which 'stimulate the energy that flows through the body'. Originated in China.

acus (ā′-kūs): 1. A needle, particularly a surgical needle. 2. A sharp needle-like process.

acusector (ak′-ū-sek-tor): A surgical needle that operates on a high frequency current; used for cutting tissue.

acusis (a-kū′-sis): Normal perception of sound. Also called *acousis*.

acute (a-kūt′): Short, sharp, severe, with definite symptoms, and of sudden onset. A. ABDOMEN term for a serious condition that may be due to inflammation, ulceration, obstruction, or perforation of an abdominal organ, or some other pathological condition; requires immediate surgery; A. BRAIN SYNDROME an acute state of delirium or confusion, assumed to be of structural origin; affects individuals of all ages; may be brief and reversible, or may progress to chronic brain syndrome; A. COMPARTMENT SYNDROME a condition occurring in a compartment of the hand, forearm, shoulder, buttock, thigh, or leg, most often in the leg; usually follows trauma caused by fracture or surgery that results in swelling of the muscle tissue, causing constriction of a nerve or tendon and severe ischaemia and pain that increases when the person is at rest or on passive stretch of the part. A. HEART FAILURE serious impairment or failure of heart function in an individual not previously diagnosed as having heart disease; A. RENAL FAILURE sudden decrease in output of urine resulting in rapid accumulation of metabolic waste products in the body; may be a postoperative complication or due to ingestion of toxic material; A. RESPIRATORY DISTRESS SYNDROME see under RESPIRATORY DISTRESS SYNDROME; A. YELLOW ATROPHY diffuse necrosis of the liver, often a result of viral hepatitis.

acute care (a-k-ut'): Care rendered to a person whose illness is characterized by sudden onset and brief duration. A. C. FACILITY a hospital department or medical centre for diagnosis and management of short-term illnesses and emergency health problems.

acyesis (a-sī-ē'-sis): 1. Absence of pregnancy. 2. Sterility in the female. 3. Inability of a woman to have a normal delivery. — acyetic, adj.

Acystosporidia (a-sis'-tō-spō-rid'-i-a): An order of parasitic sporozoa that includes the genus *Plasmodium*, the causative organism in malaria.

ad-: Prefix denoting to, towards, before, near, adjacent. May change to ac- before c, k, or q; af- before f; ag- before g; al- before l; ap- before p; as- before s; at- before t.

-ad: Suffix denoting towards, in the direction of.

adacrya (a-dak'-ri-a): The absence of tears.

adactylia (a-dak-til'-i-a): A congenital anomaly characterized by absence of fingers or toes, or both. Also called *adactylism, adactyly.* — adactylous, adj.

adamantine (ad-a-man'-tin): 1. Relating to a hard, unbreakable substance. 2. Relating to dental enamel.

adamantinoma (ad'-a-man-ti-nō'-ma): See AMELOBLASTOMA.

Adam's apple: Common name for the laryngeal prominence in the front of the neck, formed by the junction of the two wings of the thyroid cartilage.

Adams–Stokes disease, syndrome, or syncope: A disease condition characterized by sudden attacks of unconsciousness or convulsions, due to inadequate blood flow to the cerebrum; often associated with heart block.

adaptation (ad-ap-tā'-shun): 1. Mental and physical change that results in adjustment to a situation or condition in the environment. 2. Any beneficial change made to meet environmental change. 3. The ways in which the body counteracts stress. 4. The action of the eye in adjusting to variations in the intensity of light. 5. The decline in receptivity of a receptor when a stimulus is delivered constantly. 6. The development, in microorganisms, of resistance to antibiotic agents. DARK A. the adaptation of the eye to vision in conditions of darkness.

adapter, adaptor (a-dap'-ter): 1. A device that makes it possible to fit two instruments or pieces of apparatus together. 2. A device that converts electric current from one form to a different form, required by certain electrical appliances.

adaptibility (ad-ap-ta-bil'-i-ti): The ability to adjust mentally and physically to new or changed circumstances.

adaptive (a-dap'-tiv): Having a tendency towards, or the capacity for adaptation. A. BEHAVIOUR beneficial or appropriate behaviour in response to a change.

addict (ad'-ikt): 1. One who is physically dependent on, or unable to resist indulgence in some practice or habit, such as the use of alcohol. 2. To devote oneself to something obsessively, *e.g.*, gambling, or to cause someone else to become addicted to a practice or habit. — addiction, n.; addictive, adj.

addiction (a-dik'-shun): The condition of having established the practice of yielding to something that is habit-forming to the extent that discontinuing the practice causes severe-physiological and psychological symptoms. In healthcare, a state in which therapeutic use of an addictive drug to control such symptoms as intractable pain has created a dependence wherein discontinuing the drug would result in severe distress symptoms. ENDEMIC A. occurs in groups wherein addiction to certain substances is socially acceptable; EPIDEMIC A. refers to a situation in which a high rate of A. occurs at a specific time and place; IATROGENIC A. results from the regular use of drugs for the relief of severe or intractable pain; POLYSURGICAL A. the habitual seeking of surgical treatment.

Addis count method: A laboratory method of counting the red and white blood cells, epithelial cells, casts, and protein content in a specific amount of a 12-hour urine specimen; useful in making diagnoses and in assessing prognoses and treatment.

Addison's anaemia: Pernicious anaemia. See ANAEMIA.

Addison's disease: Chronic adrenocortical insufficiency; characterized by reduced adrenal steroid production resulting from slowly progressive destruction of the adrenal cortex which may occur as a sequel to tuberculosis or some other systemic infection or disorder, or it may be idiopathic in origin. Characteristic symptoms include electrolytic upset, diminution of blood volume, hypotension, marked anaemia, high serum potassium, bronze-like pigmentation of the skin, anorexia, gastrointestinal upsets, weight loss with emaciation, weakness, fatigability, decreased tolerance to cold, emotional disturbances, depression. [Thomas Addison, English physician, diagnostician, teacher 1763–1860.]

additive (ad´-i-tiv): Any substance added to another to strengthen, improve, or diversify its action.

adduct (ad-dukt´): To draw towards the midline of the body or towards a neighbouring part. Opp. to abduct. In optics, to turn the eyes inward.

adduction (ad-duk´-shun): 1. The drawing of a part of the body towards the midline, or of a part towards an adjacent part, or the result of such motion. Opp. to abduction. 2. The act of turning inward. 3. In optics, the turning of the eyes inwardly; may be a voluntary act or occur unconsciously as in accommodation. — adductent, adj.

adductor (ad-duk´-tor): Any muscle that moves a part towards the median axis of the body. Opp. to abductor.

aden-, adeno-: Combining form denoting gland or glands.

adenectomy (ad-e-nek´-to-mi): 1. Surgical removal of a gland or lymph node. 2. Surgical removal of an adenoid growth.

adenitis (ad-e-nī´-tis): Inflammation of a gland or lymph node. CERVICAL A. inflammation of lymph nodes in the neck; HILAR A. inflammation of bronchial lymph nodes; MESENTERIC A. inflammation of lymph nodes in the mesenteric portion of the peritoneum; symptoms include pain resembling that of appendicitis but is less localized; TUBERCULOSIS A. swelling and induration of lymph nodes, usually cervical and most often painless; occurs in children more often than adults; caused by certain strains of the tubercle bacillus; may result in a chronic draining fistula.

adenocarcinoma (ad´-e-nō-kar-sin-ō´-ma): A malignant growth of glandular tissue.

ENDOMETRIAL A., A. of the lining of the uterus; fairly common in women 55–65 years of age and those who have had few or no children; VAGINAL A. usually an extension of cervical or endometrial carcinoma; has been found in young women whose mothers were treated with diethylstilboesterol for threatened abortion; extensive involvement of the lymphatics often results in death in about 5 years. — adenocarcinomata, pl.; adenocarcinomatous, adj.

adenocele (ad´-e-nō-sēl): A benign cyst-like tumour of glandular origin.

adenochondroma (ad´-e-nō-kon-drō´-ma): A mixed tumour made up of both glandular and chondromatous tissue, as sometimes occurs in a salivary gland.

adenohypophysis (ad´-e-nō-hī-pof´-i-sis): The anterior lobe of the pituitary gland. It secretes several important hormones: growth hormone, which helps control the metabolism of proteins, fats, and carbohydrates, and influences normal growth; thyrotrophin, which stimulates thyroid activity; adrenocorticotrophic hormone, which stimulates activity of the adrenal cortex; and the gonadotrophic hormones including (1) follicle-stimulating hormone; (2) luteinizing hormone, and (3) lactogenic hormone; all of which help control the development and functioning of the sex glands.

adenoid (ad´-e-noid): 1. Resembling a gland. 2. In the plural, refers to overgrowth of lymphoid tissue (the pharyngeal tonsil) in the nasopharynx. A. FACIES the facial expression characteristic of a person with enlarged adenoids; the mouth is open, the nose appears pinched due to interference with nasal breathing.

adenoidectomy (ad´-e-noyd-ek´-to-mi): Surgical removal of adenoid tissue from the nasopharynx.

adenoma (ad-e-nō´-ma): A tumour of glandular epithelial tissue; usually benign, but when occurring in the thyroid gland may be associated with carcinoma. A. SEBACEUM a manifestation of tuberous sclerosis in the facial skin, chiefly of the fibrovascular tissue; ADRENAL CORTICAL A. a benign tumour of adrenal cortical cells; may be associated with Cushing's disease or be symptomless; BRONCHIAL A. a circumscribed A. occurring in the submucosal tissue of the large bronchi; now considered to be a low-grade malignancy; EOSINOPHILIC A. a tumour of the anterior lobe of the pituitary gland; it results in acromegaly and gigantism; associated with bone weakness and sterility; HEPATIC A. a benign neoplasm of the liver, sometimes seen in the newborn; associated with the use of oral contraceptives; because the tumour is highly vascular, there is danger of rupture of the liver and haemoperitoneum; VILLOUS A. a large polyp (*q.v.*) on the mucosa of the large intestine.

adenomyoma (ad'-en-ō-mī-ō'-ma): A tumour, usually benign, composed of muscle and glandular elements of the endometrium of the uterus. — adenomyomata, pl.; adenomyomatous, adj.

adenomyosarcoma (ad'-e-nō-mī'-ō-sar-kō'-ma): A malignant tumour of glandular tissue that contains striated muscle tissue.

adenomyosis (ad'-en-ō-mī-ō'-sis): The benign overgrowth of glands and muscular tissue. A. UTERI a general enlargement of the uterus due to overgrowth of the myometrium.

adenomyositis (ad'-e-nō-mī-ō-sī'-tis): Endometriosis (*q.v.*).

adenose (ad'-e-nōz): Relating to or resembling a gland.

adenosine (a-den'-ō-s-ēn): A nucleoside (*q.v.*). A. MONOPHOSPHATE an ester that has important influence on the release of energy by cells for muscular activity; abbreviated AMP; A. DIPHOSPHATE a compound derived from adenosine triphosphate; a necessary substance for the production of energy by cells and needed for a variety of physical processes; abbreviated ADP; A. TRIPHOSPHATE coenzyme produced by cells and used by cells to release energy for a variety of energy-requiring activities, chiefly muscular activities; abbreviated ATP.

adenosis (ad-e-nō'-sis): 1. Any disease of a gland, especially of a lymph gland. 2. Development of an unusually large number of glandular elements without formation of a tumour.

adenotonsillectomy (ad'-en-ō-ton-sil-ek'-to-mi): Surgical removal of the adenoids and tonsils.

adenovirus (ad'-e-nō-vī'-rus): Many types have been isolated. Some cause upper respiratory infection, others pneumonia, others tumours.

adermia (a-der'-mi-a): 1. Congenital absence of skin. 2. A defect in the skin.

ADH: Abbreviation for antidiuretic hormone (*q.v.*).

ADHD: Abbreviation for attention deficit hyperactivity disorder (*q.v.*).

adhesion (ad-hē'-zhun): 1. The holding together, or adhering of two substances that may be of similar or dissimilar nature. 2. In physics, the force exerted between the molecules of two substances that are in contact. 3. The joining together by fibrous tissue of

bodily parts or tissues that are normally separate. 4. A band of fibrous tissue that holds together two body tissues or surfaces that are not normally in contact. 5. In the plural, the fibrous bands that may develop following surgery or inflammation; in the abdomen they may cause obstruction; in the joints they cause restriction of movement. — adherent, adj.; adherence, n.; adhere, v.

adhesiotomy (ad-hē-zi-ot'-o-mi): The surgical division or removal of adhesions.

adhesive (ad-hē'-siv): 1. A substance that causes two substances or materials to adhere to each other. 2. Sticky. 3. Tending to cling or stick together. A. TAPE tape with a sticky substance on one side; has many uses including holding bandages and dressings in place.

adiadochokinesia (a-dī'-ō-dō-kō-kī-nē'-zi-a): Inability to perform fine coordinated movements in rapid succession, *e.g.*, pronation and supination of the hand. Usually indicates cerebellar disturbance.

Adie's syndrome: A condition in which one pupil reacts more slowly than the opposite one, and only after prolonged stimulation. Also called *Adie's tonic pupil*, and *pseudo-Argyll-Robertson pupil*. [W.J. Adie, English physician, 1886–1935.]

adipectomy (ad-i-pek'-to-mi): The surgical removal of adipose tissue. See LIPECTOMY.

adipo-: A combining form denoting fat, fatty tissue.

adipocele (ad'-i-po-sēl): A hernia in which the sac contains only fat or fatty tissue.

adipofibroma (ad'-i-pō-fi-brō'-ma): A lipoma that contains some fibrous elements.

adipokinin (ad'-i-pō-kī'-nin): A hormone secreted by the anterior pituitary that mobilizes fat, causing an increase in the serum level of fatty acids.

adiponecrosis (ad'-i-pō-nē-krō'-sis): The necrosis of fatty tissue.

adipose (ad'-i-pōz): 1. Relating to fat. 2. Fat, fatty, or of a fatty nature. A. TISSUE connective or areolar tissue containing masses of stored fat cells.

adiposuria (ad-i-pō-sū'-ri-a): The presence of fat in the urine.

adipsia (a-dip'-si-a): Absence of the sensation of thirst; avoidance of taking fluid by mouth.

adjunct (ad'-junkt): Something attached to another thing but in a dependent or helping position; may be a procedure, a substance such as a drug, or a treatment mode. — adjunctive, adj.

adjustment: 1. The mechanism by which the tube of a microscope is raised or lowered thus bringing the object into focus. 2. In psychology, the alteration or accommodation by which an individual adapts himself and his actions to the environment.

adjuvant (ad′-joo-vant): That which aids, assists, or supports. In pharmacology, a substance included in a prescription that enhances the action of the principal constituent. A. THERAPY therapy that utilizes supportive measures or substances that enhance the effects of the main treatment.

ADL: Abbreviation for activities of daily living (*q.v.*).

Adler's theory: Holds that neuroses arise as a result of the individual's drive to overcome feelings of inferiority, either social or physical, through compensation.

ad lib: Abbreviation for *ad libitum* [L.], meaning at pleasure, without restraint, as much as desired.

ad nauseam (ad naw′-sē-am): To the point of nausea or producing nausea.

adolescence (ad-ō-les′-sens): The age that begins with puberty, extends through the years of physical and psychological maturation and ends with the completion of bone growth; often referred to as the *teens*. — adolescent, adj.

adolescent (ad-ō-les′-ent): 1. A person in the period between childhood and adulthood, who has reached puberty but has not fully matured; usually referred to as a teenager. 2. Relating to adolescence.

ADP: Abbreviation for adenosine diphosphate. See under ADENOSINE.

adrenal (ad-rē′-nal): 1. Near the kidney. 2. One of two small triangular hormone-secreting glands that lie on the superior surface of each kidney, consisting of two parts: (a) the medulla, the inner part, which secretes adrenaline and noradrenaline; and (b) an outer part, the cortex, which secretes cortisone, aldosterone and testosterone. The cortical secretions have important actions in the control of many body functions including growth and weight changes, basal metabolism regulation, neuromuscular activity, gastrointestinal function, maintenance of body fluid balance, reproduction. Functionally, the A. glands are closely related to the pituitary and other endocrine glands. A. CRISIS acute adrenal failure, *e.g.*, a severe exacerbation of Addison's disease; A. INSUFFICIENCY hypofunction of the adrenal gland; Addison's disease (*q.v.*); A. STEROIDS

hormones secreted by the adrenal cortex. See also ADRENALINE, NORADRENALINE, CORTISONE, ALDOSTERONE, TESTOSTERONE

adrenal cortical hyperplasia: See ADRENOGENITAL SYNDROME.

adrenal cortical insufficiency: Failure of secretion of glucocorticoid and mineralocorticoid hormones by the adrenal cortex.

adrenalectomy (ad-rē-na-lek′-to-mi): Surgical removal of all or part of one or both adrenal glands for treatment of Cushing's syndrome (*q.v.*), phaeochromocytoma (*q.v.*), hypertension (*q.v.*), malignant disease of the breast, or other adrenal disorder; if bilateral, requires replacement administration of cortical hormones.

adrenaline (a-dren′-a-lēn): The chief hormone of the normal adrenal medulla; is also produced synthetically. A powerful vasopressor substance. Contracts arterioles of skin, mucous membrane and viscera; dilates arterioles of skeletal muscles and brain; increases strength and rate of heartbeat; increases heart output, blood pressure, blood sugar and metabolism; speeds blood clotting; relaxes bronchial muscles. Used therapeutically to control local bleeding as in epistaxis (*q.v.*), and to relieve anaphylaxis (*q.v.*), allergic conditions, asthmatic attacks, heart and circulatory failure, also in treatment of open-angle glaucoma (*q.v.*).

adrenergic (ad-re-ner′-jik): Relates to (1) sympathetic nerve fibres that release adrenaline at their endings when stimulated, or (2) the chemical activity characteristic of adrenaline and like substances on nerve endings. A. BLOCKING AGENTS compounds that inhibit responses to adrenergic nerve activity and to noradrenaline and like substances; classified according to their selective activity as alpha and beta, the beta group being in most common use. A. CRISIS a condition characterized by overactivity of the part of the sympathetic system that is activated by adrenaline, causing adrenaline intoxication with symptoms of arrhythmia, tachycardia, hypertension, anxiety, dilated pupils, and often psychotic behaviour.

adrenocortical (ad-rē′-nō-kor′-ti-kal): Relating to or originating in the adrenal cortex.

adrenocorticoid (ad-rē′-nō-kor′-ti-koyd): 1. Relating to the adrenal cortex or its hormonal secretion. 2. An adrenal cortical hormone. A. STEROIDS endocrine secretions of the adrenal cortex; see ALDOSTERONE, CORTISONE, DEOXYCORTICOSTERONE.

adrenocorticosteroid (ad-rē′-nō-kor′-ti-kō-stē′-roid): A hormone that is elaborated in the cortex of the adrenal gland. See CORTICOSTEROID.

adrenocorticotrophic hormone (ad-rē′-nō-kor′-ti-kō-trōp′-ik hor′-mōn): A secretion of the anterior lobe of the pituitary gland; it stimulates the release of the corticoid steroids from the adrenal cortex. Abbreviated ACTH. Also called *adrenocorticotrophin*.

adrenogenic (a-drē-nō-jen′-ik): Produced or originating in the adrenal glands.

adrenogenital syndrome (ad-rē′-nō-jen′-i-tal sin′-drōm): A congenital or acquired condition resulting from overproduction of androgenic hormones by the adrenal cortex; may be due to hyperplasia (*q.v.*) or tumour. In female children it is usually evident at birth by pseudohermaphroditism (*q.v.*); in male children it is not usually evident until the child is three or four years old and is represented by precocious sexual development. In adults the syndrome is characterized by masculinization in women and feminization in men. Also called *adrenal cortical hyperplasia*.

adrenoleukodystrophy (ad-rē′-nō-lū′-kō-dis′-tro-fi): A progressive, inherited, metabolic disorder of children; characterized by bronzing of the skin, adrenal insufficiency, and degeneration of the white matter in various parts of the central nervous system.

adrenolytic (ad′-ren-ō-lit′-ik): 1. Inhibiting or antagonizing the action or secretion of adrenaline. 2. Having a depressing effect on sympathetic (adrenergic) nerve fibres.

adrenosterone (ad-rēn-os′-ter-ōn): A male sex hormone present in the adrenal cortex.

adsorbate (ad-sor′-bāt): A substance that adheres to the surface of another substance by adsorption.

adsorbent (ad-sorb′-ent): 1. Having the quality of adsorption (*q.v.*). 2. An agent that has the quality of adsorption, *e.g.*, charcoal, which adsorbs gases and acts as a deodorant.

adsorption (ad-sorp′-shun): The process by which a gas, liquid, or other substance is collected and concentrated at the surface of another substance.

adtorsion (ad-tor′-shun): Inward turning of both eyes simultaneously.

adult (ad′-ult, a-dult′): 1. A person who is fully developed and mature. 2. Relating to persons who are fully developed and mature. 3. Having attained full growth, maturity, and reproductive ability.

adulteration (a-dul-ter-ā′-shun): The addition of an impure, cheap, or inferior substance to another substance in deliberate attempt to alter that substance and to deceive the user; the usual implication is that the original substance is thereby rendered less effective, less desirable, weaker, or cheaper.

adulthood (a-dult′hood): The state of being fully developed, mature, and capable of reproduction.

advanced directive: A written statement made by a competent individual, giving his or her wishes with regards to treatment should he or she become incapable of expressing these wishes to healthcare professionals. Also known as a *living will*.

advanced life support: Resuscitation technique used when there is a cardiac arrest; it follows on from basic life support (*q.v.*). Includes the administration of drugs and defibrillation.

advanced practice: a nurse who has acquired the expert knowledge base, complex decision-making skills, and clinical competencies for expanded practice, the characteristics of which are shaped by the context and/or country in which he or she has the credentials to practise.

advancement (ad-vans′-ment): In surgery, an operation in which a muscle or tendon is severed and reattached farther forward. Specifically, the operation to remedy strabismus; the muscle tendon opposite to the direction of the squint is detached and sutured to the sclera at a point farther from its origin.

adventitia (ad-ven-tish′-i-a): The external coat of an organ or structure, especially that of an artery or vein. — adventitiae, pl.; adventitious, adj.

adventitious (ad-ven-tish′-us): 1. Coming from the outside; external; not inherent. 2. Appearing sporadically in other than the usual location. 3. Relating to adventitia. A. SOUNDS abnormal sounds, as in the lungs, *e.g.*, rales, rhonchi.

adverse drug reaction: An unwanted effect of a drug; ranging from a minor side effect to a severe, harmful effect.

advocacy (ad′-vō-ka-si): The act or process of defending or supporting a cause or proposal.

advocate (ad′-vō-kāt): A person who acts for or defends the rights of another person who is unable or unwilling to act for himself. PATIENT A. an individual who becomes the patient's advocate through representing his or her needs and wishes.

-aemia: Combining form denoting (1) blood, (2) a condition of blood.

aer-, aero-: Combining form denoting relationship to: (1) air or atmosphere (2) gas, (3) aviation.

aerate (air' -āt): 1. To charge a substance with air or a gas such as carbon dioxide or oxygen. 2. To supply the blood with oxygen, by respiration, or by artificial ventilation. — aerated, adj.

aeration (air' -a' -shun): 1. Exposing to or supplying with air. 2. Charging a fluid with gas or air. 3. The process, which occurs within the lungs, whereby the carbon dioxide in the blood is exchanged for oxygen.

aerobe (air' -ōb): A microorganism that requires oxygen for growth and life. FACULTATIVE A. a microorganism that can grow and live either with or without oxygen; OBLIGATE A. a microorganism that can grow and live only in the presence of free oxygen. — aerobic, adj.

aerobic (air' -ō' -bik): 1. Relating to an aerobe. 2. Relating to the utilization or requirement of oxygen in order to live and grow. A. EXERCISE steady, continuous movement of the arms, legs, and trunk which forces a continuous flow of blood (and oxygen) through the heart and muscles but which is not vigorous enough or continued long enough to produce metabolic acidosis; includes jogging, walking, dancing, swimming, bicycling. See ANAEROBIC EXERCISE under ANAEROBIC.

aerocele (air' -ō-sēl): A tumour or swelling consisting of air that has collected in an abnormally formed sac or pouch, most often occurring in the trachea or larynx. INTRACRANIAL A. and A. formed in the cranium; may occur following compound fracture of the skull.

aerodermectasia (air' -ō-der-mek-tā' -zi-a): Subcutaneous emphysema; see EMPHYSEMA.

aerodynamics (air'ō-dī-nam' -iks): The science and study of air and gases in motion.

aeroembolism (air-ō-em' -bō-lizm): A condition that occurs particularly in aviators, when it is caused by rapid ascent to great heights, and in deep sea divers when returning to the surface from great depths. See also CAISSON DISEASE and BENDS. Nitrogen bubbles form in body tissues and fluids, causing symptoms that include rash, pain in the joints and lungs, itching, neuritis, paraesthesia, sometimes paralysis and coma. Patients having head, neck, or heart surgery may also exhibit these symptoms.

aerogen (air' -ō-jen): Any gas-producing microorganism.

aerogenesis (air-ō-jen' -e-sis): The production of gas. — aerogenic, adj.

aerogenous (air-oj' -e-nus): 1. Gas producing. 2. Descriptive of organisms that produce gas; e.g., Welch's bacillus (q.v.).

aerogram (air' -ō-gram): An x-ray of a hollow organ or structure after it has been filled with air or gas.

aeroneurosis (air' -ō-nū-rō' -sis): A chronic functional psychoneurosis, occurs in aviators; caused by prolonged periods of anoxia and stress; characterized by gastric distress, insomnia, worry, loss of self-confidence, and various other physical and emotional symptoms.

aero-otitis media (air' -ō-ō-tī' -tis mē' -di-a): Inflammation of the middle ear due to trauma caused by the difference between atmospheric and intratympanic pressure that develops when an aircraft descends rapidly from a high altitude.

acropathy (air' op' a thi): Any pathological condition caused by change in atmospheric pressure, e.g. decompression sickness, commonly called 'the bends'.

aerophagia (air' ō fa' ji a): Air swallowing followed by belching and distension of the stomach and colon; a habit associated with nervous or digestive disorders. Also called aerophagy.

aerophil (air' -ō-fil): An organism that requires air or oxygen for growth and life. Also said of an individual who loves to be in the open air.

aerophobia (air' -ō-fō' -bi-a): 1. Abnormal dread of air, particularly fresh air, draughts of air, or bad air. 2. Abnormal dread of being up in the air, as of flying.

aerophyte (air' -ō-fīt): An organism that lives on air or oxygen.

aeroplethysmograph (air' -ō-ple-thiz' -mo-graf): An apparatus for measuring and registering the amount of air inspired and expired.

aerosol (air' -o-sol): A suspension of atomized solid or liquid particles in air or a gas which is dispensed in a fine mist. Aerosols containing drugs are used in inhalation therapy for several pulmonary conditions. Bacteriocidal aerosols are sprayed into a room as a disinfectant. Aerosols containing chemicals are used in mosquito and insect control projects, and as deodorants. A. SEAL plastic resin dissolved in ether; when sprayed onto a wound it forms a flexible adhesive seal; A. THERAPY the use of aerosol or of a nebulizer that creates a vapour containing particles of a drug in a gas stream to help liquefy secretions and aid in their removal from the bronchial tree.

aerosol sniffing: The inhalation of hair spray, deodorants, household cleansers or other aerosol sprays by spraying them into a bag which is held over the head or face to be inhaled; causes a strange floating kind of high; has been known to cause death from cardiac arrest; most victims are teenagers.

aerotitis (air′-ō-tī′-tis): See BAROTITIS. A. MEDIA inflammation of the middle ear, caused by the difference between the atmospheric pressure and the air pressure in the middle ear, or by rapid descent in an aeroplane.

aesthetic (es-thet′-ik): 1. Relating to sensation or feeling. 2. Relating to beauty.

aetiology (ē-ti-ol-ji): The science that deals with causation of diseases and their modes of introduction into the host. — aetiologic, aetiologic, adj.; aetiologically, adv.

AF: Abbreviation for atrial fibrillation, see under ATRIAL.

afebrile (a-feb′-ril): Without fever.

affect (af′-ekt): The outward manifestation of a feeling or mood evoked by a stimulus; may be directed towards anything. In psychiatry, that aspect of the mind that is concerned with emotions, mood, or the external representation of mood. The term is often used interchangeably with emotion or feeling. — affective, adj.

affection (a-fek′-shun): 1. An emotional or feeling state. 2. Any disease or disorder, physical or mental. See AFFECT.

affective (a-fek′-tiv): Relating to affect.

affective disorders: Categorized as neurotic, this group includes as the major affective disorders the bipolar disorders (mixed, manic, and depressed), as well as major depression, both single episodic and recurrent. The specific affective disorder group includes CYCLOTHYMIC DISORDER which is characterized by periods of hypomania and depression which may be mixed or alternating, and DYSTHYMIC DISORDER in which there is a chronic depressed mood that may be persistent or intermittent. The atypical affective disorder group includes ATYPICAL BIPOLAR DISORDER in which the manic features cannot be classified under bipolar disorder or cyclothymic disorder, and ATYPICAL DEPRESSION in which the individual has depressive symptoms that cannot be classified under other affective disorders.

afferent (af′-er-ent): Conveying a fluid or impulse to or towards a centre; term used to designate nerves, blood vessels and lymphatics that perform this function. Opp. to efferent. A. NERVE a bundle of nerve fibres that carry impulses from the periphery to the central nervous system; receptors connect directly to

them. Often synonymous with sensory nerve; A. PATHWAYS neural structures that conduct information from the periphery to the central nervous system.

affiliation (a-fil-i-ā′-shun): 1. Close connection as a member, associate, or branch of an association or society 2. Membership. 3. The origin of an association.

affinity (a-fin′-i-ti): Attraction, or a common inherent relationship. In chemistry, the attractive force between two substances. In immunology, the attractive force between antibody and antigen.

afflux (af′-luks): The rush of blood or other body fluid to a part, causing congestion.

affusion (a-fū′-zhun): The act of pouring water on the body or a part of it; usually to reduce fever or nervousness.

afibrinogenaemia (a-fī′-brin-ō-jen-ē′mi-a): A rare congenital or acquired blood disorder characterized by a deficiency or absence of fibrinogen (*q.v.*) in the blood plasma. More correctly, hypofibrinogenaemia. — afibrinogenaemic, adj.

AFP: Abbreviation for alpha-fetoprotein (*q.v.*).

African trypanosomiasis (trip′an-ō-sō-mī′-a-sis): An acute, infectious, highly fatal disease, particularly of tropical Africa; caused by *Trypanosoma gambiense*; transmitted to humans by the bite of a tsetse fly which has become infected by having previously bitten an infected person or animal. Often called *African sleeping sickness* and *Gambian trypanosomiasis*.

afterbirth (af′-ter-berth): The placenta, umbilical cord, and fetal membranes that are expelled from the uterus following the birth of a child.

aftercare (af′-ter-kair): Care, including but not confined to medical care, that is given during and after convalescence and rehabilitation following hospitalization.

afterpains (af′-ter-pāns): The cramp-like pains felt during the first few days following childbirth and the expulsion of the afterbirth; due to contraction of the uterine muscle fibres.

aftertaste (af′-ter-tāst): Persistence of the sensation of taste after cessation of the stimulus that initiated it.

A/G ratio: See ALBUMIN–GLOBULIN RATIO.

agalactia (a-ga-lak′-shi-a): Lack of secretion, or imperfect secretion of milk following childbirth. — agalactic, adj.

agalorrhoea (a-gal-ō-rē′-a): Absence or arrest of the flow of milk.

agar, agar-agar (āg′-ar): A gelatinous substance obtained from certain marine algae (*q.v.*). It is used as a bulk-increasing laxative, a bacterial culture medium, and a suspending agent in emulsions. A. STREAK SLANT, agar slanted in a test tube on which bacteria are planted for culture; BLOOD A. nutrient agar to which blood has been added; CHOCOLATE A. agar or a nutrient bouillion to which heated blood is added, turning the blood brown; it does not contain chocolate; NUTRIENT A. a straw-coloured culture medium composed of peptone, meat extract, sodium chloride, and agar.

age: Length of time that a person or thing has existed. OLD A. ageing, to show or cause to show signs of advancing age. CHRONOLOGICAL A. arranged or regarded in the order of age.

aged (ā′-jed): **1.** Relating to a person of old age. **2.** Persons of old age.

ageing (ā′-jing): In the human, the gradual physical and psychological changes in the body and mind that are not due to disease or accident, and do not proceed at the same rate in all, but which are universal and inevitable and eventually terminate in death. TIME-CLOCK THEORY OF A. the theory that nature endows every individual with a time clock (the ageing process) set to run down so that everyone is programmed to self-destruct.

ageism (ā′-jism): **1.** The tendency to draw conclusions or formulate beliefs about a person on the basis of his chronological age alone. **2.** The systematic negative stereotyping of the elderly as being unhealthy, helpless, mentally confused, and in need of supportive services. This approach ignores the mental and physical potentialities of the elderly and often results in irreversible mutual withdrawal, the development of poor interrelationships, and eccentricities in older people. **3.** Prejudice or discrimination on grounds of age. — ageist, adj.

agenesis (a-jen′-e-sis): **1.** Incomplete and imperfect development of a body organ or part. **2.** Congenital absence of a body organ or part. **3.** Impotence or sterility due to lack of gonadal development. Also *agenesia*.

agenitalism (a-jen′-i-tal-izm): A congenital absence of genitalia.

agent (ā′-jent): A person, substance, or force that acts, or is capable of acting, on something else, thereby producing an effect. CATALYTIC A. a substance that enhances or speeds a reaction without itself being affected.

age spot: Senile lentigo; see under LENTIGO.

ageusia (a-gū′-si-a): Impairment or loss of the sense of taste.

agglutination (a-gloo-ti-nā′-shun): **1.** A phenomenon characterized by the clumping together of insoluble particles (bacteria or cells) distributed in a fluid, which is effected by specific immune antibodies (agglutinins) that develop in the blood of a previously infected or sensitized person. **2.** The clumping together of blood cells when incompatible bloods are mixed in transfusion. **3.** The joining together of surfaces in the healing of wounds. — agglutinate, v.

agglutinins (a-gloo′-ti-ninz): Specific substances (antibodies) that are formed in blood serum in the presence of particular invading bacteria or other cells causing them to adhere to one another forming a clump. COLD A., A. that will act only at low temperatures (0° to 20°C).

agglutinogen (a-gloo-tin′-ō-jen): A protein substance that stimulates the production of a specific agglutinin when introduced into the body, *e.g.*, dead bacteria in a vaccine.

aggregate (ag′-grē-gāt): **1.** To clump, gather, or crowd together in a mass. **2.** The mass formed by substances or cells clumping together.

aggressin (a-gres′-in): A metabolic substance believed to be produced by certain bacteria; promotes infection by enhancing aggressive action of the bacteria against the host. Also called *virulin*.

aggression (a-gresh′-un): An attitude of animosity or hostility, or an assaultive action, usually resulting from frustration, fear, or a threatening situation. May be justified and self-protective. May be directed outwards towards the environment and expressed in explosive actions, or inward towards the self, as occurs in depression.

agitation (aj-i-tā′-shun): Excessive chronic restlessness; with constant purposeless physical activity, distractibility, limited concentration, sometimes as with mental disturbances and intellectual ineffectiveness; usually due to feelings of apprehension; seen in patients with severe depressive states, presenile dementia, or as a sequela of brain injury.

aglutition (ag-loo-tish′-un): See DYSPHAGIA.

aglycaemia (a-gl-ī-sē′-mi-a): Absence of sugar from the blood.

aglycosuria (a-glī-kō-sū′-rē-a): Absence of glucose from the urine.

agnogenic (ag-no-jen′-ik): Of unknown source, cause, or origin; idiopathic (*q.v.*).

agnosia (ag-nō′-si-a): Inability to recognize certain sensory impressions although recognition of other impressions is normal. Several types are distinguished, according to the sense organ(s) involved, *e.g.*, visual, auditory, gustatory, tactile. TIME A. loss of comprehension of the passage of time.

-agog,-agogue: Combining form denoting an agent that leads, incites, incites, induces, or produces.

agonad (a-gō´-nad): An individual who has no sex glands.

agonal (ag´-o-nal): 1. Associated with agony, particularly the death agony or struggle. 2. Occurring at the time of death or just preceding it.

agonist (ag´-on-ist): 1. A muscle which contracts and shortens to perform a movement that opposes the action of another muscle which is in a state of relaxation at the same time; see ANTAGONIST. 2. A drug or other agent that can interact with receptors to produce an effect or response.

agony (ag´-o-ni): 1. Intense pain of mind or body. 2. Anguish, distress, or torture. 3. A violent struggle. 4. The death struggle.

agoraphobia (ag-o-ra-fō´-bi-a): Morbid fear of being alone in large open spaces; of being away from home; of lakes and oceans; of crowds, stores, tunnels, bridges, theatres, or public transportation vehicles from which it might be difficult to escape.

agranular (a-gran´-ū-lar): Without granules; often refers to certain leukocytes.

agranulocyte (a-gran´-ū-lō-sīt): A leukocyte in which the cytoplasm contains no granules.

agranulocytosis (a-gran´-ū-lō-sī-tō´ sis): An acute, serious condition, characterized by sudden marked reduction or complete absence of granulocytes or polymorphonuclear leukocytes, fever, and ulceration of mucous membranes, especially those of the mouth, gastrointestinal tract, and vagina. May be idiopathic, or may result from the use of certain drugs, chemicals, or radiation therapy.

agraphia (a-graf´-i-a): Partial or total loss of the ability to express one's thoughts coherently in writing; writing is characterized by omission or repetition of words or parts of words, incorrect usage, faulty grammar; due to pathology or injury to the cerebral cortex. — agraphic, adj.

AHF: Abbreviation for antihaemophilic factor (*q.v.*).

ahypnia (a-hip´-ni-a): Insomnia.

AI: Abbreviation for: 1. Aortic insufficiency, see under AORTIC. 2. Artificial insemination, see under INSEMINATION.

AID: Abbreviation for artificial insemination (*q.v.*) by donor, see also INSEMINATION.

aid (ād): 1. Help given by one person to another. 2. Any of the various objects and appliances that help a disabled person to walk, hear, see, etc. FIRST A. care or treatment given to a person who has been injured or become suddenly ill pending further medical or surgical treatment.

aide (ād): In health-care, a non-professional person who acts as assistant to a professional care giver.

AIDS (ādz): Abbreviation for acquired immunodeficiency syndrome (*q.v.*). A.-RELATED COMPLEX (1) a group of common complications found in early stage HIV infection; they include progressive generalized lymphadenopathy, recurrent fever, unexplained weight loss, swollen lymph nodes, diarrhoea, herpes, hairy leukoplakia, fungal infection of the mouth and throat and/or the presence of HIV antibodies; (2) symptoms that appear to be related to infection by HIV; they include an unexplained, chronic deficiency of white blood cells (leukopenia) or a poorly functioning lymphatic system with swelling of the lymph nodes (lymphadenopathy) lasting for more than 3 months without the opportunistic infections required for a diagnosis of AIDS.

AIH: Abbreviation for artificial insemination (*q.v.*) with the husband's semen.

ailment (āl´-ment): A complaint, infirmity, or sickness. The term is usually applied to a physical or mental disorder of a mild nature.

air: The colourless, odourless, tasteless gaseous mixture that surrounds the Earth. It consists of approximately four parts of nitrogen by volume to one part of oxygen, and small amounts of such other substances as carbon dioxide, hydrogen, helium, ozone, neon, argon, krypton, xenon, ammonia, and varying amounts of water vapour. Also called *atmosphere*. A. BATH see under BATH; A. BOOT a pneumatic splint or prosthesis for the lower extremity; reaches from the ankle to the knee; used to eliminate pressure by holding the foot off the bed; A. EMBOLUS a bubble of air constructing a blood vessel; A. ENCEPHALOGRAPHY see PNEUMOENCEPHALOGRAPHY; A. HUNGER shortness of breath, with inspiratory and expiratory distress; characterized by rapid breathing, sighing, and gasping; due to anoxia; A. MATTRESS one filled with air; supports the body uniformly with a minimum amount of pressure on the skin; A. RING an inflated rubber or plastic ring, covered with bandage and placed under pressure points to prevent development of decubitus ulcers; A. SAC an alveolus in the lung; A. SICKNESS motion sickness occurring in aeroplane flights; symptoms include nausea, vomiting, dizziness; A. SWALLOWING aerophagia (*q.v.*); COMPLEMENTAL A. the extra air, over and above the volume of tidal air, that can be drawn into the lungs by the deepest possible inspiration; RESIDUAL A. that which remains in the lungs after the fullest possible forced expiration; STATIONARY A. that which remains in the lungs after normal expiration; SUPPLEMENTAL A. the expiratory reserve volume; see under EXPIRATORY; TIDAL A. that which passes in and out of the lungs in normal breathing.

airborne (air' -born): In microbiology, refers to the transmission of infection from one person to another by means of droplets of moisture that contain the causative organism.

airway (air' -way): 1. The natural passageway for air into and out of the lungs. 2. Any of the several kinds of devices for maintaining a clear and unobstructed passageway for air to enter and leave the lungs. The most common types of artificial airway are: (1) OROPHARYNGEAL in which a rubber or plastic tube is inserted through the mouth into the pharynx to prevent the tongue from forming an obstruction in the pharynx; (2) ENDOTRACHEAL A. in which a rubber or plastic tube is inserted through the mouth or nose and passed through the larynx into the trachea; used for the administration of anaesthesia and for prevention and treatment of acute respiratory failure in patients with pulmonary disease; also provides a route for ventilation with a respirator; (3) TRACHEOSTOMY in which a tube is inserted into the trachea, below the larynx through an incision in the neck; used when there is an obstruction in the upper respiratory tract, or to prevent aspiration of secretions from the bronchial tract, or to provide a route for mechanical ventilation.

akaryocyte (a-kar' -i-ō-sīt): 1. A cell that has no nucleus. 2. Erythrocyte.

akaryote (a-kar' -i-ōt): Non-nucleated, referring usually to cells. Also spelled *acaryote*.

akathisia (ak-a-thiz' -i-a): Inability to sit still or to lie quietly; a state in which the individual feels an inner restlessness that results in motor restlessness; may be due to an emotional disturbance or be a side effect of certain drugs, particularly the antipsychotic drugs.

akeratosis (a-ker-a-tō' -sis): A deficiency of horny tissue, of the nails in particular.

akinesia (a-kī-nē' -si-a): Inability to initiate or sustain voluntary muscular action; may be due to the side effects of certain drugs; also some-

times seen in post-encephalitic parkinsonism. — akinesic; akinetic, adj.

akinetic (a-kī-net' -ik): Without movement. A. CATATONIA occurs in schizophrenia; see CATATONIA; A. EPILEPSY a form of epilepsy in which the individual remains limp throughout the period of unconsciousness. A. MUTISM a state in which the individual appears to be relaxed and asleep, makes no movements or sounds, and can be roused only with difficulty; due to a neurological or psychological disturbance.

Al: Chemical symbol for aluminium.

-al: A suffix denoting connection with, *e.g.*, abdominal.

alanine transaminase (gloo-tam' -ik pī-roo' -vik trans-am' -i-nās): An enzyme found in high concentrations in the liver, and in lesser amounts in the kidney, heart, and muscle tissue; used in laboratory tests for diagnosis of liver disease. Essential in the hydrolysis of protein.

Al-Anon: A worldwide self-help group for relatives and friends of alcoholics; based on the principles of Alcoholics Anonymous (*q.v.*) and adapted for non-alcoholics.

alaryngeal (a-la-rin' -jē-al): Without a larynx. A. SPEECH usually refers to oesophageal speech developed following total laryngectomy (*q.v.*).

alb-, alba-: A combining form meaning white, whitish.

albedo (al-bē' -dō): 1. Whiteness or paleness. 2. Reflected light from any surface. A. RETINAE paleness of the retina due to oedema.

albicans (al' -bi-kans): White or whitish.

albinism (al' -bi-nizm): A recessive genetic condition in which the inability to produce melanin results in lack of normal pigmentation of the skin, hair, and eyes. OCULAR A. absence of pigmentation in the tissues of the eye; PARTIAL A. lack of pigmentation in a local area only; TOTAL A. lack of any pigmentation in the skin, hair, and eyes; often accompanied by photophobia (*q.v.*), astigmatism (*q.v.*), and nystagmus (*q.v.*). In black people the skin is tan or cream coloured, sometimes freckled, the hair is brownish-yellow; the eye symptoms are similar to those in white people.

albino (al-bī' -nō): A person affected with albinism (*q.v.*); strictly speaking, a male person so affected. — albinotic, adj.

Albright's syndrome: A group of symptoms including overgrowth of several parts of the skeleton with formation of multiple cysts, the appearance of dark pigmented spots on the skin tending to occur on one side of the body, and, in females, sexual precocity. [Fuller Albright, American physician 1900–1969]

albugo (al-bū' -gō): An opaque white spot that develops on the cornea.

albumin (al-bū' -min): A variety of protein found in all animal tissues and in many vegetable tissues; is soluble in water and coagulates on heating. SERUM A. the chief protein in blood plasma and other serous fluids. — albuminous; albuminoid, adj.

albuminaemia (al-bū-mi-nē' -mi-a): The presence of an abnormal amount of albumin in the blood plasma.

albumin–globulin ratio (al-bū' -min-glob' -ū-lin): The ratio of albumin to globulin in the blood serum. Normally the ratio is from 1:3 to 1:8; lower ratios usually indicate the present of pathology. Abbreviated A/G ratio.

albuminoid (al-bū' -mi-noyd): 1. Having the characteristics of albumin. 2. A protein. 3. Any of a group of proteins that are not soluble in aqueous solutions and which have a structural or protective function in the body, e.g., collagen (q.v.), keratin (q.v.), or elastin (q.v.), found in hair, nails, cartilage, and the lens of the eye.

albuminuria (al-bū' -mi-nū' -ri-a): The presence of albumin in the urine. Temporary albuminuria may occur in fevers, pregnancy, or after exercise; it usually clears up completely after the cause is removed. It may also be the result of renal impairment caused by kidney disorders, malignant hypertension, congestive heart failure. CHRONIC A. leads to a deficiency of protein in the blood plasma. ORTHOSTATIC or POSTURAL A. occurs only when the person is standing; is absent during sleep; not due to renal disease.

alcohol (al' -ko-hol): 1. Ethyl alcohol, a colourless, volatile, flammable liquid produced by fermentation of carbohydrates by yeast. The principal constituent of wine and spirits. Taken in small quantities it is a nervous system stimulant; in larger quantities it is a nervous system depressant. It enhances the action of barbiturates and tranquillizers. Medicinal uses include local application as an antiseptic or astringent; internal use as a cardiac stimulant and for its euphoric effect; as a base for tinctures and extracts; to preserve anatomical specimens. As a food, alcohol furnishes about 110 kilocalories of heat per 25 millilitres. ABSOLUTE A. contains at least 99% pure alcohol and is free of water and any impurities; sometimes used by injection for relief of trigeminal neuralgia and other intractable pain; A. PSYCHOSIS see KORSAKOFF'S SYNDROME;

DENATURED A. has had some substance added to it to make it unfit for internal use; used externally on the skin as a cooling agent and disinfectant. 2. Any of a series of volatile hydroxyl compounds that are made from hydrocarbons by distillation. BENZYL A. used as a local anaesthetic, ISOPROPYL A. used externally for rubbing and as a disinfectant; not used internally; METHYL or WOOD A. made by distilling wood; for external use only.

alcohol-fast: A bacteriological term describing a stained bacterium that resists discoloration by alcohol.

alcoholic (al-kō-hol' -ik): 1. Relating to or containing alcohol. 2. A person who habitually uses alcoholic beverages to excess. A. AMNESTIC SYNDROME Korsakoff's syndrome (q.v.). A. DEMENTIA a non-hallucinatory dementia associated with alcoholism but not having the features of Korsakoff's syndrome; A. HALLUCINOSIS a psychosis characterized by anxiety, restlessness, hallucinations of voices uttering threats, etc.; may be a withdrawal symptom in persons who have been heavy drinkers; A. PARANOIA chronic paranoid psychosis characterized by delusional jealousy, delusions of persecution, and aggressive, violent behaviour; A. PSYCHOSIS any of a group of mental disorders caused by excessive use of alcohol; associated with brain damage; symptoms include delirium tremens and hallucinosis.

Alcoholics Anonymous: A fellowship of alcoholics and former alcoholics who seek to control their compulsive urge to drink and to help others to do likewise through the group process.

alcoholism (al' -kō-hol-izm): 1. Alcohol poisoning. 2. Physical dependence on alcohol and its uncontrollable overuse; now recognized as a disease with physiological, psychological, and sociological aspects; may be acute or chronic.

alcoholuria (al-ko-hol-ū' -ri-a): Alcohol in the urine. Basis of one test for fitness to drive a car after drinking alcohol.

alcohol withdrawal: The diagnosis now given for the condition occurring when alcohol is withdrawn after one has been drinking alcohol for several days or longer; symptoms include coarse tremor of the hands, tongue, and eyelids, nausea and vomiting, malaise, anxiety, and depression. Symptoms usually disappear within a week unless alcohol withdrawal delirium develops.

alcohol withdrawal delirium: Delirium following recent reduction or cessation of alcohol consumption. Symptoms include tachycardia, sweating, elevated blood pressure, delusions, agitated behaviour, and hallucinations. Has been referred to as *delirium tremens*.

aldosterone (al-do'-ster-ōn): A potent adrenocortical hormone that has an electrolyte-regulating function; it enhances the reabsorption of sodium by the kidney tubules and functions in the metabolism of sodium, chloride, and potassium; is described as a mineralocorticoid.

aldosteronism (al-do'-ster-o-nizm): A condition of electrolyte imbalance caused by excessive secretion of aldosterone; may be called primary when it is associated with tumour of the adrenal cortex, or secondary when it is associated with hypertension or oedema, as occur in hepatic disease and kidney or cardiac failure.

aleukaemia (a-lū-kē'-mi-a): Lowered proportion of white blood cells in the circulating blood; aleukaemic leukaemia. — aleukemic, adj.

aleukia (a-lu'-ki-a): Lack of or abnormal decrease in the number of white blood cells, or of blood platelets.

alexia (a-leks'-i-a): Word blindness; a type of aphasia with loss of ability to interpret the significance of printed or written words, but without loss of visual power or intelligence. Due to a lesion in the central nervous system. — alexic, adj.

ALG: Abbreviation for antilymphocyte globulin (*q.v.*).

algae (al'-jē): A large group of simple, unicellular marine plants, containing chlorophyll, including seaweed and freshwater plants, varying in size from microscopic to some metres in length. Some are useful as food, others in the preparation of medicinal substances, see AGAR. Algae collect on the top of sand filters and are effective in screening out bacteria, thus helping in the purification of water. — alga, sing.

alge-, algesi-, algo: Combining forms denoting relationship to pain.

algesia (al-jē'-zi-a): Hyperaesthesia; excessive sensitivity to pain. Opp. of analgesia. — algesic, adj.

algesimeter (al-je-sim'-e-ter): An instrument used for determining the degree of sensitivity to pain by pricking the skin with a sharp point.

algesthesia (al-jes-thē'-zi-a): Perception of pain.

-algia: Combining form denoting pain.

algid (al'-jid): 1. Cold. 2. Condition after a severe attack of fever, especially malaria,

with collapse, extreme coldness of the body, suggesting a fatal termination. During this stage the rectal temperature may be high.

alginates (al'jin-ātz): Seaweed derivatives which, when applied locally, encourage the clotting of blood. They are available in solution and in specially impregnated gauze used in making surgical dressings. Also used for making dental impressions after being converted into a gel by combination with certain chemicals.

algogenesis (al-gō-jen'-e-sis): The origin of pain.

algogenic (al-gō-jen'-ik): 1. Producing pain. 2. Producing cold. 3. Lowering the body temperature.

algolagnia (al-gō-lag'-ni-a): A sexual perversion in which the person achieves sexual gratification from inflicting or experiencing pain; masochism, sadism.

algophily (al-gof'-i-li): Sexual perversion characterized by a morbid love of inflicting, experiencing, or thinking about pain.

algophobia (al-gō-fō'-bi-a): Morbid dread of witnessing or experiencing pain.

algor (al'-gor): Coldness, rigor, a chill. A. MORTIS the gradual cooling of the body after death.

algorithms (al'-go-rith-ems): Procedures consisting of sequences of algebraic formulas and/or logical steps to calculate or determine tasks, such as those used by NHS Direct.

alienation (āl-i-en-ā'-shun): 1. In psychology, the term is used in several ways: (a) to express feelings of unreality or strangeness; (b) the fear felt when one views a situation as foreign or unpredictable; (c) the inability to think that a meaningful life is possible. 2. Insanity. 3. Mental illness. 4. In physiology, the state of a muscle that has been paralysed and has regained some but not all of its ability to contract.

aliform (āl'-i-form): Wing-shaped.

alignment (a-līn'-ment): Arrangement in a straight line, as bones after a fracture. Also called *alinement*.

aliment (al'-i-ment): Food.

alimentary (al-i-men'-tar-i): Relating to food. A. CANAL or TRACT the passage down which the food goes during the process of digestion; it begins at the mouth and ends at the anus; the structures forming it are the mouth, pharynx, oesophagus, stomach, small intestine, colon and rectum; A. SYSTEM the alimentary canal and those organs connected with it that are concerned with digestion and absorption of food and the elimination of residual waste; A. TUBE A. tract or canal.

alimentation (al'-i-men-tā'-shun): The act of providing or receiving nourishment; feeding. ARTIFICIAL A. providing nourishment in some way other than normal, usually referring to intravenous feeding; FORCED A. forced feeding of a person against his or her will; PARENTERAL A. providing nourishment intravenously when the individual cannot take food orally; PERIPHERAL A. utilizing peripheral veins for feeding intravenously; RECTAL A. providing nourishment by injection into the rectum; TOTAL PARENTERAL A. providing nutrients through a large central vein, *e.g.*, the subclavian.

aliphatic (al-i-fat'-ik): Relating to an oil or fat. Fatty. A. ACIDS the so-called fatty acids, including acetic, butyric, and proprionic acids.

aliquot (al'-i-kwot): **1.** A number that will divide evenly into a large number. **2.** A fraction of a larger sample used for analysis; in urinalysis the sample is taken from a 24-hour urine specimen.

alkalaemia (al-ka-l-ē'-mi-a): An increase in the alkalinity of the blood. See ALKALOSIS. — alkalaemic, adj.

alkali (al'-ka-lī): Any one of a class of soluble bases that neutralize acids to form salts, combine with fatty acids to form soaps, and have a pH above 7; many are corrosive. Alkaline solutions turn red litmus paper blue. A. RESERVE a biochemical term denoting the amount of buffered alkali (normally bicarbonate) available in the blood for the neutralization of acids formed in, or introduced into, the body. When the alkali reserve falls, acidosis results; when it rises above normal, alkalosis results.

alkaline (al'-ka-l-īn): **1.** Possessing the properties or reactions of an alkali. **2.** Containing an alkali.

alkalinity (al-ka-lin'-i-ti): The quality or condition of being alkaline.

alkaloid (al'-ka-loyd): **1.** Resembles an alkali. **2.** Any of a large group of nitrogenous bases obtained from the leaves, seeds, bark or other part of certain plants; characteristically, alkaloids have a bitter taste and important physiological actions; those widely used in medicine include morphine, atropine, caffeine, and quinine. Some alkaloids are also produced synthetically.

alkalosis (al-ka-lō'-sis): A pathological condition in which the alkalinity of the body tends to increase; results from an excess of alkali intake or reduction of acid in the body. METABOLIC A. often results from loss of body acid through vomiting and diarrhoea, and is associated with an increase in pCO_2 in the blood; RESPIRATORY

A. usually results from hyperventilation and is associated with a decrease in pCO_2 in the blood.

alkapton (al-kap'-ton): Homogentistic acid (*q.v.*). An abnormal product of protein metabolism.

alkylating agents (al'-ki-lā-ting): Compounds containing two or more alkyl groups (see under ALKYLATION) that readily combine with other molecules, their chief action being damage to the DNA in the nucleus of cells; includes the nitrogen mustards (*q.v.*) used in chemotherapeutic treatment of cancer.

alkylation (al-ki-lā'-shun): In organic chemistry, the substitution of an alkyl group (a radical that is formed when certain hydrocarbons lose one hydrogen atom) for an active hydrogen atom in an organic compound.

ALL: Abbreviation for acute lymphocytic leukaemia. See under LEUKAEMIA.

allaesthesia (al-es-thē'-zi-a): A disorder of the discriminatory sense in which the person perceives a stimulus at a point far removed from the point that is stimulated; usually indicative of a lesion in the parietal lobe.

allantois (al-an'-tō-is): A tubular diverticulum of the posterior part of the yolk sac of the embryo, passing into the body stalk, thus taking part in the formation of the umbilical cord and, later, the placenta. — allantoic, allantoid, adj.

allay (a-lā'): **1.** To lessen or relieve. **2.** To calm or pacify.

allele (a-lēl'): One of two or more variants of a gene that occur at the same position on homologous chromosomes; alleles account for the inheritance of particular traits. Also called *allelomorph.*

allergen (al'-er-jen): Any substance capable of inducing an allergic state, *e.g.*, foods, drugs, animal fur or hair, feathers, pollens, smoke, dust, fungi, bacteria, viruses, animal parasites. — allergenic, adj.; allergenicity, n.

allergic (al-er̆'-jik): **1.** Relating to or associated with an allergy. **2.** Being affected with an allergy. A. ASTHMA see under ASTHMA; A. DERMATITIS see DERMATITIS, CONTACT; A. REACTION see ALLERGY; A. RHINITIS rhinitis (*q.v.*) caused by an inhalant such as pollen.

allergist (al'-er-jist): A physician who specializes in diagnosing and treating allergies.

allergy (al'-er-ji): A hypersensitive reaction to a particular allergen (*q.v.*) or a foreign substance (which is harmless to the great majority of individuals), following initial sensitizing contact, as in hay fever, asthma, urticaria, vasomotor rhinitis, reactions to certain drugs or foods, contact dermatitis. It is due to an antigen–antibody reaction, though the antibody formed is not always demonstrable. A. SKIN TESTING see SENSITIVITY TESTS. See also ANAPHYLAXIS, SENSITIVITY, SENSITIZATION.

alleviate (a-lē'-vē-at): To lessen, mitigate, or make it easier to endure.

Allitt Inquiry (Clothier Report) (al'-lit): A report published in 1994 which examined the events surrounding the deaths and injuries caused by Beverley Allitt, a nurse at Grantham and Kesteven Hospital. It put forward recommendations for the screening of people entering the nursing profession, including screening out applicants 'with excessive absence through, sickness, excessive use of counselling or medical facilities, or self-harm behaviour such as attempted suicide, self-laceration or eating disorder'.

alloarthroplasty (al-lō-arth'-rō-plas-ti): The surgical creation of a new joint using materials from sources other than the human body.

allocheiria (al-ō-ki'-ri-a): A disorder of the tactile sense wherein the individual responds to a stimulus in a part of the body opposite to that where the stimulus was applied; often associated with a lesion of the parietal lobe. Also called *allochiria*.

allochezia (al-ō-kē'-zi-a): 1. The elimination of faeces through an abnormal opening in the body. 2. The elimination of non-faecal matter through the anus.

allodromy (a-lod'-ro-mi): A disturbance in the rhythm of the heartbeat.

allograft (al'-ō-graft): Homograft; a graft of tissue from one individual to another of the same species but of a different genotype.

allolalia (al-ō-lā'-li-a): Any speech defect that has its origin in the central nervous system.

allopathy (al-lop'-a-thi): A system of medical treatment in which the therapies used are intended to produce a condition that is different from or incompatible with an existing pathological condition. Opp. of homeopathy. — allopathic, adj.

alloplasty (al'-lō-plas-ti): In plastic surgery; the use of non-human material, *e.g.*, stainless steel. In psychiatry, a process of fitting one's inner needs to the external environment through adaptation involving alteration in that environment.

allopurinol (al-ō-pū'-ri-nol): A pharmaceutical substance that inhibits the production of uric acid and reduces the level of uric acid in the blood and urine: frequently used in treatment of gout.

allorhythmia (al-ō-rith'-mi-a): Irregularity of the pulse beat.

all-or-none law: States that when a nerve fibre or muscle fibre is stimulated it responds to its fullest extent or not at all.

allotherm (al'-ō-therm): An organism whose body temperature changes as the temperature of the environment changes.

allotriophagy (a-lot-ri-of'-a-ji): The eating of injurious substances or substances not fit for food. See PICA, GEOPHAGIA.

allotropism (a-lot'-rō-pizm): The existence of an element in more than one form with each form having its individual characteristics and properties.

Alma Ata Declaration (al'-ma-ā'-ta): Declaration, comprising 12 points, drawn up by the International Conference on Primary Health Care meeting in Alma-Ata (1978), expressing the need for urgent action by all governments, health and development workers, and the world community to protect and promote the health of all the people of the world.

aloe (al'-ō): The dried juice from the leaves of several species of *Aloe*, a tropical plant; a powerful purgative with a very bitter taste.

alogia (a-lō'-ji-a): Inability to speak; may be physical or psychological in origin; usually due to a lesion in the central nervous system.

alopecia (al-ō-pē'-shi-a): Complete or partial baldness which may be congenital, premature, or due to the ageing process; may be localized or general and result from systemic disease, febrile disease, extensive surgery, use of certain drugs, hormonal changes, emotional stress, radiotherapy. A. AREATA a patchy baldness affecting primarily the scalp or beard but may also affect the eyebrows and lashes; cause unknown, but shock and anxiety may be precipitating factors; exclamation point hairs are diagnostic; A. CICATRISATA progressive, permanent A. of the scalp associated with scarring and in which tufts of normal hair occur between many circular bald patches; A. SENILIS baldness in the elderly, resulting from the gradual loss of hair; A. SYPHILITICA transient baldness occurring in the secondary or tertiary stage of syphilis; bald patches occur chiefly over temporoparietal area giving the individual's head a 'motheaten' appearance; A. TOTALIS complete baldness of the scalp; A. UNIVERSALIS loss of hair from all parts of the body.

alpha (al'-fa): First letter of the Greek alphabet; often used as part of a chemical name to indicate the first of a series of compounds; A. CELLS found in the islands of Langerhans (see under ISLAND); they secrete glucogen which stimulates glycogenolysis in the liver; A. RAYS, see under RAY; A. RECEPTOR see ALPHA-ADRENERGIC RECEPTOR; under RECEPTOR; A. RHYTHM see under RHYTHM; A. TEST designed for use by the U.S. Army in World War I; consists of a series of intelligence tests that can be given to large groups and scored quickly; used to determine the subjects' ability to read and write; A. WAVE see under WAVE.

alpha-adrenergic receptor (ad-re-ner′ -jik): A site in the autonomic nervous system with which adrenergic agents, such as norepinephrine and epinephrine, combine, leading to physiological reactions including the stimulation of associated muscles and the constriction of blood vessels. Also called *alpha receptor* — see under RECEPTOR.

alpha-antitrypsin (al′ -fa-an-tī-trip′ -sin): A protein found in blood plasma that inhibits the action of trypsin; deficiency of this protein is an inherited defect associated with liver disease and pulmonary emphysema.

alpha-fetoprotein (al′ -fa-fē-tō-prō-tē-in): A protein found in elevated amounts in the amniotic fluid in the second trimester of pregnancy if the fetus has an open neural defect such as anencephaly (*q.v.*) or spina bifida (*q.v.*); can be detected and measured by amniocentesis. Also sometimes appears in elevated amounts in the sera of adult individuals with certain malignant conditions.

ALP test: A test to determine the amount of the enzyme alkaline phosphatase in the blood. Elevated levels occur in hyperthyroidism, hyperparathyroidism, Paget's disease, leukaemias, various types of carcinoma, osteogenesis imperfecta, osteitis deformans, Gaucher's disease, rickets, liver and kidney diseases. May also occur following intake of large amounts of vitamin D.

ALS: Abbreviation for 1. advanced life support (*q.v.*). 2. Amyotrophic lateral sclerosis (*q.v.*). 3. Antilymphocyte serum (*q.v.*).

altered consciousness: A level of consciousness associated with sleep. Can be effected by alcohol, drugs, anaesthesia, and head injuries. See GLASGOW COMA SCALE.

alter ego (al-ter-ē′ -gō): 1. An individual so close to one's own character as to seem a second self. 2. Another side of oneself. 3. An intimate friend or constant inseparable companion.

alteregoism (al-ter-ē′ -gō-izm): Having an interest only in those persons whose situation is similar to one's own.

alternans (al′ -ter-nans): Alternating. AUSCULTATORY A. occurs when the heartbeats are heard to alternate in intensity; PULSUS A. occurs when the pulse alternates in strength but remains regular; may indicate myocardial disease.

alternating pressure mattress: See PULSATING MATTRESS.

alternating pressure pad: A segmented inflatable pad with an electrically operated pressure system that changes the thickness of the various segments at regular intervals; fits over a regular mattress; used to prevent decubitus ulcers (*q.v.*).

alternative medicine: A system of treatment of illness used as an alternative to that of orthodox medicine. Known also as *complementary*, *natural*, and *unorthodox medicine*, its recent growth is undoubtedly due to the fact that many diseases, such as allergies, arthritis, cancer, and depression, often fail to respond to conventional treatment. It includes such specialities as osteopathy, homeopathy, acupuncture, aromatherapy, and reflexology. See COMPLEMENTARY MEDICINE, COMPLEMENTARY THERAPIES, HOLISTIC.

alternative therapies: See COMPLEMENTARY THERAPIES.

altitude sickness: 1. ACUTE A.S. occurs during aeroplane flights or other ascent to high altitudes, due to lessened oxygen pressure; symptoms include incapacitating headache, dyspnoea, lassitude, weakness, fatigue, breathlessness, palpitation, anorexia, nausea, vomiting, nosebleed, abdominal pains, diarrhoea, disturbances of vision, mental confusion, sometimes depression. Also called *acute mountain sickness, hypobarism, Acosta's syndrome*. 2. CHRONIC A.S. occurs in people who remain in altitudes of 15,000 feet and over, the Andean region in particular; the main symptom is secondary polycythaemia, which results in viscosity of the blood, cyanosis, abdominal tumour, hepatomegaly, heart failure, pulmonary disorders such as emphysema or chronic bronchitis, ulceration and haemorrhage of the gastrointestinal mucosa, obesity; the symptoms are usually relieved when the individual is moved to a lower altitude. Also called *chronic mountain sickness, Monge's disease*, or *Andes disease*.

altruism (al′ -troo-izm): Thoughtful behaviour aimed at helping other people; a tendency to see the needs of others as more important than one's own and willingness to sacrifice for others.

aluminium (a-lū-min′ -i-um): An element occurring freely in nature in the form of a silvery white, light, malleable metal. Used medicinally in various forms and preparations as an astringent, styptic, demulcent, protective, antiperspirant, antacid; also for making surgical instruments and dental prostheses. A. ACETATE a compound containing A. in solution; has mild astringent and antiseptic action on the skin; also called *Burow's solution*; A. HYDROXIDE a mildly astringent white, tasteless powder, used externally as a dusting powder and internally for its antacid properties; A. HYDROXIDE GEL a preparation of A. used to reduce stomach acidity and in treatment of peptic ulcer.

alum-precipitated diphtheria toxoid: a diphtheria prophylactic used mainly for immunization of children.

alveoalgia (al′ -vē-ō-al′ -ji-a): Pain in the alveolus of a tooth; may occur when the clot that forms following extraction of a tooth is dislodged causing a 'dry socket' with exposure of the bone. Also called *alveolalgia*.

alveolar (al-ve′ -ō-lar): Relating to an alveolus. A. DUCT any of the minute passages which branch from the terminal bronchioles to the A. sacs; A. PROCESS a bony ridge in the maxillae and mandibles which contain the alveoli of the teeth; A. SAC any of the sac-like structures at the terminus of the A. ducts; they are surrounded by a network of capillaries in which the exchange of oxygen in the alveoli and the carbon dioxide in the blood takes place; A. VENTILATION the exchange of gases between the inspired air and the blood in the alveoli of the lung.

alveolitis (al-vē-ō-lī-tis): Inflammation of an alveolus or alveoli. A. SICCA DOLOROSA dry socket; see ALVEOALGIA; EXTRINSIC ALLERGIC A. an occupational disease due to inhalation of organic particles; as occurs in bagassosis and farmers' lung. Characterized by a feeling of tightness in the chest, fever, chills, malaise, headache, cough, tachypnoea, occurring soon after exposure; later symptoms include dyspnoea, cyanosis, clubbing, thickened alveolar walls.

alveolus (al-vē′ -ō-lus): In anatomy, a term used to designate: 1. A small cavity or sac-like dilatation. 2. The termination of a bronchiole in a microscopic sac-like vesicle of the lung where the exchange of oxygen and carbon dioxide takes place. 3. A gland follicle or acinus. 4. A tooth socket.

alymphia (a-lim′ -fi-a): Lack or absence of lymph.

alymphocytosis (a-lim-fō-sī-tō′ -sis): A deficiency or complete absence of lymphocytes from the circulating blood.

alymphoplasia (a-limf′ -ō-plā′ -zi-a): Imperfect development or failure of development of lymphoid tissues; may be due to incomplete or imperfect development or functioning of the thymus gland.

Alzheimer's disease: The most common form of dementia (*q.v.*), making up 55% of all cases.

amalgam (a-mal′ -gam): 1. A combination, mixture, blend. 2. A mixture of an alloy of mercury and other metals, used for filling dental cavities. Also called *dental amalgam*.

amarilla (am-a-ril′ -a): The international term for yellow fever (*q.v.*).

amasesis (am-a-sē′ -sis): Inability to chew food, for any reason.

amastia (a-mas′ -ti-a): Absence of the breasts; may be a congenital condition, or due to surgical removal, or to an endocrine disturbance that inhibits development.

amaurosis (am-aw-rō′ -sis): Partial or total blindness, particularly that which occurs without apparent disease or lesion of the eye; often temporary. A. FUGAX sudden transient partial or complete blindness in one eye; may occur in transient ischaemic attack, alcoholic poisoning, emotional shock, or from sudden acceleration as in an aeroplane flight.

ambi-: A prefix denoting both, or on both sides.

ambidextrous (am-bi-deks′ -trus): Ability to use both hands with equal facility.

ambient (am′ -bi-ent): Surrounding; encompassing; present everywhere; moving freely or circulating, as A. air.

ambilateral (am-bi-lat′ -er-al): Relating to both right and left sides, or affecting both sides.

ambivalence (am-biv′ -a-lens): The coexistence of conflicting attitudes and feelings towards a particular situation, object, or person, *e.g.*, love and hate.

ambivalent (am-biv′ -a-lent): 1. Relating to ambivalence. 2. Relating to a type of personality that has both introversive and extroversive characteristics.

ambivert (am′ -bi-vert): One who is neither an extrovert nor an introvert; a person between these two extremes.

amblyacousia (am-bli-a-koo′ -si-a): Dullness of the sense of hearing.

amblygeustia (am-bli-gūs-′ti-a): Temporary or permanent dullness of the sense of taste.

Ambu bag: A hand-operated resuscitator which delivers about 40% oxygen.

ambulance (am'-bū-lans): A vehicle used for transporting the sick or injured.

ambulant (am'-bū-lant): Able to walk and move about; not confined to bed.

ambulation (am-bū-lā'-shun): The act of walking or moving about.

ambulatory (am'-bū-la-tor-i): Mobile. Able to walk. A. TREATMENT in which the patient is kept on his or her feet as much as possible.

amelioration (a-mē-li-or-ā'-shun): Reduction of the severity of symptoms. Improvement in the general condition.

ameloblast (a-mel'-ō-blast): An epithelial cell that has a function in the production of dental enamel.

ameloblastoma (a-mel'-ō-blas-tō'-ma): A rapidly growing, aggressive tumour of the jaw, usually in the molar region; begins in the epithelium at the origin of the teeth; apt to be recurrent; may cause dysphagia and blockage of the airway; haemorrhage due to erosion of blood vessels may result in death. Seen chiefly in certain areas of Africa and Asia. Also called *adamantinoma*.

amelogenesis (am-e-lō'-jen'-e-sis): The formation of dental enamel. A. IMPERFECTA an inherited condition in which there is deficient or imperfect development of tooth enamel resulting in brownish discoloration and friability of the teeth.

amenorrhoea (a-men-ō'-rē'-a): Abnormal absence or cessation of the menses. PRIMARY A. failure of menstruation to become established at puberty; SECONDARY A. absence of the menses after they have once commenced; occurs in some women after they cease taking contraceptive pills.

ametropia (am-e-trō-pi-a): Defective vision due to imperfect refractive power of the eye that prevents proper focusing of parallel rays on the retina, and which results in such conditions as myopia, hyperopia, and astigmatism.

amide (am'-īd): An organic compound derived from ammonia by chemical reaction in which an acid radical is substituted for one of the hydrogen atoms.

amidone (am'-i-dōn): Methadone.

amines (am'ēns): Name given to organic compounds that contain the amino group (NH_2). They are derived from ammonia; important in biochemistry.

amino-: Prefix denoting a compound that contains the radical group (NH_2).

aminoacidaemia (a-mē'-nō-as-id-ē'-mi-a): An excess of amino acids in the blood.

aminoacidopathy (a-mē'-nō-as-i-dop'-a-thi): Any disorder involving an imbalance of amino acids in the body.

amino acids (a-mē'-no): Organic acids that contain one or more amine groups (NH_2) and a carboxyl group (CO_2H); the structural units of protein, occurring naturally in foods of animal origin and plant origin. In the body they are the end products of protein hydrolysis and from these the body resynthesizes its protein. Classified as (1) endogenous, those amino acids that are made within the body; and (2) exogenous, those found in sources outside the body. Also classified as (1) essential, those amino acids that cannot be made within the body (exogenous) and must come from the outside; and (2) non-essential (endogenous). Foods that contain large amounts of amino acids are known as complete or HBV (high biological value) proteins, *e.g.*, meat, fish, eggs, milk; and those that contain lesser amounts are known as incomplete or LBV (low biological value) proteins, *e.g.*, vegetables such as peas, beans, and wheat.

aminoaciduria (a-mē'-nō-as-i-dū'-ri-a): An excess of amino acids in the urine.

aminocaproic acid (am'-ē-nō-kā-prō'-ik): An agent used as an antifibrinolytic to control excessive bleeding in haemophilia and in certain post-surgical patients.

aminoglycoside (am'-ē-nō-glī'-ko-sīde): Any of the bacterial antibiotics which act by inhibiting protein synthesis; includes streptomycin, neomycin, kanamycin, gentamycin, tobramycin.

amino group: The NH_2 group in a protein compound; it is a portion of all amino acids and is the basic building block of proteins. Also called the *amino acid radical*.

amitosis (am-ī-tō'-sis): Multiplication of a cell by direct fission, without change in either the nucleus or the protoplasm.

AML: Abbreviation for acute myelogenous leukaemia. See under LEUKAEMIA.

ammoaciduria (am'-ō-as-i-dū'-ri-a): The presence of an excess of both amino acids and ammonia in the urine.

ammonia (a-mō'-ni-a): A colourless, volatile, alkaline gas with a penetrating pungent odour, formed by decomposition of nitrogenous matter; contains hydrogen and nitrogen. Highly soluble in water; widely used in industry and as a detergent. AROMATIC SPIRIT OF A. solution of ammonia, water and aromatic oils; has fleeting action as a circulatory and respiratory stimulant; used in cases of fainting. Also called *sal volatile*.

Ammon's horn: See HIPPOCAMPUS.

amnalgesia (am-nal-j-ē'-zi-a): The abolition of pain or the memory of pain; may be brought about by the use of certain drugs or by hypnosis.

amnemonic (am-nē-mon'-ik): Relating to or causing impairment of memory.

amnesia (am-nē'-zi-a): Partial or complete loss of memory and of the ability to recall one's identity. May be caused by concussion, electroshock, dementia, hysteria, senility, alcoholism; or it may be a defence mechanism against anxiety-provoking situations. ANTEROGRADE A. loss of memory for recent events, especially for events since the accident causing the A.; CIRCUMSCRIBED A. loss of memory for a limited time; may occur after an epileptic or hysterical episode; memory before and after the episode is intact; NEUROTIC A. occurs when a person consciously or unconsciously wishes to forget his or her memories and does not wish to recover them; POST-TRAUMATIC A., A. for a short time following severe head injury; RETROGRADE A. loss of memory for events that occurred before an accident which caused amnesia. TRAUMATIC A. occurs after a sudden injury; VERBAL A. loss of memory for words; VISUAL A. inability to recognize familiar objects. — amnesic, adj.

amnesic (am-nē'-zik): 1. Relating to or suffering from amnesia. 2. A drug that causes loss of memory for pain.

amniocentesis (am'-ni-ō-sen-tē'-sis): Removal of a small amount of fluid from the amniotic sac by aspiration through the abdominal wall for diagnostic purposes; usually done during or after the 15th week of pregnancy. Analysis of the chromosomes or enzyme production of the fetal cells can determine certain structural disorders and many disorders of the fetus's body chemistry that may lead to mental or physical retardation and sometimes death, e.g., Down's syndrome or the presence of a deforming virus infection such as German measles. The fluid contains increased haemoglobin products in cases of Rhesus incompatibility.

amniogenesis (am-ni-ō-jen'-e-sis): The formation of the amnion.

amniography (am-ni-og'-ra-fi): X-ray of the gravid uterus after injection of the amniotic sac with an opaque medium; it outlines the amniotic cavity, the fetus, and the umbilical cord and placenta; a diagnostic procedure when placenta praevia (q.v.), hydatidiform mole, or choriocarcinoma (q.v.) is suspected. — amniogram, n.; amniographical, adj.; amniographically, adv.

amnion (am'-ni-on): The innermost of the fetal membranes; a thin transparent sac that holds the fetus suspended in the liquor amnii (amniotic fluid); commonly called the *bag of waters.* — amnionic, amniotic, adj.

amniorrhexis (am-ni-ō-rek'-sis): Rupture of the amnion.

amniorrhoea (am-ni-ō-rē'-a): Escape of amniotic fluid prematurely.

amnioscopy (am-ni-os'-ko-pi): Direct observation of the amniotic sac, the fetus, and the colour and amount of amniotic fluid through the intact membrane using a specially designed optical instrument inserted through the uterine cervix; is usually done during the last trimester of pregnancy. TRANSABDOMINAL A. direct examination of the fetus and amniotic fluid through the abdominal wall; usually done during the second trimester of pregnancy.

amniotic (am-ni-ot'-ik): Of or relating to the amnion (q.v.). A. CAVITY the fluid-filled amnion; A. FLUID the transparent fluid that is secreted rapidly and resorbed by the amniotic sac; composed of water, urea, albumin, cells and various salts; A. FLUID EMBOLISM occurs when an embolus forms in the amniotic sac, enters the maternal circulation and is transported to the mother's lung or brain; a rare occurrence, happens after the membranes rupture; A. FLUID INFUSION the escape of amniotic fluid into the maternal circulation; A. SAC the sac formed by the amnion; contains amniotic fluid.

amniotitis (am-ni-ō-tī'-tis): Inflammation of the amnion (q.v.).

amniotomy (am-ni-ot'-o-mi): Surgical rupture of the fetal membranes to induce or expedite labour.

amoeba (a-mē'-ba): A microscopic, elementary, one-celled protozoan of the genus *Amoeba* that moves by extruding pseudopodia (q.v.) is capable of ingestion, absorption, respiration, excretion, and reproduction by simple fission. Many species are pathogenic to man, especially *Entamoeba histolytica,* the causative organism of amoebic dysentry. — amoebae, amoebas, pl.; amoebic, amoeboid, adj.

amoebiasis (am-ē-bī'-a-sis): Infestation with *Entamoeba histolytica* affecting chiefly the mucosa of the large intestine but also often involving the liver; the organism enters the body through food or water that is contaminated by faeces. Symptoms include acute abdominal pain, anorexia, severe diarrhoea with stools containing mucus and, sometimes, flecks of blood, jaundice, emaciation. Particularly serious in infants, older people, and the debilitated. Diagnosis is confirmed by isolating the causative organism in the stools.

amoeboid (a-mē'-boyd): Resembling an amoeba in shape or mode of movement, *e.g.*, white blood cells. A. MOVEMENT, M. that progresses by diapedesis, *i.e.*, the alternate projection and retraction into the cell 'legs' of cytoplasm called pseudopodia.

amok (a-mok', a-muk'): A wild, frenzied, maniacal manner of behaviour that threatens harm to others.

amorph (a'-morph): An inactive gene; one that has no action at all. — amorphic, adj.

amorphous (a-mor'-fus): Having no definite structure; formless — amorphia, amorphism, n.

AMP: Abbreviation for adenosine monophosphate. See under ADENOSINE.

ampere (am'-pair): The standard intensity of electrical current. The unit is known informally as the amp, but A is its official symbol. It is the International System of Unit (SI unit) of electric current.

amph-, amphi-: Prefixes denoting around; on both sides; both.

amphetamine (am-fet'-a-mēn): Any of a group of chemical substances in the form of a white crystalline powder, odourless and tasteless, used as a nervous system stimulant; highly addictive. Used therapeutically in treatment of narcolepsy, depression, low blood pressure, obesity. Often misused by both adolescents and adults to produce euphoria and control fatigue. Also called *speed* (slang).

amphiarthrosis (am'-fi-arth-rō'-sis): A slightly movable joint. The articulating surfaces are separated by fibrocartilage or ligaments that permit only slight movement, as between the vertebrae. — amphiarthroses, pl.

amphithymia (am-fi-thī'-mi-a): An emotional state in which periods of depression and elation alternate.

amphitrichate (am-fi-trī'-kāt): Descriptive of a microorganism that has a flagellum or flagella at both ends.

amphodiplopia (am'-fō-di-plō'-pi-a): Double vision in both eyes.

amphophilic (am-fō-fil'-ik): Relating to cells that stain with either acidic or basic dyes.

amphoteric (am-fō-ter'-ik): Having two opposite characteristics; said especially of a substance that reacts as either an acid or base.

ampule (am'-pūl): A small, hermetically sealed glass vial containing a single dose of a drug. Also called *ampul, ampoule.*

ampulla (am-poo'-la): Any flask-like dilatation. In anatomy, a flask-like dilatation of a tubal structure. A. OF THE BREAST a widened portion of the lactiferous duct near its opening on the nipple; A. OF THE UTERINE TUBE a widened area of the tube where fertilization is thought to occur; A. OF VATER the enlargement formed by the union of the common bile duct with the pancreatic duct where they enter the duodenum. [Abraham Vater, German anatomist, 1684–1751.] — ampullae, pl.; ampullar, ampullary, ampullate, adj.

amputation (am-pū-tā'-tion): 1. Removal of an appending part by surgery, *e.g.*, a breast, or limb. 2. Lack or loss of a limb or limbs due to heredity or trauma, or occurring spontaneously as a result of gangrene.

amputee (am-pū-tē'): A person who has lost a limb or limbs or had one or more limbs amputated by surgery.

amydriasis (am-i-drī'a-sis): Contraction of the pupil.

amyelia (a-mī-ē'-li-a): A congenital anomaly marked by the absence of the spinal cord.

amygdala (a-mig'-da-la): 1. An almond-shaped mass of grey matter in the lateral ventricle of the brain. 2. A tonsil. 3. An almond.

amygdaloid (a-mig'-da-loyd): 1. Almond-shaped. 2. Resembling an almond or a tonsil.

amygdalolith (a-mig'-da-lō-lith): A stone or a concretion in a tonsillar crypt.

amylaceous (am-i-lā'-shē-us): Starchy. Containing or resembling starch.

amylase (am'-i-lās): An enzyme of the saliva (salivary amylase), pancreatic juice (amylase), or intestinal juice that converts starches into sugars. A. TEST a test to determine the amount of starch in the urine; less than normal indicates a disorder of kidney function; SERUM A. TEST test to measure the amount of amylase in the circulating blood; it is elevated notably in pancreatitis.

amylogenesis (am'-i-lō-jen'-e-sis): The formation of starch.

amyloid (am'-i-loyd): 1. Starch-like. 2. A starchy food or substance. 3. A wax-like protein complex that has some starch-like qualities; may be deposited in tissues in certain pathological states.

amylolysis (am-i-lol'-is-is): The conversion of starch to sugar by the action of enzymes during digestion.

amylose (am'-i-lōs): A component of starch; composed of a polymer of glucose.

amylum (am'-i-lum): 1. Starch 2. Corn starch.

amyoplasia (a-mī-ō-plā'-zi-a): Lack of formation and development of muscle tissue. A. CONGENITA see ARTHROGRYPOSIS.

amyostasia (a-mī-ō-stā′-zi-a): Nervous shaking or tremor of the muscles with incoordination, which makes standing difficult; often seen in locomotor ataxia.

amyotonia (a-mī-ō-tō′-ni-a): Myatona. Lack or loss of muscle tone. A. CONGENITA any one of several congenital conditions of infants that are characterized by pronounced muscular weakness and flaccidity; also called *floppy-infant syndrome* and *Oppenheim's disease.*

amyotrophic lateral sclerosis (a-mī-ō-trōf′-ik lat′ -er-al skle-rō′-sis): A progressive degenerative disease that affects the motor system; cause unknown. Usually occurs in the fifth to seventh decade with death in about 3 years. Chief symptom is muscular wasting with associated weakness and difficulty in swallowing and talking. Also called *Lou Gehrig's disease.* See ECLEROSIS.

amyotrophy (a-mi-ot′-rō-fi): Progressive muscle wasting or atrophy. Also called *amyotrophia.* — amyotrophic, adj.

amyxia (a-mik′-si-a): Deficiency or absence of mucus.

ana-: Prefix denoting up, upwards, back, backward, excessive, again, throughout.

anabolic (an-a-bol′-ik): Relating to or promoting anabolism. A. COMPOUND a chemical substance that causes a synthesis of body protein. A. STEROIDS androgens that increase protein synthesis and muscle mass and weight; used therapeutically to improve appetite and well-being; have been misused by body builders and athletes. See STEROID.

anabolism (an-ab′ō-lizm): The constructive phase of metabolism during which foods are converted into complex body substances such as hormones, enzymes, cell glycogen and cell protein; the reverse of catabolism. — anabolic, anabolistic, adj.

anacidity (an-asid′-i-ti): Lack of or deficiency in normal acidity, especially of hydrochloric acid in gastric juice.

anaclitic (an-a-klit′-ik): Being psychologically dependent on others; refers especially to the infant. A. DEPRESSION that occurs in all aspects of an infant's development following sudden separation from its mother or mother surrogate; A. THERAPY in psychiatry, a therapy that fosters dependency needs and nurtures the relationship between patient and therapist; used to reduce feelings of anxiety and guilt.

anacroasia (an-a-krō-ā′-zi-a): Inability to understand language; auditory aphasia.

anacusis (an-a-kū′-sis): Absence or total loss of hearing. Also called *anacusia, anacousia, anakusis.*

anadipsia (an-a-dip′-si-a): Excessive thirst.

anadrenalism (an-a-drē′-nal-izm): Absence of or defective function of the adrenal glands.

anaemia (a-nē′-mi-a): Term applied to a large group of disorders that result from deficiency in the number of red blood cells or their haemoglobin content, or both, or the volume of packed red blood cells. Types are differentiated on the basis of cause, hereditary factors, size, shape and haemoglobin content of the red blood cells, response to therapy, etc. Also classified as primary when due to disease of the blood or blood-producing organs; secondary when it is the result of another pathological condition such as cancer, bleeding ulcers, etc. Clinical features include pallor, easy fatigue, breathlessness on exertion, giddiness, palpitations, loss of appetite, gastrointestinal disorders and amenorrhoea. ADDISONIAN A. pernicious A.; ANAPLASTIC A. secondary A., may follow use of certain chemicals, x-ray or other ionizing radiation, infection, or metastatic bone cancer; the bone marrow is replaced by fibrous tissue which results in pancytopenia (*q.v.*); APLASTIC A., A. from failure of the bone marrow to produce blood cells; usually fatal; CONGENITAL HAEMOLYTIC A. usually not recognized until late in life; may follow transient jaundice; cholelithiasis often present; may require splenectomy to prevent haemolytic crisis; COOLEY'S A. thalassaemia (*q.v*); FOLIC ACID A. an anaplastic A. due to deficiency of folic acid in the diet; GENETIC ANAEMIAS include sickle cell A., thalassaemia, and congenital haemolytic A.; HAEMOLYTIC A. a type characterized by excessive destruction of red blood cells; see ACHOLURIC JAUNDICE under JAUNDICE; HYPERCHROMATIC A. characterized by red cells that are deeply coloured; HYPOCHROMIC A. characterized by low haemoglobin content of red blood cells; HYPOCHROMIC MICROCYTIC A. hypochromic A. in which the red cells are small and the haemoglobin content reduced; IRON DEFICIENCY A. the commonest type of A. due to poor uptake of iron resulting from inadequate or ill-balanced diet, poor absorption, increased bodily needs as in pregnancy, or to excessive blood loss; MACROCYTIC A. a group of A.s characterized by very large blood cells and splenomegaly; MEGALOBLASTIC A., A. characterized by the presence of megaloblasts in the blood; MICROANGIOPATHIC A. haemolytic A.; MICROCYTIC A. characterized by the formation of abnormally small red blood cells; NORMOCYTIC A., A. in which the red blood cells are of normal size and haemoglobin content; NUTRITIONAL A. due to faulty nutrition; PERNICIOUS A. a chronic disorder primarily of middle and old age, and especially in blue-eyed, fair-haired, prematurely grey people; the red blood cells are enlarged and often of bizarre shapes; symptoms include enlargement of the liver and spleen, icterus, glossitis, tachycardia, and such neurological symptoms as confusion, numbness, loss of muscle coordination and position sense; caused by atrophy of the stomach mucosa and its consequent failure to produce the intrinsic factor necessary for absorption of vitamin B_{12}; treated by lifelong injections of the vitamin; POSTHAE-MORRHAGIC A., A. which follows a haemorrhage; SICKLE CELL A. a hereditary and familial type of A. occurring most commonly in Afro-Caribbeans; the red blood cells have a short lifespan, acquire a characteristic crescent or sickle shape, and tend to clog the small capillaries, causing clots. Children become barrelchested with protruding abdomens; SIDERO-BLASTIC A. may be hereditary or acquired; often develops from use of certain drugs; marked by elevated serum level of iron due to a derangement of haem synthesis; SPHEROCYTIC A. hereditary spherocytosis; see SPHERO-CYTOSIS.

anaemic (a-nē'-mik): Relating to, affected with, or characteristic of anaemia.

anaerobe (an'-er-ob): A microorganism that grows and thrives best in an oxygen-free environment. When this is strictly so, the organism is termed obligatory. Most pathogens will flourish in either the presence or absence of oxygen and are, therefore, termed facultative.

anaerobic (an-er-ō'-bik): 1. Without oxygen. 2. Able to grow and thrive in the absence of oxygen. A. EXERCISE short bursts of vigorous exercise which rely for oxygen on its release from compounds in the body; continuation produces metabolic acidosis. See AEROBIC EXERCISE under AEROBIC.

anaesthekinesis (an-es'-thē-ki-nē'-zi-a): Sensory and motor paralysis occurring together.

anaesthesia (an-es-thē'-zi-a): Absence of feeling or sensation in a part of the body or the whole of it. May be induced by a drug, trauma, disease, or hypnosis. BASAL A. a preliminary anaesthesia, usually not complete, often produced by narcosis and requiring supplementation to produce surgical anaesthesia; CAUDAL A. produced by injection of an anaesthetic into the space outside the dura mater between the fifth sacral vertebrae and the coccyx or between the first and third lumbar vertebrae; used chiefly in childbirth; CUTANEOUS A. pro-

duced by spraying an anaesthetic into or onto the skin in a particular area; DISSOCIATED A. loss of sensation for pain and temperature but without loss of touch sensation or proprioception; occurs in patients with syringomyelia (q.v.); ENDOBRONCHIAL A. produced by administering a gaseous mixture through a slender tube into a large bronchus of one lung to exclude the anaesthetic from one lung during thoracic surgery; ENDOTRACHEAL A., A. administered through an endotracheal tube; EPI-DURAL A. see EPIDURAL BLOCK; under EPIDURAL GENERAL A. loss of sensation with loss of consciousness; INFILTRATION A. local anaesthesia induced by injection of an anaesthetic solution directly into the tissues to be anaesthetized; INHALATION A. the oldest and most common form of administration; any one of, or a combination of, several gases and vapours is introduced through the nose, endotracheal tube, or tracheostomy tube; INTRAVENOUS A. produced by the introduction of an anaesthetic drug into a vein to induce general A.; LOCAL A. produced by nerve blocking to prevent impulses from a limited area from reaching the brain; NERVE-BLOCK A. injection of an anaesthetic drug into a nerve or nerve root to anaesthetize a specific area; ORAL A., A. produced by drugs and administered by mouth; RECTAL A., A. produced by injection of an anaesthetic drug into the rectum; REFRIGERATION A. produced by use of ethyl chloride spray or cracked ice locally for several hours to produce anaesthesia of an extremity in amputation cases; RE-GIONAL A., A. producing insensitivity over a certain area by injection of an anaesthetic into tissues in the immediate vicinity of the nerve to be blocked; it affects the smallest area necessary to accomplish the particular procedure; SADDLE-BLOCK A., A. limited to the buttocks, perineum, and inner surfaces of the thighs; SPINAL A. produced by injection of an anaesthetic in the spinal subarachnoid space; may also be produced by a lesion in the spinal cord; SUBARACHNOID A. spinal A.; SUR-FACE A. produced by the application of an anaesthetic to a particular body surface, as with a swab; TACTILE A. see under TACTILE; TOP-ICAL A. produced by applying a local anaesthetic directly to the area to be operated on e.g., the cornea, mucous membrane or the skin.

anaesthesiology (an'-es-thē-zi-ol'-ō-ji): The science concerned with the uses, administration, and effects of anaesthetic agents, and the care of the patient under anaesthesia.

anaesthetic (an-es-thet′-ik): 1. Relating to anaesthesia. 2. An agent that produces loss of sensibility to pain and/or loss of consciousness. GENERAL A. a drug or agent that produces unconsciousness; LOCAL A. a drug or agent that produces local insensitivity to pain when injected into the tissues or applied topically.

anaesthetist (a-nēs′-the-tist): A physician who specializes in anaesthesiology and the care of the patient under anaesthesia.

anaesthetization (a-nes′-the-tī-zā′-shun): The act of producing insensibility to pain through the administration of an anaesthetic (q.v.). — anaesthetize, v.

anagenesis (an-a-jen′-e-sis): Regeneration or repair of tissue or structure.

anakastia (an-a-kas′-ti-a): Any psychopathological disorder that causes the individual to act compulsively or to react emotionally against his will. — anakastic, adj.

anal (ā′-nal): Relating to or near the anus. A. CANAL the lower end of the digestive tube; extends from the rectum to the anus; A. CHARACTER a personality characterized by persistence of the erotic traits of the anal phase of childhood into adult life and behaviour; A. CRYPT one of the small culs-de-sac between the folds of the mucous membrane in the anal canal; A. EROTICISM deriving sexual pleasure from anal functions; A. FISSURE a crack or slit in the mucous membrane at the margin of the anus; A. FISTULA an abnormal opening in the skin or mucous membrane near the anus; A. PHASE or STAGE the period in a child's development usually from one to three years of age, when he is intensely interested in the process and products of defecation; A. SPHINCTER either the external or internal sphincter muscle of the anus. See SPHINCTER.

analeptic (an-a-lep′-tik): 1. Having restorative properties. 2. A drug that acts as a restorative by stimulating the central nervous system; often used in medicine to counteract drowsiness or the effects of barbiturates.

analgesia (an-al-jē′-zi-a): Lack of sensitivity to pain without loss of consciousness; may be produced by a drug or occur as a symptom of a nervous disorder. HYPNOTIC A. the production of analgesia through hypnosis; sometimes used in treatment of severe burns, migraine headache, and asthma; WAKING IMAGED A. a psychological technique whereby the patient is asked to think and talk about an earlier experience that was pleasurable; sometimes succeeds in reducing moderate pain.

analgesic (an-al-jē′-zik): 1. Insensible to pain. 2. Alleviating pain. 3. a drug that relieves pain. — Also called anodyne.

analogous (a-nal′-o-gus): Similar in function and/or appearance, but not in structure. — analogue, n.

analogue (an′-a-log): An organ or part that serves the same function as another but has a different structure. In chemistry, a compound that has a structure similar to that of another but with one component that is different.

analysis (a-nal′-i-sis): 1. The separation of substances into their components for examination and determination of their properties. 2. In chemistry, a term used to describe the procedure for determining the composition and properties of the components of a compound. 3. In psychiatry, psychoanalysis (q.v.). — analyses, pl ; analytic, adj. A. OF VARIANCE a statistical test used to compare more than two groups of data.

analyst (an′-a′-list): A person experienced in performing analyses. In psychiatry, a psychoanalyst (q.v.). 'LAY' A. a person outside of the medical profession who has undergone training in analysis in preparation for performing analyses.

anamnesis (an-am-nē′-sis): 1. The act of remembering or recalling to mind. 2. That which is recollected. 3. A patient's medical history, particularly that part recalled by the patient and others. 4. In immunology, a rapid and unexpectedly strong antibody response in an individual to the administration of what was assumed to be an initial dose of an antigen.

ananabolic (an-an-a-bol′-ik): Lack of anabolism (q.v.).

anandria (an-an′-dri-a): Absence or loss of virility or masculinity. Impotence.

anaphase (an′-a-fāz): A phase in mitosis (q.v.), when the divided chromosomes are drawn apart and collected at the opposite poles of the cell to form two separate nuclei.

anaphrodisiac (an-af-rō-diz′-i-ak): 1. Lessening sexual desire. 2. A drug that lessens sexual desire.

anaphylactic (an-a-fi-lak′-tik): Relating to anaphylaxis. A. SHOCK a condition of extreme hypersensitivity to a foreign protein or other substance induced in a person who has had a previous exposure to the same substance; an emergency condition requiring immediate medical attention. Symptoms include breathlessness, dyspnoea, cyanosis, pallor, weakness, fever, vascular collapse, sometimes convulsions and unconsciousness.

anaphylaxis (an-a-fi-lak'-sis): Extreme hypersensitivity reaction to a foreign protein after a previous exposure to the same substance; symptoms are as for anaphylactic shock; see ANAPHYLACTIC.

anaplasia (an-a-plā'-zi-a): Loss of the distinctive characteristics of a cell, with reversion to a more primitive type, often associated with proliferative activity as in cancer. — anaplastic, adj.

anaptic (an-ap'-tik): Relating to the loss of the sense of touch.

anarthria (an-ar'-thri-a): Loss of ability to pronounce words distinctly, due to muscle dysfunction; thought to result from a brain lesion. — anarthric, adj.

anasognosia (an-a-sog-nōz'-ē-a): Inability of a hemiplegic patient to recognize his disability; or his denial of it.

anastalsis (an-a-stal'-sis): Antiperistalsis (*q.v.*).

anastomosis (a-nas-tō-mō'-sis): 1. The joining together of two hollow organs or of two or more arteries or veins, *e.g.*, the two vertebral arteries join to form the basilar artery. 2. The surgical establishment of an artificial connection between two hollow organs, nerves, or blood vessels; may be done to bypass a vascular obstruction or aneurysm. — anastomoses, pl.; anastomotic, adj., anastomose, v.

anatomic (an-a-tom'-ik): Relating to the structure of the body or a body part. A. SNUFF BOX the hollow triangular space at the base of the metacarpal of the extended thumb.

anatomical (an-a-tom'-i-kal): Relating to the anatomy or structure of the body. A. NECK often refers to the constricted part of the humerus just below the head; A. POSITION see under POSITION.

anatomist (a-nat'-o-mist): One who specializes in the study of anatomy or who performs dissections.

anatomy (a-nat'-o-mi): The science that deals with the structure and composition of the body; it is largely based on dissection. — anatomical, adj.; anatomically, adv.

anatripsis (an-a-trip'-sis): The use of rubbing or friction as a treatment. May or may not include the simultaneous application of a medicament.

anatriptic (an-a-trip'-tik): 1. Relating to anatripsis. 2. The application of an ointment or a medication by rubbing it into the skin.

anatropia (an-a-trō'-pi-a): The tendency for the eyeballs to turn upwards when the individual is at rest.

anchylo-: See ANKYLO-.

ancillary (an'-si-ler-i): Auxiliary; supplementary.

Ancylostoma (an-si-los'-tō-ma): A genus of nematodes, including the hookworms. A. *DUODENALE* the Old World hookworm of man, a species found chiefly in temperate areas in contrast to the species *Necator americanus*, the New World hookworm which is found chiefly in tropical areas.

ancylostomiasis (an'-si-los-tō-mī'-a-sis): See HOOKWORM DISEASE under HOOKWORM.

andr-, andro-: Combining forms denoting man, male, having the characteristics of a man.

androblastoma (an'-drō-blas-tō'-ma): A tumour of the ovary or testis, composed of stromal cells; may cause development of feminization or masculinization.

androgen (an'-drō-jen): Any substance that stimulates and preserves the secondary male characteristics and structure; usually a hormone secreted by the testes or adrenal cortex, also prepared synthetically. When given to a female these substances have a masculinizing effect. — androgenic, adj.

androgy (an'-drō-gō-ji): The teaching of adults as opposed to pedagogy (the teaching of children).

androgyne (an'-drō-jīn): A person in whom the female characteristics are most prominent; a female pseudohermaphrodite.

androgyny (a-droj'-i-ni): 1. Hermaphroditism. 2. Female hermaphroditism.

android (an'droyd): Resembling a man. A. PELVIS, see under PELVIS.

andromorphous (an-drō-mor'-fus): Having the form or appearance of a male individual.

androsterone (an-dros'-ter-ōn): An androgenic hormone secreted in the urine; derived from testosterone metabolism; also produced synthetically; influences the development of secondary male sex characteristics.

anencephaly (an-en-kef'-a-li,-sef'-): A congenital anomaly in which there is an absence of the flat bones of the skull and absence of the brain and spinal cord; the condition is incompatible with life. Also called *anencephalia*. — anencephalous, anencephalic, adj.

anenzymia (an-en-zī'-mi-a): Lack of sufficient secretion, or the absence of, an enzyme in the body.

anephric (a-nef'-rik): 1. Refers to a person who lacks both kidneys, either as a congenital defect or because of surgical removal. 2. A person who has lost all kidney function due to either surgical removal or nephritic pathology.

anepia (a-nē'-pi-a): Lack of ability to speak.

anergy (an'-er-ji): 1. Lethargy; inactivity; sluggishness; lack of energy. 2. Decreased or absence of sensitivity to specific antigens. Also called *anergia*. — anergic, adj.

anerythrocyte (an-ē-rith'-rō-sīt): A red blood cell containing no haemoglobin.

anerythroplasia (an-ē-rith'-rō-plā'-zi-a): Incomplete or inadequate formation of erythrocytes.

aneuploid (an'-ū-ployd): Having an abnormal number of diploid chromosomes.

aneurin (e) hydrochloride (an'-ū-rin hī-drO-klō'-rīd): Thiamin hydrochloride; see THIAMIN. Also called *vitamin B₁*.

aneurysm (an'-ū-rizm): Permanent, abnormal, local dilatation or ballooning out of a blood vessel wall, most commonly in the aorta; the result of a congenital defect or of degeneration and weakening of the wall due to injury or disease, which produces a pulsating swelling over which a murmur may be heard. ABDOMINAL AORTIC A. common in the elderly; usually associated with degenerative atherosclerosis; AN TERIAL A. an A. in an artery; may be due to a congenital defect or to hypertensive atherosclerosis; ARTERIOVENOUS A. an abnormal direct connection between an artery and a vein, often follows an injury; ARTERIOSCLEROTIC A. the commonest type of abdominal A.; occurs chiefly in the elderly, due to atherosclerosis; BERRY A. a small thin-walled A. often occurring at the junction of a cerebral artery; likely to rupture, causing haemorrhage into the subarachnoid space; CARDIAC A. thinning and bulging of a weakened ventricular wall, usually the result of a myocardial infarction; CEREBRAL A. BERRY A., CHARCOT–BOUCHARD A. a small A. of an artery or arteriole; may be the cause of a massive cerebral haemorrhage; CIRCOID A. a tangled mass of pulsating blood vessels, appearing as a subcutaneous tumour, often of the scalp; DISSECTING A. one that is formed by a longitudinal tear or break in the intima, usually of the aorta, which allows blood to collect between the intima and the other layers of the vessel wall; FALSE A. one in which all the coats of the vessel rupture and the blood is retained by the surrounding tissue; FUSIFORM A. an elongated spindle-shaped A. that involves the entire circumference of the arterial wall; INTRACRANIAL A. one within the cranium; MYCOTIC A. an A. produced by the growth of microorganisms in the vessel wall; often the sequela of bacterial endocarditis; also called *bacterial aneurysm*; POSTERIOR-COMMUNICATING A. an A. in the artery that passes from the internal carotid to the posterior cerebral artery; SACCULAR A. a localized outpouching of an

artery that does not affect the entire circumference of the artery, often occurring in an artery of the circle of Willis; does not usually produce symptoms unless it ruptures; THORACIC AORTIC A. an A. in the thoracic aorta that develops slowly and is less apt to rupture than an abdominal aortic A.; usually seen in the elderly.

aneurysmoplasty (an-ū-riz'-mō-plas-ti): Plastic repair of an artery damaged by an aneurysm.

ANF: Abbreviation for antinuclear factor, see ANTINUCLEAR FACTOR TEST.

angi-, angio-: Combining forms denoting a vessel(s), particularly a blood or lymph vessel.

angiectasis (an-ji-ek'-ta-sis): Abnormal dilatation of blood vessels; seen mostly in older people as red or purplish areas usually on the chest or trunk. See TELANGIECTASIS — angiectatic, adj.

angiectomy (an-ji-ek'-tō-mi): Surgical excision of part or all of a blood or lymph vessel.

angina (an-jī'-na): A sense of suffocation, choking or constriction; or a disease characterized by spasmodic suffocative attacks. A. DECUBITIS attacks of A. occurring when the person is sleeping or in the recumbent position; INTESTINAL A. cramping pain in the abdomen following a meal; caused by ischaemia of the musculature of the intestine. LUDWIG'S A. a severe, acute, purulent infection of the floor of the mouth, particularly around the submaxillary gland, usually caused by streptococcus; may originate with a dental infection; see CELLULITIS. PREINFARCTION A., A. characterized by severe abrupt onset of chest pain that lasts longer than usual anginal pain; may be precipitated by situations of minimal stress; symptoms include severe dyspnoea, and unless the patient is treated, heart failure may ensue; PRINZMETAL'S A. a type of A. that is caused by spasm of one of the large coronary vessels; may occur during normal activity or during rest; tends to occur at one time of day or night and the pain is severe and long-lasting; sudden death may occur as a result of severe dysrhythmia; VINCENT'S A. a bacterial infection of the mucous membranes of the mouth, especially of the gums but may extend to the tonsils and pharynx, with necrosis of the gingivae, causing bleeding, tenderness, offensive breath, fever, swelling of the cervical lymph glands; seen mostly in adolescents. Also called *trench mouth*. — anginal, anginoid, adj.

angina pectoris (an-jī'-na-pek'-tor-is): Severe but temporary paroxysmal attack of cardiac pain which may radiate to the shoulder, arm, or epigastrium; accompanied by a feeling of suffocation and impending death; caused by inadequate supply of oxygen to the heart muscle; may be precipitated by exercise or emotional stress. INTRACTABLE A.P. can become quite crippling; treatment includes use of antihypersensitives if indicated and eliminating stressors as much as possible as well as giving up smoking; STABLE A.P. the causes, frequency, and severity of attacks are all predictable; STATUS ANGIOSUS a type of A.P. in which the pain lasts an hour; due to coronary insufficiency.

angioblast (an'-ji-ō-blast): 1. The embryonic tissue from which the blood vessels and the blood cells in the early embryo develop. 2. A blood vessel-forming cell.

angioblastoma (an'-ji-ō-blas-tō'-ma): A tumour arising in a blood vessel of the meninges of the brain or spinal cord; also called *angioblastic meningioma*.

angiocardiogram (an-ji-ō-kar'-di-ō-gram): An x-ray film of the heart and great vessels after the intravenous injection of an opaque medium.

angiocardiography (an'-ji-ō-kar-di-og'-ra-fi): A radiographic procedure for demonstrating the chambers of the heart and the great blood vessels after injection of a radiopaque medium. — angiocardiographic, adj.; angiocardiographically, adv.

angiocardiopathy (an'-ji-ō-kar-di-op'-a-thi): Any disorder of the heart and blood vessels.

angiocarditis (an'-ji-ō-kar-dī'-tis): Inflammation of the great vessels and the heart.

angiofibroma (an'-ji-ō-fī-brō'-ma): 1. A fibroma that contains numerous blood vessels: often appears as a skin tag. 2. Benign tumour in the nasopharynx.

angiogenesis (an'-ji-ō-jen'-i-sis): Formation of new blood vessels, often seen in wound healing.

angiogram (an'-ji-ō-gram): A series of x-ray pictures of blood vessels, especially arteries, after injection of a radiopaque medium.

angiography (an-ji-og'-ra-fi): Radiography of the blood vessels following the injection of a radiopaque material. — angiogram, n.; angiographic, adj.; angiographically, adv.

angiolith (an'-ji-ō-lith): A calculus in the wall of a blood vessel.

angiology (an'-ji-ol'-o-ji): The science of blood and lymphatic vessels.

angioma (an-ji-ō'-ma): An innocent tumour formed of the blood vessels. See HAEMANGIOMA; LYMPHANGIOMA. CAVERNOUS A. a benign tumour present at birth, consisting of a spongy, bluish red mass made up of many large cavernous spaces filled with blood and blood vessels; CHERRY A. raised bright red vascular papules containing many vascular loops, usually appearing on the trunk; often seen in the middle-aged and elderly; SPIDER A. spider naevus; characterized by a small central elevated red dot from which tiny blood vessels radiate like a spider's web; usually appears on the face, neck, arms, and upper trunk; STRAWBERRY A. a cavernous A. the size and colour of a strawberry. — angiomata, angiomas, pl.; angiomatous, adj.

angiomegaly (an-ji-ō-meg'-a-li): Enlargement of one or more blood vessels, particularly when it occurs in the eyelid.

angiomyolipoma (an'-ji-ō-mī'-ō-lī-pō'-ma): A benign tumour having vascular and adipose tissue elements.

angiomyoneuroma (an'-ji-ō-mī'-ō-nū-rō-ma): A glomus tumour; see under GLOMUS.

angiomyopathy (an'-ji-ō-mī-op'-a-thi): Any disorder of the muscular walls of the blood vessels.

angioneuroma (an'-ji-ō-nū-rō'-ma): A benign tumour containing elements of vascular and nerve fibre tissue.

angioneurotic oedema (an'-ji-ō-nū-rot'-ik ē-dē'-ma): An acute condition characterized by the sudden development of large painless, localized, oedematous, itchy lesions; may involve the face, lips, larynx, neck, hands, feet, or genitalia; is accompanied by swelling of subcutaneous and submucous tissues; oedema of the glottis may be fatal; may be caused by an allergy, usually a food allergy, or by infection, emotional stress, insect bites, parasitic infestation; may also be a congenital condition.

angiopathy (an-ji-op'-a-thi): Any disease of the blood vessels or lymph vessels — angiopathic, adj.

angiophilia (an-ji-ō-fil'-i-a): Haemophilia, with bleeding from the skin and mucous membranes, a condition characterized by increased bleeding time and low activity of Factor VIII (*q.v.*).

angioplasty (an'-ji-ō-plas-ti): 1. Plastic surgery of blood vessels. 2. A surgical procedure to restore blood flow in an artery by threading a balloon-tipped catheter into the vessel and then inflating it, thus pressing the atherosclerotic plaque causing the obstruction against the walls of the vessel, widening its lumen.

angiopoiesis (an'-ji-ō-poy-ē'-sis): The process of developing blood vessels in new tissue.

angiosclerosis (an'-ji-ō-sklē-rō'-sis): Hardening and thickening of the blood vessel walls.

angiospasm (an'-ji-ō-spazm): Local, intermittent constriction of the walls of a blood vessel.

angiotensin (an-ji-ō-ten'-sin): A polypeptide formed in the blood plasma by the action of the enzyme renin on a globulin in the plasma; a potent vasoconstrictor; stimulates release of aldosterone from the kidney cortex. A.-CONVERTING ENZYME (ACE) INHIBITORS drugs that block the angiotensin–aldosterone response; used in the treatment of heart failure and hypertension.

angiotomy (an-ji-ot'-o-mi): Surgical excision into a blood or lymph vessel, or the severing of a vessel.

angiotonin (an-ji-ō-tō'-nin): Angiotensin (*q.v.*).

angle of Louis: A landmark on the anterior chest wall; it is a projection formed at the junction of the manubrium and the body of the sternum at the level of the fifth thoracic vertebra.

Angstrom unit: An internationally adopted unit of measurement; used primarily to express electromagnetic wavelengths. Equals one ten thousandth of a micron; one-tenth of a millimicron; one-ten millionth of a millimetre; one hundred millionth of a centimetre; or 1/ 254,000,000 of an inch. Ten million angstroms equal 39.37 inches.

angulation (ang-ū-lā'-shun): 1. The bending of a hollow structure to form an abnormal angle, as may occur in the intestine or ureter; may become the site of an obstruction. 2. A deviation from the normal axis of a structure, as may occur in fracture of a long bone.

anhaematopoieses (an-hē'-ma-tō-poy-ē'-sis): Defective or deficient formation of blood.

anhaemolytic (an-hē-mō-lit'-ik): Not destructive to red blood cells by lysis; opp. of haemolytic.

anhydraemia (an-hī-drē'-mi-a): Decreased fluid content of the blood. — anhydraemic, adj.

anhydrase (an-hī'-dras): An enzyme that acts as a catalyst in removing water from a compound.

anhydride (an-hī'-drid): A chemical compound that results when water is removed from a substance, particularly from an acid, base, or alcohol.

anhydrochloria (an-hī-drō-klo'-ri-a): Deficiency or absence of hydrochloric acid in the gastric secretion. Also called *achlorhydria*.

anima (an'-i-ma): In Jungian psychiatry, the soul, inner being, or personality as contrasted with the persona or outer character of a person.

animate (an'-i-mat): Having life.

animation (an-i-mā'-shun): The quality of being alive. SUSPENDED A. a temporary condition marked by suspension of normal vital functions.

animism (an'-i-mizm): 1. The tendency to ascribe qualities of life to inanimate objects; occurs normally in children. 2. The belief that all animals and inanimate objects possess souls; basic to many primitive religions. 3. An ancient doctrine which, among other theories, held that the soul is the vital principle governing all life phenomena, both normal and abnormal.

animus (an'-i mus): 1. A feeling of hostility or hatred. 2. In Jungian psychology, the masculine as compared to the feminine aspect of the inner self.

anion (an'ī-on): A negatively charged ion that is attracted to and moves towards the positively charged anode during electrolysis (*q.v.*). In physiological chemistry, the important ions are bicarbonate, chloride, and phosphate. A. GAP the difference between the serum sodium concentrates and the sum of the bicarbonate and chloride concentrates.

aniridia (an i-rid'-i-a): Lack or defect of the iris; usually congenital and usually bilateral. Also called *irideremia*.

anis-, aniso-: Combining forms denoting irregular or unequal.

anisakiasis (an-i-sak-ī'-a-sis): An infection caused by a parasitic worm that thrives on saltwater fish; is not communicable; occurs in those who eat raw infected fish; causes severe acute abdominal symptoms resembling those of appendicitis or intestinal blockage. The parasite survives smoking but is killed by heat and freezing. Also called *herring worm disease*.

anisocoria (an-ī'sō-kō'-ri-a): Inequality in the diameter of the pupils, frequently seen in older people and those with nervous system disorders or head trauma.

anisodactyly (an-ī-sō-dak'-ti-li): Unequal length in corresponding digits. — anisodactylous, adj.

anisodont (an-ī'-sō-dont): Having teeth that are irregular or uneven in length, shape, or spacing.

anisognathous (an-ī-sog'-na-thus): Having jaws of unequal size, with the upper one usually being the larger.

anisoleukocytosis (an-ī'-sō-lū'-kō-sī-tō'-sis): Abnormality in the ratio of the various forms of leukocytes in the blood.

anisometropia (an-i'-sō-mē-trō'-pi-a): A condition in which light rays are refracted differently in two eyes; usually correctable by ordinary lenses.

anisopiesis (an-ī-sō-pī-ē′ -sis): Inequality of arterial blood pressure in different or paired parts of the body as registered by a sphygmomanometer.

anisuria (an-i-sū′ -ri-a): A condition marked by changes in the amount of urine excreted, alternating between polyuria and oliguria.

ankle (an′ -kl): A synovial hinge joint, the distal ends of the tibia and fibula articulating with the talus (astragalus); the joint between the lower leg and the foot. A. CLONUS a series of rapid muscular contractions of the calf muscle when the foot is dorsiflexed by pressure upon the sole; A. JERK contraction of the calf muscles causing extension of the foot, elicited by tapping the tendon of Achilles.

ankyl-, ankylo-: Combining forms denoting (1) crooked, curved; (2) stiff, immobile, constricted or closed because of adhesion.

ankylodactylia (an′ -ki-lō-dak-til′ -i-a): A deformity in which two or more fingers or toes are in adhesion with each other; a fairly common congenital anomaly.

ankylosing spondylitis (an′ki-lō-sing spon-di-lī′ -tis): See SPONDYLITIS.

ankylosis (an′ -ki-lō′ -sis): Immobility or fixation of a joint; may result from trauma or a pathological condition, or be produced by surgery.

ankylotia (an-ki-lō′ -shi-a): Closure or occlusion of the external auditory canal.

ankyroid (an′ -ki-royd): Hook-shaped.

'anniversary' phenomenon: The occurrence or deepening of depression, associated with an exacerbation of any physical symptoms, coinciding with the anniversary of the death or loss of a loved one; commonly seen in the elderly.

annual budget: Amount of money allocated at the start of the financial year, for example to a hospital, department, or ward.

annular (an′ -ū-lar): Ring-shaped. A. LIGAMENTS surround adjoining parts and bind them together; e.g., A. L. of the wrist and of the ankle.

annulus, anulus (an′ -ū-lus): A ring, ring-like or encircling structure, e.g., the tough fibrocartilaginous ring that joins the borders of the vertebrae and holds them together, or the dense fibrous rings around the four major orifices of the heart. A. OF ZINN the circular fibrous ligament at the back of the orbit that gives rise to the extraocular muscles.

ano-: Combining form denoting (1) anus; (2) upper or upwards.

anochromia (an-ō-krō′ -mi-a): The concentration of the haemoglobin of the erythrocytes around the edges of the cells, leaving the centres pale; occurs in certain types of anaemia.

anoci-association (a-nō′ -si-a-sō-si-ā′ -shun): A method of preventing or minimizing surgical shock by allaying the patient's anxiety, fear, or apprehension through the use of sedatives and hypnotics previous to anaesthesia, and by measures that reduce postoperative discomfort.

anococcygeal (ā-nō-kok-sij′ -ē′ -al): Relating to the anus and the coccyx.

anocutaneous (ā-nō-kū-tā′ -nē-us): Relating to the anus and the skin around it.

anode (an′ -ōd): The positive pole or terminus of an electric source such as the galvanic battery. — anodal, anodic, adj.

anodontia (an-ō-don′ -shi-a): Absence of some or all of the teeth; may be congenital and affect both deciduous and permanent teeth, or may occur in an older person who has had teeth extracted.

anodyne (an′ -ō-dīn): An agent that relieves pain. *Analgesic.*

anogenital (ā-nō-jen′ -i-tal): Relating to the anal and genital regions.

anomalous (a-nom′ -a-lus): Abnormal, irregular; out of the ordinary.

anomaly (a-nom′ -a-li): That which is unusual, abnormal or unconforming; that in which there is marked deviation from the normal in form, structure, or location. — anomalous, adj.

anomia (an-ō′ -mi-a): Inability to name objects or persons. Same as *nominal aphasia.* — anomic, adj.

anomie (an′ -ō-mē): In society, refers to a state characterized by lack or loss of normative standards of conduct. In individuals, refers to a person who lacks normal standards of conduct, is disoriented, anxious, isolated, and cannot relate to others.

anonychia (an-ō-nik′ -i-a): Absence of a nail or nails.

anoopsia (an-ō-op′ -si-a): Strabismus, accompanied by a tendency for one eye to turn upwards.

anoperineal (ā′ -nō-per-i-nē′ -al): Relating to the anus and perineum.

Anopheles (a-nof′ -e-lēz): A genus of mosquitoes; many of the several species are vectors of disease, e.g., malaria, dengue, filariasis. The females are the vectors of the malarial parasite, and their bite is the means of transmitting the disease to humans.

anophoria (an-o-fō′ -ri-a): The condition in which one eye turns upwards because its visual axis rises above that of the other eye which is normal. Also called *anopia, anotropia, hyperphoria.*

anophthalmia			39			anterior tibial

anophthalmia (an-of-thal′-mi-a): A congenital anomaly characterized by the absence of one or both eyes. Also called *anophthalmos*.

anorectal (ā-nō-rek′-tal): Relating to the anus and rectum, as a fissure (*q.v.*). A. AGENESIS lack of normal development of the anus and rectum.

anorectic (a′-nō-rek′-tik): 1. An appetite depressant. 2. Relating to anorexia.

anorexia (an ō-rck′-si a): Loss or lack of appetite for food. A. NERVOSA a psychosomatic disorder characterized by an aversion to food, leading to atrophy of the stomach, emaciation and, in women, amenorrhoea. — anorexic, anorectic, adj.

anorexigenic (an′-ō-rek′-si-jen′-ik): 1. Producing anorexia. 2. An agent that diminishes the appetite.

anoscopy (ā-nos′-ko-pi): Examination of the lower rectum and the anus by means of an anoscope. — anoscopic, adj.

anosmia (an-oz′-mi-a): Absence or impairment of the sense of smell; may result from a lesion of the olfactory nerve, an obstruction in the nasal passages, cerebral disease involving the olfactory centre, or there may be no apparent cause. — anosmic, anosmatic, anosmous, adj.

anosognosia (an-ō-sog-nō′-zi-a): Inability to recognize, denial of, or unawareness of loss or defect of a physical function; seen most often in patients with a lesion of the left hemisphere but may also occur in those with other brain lesions.

anostosis (an-os-tō′-sis): Defective formation or ossification of bone.

ANOVA: Abbreviation for analysis of variance, see under ANALYSIS.

anovular (an-vo′-ū-lar): Not pertaining to, associated with, or coincidental with ovulation. A. BLEEDING is uterine bleeding that has not been preceded by ovulation. Also called *anovulatory*.

anovulation (an-ov-ū-lā′-shun): Cessation or absence of ovulation.

anoxia (a-nok′-si-a): Literally, no oxygen in the tissues, which occurs when the blood supply to a part is cut off; results in injury or death of the tissues involved. More frequently used to refer to a condition in which there is less than the normal amount of oxygen in red blood cells and, consequently, reduced amounts in tissues and organs; or failure of tissues to utilize sufficient oxygen. May be due to impaired lung function, lack of haemoglobin, or circulatory disorders. — anoxic, adj.

ansiform (an′-si-form): Loop-shaped.

-ant: An adjective-forming suffix denoting (1) a thing or agent that enhances a specific action; (2) a thing or substance that is acted upon in a specific manner.

antacid (ant-as′-id): 1. Neutralizing or counteracting an acid. 2. Any substance that neutralizes or counteracts acidity, *e.g.*, that of gastric juice.

antagonism (an-tag′-o-nizm): A state of mutual opposition or force between like things that is characteristic of some muscles, drugs, and organisms. In pharmacotherapeutics, refers to a situation in which two drugs given together produce an action that is less intense than that of either of the drugs given alone.

antagonist (an-tag′-o-nist): 1. A muscle that relaxes to allow its agonist (*q.v.*) to perform a movement. 2. Any agent that opposes or nullifies the action of another agent 3 A drug that reduces or counteracts the effects of another drug.

antaphrodisiac (ant′ af-rō-diz′-i-ak): An agent that diminishes sexual desire.

ante-: Prefix denoting before, with reference to time or place.

antecedent (an-te-sē′-dent): 1. A preceding event, cause, or condition. 2. Prior in time or cause.

antecubital (an-tē-kū′-bit-al): Situated in front of the elbow. A. FOSSA or SPACE the depression on the inner aspect of the elbow.

anteflexion (an-tē-flek′-shun): The abnormal bending forward of an organ. Commonly applied to the position of the uterus. Opp. to retroflexion.

antegrade (an′-tē-grād): Extending or moving forward. Also called *anterograde*.

antenatal (an-tē-nā′-tal): Relating to any event or condition that occurs or exists in the embryo or the mother during the period between conception and delivery of the infant.

antepartum (an-te-par′-tum): In obstetrics, before parturition; generally refers to the 3 months preceding full-term delivery. A. HAEMORRHAGE bleeding from the genital tract before birth.

anterior (an-tē′-ri-or): In front of; the front surface of; ventral. Opp. of posterior. A. CHAMBER OF THE EYE the space between the posterior surface of the cornea and the anterior surface of the iris; contains aqueous humor (*q.v.*); A. PITUITARY refers to the anterior lobe of the pituitary gland.

anterior tibial compartment syndrome: A condition characterized by rapid swelling of the anterior tibial compartment, accompanied by pain in the leg, necrosis of the compartment muscle, oedema, erythema over the area; may result from local injury due to excessive exertion or arterial occlusion.

antero-: Prefix denoting before; in front of.

anteversion (an-tē-ver′-zhun): The forward tilting or displacement forward, without bending, of the whole of an organ or part. Opp. to retroversion. — anteverted, adj.; antevert, v.

anthelmintic (ant-hel-min′-tik): **1.** Destructive to intestinal worms. **2.** Any remedy for the destruction or elimination of intestinal worms.

anthracaemia (an-thra-sē′-mi-a): Anthrax septicaemia; the presence of *Bacillus anthracis* in the bloodstream. — anthracaemic, adj.

anthracosilicosis (an′-thra-kō-sil-i-kō′-sis): A disease of the lungs caused by inhalation of coal dust and particles of silica; often an occupational disease; symptoms are those of both anthracosis (*q.v.*) and silicosis (*q.v.*).

anthracosis (an-thra-kō′-sis): Black pigmentation of the lung due to inhalation of coal dust; when large amounts of coal dust are inhaled, as occurs in coal miners, pneumoconiosis (*q.v.*) may develop.

anthrax (an′-thrax): An acute infectious disease of animals, cattle and sheep especially caused by the *Bacillus anthracis*, a spore-forming organism found in soil and directly transmissible to humans through an abrasion in the skin or by inhalation or ingestion of airborne spores. An occupational disease occurring particularly in people who handle wool, fleece, hides, hair, or other animal tissues; characterized by the formation, at the site of infection, of a papule which becomes vesicular and ulcerates producing a tenacious, thick black crust with the underlying and surrounding tissues becoming very swollen and oedematous; may occur in the tongue and throat, intestine, and lung in addition to the skin. Other symptoms include headache, fever, malaise, pruritus; the acute form may be rapidly fatal. Protective measures include prophylactic immunization of cattle and humans. Also called *woolsorter's disease*.

anthro-, anthrop-, anthropo-: Combining forms denoting man or human being.

anthropogeny (an-thro-poj′-e-ni): The study of the evolution of humans.

anthropoid (an′-thro-poyd): Like a human being. A. PELVIS see under PELVIS.

anthropology (an-thro-pol′-o-ji): **1.** The study of humankind, of its societies and customs. **2.** The study of the structure and evolution of humans as animals.

anthropomorphic (an′-thro-pō-mor-fik): Having a human form.

anthropophobia (an′-thrō-pō-fō′-bi-a): A morbid dread of human society or companionship.

anthropozoonosis (an′-thrō-pō-zō′-ō-nō′-sis): A disease which may affect either animal or man and may be transmitted from one species to the other.

anti-: Prefix denoting against, effective against, opposed to, counter.

antiabortifacient (an′-ti-a-bor-ti-fā′-shent): **1.** An agent that prevents abortion or promotes normal gestation. **2.** Tending to prevent abortion.

antiacid (an-ti-as′-id): See ANTACID.

antianaemic (an-ti-a-nē′-mik): **1.** Any agent that prevents or relieves anaemia. **2.** Relieving or preventing anaemia. A. FACTOR vitamin B_{12} (cyanocobalamin) found in liver, fish meal, eggs, and some other natural products; for absorption in the body it must combine with hydrochloric acid and an intrinsic factor produced by the lining of the stomach; it is essential for proper development of red blood cells in bone marrow.

antibody (an′ti-an′-ti-bod-i): A substance that is formed in the body after the injection of an antibody which the substance is intended to counteract.

antianxiety (an′-ti-ang-zī′-i-ti): A. AGENT a drug that depresses the activity of the central nervous system through its sedative and hypnotic actions and thus reduces anxiety.

antiarrhythmic (an′-ti-a-rith′-mik): **1.** Preventing or correcting cardiac arrhythmia (*q.v.*). **2.** An agent that prevents or corrects arrhythmia.

antiarthritic (an′-ti-ar-thrit′-ik): **1.** Relieving arthritis or gout. **2.** An agent that relieves arthritis or gout.

antibacterial (an′-ti-bak-tēr′-i-al): **1.** An agent that destroys bacteria or prevents their growth and reproduction. **2.** Tending to destroy bacteria or prevent their growth and reproduction.

antibiosis (an′-ti-bī-ō′-sis): An association between organisms of different species that is harmful to one of them. Opp. to symbiosis. — antibiotic, adj.

antibiotic (an′tī-bī-ot′-ik): **1.** Relating to antibiosis. **2.** Destructive to life. **3.** Any of a group of antibacterial chemical compounds originally derived from fungi, moulds, or bacteria; many are now produced synthetically; used extensively in medicine. Some are active against only certain bacteria, fungi, or viruses; others are active against a wider range of microorganisms. Some are effective when given by injection or orally; others are rarely used internally because of their high toxicity but are effective applied topically. BROAD-SPECTRUM A. one which is effective against many different microorganisms.

antibiotic resistance: The ability of some pathogenic microorganisms to remain unaffected by antibiotics. Genes for antibiotic resistance are often carried in plasmids in transposons, which can spread across species barriers.

antibodies (an'-ti-bod'-iz): A class of specific protein substances in the blood that destroy or render inactive certain foreign substances, particularly bacteria and their products. May be developed naturally or in response to a specific antigen that has been introduced into the body parenterally or otherwise; may be transferred to the fetus *in utero*; may develop as a result of a subclinical infection with the specific agent, thus producing immunity to the specific disease. They cause agglutination, flocculation, inactivation or lysis of the antigen. A. include agglutinins, amboceptors, antienzymes, antitoxins, bacteriolysins, cytotoxins, haemolysins, opsonins, and precipitins.

anticarcinogen (an'-ti-kar-sin'-o-jen): An agent that opposes the action of carcinogens.

anticardium (an'-ti-kar'-di-um): The precordium (*q.v.*).

anticariogenic (an'-ti-kar-i-o-jen'-ik): Having the effect of retarding decay, dental decay in particular.

anticathexis (an'-ti-ka-thek'-sis): The outward expression of an emotional impulse that is the complete opposite of the emotion actually felt, *e.g.*, the expression of unconscious hate as conscious love.

anticholinergic (an'-ti-kō-lin-er'-jik): 1. Tending to inhibit the action of a parasympathetic nerve by interfering with the action of acetylcholine, a chemical by which such a nerve transmits its impulses at neural or myoneural junctions. 2. An agent that blocks the transmission of impulses across the parasympathetic ganglia or blocks the effect of acetycholine, *e.g.*, atropine.

anticholinesterase (an'-ti-kō-lin-es'-ter-ās): A substance that lessens or inhibits the enzymatic activity of cholinesterase.

anticipatory grief: A stage of bereavement engaged in by relatives who have accepted the fact that death of a loved one is inevitable.

anticoagulant (an'-ti-kō-ag'-ū-lant): 1. An agent that suppresses, prevents, or retards the clotting of blood. 2. Having the effect of suppressing, preventing or retarding the clotting

of blood. A. THERAPY the administration of an anticoagulant to prevent intravascular clotting in the treatment of coronary thrombosis, phlebothrombosis, and similar disorders.

anticonvulsant (an'ti-kon-vul'-sant): 1. An agent that stops or prevents convulsions. 2. Tending to prevent or relieve the severity of convulsions.

anti-D immunoglobulin (an'-ti dē' im-mū-nō-glob'-ū lin): An immune globulin specific for the D antigen; it is administered to Rh-negative women within 72 hours of delivery to destroy any Rh-positive cells that the mother may have received from the fetal blood during delivery; done to prevent formation of antibodies that would affect future pregnancies.

antidepressant (an'-ti-dē-pres'-ant): An agent or procedure that inhibits or alleviates depression.

antidiarrhoeal (an'-ti-dī-a-rē'-al): 1. An agent that prevents or checks diarrhoea. 2. Tending to prevent or alleviate diarrhoea. Also called *diarrhoeic*.

antidiuretic (an'-ti dī-u-ret'-ik): 1. An agent that reduces the volume of the urine secreted. 2. Tending to reduce the secretion of urine.

antidiuretic hormone: A hormone made and stored in the posterior pituitary gland, and released as required to suppress diuresis. It stimulates reabsorption of water in the kidney tubules and thus helps to regulate fluid balance. Too small an amount results in diabetes insipidus (*q.v.*); too large an amount results in oliguria and excessive fluid retention. Abbreviated ADH. Also called *vasopressin*.

antidote (an'-ti-dōt): An agent that counteracts or neutralizes the action of a poison.

antidysthanasia (an'-ti-dis-tha-nā'-zi-a): Descriptive of a belief or commitment not to utilize extraordinary measures to prolong life in a patient who faces a long and agonizing death.

antiembolism stockings (an-ti-em'-bo-lizm): Tight-fitting elastic stockings that compress the superficial veins; prescribed for immobilized patients to promote the flow of blood in the leg veins and decrease the possibility of embolus formation and other circulatory problems.

antiemetic (an'-ti-ē-met'-ik): Any agent that prevents nausea and vomiting.

antienzyme (an-ti-en'-zīm): A substance that exerts a specific inhibiting effect on an enzyme. In the digestive tract they prevent digestion of the digestive tube lining; in the blood they act as antibodies (*q.v.*).

antiepileptic (an'-tī-ep-i-lep'-tik): An agent that reduces the frequency and/or the severity of epileptic attacks.

antifebrile (an-ti-feb'-ril): 1. Reducing or abolishing fever. 2. Any agent that reduces or allays fever.

antifibrinolytic (an'-ti-fi-brin-ō-lit'-ik): Any substance that inhibits or retards the proteolytic action of fibrinolysin.

antigen (an'-ti-jen): Any substance, usually a protein, which can stimulate the production of antibodies and react specifically with those antibodies; may be a bacterium, pollen, grain, etc.; each type requires a different antibody to neutralize it. AUSTRALIAN A. an A. found in serum of patients with acute serum hepatitis and in normal inhabitants of south-east Asia and the tropics. Now called *hepatitis B surface antigen* (*q.v.*).

antigen–antibody reaction: The specific reaction of an antibody to an antigen; occurs when the antigen provokes an immunological response and antibodies are produced which try to neutralize the antigen that stimulated their production.

antigenicity (an'-ti-jen-is'-i-ti): The ability to promote antibody formation.

antigravity (an-ti-grav'-i-ti): Against or opposing the force of gravity. A. MUSCLES the muscles of the limbs which support the body in the upright position, chiefly the extensor muscles; A. POSTURE the upright position; the ability to achieve and maintain this position is usually learned by the end of the first year of life.

antihaemophilic (an'-ti-hē-mō-fil'-ik): An agent that counteracts the bleeding tendency in haemophilia.

antihaemophilic factor (an'-ti-hē-mō-fil'-ik fak'-tor): Factor VIII, required for the formation of a blood clot. Deficiency of this inherited factor causes classic haemophilia. Also called *antihaemophilic globulin (AHG)* and *thromboplastinogen*.

antihaemorrhagic (an'ti-hem-ō-raj'-ik): 1. Any drug or agent that prevents haemorrhage. 2. Tending to prevent haemorrhage. A. VITAMIN vitamin K (*q.v.*).

anti-HBc: Antibody (*q.v.*) against the hepatitis B core antigen.

anti-HBe: Antibody (*q.v.*) against the e antigen associated with the core of the hepatitis B virus.

anti-HBs: Antibody (*q.v.*) against the hepatitis B surface antigen (*q.v.*).

antihistamines (an-ti-hist'-a-mēnz): Drugs that suppress some of the effects of released hista-

mine (*q.v.*); widely used in treatment of hay fever, urticaria, angioneurotic oedema, and some forms of pruritus. Because of their antiemetic properties, are used to prevent motion and radiation sickness. Side effects include drowsiness. — antihistaminic, adj. and n.

antihuman globulin (anti-hū'-man glob'-ū-lin): Any natural or artificially produced substance which reacts with globulin that has been prepared by immunizing an animal with purified human gamma globulin. Also called *antiglobulin* and *Boombs serum.*

antihyperglycaemic (an'-ti-hī-per-glī-sē'-mik): 1. An agent that acts to reduce high levels of glucose in the blood. 2. Reducing high glucose levels in the blood.

antihypertensive (an'-ti-hī-per-ten'-siv): 1. Any drug or agent that lowers blood pressure in hypertensive patients. 2. Tending to counteract hypertension.

antihypnotic (an'-ti-hip-not'-ik): 1. An agent that prevents or hinders sleep. 2. Tending to prevent sleep.

antihypotensive (an'-ti-hī-pō-ten'-siv): 1. Counteracting abnormally low blood pressure. 2. An agent that counteracts abnormally low blood pressure.

anti-infective (an'-ti-in-fek'-tiv): 1. Counteracting infection. 2. Any agent that counteracts or prevents infection. See VITAMIN A.

anti-inflammatory (an'-ti-in-flam'-a-to-ri): 1. Counteracting or preventing inflammation. 2. An agent that counteracts or suppresses inflammation.

antilithic (an-ti-lith'-ik): 1. Tending to counteract the formation of stones or calculi. 2. An agent that helps prevent the formation of stones or calculi, or that aids in their dissolution.

antilymphocyte globulin (an'-tī-limf'-ō-sīt glob'-u-lin): The globulin fraction of antilymphocyte serum prepared by injecting the individual's lymphocytes into a different species; a powerful immunosuppressive agent used in combating the rejection reaction in persons who have had an organ transplant.

antilymphocyte serum: Serum containing antibodies that bind to lymphocytes inhibiting their function. Used in patients undergoing organ transplantation to induce immunosuppression.

antilysin (an-ti-lī'-sin): An antibody that opposes the activity of a lysin thereby protecting cells against lysis.

antimalarial (an-ti-ma-lai'ri-al): 1. Having the effect of preventing or suppressing malaria. 2. Any drug or measure taken to prevent or suppress malaria, or to destroy the causative agent in malaria.

antimetabolite (an'-tī-me-tab'-ō-līt): A drug or other agent that is similar in constituents to the chemicals needed by a cell for formation of nucleoproteins, and which interferes with cell metabolism of essential metabolites, thereby preventing further development of the cell.

antimetropia (an'-ti-me-trō'-pi-a): An ocular condition in which the two eyes present different refractive errors: *e.g.*, one eye may be myopic and the other hypermetropic.

antimicrobial resistance (an'-ti-mī-krō'-bi-al): Resistance to specific medicines developed by any type of microbe (a common misconception being that a person's body becomes resistant to specific drugs). Enables microbes to survive the use of medicines that threaten their existence. If a microbe becomes resistant to many medicines, treating the infection it causes can become difficult and sometimes impossible.

antimitotic (an'-ti-mī-tot'-ik): 1. Relating to the inhibition of mitosis. 2. An agent that inhibits or prevents reproduction of a cell by mitosis.

antimycotic (an'-ti-mī-kot'-ik): 1. Preventing or suppressing the growth of fungi. 2. An agent or measure that destroys or suppresses the growth of fungi.

antinarcotic (an'-ti-nar-kot'-ik): 1. Preventing or relieving the effects of a narcotic (*q.v.*) drug. 2. A drug or agent that counteracts the stupor produced by a narcotic drug.

antinauseant (an'-ti-naw'-sē-ant): 1. Tending to relieve or counteract nausea. 2. An agent that relieves or counteracts nausea.

antineoplastic (an'-ti-nē-ō-plas'-tik): 1. Having the effect of inhibiting or preventing the development and proliferation of malignant cells. 2. Referring to a chemically produced substance that inhibits or controls the growth of certain malignant cells.

antinuclear antibody: An antibody found in persons with any of several connective tissue disorders; its action is directed at the components of the cell nucleus.

antinuclear factor test: A screening test for the presence of antibodies against the cell nuclear material (DNA). A positive reaction is indicative of lupus erythematosus. Also known as *ANF test*.

anti-oppressive practice: Practice ensuring that peoples' rights, values, and culture are not violated or disrespected.

antioxidant (an'-tī-oks'-i-dant): Any of several substances, synthetic or natural, that prevent deterioration by the action of oxygen; commonly used in the preparation of foods for marketing, *e.g.*, vegetable oils and fats.

antiparasitic (an'-ti-par-a-sit'-ik): 1. Destructive to parasites. 2. Any agent that destroys parasites or inhibits their growth.

antiparkinsonian (an'-ti-park-in-sōn'-i-an): Effective against the symptoms of parkinsonism; said especially of certain drugs.

antipathy (an-tip'-a-thi): Incompatibility; aversion; distaste; dislike. In medicine, the mutual antagonism between two diseases. — antipathic, adj.

antiperiodic (an'-ti-pē-ri-od'-ik): Any agent or measure that prevents the periodic recurrence of symptoms of disease, *e.g.*, the use of quinine in malaria.

antiperistalsis (an'-ti-per-i-stal'-sis): A reversal of the normal peristaltic action, *i.e.*, beginning in the lower ileum the peristaltic wave proceeds from below upwards preventing the passage of intestinal contents into the caecum. — antiperistaltic, adj.

antiperistaltic (an'-ti-per-i-stal'-tik): 1. Inhibiting or diminishing peristalsis. 2. A substance that inhibits or diminishes peristalsis.

antiperspirant (an'-ti-per'-spi-rant): An agent having an inhibitory action on the secretion of sweat.

antiplatelet (an-ti-pl-āt'-let): A substance that acts to lyse or agglutinate blood platelets and thus inhibits or destroys their normal action.

antipodal (an-tip'-ō-dal): Situated exactly opposite.

antiprothrombin (an'-ti-prō-throm'-bin): An anticoagulant present in the blood or an agent that acts to prevent conversion of prothrombin into thrombin.

antipruritic (an'-ti-proo-rit-ik): 1. Any procedure or agent that relieves or prevents itching. 2. Having the action of preventing or relieving itching.

anti-psychiatry: Term used to describe a movement to denigrate psychiatry, modern psychiatric treatments, and the conduct of institutions for the care of psychiatric patients.

antipsychotic (an'-ti-sī-kot'-ik): Usually pertains to an agent that reduces psychomotor activity; a neuroleptic agent.

antipyretic (an'-ti-pī-ret'-ik): 1. Effective in reducing or relieving fever. 2. Any agent that reduces or relieves fever. — antipyresis, n.

antisepsis (an-ti-sep'-sis): 1. The prevention of sepsis (*q.v.*) by any or all of the following actions: destroying the microorganisms that produce infection; preventing their access to the site of potential infection; or inhibiting their growth and multiplication. Introduced into surgery in 1880 by Lord Lister who used carbolic acid to prevent sepsis. 2. The use of specific procedures or agents to prevent the development of sepsis.

antiseptic (an-ti-sep′-tik): 1. Tending to prevent or inhibit the growth and multiplication of microorganisms and viruses that produce disease. 2. Any agent that inhibits or prevents the growth and multiplication of microorganisms that produce disease.

antiserum (an′-ti-sē′-rum): A serum (from human or animal) that contains specific antibody or antibodies against a specific bacterium or other antigenic agent; the specific antibodies may be produced by infection with the specific bacterium or toxin, or by immunization through repeated injection of the specific bacterium or toxin into the tissues or blood. Useful in creating passive immunity (*q.v.*) or in treating such diseases as diphtheria, tetanus, meningitis. — antisera, pl.

anti-social (an-ti-sō′-shal): Against society. A term used to denote a psychopathic state in which the individual cannot accept the obligations and restraints imposed by a community on its members and, consequently, is in frequent conflict with society. The individual develops behaviour patterns characterized by callous indifference to the effect of his actions on others, and irresponsibility. A. PERSONALITY see under PERSONALITY DISORDER.

antispasmodic (an′-ti-spaz-mod′-ik): 1. Tending to prevent spasm of smooth muscle. 2. Any agent or measure used to prevent smooth muscle spasm.

antispastic (an-ti-spas′-tik): 1. Tending to prevent or relieve skeletal muscle spasm. 2. An agent or therapeutic measure that tends to prevent or relieve skeletal muscle spasm.

antistalsis (an-ti-stal′-sis): Reversed peristalsis (*q.v.*).

antistatic (an-ti-stat′-ik): Any measure taken to prevent or deal with the collection of static electricity.

antistreptolysin (an′-ti-strep-tol′-i-sin): An inhibitor of the streptolysin on group A haemolytic streptococci (see LANCEFIELD'S GROUPS); a raised titre of A. in the blood is indicative of recent streptococcal infection.

antisudorific (an′-ti-sū-dō-rif′-ik): 1. Acting to inhibit or reduce secretion of sweat. 2. An agent that inhibits or reduces the secretion of sweat.

antisyphilitic (an′ti-sif-i-lit′-ik): 1. Any measures taken or agent used to combat or treat syphilis. 2. Effective against syphilis.

antitetanus serum: Contains tetanus antibodies. Produces artificial passive immunity. A test dose must be given first. Can cause anaphylaxis.

antitetanus toxoid: Contains treated tetanus toxins. Produces artifical active immunity. Does not cause anaphylaxis.

antithrombin (an-ti-throm′-bin): Any substance that occurs naturally in the blood, *e.g.*, heparin, or is given therapeutically to inhibit clotting of blood and the formation of thrombi.

antithromboplastin (an′-ti-throm-bō-plas′-tin): A substance that interferes with the action of thromboplastin and thus inhibits normal coagulation of blood.

antithyroid (an-ti-thī′-roid): 1. Any agent or drug used to reduce the activity of the thyroid gland; *e.g.*, thiouracil. 2. Capable of counteracting the influence of the thyroid gland.

antitoxic (an-ti-tok′-sik): 1. Relating to an antitoxin. 2. Antidotal; counteracting or neutralizing the action of a toxin. A. SERA the serum of horses which have been immunized by injections of pathogenic bacterial toxins, such as tetanus and gas gangrene. Such serum contains antibodies or antitoxins, and after injection into humans confers a temporary immunity against the original toxin.

antitoxin (an-ti-tok′-sin): An antibody that neutralizes a given toxin. It is elaborated in the body in direct response to the invasion of a bacterium or toxin. Antitoxins may be prepared from the blood serum of animals or humans that have been immunized against specific toxins, and used therapeutically.

antitrismus (an-ti-triz′-mus): Inability to close the mouth due to tonic muscle spasm.

antitrypsin (an-ti-trip′-sin): A substance that inhibits the physiological action of trypsin.

antituberculin (an-ti-tū-ber′-kū-lin): An antibody developed within the body after the injection of tuberculin (*q.v.*).

antitussive (an-ti-tus′-iv): 1. Effective in relieving or suppressing cough. 2. Any measure or agent that suppresses cough.

antivenin (an-ti-ven′-in): An antiserum (*q.v.*) obtained from an animal immunized against the venom of a particular snake or insect and containing antitoxin to that venom. Used as an antidote in first aid treatment of poisoning by snake bite.

antiviral (an-ti-vī' -ral): **1.** Destructive to viruses and inhibiting their replication. **2.** An agent that is active against viruses and inhibits their replication.

antivivisection (an' -ti-viv-i-sek' -shun): Opposition to the use of living animals for experimentation or medical research.

antrobuccal (an-trō-buk' -al): Relating to the maxillary antrum and the mouth. A. FISTULA can occur after extraction of an upper molar tooth, the root of which has protruded into the floor of the antrum.

antrostomy (an-tros' -to-mi): An incision into an antrum to provide for drainage.

antrum (an' -trum): A closed or nearly closed cavity, especially in a bone, *e.g.*, the antrum of Highmore in the superior maxillary bone. [Nathaniel Highmore, British physician, 1613–1685.] The term is also used to describe the pyloric end of the stomach when it is partially shut off from the fundus, during digestion, by the contraction of the pyloric sphincter. — antra, pl.; antral, adj.

anuclear (a-nū' -klē-ar): Having no nucleus; said particularly of erythrocytes.

anulus (an' -ū-lus)· See ANNULUS.

anuresis (an-ū-rē' -sis): Failure to excrete urine. May be due to either lack of secretion or obstruction in the urinary passages. — anuretic, adj.

anuria (a-nū' -ri-a): Cessation of the production and excretion of urine. See SUPPRESSION. — anuric, adj.

anus (ā' -nus): The opening at the end of the alimentary canal; the extreme termination of the rectum; formed of a sphincter muscle which relaxes to allow faecal matter to pass through. IMPERFORATE A. a congenital anomaly in which there is no opening at the terminus of the alimentary canal.

anvil (an' -vil): The middle of the three ossicles of the middle ear which conduct sound waves from the tympanum to the inner ear; likened to an anvil in shape; also called the *incus*.

anxiety (ang-zī' -e-ti): A condition of disturbed mood and behaviour, characterized by feelings of fear, apprehension, nervousness, inadequacy, tensions, and dread; usually associated with a real or imagined threat to one's security. Signs and symptoms include increased heart rate and muscle tone, restlessness, perspiration, and agitation. A. STATE NEUROSIS see under NEUROSIS; CASTRATION A. see under CASTRATION; FREE FLOATING A., A. without any apparent or conscious cause; SEPARATION A. a state usually seen in infants from six to ten months of age; marked by apprehension when the mother or mother surrogate is not present; may continue into later life when the person is separated from his normal environment or from persons who are significant to him.

anxiolytic (ang-zi-ō-lit' -ik): An agent that helps to dispel anxiety.

aorta (ā-or' -ta): The main trunk of the arterial system of the body; it arises in the left ventricle, carries oxygenated blood away from the heart, and, along with its branches, forms the arterial system of the body. Anatomically, the aorta is divided into three main parts: (1) the ASCENDING A. that portion that arises in the left ventricle of the heart and, passing upwards, joins the heart to the arch of the aorta; (2) ARCH OF THE A. the part that passes anteroposteriorly over the base of the heart, and joins the ascending aorta to the descending aorta; (3) the DESCENDING A. extends downwards from the arch to the level of the fourth lumbar vertebra where it divides into the right and left iliac arteries. The portion of the descending A. that lies above the diaphragm is called the THORACIC A. and the portion below the diaphragm is called the ABDOMINAL A. — aortal, aortic, adj.

aortalgia (ā-or-tal' -ji-a): Pain in the area of the aorta.

aortarctia (ā-or-tark' -shi-a): Narrowing or stenosis of the aorta.

aortectasia (ā-or-tek-tā' -zi-a): Dilatation of the aorta.

aortic (ā-ōr' -tik): Relating to the aorta. A. ARCH see under AORTA. A. BODIES small neurovascular chemoreceptive structures on both sides of the aorta near the arch; they have a function in regulating respiration by responding to changes in concentrations of oxygen, carbon dioxide, and hydrogen in the blood; A. HIATUS the opening in the diaphragm through which the aorta passes from the thorax into the abdominal cavity; A. INSUFFICIENCY or INCOMPETENCE improper closing of the valve between the left ventricle and the aorta permitting the backflow of blood; A. MURMUR an abnormal sound heard as blood flows through a diseased aorta or aortic valve; A. PLEXUS important network of sympathetic nerves, extending from the coeliac (solar) plexus over the anterolateral aspect of the aorta and downwards to the hypogastric plexus; A. SINUS one of the sac-like dilatations of the aorta opposite the semilunar valve cusps; A. STENOSIS see under STENOSIS; A. VALVE a tricuspid valve at the junction of the left ventricle and the aorta.

aorticsclerosis (ā-ōr′-tik-sklē-rō′-sis): Sclerosis of the aorta.

aorticstenosis (ā-ōr′-tik-sten-ō′-sis): Narrowing of the aorta.

aortitis (ā-or-tī′-tis): Inflammation of the aorta.

aortogram (a-or′-tō-gram): An x-ray picture of the aorta made by aortography.

aortography (ā-or-tog′-ra-fi): Roentgenography of the aorta utilizing a radiopaque medium. See also ARTERIOGRAPHY.

aortotomy (ā-or-tot′-o-mi): Incision into the aorta.

ap-, apo-: Prefixes denoting: 1. Away from, detached from, separate. 2. Related to.

Apache score (a-pach′-i): A numerical system of classifying patients in the intensive care unit. Patients are evaluated by physiological scores, which correlate with the severity of illness, and chronic health status, which estimates their mortality rate during hospitalization. 'Apache' – Acute Physiology and Chronic Health Evaluation.

apareunia (a-pa-roo′-nē-a): Inability to practise sexual intercourse; usually because of an obstruction in the vagina, or an atresic vagina.

apastia (a-pas′-ti-a): Abstention from food when it occurs as a symptom of neurological or psychological disorder.

apathism (ap′-a-thizm): Indifference or sluggishness of reaction.

apathy (ap′-a-thi): Want of feeling, emotion, or concern; indifference, insensibility. Seen in patients with depression, dementia, schizophrenia, and certain organic disorders. — apathetic, apathic, adj.

APEL: Abbreviation for accreditation (assessment) of prior experiential learning, see under ACCREDITATION.

aperient (a-pē′-ri-ent): A mild laxative.

aperistalsis (a-per-i-stal′-sis): Absence of the normal contractions of the intestines as occurs *e.g.*, in paralytic ileus. — aperistaltic, adj.

aperture (ap′er-chur): An opening or orifice in an anatomical structure.

apex (ā′-peks): In anatomy, a term used to designate the top or the tip of an organ or body, or the pointed end of a cone-shaped or pyramidal structure, *e.g.*, the heart or lungs. Also applied to the end of a tooth. A. BEAT see under BEAT; A. OF THE HEART the blunt narrow end enclosing mainly the left ventricle; it rests on the diaphragm; A. OF THE LUNG that portion nearest the shoulder level. — apical, adj.; apices, pl.

Apgar score: The numerical expression of a newborn infant's well-being and ability to survive; consists of the sum of points from zero to 10, based on five signs ranked in order of importance, with assessments being made at one minute and five minutes after birth. Included are (1) heart rate; (2) respiratory effort as demonstrated by the infant's cry; (3) muscle tone, checked by flexion and response of the extremities; (4) reflex irritability, checked by flicking the sole of the foot or tickling the nostril with a wisp of cotton and noting foot or facial changes; (5) colour, check for presence or absence of cyanosis and general body colour. [Virginia Apgar, American anaesthetist 1909–1974].

aphagia (a-fā′-ji-a): Inability or refusal to swallow. — aphagic, adj.

aphalangia (a-fa-lan′-ji-a): Congenital absence of one or more of the fingers or toes.

aphasia (a-fā′-zi-a): Loss of ability to use language normally; usually due to damage to the cortex of the dominant cerebral hemisphere that results from disease or trauma. May involve impairment of ability to express ideas by speech, writing, or signs, or of the ability to

Assessing the Apgar score.

	Score		
Factors to assess	0	1	2
Heart rate	Nil	<100	>100
Respiratory effort	Absent	Gasping or irregular	Regular respiration or strong cry
Muscle tone	Limp	Reduced	Normal active movement
Response to stimulation	None	Grimace	Cry or cough
Colour of trunk	White	Blue	Pink

comprehend spoken or written language. Many types are recognized, depending on the area of the brain that has been damaged. AMNESIC A. inability to name a familiar object; ATAXIC A. see motor A.; AUDITORY A. word deafness in which the person hears spoken words but does not understand them; BROCA'S A., A. in which the person cannot speak or write although he understands spoken and written language; EXPRESSIVE A. Broca's A.; GLOBAL A. complete loss of all functions of communication even when hearing is normal; JARGON A. repetition of unfamiliar words that the person appears to understand; MIXED A. loss of voluntary speech and ability to write, and difficulty in understanding speech; MOTOR A. inability to articulate speech or to communicate by writing, gestures, or signs, although understanding remains intact; NOMINAL A. amnesic A.; OPTIC A. inability to recognize and name a familiar object; SENSORY A. loss of power to recognize the meaning of written or spoken words or phrases, gestures, or signs; WERNICKE'S A. loss of ability to comprehend language; accompanied by inappropriate use of language. — aphasic, adj.

aphlexia (a-flek'-si-a): 1. Absent-mindedness. 2. Daydreaming.

aphonia (a-fō'-ni-a): Loss of voice from a cause other than a cerebral lesion. May be due to organic causes such as disease or injury to the larynx, or to psychosomatic causes. CONVERSION A. voice disorder caused by anxiety, stress, or depression and used by a patient to meet an uncomfortable situation; HYSTERICAL A. loss of voice associated with a functional disorder; more common in women than men.

aphrasia (a-frā'-zi-a): Inability to speak or to use connected phrases in speaking. A. PARANOICA voluntary and stubborn silence in the mentally ill.

aphrenia (a-frē'-ni-a): Dementia.

aphrodisiac (af-rō-diz'-i-ak): 1. Tending to arouse the sexual impulse. 2. A drug or agent that stimulates or arouses the sexual impulse.

aphthae (af'-thē): Small whitish or greyish ulcerous areas, usually surrounded by a ring of erythema, found on mucous membrane of the mouth, sometimes also of the gastrointestinal tract. Caused by various fungi and bacteria. Characteristics of such diseases as thrush, sprue, aphthous stomatitis (q.v.). BEDNAR'S A. whitish ulcerous spots on the posterior part of the hard palate, seen in young children; CACHECTIC A. an often fatal disease characterized by lesions under the tongue and such severe constitutional symptoms as enlargement and de-

generation of liver and spleen. — aptha, sing.; aphthous, adj.

aphthous (af'-thus): Relating to or characterized by aphthae. A. FEVER see FOOT-AND-MOUTH DISEASE; A. STOMATITIS inflammation of the mucous membrane of the mouth with the formation of small painful ulcerations.

apical (ā'-pi-kal): Relating to or located at the apex of a structure. A. BEAT or PULSE heart rate taken over the apex of the heart.

APL: Abbreviation for accreditation of prior learning, see under ACCREDITATION.

aplasia (a-plā'-zi-a): 1. Incomplete development of an organ or tissue. 2. Defective cell formation. 3. Absence of growth.

aplastic (a-plas'-tik): 1. Relating to aplasia. 2. Incapable of forming new tissue. A. ANAEMIA see under ANAEMIA; A. CRISIS a type of sickle cell crisis in which the production of red cells is diminished, causing the patient to become pale, listless and dyspnoeic due to lack of sufficient oxygen in the circulating blood.

apneusis (ap-nu' sis): Continued contraction of the muscles of inspiration for an abnormally prolonged period of time; usually occurs after surgery for removal of part of the pons.

apneustic (ap-nū'-stik): Relating to or exhibiting apneusis. A. BREATHING breathing that is characterized by long inspirations, short inefficient expirations, and long pauses between breaths; the respiratory rate may become very slow and finally fade away into apnoea; A. CENTRE located in the pons; assists in controlling inspiration.

apnoea (ap'-nē-a): Temporary cessation of breathing, as seen, e.g., in Cheyne–Stokes respiration (q.v.). — apnoeic, adj.

apo-: Combining form denoting away from or derived from.

apocarteresis (ap'-ō-kar-te-rē'-sis): Suicide by voluntary starvation.

apoclesis (ap-ō-klī'-sis): Aversion to food or eating.

apocrine (ap'-ō-krīn): Designating a type of glandular secretion that contains some of the protoplasm of the cells that elaborate it. A. GLANDS modified sweat glands, especially in the axillae, genital, mammary and perineal regions; they produce both sweat and a solution that, after puberty, is responsible for body odour.

apomorphine (ap-ō-mor'-fēn): A derivative of morphine; used in medicine as a powerful emetic (q.v.).

aponeurosis (ap'-ō-nū-rō'-sis): A broad glistening sheet of tendon-like tissue that serves to invest and attach muscles to each other, and also to the parts that they move. — apo-neuroses, pl.; aponeurotic, adj.

apophysis (a-pof'-i-sis): A projection, protuber-ance, or outgrowth, usually from a bone to which it remains attached. — apophyses, pl.; apophyseal, apophysial, adj.

apoplexy (ap'-ō-pleks-i): Term formerly used to designate stroke. A sudden haemorrhage of blood into an organ, often into the brain after the rupture of an intracranial vessel. Signs in-clude stertorous breathing, unconsciousness, incontinence of urine and faeces, and usually some degree of hemiplegia. — apoplectic, adj.

aposia (a-pō-zi-a): 1. Absence of the sensation of thirst. 2. Reluctance to take fluid by mouth.

apositia (ap-ō-sish'-i-a): Disgust for and aver-sion to food.

apothecaries' system (a-poth'-e-kā-rēz): A system of weights and measures in which weights are given in grains, scruples, drams, ounces, and pounds. Capacity is given in minims, fluidrams, fluid ounces, gills, pints, and quarts.

apothecary (a-poth'-e-kā-ri): 1. A pharmacist. 2. A pharmacy.

appendage (a-pen'-dij): A subordinate attached or suspended part of an organ or structure; usually less important in function and smaller than the main structure.

appendectomy (a-pen-dek'-to-mi): 1. Surgical removal of the vermiform appendix, see under APPENDIX. 2. Surgical removal of an append-age.

appendicectomy (a-pen-di-sek'-tō-mi): Surgical removal of the vermiform appendix, see under APPENDIX.

appendicitis (a-pen-di-sī'-tis): Inflammation of the vermiform appendix (q.v.), chronic or acute; usually sudden in onset with pain over the entire abdomen but which later localizes in the lower right side. RETROCAECAL A. pre-sents the usual signs of appendicitis, except that the anterior abdominal signs are lacking due to the location of the appendix at the back of the caecum.

appendicular (a-pen-dik'-ū-lar): 1. Relating to an appendage. 2. Relating to the upper and lower extremities of the body. A. SKELETON the arms and legs.

appendix (a-pen'-diks): An appendage; A. VER-MIFORMIS a worm-like appendage of the caecum; about the thickness of a pencil and may be from two to six inches long, ending in a blind extremity. Usually extends downwards in the right iliac region but its position is vari-able. Apparently functionless. Frequently re-ferred to as the *vermiform appendix*. — appen-dices, pl.; appendiceal, appendicular, adj.

apperception (ap-er-sep'-shun): 1. Clear per-ception of sensory stimulus, particularly when there is identification or recognition. 2. Per-ception as modified by one's own emotions, memories, and experiences. — apperceptive, adj.

appetite (ap'-e-tīt): A normal desire to satisfy a natural physical or mental need; specifically, the desire to eat.

appliance (a-plī'-ans): Any device to assist an individual in the performance of a basic function.

applicator (ap'-li-kā-tor): An instrument for ap-plying local remedies, often consisting of a slender rod of wood or metal to which a cotton pledget has been attached.

appose (a-pōz'): To juxtapose or to place next to one another.

apposition (ap-ō-zish'-un): 1. The bringing of two adjacent surfaces or edges together so they are in contact. 2. Side by side.

appraisal (a-prā'-sal): An evaluation of the per-formance of an employee. The results of the appraisal may be used in deciding an employ-ee's pay, career prospects, training, or job sat-isfaction. It is usually carried out by means of an interview with the employee's immediate manager, although in some cases self-appraisal may be used. In most organizations, appraisal consists of assessing the employee's ability (or otherwise) to meet objectives and his or her general demeanour as a member of the workforce.

apprehension (ap-rē-hen'-shun): Fear; anxiety, dread.

approximate (a-prok'-si-māt): To bring close together or into apposition, as the teeth in the human jaw. — approximation, n., approximal, adj.

apraxia (a-prak'-si-a): Loss of the ability to per-form learned or purposeful movements, to maintain posture, to make proper use of objects, or to execute acts that are normally automatic, when there is no sensory loss or paralysis; many variations are described. CON-STRUCTIONAL A., A. in which the person appar-ently understands directions but cannot copy simple drawings or use building blocks to con-struct simple patterns; IDEATIONAL A. charac-terized by extreme absent-mindedness and lack of purpose of various actions; thought to be due to an affection of the ideation area of the cortex; IDEOMOTOR A. inability to execute ideas; thought to be due to disconnection between the two motor areas of the cortex; SPEECH or VERBAL A. impairment of the ability to control the positioning and sequence of the speech muscles and their movements, resulting in incorrect formation of sounds; may be due to brain injury.

aprosexia (a-prō-sek′-si-a): Inability to fix the attention or to concentrate, arising from such causes as mental deficiency or deficient hearing or vision.

aprosody (a-prōs′-o-di): The absence, in one's speech, of the normal rhythm, pitch, and variations in stress and tone.

apsychia (a-sī′-ki-a): Temporary loss of consciousness, *e.g.*, fainting.

APT: Abbreviation for alum-precipitated diphtheria toxoid (*q.v.*).

aptitude (ap′-ti-tūd): Natural ability or acquired facility in performing certain tasks, either mental or physical. In psychology, potential rather than developed ability or facility for learning a certain kind of performance; *e.g.*, musical aptitude. A. TEST one which permits evaluation of one's potential for learning certain skills or for performing tasks which may or may not have similarity to the test tasks, or for success in a particular field or profession.

APUD cells: So called because of their capability of *a*mine *p*recursor *u*ptake *d*ecarboxylation; refers to epithelial cells found in the pancreas, bile ducts, gastrointestinal tract, and bronchi, which are capable of synthesizing and secreting polypeptide hormones such as gastrin and glucagon.

apyrexia (a-pī-rek′-si-a): Absence of fever. — apyrexial, apyretic, adj.

aqua (ak′-wa): Water. A. AMNII amniotic fluid; A. DESTILLATA distilled water; A. FORTIS a solution of nitric acid; A. MENTHAE PIPERITAE peppermint water; A. OCULI the aqueous humor of the eye; A. PURA pure water; A. ROSEA rose water.

aquapuncture (ak-wa-pungk′-tūr): The hypodermic injection of water as a placebo, for counter irritation, or for any other purpose.

aqueduct (ak′-we-dukt): A canal in an organ or structure for the passage of fluid. A. OF SYLVIUS the canal connecting the third and fourth ventricles of the brain; aqueductus cerebri. [Francois Sylvius de la Boe, French anatomist 1614–1672].

aqueous (ā′-kwē-us): Watery. A. HUMOUR the clear watery fluid that fills the anterior and posterior chambers of the eye.

arachidonic acid (ar-ak-i-don′-ik as′-id): A polyunsaturated fatty acid; essential in nutrition. Found in small amounts in human and animal liver and organ fats; also synthesized from linoleic acid.

arachnidism (a-rak′-ni-dizm): Systemic poisoning resulting from the bite of a spider.

arachnoid (a-rak′-noyd): Resembling a spider's web. A. MEMBRANE a delicate membrane enveloping the brain and spinal cord, lying between the pia mater internally and the dura mater externally; the middle serous membrane of the meninges.

arachnoidea (a-rak-noyd′ē-a): The arachnoid membrane; see under ARACHNOID.

arachnoidism (a-rak′-noyd-izm): Poisoning caused by a spider bite.

arachnoiditis (a-rak′-noy-dī′-tis): Inflammation of the arachnoid. CHRONIC ADHESIVE A. thickening and adhesion of the pia mater and arachnoid membranes; may result from trauma or meningitis and cause obliteration of the subarachnoid space; symptoms vary; OPTICO-CHIASMATIC A. chronic inflammation around the optic chiasm and optic nerves; may be due to syphilis; results in impairment of vision and optic atrophy.

Aran-Duchenne disease: A chronic, progressive wasting and atrophy of muscles beginning in the extremities, usually bilateral, and gradually progressing to other parts of the body; may be familial in origin or due to infection, avitaminosis, or toxins; also known as *pseudohypertrophic muscular dystrophy* or *progressive spinal muscular atrophy*.

arbor: In anatomy, a structure or part that is tree-like in appearance. A. ALVEOLARIS the branched terminal end of an air passage in the lung; A. VITAE (1) the tree-like outline of white substance seen on a section of the cerebellum; (2) the pattern of folds and ridges seen in the mucous membrane of the uterine cervix.

arboviruses (ar′-bō-vī′rus-es): Any of a great number of viruses transmitted by bloodsucking arthropods, including mosquitoes, sandflies, fleas, ticks; the causative agent of yellow fever, plague, dengue, Rift Valley fever, sandfly fever, viral encephalitis, Rocky Mountain spotted fever.

arc (ark): REFLEX A. in anatomy, the pathway over which a nerve impulse travels in producing a reflex action; *i.e.*, the afferent nerve that carries the impulse to a nerve centre, the nerve centre, the efferent nerve that carries the impulse to a peripheral organ or structure, and the organ or structure that produces the reflex action.

ARC: Abbreviation for AIDS-related complex, see under AIDS.

arcate (ar′-kāt): Curved. In anatomy, an arch-like structure.

arch: A curve or loop; a curved or bow-like structure. A. OF THE AORTA the curved part between the ascending and descending aorta; A. OF THE FOOT (1) transverse, along the line of the tarsometatarsal joints; (2) inner longitudinal, formed by the calcaneus, talus, navicular, three cuneiform bones, and the first three toes; (3) outer longitudinal, formed by the calcaneus and cuboid bones and the fourth and fifth toes; GLOSSOPHARYNGEAL A. the posterior of two folds of mucous membrane that connect with the soft palate at either side of the oropharynx; the palatine tonsil is located between it and the palatoglossal A.; PALATOGLOSSAL A. the more forward of the two folds of mucous membrane that connect with the soft palate at either side of the oropharynx; PALMAR A. the A. formed by the union of the radial and ulnar arteries in the palm; PLANTAR A. that formed by the anastomosis of the plantar and dorsalis pedis arteries in the foot; PUBIC A. that formed by the convergence of the rami and ischium and pubis on each side; it is immediately below the symphysis pubis; ZYGOMATIC A. that formed by the malar and temporal bones.

archetype (ar′-ke-tīp): 1. The original model or pattern on which all things of the same type are copied. 2. In Jungian psychology, an inherited mode of thought, derived from the experiences of the race, which is present in the unconsciousness of the individual.

archiform (ar′-ki-form): Refers to lesions that appear in circles, arcs, or irregular combinations of both forms.

Archimedes' principle: When a body is wholly or partly immersed in a fluid it experiences an upthrust equal to the weight of the fluid it displaces.

arcus (ar′-kus): A curved bow-like structure or ring. A. SENILUS an opaque greyish white ring around the edge of the cornea; usually bilateral; does not interfere with vision; seen in the elderly.

areflexia (a-rē-flek′-si-a): The state of being without reflexes. — areflexic, adj.

arenavirus (ar-ē′-na-vī′-rus): Any of a family of RNA viruses that are characterized by the presence of fine granules in their virions; choriomeningitis is an example of diseases caused by a member of this group of viruses. Lassa fever, seen chiefly in Africa, and Argentinian and Bolivian haemorrhagic fevers, seen chiefly in Latin America, are other examples.

areola (ar-ē′-o-la): 1. The pigmented area around a part, e.g., the nipple; or around an area, e.g., around certain lesions on the skin. 2. The part of the iris immediately surrounding the pupil. 3. A minute interstice or space in a tissue. A. MAMMAE the darkened ring that surrounds the nipple; SECONDARY A. a dark circle of pigmentation that surrounds the primary areola of the nipple in pregnancy. — areolar, adj.

argent-: A combining form meaning silver.

argentaffin (ar-jen′-ta-fin): Having an affinity for silver salts or chromium salts. A. CELLS cells that are capable of being stained by silver salts.

arginase (ar′-ji-nās): An enzyme found in the liver, kidney and spleen. It splits arginine into ornithine and urea.

arginine (ar′-ji-nin): One of the non-essential amino acids (q.v.). It is obtained from animal and vegetable proteins and must be supplied in the diet. Also prepared synthetically.

argon (ar′-gon): An inert, gaseous element present in small quantity, 0.94%, in the atmosphere.

Argonz-del Castillo syndrome: Galactorrhoea, amenorrhoea, and low production of the follicle-stimulating hormone; cause unknown; may be due to overproduction of prolactin or the presence of a pituitary tumour.

Argyll Robertson pupil: A pupil that is small and does not react when a light is shone in it but contracts when shown a near object; usually bilateral; seen chiefly in diseases of the nervous system. (Douglas Argyll Robertson, Scottish ophthalmologist, 1837–1909.)

arm: In common usage, the upper extremity from the shoulder to the wrist. In anatomy, the part of the upper extremity from the shoulder to the elbow, as distinguished from the forearm.

arm board: A piece of firm, flat padded material used to keep the arm straight, usually to keep the arm extended while the patient is receiving intravenous infusion.

armpit: The axilla.

aromatherapy (a-rō-ma-ther′-a-pi): The use of aroma to enhance a feeling of well-being. More specifically, massage of the body with a preparation of fragrant essential oils extracted from herbs, flowers, and fruits. See ESSENTIAL OIL.

aromatic (ar-ō-mat′-ik): 1. Having a fragrant, spicy, or pungent odour. 2. A medicinal substance having a fragrant, spicy aroma; often of vegetable origin and used as a stimulant. — aromatic, adj.

arousal (a-row′-sal): The state of being responsive to stimuli; wakefulness.

arrector (a-rek′-tor): Refers to the minute smooth muscles of the skin that are attached to the hair follicles. See ARRECTORES PILORUM.

arrectores pilorum (a-rek-tō′-rēz pī-lō′-rum): Any of the minute internal, plain, involuntary muscles of the skin which are attached to hair follicles and which, under the stimulus of fright or cold, contract and thus erect the hair follicles causing 'goose-flesh'. — a. pili, pl.

arrest: The sudden stoppage or cessation of a physiological function or of the course of a disease. CARDIAC A. complete cessation of mechanical action of the heart, *i.e.*, the heartbeat; EPIPHYSEAL A. arrest of the growth of long bones by premature fusion of the diaphysis and epiphysis.

arrhenoblastoma (a-rē′-nō-blas-tō-ma): A relatively rare malignant tumour of the ovary that may result in production of androgen and consequent masculinization.

arrhythmia (a-rith′-mi-a): In physiology, any deviation from the normal rhythm of the heartbeat. ATRIAL A. that originates in any part of the atrium except the sinoatrial node; SINUS A., A. that originates in the sinoatrial node; the rhythm of the heartbeat varies, being slower during expiration and more rapid during inspiration; fairly common in children in whom it appears to be normal, and in the elderly; VENTRICULAR A., A. originating in an ectopic focus in the ventricle.

arrhythmogenic (a-rith-mō-jen′-ik): Producing or capable of producing arrthythmia.

arsenic (ar′-sen-ik): A metallic element. Formerly widely used in medicine; now largely replaced by penicillin. Its toxic potential is high; poisoning is recognized by the garlic odour of the breath; industrial exposure is likely to put one at risk of bronchial carcinoma A. contained in weedkiller, rat poisons and in insecticides is a frequent cause of poisoning.

artefact (ar′-ti-fakt): 1. Any artificial product resulting from a physical or chemical agency. 2. An unnatural change in a structure or tissue. 3. In electrocardiography, any wave or mark on the electrocardiograph tracing that does not represent part of the cardiac cycle; caused by the technique used. Also called *artefact*.

arteri-, arterio-: Combining forms denoting artery or arteries.

arterial (ar-tē′-rē-al): Relating to an artery or arteries. A. ANEURYSM an aneurysm occurring in an artery; may be due to a congenital defect; also caused by hypertensive athero-

sclerosis; A. BLOOD blood that has been oxygenated in the lungs and passes to the left side of the heart from which it is distributed throughout the body; A. BLOOD GASES gases dissolved in the liquid part of the blood, specifically oxygen, carbon dioxide, and nitrogen; A. THROMBOSIS the development of a thrombus in an artery; usually a slow process causing paraesthesias with coldness of the part, paralysis of muscles, and absence of pulses below the obstruction; may break away and become an embolus.

arteriectomy (ar-tēr-i-ek′-tō-mi): Excision of a segment of an artery. Also called *arterectomy*.

arteriogram (ar-tē′r-i-ō-gram): X-ray of an artery or arteries after injection of a radiopaque medium.

arteriography (ar-tēr′-i-og′-ra-fi): 1. Roentgenography of the arteries after the intravenous administration of a radiopaque substance. 2. Sphygmography (*q.v.*). COMPUTERIZED INTRAVENOUS A. direct visualization of the arterial system following injection of a contrast medium into a peripheral vein.

arteriole (ar-tēr′-i-ōl): A small artery, particularly one joining an artery to a capillary.

arterionephrosclerosis (ar-tēr′-i-ō-nef-rō-skle-rō′-sis): Gradual narrowing of the larger branches of the renal artery with hardening of the kidney, occurring in the elderly; may be due to hypertension; may also cause hypertension. Also called *arterial nephrosclerosis* and *senile nephrosclerosis*.

arteriopathy (ar-tēr′-i-op′-a-thi): Any disease of an artery or arteries. — arteriopathic, adj.

arterioplasty (ar-tēr′-i-ō-plas′-ti): Plastic surgery applied to an artery. Term often used to denote an operation for the reconstruction of an artery after an aneurysm. — arterioplastic, adj.

arteriopuncture (ar-tēr′-i-ō-pungk′-tur): The insertion of needle into an artery, usually for the purpose of withdrawing blood.

arteriorrhaphy (ar-tēr′-i-or′-a-fi): 1. Suture of an artery. 2. A plastic procedure on an artery, such as obliteration of an aneurysm.

arteriosclerosis (ar′-tēr′-i-ō-skle-rō′-sis): Name given to a group of common disorders characterized by degenerative changes in the arteries, primarily thickening and hardening of the walls with loss of elasticity and narrowing of the lumen which leads to decreased blood supply, chiefly to the brain and extremities. Although the specific cause of A. is usually unknown, it is often associated with high blood pressure, lipidaemia, kidney disease and diabetes. The usual signs and symptoms include headache, intermittent claudication, bruits over the artery. ARTERIOLAR A., A. that affects the arterioles; A. OBLITERANS, A. in which the lumen of the artery is obliterated by thickening of the intima; usually affects the smaller vessels; CEREBRAL A., A. involving the arteries of the brain; most often seen in men and those over 50 years of age; patients are usually also hypertensive; CORONARY A., A. that involves the coronary arteries; MÖNCKEBERG'S A., A. characterized by calcification and thickening of the medial (muscular) coat in arteries, affecting especially the extremities; may lead to intermittent claudication or gangrene; also called *medial* A.; SENILE A. occurs as a natural process during ageing. See also ATHEROSCLEROSIS — arteriosclerotic, adj.

arteriosclerotic (ar-tēr′i-ō-skle-rot′ -ik): Relating to or associated with arteriosclerosis. A. DEMENTIA impairment of mental functions, due to occlusion of blood vessels in the brain, and ischaemic infarction. A. HEART DISEASE common in the elderly; characterized by arrhythmias, angina pectoris, infarction, sudden death.

arteriostenosis (ar-tēr′ -i-ō-stē-nō′ -sis): A temporary or permanent decrease in the size of the lumen of an artery or arteries.

arteriotomy (ar-tēr′ -i-ot′ -o-mi): The surgical opening of an artery.

arteriovenous (ar-tēr′ -i-ō-vē′ -nus): Relating to both an artery and a vein. A. FISTULA an abnormal direct connection between the arteriole and a venule; A. SHUNT see under SHUNT.

arterioversion (ar-tēr-i-ō-ver′ -shun): A turning back or eversion of the walls of the cut end of an artery to arrest haemorrhage.

arteritis (ar-te-rī′ -tis): A general term for inflammation of one or more of the arterial coats. May be secondary to some underlying condition, or primary. GIANT CELL A. affects particularly the temporal and cranial arteries; characterized by headache, fever, pain, and neurological disturbances including blindness; occurs mostly in the elderly. Also called *Takayasu′s A.; pulseless disease.* — arteritides, pl.

artery (ar′ -ter-i): A large vessel carrying blood from the heart to supply the various organs and tissues of the body. With the exception of the pulmonary artery, the arteries carry blood that has been oxygenated in the lungs. Arteries are tubular structures with three coats: (1) the internal endothelial lining (tunica intima) which provides a smooth surface to prevent clotting of blood; (2) the middle layer of plain muscle fibres (tunica media) which allows for distension as blood is pumped from the heart; and (3) the outer, mainly connective tissue layer (tunica adventitia), which prevents overdistension. The lumen is largest near the heart; it gradually decreases in size. — arterial, adj.

arthr-, arthro-: Combining forms denoting joint(s).

arthralgia (ar-thral′ -ji-a): Pain in a joint especially when there is no inflammation. Also called *arthrodynia.* — arthralgic, adj.

arthrectomy (ar-threk′ -to-mi): Excision of a joint.

arthritic (ar-thrit′ -ik): 1. Relating to or affected by arthritis. 2. An individual suffering from arthritis.

arthritis (ar-thrī′ -tis): Inflammation of a joint, often accompanied by pain, swelling, stiffness, and structural changes. May be caused by a variety of factors including infection, neurological disorders, metabolic disturbances, neoplasms, bursitis, acromegaly, trauma. ACUTE A. marked by pain, heat, redness, swelling; may be due to gout, rheumatism, gonorrhoeal infection, trauma; may occur after surgical procedures, particularly parathyroidectomy; ACUTE RHEUMATIC A. rheumatic fever; ACUTE SEPTIC A. may follow the same course as acute osteomyelitis; A. DEFORMANS rheumatoid A. usually begins in the fingers and is progressive, resulting in deformity; A. DEFORMANS JUVENILIS Still's disease (*q.v.*); see also PERTHES′ DISEASE; A. DEFORMANS NEOPLASTICA osteitis fibrosa (*q.v.*); A. NODOSA (A. URATICA) gout (*q.v.*). DEGENERATIVE A. osteoarthritis (*q.v.*); GONOCOCCAL A. severe pain and swelling of the joints resulting from an infection with the *Neisseria gonorrhoeae* organism; GOUTY A., A. in which uric salts are deposited in cartilage, bursae, and ligaments; INFECTIOUS or INFECTIVE A., A. in which microorganisms enter the joint from the bloodstream, or from a wound, or from osteomyelitis already present; acute or insidious onset; marked by acute or chronic inflammation of a joint or joints; organisms involved are usually staphylococcus, streptococcus, gonococcus, or meningococcus; most often affects joints already damaged by osteoarthritis, but may attack normal joints; NEUROPATHIC A. a condition that may accompany neurological disorders that interfere with deep pain impulses; the joints become disorganized from repeated minor injuries; POLYARTICULAR A., A. affecting several joints; PSORIATIC A. rheumatoid A. associated with psoriasis, affecting chiefly the distal interphalangeal joints; PYOGENIC A. caused by infection of a joint with pyogenic bacteria; characterized by severe pain on movement, swelling, and fever; may result in ankylosis; RHEUMATOID A. chronic, mild, non-bacterial A.; usually affects several joints at one time; occurs chiefly in young adults; see under RHEUMATOID; SEPTIC A. pyogenic A.; TUBERCULOUS A. caused by infection of a joint with tubercle bacilli from a focal infection elsewhere; affects mostly the intervertebral, hip, and knee joints; causes erosion of cartilage and bone with formation of cold abscess which may rupture and create a tuberculous fistula; occurs most often in children and young adults. See OSTEOARTHRITIS.

arthrocele (ar'-thrō-sēl): 1. A swollen joint. 2. A hernia of the synovial membrane into the joint capsule.

arthrochondritis (ar'-thrō-kon-drī'-tis): Inflammation of the cartilages within and around a joint. Also called osteochondritis.

arthrodesis (ar-throd-e'-sis): The fixation or stiffening of a joint by surgical means.

arthrodia (ar-thrō'-di-a): A joint permitting gliding movement. — arthrodial, adj.

arthrodysplasia (ar'-thrō-dis-plā'-zi-a): Hereditary deformity of various joints; the patella is usually affected and the nails are absent; also called nail patella syndrome.

arthroendoscopy (ar'-thrō-en-dos'-ko-pi): Visualization of the interior of a joint using an endoscope (q.v.). — arthroendoscopic, adj.; arthroendoscopically, adv.

arthrogram (ar'-thrō-gram): A roentgenogram of a joint, often after injection of a contrast material, which demonstrates the internal structure of the joint.

arthrography (ar-throg'-raf-i): X-ray of a joint, sometimes after injection of air or radiopaque material. — arthrographic, adj.; arthrographically, adv.

arthrogryposis (ar'-thrō-grī-pō'-sis): The permanent retention of a joint in a flexed position as a result of muscular contractions and adhesions about the joint capsule. A. MULTIPLEX CONGENITA a congenital syndrome characterized by contractures, ankylosis, deformities of many joints, limitation of motion, and lack of muscle development.

arthropathy (ar-throp'-a-thi): Any joint disease. NEUROGENIC and NEUROPATHIC A. chronic degenerative joint disease seen in persons with neurologic disease, particularly tabes dorsalis; characterized by loss of sensation and joint fusion; see also CHARCOT'S JOINT; OSTEOPUL-

MONARY A. clubbing of fingers and toes and enlargement of ends of long bones; usually occurs in persons with chronic cardiac or pulmonary disease; PSORIATIC A. see under ARTHRITIS; TABETIC A. neuropathic A.

arthroplasty (ar'-thrō-plas-ti): Plastic surgery on a joint; the repair, reconstruction, reformation, or replacement of a diseased or damaged joint. CUP A. plastic surgery on a ball and socket joint, now usually consists of replacement of the ends of the articulating bones with an inert prosthesis; most often used for repair of hip and knee joints.

arthropod (ar'thro-pod): Any of the many invertebrate organisms of the family Arthropoda.

arthrosclerosis (ar'-thrō-sklē-rō'-sis): Stiffening of the joint(s), particularly in the aged.

arthroscope (ar'-thro-skōp): A self-illuminating and magnifying endoscope for visualizing the interior of a joint cavity. See ENDOSCOPE. — arthroscopic, adj.

arthroscopy (ar-thros'-kō-pi): The act of visualizing the interior of a joint with an arthroscope. — arthroscopic, adj.

arthrosis (ar-thrō'-sis): 1. A joint or articulation. 2. Degeneration or disease of a joint. See AMPHIARTHROSIS, DIARTHROSIS, SYNARTHROSIS, SYNCHONDROSIS. — arthroses, pl.

arthrostomy (ar-thros'-to-mi): The surgical establishment of an opening into a joint, usually for the purpose of drainage.

arthrosynovitis (ar'-thrō-sin-ō-vī'-tis): Inflammation of the synovial membrane of a joint.

Arthu's reaction: A severe hypersensitive reaction with inflammation and oedema at the site of repeated injections of an antigen, but may also present as a generalized anaphylactic (q.v.) reaction. Also called Arthu's phenomenon.

articular (ar-tik'-ū-lar): Relating to a joint or articulation. Applied to cartilage, surface, capsule, disc, fracture, process, etc.

articulate (ar-tik'-ū-lāt): 1. To join together, as in a joint. 2. Articulated; jointed. 3. To enunciate words and sentences distinctly. 4. In dentistry, to adjust teeth so they are in correct relationship to each other.

articulated (ar-tik'-ū-lāt-ed): The state of being joined together. In anatomy, the connection of separate parts in such a way as to permit motion.

articulation (ar-tik-ū-lā'-shun): 1. The junction of two or more bones; a joint. 2. Enunciation of speech. — articular, adj.

articulus (ar-tik'-ū-lus): 1. A joint. 2. A knuckle.

artificial (ar-ti-fish'-al): 1. Imitated by art; not natural; invented, or performed by humans. 2. Relating to an apparatus designed to take over the function of a diseased organ such as the eye, kidney, larynx, or heart, or of a disordered function such as feeding or respiration. A. IN-SEMINATION, see under INSEMINATION. A. KIDNEY, see under HAEMODIALYSIS; A. PACE-MAKER see under PACEMAKER; A. RESPIRATION see under RESPIRATION.

art therapy: The use of various art forms in therapy. — drawing, painting, sculpture, music, dancing, writing.

As: Chemical symbol for arsenic.

asaphia (a-saf'-i-a): Indistinct speech or pronunciation as occurs particularly in patients with cleft palate.

asbestos (as-bes'-tos): A fibrous, incombustible, mineral substance of magnesium and calcium silicone; has many uses in industry. Small spicules may cause keratotic papules on hands of industrial workers. Inhalation of asbestos dust or spicules is a serious occupational hazard, and for the same reason, the use of asbestos as fireproofing in the construction of schools and public buildings is an important public health issue.

asbestosis (as-bes-tō'-sis): A form of chronic lung disease resulting from prolonged inhalation of fine asbestos dust and fibrils. Manifested in several forms and may be related to lung cancer, particularly diffuse malignant mesothelioma; sometimes occurs in more than one form in the same individual. Asbestos miners and workers are most often affected, but schoolchildren and others exposed to asbestos building materials are also at risk.

ascariasis (as-ka-rī'-a-sis): Infestation with worms of the genus *Ascaris* (*q.v.*). The bowel is most often affected, but in the case of round worms, infestation may spread to the stomach, liver, and lungs. Also *ascaridiasis, ascaridosis, ascariosis.*

Ascaris (as'-kar-is): A genus of nematode worms which includes the round worm (*Ascaris lumbricoides*) and the threadworm (*Enterobius vermicularis*). — ascarides, pl.

ascending: Rising; taking an upwards course. In the nervous system refers to impulses that move from the periphery up the spinal cord to the central nervous system via the afferent fibres. A. AORTA the first part of the aorta between its origin at the heart and its arch; A.

COLON the part of the large intestine between the caecum and the hepatic flexure; A. PAR-ALYSIS Guillain–Barré syndrome (*q.v.*); A. POLIOMYELITIS see under POLIOMYELITIS.

Aschoff: A's. BODIES, a group of cells and leukocytes appearing as nodules in the interstitial tissues of the heart in patients with rheumatic myocarditis; also called A.'s *nodules.* A's. NODE a flat white microscopic mass of Purkinje fibres found beneath the endocardium of the right atrium of all mammalian hearts and continuous with the muscle fibres of the atrium and the atrioventricular bundle of His. [Ludwig Aschoff, German pathologist, 1866–1942.]

ascites (as-sī'-tez'): Accumulation of excess free serous fluid in the peritoneal cavity. Causes include cirrhosis of the liver, tumour, tuberculosis peritonitis, interference in venous circulation, cardiac or renal failure. MALIG-NANT A. a condition sometimes occurring in the end stage of cancer with metastasis to the peritoneum; treatment may consist of peritoneovenous shunt. Also called *hydroperitoneum, abdominal dropsy.*

ascorbic acid (as-kor'-bik): Vitamic C (*q.v.*). Essential element of diet; not stored in the body so needs to be supplied regularly. Occurs naturally in citrus fruits, green leafy vegetables, tomatoes, potatoes, berries; also prepared synthetically. Used in treatment of anaemia and to promote healing.

ASD: Abbreviation for atrial septal defect.

ase: Suffix denoting: 1. An enzyme. 2. A destroying substance.

asepsis (ā-sep'-sis): The state of being free from living pathogenic microorganisms. MEDICAL A. reduction in the number and possibility of transfer of pathogenic organisms in a particular area or environment; involves proper handwashing, and use of clean articles such as gowns, masks, gloves, etc.; SURGICAL A. the elimination of all microorganisms from a particular field or area; involves the use of sterile gloves, gowns, masks, etc., and use of proper methods to protect the sterile area or field. — aseptic.

aseptic (ā-sep'-tik): Relating to asepsis. A. MEN-INGITIS a condition usually caused by a virus with the spinal fluid showing an increase in white blood cells but being bacteriologically sterile; A. NECROSIS necrosis that occurs without infection; A. TECHNIQUE a precautionary method used in any procedure in which there is a possibility of introducing pathogenic organisms into the patient's body; every article used must have been sterilized.

asexual (ā-seks'-ual): Without sex or without reference to sex. A. REPRODUCTION reproduction without sexual union.

Asherman's syndrome: Adhesions within the endometrial cavity; a frequent cause of amenorrhoea and infertility.

Ashman's phenomenon: In the electrocardiogram, an aberrant beat of the ventricle at the end of a short cycle that follows a long cycle; seen in atrial fibrillation and some other arrhythmias.

ASO: Abbreviation for antistreptolysin O (*q.v.*).

asocial (ā-sō'-shul): Unable or unwilling to conform to the social demands of the environment; selfish; indifferent, withdrawn from normal social intercourse.

asparaginase (as-par'-a-jināse): An enzyme present in liver and other animal tissues, yeast, and some bacteria; has some antileukaemic activity and may be used in chemotherapeutic treatment of acute lymphoblastic leukaemia.

aspartate transaminase (gloo-tam'-iks oks'-a-lō-a-se'-tik trans-am'i-nās): An enzyme that catalyses the transfer of the amino group of glutamic acid to oxloacetic acid; tests for measuring the levels of this enzyme in the blood serum give useful information in diagnosing myocardial infarction and certain liver diseases. Found in varying concentrations in heart and skeletal muscle, liver, pancreas, and kidney tissue.

aspartic acid (as-par'-tik as'-id): One of the non-essential amino acids; found in certain animals and plants, especially in molasses from sugar cane and sugar beet.

Asperger's syndrome (as'-per-jerz): A neurobiological disorder, a milder form of autistic (*q.v.*) disorder. Affected individuals are characterized by social isolation, repetitive patterns of behaviour, and non-verbal communication. Sufferers have difficulty in dealing with change, they often have obsessive routines, and may be preoccupied with a particular subject of interest.

aspergilloma (as-per-jil-ō'-ma): A tumour-like mass that forms in a bronchus or a pulmonary cavity; caused by the fungus *Aspergillus*.

Aseptic technique: areas most commonly missed following handwashing.

aspermia (ā-sperm'-i-a): Inability to form or to ejaculate semen, or absence of sperm in the semen.

aspheric (a-sfēr'-ik): In anatomy, refers to a structure that varies slightly from complete roundness; usually refers to lenses of the eyes.

asphyxia (as-fik'-si-a): Suffocation, local or systemic lack of oxygen and increase in carbon dioxide in the blood as a result of interruption in breathing. This occurs when not enough oxygen is taken in or when the tissues are unable to utilize what is taken in; *e.g.*, in drowning, electric shock, chest injury, poisoning by a gas such as carbon monoxide, or by a substance such as cyanide. A. NEONATORIUM A. occurring in the newborn; among the causes are prolapsed cord, immaturity, intracranial damage, blockage of an airway; BLUE A. or A. LIVIDA a

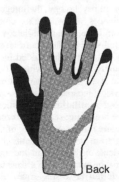 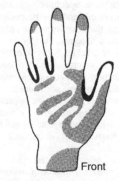

Back   Front

■ Most frequently missed
▨ Less frequently missed
□ Not missed

Aseptic technique: areas most commonly missed following handwashing.

condition of the newborn when the skin colour is deep blue but there is good muscle tone and responsiveness to stimuli; SECONDARY A., A. caused by haemorrhage or oedema of the lung, pneumothorax, narcotic drugs, tumour, aspiration of vomitus or a foreign body; WHITE A. or A. PALLIDA a serious condition of the newborn; the skin is pale and there is flaccidity and unresponsiveness to stimuli.

asphyxiant (as-fik′ -si-ant): Producing asphyxia or an agent that is capable of producing asphyxia.

asphyxiate (as-fik′ -si-āt′): To deprive the body of oxygen and thus cause asphyxiation.

asphyxiation (as-fik′ -si-ā′ -shun): Suffocation.

aspirate (as′ -pi-rāt): 1. To remove gas or fluid by suction or negative pressure. 2. Fluid drawn off from a body cavity by means of suction. 3. To pronounce a vowel or a word with release of breath, as in pronouncing the letter *h*. 4. A fluid or foreign body that is sucked into the airway, *e.g.*, vomitus.

aspiration (as-pi-rā′ -shun): 1. The act of drawing in breath; inspiration. 2. The withdrawal of fluids from a body cavity by means of a suction or siphonage apparatus. 3. The sucking of fluid into the airway. A. BIOPSY, NEEDLE BIOPSY, see under BIOPSY; A. PNEUMONIA inflammation of the lung from inhalation of a foreign body, usually fluid or food particles. NEEDLE A. removal of fluid with a long slender needle; PATHOLOGICAL A. the drawing into the respiratory tract of food particles or mucus during unconsciousness or anaesthesia; SUPRA-PUBIC A. a needle is inserted above the symphysis pubis into the bladder to collect an uncontaminated urine specimen; TRANSLAR-YNGEAL A. is accomplished by a percutaneous puncture through the cricothyroid membrane; TRANSTRACHEAL A. accomplished by puncture of the wall of the trachea below the larynx; done to obtain a sputum specimen needed for diagnosis of primary pneumonias when a normal cough does not produce enough.

aspirator (as′ -pi-rā-tor): A negative-pressure apparatus for collecting material by suction, specifically for withdrawing fluid or gas from a cavity for diagnostic or therapeutic purposes.

aspirin (as′ -pi-rin): Acetylsalicyclic acid.

asplenia (a-splē′ -ni-a): 1. Absence of the spleen. 2. Impaired splenic function.

asporogenic (as-po-rō-jen′ -ik): Not sporeproducing, or not produced by spores.

assay (as′ -sā): The use of physical, chemical, or biological methods to analyse, test, or examine a substance to determine its purity or the relative proportion of its constituents, or the potency of a drug. — assay, v.

assertiveness (a-ser′ -tiv-nes): A communication technique utilizing statements and actions forcefully and positively to compel recognition of one's position, rights, and status. A. TRAINING a technique that teaches one to make appropriate responses to others, and to express one's feelings openly and honestly in a manner that is both satisfying and respectful while taking into consideration the rights of others as well as one's own.

assessment (a-ses′ -ment): 1. A judgement made after evaluating or examining a situation or condition. 2. Any method of measuring the degree of competence of another person's ability to perform physical and/or intellectual skills. NURSING A. involves gathering information from and about a patient, identifying his or her health-care problem and needs, and stating these in terms that relate to the particular problem or condition.

assessor (a-ses′ -ser): The individual appointed to carry out the formal testing of a candidate's performance against the standards for a qualification. Assessors must be competent in the areas they are testing and be qualified and registered with an approved centre or educational establishment. An assessor would be expected to work with the candidate/student in normal work situations to observe practice.

assimilation (a-sim-i-lā′ -shun): The process whereby the already digested foodstuffs are absorbed and utilized by the tissues. The constructive phase of metabolism. Syn., *anabolism*. In psychology, the integration of new experiences into one's consciousness. — assimilable, adj., assimilate, v.

assisted suicide: The act of an individual taking his or her own life, aided by another person. Usually associated with individuals who are unable to do this themselves because of a physical incapacity.

assisted ventilation: Intermittent positive pressure breathing; see under INTERMITTENT.

associate nurse: A member of the primary nursing team who implements a care plan for a patient on behalf of the patient's primary nurse or in that nurse's absence.

association (a-sō-si-ā′ -shun): A union or close relationship of ideas, things, or persons. A. AREAS or CORTEX areas in the cortex of the brain that serve to integrate motor and sensory input; A. OF IDEAS in psychology, the connection between ideas in the cortex so that one idea calls up another that was previously linked with it; A. TEST the subject responds immediately with another word when the examiner speaks a word; the nature of the response and the time it takes for the response are used in diagnosis; FREE A. ideas arising spontaneously when censorship is removed.

assumption: 1. The act of taking to or upon oneself. 2. The act of taking a fact or statement (as a proposition, postulate, or notion) for granted. 3. The act of laying claim to, or taking possession of, something.

astasia (as-tāz-i-a): Inability to stand erect due to muscle incoordination which is not of physical origin. A. ABASIA hysterical inability to stand, walk, or perform movements while erect; there is no paralysis or organic pathology; considered a sign of neurosis or of disease of the frontal lobe.

asterixis (a-stēr-ik'-sis): Intermittent, involuntary jerking contractions of muscle groups, those of the wrist and fingers in particular; due to any of several pathological conditions; manifested by flapping tremor of the outstretched hand.

asteroid (as'-ter-oyd): Star-shaped.

asthenia (as-thē'-ni a): Thinness, weakness, debility, and lack of strength, particularly muscle strength. The term often forms part of combination words, e.g., neurasthenia. NEUROCIRCULATORY A. an anxiety neurosis associated with chest pains, faintness, palpitation, and extreme fatigue.

asthenic (as-then'-ik): Relating to asthenia. A. PERSONALITY see under PERSONALITY DISORDER.

asthenopia (as-the-nō'-pi-a): 1. Poor vision. 2. Eye-strain or speedy tiring of the eyes, usually due to weakness of the visual organ or muscles and attended by headache, sometimes pain in the eyes, dimness of vision.

asthenospermia (as'-the-nō-sper'-mi-a): Weakness or reduced motility of the spermatozoa in the semen.

asthma (as'-ma): A disease characterized by recurrent paroxysmal attacks of difficulty in breathing which may be associated with wheezing, cough, sense of suffocation or constriction in the chest; due to bronchiolar constriction and inflammation, often allergic in origin. Occurs most often in children or young adults. Often caused by inhalation or ingestion of substances to which the patient is hypersensitive. A family history of asthma is often present. ALLERGIC A. reaction to a specific allergen such as pollen, dust; attacks are of

sudden onset and brief duration; BRONCHIAL A. attacks of breathlessness associated with bronchial obstruction or spasm; characterized by expiratory wheeze; CARDIAC A. paroxysmal dyspnoea often seen in left ventricular failure; EXTRINSIC A. caused by something in the environment; allergic A.; FOOD A. caused by ingestion of certain foods; characterized by diaphoresis, diminished breath sounds, diffuse prolonged expiratory wheezes, respiratory distress; GRINDERS' A. popular name for silicosis that arises from inhalation of metallic dust; INTRINSIC A. due to some particular physiological disturbance; OCCUPATIONAL A. seen in persons who are exposed in their work environments to grain dust, wood dust, asbestos, enzymatic detergents. See STATUS ASTHMATICUS under STATUS.

asthmatic (as-mat'-ik): 1. Relating to asthma. 2. A person suffering from asthma.

astigmatism (a-stig'-ma-tizm): Defective vision caused by inequality of one or more of the refractive surfaces of the eye, usually the corneal, so that the light rays do not converge to a single point on the retina. May be congenital or acquired. Syn., *astigmia.* — astigmatic, astigmic, adj.

astragalus (as-trag'-a-lus): The ankle bone or talus upon which the tibia rests. — astragalar, adj.

astringent (as-trin'-jent): An agent that contracts organic tissue, thus lessening secretion, arresting haemorrhage, diarrhoea, etc. — astringency, n.; astringent, adj.

astro-: Combining form denoting star or star-shaped.

astroblast (as'-trō-blast): A cell from which an astrocyte develops.

astroblastoma (as'-trō-blas-tō'-ma): A relatively rare rapidly growing brain tumour arising from and composed of astroblasts.

astrocyte (as'-trō-sīt): A star-shaped cell, particularly a neuroglial or brain cell. See NEUROGLIA.

astrocytoma (as-trō-sī-tō'-ma): A relatively common slow-growing primary tumour of the brain and spinal cord tissue; formed from astrocytes; characteristically invades surrounding structures. Usually graded I to IV, depending on the degree of potential malignancy of the tumour. Grades I and II occur most often in children; grades III and IV are the most common of all gliomas, occurring most often in middle or old age. See GLIOMA.

Astrup technique: A technique for measuring the pH of arterial and capillary blood with a micro-electrode; allows for calculation of pCO_2 and bicarbonate concentration.

asyllabia (a-sil-lā′-bi-a): A form of asphasia in which one recognizes individual letters of the alphabet but cannot form them into syllables or comprehend them when combined to form syllables.

asylum (a-sī′-lum): An old term for: (1) an institution for housing aged or debilitated persons who, for some reason, cannot care for themselves; (2) a mental hospital. A. SEEKERS foreign nationals who, because of political, economic, or ethnic pressures in their home country, seek sanctuary in another host country.

asymmetry (a-sim′-e-tri): In anatomy, uneven or unequal in size, shape, or placement of paired organs or parts on opposite sides of the body. — asymmetric, asymmetrical, adj.

asymptomatic (a-simp-tō-mat′-ik): Exhibiting no symptoms.

asynchronous (a-sin′-krō-nus): **1.** A disturbance in coordination. **2.** Relates to the occurrence, at different times, of events that normally occur at the same time. A. PACEMAKER see under PACEMAKER.

asynclitism (a-sin′-kli-tizm): The condition existing when the planes of the presenting parts of the fetal head and the mother's pelvis are not parallel; the skull bones overlap as a result of labour; Caesarean section is usually indicated.

asynergy (a-sin′-er-ji): Failure of organs or parts which normally work together to do so; pertains to muscle groups especially. Also called *asynergia*. — asynergic, adj.

asystemic (a-sis-tem′-ik): Not confined to a specific system.

asystole (a-sis′to-li): Imperfect, incomplete, or no contractions of the ventricles of the heart during the systolic phase of the cardiac cycle. Cardiac standstill.

atactic (a-tak′-tik): Ataxic. See ATAXIA.

atactilia (a-tak-til′-i-a): Loss of ability to recognize impressions received through the sense of touch.

ataractic (at-a-rak′-tik): **1.** Relating to a state of mental calmness or tranquility. **2.** An agent that helps to relieve anxiety thus providing emotional equilibrium and tranquility without causing drowsiness. Syn., *tranquilizer, neuroleptic*.

ataralgesia (at-ar-al-jē′-zi-a): A method of allaying mental distress and pain associated with certain surgical procedures by sedation combined with analgesia which makes it possible for the patient to remain conscious and alert.

ataraxia (at-a-rak′-si-a): A state of tranquility or calmness in which neither consciousness

nor mental faculties are interfered with. — ataractic, adj.

atavism (at′-a-vizm): The reappearance of a hereditary trait which has skipped one or more generations. — atavic, atavistic, adj.

ataxia, ataxy (a-taks′-i-a, a-tak′-si): Defective control and coordination of voluntary muscles; due to a lesion in the central nervous system which may be hereditary or caused by infection, the presence of a tumour, trauma, or atrophy of nervous system tissues. ACUTE CEREBELLAR A. usually unilateral, with hypotonia of muscles on the affected side causing a characteristic posture; FRIEDREICH'S A. occurs in children and young adults; affects chiefly the lower extremities; marked by lateral curvature of the spine, swaying movements, and speech difficulties; HEREDITARY CEREBELLAR A. occurs chiefly in young adults; marked by speech defects and nystagmus; also called *Marie's ataxia*; LOCOMOTOR A. see TABES DORSALIS.

ataxiaphasia (a-tak′-si-a-fā′-zi-a): A speech disorder in which the person has the ability to utter words but cannot speak in sentences.

ataxia-telangiectasia (a-taks′-i-a tē-lan′-ji-ek-tā′-si-a): An inherited disorder with onset in infancy or early childhood, characterized by progressive cerebellar ataxia, abnormal eye movements, recurring lung and sinus infections. Syn., *Louis-Bar syndrome*. See ATAXIA; TELANGIECTASIA.

ataxic (a-taks′-ik): Relating to or affected by ataxia. A. GAIT an awkward gait, characterized by walking with the legs far apart, lifting the leg high and then bringing it down so that the entire foot strikes the ground at once; indicative of a spinal cord lesion; A. TREMOR intention tremor; see under TREMOR.

ataxiophemia (a-tak′-si-ō-fē′-mi-a): Lack of coordination of the muscles involved in producing speech.

atel-, atelo-: Combining forms denoting incomplete or imperfect.

atelectasis (at-e-lek′-ta-sis): **1.** Imperfect expansion of the lungs at birth. **2.** Collapse of a lung or part of it, resulting in a partial or complete airless state of a lung; due to occlusion of a bronchus or bronchiole caused by tumour, aneurysm, mucous plug, certain drugs, inspiration of a foreign object, a disease such as tuberculosis. Also, a complication following abdominal surgery. — atelactatic, adj.

atelencephalia (at-el′-en-ke-, se-fā′-li-a): A congenital anomaly consisting of imperfect or incomplete development of the brain.

atelia (a-tē′-li-a): A congenital anomaly consisting of imperfect or incomplete development of the body or any of its parts. Also called *ateliosis*.

atelocardia (at-el-ō-kar′-di-a): A congenital anomaly consisting of underdevelopment or imperfect development of the heart.

athermia (a-ther′-mi-a): 1. Lacking warmth. 2. Without fever.

atheroembolization (ath′-er-ō-em-bō-lī-zā′-shun): A condition in which an embolus consisting of atheromatous intima breaks off from an artery and is carried by the bloodstream to a smaller distal branch.

atheroma (ath-er-ō′-ma): 1. Disposition of hard yellow plaques of lipoid material in the intimal layers of the arteries; the primary lesion in atherosclerosis (*q.v.*). May be related to high level of cholesterol in the blood. Of great importance in the coronary arteries in predisposing to coronary thrombosis. 2. A sebaceous cyst, see under CYST. — atheromata, pl.; atheromatous, adj.

atherosclerosis (ath′-e-rō-sklē-rō′-sis): The most frequently occurring form of arteriosclerosis, coexisting with atheroma; a disease process that causes thickening of arterial walls and loss of their elasticity; affects chiefly the large and medium-sized arteries, especially the aorta, coronary arteries, and peripheral vessels. The WHO definition calls A. a complex chemical process involving 'a combination of changes in the intima and media, including accumulation of lipids, haemorrhage, fibrous tissue and calcium deposits.' — atherosclerotic, adj.

atherosis (ath-er-ō′-sis): Atherosclerosis (*q.v.*).

athetosis (ath-e-tō′-sis): A condition marked by slow, purposeless, involuntary, repeated, sinuous, writhing movements of the fingers and hands, toes and feet; sometimes involving most of the body. Generally due to a brain lesion. Seen chiefly in children in whom it is usually congenital; in older patients it is usually associated with cerebrovascular disease. — athetoid, athetotic, adj.

athlete's foot: See TINEA PEDIS under TINEA.

athrombia (a-throm′-bi-a): Lack of, or defect in, the clotting of blood.

athymia (a-thī′-mi-a): 1. Congenital absence of the thymus gland. 2. Without spirit or feeling. 3. Dementia.

athyroidism (a-thī′-mi-a): Lack of thyroid secretion because of absence or dysfunction of the gland. May be congenital or acquired; when congenital it produces cretinism (*q.v.*); when acquired in maturity it produces myxoedema (*q.v.*).

atlas: The first cervical vertebra which supports the head; so called because the Greek hero Atlas was supposed to carry the Earth on his shoulders. It articulates with the occipital bone above and the second cervical vertebra (axis) below. — atloid, adj.

atmosphere (at′-mos-fēr): See AIR.

atmospheric (at-mos-fēr′-ik): Relating to the atmosphere. A. PRESSURE the pressure exerted by the weight of the atmosphere (in every direction); it is the sum of the pressures of oxygen, nitrogen, carbon dioxide, and other gases in proportion to their fractional concentration in the air; this amounts to approximately 15 pounds per square inch ($101.325 \, kN/m^2$) at sea level, and increases below that level and decreases above it; is also affected by humidity, moist air being lighter than dry air; also known as *barometric pressure*.

atocia (a-tō′-si-a): Sterility in the female.

atom (at′om): In physics, the smallest particle of an element capable of existing individually and of taking part in a chemical reaction without losing its identity. In combination with one or more atoms of the same or another element, it makes up all the known kinds of matter. Has a dense central nucleus containing positively charged protons, which is surrounded by negatively charged electrons, equal in number to the nuclear protons, and which move in an orbit around the nucleus. — atomic, adj.

atomic (a-tom-ik): Relating to an atom. A. NUMBER the number of protons in the nucleus of an atom; it is the same for every atom of a given element, and each element has a characteristic number; A. THEORY a theory that the basic unit of all types of matter is the atom; RELATIVE A. MASS the average weight of the atoms of an element compared with that of the atoms of carbon; formerly *atomic weight*.

atomization (at-om-ī-zā′-shun): A mechanical process whereby a liquid is divided into a fine spray. — atomizer, n.

atomizer (at′-o-mīz-er): A device for converting a liquid into a spray and for throwing a jet of the spray.

atonia, atony (a-tō′-ni-a, at′-ō-ni): Lack of normal tone; refers particularly to muscles.

atonic (a-ton′-ic): Without tone; weak. — atonia, atony, atonicity, n.

atopens (at′-ō-pens): Soluble antigens which function as allergens; found as part of the total protein in many foods including milk, eggs, tomatoes, wheat.

atopic (a-top′-ik): **1.** Relating to atopy (*q.v.*). **2.** Out of place; displaced. A. ALLERGY atopy (*q.v.*).

atopy (at′-op-i): Allergy which is hereditary. Term covers diseases such as hay fever, asthma, urticaria, and eczema where there is a clear family history of these conditions. — atopic, adj.

atoxic (ā-toks′-ik): **1.** Not poisonous. **2.** Not caused by poison.

atoxigenic (ā-tok-si-jen′-ik): Not producing toxin(s).

ATP: Abbreviation for adenosine triphosphate. See under ADENOSINE.

atraumatic (ā-traw-mat′-ik): Not producing or inflicting damage or injury.

atremia (a-trē′-mi-a): **1.** Absence of tremor. **2.** An hysterical condition in which the patient is unable to walk although the movement of walking can be performed without discomfort while lying down.

atresia (a-trē′-zi-a): Imperforation or closure of a normal body opening or canal; often congenital. A. ANI imperforate anus; BILIARY A. closure of one or more of the bile ducts; results in jaundice, liver damage, splenomegaly; CONGENITAL CHOANAL A. failure of the sides of the nose to communicate with each other; DUODENAL A. congenital closure of the duodenum or absence of part of it; characterized by vomiting, distension of the epigastrium, may be associated with Down's syndrome (*q.v.*), FOLLICULAR A. a normal process occurring in the ovarian follicle when the ovum dies and cyclic degeneration and scar formation occur; INTESTINAL A. a congenital obstruction; may occur at any level, but usually in the ileum; OESOPHAGEAL A. congenital failure of the lumen of the oesophagus to develop fully; characterized by persistent vomiting, dyspnoea, cyanosis; often associated with a fistula between the oesphagus and the trachea; TRICUSPID A. a complex congenital anomaly in which the tricuspid valve fails to develop; the right ventricle and the pulmonary artery are underdeveloped, and there is usually an atrial and ventricular septal defect.

atrial (ā′-tri-al): Relating to an atrium. A. FIBRILLATION chaotic cardiac irregularity without any semblance of order; the fibres of the atria contract rapidly and convulsively, independently of each other and of the contraction of the ventricles; commonly associated with mitral stenosis and nodular toxic goitre, but also with other diseases of the heart; sometimes seems in general toxic conditions; A.

FLUTTER rapid regular cardiac rhythm caused by an irritable focus in the atrial muscle; usually associated with organic heart disease; speed of atrial beats may be between 200 and 350 per minute; A. GALLOP extra presystolic sounds heard in the atrium just after atrial contraction and during diastole; A. SEPTAL DEFECT continued patency of the foramen ovale (*q.v.*) after birth; A. SEPTUM the muscular wall that separates the right and left upper chambers of the heart; A. TACHYCARDIA the condition when the atrium has spasms of contracting more frequently than the ventricles; usually referred to as *paroxysmal atrial tachycardia*.

atrichia (a-trik′-i-a): Lack or loss of hair. Also called *atrichosis*. — atrichous, adj.

atrioseptal (ā-tri-ō-sep′-tal): Relating to an atrium of the heart and the septum between the two atria.

atrioseptopexy (ā′-tri-ō-sep′-tō-pek-si): A surgical procedure for correction of an interarterial septal defect.

atrioventricular (ā′-tri-ō-ven-trik′-ū-lar): Relating to the atria and ventricles of the heart. Also called *auriculoventricular*. A. BLOCK the closing or stopping of the transmission of the circulatory impulse from the atrium to the ventricle through the A-V node; A. BUNDLE see BUNDLE OF HIS; A. DISSOCIATION refers to a condition in which the atria and ventricles beat independently, each in response to its own pacemaker; A. NODE see under NODE; A. VALVES the valves between the atria and ventricles of the heart; they control the flow of blood through the heart; see under MITRAL and BICUSPID.

at risk: In healthcare, at-risk situations are those involving possible problems that often can be prevented but which will require therapeutic intervention if allowed to occur.

atrium (ā′-tri-um): A chamber. In anatomy, refers to either of the upper two chambers of the heart; the right atrium collects venous blood from the vena cava and forces it into the right ventricle; the left atrium receives arterial blood from the pulmonary veins and forces it into the left ventricle. — atria, pl.; atrial, adj.

atrophy (at′-rō-fi): Wasting, emaciation, diminution in size and function of an organ or part that had previously reached mature size. May result from a pathological condition or a physiological cause such as ageing or disuse. — atrophied, atrophic, adj. ACUTE YELLOW A. massive necrosis of the liver associated with severe infection, toxaemia of pregnancy, or ingested poisons; HEMIFACIAL A. may be unilateral or bilateral and involve bones and cartilage as well as muscle; may be congenital or caused by a pathological process; see ROMBERG'S DISEASE; MUSCULAR A. affects primarily the skeletal muscles, may result from interruption of nerve supply, disuse, or pathology of muscle tissue; PROGRESSIVE MUSCULAR A. a chronic disease marked by progressive wasting of the muscles, beginning with those of the upper extremities; SUDEK'S A. a syndrome occurring in a limb a few weeks after fracture, usually of the hand; the part becomes painful, the fingers stiff, warm, and shiny as the bones of the hand become rarefied.

atropine (at'-rō-pēn): A drug derived from the belladonna plant or produced synthetically; used in medicine as a smooth muscle relaxant, to increase the heart rate, and as a mydriatic, also used in treating parkinsonism and frequently given before anaesthesia to decrease salivary and bronchial secretions.

ATS: Abbreviation for antitetanus serum (*q.v.*).

ATT: Abbreviation for antitetanus toxoid (*q.v.*).

attachment (a-tach'-ment): 1. Something that serves to attach one thing to another. 2. In anatomy, the place or means by which one structure or body part is fixed to another. 3. Affection or fond regard. 4. In psychology, the attitude or feeling that develops in interpersonal relationships in critical periods of life when one individual is in a dependent situation to another, as occurs in bonding between an infant and its mother, an important experience in development of personality and in one's ability to adapt to the environment.

attempted suicide: An act of self-harm with the intention of ending life, which does not succeed. See also PARASUICIDE.

attendance allowance: Benefit paid by the Department of Work and Pensions (UK) available to those who need a carer. It is paid at different rates depending on whether care is needed during the day, during the night, or both.

attendant: A non-professional person who performs many different kinds of services in assisting the professional nurse to care for the sick.

attention: The focusing of one's listening, seeing, and thinking on a certain person, thing, or idea to the exclusion of any non-pertinent stimuli; A. SPAN the time interval during which one's attention is centred on a single person, object, idea, or situation.

attention deficit hyperactivity disorder (def'-i-sit, hī'-per-ak-tiv'-i-ti): A behavioural disorder usually seen in childhood. Characterized by poor attention and concentration, impulsive behaviour, and increased activity. It is more often associated with boys than girls, and is managed using behaviour modification and medication. Abbreviated ADHD.

attenuate (a-ten'-ū-āt): To modify, change, or cause to lose virulence.

attenuation (a-ten-ū-ā'-shun): A bacteriological process by which organisms are rendered less virulent by exposure to an unfavourable environment such as drying, heating, or being passed through another organism. They can then be used in the preparation of vaccines. — attenuant, attenuated, adj.; attenuate, v.

attic (at'-ik): The upper part of the cavity of the middle ear.

atticotomy (at-i-kot'-o-mi): A surgical opening of the attic of the middle ear cavity.

attitude: 1. A settled mode of thinking. 2. Posture; position of the body or limbs, particularly a position assumed in illness or abnormal mental states such as catatonia (*q.v.*).

attraction: The force or influence existing mutually between particles or masses which causes them to be drawn towards each other. Opposite of repulsion. CAPILLARY A. the force which causes a fluid to be drawn into and to rise in a tube of fine calibre.

attrition (a-trish'-un): 1. The process of eroding or abrading the skin or other body surface. 2. The normal wearing away of tissue or a structure by use.

at. wt.: Abbreviation for atomic weight, see RELATIVE ATOMIC MASS, under ATOMIC.

atypical (ā-tip'-i-k'l): Not typical; unusual, irregular; not conforming to type, *e.g.*, A. pneumonia. A. MEDICATION unconventional medication or treatment for the condition or illness.

Au, au: Chemical symbol for aurum [L.], meaning gold.

audio-, audito-: Combining forms denoting (1) sound; (2) hearing.

audioanalgesia (aw'-di-ō-an-al-jē'-zi-a): The abolition or control of pain by listening to specially recorded music.

audiofrequency (aw'-di-ō-frē'-kwen-si): Any frequency within the normal range of human hearing.

audiogenic (aw-di-ō-jen'ik): Caused or produced by sound.

audiogram (aw-di-ō-gram): A graph showing the variations in acuteness of hearing; utilizes a standardized test that determines the individual's hearing threshold at various frequencies and using an audiometer.

audiologist (aw-di-ol'ō-jist): One skilled in audiology and who specializes in treating persons with impaired hearing.

audiology (aw-di-ol'-o-ji): The science dealing with the evaluation and treatment of hearing impairment. — audiological, adj., audiologically, adv.

audiometer (aw-di-om'-i-ter): A delicate electrical instrument for measuring the sharpness and range of hearing for pure tones, speech, and bone and air conduction.

audiometry (aw-di-om'-i-tri): The testing and measuring of hearing acuity by use of an audiometer.

audiovisual (aw'-di-ō-viz'-ū-al): Relating to both sight and sound; usually refers to communication or teaching techniques.

audit (aw'-dit): 1. A formal examination of an organization's or individual's accounts or financial situation. 2. A methodical examination and review. See NURSING AUDIT. 3. The final report of such a formal examination.

Audit Commission: An independent body responsible for ensuring that public money is used economically, efficiently, and effectively.

audit trail: A record of a sequence of events (for example, actions performed by a computer) from which a history may be constructed.

auditory (aw'-di-to-ri): Relating to the sense or the organs of hearing. A. AREA that portion of the temporal lobe cortex which interprets sound; A. CANAL or MEATUS the canal between the pinna and the ear drum; about 3 cm long, the outer part is made up of cartilage; the inner one-third has a bony wall and contains wax-secreting glands; A. FATIGUE a temporary shift of one's sensitivity threshold for a certain sound following exposure to the sound for a period of time; A. NERVES the eighth pair of cranial nerves; they relay information from the ear to the brain; A. OSSICLES three tiny bones (malleus, incus, and stapes) stretching from the tympanum across the cavity of the middle ear to a membrane that separates the middle from the inner ear; A. TUBE the canal that connects the pharynx with the tympanic cavity; it is partly bony, partly cartilaginous, and lined with mucous membrane. The Eustachian tube (*q.v.*).

aur-, auri-: Combining forms denoting the ear.

aura (aw'-ra): A premonition; a peculiar sensation or warning, recognized by the patient, of an impending convulsion or seizure such as occurs in migraine and epilepsy. May be auditory, optic, kinaesthetic, epigastric, etc. in nature.

aural (aw'-ral): 1. Relating to the ear. 2. Relating to an aura.

auricle (aw-ri-k'l): 1. The pinna or flap of the external ear. 2. An ear-shaped appendage to either cardiac atrium. 3. Formerly used to refer to the cardiac atrium. — auricular, adj.

auricular (aw-rik'-ū-lar): 1. Relating to the ear. 2. Relating to an auricle. A. FIBRILLATION see ATRIAL FIBRILLATION, ATRIAL FLUTTER, under ATRIAL.

auriculoventricular: See ATRIOVENTRICULAR.

auriculoventriculostomy (aw-rik'-ū-lō-ven-trik'-ū-los'-to-mi): A surgical procedure utilized in the treatment of certain forms of hydrocephalus; consists of a polyethylene tube inserted into the lateral ventricle of the brain through a burr hole in the skull and which leads to the right atrium or the superior vena cava; the purpose is to drain excessive cerebrospinal fluid from the ventricle into the general circulation.

auripuncture (aw-ri-pungk'-tur): Puncture of the tympanic (*q.v.*) membrane.

auris (aw'-ris): The ear.

auriscope (aw'-ris-kōp): An instrument for examining the ear; a type of otoscope.

auscultation (aws-kul-tā'-shun): A method of examining internal organs by listening to the sounds they produce; a diagnostic procedure used particularly in examining the heart, lung, pleura, and intestine, and the fetal circulation. It may be (1) immediate, by placing the ear directly against the body; or (2) mediate, by use of the stethoscope. — auscultatory, adj.; auscult, auscultate, v.

auscultatory (aws-kul'-ta-tō-ri): Of, or relating to, ascultation. A. GAP a zone of silence sometimes noted when measuring blood pressure by the auscultatory method; occurs chiefly in patients with hypertension or in cases of aortic stenosis.

Australia antigen: Hepatitis B surface antigen; found in the serum of individuals with acute or chronic serum hepatitis, or in carriers of that disease; is easily transmitted by blood, needles, or other instruments; blood for transfusion is screened for this antigen.

autacoid (aw'-ta-koyd): See AUTOCOID.

autemesia (aw-te-mē'-zi-a): Idiopathic or self-induced vomiting.

authenticity (aw-then-ti'-si-ti): 1. The quality of being genuine and valid. 2. In psychological functioning and personality, the quality of conscious feelings, perceptions, and thoughts that one expresses and communicates honestly and genuinely.

autism (aw'tizm): **1.** Usually appears during first three years of life; marked by poor development of language and social skills and abnormal relationships to persons and the environment. **2.** A state of morbid self-absorption in which one is dominated by self-centred thoughts that are wishful, symbolic, delusional, hallucinatory, or irrational; and by daydreaming, fantasizing, and detachment from reality, with excessive concentration on oneself.

autistic (aw-tis'-tik): Morbidly self-centred thinking, governed by the wishes of the individual; wishful thinking (fantasy), in contrast to reality thinking. Occurs in schizophrenia (*q.v.*). A. BEHAVIOUR self-absorption, refusal to use language or to speak, isolation of self from others, repetitive actions; inability to relate realistically with people in one's environment; A. LANGUAGE sounds invented by a person to express meanings but which are unintelligible to others.

auto-: Combining form denoting relationship to self.

autoagglutination (aw'-tō-a-gloo-ti-nā'-shun): Agglutination of an individual's red blood corpuscles by a factor in his own serum, in the absence of a specific antibody.

autoagglutinin (aw'-tō-a-gloo'-ti-nin): A factor in the blood serum that causes a clumping together of an individual's own cells.

autoanalysis (aw'-tō-a-nal'-i-sis): A psychotherapeutic method wherein the individual analyses his own mental disorder.

autoantibody (aw'-tō-an'-ti-bod-i): An antibody formed in an individual and which reacts against other antigenic substances in the same individual.

autoantigen (aw'-tō-an'-ti-jen): A normal tissue constituent within the body that is capable of stimulating the production of antibody in the tissues of the individual in which it occurs.

autoantitoxin (aw'-tō-an-tī-tok'-sin): An antitoxin produced by the body itself.

autoclave (aw'-tō-klāv): **1.** An apparatus for sterilizing articles by steam under high pressure. **2.** To sterilize articles in an autoclave.

autocoid (aw'-tō-koyd): In biochemistry, any organic substance such as a hormone that is secreted into the bloodstream directly and carried by the blood or lymph to the part of the body where its primary action takes place.

autodigestion (aw'-tō-di-jest'-shun): Self-digestion of body tissues by their own secretions. *Autolysis* (*q.v.*).

autoechopraxia (aw'-tō-ek-ō-park'-shi-a): The continual repetition of some action the individual has previously performed.

autoepilation (aw'tō-ep-i-lā'-shun): The spontaneous loss of hair.

autoeroticism (aw'tō-e rot'-i-sizm): Sensual arousal and self-gratification of sexual desire obtained by manipulation of or looking at or touching one's genitalia or other erotic zones, masturbation, or fantasy. Often a characteristic of the period of early emotional development of the child but not limited to this age group.

autogenesis (aw'-tō-jen'-es-is): Originating within the organism; spontaneous generation.

autogenous (aw-toj'-e-nus): Self-generated; endogenous; originating within the body and not acquired from any outside source. Applied to bone graft, skin graft, etc. Opp. to heterogenous (*q.v.*). A. VACCINE one prepared from the bacteria from the patient's own infection. Also called *autogenetic, autogenic.*

autograft (aw'-tō-graft): A graft in which the tissue is taken from another part of the body which is to receive it.

autohaemolysis (aw-tō-hē-mol'-i-sis): Destruction of an individual's red blood cells by a factor in the person's own serum.

autohaemotherapy (aw'-tō-hē-mō-ther'-a-pi): The treatment of a person with his or her own blood which is withdrawn from a vein and reinjected intramuscularly; may be used in cases of recurring urticaria (*q.v.*).

autohypnosis (aw-tō-hip-nō'-sis): A state of hypnosis that is self-induced.

autoimmune (aw-tō-im-mūm): Refers to a disease condition in which the body produces an immunological reaction to its own cells or tissues; includes such diseases as rheumatoid arthritis, myasthenia gravis, lupus erythematosus, haemolytic anaemia.

autoimmunity (aw'-tō-im-mū'-ni-ti): The condition of being allergic to one's own tissues.

autoimmunization (aw'-tō-im-mū-nī-zā'-shun): Immunization obtained by having an attack of a disease or by processes occurring naturally in the body.

autoinfection (aw-tō-in-fek'-shun): Infection arising from an organism already present within the body or transferred from one part of the body to another by fingers, etc.; self-infection.

autokinesis (aw-tō-kī-nē'-sis): Voluntary movement. — autokinetic, adj.

autologous (aw-tol′-ō-gus): **1.** Belonging to or part of the same organism; related to self. **2.** Derived from the subject itself.

autolysin (aw-tol′-i-sin): A lysin that originates within an organism and is capable of destroying its own tissues and parts.

autolysis (aw-tol′-i-sis): The destruction of tissues or cells by the action of their own enzymes. — autolytic, adj.

automatic (aw-tō-mat′-ik): That which is performed independently of the will; self-regulating; involuntary; spontaneous. A. BLADDER, see AUTONOMOUS BLADDER under BLADDER.

automaticity (aw-tom-a-tis′-i-ti): The state or condition of being automatic.

automatism (aw-tom′-a-tizm): The involuntary performance of actions that are normally voluntary, without purpose or intention on the part of the individual, and often without the knowledge that they are taking place. May occur in somnambulism (q.v.), hysteria (q.v.), and post-epileptic (q.v.) states.

automaton (aw-tom′-a-ton): **1.** An apparatus that automatically follows programmed instructions; a robot. **2.** Anything that moves or acts of itself. **3.** A person who acts or reacts in a predictable or mechanical manner.

automysophobia (aw′-tō-mis-ō-fō′-bi-a): A manic dread of personal uncleanliness.

autonomic (aw-to-nom′-ik): Independent; involuntary; automatic. A. NERVOUS SYSTEM see under NERVOUS SYSTEM; A. SPEECH see under SPEECH.

autonomous (aw-ton′-o-mus): Self-directing freedom and especially moral independence.

autonomy (aw-ton′-o-mi): The quality or state of being self-governing; especially the right of self-government.

autopathy (aw-top′-a-thi): A disease that has no observable external causation; an idiopathic (q.v.) condition.

autopepsia (aw-tō-pep′-si-a): The destruction of the stomach wall by the action of the gastric secretion; autodigestion.

autophagia (aw-tō-fā′-ji-a): The biting of one's own flesh; occurs sometimes in persons with dementia.

autophilia (aw-tō-fil′-i-a): Narcissism; self-love to a pathological degree.

autoplasty (aw′ tō-plas-ti): Replacement or repair of injured or diseased tissues by a graft of healthy tissues from another area of the same body. — autoplastic, adj.; autoplast, n.

autopsy (aw′-top-si): The examination of the organs of a dead body for the purpose of determining the cause of death or of studying the

pathological conditions of the organs. Also called *postmortem examination; necropsy.*

autoregulation (aw′-tō-reg-ū-lā′-shun): **1.** The action of inherent factors and inhibitory feedback systems to largely or completely counteract internal or external changes and stresses; said especially of the circulatory physiology. **2.** The tendency of blood flow to an organ or part to remain at or return to the same level regardless of changes in the artery conveying blood to it.

autosensitization (aw′-tō-sen-si-ti-za′-shun): Sensitization to one's own serum or body tissues. — autosensitize, v.

autoserous (aw-tō-sē′-rus): Relating to autoserum (q.v.). A. TREATMENT treatment by inoculation of an individual with serum obtained from his or her own blood.

autoserum (aw-tō-sē′-rum): Serum to be administered to the individual from whose blood it was derived.

autosomal (aw-tō-sō′-mal): Relating to an autosome (q.v.). A. DOMINANT INHERITANCE (or disease) an inherited disease which may affect only one of the parents of the person having it; affects either sex; less serious than recessive inherited disease; A. RECESSIVE INHERITANCE affected individuals tend to be in the same-generation; normal parents are the carriers; rare but more severe than dominantly inherited conditions.

autosome (aw-tō-sōm): One of the ordinary chromosomes, i.e., any chromosome other than the X or Y; autosomes are equally distributed among the germ cells — autosomal, adj.

autosplenectomy (aw′-tō-splē-nek′-tō-mi): A pathological condition in which the tissues of the spleen shrink and are replaced by fibrous tissue; occurs in sickle cell anaemia.

autosuggestion (aw′tō-sug-jest′-yun): **1.** Self-suggestion; uncritical acceptance of ideas arising in the individual's own mind. Occurs in hysteria. **2.** The technique of trying to improve health or change behaviour by constant repetition of certain phrases; e.g., 'Every day in every way I am getting better and better.'

autotherapy (aw-tō-ther′-a-pi): **1.** Treatment by administration of filtrates of the patient's own secretions. **2.** Cure of disease without medical supervision; self-cure.

autotopagnosia (aw′-tō-tōp-ag-nō′si-a): Loss of the ability to identify various parts of one's own body; a type of agnosia (q.v.).

autotransfusion (aw′-tō-trans-fū′-shun): **1.** The infusion into the patient of actual blood lost by haemorrhage. **2.** Binding the lower extremities and, sometimes, the lower abdomen, to force blood from them to the vital organs.

autotransplantation (aw′-tō-trans-plan-tā′-shun): The surgical procedure of transplanting a graft of tissue from one part of the body to another site on the same person.

aux-, auxe-, auxo-: Combining forms denoting (1) growth, enlargement; (2) accelerating, stimulating.

auxesis (awk-sē-sis): An increase in size or bulk due to growth or expansion of the cells rather than an increase in their numbers.

A-V: Abbreviation for atrioventricular (*q.v.*) or atriovenous. A-V BLOCK a type of heart block in which the impulse between the atria and the ventricles of the heart is either slowed down or blocked; A-V DISSOCIATION independent action of atria and ventricles; a form of heart block.

avascular (ā-vas′-kū-lar): Bloodless; not vascular; *i.e.*, without blood vessels. May be normal, as in cartilaginous tissue, or pathological. A. NECROSIS death of tissue from deficient blood supply following injury or disease. It is often a precursor of osteoarthritis.

avascularization (ā-vas′-kū-lar-ī-zā′-shun): The act of expelling blood from a part as by application of elastic bandage, by posture, or by ligation.

aversion (a-ver′-zhun): A method of treatment by deconditioning. Effective in some forms of addiction or other abnormal behaviour. A. THERAPY involves the use of punishment or unpleasant stimuli to weaken and ultimately eliminate the particular behaviour or habit that is unacceptable; also called *negative reinforcement* and *aversive conditioning*.

Avery's syndrome: Transient tachypnoea of the newborn, with grunting; sometimes seen in full-term infants; usually resolves within two days; may represent a mild form of respiratory distress syndrome.

avian (ā′-vi-an): Relating to birds. A. TUBERCLE BACILLUS resembles other types of tubercle bacilli but attacks primarily birds, including chickens and ducks; occasionally causes disease in man.

avidin (av′-i-din): An antivitamin; a specific protein found in raw egg white. It interferes with the absorption of biotin (*q.v.*), thus producing biotin deficiency.

avirulent (a-vir′-ū-lent): Without virulence (*q.v.*).

avitaminosis (ā-vī′-ta-min-ō-sis): Any disease resulting from a deficiency of one or more essential vitamins in the diet; includes such disease conditions as scurvy, beri beri, and rickets.

avulsion (a-vul′-shun): A forcible wrenching or tearing away of a body part or structure; surgical repair is often possible and, if the avulsion is complete, certain body parts may be successfully rejoined.

awarding body: An organization that is accredited by the Qualifications and Curriculum Authority (*q.v.*) to give qualifications. This term is used primarily within the NVQ/SVQ (*q.v.*) system, although it also applies in other educational sectors such as further and higher education. A.B.s register organizations as approved centres, award NVQs/SVQs, and maintain external quality control.

awareness (a-wair′-nes): Consciousness. Being awake, conscious, and cognizant of one's self and one's surroundings.

axial (ak′-si-al): In anatomy, pertaining to the axis of a body part or structure. A TOMOGRAPHY a type of radiology in which a series of cross-sectional images along an axis are combined to make a three-dimensional scan. See COMPUTERIZED AXIAL TOMOGRAPHY.

axilla (ak-sil′-a): The armpit — axillae, pl.; axillary, adj.

axillary (aks′-i-lar-i): Relating to the axilla. Term is applied to nerves, blood vessels, lymphatics, nodes.

axion (ak′-sē-on): The brain and spinal cord.

axis (ak′-sis): 1. The second cervical vertebra. 2. An imaginary line passing through the centre of a structure, *e.g.*, the median line of the body. A. CYLINDER the axon of a cell. — axes, pl.; axial, adj.

axodendritic (ak′-sō-den-drit′-ik): Relating to an axon and to dendrites. A. SYNAPSE a synapse between two neurons wherein the fibres of the axon are in direct contact with the dendrites of another neuron.

axon (ak′-son): That process of a nerve cell conveying impulses away from the cell body and towards the next nerve; the essential part of the nerve fibre and a direct prolongation of the nerve cell. Also called *axis-cylinder, axis-cylinder process, neuraxon, neurite*. — axonal, adj.

axoneuron (ak-sō-nū′-ron): A nerve cell of the central nervous system.

axonotmesis (ak-son-ot-mē′-sis): Peripheral degeneration as a result of damage to the axon of a nerve. The internal architecture is preserved and recovery depends upon regeneration of the axon, and may take many months (about 2.5 cm a month is the usual period of regeneration). Such a lesion may result from pinching, crushing, or prolonged pressure on a nerve without severing it.

axoplasm (aks'-ō-plazm): The cytoplasm of an axon. — axoplasmic, adj.

azo-: Prefix indicating the presence of nitrogen in a substance.

azoospermia (a-zō-ō-sperm'-i-a): Sterility in the male through absence of motile spermatozoa in the semen.

azotaemia (az-ō-tē'-mi-a): The presence of pathological amounts of nitrogenous products, principally urea, in the blood. Seen in such conditions as circulatory or renal failure, gastrointestinal haemorrhage, dehydration. Often used synonymously with uraemia. — azotaemic, adj.

azotometer (az-ō-tom'-e-ter): An instrument used to measure the amount of nitrogen compounds in a solution, particularly the amount of urea in urine.

azygos, azygous (az'-i-gus): Occurring singly; unpaired, as the A. vein.

azymia (a-zim'-i-a): Absence of an enzyme or enzymes.

B

B: Chemical symbol for boron.z

Ba: The chemical symbol for barium (*q.v.*).

BA: Abbreviation for Bachelor of Arts.

Babcock sentence test: A test for dementia in which the patient is asked to repeat a complicated sentence.

babesiasis (ba-bē-sī´-a-sis): A malaria-like disease caused by the protozoan parasite *Babesia* which is widely distributed in nature, and is transmitted to man by the bite of an infected wood tick; rodents and other animals harbour the parasite in their red blood cells. Symptoms include nausea and vomiting, fever, sweating, chills, myalgia, arthralgia, haemolytic anaemia. There is no known cure; the disease is apparently self-limited. Also called *babesiosis*.

Babinski (ba-bin´ ski): B.'S REFLEX see under REFLEX. B.'S SIGN a diminishment or loss of the Achilles tendon reflex, as occurs in sciatica. [Joseph François Felix Babinski, French neurologist, 1857–1932.]

baby: An infant from birth to about two years of age or until the child is able to walk and talk. B. BATTERING term sometimes used to describe child abuse when the victim is under two years of age; includes such abuses as throwing, banging, or violently shaking the infant, which may cause bleeding in and around the brain and lead to mental handicap; B. BLUES colloquial term for transient mild depression occurring after childbirth.

baccalaureate degree nurse (bak-a-law´ -rē-at): A nurse who holds a bachelor's degree in nursing from an accredited college or university in the USA.

baccate (bak´ -āt): Resembling a berry in form or structure.

bacillary (bas´ -i-lar-i): 1. Relating to bacilli. 2. Having a rod-like structure. B. DYSENTERY a severe form of enteritis marked by abdominal pain, fever, severe diarrhoea, sometimes bloody stools. Caused by a bacteria of the *Shigella* genus. Especially prevalent in tropical climates. Also called *shigellosis*.

bacilliform (ba-sil´ -i-form): Shaped like a bacillus; rod-shaped.

Bacillus (ba-sil´ -us): A term now restricted to a genus of rod-shaped microorganisms of the family *Bacillaceae*, consisting of aerobic, Gram-positive, spore-producing organisms; the majority are saprophytic and non-pathogenic; their spores are commonly only found in soil and dust. B. ANTHRACIS the cause of anthrax in humans and animals; B. CEREUS an aerobic bacillus, often causes food poisoning; B. SUBTILIS a common organism in soil and water; occurs frequently as a laboratory contaminant and occasionally causes disease in humans.

bacillus (ba-sil´ -us): 1. An organism of the class Schizomycetes. 2. A general term loosely employed to designate any rod-shaped microorganism. — bacilli, pl,; bacillary, adj.

bacillus Calmette–Guérin (kal´ -met-gair´ -an): A vaccine prepared from the bovine tubercle bacilli; intended for use in producing active immunity to tuberculosis in children and young adults. Originally given by mouth, now subcutaneously. Abbreviated BCG.

back: In anatomy, refers to the posterior part of the body from the neck to the pelvis. FLAT B. a B. that appears flat because of a reduction in the normal thoracic and lumbar curves; HOLLOW B. lordosis (*q.v.*) that extends to part or all of the lumbar spine; HUMP B. kyphosis (*q.v.*), also called *hunchback*; POKER B. rigidity of the spine caused by ankylosis (*q.v.*) commonly associated with rheumatoid arthritis, also called *poker spine* and *bamboo spine*; SWAY B. lordosis (*q.v.*) that extends to all or part of the spine.

backache (bak´ -āk): Any pain in the back, especially the lower back.

backbone: The spine or vertebral column.

backflow: The flowing of a current or substance in a direction opposite to that it usually takes, *e.g.*, regurgitation.

back rest: A device used to support a bed patient in a semi-reclining or sitting position.

BACP: Abbreviation for British Association of Counselling and Psychotherapy (*q.v.*).

bacteraemia (bak-ter-ē´ -mi-a): The presence of bacteria in the bloodstream. May be primary,

bacteraemia   68   **balance**

or secondary when it is associated with the use of an intravascular device or when it develops as a nosocomial (*q.v.*) infection in a hospitalized patient. — bacteraemic, adj.

bacteri-, bacterio-: Combining forms denoting bacteria.

bacteria (bak-tēr-i-a): One-celled, microorganisms, visible only under the microscope. A great many varieties are found in the human environment; the majority are not disease producing. B. are recognized according to shape, growth needs, staining reactions, and loci of infection in the body. Structurally, there is a protoplast containing cytoplasmic and nuclear material (not seen by ordinary methods of microscopy) within a limiting cytoplasmic membrane, and a supporting cell wall. Other structures such as flagella, fimbriae and capsules may also be present. Individual cells may be spherical (cocci), straight, or curved rods (bacilli), or spiral (spirilla); they may form chains or masses, and some show branching with mycelium (*q.v.*) formation. They may produce various pigments, including chlorophyll. Reproduction is chiefly by simple binary (*q.v.*) fission. Some live on dead organic matter and so are saprophytes; others live in living tissue and so are parasites. Each variety has its own requirements as to nourishment, light, moisture, pH, etc. Some are pathogenic to humans and other animals; some cause plant diseases. — bacterium, sing.; bacterial, adj.

bacterial (bak-tēr-i-al): Relating to or caused by bacteria. B. ENDOCARDITIS see ENDOCARDITIS; B. RESISTANCE the resistance that some organisms, particularly pathogenic organisms, develop for a drug to which they were originally susceptible.

bactericide (bak-tēr-i-sīd): Any agent that destroys bacteria. — bactericidal, adj.; bactericidally, adv.

bacterid (bac'-ter-id): A skin condition characterized by a recurring or persistent eruption of lesions, particularly on the palms and soles; thought to be due to sensitivity to the bacterial products from an infection elsewhere in the body.

bacteriofluorescein (bak-tē'-ri-ō-floo-ō-res'-ē-in): A fluorescent material produced by certain bacteria.

bacteriology (bak-tēr-i-ol'-ō-ji): The science and study of bacteria. — bacteriologically, adv.

bacteriolysin (bak-tēr-i-ol'-i-sin): A specific antibody (*q.v.*) produced in the blood after an infection with an organism and which is

capable of destroying the invading organism by lysis. — bacteriolytic, adj.

bacteriolysis (bak-tēr-i-ol'-sis): The disintegration and dissolution of bacteria. — bacteriolytic, adj.

bacteriophage (bak-tēr-i-ō-fāj): A filterable virus that destroys bacteria; usually each of several varieties acts against only one specific type of bacteria.

bacteriostat (bak-tēr'-i-ō-stat): An agent that prevents or inhibits the growth of bacteria. — bacteriostatic, adj.

bacterium (bak-tēr'-i-um): Singular of bacteria (*q.v.*).

bacteriuria (bak-tēr-i-ū'-ri-a): The presence of bacteria in the urine. Also called *bacteruria*. — bacteriuric, adj.

Bacteroides (bak'-tēr-oy'-dēz): A genus of non-spore-forming anaerobic bacteria normally present in the mouth and large intestine. *B. fragilis* the most common and most virulent B. found in septicaemia, appendicitis, and metastatic abscesses of the lung, liver, and pelvis; also called *Bacillus fragilis*; *B. melaninogenesis*, found in abdominal wounds, kidney infections, puerperal sepsis.

bactometer (bak-tom'-e-ter): A laboratory device for detecting the density and growth of bacteria in urine specimens.

bag: A pouch or sac. COLOSTOMY B. one worn over the stoma after a colostomy. B. OF WATERS the membranous sac that contains the amniotic fluid and the fetus. In obstetrics, a silk or rubber B. that is inserted into the uterine cavity and then inflated to induce labour or dilate the cervix; common types are Barnes and Voorhees. See also AMBU BAG and POLITZER'S BAG.

bag of waters: The amnion and amniotic fluid.

bagging: A relatively easy method of providing positive pressure during suctioning and intermittent sighing; apparatus consists of a Huested valve and an attached bag which is squeezed to deliver air to the lungs.

BAI: Abbreviation for Beck anxiety inventory (*q.v.*).

Baker's cyst: A cyst in the popliteal space; formed of synovial fluid that has escaped from the bursa; usually secondary to some other disease; symptoms include pain, swelling, limitation of movement.

baking soda: Sodium bicarbonate; see under SODIUM.

balance (bal'-ans): In physiology, the harmonious relation between the parts and organs of the body and their functions, or between substances in the body. ACID–BASE B. a normal equilibrium or ratio between the acid and base elements of the blood and body fluids, expressed as pH; ELECTROLYTE B. is associated with water B. since the electrolytes are the ions present in body water; term refers to the concentration of ions of electrolytes in the interstitial fluid and the blood plasma, which are normally essentially the same; FLUID B. term commonly used to express the concept of both water balance and electrolyte balance in the body; NITROGEN B. balance between the intake and output of nitrogen. NEGATIVE NITROGEN B. occurs when more nitrogen is lost than is taken into the body; may happen in such conditions as burns, starvation, fevers, malnutrition. POSITIVE NITROGEN B. occurs when more nitrogen is taken into than is lost from the body; happens in pregnancy, repair of tissues, and during growth of infants and children; WATER B. (1) the condition in which water intake equals water excreted; or (2) the proper distribution of water between the intercellular and extracellular compartments of the body.

balani-, balano-: Combining forms denoting relationship to the glans penis or glans clitoridis. See GLANS.

balanic (bal-an'-ik): Relating to the glans penis or glans clitoridis.

balanitis (bal-a-nī'-tis): Inflammation of the glans penis, often associated with phimosis. B. GANGRENOSA destruction of part or all of the male external genitalia by infection, thought to be due to a spirochete; B. XEROTICA OBLITERANS inflammation of the glans penis with scarring and white induration; the meatus may be stenosed; often occurs in men with diabetes. — balanitic, adj.

balanoplasty (bal'a-nō-plas-ti): Plastic surgery of the glans penis.

balantidiasis (bal'-an-ti-dī'-a-sis): A disease caused by infection by the *Balantidium coli* organism; symptoms vary from those of mild colitis to acute dysentery and include nausea, vomiting, diarrhoea, headache, fever, weakness, abdominal pain, weight loss and, sometimes, ulceration of the colon.

balanus (bal'-an-us): The glans of the penis or clitoris.

baldness: Partial or complete lack of hair on the scalp. See ALOPECIA.

Ballance's sign: The presence of a dull sound heard on percussing the right flank when the patient lies on the left side; said to indicate a ruptured spleen.

ball-and-socket joint: A joint in which the round head of one bone fits into a cup-like cavity of another bone, permitting full freedom of movement or circumduction (*q.v.*), *e.g.*, the shoulder or hip joint.

ballismus (ba-liz'-mus): The occurrence of violent, quick, jerking, or twisting movements, caused by contraction of arm or leg muscles and seen in Sydenham's chorea. May be bilateral; when it occurs in only one side it is called hemiballism. Also called *ballism*.

ballistocardiograph (ba-lis'-tō-kar'-di-ō-graf): An apparatus for estimating the volume of cardiac output by recording the movement of the body resulting from the contraction of the ventricles and ejection of blood into the aorta. The record of this movement is called a ballistocardiogram.

balloon or balloon-tip catheter: See FOLEY CATHETER under CATHETER.

ballooning (ba-loon'-ing): Distending a body cavity by the introduction of air or other agent to facilitate its examination or for therapeutic purposes.

ballottement (ba-lot'-ment): 1. Palpation to detect a floating enlarged organ when abdominal ascites is present. 2. Testing for a floating object, especially used to diagnose pregnancy after the sixteenth week and before the twenty-eighth week. A finger is inserted into the vagina and the uterus is pushed forward; if a fetus is present it will fall back, bouncing in its bath of fluid. RENAL B. palpation of the kidney by pushing it suddenly and firmly forward from the back with one hand while the other hand is pressed firmly into the abdominal wall. — ballottable, adj.

ball squeezing: An exercise for strengthening hand and arm muscles; a rubber ball or wad of crumpled newspaper is held in the hand and squeezed at a regular rate several times a day.

balm (bahm): A healing or soothing medication, usually an ointment. Syn., *balsam* (*q.v.*).

balsam (bawl'-sam): A pharmaceutical preparation containing resinous substances; used topically for its healing and soothing qualities.

bandage (ban'-dij): A piece of cloth or other material, of varying size and shape, applied to some part of the body to hold a dressing or splint in place; to support, compress or immobilize a part; prevent or correct a deformity; or to aid in the arrest of haemorrhage. Depending on its purpose and the part to which it is applied, a B. can be made of gauze, muslin, flannel, elastic webbing, rubber, adhesive plaster or moleskin, paper, cohesive material which adheres to itself but not to any other substance, and wide-mesh material impregnated with such substances as plaster of Paris, waterglass, chalk, dextrin, starch, etc., which harden or solidify after application. Shapes of bandages are: ROLLER a continuous strip of material of varying length and width, which has been tightly wound; TRIANGULAR half of a piece of material about 1 metre square.

band cells: See under CELL.

Bandl's ring (band'-lz): Name given to the ridge that develops when the fibrous tissue that divides the upper muscular segment from the lower fibrous segment of the uterus pulls over the presenting part in prolonged labour and interferes with expulsion of the fetus.

bandy leg: Bowleg (also called *genu varum*).

bank: 1. In medicine, a place for storage of such materials as whole blood, plasma, bone, skin, cornea, or other human tissue, to be used therapeutically, often in reparative surgery. 2. A reserve supply of certain human tissue or blood to be used therapeutically in another person, *e.g.*, eye B. or blood B., human milk B.

Banting: Sir Frederick Grant Banting, Canadian scientist 1891–1941; with Charles Herbert Best, American-born physiologist in Canada, and John J. R. Macleod, a Scot who lived and worked in Canada, discoverers of insulin (1922).

BAOT: Abbreviation for British Association of Occupational Therapists (*q.v.*).

baraesthesia (bar-es-thē'-zi-a): The pressure sense.

Barbados leg (bar-bā'-doz): See ELEPHANTIASIS.

barbituism (bar-bit'-ū-izm): Acute or chronic poisoning caused by excessive use of any of the barbiturates; symptoms include fever, chills, headache, skin eruptions, psychological changes. Also spelled *barbiturism.*

barbiturates (bar-bit'-ū-rātz): A large group of synthetic compounds derived from barbituric acid and widely used for the hypnotic or sedative effects through depressing the central nervous system. Small changes in the basic structure result in the formation of rapid-, medium-, or long-acting drugs, and a wide range is available. Continued use may lead to tolerance and dependence, hence addiction. Action is potentiated in the presence of alcohol. Overdosage may lead to profound narcosis, respiratory depression, and death. Allergic skin conditions may develop in some patients.

bargaining: A technique sometimes used by very ill patients who try to trade off their present unfavourable condition for a situation that is less serious.

barium (bair'-i-um): A metallic element with several uses in medicine. B. SULPHATE a bulky, fine white powder that is tasteless and odourless; used in solution as a radiopaque substance to outline internal structures on x-ray; B. ENEMA injection of barium sulphate into the rectum; allows for x-ray visualization of the large intestine; B. MEAL a large amount of barium sulphate is swallowed; allows for x-ray visualization of the action of the oesophagus and stomach; B. SWALLOW a small amount of barium sulphate is swallowed to allow for x-ray visualization of the action of the oesophagus.

Barlow: B.'S DISEASE infantile scurvy, a deficiency of vitamin C; B. 'S SYNDROME a condition characterized by an apical systolic murmur and a lick, resulting from mitral regurgitation due to prolapse of the mitral valve; B. 'S TEST or SIGN the newborn child is placed in supine position, the hips and knees are flexed to 90°, and the hips abducted; if a jerk is felt and a click is heard, the test is a positive sign of congenital dislocation of the hips. [Thomas Barlow, English physician, 1845–1945.]

barometer (ba-rom'-e-ter): An instrument used to measure atmospheric pressure.

baroreceptor (bar'-ō-re-sep'-tor): A sensory nerve receptor that is sensitive to changes in pressure; chiefly those receptors in the ascending aorta and at the bifurcation of the external and internal carotid arteries which, when stimulated, cause vasodilatation, decreased blood pressure, bradycardia, and decrease in cardiac output.

barosinusitis (bar'-ō-sī-nus-ī'-tis): Inflammation of the frontal sinuses accompanied by oedema and haemorrhage; caused by rapid changes in atmospheric pressure, as occur in flying and deep-sea diving. Also called *aerosinusitis.*

barotalgia (bar-ō-tal'-ji-a): Pain in the middle ear caused by a difference between the air pressure in it and in the surrounding atmosphere.

barotitis (bar-ō-tī'-tis): Inflammation of the ear caused by rapid changes in atmospheric pressure. B. MEDIA inflammation of the middle ear caused by a difference between the air pressure in the middle ear and that in the environment.

barotrauma (bar-ō-traw'-ma): Injury to the middle ear, ear drum, auditory tube, or the paranasal sinuses; often caused by blunt chest injury when the glottis is closed and pressure in the airways is increased, causing an imbalance between the atmospheric pressure and that within the affected cavity. Trauma to lung tissue may result from the high pressure employed in ventilating patients with positive and expiratory pressure (PEEP) (*q.v.*).

Barr body: Sex chromatin; a small mass of chromatin in the nucleus of all non-dividing cells of females. The sex of a fetus can be determined by examination of the amniotic fluid for the presence or absence of this body.

Barré–Guillain syndrome: Guillain–Barré syndrome (*q.v.*).

barrel chest: An enlarged thorax which appears rounded and with a widened anterior–posterior measurement; may be normal in some persons, as in those living in high altitudes, or pathological, as seen in persons with chronic pulmonary emphysema or some other chronic obstructive pulmonary disease; may also be seen in those with kyphosis or asthma.

Barr–Epstein virus: Epstein–Barr virus (*q.v.*).

barrier (bar'-ē-er): An obstruction, obstacle, blocking agent. BLOOD–BRAIN B. the mechanism that prevents certain substances, such as bacteria, their toxins, or drugs, from passing from the blood to the cerebrospinal fluid or brain; PLACENTAL B. the tissue in the placenta that prevents certain substances from passing from the mother's blood to that of the fetus; B. NURSING a method of preventing the spread of infection from an infected patient to others in the area by use of isolation technique; see under NURSING.

Barthel index of activities of daily living (bar-tel'): A numerical index that aims to record what a patient does in daily life, not what he or she can do. The patient is assessed and scored (from 0 to 3) using the following categories: bowels, bladder, feeding, grooming, dressing, transfer, toilet use, mobility, stairs, and bathing. The score reflects the degree of independence from help provided by another person: if supervision is required, the patient is not independent; if aids and devices are used but no help is required, the patient is independent.

bartholinitis (bar-tō-lin-ī'-tis): Inflammation of a vulvovaginal gland (Bartholin's gland).

Bartholin's duct (bar'-to-linz): 1. The major duct draining the sublingual fluid. 2. The ducts that lead from Bartholin's gland to the vulva.

Bartholin's gland (bar'-to-linz): Two small, bean-shaped mucus-secreting glands situated at either side of the vagina at the base of the

labia minora. [Caspar Bartholin Jr, Danish anatomist, 1655–1738.]

basal (bā'-sal): 1. Relating to a base. 2. Fundamental.

basal body temperature: The lowest temperature reached by the body during one's waking hours; usually occurs immediately upon wakening in the morning.

basal cell: A cell of the deepest layer of stratified epithelium; see EPITHELIUM. B.C. CARCINOMA see under CARCINOMA; B.C EPITHELIOMA see under EPITHELIOMA.

basal ganglia (bā'-sal gan'-gli-a): Four small islands of grey matter located in the white matter at the base of the cerebrum. The lentiform nucleus, comprising globus pallidus and putamen, together with the caudate nucleus make up the corpus striatum, which along with the claustrum make up the four B.G. Concerned with modifying and coordinating voluntary muscle movement. Site of degeneration in Parkinson's disease (*q.v.*).

basal metabolic rate: The rate at which energy is expended by an individual during digestive, physical, and emotional rest, as estimated by measuring the amount of O_2 intake and CO_2 output during a specified time period. Abbreviated BMR.

basal metabolism: The amount of energy used by the body at complete rest, being the minimum necessary for sustaining life.

basal metabolism test: A test for measuring the basal metabolic rate (*q.v.*), which utilizes an apparatus that measures and records the amount of oxygen used per unit of time. The test is performed in the morning before breakfast and preferably after a good night's sleep and 18 hours after taking food. The normal rate is -10 to $+10$, and is elevated in hyperthyroidism and lowered in hypothyroidism.

base (bās): 1. the lowest part. 2. The wide or broad end of an organ. 3. The main part of a compound. In chemistry, a substance that combines with an acid to form a salt. — basal, basic, basilar, adj.

Basedow's disease: Exophthalmic goitre. See THYROTOXICOSIS.

basement membrane: A thin, delicate, transparent layer of connective tissue underlying the epithelium of mucous membranes and glands.

basi-, basio-: Combining forms denoting base, basic, basis, basilar.

basic (bā'-sik): 1. Fundamental. 2. Having properties of a base; alkaline.

Basic Four, the: A nutrition guide that classifies the foods needed to provide an adequate diet into four basic groups: the milk group, the meat group, the vegetable–fruit group, and the bread–cereal group.

basicity (bā-sis′-i-ti): **1.** The quality or state of being a base. **2.** The power of a base to unite with one or more atoms or equivalents of an acid, as indicated by the number of replaceable hydrogen atoms contained in the acid.

basicranial (bā′-si-krā-ni-al): Relating to the base of the skull.

basic life support: A system of resuscitation of the collapsed patient which comprises the elements: initial assessment, then airway maintenance, expired air ventilation (rescue breathing), and chest compression. Basic life support implies that no equipment is employed. Its purpose is to maintain adequate ventilation and circulation until means can be obtained to reverse the underlying cause of the patient's condition. See also APPENDIX 5.

basilar (bas′-i-lar): Situated at or relating to a base. B. ARTERY artery at the base of the skull, formed by the junction of the right and left vertebral arteries; B. MEMBRANE the structure that forms the floor of the cochlear duct and supports the spiral organ of Corti (q.v.).

basilar artery insufficiency syndrome: Occurs in patients with sclerosis of the basilar artery but no occlusion. There is insufficient flow of blood through the artery, with slow pulse rate, low blood pressure, and symptoms of cardiovascular accident including diplopia, vertigo, numbness, dysarthria, weakness of one side of the body, depressed consciousness.

basilic (ba-sil′-ik): Prominent B. VEIN a large vein on the inner side of the arm. The MEDIAN B. VEIN at the bend of the elbow, is generally chosen for venepuncture.

basiloma (bās-i-lō′-ma): A basal cell carcinoma.

basioccipital (bā-si-ok-sip′-i-tal): Relating to the basilar part of the occipital bone.

basis (bā′-sis): A base or foundation. Opp. of apex.

basocyte (bā′-sō-sīt): A basophil or leukocyte cell.

basoerythrocyte (bā-sō-ē-rith′-rō-sīt): An erythrocyte that contains basophil granules.

basophil (bā′-sō-fil): **1.** A substance, cell, or tissue that stains well with basic dyes. **2.** A polymorphonuclear leukocyte distinguished by the presence of large granules which stain intensely with basic dyes and have a relatively lightly staining nucleus; they make up approximately 0.5–1.0% of the polymorphonuclear leukocytes in the circulating blood; they contain heparin and histamine and are increased in numbers in such pathological conditions as Hodgkin's disease, chickenpox, myelotic leukaemia.

basophilia (bā-sō-fil′-i-a): **1.** Increase of basophils in the circulating blood. **2.** A condition in which red blood cells develop basophilic-staining granules; seen in leukaemia, advanced anaemia, malaria, lead poisoning and some other toxic states.

basophilic (bās-ō-fil′-ik): Relating to an organism that stains readily with basic dyes.

basophobia (bā-sō-fō′-bi-a): Morbid fear of walking.

basoplasm (bā′-sō-plazm): That part of the cytoplasm of a cell that takes an alkaline dye stain readily.

Bateman's needle: A special needle that has two cannulae; used for giving intravenous injections to infants.

bath: **1.** The immersion of all or any part of the body into water or other substance, or the application of a spray, jet, or vapour from a fluid, for cleansing purposes or therapy. **2.** The apparatus or place used for bathing. **3.** The substance used for bathing. The term is modified according to (a) temperature, e.g., cold (18°C), hot (40°C), warm (38°C), tepid (29°C); (b) medium used, e.g., milk, mud, brine (water rich in salt), starch, wax, water; (c) medicament added, e.g., sodium chloride; (d,) function of the medicament, e.g., astringent; (e), part bathed, e.g., arm; (f) environment, e.g., bed. AIR B. the therapeutic exposure of the unclothed body to flowing warm moist air; CHARCOT'S B. bathing the body with cold water while standing in hot water; CONTRAST B. immersion of an extremity in hot and cold water alternately; FINNISH B. a sauna B.; see SAUNA; FOOT B. a B. for one or both feet; HALF B., B. of the hips and lower part of the body; HIP B. the body is immersed in water from the waist down for therapeutic purposes; LIGHT B. exposure of the body or part of it to heat from an electric light bulb in a box or cabinet or under a cradle; NAUHEIM B. one in which the patient is immersed in warm carbonated water; NEEDLE B. one in which water is projected onto the body in fine streams under pressure; PARAYN B. the application of heated liquid paraffin; SAND B. a physical therapy procedure wherein the entire body is immersed in either dry or moist warm sand; SITZ B. a hip bath in which the body is immersed in water only up to and and including the hips and buttocks; SPONGE B. the body is washed with a wet cloth but is not immersed in water; SWEAT B. warm bath to promote sweating; TURKISH B. a steam B. in a cabinet where the temperature becomes increasingly hotter, followed by a rub and massage and then a cold shower; WAX B. paraffin B.; WHIRLPOOL B. a B. in which the water is whirled by a powered device.

bathy-: Combining form denoting deep.

battery: 1. The touching or beating of one person by another without permission, either directly or by use of an object. 2. A series of tests given for a specific purpose. 3. Two or more cells grouped together to furnish a source of electric current.

battledore (bat' -el-dōr): B. PLACENTA a placenta in which the umbilical cord is attached to its margin rather than the centre.

Baxter pump: An infusion device used for the administration of intravenous (IV) infusions.

Baxter's formula: Used for calculating fluid replacement, particularly in burn victims; based on percent of burned area; 4 ml of Ringer's lactate per kilogram of body weight per percent of body surface burned.

bayonet (bā-ō-net'): B. FORCEPS a forceps that has the blades offset from the handle. B. LEG refers to a backward dislocation of the knee joint.

BBB: Abbreviation for blood–brain barrier; see under BARRIER.

BCC: Abbreviation for basal cell carcinoma; see under CARCINOMA.

B cell: A lymphocyte (q.v.) that originates in the bone marrow; a precursor of the plasma cell, and one of two types of lymphocytes that have important roles in the body's immunological response.

BCG: Abbreviation for bacillus Calmette–Guérin (q.v.).

bd: Abbreviation for the Latin bis die, used in prescriptions; means twice daily.

BDI: Abbreviation for Beck depression inventory (q.v.).

beacon sites: Hospitals or trusts within a scheme identifying examples of best practice in the NHS with the intention of facilitating the sharing of that practice so that other organizations can develop similar schemes of their own.

bead (bēd): A small, usually spherical projection. RACHITIC B.S a series of small, rounded prominences at the points where the ribs join their cartilages; sometimes seen in rickets; also called rachitic rosary.

bearing down: 1. Colloquial term for the expulsive pains in the second stage of labour. 2. A feeling of weight and descent in the pelvis associated with uterine prolapse or pelvic tumour.

beat: A throb or pulsation as of the heart or an artery. APEX B. in a heart of normal size the apex beat can be seen or felt in the fifth left intercostal space in the midclavicular line; it is the lowest and most lateral point at which an impulse can be detected and provides a rough indication of the size of the heart; DROPPED B. refers to the loss of an occasional ventricular beat; ECTOPIC B. one that does not originate in the sinus node; PREMATURE B. an early beat not in the normal sequence of cardiac impulses.

beating: A massage manoeuvre consisting of percussion with the ulnar border of the hand and little finger.

bechic (bek' -ik): 1. A cough remedy. 2. Acting to control coughing. 3. Relating to cough.

Beck anxiety inventory: A questionnaire that measures a client's anxiety.

Beck depression inventory: A self-administered tool for measuring depression.

Beck hopelessness scale: A scale for identifying suicide risk.

Beck scale of suicide ideation (ī-dē-ā' -shun): An assessment scale for identifying suicide risk.

BEd: Abbreviation for Bachelor of Education.

bed: 1. CAPILLARY B. the total mass of capillaries in the body. 2. NAIL B. the modified epidermis lying underneath the fingernails and toenails. 3. A couch or other article of furniture to sleep or rest in or on; the term generally is used to include the frame, springs, mattress, and bed linen. AIR B. one with an inflatable mattress, usually rubber; ANAESTHETIC B. one that is prepared to receive a patient who has had a general anaesthetic; CIRCOELECTRIC B. a hospital B. that permits vertical turning of the patient; an electric motor turns the entire bed frame which is suspended between hoop-like supports; can be operated by the patient or nurse and permits different positions; CLOSED B. a B. that is unoccupied but is prepared to receive a new patient; FLOTATION B. one that has a mattress filled with water or some other substance through which air can be circulated; FRACTURE B. one with an overhead frame for the attachment of fracture appliances; OSCILLATING B. a B. that oscillates around its transverse axis as a ROCKING B. or around its longitudinal axis; ROCKING B. one with a motor attachment which causes it to rock at a regular rate; used as a means of performing artificial respiration; WATER B. one with a rubber mattress partly filled with water; used to prevent bedsores.

bedbug: A blood-sucking insect, *Cimex lectularis*; small, wingless, reddish-brown in colour, hard and smooth in appearance, and with a distinctive odour. Bedbugs live and lay eggs in cracks and crevices of furniture and walls, and can survive long periods without food. They are nocturnal in habit, and an irritating substance in their saliva causes their bites to produce weals with a central haemorrhagic point. They apparently are not vectors of disease but their bites leave a route for secondary infection.

bed occupancy: The number of hospital beds occupied by patients expressed as a percentage of the total beds available in the ward, speciality, health authority, or region. The calculation is used to assess demand for hospital beds in relation to speciality and regional availability.

bedpan: A special, appropriately shaped receptacle used to receive faecal and urinary waste from patients who are bedridden.

bedrail: A device which is fastened to the side of the bed to prevent the patient from falling or getting out of bed.

bedrest: 1. A device used for propping a patient up in bed. 2. Continuous confinement to bed for the purpose of rest.

bedridden (bed′-rid-den): Confined to bed for a prolonged period.

bedsore (bed′-sōr): Decubitus ulcer (*q.v.*).

bedwetting: See ENURESIS.

bee: An insect of the genus *Apis*; the honeybee. B. STING causes redness, pain, local swelling; hypersensitive individuals may have severe anaphylactic reactions and must be treated immediately (usually with adrenaline).

beef tapeworm: *Taenia saginata*; see under TAENIA.

Beer's knife: Delicate instrument with triangular blade used in cataract operations for incision of cornea preparatory to removal of lens. [Georg Joseph Beer, Austrian ophthalmologist, 1763–1821.]

beeswax (bēz′-waks): Wax derived from honeycomb; used in preparation of ointments.

behaviour (bē-hāv′-yor): In the general sense, conduct, *i.e.*, any observable action or response of an individual. In psychology, the meaningful response of an organism to its environment. ANTI-SOCIAL B., B. that ignores or violates the customs and laws of society; B. DISORDER, B. that (1) deviates noticeably from one's normal

B. or (2) is marked by abnormal conduct or mode of action; B. MODIFICATION the use of rewards or punishment of a response to a stimulus, as an approach to maximize learning. B. REFLEX one acquired through training or repetition; B. THERAPY any treatment that attempts to modify one's behaviour by any of several techniques, *e.g.*, aversion therapy (*q.v.*) or flooding (*q.v.*); INCONGRUOUS B., B. that is inconsistent with the individual's usual behaviour; INVARIABLE B., B. that is determined by nature, *e.g.*, reflex actions; OPERANT B. (1) B. that involves specific responses to stimuli that previously did not provoke a response; or (2) B. that seeks to change the environment to produce a desired effect; PASSIVE–AGGRESSIVE B. marked by aggression expressed passively as in pouting, procrastinating, or obstructing; REGRESSIVE B. immature B. patterns characterized by partial or complete return to infantile B.; RITUALISTIC B. a pattern of behaviour marked by the performance of certain motor activities in a mechanical, consistent manner to relieve anxiety; sometimes used by children to provide security; SOCIOPATHIC B., B. characterized by a disregard for the usual social rules and constraints.

behavioural (bē-hāv′-yor-al): Relating to behaviour. B. CONTRACTING a clinical management tool consisting of a written contract, prepared jointly by the patient and the therapist or healthcare team, which commits the patient to specific behaviours, states the input expected from the worker or team, and outlines the consequences of behavioural outcomes at various stages during the term of the contract; B. DISORDERS see BEHAVIOUR DISORDER under BEHAVIOUR; B. SCIENCES those areas of study that are devoted to the development of man's interpersonal relationships and activities, as well as his beliefs and values; includes such widely diverse fields as cultural anthropology, political science, sociology, psychology and psychiatry; B. STATUS INDEX a model developed in the UK to assess patient dangerousness and risk in relation to his or her mental illness.

behaviourism (bē-hāv′-yor-ism): A psychological term that denotes an approach to psychology through the study of measurable responses and reactions, *i.e.*, objective, observable behaviour, rather than through such subjective phenomena as ideas or emotions. Developed by Watson, who insisted that human behaviour is predictable, controllable, influenced primarily by the environment, and accessible to understanding chiefly through observation. [John B. Watson, American psychiatrist, 1878–1958.]

behaviourist (bē-hāv´ -yor-ist): One who is concerned with the description, prediction, and, sometimes, the control of behaviour.

bejel (bej´ -el): An endemnic, non-venereal, infectious disease found in Arabs of the Near and Middle East, mostly in children; the causative organism is indistinguishable from that which causes syphilis.

bel: A term used to express the relative intensity of a sound. See DECIBEL.

belch: 1. An eructation (*q.v.*). 2. To eructate, or allow gas from the stomach to escape noisily through the mouth.

beliefs: Thoughts, ideas and concepts moulded by education, culture, religion, and parental and family influence, which play a major role in opinion and behaviour. FALSE B S ideas that are patently untrue. When shared by a group, superstitions; when singular in a mentally ill person, delusions.

Bell: B.'S PALSY unilateral or bilateral pain and paralysis of the muscles of facial expression, due to a lesion of the seventh cranial nerve; of unknown origin; results in distortion of the face; B.'S PHENOMENON under normal circumstances, the eyes turn sharply upwards when the eyelids are closed intentionally, but in individuals with facial palsy the eye on the affected side will turn upwards but the lid that should close remains widely open.

belladonna (bel-a-don´ -a): A substance obtained from the dried leaves and flowers of a common poisonous plant, the deadly nightshade; the source of atropine, used in medicine for its powerful antispasmodic effect, as a cardiac and respiratory stimulant, for treatment of parkinsonism, as an adjunct to general anaesthesia, and to check certain secretions. B. is also the source of hyoacyamine, an anticholinergic substance used in the treatment of certain gastrointestinal disorders.

belle indifference: The incongruous unconcern and lack of emotion or anxiety despite incapacitating symptoms, commonly shown by patients with hysteria. [First noted in 1893 by Pierre Marie Felix Janet, French psychiatrist, 1859–1947.]

Bellevue bridge: A device used to keep the scrotum elevated when the patient is in the supine position; useful in treatment of epididymitis.

belly: 1. The abdomen. 2. The fleshy, prominent part of a muscle. B. ACHE colic, B. BUTTON the navel or umbilicus.

benchmark: 1. A point of reference from which measurements may be made. 2. Something that serves as a standard by which others may be measured or judged.

benchmarking: A process whereby organizations identify best performers in order to improve their own performance using a set of standards (or 'benchmarks') that are used for continuous improvement through comparison and sharing. Benchmarking statements set out the nature and characteristics of programmes of study and represent the general expectations of the attributes and capabilities that those possessing a qualification should be able to demonstrate. They are used when new courses are being designed and developed for internal quality assurance and external review.

bends: Decompression sickness. Severe pains in the bones, joints, muscles and abdomen, and general weakness often experienced by a person who goes too quickly from a place of abnormal atmospheric pressure to one of normal pressure; observed in aviators and divers. See CAISSON DISEASE.

beneceptor (ben´ -e-sep-tor); A nerve organ or receptor that receives and transmits stimuli of a beneficial nature. See also NOCICEPTOR.

benign (bē-nīn´): Innocent; mild; non-recurring; favourable for recovery; the opposite of malignant. B. POSITIONAL VERTIGO see under VERTIGO; B. PROSTATIC HYPERTROPHY enlargement of the prostate gland, a fairly common condition which may interfere with the flow of urine; B. TUMOUR a neoplasm that does not metastasize or invade other tissues but which may, nevertheless, require removal because it presses on an organ and interferes with its function or occupies space needed by other structures.

Benjamin's operation: Osteotomy (*q.v.*) of the femur and tibia, or double osteotomy of these bones, to alter the weight-bearing surfaces; sometimes performed in treatment of osteoarthritis of the knee.

Benner, Patricia: A nursing theorist who studied the nature of nursing expertise and nursing knowledge. Benner believes that knowledge embodied in the practice of nursing is important for the development of nurses' ability to care. Thus her area of interest is not how to do nursing, but how do nurses learn to do nursing.

Benzedrene (ben´ -ze-drēn): Proprietary name for one of the amphetamines popularly used to stave off sleepiness in people who work long hours; a nervous stimulant that may lead to hyperactivity, paranoid thinking, and other psychotic symptoms; there is a tendency to escalate the dosage and to become addicted.

benzene (ben'zēn): A colourless, inflammable liquid obtained from coal tar. Extensively used as a solvent. Its chief importance in medicine is in industrial toxicology. Continued exposure to it results in leukopenia, anaemia, and purpura.

benzidine (ben'-zi-dēn): A chemical compound used for detecting traces of blood and in testing for sulphates in water.

benzocaine (ben'-zō-kān): A chemical substance consisting of white crystals or powder; used in solution as a non-toxic local anaesthetic; also used as a dusting powder or in ointment form for pruritis.

benzodiazepines (ben-zō-dī-az'-e-pēns): A group of drugs used as major tranquillizers, e.g., Librium, Valium; administered orally; used in treatment of anxiety states without depression; habit-forming and widely abused.

benzoin (ben'-zō-in): A balsamic resin; has several uses in medicine including use as a stimulating expectorant, with administration by inhalation to patients suffering from bronchitis or laryngitis; also used as a topical protectant.

benzyl benzoate (ben'-zil ben'-zō-āt): A clear, odourless, aromatic liquid; often used as an active ingredient of a lotion for treatment of scabies (q.v.).

bereavement (be-rēv'-ment): The state or fact of being bereaved; especially the loss of a loved one by death. Increasing interest in the topic for nurses has developed with the growth of the hospice movement and sociological interest in death and dying, along with the expansion of the nursing role to include comprehensive care of both the dying patient and his or her family.

beriberi (ber'-ē-ber'-ē): A deficiency disease caused by lack of thiamine (vitamin B$_1$). Occurs mainly in the Orient where the staple diet is polished rice; also occurs in areas where there is famine for any length of time; rare in the UK. The symptoms are pain from neuritis, paralysis, muscular wasting, chronic constipation, progressive oedema, mental deterioration and, finally, heart failure.

Berkow's method: A method of determining the size of a burn injury in children; more accurate than the rule of nines (q.v.). It takes into account the difference in body proportions of children according to their ages; e.g., in infants the head is considered to account for

18% of total body surface and the legs for 14%. These proportions change until the age of 15; from then on the rule of nine applies.

bestiality (bēs'-ti-al-i-ti): 1. Any animal-like behaviour. 2. Sexual intercourse between a human and an animal.

best practice statements: Statements derived in partnership by practitioners, educators, and service users to develop, promote, and disseminate clinical evidence. The statements relate to a variety of nursing interventions and are reviewed regularly to ensure currency and validity.

beta (bē-ta): The second letter of the Greek alphabet; in chemistry and other types of series, often used to designate the chemical position of a substance in certain compounds. B. CELLS see under CELL; B. RAYS see under RAY; B. RECEPTOR see under RECEPTOR; B. RHYTHM see under RHYTHM; B. WAVE see under WAVE.

beta-adrenergic receptor: Any of the adrenergic parts of a receptor of a stimulus that react to noradrenaline and certain other blocking agents by causing relaxation of bronchial muscles, elevated blood pressure and heart rate, and strengthened contraction of cardiac muscle. The opposite of alpha-adrenergic receptor, see under RECEPTOR.

beta-blocking agent: An agent that blocks the action of a beta-adrenergic receptor; relieves symptoms of anxiety, diminishes heart rate and cardiac output; may be used in treatment of withdrawal symptoms in alcoholism and drug addiction; some are used in treatment of hypertension and angina pectoris.

beta-endorphin (bē-ta en-dor'-fin): An amino acid peptide involved in many body processes, especially the relief of pain; has a morphine-like activity.

betel (bē'-tel): A climbing plant of southern Asia; the seed of the fruit, or nut, is wrapped in a leaf of the plant, along with lime, and chewed to produce both stimulating and narcotic effects; continued use causes black discoloration of the teeth; formerly used in Asiatic medicine as a stimulant, astringent, tonic, and counterirritant.

bezoar (bē'-zor): A ball or concretion found in the alimentary tract of certain animals and sometimes in the stomach of humans, particularly in psychiatric patients; usually made up of ingested hair and vegetable fibres. In the past thought to have magical therapeutic value, and still used in some parts of the world as a medicament with mystical properties.

bhang (bang): *Cannabis sativa*. See under CAN-NABIS.

BHS: Abbreviation for Beck hopelessness scale (*q.v.*).

Bi: The chemical symbol for bismuth.

bi-: Prefix denoting (1) two, twice; (2) between; (3) affecting two similar parts. In chemistry, double.

biarticular (bī-ar-tik'-ū-lar): Relating to or affecting two joints.

bias (bī'-as): 1. An inclination of temperament or outlook; especially a personal and some-times unreasoned judgement, such as preju-dice. 2. Deviation of the expected values of a statistical estimate from the quantity it esti-mates: systematic error introduced into sam-pling or testing by selecting or encouraging one outcome or answer over others.

biauricular (bī-aw-rik'-ū-lar): Relating to or affecting the auricles of both ears.

bibulous (bib'-ū-lus): Absorbent; spongy.

bicameral (bī-kam'-er-al): Consisting of two chambers or hollows; term often used to de-scribe an abscess which is divided into two cavities by a septum.

bicarbonate (bī-kar'-bō-nāt): A salt of carbonic acid; formed by the combination of water and carbon dioxide under the influence of carbonic anhydrase. BLOOD B. that in the blood, indicat-ing the alkaline reserve; also called *plasma* B.; SODIUM B. a white crystalline powder, used in medicine chiefly as a gastric antacid; also used in solution as a dressing for wounds, for cleansing the mouth, nose, and vagina, as an enema, or as an emollient in bathwater.

biceps (bi'-seps): A muscle possessing two heads or points of origin. B. BRACHII the flexor muscle at the front of the humerus; B. FEMORIS the flexor muscle at the back of the thigh; B. REFLEX contraction of the biceps muscle when its tendon is tapped; this is normal but when greatly increased indicates some pathology.

bichloride (bī-klō'-rīd): A compound, particu-larly a salt, in which the molecules contain two equivalents of chlorine to one of another element. B. OF MERCURY a corrosive antisep-tic, formerly used both as a germicide and as an antisyphilitic; highly toxic.

bicipital (bī-sip'-i-tal): 1. Two-headed. 2. Relat-ing to a biceps muscle. B. TENDINITIS see under TENDINITIS.

biconcave (bī-kon'-kāv): Being concave or hollow on two surfaces; said of lenses.

biconvex (bī-kon'-veks): Being convex or curving outwardly on two surfaces; said of lenses.

bicornuate (bī-kor'-nū-āt): Having two horns, generally referring to a double uterus or a single uterus possessing two horns. Also called *bicornate*.

biscuspid (bī-kus'-pid): Having two cusps or points. B. TEETH the premolars; B. VALVE the mitral valve between the left atrium and ven-tricle of the heart; it allows blood to flow freely from the left atrium into the left ventricle and prevents backflow from the ventricle to the atrium during ventricular contraction.

bidactyly (bī-dak'-ti-li): Absence of all fingers or toes except the first and fifth. See LOBSTER-CLAW HAND.

bidet (bē-dā'): A low-set, trough-like basin or sitz bath in which the perineum can be im-mersed while the legs are outside and the feet on the floor. Can have attachments for douch-ing the vagina or rectum.

Bielchowsky's disease: Cerebral sphingolipido-sis, see under SPHINGOLIPIDOSIS. Also called *Bielchowsky–Jansky disease*.

Bifid (bī-fid): Divided into two parts. Cleft. Forked.

bifocal (bī-fō'-kal): Having two foci; term used especially in reference to eyeglasses that have a lens that corrects for near vision set into a lens that corrects for distant vision.

bifurcation (bī-fur-kā'-shun): A division or fork-ing into two branches, or the site where such division occurs, *e.g.*, the B. of a blood vessel. — bifurcate, adj. and v.

bigeminal (bī-jem'-i-nal): Paired; double. B. PREGNANCY twin pregnancy; B. PULSE two heartbeats followed by a pause before the next two beats; also called *pulsus bigeminus*; may originate in the atria, the A–V node, or the ventricles.

bigeminy (bī-jem'-i-ni): 1. The condition of oc-curring doubly or in pairs. 2. A type of heart-beat in which two beats occur close together, with the third beat being skipped; a regularly occurring irregularity. Also called *bigeminus*.

biguanides (bī-gwan-īds): A group of synthetic drugs given orally in treatment of non-insulin-dependent diabetics, particularly the obese; thought to stimulate the uptake of glucose in the absence of insulin.

bilateral (bī-lat'-er-al): 1. Having two sides. 2. Pertaining to both sides of a structure or the body. 3. Occurring on both sides of the body or on right and left structures, as bilateral cat-aracts. — bilaterally, adv.

bile (bīl): A bitter, alkaline, viscid, greenish-yellow to golden brown, slightly antiseptic fluid secreted by the liver and stored in the gall bladder from which it is released into the duodenum via the common bile duct and where it aids digestion by emulsifying fats, stimulating peristalsis, and preventing putrefaction. It contains water, mucin, lecithin, cholesterol, B. salts and the pigments bilirubin and biliverdin. B. DUCTS the hepatic and cystic, which join to form the common B. duct. — biliary, bilious, adj.

Bilharzia (bil-har′ -zi-a): *Schistosoma* (*q.v.*).

biliary (bil′i-ar-i): Relating to bile, the bile ducts, or the gall bladder. B. CALCULUS a gallstone; B. COLIC excruciating, paroxysmal pain in the upper right quadrant of the abdomen and referred to the shoulder, due to smooth muscle spasm arising in the bile passages; often caused by pressure of a stone in the gall bladder or its passage through the ducts; B. DUCTS passages in the liver which join the duct from the gall bladder to form the common bile duct; B. FISTULA an abnormal tract conveying bile to the surface or to some internal organ; B. SYSTEM the heptic (biliary) ducts, gall bladder, cystic duct, and common bile duct; also called the *biliary tract* or *tree*.

bilin (bī′ -lin): The chief ingredient of bile, consisting mostly of sodium salts of normal bile acids.

bilious (bil′ -ius): 1. Relating to bile. 2. Relating to excess of bile. 3. A popular non-medical word signifying a digestive upset, often with headache and constipation, and attributed to excess secretion of bile.

bilirubin (bil-i-roo′ -bin): A reddish-yellow crystalline pigment that gives bile its orange colour; it is a waste product from the normal breakdown of old red blood cells which passes through the liver where it is changed chemically and is excreted chiefly in the faeces.

bilirubinaemia (bil-i-roo-bi-nē′ -mi-a): The presence of more bilirubin in the blood than the slight amount normally found there.

biliuria (bil-i-ū′ -ri-a): The presence of bile or bile salts in the urine. — biliuric, adj.

biliverdin (bil-i-ver′ -din): The green pigment occurring in bile, an oxidation product of bilirubin.

bill: A draft of a law presented to a legislature for enactment; also the law itself, the Bill.

Billing's ovulation method: A birth control method based on a daily examination by the woman of her cervical mucus, which varies in consistency and colour during the menstrual cycle. The method relies on her interpretation of the changes that accompany the menstrual cycle, particularly those which occur around the time of ovulation, and the avoidance of sexual contact from the time she recognizes the approach of ovulation until three days following ovulation.

bilobate (bī-lō′ -bāt): Having two lobes.

bilobular (bī-lob′ -ū-lar): Having two little lobes or lobules.

bimanual (bī-man′ -ū-al): 1. Relating to both hands. 2. Performed with both hands, *e.g.*, in gynaecology, the method of examining internal female genitalia with one hand on the abdomen and the finger or fingers of the other hand in the vagina. — bimanually, adj.

binary (bī′ -na-ri): Made up or consisting of two things; characterized by two. In chemistry, a compound made up of two elements. In anatomy, dividing or separating into two. B. DIGIT a bit (short for binary digit) is the smallest unit of data in a computer; it has a single binary value, either 0 or 1; in most computer systems there are 8 bits to a byte; B. FISSION reproduction of cells by division into two approximately equal parts.

binaural (bī-naw′ -ral): Relating to, or having, two ears. Applied to a type of stethoscope (*q.v.*).

binder (bīn′ -der): A broad bandage, applied about the abdomen or breasts; often used following surgery or childbirth. T-BINDER a B. patterned after the letter T; used to hold perineal or rectal dressings in place.

binge (binj): Heavy continuous drinking leading to a sustained high blood alcohol; may last an evening or a month, but has a beginning and an end. Also used to describe periodic excessive food intake.

binocular (bin-ok′ -ū-lar): 1. The use of both eyes in vision. 2. Relating to both eyes. 3. Describing an optical instrument requiring both eyes for its use.

binovular (bin-ov′ -ū-lar): Derived from two separate ova; B. twins may be of different sexes. Cf. UNIOVULAR.

binuclear (bī-nū′ -klē-ar): Having two nuclei.

bio-: Combining form denoting (1) life; (2) living organism or tissue.

bioassay (bī-ō-as′ -sā): Assessing the potency or strength of a substance by comparison of the effects it has on living organisms, *e.g.*, animals, with the effects of a standardized preparation. Also called *biological assay*.

bioavailability (bī′ -ō-ā-vāl-a-bil′ -i-ti): The degree to which a drug, other medication, or other substance becomes available for use by the body after administration.

biocatalyst (bī-ō-kat′ -a-list): An enzyme.

biochemistry (bī-ō-kem′-is-tri): The branch of chemistry that deals with the changes of organic compounds as they occur in living organisms. — biochemical, adj.

biocidal (bī-ō-sī′-dal): Active against life; causing death, particularly of living microorganisms.

bioelectricity (bī′-ō-ē-lek-tris′-i-ti): 1. Electric phenomena that occur in living tissues. 2. Effects of electric current on living tissue. B. TESTS tests that detect and record electric currents generated within the body.

bioengineering (bī′-ō-en-jin-ēr′-ing): The application of engineering principles to the biological sciences, especially to medicine and surgery, in the designing of sophisticated mechanical or microelectric devices that are safe for patient use; e.g., renal dialysis machines, cardiac pacemakers, electronic monitors.

bioequivalent (bī-ō-ē-kwiv′-a-lent): In pharmacology, refers to the relative equivalency of effect of different forms of a drug; for example, generic and brand-name preparations.

bioethics (bī-ō-eth′-iks): The principles that govern the uses of medical and biological technology, particularly when they have a bearing on human life. Is concerned with the social, ethical, legal, and even theological ramifications of the effects of biomedical research and technology. The term is often used synonymously with medical ethics.

biofeedback (bī-ō-fēd′-bak): A combination of meditation and technology (including monitoring devices) utilized for controlling states of mind to help the person identify, monitor, and even control certain body functions; used in treating stress, neurological disorders, certain psychological disturbances such as tension headache. B. TRAINING learning to control body processes such as breathing, heartbeat, and other involuntary body functions including muscle contraction; consists of learning a series of deep relaxation exercises.

bioflavonoids (bī-ō-flā′-vo-noyds): Any of a group of compounds obtained from the rinds of citrus fruits and from many plants; their action in the body is to maintain a normal state of the walls of small blood vessels.

biogenesis (bī-ō-jen′-e-sis): 1. The origin of living organisms. 2. Term used to describe the theory that living organisms can be produced only by organisms already living; opp. to the theory of spontaneous generation. — biogenetic, adj.

biogenics (bī-ō-jen′-iks): A system of self-education achieved by practising exercises in relaxation and focusing the attention, along with concentration, on spiritual matters; utilizes techniques developed by Coué, Jung, the gestaltists and others.

biographical research (bī-ō-graf′-i-kal): The process of collecting oral accounts through interview. May also include the use of personal documents, such as letters or diaries, to construct accounts of individual experiences/lives. The data require careful appraisal for reliability and representativeness.

biographical therapy: Therapy that uses understanding of the past and self-knowledge to help patients make choices and to steer their lives. The individual's life is mapped and, through questioning, personal development, people who have made an impact, and recurring issues are identified.

biohazard (bī′-ō-haz-ard): Any hazard arising from inadvertent human biological processes, e.g., needlestick injuries or spillages.

biologic (bī-ō-loj′-ik): Relating to biology. B. RHYTHMS, see under RHYTHM.

biological (bī-ō-loj′-i-kal): 1. Relating to biology. 2. In pharmacy, a preparation made from living organisms or their products and used in the diagnosis, treatment, or prevention of disease; includes the serums, vaccines, antitoxins and antigens. B. AGE see under AGE; B. CLOCK the mechanism of a learned 24-hour pattern of sleep and wakefulness; see CIRCADIAN RHYTHM; B. CLOCK THEORY holds that ageing is due to the running down of an inherent biological clock located in the nucleus of cells that determines the number of divisions a normal cell can undergo before it dies; B. HALF-LIFE the time it takes the body to excrete or eliminate one-half of a dose of an administered substance; it is the same for all isotopes of a given element; see HALF-LIFE.

biological engineering: The creation of electronic or electrical aids to assist function, such as pacemakers, hearing aids.

biologicals (bī-ō-loj′-i-kalz): Complex substances from living organisms and their products, including antigens, antitoxins, serums, and vaccines.

biological warfare: The use of disease-causing agents such as bacteria, viruses, etc., against both military forces and civilians during the conduct of war.

biology (bī-ol′-ō-ji): The science of life, dealing with the structure, function, and organization of all living things including plants and animals. — biologic, biological, adj.; biologically, adv.

biomechanics (bī-ō-me-kan-iks): The science that deals with the mechanics of the human body, based on the application of principles of physics and engineering to the action of biological systems; includes the study of the environment required by astronauts when in space.

biomedical (bī-ō-med′-i-kal): Relating to both biology and medicine.

biomedicine (bī-ō-med′-i-sin): Clinical medicine that utilizes in practice the principles of such natural sciences as biology and biochemistry.

biometry (bī-om′-e-tri): The application of statistical methods in the study of biology. Biostatistics.

biomicroscope (bī-ō-mī′-kro-skōp): A special microscope with a thin beam of light which permits the examiner to observe minute details within living tissue or organs, *e.g.*, the eye. See SLITLAMP.

biomicroscopy (bī-ō-mī-kros′-ko-pi): 1. The microscopic study of the structure of living cells. 2. The microscopic examination of living tissue in the body. 3. Examination of the cornea, lens, vitreous body, and retina with a slitlamp (*q.v.*).

bion (bī′-on): An individual living thing.

bionics (bī-on′-iks): The science of developing models that parallel the human vertebrate nervous system; may be mathematical, electronic, or physical; applied in cybernetic engineering. See CYBERNETICS.

bionosis (bī-ō-nō′-sis): Any disease caused by a living agent such as a bacterium or a virus.

bionursing (bī′-ō-nur-sing): The application of life sciences to the theory and practice of nursing.

biophage (bī′-ō-fāj): A parasite. Any living organism that derives its nourishment from another living organism.

biophilia (bī-ō-fil′-i-a): The instinct of self-preservation.

biophysics (bī-ō-fiz′-iks): The branch of knowledge that deals with (1) the physics of living organisms; (2) the applications of the principles and methods of physics to the problems of living organisms.

bioplasm (bī′-ō-plazm): The essential or vital part of the protoplasm of living cells. Protoplasm.

biopsy (bī′-op-si): 1. Observation or examination of a living subject or of tissue taken from a living body, as opposed to a postmortem observation. 2. Term used to describe the removal of a small piece of tissue from a living body for histologic examination needed to establish an accurate diagnosis. ASPIRATION or NEEDLE B. examination of tissue removed by a hollow needle; BIOCHEMICAL B. a combination of histological and chemical examination of tissue for diagnostic purposes; CONE B. examination of a cone-shaped piece of tissue; in a CERVICAL C. B. a circular tapering piece of tissue is excised from the external os of the uterus, for pathological examination; ENDOSCOPIC B. in which the specimen is obtained by a surgical instrument inserted through an endoscope; NEEDLE B. aspiration B.; OPEN B. examination of a specimen taken following a surgical incision, to be examined immediately; PUNCH B., B. in which the specimen is removed by a punch; SPONGE B., B. in which the specimen is obtained by placing a sponge over a lesion or membrane; STERNAL B. examination of bone marrow that is removed from the sternum by puncture or aspiration; SURFACE B. examination of tissue removed from a surface by scraping; used especially to diagnose cancer of the uterine cervix; TOTAL B. examination of an entire organ or part that is removed from the body; WEDGE B. examination of a wedge-shaped portion of tissue.

biopsychology (bī′-ō-sī-kol′-o-ji): See PSYCHOBIOLOGY.

biopsychosocial (bī′-ō-sī-kō-sō′-shul): Relates to the 'whole person' approach to healthcare which involves the biological, psychological, and social factors involved in an illness.

biorbital (bī-or′-bit-al): Relating to or involving the orbits of both eyes.

biorhythm (bī′-ō-rithm): A biologically regulated rhythmic pattern of change in physiological behaviour, such as occurs in the menstrual cycle, or the regular variations in body temperature, blood pressure, or mood.

biosocial (bī-ō-sō′-shul): 1. Relating to the biological and social aspects of life. 2. Relating to the human aspects of social life as they are affected by the principles of biology.

biospectroscopy (bī′-ō-spek-tros′-ko-pi): The spectroscopic examination of living tissue and/or of body fluids; clinical spectroscopy.

biosphere (bī′-ō-sfer): All areas of the known universe where life can exist.

biostatistics (bī-ō-sta-tis′-tiks): The science of statistics applied to collected numerical data concerning human populations. Vital statistics.

biosynthesis (bī-ō-sin′-the-sis): The forming of chemical compounds by synthesis within the living organism.

biotechnology (bī′-ō-tek-nol′-o-ji): Biological science when applied, especially in genetic engineering and technology.

bioterrorism (bī-ō-ter′-rer-izm): The use of biological weapons as a means of inducing fear in people; *e.g.*, the posting of letters contaminated with anthrax.

biotherapy (bī-ō-ther′-a-pi): The treatment of disease with a living microorganism or the product of a living microorganism.

biotic (bī-ot′-ik): Relating to life or living organisms.

-biotic: Combining form denoting life, or having life.

biotics (bī-ot′-iks): The study of living organisms and their qualities, functions, and activities.

biotin (bī′-o-tin): One of the water-soluble members of the vitamin B complex which acts as a coenzyme, and is presumed essential to humans. Found in varying amounts in many plant and animal foods, but chiefly in liver, kidney, egg yolk, milk, yeast, peanuts, unpolished rice; also synthesized from ingested foods in the intestine. Raw egg white in quantities interferes with its absorption. Formerly called *vitamin H.*

biotomy (bī-ot′-ō-mi): Vivisection.

biotoxicology (bī-ō-toks-ı kol′-o-ji): The study of toxins and toxic conditions produced by living organisms.

biotransformation (bī′-ō-trans-for mā′-shun): The chemical and metabolic changes that substances undergo in the body, particularly drugs.

biotripsis (bī-ō-trip′-sis): Wearing away or eroding of the skin, seen mostly in the elderly.

Biot's respiration: See BIOT'S BREATHING under BREATHING.

biotype (bī-ō-tīp): A group of organisms having the same genotype. See GENOTYPE.

biovular (bī-ov′-ū-lar): See BINOVULAR.

bipara (bī-pa′-ra): A woman who has given birth to two children in two different labours.

biparental (bī′-pa-ren′-tal): 1. Having two parents, one male and one female. 2. Derived from two parents.

biparietal (bī′-pa-rī-et-al): Relating to both parietal bones or both parietal lobes.

biparous (bī-par′-us): 1. Producing two ova or two offspring at one time. 2. Having borne twins.

bipartite (bī-par′-tīt): 1. Divided into two parts. 2. Consisting of two parts or divisions.

biped (bī′-ped): 1. Any animal with two feet, as humans. 2. Two-footed.

bipolar (bī-pō′-lar): Having two poles. B. NERVE CELL, a nerve cell with two processes, *i.e.*, an afferent and an efferent process.

bipolar disorders: Major affective neurotic disorders occurring as: B. D.S, MIXED in which alternating manic and depressive episodes occur, or have recently occurred, with the two phases being intermixed or alternating. B. D. MANIC in which a manic episode occurs or has occurred recently. B. D. DEPRESSED in which a major depressive episode occurs or has occurred recently.

biramous (bī-rā′-mus): Having two rami or branches.

birefringence (bī-rē-frin′-jens): The quality of splitting a ray of light in two, or of transmitting light unequally in different directions. Also called *double refraction.* — birefringent, adj.

Birnberg bow: An intrauterine contraceptive device.

BIT: Abbreviation for binary digit; see under BINARY.

birth: The act of expelling the young from the mother's body; delivery; being born. B. CANAL the cavity or canal of the pelvis through which the baby passes during labour; B. CERTIFICATE in the UK, a legal document given on registration, within 42 days of birth, listing date and place of birth, name and sex of child, names of parents, other pertinent information; B. CONTROL the prevention or regulation of conception by any means; contraception; B. INJURY any injury occurring during parturition, *e.g.*, fracture of a bone, subluxation of a joint, injury to a peripheral nerve, intracranial haemorrhage; B. PALSY or PARALYSIS paralysis caused by injury received at or during birth; B. TRAUMA (1) an injury sustained in the process of being born; (2) in psychiatry, a hypothesis that relates the shock of being born with the later development of anxiety or neurosis; PREMATURE B. one occurring after the seventh month of pregnancy but before term; B. RATE the number of live births per 1000 population per year.

birth control pill: A contraceptive agent in the form of a pill, taken orally. See CONTRACEPTION, CONTRACEPTIVE.

birthing: Giving birth. B. CHAIR a chair used by women in labour; may have a complicated design or be a simple chair with a large central hole in the seat; allows for the upright position and thought by some to facilitate labour, particularly in the second stage; B. BED a special bed equipped with levers that control the head, seat, and foot positions; the foot section can be adjusted to provide for Trendelenburg position; the advantage is that the patient does not have to change beds for labour, delivery, and recovery; B. ROOMS special rooms in hospitals or clinics for family-centred childbirth; husbands and children can take part in the event.

birthmark: A haemangioma or other blemish present on the skin at birth: naevus (*q.v.*).

bisect (bī´-sekt): To divide into two equal parts. — bisection, n.

bisection (bī-sek´-shun): The process of cutting into two parts.

bisexual (bī-seks´-ū-al): 1. A person who is sexually attracted to both men and women. 2. Having gonads of both sexes; hermaphrodite. 3. Relating to both sexes. 4. Consisting of both sexes.

bisferiens (bis-fē´-ri-ens): Refers to a pulse that has two palpable beats during one systole.

bisferious (bis-fē´-ri-us): Striking twice; having two beats, as a pulse; dicrotic.

bisiliac (bis-il´-i-ak): Relating to the two ilia or to two iliac parts or structures.

bisulphate (bī-sul´-fāt):A salt of sulphuric acid in which half the hydrogen is replaced by a postive element or radical.

bite: Puncture, laceration, or penetration of the skin by human teeth or by an animal or insect. In dentistry, the occlusion of the teeth.

bitemporal (bī-tem´-por-al): 1. Relating to both temporal areas of the skull. 2. Relating to both temporal lobes of the brain.

bitrochanteric (bī-trō-kan-ter-ik): Relating to (1) the greater trochanter of both femurs or (2) the greater and lesser trochanter of a femur.

bituminosis (bī-tū-mi-nō´-sis): A form of pneumoconiosis (*q.v.*) caused by inhalation of soft coal dust.

bivalent (bī-vā´-lent): 1. In chemistry, refers to a substance that has a valence of two, or one that has two valences; see VALENCE. 2. Double or paired, as two joined chromosomes.

bivalve (bī-valv): 1. Having two blades, as in a vaginal speculum. 2. To divide a plaster of Paris cast into two portions, an anterior and a posterior half. 3. Having two valves, as molluscs or clams.

biventricular (bī-ven-trik´-ū-lar): Involving or relating to both ventricles of the heart.

black damp: See under DAMP.

Black Death: An extremely virulent form of the plague that ravaged Europe and Asia in the 14th century. Named for the haemorrhagic, blackening spots which formed on the skin. Bubonic plague.

blackhead: See COMEDO.

black lung, black lung disease: Pneumoconiosis (*q.v.*). So called by coal miners because the inhalation of coal dust blackens the lungs and slowly destroys the lung tissues.

blackout: 1. A condition characterized by failure of vision and unconsciousness of short duration, caused by sudden reduction in the amount of blood reaching the brain and retina. 2. A period of time during alcoholic or other drug intoxification that the individual cannot remember afterwards.

blackwater fever: A malignant form of malaria (*q.v.*) occurring in the tropics, especially Africa. There is great destruction of red blood cells, and this causes a very dark-coloured urine. Other symptoms include high fever, vomiting, jaundice, enlarged liver and spleen, acute renal failure, tachycardia. The prognosis is poor.

bladder: A membranous sac that serves as a receptacle or reservoir for a fluid or gas. ATONIC B. a condition in which there is no sensation in the urinary bladder, with overdistension, incomplete emptying; may or may not be of neurogenic origin; seen in tabes dorsalis and pernicious anaemia; AUTONOMOUS B. a condition of the bladder in which the individual has lost control of the function of micturition due to injury of the spinal cord in the lumbosacral region; GALL B see GALLBLADDER; HYPOTONIC B. a condition of greatly decreased or absent tonus of the detrusor urinae muscle; see DETRUSOR; ILEAL B see ILEOURETEROSTOMY; IRRITABLE B. a condition in which extreme sensitivity of the bladder is accompanied by constant desire to urinate; NERVOUS B. a term describing the condition in which one has a constant desire to urinate but cannot empty the bladder; NEUROGENIC B. a term designating any dysfunction of the urinary bladder caused by a lesion in the spinal cord or peripheral nervous system; PSYCHOGENIC B. a term descriptive of a condition in which the patient empties the bladder at increasingly shorter intervals until eventually the bladder fails to fill to any degree before the need to void is felt; caused by one or more nervous and emotional factors; RECTAL B. a term used to describe the results of surgery in which the ureters are transplanted to the rectum; REFLEX B. a condition in which the sensation of the bladder distension and ability to control micturition are lost; results from a lesion in the spinal cord; seen in paraplegic patients; SPASTIC B. autonomous B.; STAMMERING B. a term describing a condition in which the stream of urine is interrupted several times during voiding; UNINHIBITED B a B. that has retained the sensation of distension but lost the ability to inhibit voiding; due to a lesion in the cerebral cortex; frequently seen in persons with cardiovascular disease; UNSTABLE B. a condition to be differentiated from stress incontinence by the fact that a cough, sneeze, or posture change may cause an uninhibited bladder contraction resulting in complete emptying of the bladder whereas in stress incontinence only part of the bladder content leaks out; URINARY B. the muscular bag in the pelvis that serves as a reservoir for urine.

blanch: 1. To become ashen or pale. 2. To take the colour out of.

bland: Mild, non-irritating, soothing. B. DIET see under DIET.

blas-, blasto-: Combining forms denoting bud, budding; used particularly in relation to a primitive cell or element in the early stage of development of the embryo.

blast: An immature stage in cell development before the distinctive characteristics of the particular cell appear.

-blast: Combining form denoting an embryonic or formative unit, especially of living matter, e.g., neuroblast.

blastema (blas-tē′-ma): The primitive material from which cells and tissues of the embryo develop.

blastocele (blas′-tō-sēl): The central cavity of the blastula of a developing embryo.

blastocyst (blas′-tō-sist): The modified blastula, consisting of an outer part the trophoblast – an inner cell mass, and the blastocele; it represents the stage in embryonic development that follows the morula (q.v.).

blastocyte (blas′-tō-sīt): An embryonic cell that has not yet become differentiated into its specific type.

blastocytoma (blas-tō-sī-tō′-ma): A neoplasm made up chiefly of immature undifferentiated embryonic tissue. Syn., blastoma (q.v.).

blastoderm (blas′-tō-derm): A delicate membranous lining of the zona pellucida of the fertilized ovum. The rudimentary structure from which the embryo is formed.

blastogenesis (blas-tō-jen′-e-sis): 1. Multiplication of an organism by asexual reproduction or budding. 2. Transmission of parental characteristics to offspring by the germ cells.

blastolysis (blas-tol′-i-sis): Dissolution and destruction of the blastocyst (q.v.).

blastoma (blas-tō′-ma): A true tumour. A tumour originating from the blastema of tissue or an organ. Syn., blastocytoma. — blastomatous, adj.

blastomere (blas′-tō-mēr): One of the cells resulting from the division of the fertilized ovum.

blastula (blas-tū-la): The stage of development at which an embryo consists of one or several layers of cells around a central fluid-filled cavity.

bleed: 1. To lose blood from a vein or artery. 2. To cause blood to be lost from a vein or artery.

bleeder: 1. A blood vessel that is severed, sometimes during surgery, and from which blood continues to escape. 2. An individual who is subject to frequent loss of blood, as one suffering from haemophilia (q.v.).

bleeding: Losing blood as a result of a severed or ruptured blood vessel. ANOVULATORY B., B. not associated with ovulation; B. TIME the time required for the spontaneous arrest of bleeding from a skin puncture; under controlled conditions this forms a clinical test and is not to be confused with clotting time; DYSFUNCTIONAL B. uterine B. usually due to an endocrine imbalance rather than a tumour or organic disease; OCCULT B. hidden or concealed B., the blood being so changed that it is not easily identifiable.

blennophthalmia (blen-of-thal′-mi-a): Catarrhal conjunctivitis. — blennophthalmic, adj.

blennorrhoea (blen-ō-rē′a): Syn., blenorrhagia. INCLUSION B. acute, purulent conjunctivitis; in infants, this is due to infection from the mother's genital tract during birth; affects both eyes; marked by red swollen lids and purulent discharge. In adults, it is less severe; often acquired venereally or in swimming pools; the discharge is less purulent; usually affects only one eye; also called inclusion conjunctivitis.

bleph-, blephar-, blepharo-: Combining forms denoting eyelid.

blepharadenitis (blef′-ar-ad-e-nī′-tis): Inflammation of the Meibomian glands. Also called blepharoadenitis.

blepharal (blef′-a-ral): Relating to the eyelids.

blepharism (blef′-a-rizm): Spasm of the eyelids.

blepharitis (blef-a-rī′-tis): Inflammation of the eyelids, particularly the edges. B. MARGINALIS chronic inflammation of the eyelid margins, the hair follicles, and the sebaceous glands; marginal B.; NON-ULCERATIVE B., B. marked by hyperaemia, thickening, and scaling of the eyelid edges; may be associated with seborrhoea of the scalp or psoriasis; ULCERATIVE B., B. resulting from bacterial infection of the sebaceous glands of the eyelids; marked by redness, swelling, ulceration with crust formation, photophobia, conjunctivitis.

blepharoconjunctivitis (blef′-a-rō-kon-junk-ti-vī′-tis): Inflammation of the eyelids and the conjunctiva.

blepharodiastasis (blef'-a-rō-dī-as'-ta-sis): Abnormally wide separation of the eyelids or inability to close them completely.

blepharoedema (blef-ar-ē-dē'-ma): Oedema of the eyelids.

blepharoplasty (blef'-a-rō-plas-ti): Plastic repair of an eyelid. Sometimes done for cosmetic purposes to remove wrinkles and bulges caused by hereditary factors and ageing.

blepharoplegia (blef-ar-ō-plē'-ji-a): Paralysis of an eyelid.

blepharoptosis (blef-a-rō-tō'-sis): Drooping of an upper eyelid. See PTOSIS. — blepharoptotic, adj.

blepharospasm (blef'-a-rō-spazm): 1. Excessive winking. 2. Spasm of the obicularis oculi muscle producing partial or complete closure of the eyelid for seconds or minutes at a time. — blepharospastic, adj.

blind (blīnd): 1. Unable to see. 2. Closed at one end, as a pouch.

blindness: Loss or lack of ability to see; may be due to disorder of the organ of sight or to a lesion in the central nervous system. COLOUR B. a term loosely applied to any deviation from the normal ability to distinguish hues accurately; CONCUSSION B. that caused by violent explosion, gunfire, etc.; DAY B. hemeralopia (*q.v.*); ECLIPSE B. may occur while watching an eclipse of the sun without proper eye protection; FUNCTIONAL B. occurs without any disorder of the organ of sight; LEGAL B. less than 20/200 vision in the better of the two eyes, or when visual acuity is restricted to 20 degrees or less; NIGHT B. nyctalopia (*q.v.*); PSYCHIC B. inability to recognize known objects; due to a lesion in the central nervous system; TOTAL B. no light perception whatever.

blind spot: The spot at which the optic nerve leaves the retina. It is insensitive to light.

blink: To close the eyelids and then open them quickly several times in succession. B. REFLEX the reflex action of closing the eyes when the cornea is touched. Also called *corneal reflex*.

blister: Separation of the epidermis from the dermis by a collection of fluid, usually serum or blood. See VESICLE. fever b., herpes simplex (*q.v.*) of the lip.

bloat (blōt): To become swollen, puffy, or oedematous. Usually refers to abdominal distension; may be caused by air swallowing or by intestinal gas from fermentation of intestinal contents.

block: 1. An obstruction or blockage of a passage. 2. Regional anaesthesia. 3. An obstruction in the path of a nerve or muscle impulse. See HEART BLOCK, NERVE BLOCK, and under SADDLE.

blood: The red, viscid fluid filling and circulating through the heart and blood vessels; supplies nutritive material to, and carries waste away from the body tissues. Consists of plasma, a clear straw-coloured fluid with particles or corpuscles immersed in it. Corpuscles (blood cells) are of two varieties: (1) red (also called *erythrocytes*) are non-nucleated, biconcave dises, present in normal blood in amounts ranging from 4,000,000 to 6,000,000 per cu mm; they transport oxygen from the lungs to

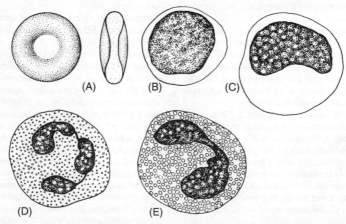

Blood Cells: (a) red cell in full face, and on section, (b) lymphocycle, (c) monocycle, (d) granulocyte with three lobes, (e) granulocyte with two lobes

the tissues and carry carbon dioxide away from the tissues; (2) white cells, or leukocytes, are nucleated, granular, motile cells; the range in normal blood is from 5000 to 10,000 per cu mm with definite percentages of each of several types; they protect the body by destroying invading organisms. Also present are minute cell fragments called platelets or thrombocytes which are important in the clotting mechanism: the normal range is 200,000 to 500,000 per cu mm. ARTERIAL B. aerated blood which carries oxygen to tissues; DEFIBRINATED B. that in which the fibrin has been removed by agitation and which therefore does not clot; LAKED B. that in which the red cells are haemolysed; OCCULT B. that which is not visible; its presence is determined by chemical tests; VENOUS B. that which has transported oxygen to the tissues and has picked up carbon dioxide which is being carried back to the lungs; WHOLE B. that from which none of its elements has been removed.

blood agar: A solid culture medium for certain microorganisms; consists of nutrient agar to which blood has been added.

blood bank: A special laboratory where whole blood or its components are collected, typed, and stored until needed for transfusion.

blood–brain barrier: See BARRIER.

blood buffers: A group of substances consisting chiefly of dissolved carbon dioxide and bicarbonate ions which function in the blood to maintain the proper pH of the blood.

blood casts: Casts that contain red blood corpuscles, formed in the renal tubules and found in the urine in certain kidney diseases.

blood clotting: The mechanism whereby a clot of blood is formed, blocking a bleeding vessel. Bleeding is stopped by the process of haemostasis (*q.v.*): platelets adhere to damaged blood vessels and then to each other, forming a plug that can stop minor bleeding. The platelets release several substances that stimulate vasoconstriction, thereby reducing the blood flow at the injury. Finally, the collecting platelets and damaged tissue initiate the formation of a clot, which is the major defence against bleeding.

blood corpuscles: Blood cells. See BLOOD, ERTHROCYTE, LEUKOCYTE, PLATELET.

blood count: Calculation of the number of red or white cells per cubic millimetre of whole blood, using a haemocytometer. COMPLETE B.C. includes, in addition to numerical and differential count of white cells, a count of red cells and estimates of haemoglobin, haemato-

crit, and platelets in a blood sample; DIFFERENTIAL B.C. an estimate of the relative number of each of the various types of white cells in a cubic millimetre of blood; DIRECT PLATELET COUNT utilizes a counting chamber and microcope to determine the number of platelets in a cubic millimetre of blood.

blood crossmatching: A technique used for determining the compatibility of bloods, done before transfusion. See BLOOD GROUPS.

blood culture: After withdrawal of blood from a vein, it is incubated in a suitable medium, at an optimum temperature, so that any contained organisms can multiply and so be isolated and identified under the microscope. See BACTERAEMIA and SEPTICAEMIA.

blood donor (dō'-nor): An individual who donates some of his blood for use by another, either directly to that person or to a blood bank.

blood gas: Refers to gases normally present in the blood serum; includes oxygen, carbon dioxide, and nitrogen. Determination of the amounts of gases present is an important procedure in evaluating for treatment patients with serious cardiac, respiratory, or kidney failure and other conditions of stress or shock.

blood groups: All human blood has been classified (by Landsteiner) as belonging to one of four groups (also called *types* or *systems*), A, B, AB, and O, the divisions being based on the presence or absence of specific, genetically determined antigens (agglutinogens) located on the surface of the red cells, and of specific antibodies (agglutinins) in the serum. The cells of groups A, B, and AB contain the corresponding agglutinogens (antigens) A, B, and AB; O contains none. The serum of A blood contains anti-B agglutinins; B blood serum contains anti-A agglutinins; O blood serum contains both, and AB contains neither. If incompatible bloods are mixed *e.g.*, A and B, the agglutinins in the serum of one type will cause agglutination (clumping) of the red cells of the other type, and this may lead to a severe, sometimes fatal, reaction in the patient. Since O blood cells contain no agglutinogens, it can safely be given to persons with any type of blood and thus is known as the universal donor. Since AB blood contains no agglutinins, persons with such blood can safely receive A, B, and O blood and thus are known as the universal recipients. In addition to the four groups, Landsteiner and Wiener discovered the Rh (Rhesus) system, which is based on the presence or absence of an hereditary factor known as the Rh

Blood-group systems: examples of antigens and antibodies.

System	Antigens	Antibodies	Antibody type[*]
ABO	A, B, H	anti-A, anti-B	N
Rhesus	C, D, E, c, e	anti-C, -D, -E, -c, -e	I
MNS	M, N, S, s	anti-M, -N, -S	N
P	P, P_1	anti-P_1	N
Lutheran	Lu^a, Lu^b	anti-Lu^a	N & I
Lewis	Le^a, Le^b	anti-Le^a	N
Kell	K, k	anti-K	I
Duffy	Fy^a, Fy^b	anti-Fy^a	I
I	I, i	anti-I	N

[*]N = naturally occurring; I = immune

factor; blood that contains this factor is called Rh-positive and that which does not is called Rh-negative. See RHESUS. Several other systems more recently identified on the basis of the reaction of cells with antibodies include *Auberger*, *Diego*, *Duffy*, *Kell*, *Kidd*, *Lewis*, *Lutheran*, *MNSs*, *P*, *Sutter*, *Xg*.

bloodletting: The removal of blood from a vein for therapeutic purposes, formerly a popular form of treatment.

blood plasma: The liquid portion of whole blood. Composed of over 90% water, 6% to 8% protein substances; mineral salts; nutrients; gases; waste products; clotting agents; antibodies; and hormones.

blood platelets: Small, circular or oval colourless discs found in the circulating blood, averaging about 250,000 in 1 cu mm of blood. Important in the clotting of blood because they release thrombokinase which, in the presence of calcium, reacts with prothrombin to form thrombin. Syn., *thrombocyte*.

blood poisoning: Septicaemia (*q.v.*).

blood pressure: The lateral pressure of the blood against the blood vessel walls as the column of blood is pumped through them; may be measured indirectly by a sphygmomanometer (*q.v.*) or directly by use of a transducer-monitor system. ARTERIAL B.P. that in the arteries; CENTRAL VENOUS P. the blood pressure in the right atrium, obtained through a procedure in which a soft pliable indwelling catheter is introduced into a suitable vein (usually the internal jugular or the subclavian) and threaded into the right atrium, with the distal end attached to a water manometer and an intravenous setup; the readings on the man-

ometer are measures of cardiac competence, atrial pressure, and ventricular functioning, as well as a guide for fluid replacement; DIASTOLIC B.P. the lowest pressure registered on the apparatus when the left ventricle is in a state of relaxation; the normal adult range is likely to be between 60 and 80 mmHg; HIGH B.P. see **hypertension**; SYSTOLIC B.P. the highest point registered on the apparatus when the heart muscle is at the maximum contraction; the normal adult range is likely to be between 110 and 145 mmHg; VENOUS B.P. that in the veins.

blood sedimentation rate: See ERTHROCYTE SEDIMENTATION RATE.

blood serum: The clear fluid which exudes when blood clots; it is plasma minus the clotting agents.

bloodshot: Congestion of blood in the small vessels of a localized area, as occurs, *e.g.*, in the conjunctiva when the small vessels dilate and become visible.

blood smear: A drop of blood, placed on a glass slide and then spread and stained for microscopic examination.

bloodstream, bloodstream: The flowing blood as it is in the body as opposed to blood that has been withdrawn from the body.

blood substitute: A substance such as human plasma, serum albumin, dextran, gum acacia, or gelatine, given by transfusion in cases of haemorrhage or shock.

blood sugar: The amount of glucose, in the circulating blood; expressed in millimoles per litre. The normal range is 3·5–5·5 mmol/l. This level is controlled by various enzymes and hormones, the most important single factor being insulin (*q.v.*). See HYPERGLYCAEMIA and HYPO-GLYCAEMIA.

blood transfusion: The intravenous replacement of lost or destroyed blood by compatible citrated human blood. Also used for severe anaemia with deficient blood production and for treatment of shock or severe infections. Fresh blood from a donor or stored blood from a blood bank may be used. It can be given whole, or with some plasma remove (packed-cell transfusion). If incompatible blood is given, severe reactions follows. See BLOOD GROUPS.

blood types: See BLOOD GROUPS.

blood typing: The determination of an individual's blood group by laboratory tests. See BLOOD GROUPS; CROSSMATCHING.

blood urea: The amount of urea (*q.v.*) in the blood; varies within the normal range of 2·5–6·7 mmol/l. The level is virtually unaffected by the amount of protein in the diet when the kidneys, which are the main organs of excretion of urea, are normal. When they are diseased, the blood urea quickly rises. See URAEMIA.

blood vessels: The tubes which transport the blood throughout the body; arteries, veins, capillaries.

blood volume: The total amount of circulating blood in the body.

blotch: A spot or blemish, or an abnormally pigmented or reddened area on the skin or a membrane.

BLS: Abbreviation for basic life support (*q.v.*).

blue baby: The appearance produced by insufficient oxygen in the blood; may be due to a congenital defect that allows the arterial and venous blood to become mixed. The appearance, by contrast, of a newborn child suffering from temporary anoxia is described as 'blue asphyxia'. B. B. OPERATION a procedure designed to ameliorate the lack of adequate oxygenation of an infant's blood caused by the tetralogy of Fallot (*q.v.*).

blues: Depression; despondency. A colloquialism.

Blumberg's sign: Pain which is produced when the examiner suddenly withdraws pressure on the abdomen; it is indicative of inflammation of the peritoneum.

B lymphocyte (limf' -ō-sīt): A lymphocyte (*q.v.*) that originates in the bone marrow; has antigenic properties; when stimulated by an antigen (*q.v.*.) it differentiates into a plasma cell and produces circulating antibody (*q.v.*).

BMA: Abbreviation for British Medical Association (*q.v.*).

BMI: Abbreviation for body mass index (*q.v.*).

BMR: Abbreviation for basal metabolic rate (*q.v.*).

BN: Abbreviation for Bachelor of Nursing.

BNF: Abbreviation for British National Formulary (*q.v.*).

body: 1. The trunk or frame of a person and the structures it contains, as differentiated from the head and extremities. 2. The largest or principal part of an organ, *e.g.*, the body of the uterus. 3. Any mass of material. B. IMAGE the image in an individual's mind of his or her own body. Distortions of this occur as a result of affective disorders, parietal lobe tumours, or trauma; B. MECHANICS the application of the principles of kinesiology (*q.v.*) to body activities so as to correlate actions of the various parts and thus prevent injuries and problems related to posture; B. TEMPERATURE that of the healthy body; 37°C (98·4°F); CAROTID B. see under CAROTID; CAVERNOUS B. one of the two erectile columns in the dorsum of the penis and in the clitoris; CILIARY B. see under CILIARY; PERINEAL B. see under PERINEAL; VERTEBRAL B. see under VERTEBRAL. For other specific bodies, see under the adjectives.

body dysmorphic disorder (dis mor' -fik): An abnormal preoccupation with a part or the whole of the body, where the individual believes that it is defective or atypical.

body language: The intentional and unintentional messages transmitted wittingly or unwittingly by facial expressions, eye contact, posture, clothing, touching, and body movements; kinesic behaviour; varies with race and culture.

body mass index: A measurement derived from weight and height. This system of measurement is used to determine whether the weight of an adult is within an acceptable range.

Bohr effect: The influence of carbon dioxide on the oxygen dissociation curve (*q.v.*), causing a shift to the right and indicating a reduction in the affinity of haemoglobin for oxygen. [Neils Bohr, Danish physicist, 1885–1962.]

boil: An acute inflammatory condition surrounding a hair follicle; a furuncle.

bolometer (bō-lom' -ēter): 1. An instrument for measuring small differences in the amount of heat radiated from a specific body area or part. 2. An instrument formerly used for measuring the force of the heartbeat as distinguished from the force of the blood in the blood vessels.

boloscope (bō' -lo-skōp): An instrument for locating metallic foreign bodies in tissues.

bolus (bō' -lus): 1. A large pill. 2. A soft, pulpy mass of masticated food ready to swallow.

bombé of the iris (bom′-bā): Forward displacement of the iris, caused by a blockage in the pupil which prevents forward flow of the aqueous humour.

bonding: 1. The unique attachment and unity of two people, most often that between an infant and parent, especially the mother, which endures as a warm, secure relationship throughout life; it is brought about by touching, fondling, speaking, and having eye-to-eye contact. **2.** The attachment of dental restorations, sealants and appliances to teeth.

bone: 1. The hard, connective tissue forming the skeleton. **2.** Any distinct piece of the skeleton. B. TISSUE may be either compact or cancellous. About one-third of the total weight is accounted for by the organic matter of the fibrous tissue and the remaining two-thirds by inorganic mineral matter deposited in it. There are 206 named bones in the body; they make up about one-seventh of the body weight. In children the proportion of organic matter is greater, giving a tendency to bend rather than break; in elderly people the mineral content is in greater proportion, causing the bones to become brittle. Bones are classified according to shape as long, short, flat, irregular and sesamoid. B. CONDUCTION usually refers to conduction of sound waves through the skull to the hearing receptors in the ear by means of a hearing device applied to the exterior of the skull; B. GRAFT transplantation of a piece of healthy bone from one part of the body to another; or from one person to another; used to repair bone defects, afford support, or to supply osteogenic tissue. See CANCELLOUS, COMPACT, BONE MARROW. — bony, adj.

bone marrow: The highly vascular, soft, pulpy, network of reticular tissue that fills the cavities of most bones. RED MARROW found in the articular ends of long bones and in the cancellous parts of flat and short bones, bodies of the vertebrae, the cranial diploë, and the sternum and ribs. The main function of red marrow is the development of erythrocytes and granular leukocytes (eosinophils, basophils, and neutrophils). Blood platelets are also formed in the red marrow by fragmentation of large cells known as megakaryocytes. YELLOW MARROW consists mostly of fatty connective tissue; it is found in the medullary cavities of the long bones, the femur and humerus in particular.

bone marrow aspiration: The withdrawal, by special needle, of a specimen of bone marrow for diagnostic purposes; usually utilizes the sternum.

bone marrow depression: Decreased or diminished production and maturation of erythrocytes and granulocytes.

bone marrow transplant: The transplantation of bone marrow from a healthy donor into the bloodstream of another; if successful, it starts producing healthy blood cells; may be used in treatment of aplastic anaemia.

Bonnevie Ullrich syndrome (bon′-vē-ul′-rik): Gonadal dysgenesis. A chromosomal disorder resulting in short stature, webbed neck, facial and other bodily deformities, cardiac anomalies, lymphoedema of the hands and feet, sexual infantilism. Also called *Turner's syndrome.*

booster dose: A later dose given to enhance the effect of an initial or previous dose; usually applied to antigens given for the purpose of producing specific antibodies.

boot: 1. A covering for the foot. **2.** A boot-shaped appliance. UNNA'S PASTE BOOT see UNNA'S BOOT.

boot therapy: Refers to the application of a plastic boot which is inflated intermittently; used to prevent postoperative thrombophlebitis.

borax (bor′-aks): A compound of boron, found in certain arid areas; chief use is as a water softener and detergent; it has mild antiseptic properties.

borborygmus (bor-bo-rig′-mus): Rumbling or gurgling noises caused by the movement of flatus in the intestines. — borborygmi, adj.

Bordetella pertussis (bor-de-tel′-la-pertus′-is): The organism that causes whooping cough. See PERTUSSIS.

boric acid (bor′-ik): A common mild antiseptic, used in the form of a solution, ointment, or powder for surface application to skin and mucous membranes of the eye, ear, nose, bladder, etc. Serious and fatal accidents have occurred from internal use or accidental poisoning. Also called *boracic acid.*

Bornholm disease: Epidemic pleurodynia (*q.v.*); probably caused by coxsackie B virus through contact infection. Symptoms include severe diaphragmatic pain, fever. Also called *epidemic myalgia.* See FIBROSITIS.

boss: 1. A rounded projection or eminence as on a bone or tumour; also called *bossing.* **2.** The projection of the spine in kyphosis (*q.v.*).

bosselated (bos′-sel-ā-ted): Having knob-like protrusions.

botryoid (bot′-rē-oid): Like a bunch of grapes in appearance.

botulin (bot′-ū-lin): A very active neurotoxin that affects the nervous system; sometimes found in imperfectly preserved or canned non-acid vegetables or meat, such as sausage; causes botulism (*q.v.*); is produced by an anaerobic organism *Clostridium botulinum*, widely distributed in soil and the intestines of domestic animals.

botulism (bot'ū-lizm): A severe type of food poisoning caused by botulin (*q.v.*). Characterized by sudden onset, vomiting, abdominal pain, malaise, dry mouth, dizziness, muscular weakness, cyanosis and ocular and pharyngeal paralysis, within 24 to 72 hours after eating improperly canned or smoked food that has been contaminated by *Clostridium botulinum*. Often fatal due to respiratory failure.

bouba (boo'-ba): Yaws (*q.v.*).

bougie (boo'-zhē): A flexible, slender cylindrical instrument of varying sizes, shapes and materials: used to explore or dilate a canal such as the anus, urethra, or oesophagus, to dilate a stricture of a canal or structure such as the cardiac sphincter, to induce labour, or as a guide for the passage of other instruments.

bouton (boo-ton'): A button; pustule; knob-like swelling or nodule.

boutonnière deformity (boo-ton-yair'): A finger deformity in which the proximal interphalangeal joint is flexed and the distal joint is hyperextended. Also called *buttonhole deformity*.

bovine (bo-vīn'): Relating to the cow or ox. The bovine type of the tubercle bacillus (*Mycobacterium tuberculosis*) may infect the bones, glands, and joints in human beings.

bovine spongiform encephalopathy: A transmissible, neurodegenerative, fatal brain disease of cattle. The disease has a long incubation period of four to five years, but ultimately is fatal for cattle within weeks to months of its onset. BSE first came to the attention of the scientific community in the United Kingdom in November 1986, with the appearance in cattle of a newly recognized form of neurological disease. See CREUTZFELDT-JAKOB DISEASE.

bowel (bow'-el): The intestine; the gut. SMALL B. the first 7 m of the intestine; the first 25 cm of which is the duodenum; the next two-fifths is the jejunum and the following three-fifths the ileum. LARGE B. measures 78 cm in length but is larger in diameter than the small intestine and has other distinguishing features such as the structure of its lining membrane. See COLON.

bowel sounds: Heard on auscultation over the abdomen; caused by air mixing with fluid during peristalsis; those heard in the small intestine are high pitched and gurgling while those in the large intestine are lower in pitch and rumbling; their intensity is an indication of peristaltic activity and strength.

bowleg: The outward curving or arching of the leg, or both legs, at and/or below the knee; genu varum.

Bowman's capsule: The expanded beginning of a renal tubule in the kidney. It and the tuft of capillaries that it surrounds make up a malpighian corpuscle.

Boyle's law: At any stated temperature, a given mass of gas varies in volume inversely in proportion to the pressure exerted upon it. [Robert Boyle, English physicist, 1627–1691.]

BP: Abbreviation for **1.** Blood pressure (*q.v.*). **2.** British Pharmacopoeia (*q.v.*).

brace: An orthopaedic appliance used to support a part of the body or to keep it in proper position for functioning.

brachi-, brachio-: Combining forms denoting the arm.

brachial (brā'-ki-al): Relating to the arm. Applied to vessels in this region and to a nerve plexus at the root of the neck; see BRACHIAL PLEXUS under PLEXUS. B. BIRTH PALSY paralysis of the arm due to injury to the brachial plexus during delivery.

brachialis (brē-ki-al'-is): A muscle of the anterior part of the upper arm; it lies immediately under the biceps brachii; acts to flex the forearm.

brachy-: Combining form denoting short, shortness.

brachycardia (brak-i-kar'-di-a): See BRADYCARDIA.

brachycephalic (brak-ē-ke-fal'-ik, se-fal'-ik): Having a short, wide head.—brachycephalia, n.

brachydactylia (brak-i-dak-til'-i-a): Abnormal shortness of the fingers and toes, a congenital anomaly. Also called *brachydactyly*.

brachygnathia (brak-i-nā'-thi-a): A congenital anomaly consisting of abnormal shortness of the mandible; a receding lower jaw.

brachymetropia (brak-i-mē-trō'-pi-a): Myopia (*q.v.*).

brachytherapy (brak-i-ther'-a'pi): Radiation therapy with the source of radiation being close to or on the surface of the area being treated.

Bradford frame: A canvas and metal device used for immobilizing the spine or pelvis, resting the trunk or back muscles, or preventing deformity in patients with certain fractures, dislocations or diseases of the spinal or pelvic bones. Consists of a tubular steel frame with two canvas slings allowing a 10–15 centimetre gap to facilitate use of the bedpan. [Edward H. Bradford, American orthopaedic surgeon, 1848–1926.]

Bradley method: A method of childbirth preparation consisting of antenatal education in physiological changes and of breathing exercises to promote relaxation during labour; involves both prospective parents.

brady-: Combining form denoting: (1) slow; (2) dull.

bradyacusia (brad-i-a-kū'-zi-a): Diminished perception of sound; dullness of hearing.

bradyaesthesia (brad-i-es-thē'-zi-a): Abnormal slowness of transmission of sensory impulses or dullness of perception of sensory input.

bradyarrhythmia (brad'-i-ar-rith'-mi-a): Bradycardia (*q.v.*).

bradyarthria (brad-i-ar'-thri-a): Abnormally slow enunciation of words.

bradycardia (brad-i-kar'-di-a): Abnormally slow rate of heart contraction, resulting in a pulse rate of less than 60 beats per minute in an adult, 70 in a child, or 120 in a fetus. In febrile states the expected increase in pulse rate is 10 beats per minute for each degree of rise in body temperature; when the pulse rate does not increase, the condition is called RELATIVE B.; SINUS B. a slow heartbeat which originates in the normal sinus pacemaker; often occurs after a myocardial infarction with reduction of the oxygen needs of the myocardium.

bradycardia–tachycardia syndrome: Arrhythmic heart action in which episodes of sinus bradycardia alternate with tachycardia; usually due to pathology of the sinus node. Also called *sick sinus syndrome* and *bradytachy syndrome*.

bradykinesia (brad-i-kī-nē'-si-a): Excessive slowness of voluntary movement and speech; a characteristic of parkinsonism and certain other nervous system disorders.

bradykinin (brad-i-kī'nin): A polypeptide formed in the blood plasma; it has vasomotor action, increases the permeability of capillary walls, and contributes to the formation of oedema.

bradyphasia (brad-i-fā'-zi-a): A form of aphasia characterized by slow utterance of speech; bradylalia.

bradypnoea (brad-ip-nē'-a): Abnormal slowness of breathing: often the result of central nervous system depression.

bradystalsis (brad-i-stal'-sis): Abnormal slowness of peristaltic movement.

Braille (brāl): A kind of writing and printing used for the blind; the letters are made up of raised points or dots that the blind person can feel.

brain: The encephalon: that part of the central nervous system contained in the cranial cavity. It consists of the cerebrum, cerebellum, pons varolii, midbrain, and medulla oblongata. B. CENTRE a group of nerve cells in a circumscribed area that is concerned with the regulation of a certain function, *e.g.*, sight, hearing, speech, etc.; B. TUMOUR see MENINGIOMA; B. WAVES see under WAVE.

brain case: The part of the skull that encloses the brain.

brain concussion: Injury to the tissues of the brain due to trauma such as a violent blow. See CONCUSSION.

brain death: Occurs when all the brain function is completely and irreversibly destroyed, as demonstrated by a 'flat' electroencephalogram and lack of brain stem and other reflexes; may result from prolonged anoxia, intracranial haemorrhage, severe head injury. See also under DEATH.

brain scan: A painless diagnostic procedure in which radioisotopes administered intravenously circulate through the brain where they can be traced and photographed by a scanner (*q.v.*); a useful technique for locating and identifying tumours or other brain lesions.

brain stem: All of the brain except the cerebrum and the cerebellum *i.e.*, the midbrain, the pons varolli, and the medulla oblongata. It extends from the cerebral hemispheres through the foramen magnum and continues as the spinal cord; contains nuclei that affect respiration, blood pressure, the heart rate, coughing, swallowing, vomiting and wakefulness.

brainstorming (brān-stor-ming): The spontaneous expression of ideas or thoughts by people meeting in a group without having previously considered the advantages, disadvantages, consequences, or practicality of the ideas or thoughts.

brainwashing: A kind of mental conditioning in which stress and mental torture are used to force a captive person to accept a set of beliefs that are contrary to his former beliefs but in accord with those of his captor.

bran The husk of grain. The coarse outer part of cereals, especially wheat; high in roughage and the vitamin B complex.

branchial (bran'-ki-al): 1. Relating to gills. 2. Relating to the fissures or clefts which occur on each side of the neck of the human embryo, and which enter into the development of the nose, ears, and mouth; B. CYST a swelling in the neck arising from the embryonic remnants of a branchial cleft.

brash: 1. A burning sensation in the stomach caused by excessive acidity and often accompanied by belching of sour, burning fluid. Syn., *heartburn, pyrosis, water brash.* **2.** An attack of illness. **3.** The appearance of a rash or eruption.

Braxton–Hicks contractions: Intermittent contractions of the uterus during pregnancy; painless but can be felt after about the 16th week; they occur about every 15 or 20 minutes, and are not labour pains. Also called *Braxton–Hicks sign, Hicks sign.*

breach of duty: A legal term denoting behaviour that is not considered 'reasonable'. In nursing it usually means that a patient was injured or harmed in some way by something that the nurse did, *e.g.*, causing someone to be burned by a too hot-water bottle.

break-bone fever: See DENGUE.

breast: The anterior part of the thorax; the mammary gland. B. AMPUTATION mastectomy (*q.v.*); B. BONE the sternum; B. PROTHESIS utilized following mastectomy; may be made of foam or filled with air, liquid, or silicone; B. PUMP a hand operated or electric device for withdrawing milk from the female breast; B. RECONSTRUCTION possible following some operations for breast removal; done to remove scar, replace the nipple and areola, or to introduce a Silastic implant to replace removed breast tissue; FUNNEL B. deformity caused by abnormal depression of the sternum; PIGEON B. deformity resulting from prominent sternum, often caused by rickets.

breast awareness: A woman examining her breasts visually for changes in appearance. Self-examination technique taught as part of health prevention programmes.

breast care nurse: A nurse who specializes in the care of women with breast cancer or a family history of breast cancer.

breast screening: The screening of individuals for the presence of breast cancer, by taking mammograms of the breast. In the UK breast screening is offered to women aged 50–70 years. See MAMMOGRAPHY.

breath: The air inhaled and exhaled during respiration. B. HOLDING a phenomenon seen in young children, usually precipitated by anger, fear, or frustration; the child becomes cyanotic and sometimes loses consciousness briefly and breathing is resumed automatically.

Breathalyser (brēth′-a-lī-zer): An instrument used for analysing a person's breath to determine whether the person has imbibed alcohol within a certain period of time, and how much. B. TEST measures expired air to determine the blood alcohol level in percent by weight.

breathe: The act of alternately inhaling air into and exhaling air from the lungs.

breathing (brēth′ing): The alternate inhalation and exhalation of air to and from the lungs. APNEUISTIC B., B. characterized by long inspirations; occurs in severe hypoxia, hypoglycaemia, meningitis; ASTHMATIC B. a harsh breathing accompanied by a wheezing sound, especially on expiration; BIOT'S B., B. in a random pattern of deep and shallow respirations occurring irregularly; CLUSTER B., B. characterized by clusters of breaths occurring in a disorderly fashion with pauses between the clusters; COGWHEEL B. jerky B.; CONTINUOUS POSITIVE PRESSURE B., B. that is assisted by a ventilator that administers air or a mixture of gases under continuous positive pressure which fluctuates to permit air to flow into and out of the lungs; also called *continuous positive pressure ventilation*; DIAPHRAGMATIC B. that accomplished chiefly by movements of the diaphragm; also called *abdominal* B., EUPNIC B. free easy breathing; the type observed in normal persons at rest; GLOSSOPHARYNGEAL B., B. accomplished by gulping air rapidly and using the tongue and muscles of the pharynx to force the air into the respiratory tract; neither the main muscles of respiration nor the accessory muscles are involved; also called *frog* B. INTERMITTENT POSITIVE PRESSURE B., B. with the assistance of a respirator that administers air or a mixture of gases under positive pressure during inspiration until a preset pressure is reached; also called *intermittent positive pressure ventilation*; PARADOXICAL B. seen after severe chest injury; the injured part bulges during exhalation and is sucked in during inspiration; see FLAIL CHEST; PERIODIC B. see CHEYNE–STOKES RESPIRATION under RESPIRATION; POSITIVE PRESSURE B. the breathing of air or oxygen that is under a constant pressure relative to the ambient pressure; PURSED-LIP B. exhaling slowly through the mouth with the lips 'pursed' as for whistling; it prolongs the exhalation, increases the pressure in the airway, less air is trapped in the alveoli, and more carbon dioxide is eliminated; STERTOROUS B. characterized by a snoring sound on expiration.

breathlessness (breth′-les-nes): **1.** Not breathing. **2.** Panting or gasping for one's breath. **3.** Holding one's breath when deeply disturbed emotionally. PSYCHOGENIC B. abnormal or bizarre breathing patterns; seen in the elderly or the demented.

breath sounds: Sounds of air going in and out of the lungs that can be heard with a stethoscope during respiration; AMPHORIC B.S. harsh, high pitched sounds heard in open pneumothorax; ASTHMATIC B.S. characterized by short gasping inspirations and prolonged expirations; high-pitched and wheezing due to narrowing of the airway; BRONCHIAL B.S. high pitched, loud hollow sounds heard over the trachea in the presence of atelectasis and pleural effusion; BRONCHOVESICULAR B.S. blowing sounds of moderate pitch and loudness heard over the scapulae in the back; CAVERNOUS B.S. resemble amphoric B.S., but the sounds are low pitched and hollow; VESICULAR B.S. originate in the alveoli and can be heard over the normal lung.

breath test: A test performed on a person's breath to determine whether he is alcoholically intoxicated. See BREATHALYSER.

breech (brēch): The buttocks (q.v.) B. PRESENTATION the position of the fetus during labour in which the buttocks instead of the head is present at the uterine orifice.

Brennerman's ulcers: Ulceration of the urinary meatus in the male. Seen primarily in boys in whom the foreskin has been removed by circumcision, leaving the area open to infection.

Brenner tumour: A tumour of the ovary; may be solid or cystic and contain groups of epithelial cells and connective tissue stroma; usually benign.

bridge: A structure that joins two parts or organs. In dentistry, a device bearing one or more artificial teeth which is anchored to the natural teeth. B. OF NOSE the upper part of the external nose, formed by union of the nasal bones.

bridging: Providing relief from pressure by suspending the affected area while supporting the surrounding areas.

Bright's disease: Inflammation of the kidney; nephritis. Term formerly often used to describe glomerulonephritis and other kidney diseases marked by proteinuria. [Richard Bright, English physician, 1798–1858.]

brilliant green: An analine dye that is used as (1) a topical antiseptic and bacteriostatic, or (2) an indicator dye that changes from yellow to green when the pH of the substance is below pH 2.6.

brim: The edge or margin of a part. B. OF THE PELVIS the bony ring that divides the true from the false pelvis.

brisement (brēz'-mon): A crushing; refers particularly to the breaking up by force of the adhesions in ankylosis.

British Association of Counselling and Psychotherapy: The UK professional membership association for Counsellors and Psychotherapists. Abbreviated BACP.

British Association of Occupational Therapists: The professional, educational and trade union organization for occupational therapists and support staff in the UK. Abbreviated BAOT.

British Medical Association: An independent trade union representing all doctors from all branches of medicine throughout the UK, for negotiation on pay and conditions. Abbreviated BMA.

British National Formulary (for'-mū-la-ri): Details of the majority of drugs available on prescription in the United Kingdom, published twice a year by the British Medical Association and The Pharmaceutical Society of Great Britain. Abbreviated BNF.

British Pharmacopoeia (far'-ma-kō-pē'-a): A list of 'official' drugs published regularly by HMSO (q.v.) on behalf of the Department of Health. The drugs included are listed according to the recommendations of the Medicines Commission.

British thermal unit: See BTU.

brittle bones: See OSTEOGENESIS IMPERFECTA.

broad ligament: Lateral ligament; double fold of parietal peritoneum which hangs over the uterus and outstretched uterine tubes, forming a lateral partition across the pelvic cavity.

broad-spectrum: A term used to describe an agent, particularly an antibiotic, that is effective against a wide variety of microorganisms.

Broca's area (brok'-a): The motor centre for speech; situated at the commencement of the sylvanian fissure in the left hemisphere of the cerebrum. Injury to this centre results in inability to speak. [Pierre Paul Broca, French surgeon, 1824–1880.]

Brock's operation: An operation for the relief of pulmonary valve stenosis.

Brodie's abscess: See under ABSCESS.

bromides (brō'-mīdz): A small group of drugs, compounds of bromine and another element, that have a mild depressant action on the central nervous system; elimination is slow and the drug accumulates in the body causing a toxic condition marked by skin eruptions and mental disturbances; once used extensively as a sedative and in treatment of certain forms of epilepsy but now replaced by agents with less objectionable side effects.

bromine (brō'-mēn): A non-metallic volatile, reddish liquid element; unites with hydrogen to form hydrobromic acid which combines with many metals to form bromides.

bromoderma (brō-mō-der'-ma): Skin eruption resembling acne, caused by use of bromine or its compounds. NODOSE B. the occurrence of nodular lesions on the legs in association with bromoderma.

bromomania (brō'-mō-mā'-ni-a): Psychosis or delirium caused by overuse of bromides.

Brompton's cocktail: A analgesic mixture given on a regular basis to patients with advanced cancer to relieve pain that cannot be controlled by ordinary analgesics without clouding the sensorium. The original recipe called for heroin, cocaine, chloroform water, and ethanol; today it is usually simply an elixir of morphine, and has largely been superseded by slower-release morphines.

Bromsulphalein (brōm-sul'-fa-lē-in): A preparation of sulphobromophthalein, a dye used in liver-function tests; it is injected intravenously. Normally 80% of the dye is removed by the liver and the rest by other organs; in pathological conditions, when the liver is not functioning properly, it removes less of the dye, which then remains in the blood.

bronch-, bronchi-, bronchio-, broncho-: Combining forms denoting: (1) bronchus; (2) bronchiole.

bronchial (bron'-ki-al): Relating to or affecting the bronchi, B. ASTHMA see under ASTHMA; B. BREATH SOUNDS see under BREATH SOUNDS; B. HYGIENE the maintenance of a clear airway and removal of secretions from the tracheobronchial tree; B. PNEUMONIA see BRONCHOPNEUMONIA; B. TREE the bronchi and all their branching structures; B. TUBES subdivisions of the bronchi after they enter the lungs.

bronchiectasis (bron-ki-ek'-ta-sis): Chronic dilatation of the bronchioles; the alveolar sacs become dilated and filled with large quantities of offensive pus. Characterized by productive cough, expectoration of mucopurulent material, fetid breath, and enlargement of the air passages. Usually follows such infection as bronchopneumonia with lobular collapse, which may have occurred in infancy. May lead to greatly limited ventilatory capacity and recurrent infection of the lungs, lung abscess, or amyloid disease. Also called *bronchiectasia*. — bronchiectatic, adj.

bronchiocele (bron'-ki-ō-sēl): A circumscribed area of dilatation in a bronchiole. Bronchocele.

bronchiole (bron'-ki-ōl): One of the minute subdivisions of the bronchi which terminate in the alveoli or air sacs of the lungs. — bronchiolar, adj.

bronchiolectasis (bron-ki-ō-lek'-ta-sis): Dilatation of the bronchioles.

bronchiolitis (bron-ki-ō-lī'-tis): An acute infection of the lower respiratory tract, usually caused by a parainfluenza virus or respiratory syncytial virus, may be extremely serious in children under three, but in older children the symptoms are usually those of a simple cold. It is spread by contact and by air-borne particles. B. OBLITERANS a complication of inhalation of smoke or other irritating fumes; exudate that forms in the bronchioles obliterates the lumen, resulting in chest pain, unproductive cough, shortness of breath; may be fatal due to respiratory insufficiency. Also called *capillary bronchitis* and *bronchopneumonia*. — bronchiolitic, adj.

bronchiolus (bron-ki-ō'-lus): One of the smaller subdivisions of the bronchus. — bronchioli, pl. Syn., *bronchiole*.

bronchitis (bron-kī'-tis): Inflammation of the bronchial mucous membrane; may be primary or secondary, acute or chronic. ACUTE B. occurs chiefly in young children or elderly persons; usually an extension of infection following a common cold, upper respiratory infection, measles, or influenza. ACUTE LARYNGEAL B. a form of winter croup that resembles diptheria except that no membrane forms; occurs chiefly in infants under one year of age. ASTHMATIC B. symptoms of asthma associated with an apparent bronchial infection. CHRONIC B. occurs chiefly in older persons; may follow acute B. develop gradually, or be secondary to another condition such as sinusitis, or to cigarette smoking; tends to recur and to be worse in cold, foggy weather; can cause right-sided heart failure, especially when associated with gross emphysema. See COR PULMONALE. — bronchitic, adj.

bronchocele (bron'-kō-sēl): **1.** A circumscribed swelling or dilatation of a bronchus. **2.** A goitre.

bronchoconstriction (bron'-kō-kon-strik'-shun): Bronchostenosis (*q.v.*).

bronchoconstrictor (bron'-kō-kon-strik'-tor): Any agent that causes constriction of the bronchi, thus decreasing the calibre of the pulmonary air passages.

bronchodilator (bron-kō-dī'-lā-tor): Any agent or surgical instrument that is used to dilate the bronchi, thus increasing the calibre of the pulmonary air passages.

bronchofibrescope (bron-kō-fi'-ber-scōp): A specially designed fibrescope for visualization of the trachea and the bronchi.

bronchogenic (bron-kō-jen'-ik): Arising from a bronchus. B. CARCINOMA any of several types of carcinoma that arise in the bronchi.

bronchogram (bron´-kō-gram): Radiological picture of the bronchial tree after the introduction of a radiopaque material.

bronchography (bron-kog´-raf-i): Preparation of x-ray film after introduction of radiopaque substance into the bronchial tree. — bronchographic, adj.; bronchographically, adv.

broncholith (bron´-kō-lith): A stone or concretion in a bronchus or bronchial tube.

bronchomalacia (bron´-kō-ma-lā´shi-a): Softening and degeneration of the elastic and connective tissues of the trachea and bronchi; the condition may be congenital or acquired, and may result eventually in obstructive emphysema or atelectasis.

bronchomycosis (bron-kō-mī-kō´-sis): General term used to cover a variety of fungus infections of the bronchi and lungs, *e.g.*, pulmonary candidiasis, aspergillosis. — bronchomycotic, adj.

broncophony (bron-kof´-o-ni): Abnormal voice sounds as heard through the stethoscope when applied over consolidated lung tissue. See also PECTORILOQUY.

bronchopneumonia (bron´-kō-nū-mō´-ni-a): Inflammation of the bronchi and lungs; small areas of the lungs are consolidated and coalesce but do not have a lobular distribution; usually begins at the termini of bronchioles and alveoli and spreads throughout the lungs. Caused by a number of microorganisms, including *Streptococcus pneumoniae, Staphylococcus pyogenes,* and *Mycoplasma pneumoniae*; may occur as a primary infection in infants and the aged, in whom it is relatively common, but may also be secondary to measles, whooping cough, upper respiratory infections, and debilitating diseases; may also result from inhalation of noxious gases or dusts or from aspiration of infected material from the respiratory or gastrointestinal tract; in young children the cause is often the respiratory syncytical virus (*q.v.*). Symptoms include chest pain, cough with purulent (sometimes bloody) sputum, chills, fever; high pulse and respiration rates; weakness. Complications include pulmonary abscess, empyema, peripheral thrombosis, jaundice, congestive heart failure. Also called *lobular pneumonia, bronchial pneumonia, bronchiolitis,* and *bronchioalveolitis.*

bronchopulmonary (bron-kō-pul´-mō-nar-i): Relating to the bronchi and the lungs. B. DYSPLASIA a condition that exists throughout life in persons who received oxygen therapy as infants; lungs are overinflated, areas of the lobes are emphysemic, and there is damage to bronchioles and alveoli.

bronchorrhagia (bron-kō-rā´-ji-a): Haemorrhage from the bronchi; see HAEMOPTYSIS.

bronchoscope (bron´-kō-skōp): A curved, lighted, flexible endoscope (*q.v.*) used for examining the interior of the bronchi, removing a foreign body, or taking a specimen for biopsy, etc. — bronchoscopy, n.; bronchoscopic, adj.; bronchoscopically, adv.

bronchoscopy (bron-kos´-kō-pi): Direct visualisation of the bronchi with a bronchoscope. Most often done for patients with persistent cough, wheezing, haemoptysis, or with signs of tumour; for viewing or removing an obstruction; to create an airway; or to obtain material for biopsy. FIBRE-OPTIC B. can be done at the bedside using a local anaesthetic; RIGID B. utilizes a rigid scope; is done in the operating room under general anaesthesia.

bronchospasm (bron´-kō-spazm): Sudden, temporary constriction of the bronchial tubes due to contraction of involuntary plain muscle in their walls; the chief characteristic of asthma and bronchitis.

bronchospirometer (bron´-kō-spī-rom-e-ter): An instrument used to measure the oxygen intake and carbon dioxide output of a lung, or of each lung separately. — bronchospirometric, adj.; bronchospirometry, n.

bronchostenosis (bron-kō-ste-nō´-sis): Narrowing of a bronchus. — bronchostenotic, adj.

bronchostomy (bron-kos´-to-mi): The surgical procedure of creating an opening through the chest wall into a bronchus.

bronchus (bron´-kus): One of the two tubes into which the trachea divides; each tube enters a lung, where it divides and subdivides. The bronchi serve as passageways for air going into and out of the lungs; they are made up of three coats – an outer fibrous coat, a middle coat of smooth muscle, and an inner coat of ciliated mucous membrane.—bronchi, pl.; bronchial, adj.

Brooke formula: A widely used formula for estimating the amount of fluid to be replaced during the first 24 hours of therapy for patients with burns of up to 50% of body surface area. It calls for: (1) lactated Ringer's solution, 1.5 ml per kg of body weight per percent of body area burned; (2) colloid (blood, dextran, plasma), 0.5 ml per kg of body weight per percent of area burned; and (3) water (glucose in water), the amount dependent on weight and size of the patient (2000 ml for an adult). One-half of the patient's estimated requirement for the first 24 hours is given during the first eight hours and one-quarter during each of the two following eight-hour periods.

Brothers Hospitallers of St. John of God: A religious order founded in Spain in 1538 and spread throughout the world; members were chiefly interested in caring for the mentally ill, but cared for other patients as well; established and maintained hospitals wherever they worked.

brow: The forehead; the region of the supraorbital ridge. B. PRESENTATION the position of the fetus during labour in which the brow presents at the uterine orifice making normal delivery almost impossible.

brown atrophy: Descriptive of changes in the myocardium of ageing patients; there is loss of heart weight and infiltration of the muscle cells by lipofuscin (*q.v.*); may or may not be significant.

brown fat: A mass of tissue in the neck and scapular region of the newborn; its function is thought to be the storage of fat and formation of blood. Also called *interscapular gland*.

Brown–Séquard's syndrome: Hemiplegia caused by damage to a lateral half of the spinal cord; associated with ipsilateral motor paralysis, loss of joint and tendon sensation, decreased tactile determination, contralateral anaesthesia, and loss of temperature sense.

Brucella (broo-sel'-la): A genus of bacteria causing brucellosis (undulant fever in humans; contagious abortion in cattle). B. ABORTIS is the bovine strain, B. MELITENSIS, the goat strain; both transmissible to humans via infected milk. B. SUIS a species of B. found in swine; capable of producing severe infection in humans; B. TEST a test for undulant fever.

Brucellaceae (broo-sel-lā'-sē-ē): A large family of rodshaped, Gram-negative bacteria that are pathogenic to humans and other animals; includes *Brucella, Bordetella, Francisella, Haemophilus,* and *Pasteurella*.

brucelliasis (broo-sel-lī'-a-sis): Infection with the *Brucella* group of organisms; brucellosis.

brucellosis (broo-sel-lō'-sis): A generalized acute or chronic infection of animals and humans; caused by one of the species of *Brucella*; rarely transmitted from person to person but spreads from animal to animal and from animal to humans. In humans, characterized by recurrent attacks of fever and mental depression, headache, malaise, anorexia, weight loss, weakness, sweating, constipation, muscle and joint pain, splenomegaly. Complications include pneumonia, arthritis, endocarditis, peripheral neuritis, cirrhosis of the liver, cystitis.

Bruce treadmill test: An exercise to assess the patient's tolerance for increased exercise or physical activity after myocardial infarction; consists of walking on a slowly moving, slightly tilted treadmill which gradually goes faster; the patient is attached to an electrocardiograph machine that measures and records blood pressure at the various speeds.

Brudzinski's sign: Either of two reflexes seen in patients with meningitis. 1. Neck sign; immediate flexion of knees and hips on raising head from pillow. 2. Leg sign; when one leg is flexed onto the abdomen, the other knee and leg tend to flex also. [Josef von Brudzinski, Polish physician, 1874–1917.]

bruise (brooz): A discoloration of the skin due to an extravasation of blood into the underlying tissues; caused by an impact injury; there is no abrasion of the skin A contusion.

bruit (broo'-ē): An extracardiac diagnostically important whooshing sound heard on auscultation over a blood vessel, gland, or organ When heard over an artery it is produced by the passage of blood over an irregular surface or through a narrowed portion of the vessel; when heard over the aorta it may indicate the presence of an aneurysm; when heard over the abdomen it may indicate a constricted or dilated vessel. DIASTOLIC B. a B. heard after the second heart sound; usually indicates abnormal valve function; SYSTOLIC B. a B. heard between the first and second sounds during the systolic phase of the cardiac cycle.

Brunner's glands: Compound glands in the submucous layer of the duodenal wall.

Brun's syndrome: Paroxysmal headache, with visual symptoms, vertigo, vomiting, and sometimes syncope, when the position of the head is suddenly changed; one cause is thought to be a lesion in the third or fourth ventricle of the brain which interferes with the flow of cerebrospinal fluid.

bruxism (bruks'-izm): Grinding of the teeth, especially during sleep.

BS 5750: A British standard specifying the requirements for a quality management system (*q.v.*) overseeing the production of a product or service.

BSc: Abbreviation for Bachelor of Science.

BSE: Abbreviation for bovine spongiform encephalopathy (*q.v.*).

BTU: Abbreviation for British thermal unit; the amount of heat required to raise the temperature of one pound of water by one degree Fahrenheit.

bubo (bū'-bo): An inflammatory swelling of a lymph node, especially in the groin or axilla, due to absorption of infective material, often proceeding to suppuration. A feature of soft sore (chancroid), lymphogranuloma, inguinale, and plague. — bubonic, adj.

bubonalgia (bū-bō-nal'-ji-a): Pain in the groin or inguinal region.

bubonic plague (bū-bon'-ik plāg): An acute, infectious, frequently fatal disease caused by *Yersinia pestis* which is carried in infected rats and transmitted to humans by the bite of rat fleas; characterized by chills, fever, and formation of buboes. This was the Black Death of the Middle Ages. See PLAGUE.

bubonocele (bū-bon'-o-sēl): An inguinal hernia, particularly one in which the knuckle of intestine has not yet pushed through the external abdominal ring.

bucardia (bū-kar'-di-a): Extreme enlargement of the heart.

bucca (buk'-a): The cheek.

buccal (buk'-al): Relating to the cheek or mouth. B. ADMINISTRATION administration of a medication by placing it in the cheek and allowing absorption of it through the oral mucosa; B. CAVITY the part of the oral cavity between the inner surface of the cheek and the teeth; B. SMEAR see under SMEAR.

buccula (buk'-ū-la): Double chin.

bucking: An informal term referring to gagging on an endotracheal tube.

bud: In anatomy, a small protuberance on a part resembling the bud of a plant. TASTE B. one of the many end organs for the sense of taste; minute flask-shaped structures located on the tongue, the surface of the soft palate, and posterior part of the epiglottis; contain specialized epithelial cells and fibrils of the nerves of taste.

budding (bud'-ing): Asexual reproduction by division into two unequal parts.

Buerger–Allen exercise: Buerger's exercise (*q.v.*) plus active exercise of the feet.

Buerger's exercise: Designed to treat arterial insufficiency of the lower limbs; consists of alternate elevation and dependence of the legs; a rest period, and then repetition of the exercise. [Leo Buerger, American physician, 1879–1943.]

buffalo hump: A deposit of fatty tissue in the interscapular area; seen in persons with Cushing's syndrome. Informal.

buffer: 1. A chemical substance which, when present in a solution, causes resistance to pH (*q.v.*) change when acids or alkalis are added. Sodium bicarbonate is one of the chief buffers

of the blood and tissue fluids. **2.** A substance that tends to offset the reaction of another agent when given in conjunction with it. B. SYSTEM in the blood, keeps the pH of the blood serum at normal levels, chiefly by the actions of bicarbonate ions and dissolved carbon dioxide on each other.

bulb: 1. A rounded, globular part of a vessel or tube. **2.** Old name for the medulla oblongata. OLFACTORY B. the bulbous end of each olfactory tract; situated on the underside of the anterior lobe of the cerebrum, one on each side of the longitudinal fissure; VESTIBULAR B. the paired masses of erectile tissue at each side of the vaginal opening, joined by a thin strand below the clitoris.

bulbar (bul-bar): **1.** Relating to a bulbous structure. **2.** Relating to the medulla oblongata.

bulbitis (bul-bī-tis): Inflammation of the bulbous part of the urethra.

bulbocavernosis (bul'-bō-kav-er-nō'-sis): One of the muscles of the female pelvic floor; extends from the perineum to the clitoris, one on each side.

bulbourethral (bul-bō-ū-rē'-thral): Applied to two racemose glands (Cowper's) which open into the bulb of the male urethra.

bulbous (bul'-bus): Resembling a bulb.

bulimia (bū-lim'-i-a): Insatiable appetite or hunger, usually experienced soon after a meal; seen in some cerebral lesions, diabetes mellitus and psychotic states. B. NERVOSA refers to the uncontrollable urge to overeat followed by induced vomiting or purging.

bulkage (bulk'-ij): A material such as agar which increases the volume of the intestinal content, thereby stimulating peristalsis.

bulla (bul'la): A large watery vesicle; a bleb. In dermatology, bulla formation is characteristic of the pemphigus group of dermatoses, but it also occurs in contact dermatides such as those caused by burns, sunburn; in bullous impetigo and dermatitis herpetiformis; and on the palms and soles in scarlet fever and congenital syphilis. — bullae, pl.; bullate, bullous, adj.

bullous pemphigoid (bul'-us pem'-fi-goyd): A chronic skin condition in which large bullae occur over a wide area, especially on the lower abdomen, groin, and inner aspect of the thigh; the tendency to occur increases with age.

bundle branch block: See under HEART BLOCK.

bundle of His (hiss): Consists of neuromuscular fibres that arise at the atrioventricular node, pass along the intraventricular septum, and finally divide into right and left branches that are distributed throughout the ventricular walls. They transmit the impulse for ventricular contraction; failure to do so produces heart block (*q.v.*). [William His, German physician, 1863–1934.]

bundle of Kent: A bundle of modified cardiac muscle tissue which begins at the atrioventricular node, extends into the intraventricular septum, with its branches terminating in the subendocardium of the right and left ventricles.

bunion (bun-yun): Syn., *hallux valgus*. A deformity of the head of the metatarsal bone at its junction with the great toe. Friction and pressure of shoes at this point cause the bursa to become inflamed and enlarged, thus causing enlargement of the joint and lateral displacement of the great toe. The prominent bone with its bursa is called a bunion. TAILOR'S B. inflammation and enlargement of the fifth metatarsal bone.

bunionectomy (bun-yun-ek'-tō-mi): The surgical removal of a bunion.

buphthalmos (boof-thal'-mos): A condition of infants in which there is an increase in intraocular fluid with consequent increase in the size of the eyeball. Also called *congenital glaucoma*.

burden of proof: The duty to establish the facts; usually associated with litigation or criminal proceedings.

buret, burette (bū-ret'): A graduated glass tube fitted with a stopcock, used for measuring liquids and for delivering an accurately measured amount of a liquid.

Burkitt's tumour: Primary malignant lymphoma occurring chiefly in male children between two and 14 years of age and living in a geographical area of Africa where malaria and other mosquito-borne diseases are endemic; thought to be caused by the Epstein–Barr virus. The rapidly growing tumour occurs most often in the jaw bone and orbit of the eye, but may also occur in abdominal and other organs. [Denis Burkitt, 20th century surgeon working in Uganda.]

burn: 1. A lesion of tissues due to chemicals, dry heat, electricity, flame, friction, or radiation; usually classified in three degrees: (a) first degree, erythema; (b) second degree, vesiculation; and (c) third degree, destruction of epidermis and dermis, and damage to underlying tissues. A fourth degree is recognized when the burn is deep enough to involve fascia, muscle, and bone. **2.** In chemistry, to oxidize. **3.** To feel the sensation of heat. CHEMICAL B. one due to a caustic chemical; FLASH B. one due to a sudden brief exposure to radiant heat, as that caused by an atomic explosion; FRICTION B. one caused by friction or rapid movement of skin over an abrasive substance or of an abrasive substance over the skin; also called *brush burn*; RADIATION B. overexposure to x-rays, ultraviolet rays, radium or atomic energy. See WALLACE'S RULE OF NINES.

burning foot syndrome: The sensation of burning and other abnormal sensations in the feet sometimes in the hands; occurs in the elderly, persons with various neurological disturbances, alcoholics, and diabetics.

burnout (burn'-owt): A psychological and physical state characterized by listlessness, pessimism, apathy, and lack of motivation, interest, and energy, particularly in relation to one's work; often appears to be a result of career-related stress such as excessive demands on a person's strength, energy, and resources, disappointment in lack of advancement, or conflict between the job and family responsibilities.

burping (burp'-ing): Belching.

burr: 1. B. CELLS red blood cells with blunt cytoplasmic projections like those of acanthocytes; may be seen in the cells of persons with various disorders of the blood, cancer of the stomach, and gastric ulcers, or extensive burns. **2.** A rotary cutting instrument used: (a) in operations on bones, or (b) in dentistry, to open and prepare tooth cavities. B. HOLES holes made in the skull with a burr; for diagnostic purposes, for removing a clot, to aspirate an abscess or cerebrospinal fluid, to permit removal of a brain tumour, or to relieve intracranial pressure. Cranial trephination.

bursa (bur'-sa): A fibrous sac lined with synovial membrane and containing a small quantity of synovial fluid. Bursae are found between (1) tendon and bone; (2) skin and bone; (3) muscle and muscle. Their function is to facilitate movement without friction between these surfaces. — bursae, pl.

bursitis (bur-sī'-tis): Inflammation of a bursa; may be acute or may develop slowly after repeated injuries or strain. Characterized by pain, swelling, and tenderness. Prominent locations are the deltoid bursa of the shoulder; the radiohumeral bursa of the elbow, as in miner's, student's, or tennis elbow; and the metatarsophalangeal bursa of the great toe where it becomes the cause of a bunion. ACHILLES B. involves the bursa between the A. tendon and the posterior surface of the calcaneus; characterized by heel pain; frequently occurs in the elderly and often due to ill fitting shoes; also called *Haglund's disease*; ISCHIAL B.

inflammation of the bursa over the tuberosity of the ischium, caused by prolonged sitting; also called *weaver's bottom*; PREPATELLAR B. inflammation of the large bursa in front of the patella; also called *housemaid's knee*.

butterfly: B. NEEDLE an intravenous needle with plastic side wings used to guide the needle into a vein and provide anchorage when in position; B. RASH a rash in the shape of a butterfly extending over the nose and cheeks; seen in lupus erythematosus and certain skin disorders; B. TAPING a technique utilizing a butterfly-shaped piece of adhesive material to hold the edges of a wound together instead of stitching them, or to hold a tracheostomy tube in place.

buttock (but' -ok): One of the two fleshy projections posterior to the hip joints. Formed mainly of the gluteal muscles.

button (but' -on): A small round plastic device used to plug an opening such as a tracheostomy opening.

bypass (bī' -pas): An auxillary flow, or shunt. Often applies to a temporary or permanent surgical grafting of blood vessels to detour blood around occluded segments of arteries or veins. CARDOPULMONARY B. exclusion of the heart and lungs from the circulation; blood is diverted from the right atrium via a pump-oxygenator, and returned to the aorta; CORONARY B. surgical construction of a detour, usually consisting of a graft utilizing a strip from the saphenous vein, through which blood can bypass narrowed or occluded portions of a coronary artery. See also SHUNT.

byssinosis (bis-in-ō-sis): A chronic industrial disease of the lungs occurring in cotton workers especially, due to inhalation of cotton dust. Also occurs in those working with hemp or flax. Characterized by tightness in the chest, dyspnoea, coughing, wheezing; may lead to bronchitis, emphysema, respiratory failure.

C

C: 1. Abbreviation for: (a) calorie (large); (b) centigrade or Celsius; (c) contraction. **2.** Chemical symbol for carbon.

Ca: 1. Abbreviation for: (a) carcinoma; (b) cathode. **2.** Chemical symbol for calcium.

cabinet: A body of advisers to the head of state. SHADOW C. a group of leaders of a parliamentary opposition who constitute the probable membership of the cabinet when their party comes into power.

Cabot's ring bodies; Bluish lines in the form of figures of eight or loops, seen in the stained red blood cells of individuals with severe anaemia, especially the anaemia that occurs in lead poisoning.

cac-, caco-: Combining form denoting bad, abnormal, defective, deformed, diseased.

cacao (ka-kā'-o): The seeds from a South American tree, *Theobroma cacao*, from which cocoa, chocolate, and cocoa butter are prepared.

cachet (ka-shā'): **1.** A lens-shaped absorbable capsule for enclosing a dose of medicine to be taken orally. **2.** A flat capsule made of circles of rice paper sealed together and enclosing a dose of any bitter powdered drug to be taken orally. **3.** A cone-shaped piece of equipment made of lead, used in application of a radioactive substance.

cachetic (ka-kek'-tik): Relating to or characterized by cachexia (*q.v.*).

cachexia (ka-kek'-si-a): A term denoting a state of constitutional disorder, malnutrition, general ill health, and wasting away of body tissue. The chief signs are pale mucous membranes, anaemia, emaciation, sallow unhealthy skin, and heavy lustreless eyes. — cachectic, adj.

cachinnation (kak-i-nā'-shun): Hysterical or immoderate laughter without any apparent cause; often seen in certain psychoses including schizophrenia.

cacogenesis (kak-ō-jen'-e-sis): **1.** Abnormal growth or development. **2.** Congenital malformation.

cacoguesia (kak-ō-gū'-si-a): Term usually applies to a bad taste not necessarily due to anything ingested; often occurs with the aura that precedes some epileptic seizures.

cacomelia (kak-ō-mē'-li-a): Congenital deformity of a limb or limbs.

cacoplastic (kak-ō-plas'-tik): **1.** Defective growth or development. **2.** Lacking ability to grow or develop normally.

cacosmia (kak-oz'-mi-a): **1.** A foul odour. **2.** A hallucination of an odour, particularly of putrefaction.

cacumen (kak-ū'-men): The top or apex of a body part or structure.

cadaver (ka-dav'-er): A corpse or dead body. — cadaveric, cadaverous, adj.

cadmium (kad'-mi-um): A metallic element formerly used in medications but now used chiefly in industry, of importance because of its potential for causing poisoning due to inhalation of cadmium fumes by workers in such industries as electroplating, or from eating foods stored in cadmium-lined containers. Symptoms include nausea, vomiting, dyspnoea, prostration, headache, pulmonary oedema.

caduceus (ka-dū'-sē-us): The wand of Hermes or Mercury entwined with two serpents, often used as a symbol of the medical profession. The insignia of the medical profession is the staff of Aesculapius which has one serpent twined about it.

caecal (sē'-kal): Relating to the caecum.

caecectomy (sē-sek'-to-mi): Operation for removal of the caecum or part of it, or an incision into it.

caecocolic (sē-kō-kol'-ik): Relating to the caecum and the colon.

caecorectostomy (sē'-kō-rek-tos'-to-mi): A surgically created anastomosis between the caecum and the rectum.

caecosigmoidostomy (sē'-kō-sig-moid-os'-to-mi): A surgically created anastomosis between the caecum and the sigmoid flexure of the colon.

caecostomy (sē-kos'-to-mi): A surgically established fistula between the caecum and the anterior abdominal wall, done to bypass an area of the caecum that is diseased, obstructed, or congenitally absent; the bowel content is voided into a collection bag attached to the skin.

caecum (sē'-kum): The blind, pouch-like commencement of the colon in the right iliac fossa; it is separated from the ileum by the ileocaecal valve; the vermiform appendix is attached to it. — caecal, adj.

Caesarean section (se-sar'-ē-an): Delivery of a fetus via an incision through the abdominal and uterine walls. From the Latin verb '*caedere*', to cut.

caesium (sē'-zi-um): A rare metallic element in the alkali group. Several of its salts have actions similar to those of potassium and have been used experimentally in medicine. C. BROMIDE used in infrared spectrometry; C-137, has a half-life of 30 years; encapsulated, it is used as a source of radiation for therapeutic purposes. Chemical symbol, Cs.

caffeine (kaf'-ēn): An odourless, white, bitter powder obtained from the leaves and beans of tea, coffee, maté, and guarana; used medically as a central nervous system stimulant, a cardiac stimulant, a diuretic, and in headache remedies.

Caffey's disease: A type of hyperostosis (*q.v.*) of infants in which there is swelling of the tissues over the affected bone, fever, irritability, and periods of exacerbation and remission. Also called *infantile cortical hyperostosis*.

cage: THORACIC C. the bony structure that encloses the organs of the thorax (*q.v.*); is made up of the sternum, ribs, and part of the vertebral column.

caisson disease (kā'-son): A condition variously called decompression illness, the bends, vascular necrosis of bone, divers' disease. Results from sudden reduction in atmospheric pressure as occurs, *e.g.*, in divers returning to the surface, or airmen ascending to great heights. Due to bubbles of nitrogen which are released from solution in the blood; symptoms vary according to the site of these. The condition is largely preventable by proper and gradual decompression technique. See BENDS.

Cal: Abbreviation for large calorie (*q.v.*).

CAL: Abbreviation for computer-assisted learning (*q.v.*).

calabar (kald'-a-bar): A disease seen chiefly in Africa; caused by a parasite worm that enters through the skin and causes the development of lumps in the subcutaneous tissue; may also enter the anterior chamber of the eye.

calamine (kal'-a-mīn): 1. Zinc carbonate. 2. A preparation of zinc oxide and ferric oxide, a pink powder used in treatment of certain skin diseases; also used in ointments and lotions as a protective and astringent in treating a variety of skin conditions.

calcaneal (kal-kā'-nē-al): Relating to the calcaneus or the heel. C. SPUR a bony outgrowth on the lower surface of the calcaneus; caused by repeated traumatic pressure on the heel; C. TENDON REFLEX Achilles reflex; see under REFLEX.

calcaneoapophysitis (kal-kā'-nē-ō-a-pof-i-sī'-tis): Pain, swelling, and inflammation of the posterior part of the calcaneus at the insertion of the tendon of Achilles.

calcaneodynia (kal-kā'-nē-ō-din'-i-a): Pain in the heel, especially when standing or walking.

calcaneus (kal-kā'-nē-us): The heel bone, os calcis; the largest and strongest of the tarsal bones.

calcar (kal'-kar): A spur or spurlike projection. In biology, a pointed, projecting outgrowth of a part, often calciferous.

calcicosis (kal-si-kō'-sis): A lung disease, often occupational, due to inhalation of marble dust (calcium carbonate).

calciferol (kal-sif'-e-rol): Vitamin D_2. Produced synthetically by ultraviolet radiation of ergosterol; has the most vitamin D activity of any substance produced in this way; occurs also in milk and fish liver oils. Used in treatment of rickets, parathyroid deficiency, lupus vulgaris (*q.v.*), and osteomalacia (*q.v.*); also used prophylactically.

calciferous (kal-sif'-er-us): Containing calcium, lime, or chalk.

calcification (kal-sif-i-kā'-shun): The hardening of an organic substance by a deposit of calcium salts within it. May be normal, as in bone, or pathological, as when it occurs in arteries or other tissues.

calcify (kal'-si-fī): To deposit mineral salts in the body organs or tissues.

calcipenia (kal-si-pē'-ni-a): Deficiency of calcium in the body.

calcitonin (kal-si-tō' nin): See THYROCALCITONIN.

calcium (kal'-si-um): A soft, white, metallic element, essential for the formation and maintenance of bone; 2% of body weight is calcium, of which 97% is in the bones and teeth. Its deposition in the bones is controlled by the parathyroid gland and its utilization by bone is dependent on vitamin D (*q.v.*). It is a vital electrolyte in the blood, especially in relation to clotting, and to neuromuscular activity. Several of its salts are used in medicine. C. CARBONATE a C. compound occurring naturally in bone; also prepared artificially for use in therapy as a source of C. and as an antacid; C. CHLORIDE an odourless, white, granular compound used in medicine as a diuretic and urine acidifier, and as an antiallergenic; in solution it is used to correct electrolyte imbalance; C. GLUCONATE an odourless, tasteless salt of calcium; used in tablet and liquid form as a source of C.; C. LACTATE a white powder soluble in water; used as a source of C. and as a blood coagulant; C. TEST see SULKOWITCH'S TEST.

calculosis (kal-kū-lō'-sis): The presence of a calculus or of calculi.

calculus (kal'-kū-lus): An abnormal concretion composed chiefly of mineral substances and formed usually in the passages that transmit secretions, or in the cavities that act as reservoirs for them. Commonly called *stones*. ARTHRITIC C. a deposit of urates in or around a joint; BILIARY C. one formed in a bile duct or gall bladder; a gallstone; RENAL C. one formed in the kidney, URINARY C. one formed in any part of the urinary tract. — calculi, pl.; calculous, calculary, adj.

Caldicott guardians: Individuals within an organization who have responsibility for ensuring that the Caldicott Principles (*q.v.*) of confidentiality and security of information relating to patients are maintained.

Caldicott Principles: Six guidelines for the maintenance of confidentiality and security of information relating to patients: valid reasons for the use or transfer of information should be given; patient information should not be used unless it is absolutely necessary; use the minimum necessary patient information; access to patient information should be on a strict need-to-know basis; all staff must be aware of their responsibilities; and all staff must understand and comply with this law.

Caldwell–Luc operation: The surgical procedure of creating an opening through the canine fossa into the maxillary sinus to facilitate drainage of the sinus.

calefacient (kal-e-fā'-shent): An agent that produces a feeling of warmth in the part to which it is applied.

calf (kaf): The muscular portion at the back of the leg below the knee, formed principally by the bellies of the soleus and gastrocnemius muscles. C. BONE the fibula. — calves, pl.

calibrate (kal'-i-brāt): To determine, by measurement or by comparison to a standard, the correct value of each unit of measurement on the scale of an instrument or apparatus. — calibrated, adj.; calibration, n.

calibre (kal'-i-ber): The diameter of a round structure such as a tube or canal.

caligo (ka-lī'-gō): Dimness or obscurity of vision.

calliper (kal'-i-per): 1. A measuring instrument with two adjustable legs for determining thickness, diameter, or distance. 2. In orthopaedics, a splint or brace. SKIN C. a C. for measuring the thickness of a skinfold; WALKING C. a splint for the lower extremity; two metal legs extend from the posterior of the thigh to a metal plate attached to the sole of the shoe.

callisthenics (kal-is-then'-iks): Systematic light exercises to preserve health, develop muscles and gracefulness.

callous (kal'-us): Resembling callus. Hard.

callus (kal'-us): 1. A localized area of thickened skin, the stratum corneum of the palms and soles in particular, resulting from trauma caused by continual friction or pressure. 2. The fibrous tissue that forms at the end of bone in a fracture and which eventually becomes bone.

calor (ka'-lor): Heat, one of the classic signs of inflammation. In physiology, the heat generated by metabolic processes.

caloric (kal-or'-ik): Relating to: (1) heat; (2) calories.

caloric test: A test for assessing vestibular function. When a normal ear is irrigated with hot water, there is rotary nystagmus towards that ear; if irrigated with cold water, there is rotary nystagmus towards the opposite ear. In vestibular disease, there is no nystagmus with either hot or cold water irrigation of an affected ear.

calorie (kal'-o-ri): The unit of measure of heat energy; usually designates the small calorie which is the amount of heat required to raise the temperature of one gram of water 1°C. Usually written with a small *c* and may be abbreviated to cal.; sometimes called *gram calorie*. The large calorie is the amount of heat required to raise the temperature of 1 kilogram of water 1°C. Thus it is 1000 times as large as the small calorie; usually written with a capital C. and may be abbreviated to Cal.; sometimes called *kilogram calorie* or *kilocalorie*; is used in the study of metabolism. Sometimes called *calory*.

calorific (kal-o-rif'-ik): Heat-producing. C. VALUE the number of calories produced by a given amount of food, *e.g.*, 1 gram of protein and carbohydrate each liberate 4 calories, 1 gram of fat liberates 9 calories.

calorigenic (ka-lor-i-jen'-ik): 1. Heat-producing. 2. Energy-producing.

calorimeter (kal-ō-rim′-i-ter): An apparatus for measuring heat production. The respiration C. is used for determining the body's basal metabolic rate by measuring the heat produced by gaseous exchange in the lungs.

calorimetry (kal-ō-rim′-i-tri): The measurement of the amount of heat given off in a chemical reaction.

calvities (kal-vish′-i-ēz): Baldness.

calyx (kā′-liks): In anatomy, one of the cup-like structures in the renal pelvis into which the pyramids of the renal medulla project. — calices, pl.; caliceal, adj.

camphor (kam′-for): A colourless white compound occurring as crystals, granules, or a gum; has a characteristic penetrating odour; obtained from an Asian shrub or tree; used locally as an antipruritic, antiseptic, analgesic, rubefacient, and as a carminative and toothache remedy.

camphorated oil: Cottonseed oil with camphor added; used externally as a counterirritant.

camphorated tincture of opium: A solution of alcohol and water containing opium, anise oil, camphor, benzoic acid, and glycerin; used chiefly as an antidiarrhoetic. Syn., *paregoric.*

Campylobacter (kam-pi-lō-bak′-ter): A genus of Gram-negative bacteria; spirally curved rods with a flagella at one or both ends and which move with a corkscrew-like motion. Various species affect humans as well as domestic animals. In humans symptoms include fever, night sweats, enteritis, headache, and bloody stools. May be transmitted by drinking water.

canal (ka-nal′): In anatomy, a relatively straight narrow tube, channel, or duct in bone or tissue. For particular canals see under ALIMENTARY, AUDITORY, BIRTH, HAVERSIAN, INGUINAL, NUCK, SEMICIRCULAR, VERTEBRAL.

canaliculus (kan-a-lik′-ū-lus): 1. A minute capillary passage. 2. Any small canal, such as the passage leading from the edge of the eyelid to the lacrimal sac, or one of the numerous small canals that lead from the Haversian canals and terminate in the lacunae of bone. — canaliculi, pl.; canalicular, adj.; canaliculization, n.

canalization (kan-a-lī-zā′-shun): 1. Formation of a new channel in tissue. 2. A surgical procedure that provides for drainage of wounds without the use of tubes.

cancellate, cancelled (kan′-sel-āt, -ed): Having a structure that resembles latticework.

cancellous (kan′-sel-us): Resembling latticework; light and spongy, like a honeycomb. Refers particularly to bony tissue that underlies or lies between layers of compact bone in epiphyses, sternum, ribs, vertebrae, and diploë of the skull; the interstices are filled with red bone marrow.

cancer (kan′-ser): A general term for a variety of malignant growths in many parts of the body; often used synonymously with tumour, neoplasm, or malignancy. The growth is purposeless, parasitic, invasive, and flourishes at the expense of the human host. Although the basic aetiology is not known, cancer is considered curable if discovered early and if all cancer cells are removed by surgery or destroyed by radiation. Characteristics are the tendency to cause local destruction, to spread by metastasis, to recur, and to cause toxaemia. Cancer is broadly classified as either carcinoma, which includes malignant tumours of the skin or mucous membranes, or as sarcoma, which includes tumours of connective tissue. — cancerous, adj.

cancericidal (kan-ser-i-sī′-dal): Destructive to the cells of cancer.

cancerigenic (kan-ser-i-jen′-ik): Giving rise to a malignant neoplasm. See CARCINOGEN.

cancer *in situ*: Carcinoma *in situ*; see under CARCINOMA.

cancerous (kan′-ser-us): Relating to, of, or resembling a cancer.

cancroid (kang′-kroid): 1. Squamous cell carcinoma. 2. Relating to squamous cell carcinoma. 3. Resembling cancer. 4. Cancer of moderate degree; may be said of skin cancer in particular.

cancrum oris (kan′-krum-or′-is): Gangrenous stomatitis (*q.v.*), occurring in malnourished children; also seen in such debilitating conditions as leukaemia, Hodgkin's disease, and severe cases of mealses, tuberculosis, malaria or kala-azar. Also called *noma.*

Candida (kan′-di-da): A genus of yeast-like fungi; widespread in nature. *Candida* (*Monilia* or *Oidium*) *albicans* is a commensal of the mouth, throat, vagina, intestinal tract, and skin. Becomes pathogenic in some physiological and pathological states. May produce such infections as thrush, vulvovaginitis, balanoposthitis, and pulmonary disease. C. VAGINITIS inflammation of the vagina, often recurrent, caused by any of the several species of the *Candida* genus; characterized by pruritis, swelling of the vulva, and a thick, whitish discharge that adheres to the vaginal walls and is difficult to remove. Treatment includes the topical administration of medicated creams or suppositories; preventive measures include avoidance of tight undergarments and treatment of such underlying conditions as diabetes.

candidiasis (kan-di-dī´-a-sis): Infection with a fungus of the genus *Candida*, syn., *moniliasis, thrush.* Characterized by formation of pseudo-membranes on mucous surfaces of the respiratory and intestinal tracts and the vagina, skin lesions that resemble eczema, sometimes granulomata. Skin and local infections are usually benign; systemic infections, which may involve the kidney, may be fatal. ORAL C. thrush (*q.v.*).

canicola fever (kan-i-kō´-la): Infection of humans by the *Leptospira canicola* from rats, dogs, pigs, foxes, mice, voles, and possibly cats. There is high fever, headache, conjunctival congestion, jaundice, severe muscular pains, rigors and vomiting. As the fever abates in about one week, the jaundice disappears. See WEIL'S DISEASE.

canine (kā´-nīn): 1. Resembling a dog. 2. Relating to certain teeth, four in all, two in each jaw, situated between the incisors and the premolars, and called cuspids. Those in the upper jaw are commonly known as eye teeth; those in the lower jaw as stomach teeth; C. FOSSA a depression in the maxilla above the canine teeth; C. SPASM see RISUS SARDONICUS.

canities (ka-nish´-i-ēz): Greyness or whiteness of the scalp hair.

canker sore: Small, white ulcerative sores occurring chiefly on the lips, mouth, and inside of the cheek. See APHTHAE, NOMA, THRUSH, and APHTHOUS STOMATITIS.

cannabis (kan´-a-bis): The hemp plant *Cannabis sativa,* the buds and leaves of which are prepared as marijuana. It is any of several different species of mildly hallucinogenic plants, the main active ingredient of which is tetrahydrocannabinol. The drugs obtained from this plant are also referred to as *dope, weed, grass, herb, ganja* (traditional in Rastafarian religion), *the good herb, pot, skunk, chronic, hash, hemp. smoke, splifs, blunts, roaches* or *whacko-tobacco.*

cannon wave: In electrocardiography, a large positive wave that occurs when the right atrium contracts but, for some anatomical or pathological reason, cannot empty its contents.

cannula (kan´-ū-la): A hollow tube contained in a trocar that is introduced into a body cavity after which the trocar is withdrawn and the tube remains in place, where it is used to introduce or withdraw fluid from a cavity, to irrigate a cavity, or to instil medication into a cavity. BELLOCQ'S C. a hollow sound (*q.v.*) used to pass a thread through the nose and mouth to pull in a plug in treatment of epistaxis; NASAL C. a

double-pronged device that is placed in the nostrils; has an extension that goes behind the ears and is secured under the chin; a common method of administering oxygen. — cannulas, cannulae, pl.

cannulate (kan´-ū-lāt): To introduce a cannula into a body cavity or tube-like organ. — cannulation, n.

cantharides (kan-thar´i-dēz): A substance formerly much used externally as a rubefacient or vesicant and internally as an aphrodisiac and diuretic; made from the dried insect, *Cantharis vesicatoria,* a kind of beetle. See SPANISH FLY.

canthitis (kan-thī´-tis): Inflammation of the tissues at a canthus (*q.v.*) or canthi.

canthus (kan´-thus): The angle formed by the junction of the eyelids. The inner one is known as the nasal C. or the medial palpebral commissure, and the outer one as the temporal C. or the lateral palpebral commissure. — canthal, adj.; canthi, pl.

cap: In anatomy, a cap-shaped protective cover-like structure. CERVICAL C. a thimble-shaped cap that fits over the cervix; a birth control device.

capable practitioner: A health-care professional who is able to provide both effective and reflective practice. Such practice requires the practitioner to have an underpinning framework of values, attitudes, and knowledge centred on his or her ability to reflect in and on action. See REFLECTION IN ACTION; REFLECTION ON ACTION; SAINSBURY CENTRE FOR MENTAL HEALTH.

capacity (ka-pas´-i-ti): The ability to hold, receive, or store something. INSPIRATORY C. the volume of air that can be inspired following a normal exhalation; FUNCTIONAL RESIDUAL C. the amount of air that remains in the lung after a normal expiration; RESIDUAL C. the amount of air that remains in the lung after a maximal respiratory effort; TOTAL LUNG C. the sum of the functional residual capacity and the inspiratory capacity; VITAL C. the greatest volume of air that can be expired after a maximum inspiration.

CAPD: Abbreviation for continuous ambulatory peritoneal dialysis, see under DIALYSIS.

capillaritis (kap-i-lar-ī´-tis): 1. Inflammation of the capillaries. 2. A skin disorder characterized by rupture of superficial capillaries and the consequent development of pigmented spots on the skin; cause unknown.

capillary (kap´-i-lar-i): 1. Hair-like. 2. A tiny thin-walled vessel, forming part of the network which facilitates rapid exchange of substances between the contained fluid and the surrounding tissues. ARTERIAL C. a minute vessel distal to an arteriole; carries arterial blood; BILE C. begins in a space in the liver and joins others to form a bile duct; BLOOD C. unites an arteriole and a venule; C. FRAGILITY refers to a high potential for rupture of the blood capillaries; LYMPH C. begins in the tissue spaces throughout the body and joins others, eventually forming a lymphatic vessel; C. MEMBRANE the basement membrane (*q.v.*) which allows diffusion of oxygen and nutrients and osmosis of water; VENOUS C. a tiny vessel proximal to a venule; carries venous blood.

capillary fragility test: A test to evaluate the ability of the capillaries to resist conditions of increased pressure or anoxia.

capillus (ka-pil′-lus): A hair, specifically of the head. — capilli, pl.

capitalism (kap′-i-tal-izm): An economic system characterized by private or corporate ownership of capital goods. In such a system investments are determined by private decision, and prices, production and the distribution of goods are determined mainly by competition in a free market.

capitate (kap′-i-tāt): 1. Head-shaped; having a rounded extremity. 2. The largest of the eight carpal bones, so called because it has a head-shaped process.

capitation (kap-i-tā-shun): Any uniform payment or fee payable per capita.

capitulum (ka-pit′-ū-lum): A small, rounded head or prominence on a bone by which it articulates with another bone.

Caplan's syndrome: A form of pneumoconiosis (*q.v.*) associated with rheumatoid arthritis; characterized by the formation of numerous nodular lesions throughout the lungs.

-capnia: A combining form denoting the presence of carbon dioxide.

capsid (kap′-sid): The protective protein coat that surrounds the nucleic acid component of viruses.

capsitis (kap-sī′-tis): Inflammation of the capsule that encloses the crystalline lens.

capsulated (kap′-sū-lā-ted): Enclosed within a capsule.

capsulation (kap-sū-lā′-shun): To surround a part with a capsule. Encapsulation.

capsule (kap′-sul): 1. The ligaments that surround a joint. 2. An absorbable gelatinous or rice paper container for a dose of oral medicine. 3. The outer membranous covering of certain

organs, such as the kidney, liver, spleen, adrenal glands. — capsular, adj.

capsulitis (kap-sū-lī′-tis): Inflammation of a capsule of an organ or joint. ADHESIVE C. inflammation of a joint that results in limited motion; when it occurs in the shoulder is often referred to as frozen shoulder.

capsuloplasty (kap′-sū-lō-plas-ti): Plastic surgery for repair of a joint capsule.

capsulorrhaphy (kap-sū-lor′-a-fi): Suture of a capsule; usually refers to the surgical repair of a torn joint capsule.

capsulotomy (kap-sū-lot′-o-mi): Incision of a capsule, usually referring to that surrounding the crystalline lens of the eye.

caput (kap′-ut): 1. A general term applied to the superior extremity of an organ or other body part. 2. The superior extremity of the body; the head. C. MEDUSAE dilated veins in the area immediately surrounding the umbilicus, with blood flowing away from the umbilicus; seen in the newborn and in patients with cirrhosis of the liver; so called because the pattern of the veins resembles the snake-haired Medusa; also called *caput medusae syndrome*; C. SUCCEDANEUM a serous effusion or oedema overlying the scalp periosteum on an infant's head; the result of pressure during labour; disappears quickly.

carative factors (kair′-a-tiv): Items in the philosophy and theory of human caring devised by Professor Jean Watson, which gives nursing its unique disciplinary, scientific, and professional standing. The ten factors are: a humanistic–altruistic system of values; faith–hope; sensitivity to self and others; helping–trusting, human care relationship; expressing positive and negative feelings; creative problem-solving caring process; transpersonal teaching-learning; supportive, protective and/or corrective mental, physical, societal and spiritual environment; human needs assistance; and existential–phenomenological–spiritual forces.

CARATS: Abbreviation for Counselling, Assessment, Referral, Advice and Throughcare Scheme (*q.v.*).

carbamide (kar′-bam-īd): A product of protein metabolism; urea (*q.v.*); produces diuresis when used intravenously with dextrose solution.

carbaminohaemoglobin (kar-bam′-i-nō-hē-mō-glō′-bin): Haemoglobin united with carbon dioxide; one of the forms in which carbon dioxide exists in the blood.

carbohydrase (kar-bō-hī′-drās): Any of several enzymes that act as a catalyst in the hydrolysis of carbohydrates to simple sugars.

carbohydrate (kar-bō-hī-drāt): An organic compound containing carbon, hydrogen, and oxygen, the latter two usually present in the same proportion as in water. Formed in nature by photosynthesis in plants. Carbohydrates are energy sources; they include starches, sugars, and cellulose and are classified as monosaccharides, disaccharides, and polysaccharides. They make up about half of our food intake and are included in such foods as cereals, rice, breads, most vegetables, especially the legumes and potatoes, and most fruits. A deficiency of c. in the diet leads to fatigue and electrolyte imbalance; excessive consumption may lead to obesity, dental decay, and, possibly, hypertension, diabetes, or kidney disorders.

carbohydraturia (kar'-bō-hī-dra-tū'-ri-a): The presence of an excess of carbohydrates in the urine; glycosuria.

carbolfuchsin (kar'-bol-fook'-sin): A dark purple solution containing phenol, resorcinol, acetone, alcohol, and distilled water; used externally as an antifungal preparation. C. STAIN a solution used for staining certain acid fast bacteria including the tubercle bacillus; contains phenol and basic fuchsin in distilled water.

carbolic acid (kar-bol'-ik as'-id): Phenol (q.v.). Formerly much used as an antiseptic and germicide. Irritating to the skin and highly poisonous.

carbometer (kar-bom'-i-ter): An instrument for determining the amount of carbon dioxide that is given off with the breath. Also carbonometer.

carbon: A non-metallic element present in all organic compounds. C. DIOXIDE a tasteless, colourless gas; a waste product of many forms of combustion and metabolism, excreted by the lungs. When dissolved in a fluid, carbonic acid is formed; a specific amount of this in the blood produces inspiration; in cases of insufficiency, inhalations of C.D. act as a respiratory stimulant. It is also mixed with O_2 in anaesthetic gases to stimulate respiration. In its solid form C.D. snow it is used as an escharotic and refrigerant; C. MONOXIDE an insidious, colourless, odourless gas, present in illuminating gas, the exhaust of combustion motors and the products of incomplete combustion of wood and coal. It forms a stable compound with haemoglobin, thus robbing the body of its oxygen-carrying mechanism; signs of hypoxia ensue; C. TETRACHLORIDE a colourless liquid with an odour similar to that of chloroform. Used chiefly as a solvent and detergent. No longer used in medicine.

carbonaemia (kar-bō-nē'-mi-a): An excessive amount of carbon dioxide in the blood.

carbonate (kar'-bon-āt): 1. To charge with carbon dioxide. 2. Any salt of carbonic acid. — carbonated, adj.

carbon dioxide: See under CARBON.

carbon dioxide snow: Dry ice: solid carbon dioxide with a temperature of −79° Centigrade; in medicine, used to destroy certain skin lesions.

carbonic acid: A solution of carbon dioxide in water; often called carbonated water.

carbonic anhydrase (kar-bon'-ik an-hī'-drās): An enzyme that acts as a catalyst in the synthesis and decomposition of carbonic acid from and to carbon dioxide and water, a step in the removal of carbon dioxide from the tissues and into the blood and alveolar air.

carbon monoxide: See under CARBON.

carbonuria (kar-bo-nū'-ri-a): An excess of carbon dioxide or other carbon compounds in the urine.

carbonyl (kar'-bo-nil): CO a bivalent organic radical characteristic of aldehydes, ketones, carboxylic acid and esters.

carboxyhaemoglobin (kar-bok'-si-hē-mō-glō'-bin): A stable compound formed by the union of carbon monoxide and haemoglobin; the red blood cells thus lose their respiratory function, as occurs in carbon monoxide poisoning.

carboxyhaemoglobinaemia (kar-boks'-i-hēm-ō-glō-bin-e'-mi-a): The presence of carboxyhaemoglobin in the blood.

carbuncle (kar'-bung-k'l): An acute, circumscribed, painful, suppurative inflammation (usually caused by a staphylococcal organism) involving several hair follicles and surrounding subcutaneous tissue, forming an extensive slough with several discharging sinuses. Frequently occurs on the back of the neck and most often in men; diabetics are particularly susceptible. — carbuncular, adj.

carcin-, carcino-: Combining forms denoting cancer.

carcinoembryonic antigen (kar'sin-ō-em-brē-on'-ik): An antigen normally present in the fetus and, in very small amounts, in the adult; tests for its presence are of use in determining the existence of a malignancy, or of metastasis of a malignant tumour, and whether surgical removal of a malignant tumour is advisable.

carcinogen (kar'-sin-ō-jen): Any cancer-producing substance or agent, e.g., friction, injury, pressure, coal tar and its products, prolonged exposure to heat, sun, or radiation. — carcinogenic, adj.; carcinogenicity, n.

carcinogenesis (kar' -si-nō-jen' -e-sis): 1. The production or origin of cancer. 2. The process by which normal cells are transformed into cancer cells. — carcinogenic, adj.; carcinogenicity, n.

carcinogenicity (kar' -sin-ō-jen-is' -i-ti): The ability to cause cancer.

carcinoid (kar' -sin-oyd): Refers to a circumscribed tumour, usually benign and occurring in the gastrointestinal tract. C. SYNDROME a condition thought to be due to secretion of serotonin from C. tumours that have metastasized to the liver; characterized by intense flushing of the face, angiomas of the skin, watery diarrhoea, oedema, ascites, bronchial spasm, sudden drop in blood pressure, stenosis of the tricuspid and pulmonary valves, and right heart failure.

carcinolytic (kar' -si-nō-lit' -ik): Destructive of carcinoma cells or pertaining to such destruction.

carcinoma (kar-si-nō' -ma): A malignant new growth derived from epithelial and glandular tissues, which tends to infiltrate into surrounding tissues and to spread by metastasis; the cells resemble those of the tissue where the growth is found. ADENOSQUAMOUS C. a type of adenocarcinoma composed of both glandular and squamous malignant elements; occurs as an endometrial C., most often seen in older women; BASAL CELL C. a slow-growing, usually painless ulcer, usually occurring on the upper part of the face of older persons; may start as only a scaly patch or as a pearly raised papule with small capillaries; seldom metastasizes; highly curable. Occasionally seen also on the vulva of women over 60, where it begins as a small nodule, grows steadily and slowly, and eventually ulcerates; BRONCHOGENIC C., C. of the lungs; arises in the epithelium of the bronchial tubes; C. IN SITU an asymptomatic condition; cells resembling cancer cells grow from the basal epithelial layer and finally involve the whole epithelium so that its layers can no longer be recognized; the term is often applied to C. of the cervix; also called *preinvasive* C.; CHORIONIC C., C. composed of cells that are characteristic of the chorion of the embryo; occurs in the testes and ovaries and sometimes in other parts of the body; see CHORIOCARCINOMA; EPIDERMOID C. squamous cell C.; MEDULLARY C. a poorly differentiated malignant neoplasm composed mostly of epithelial cells with little or no stroma; often occurs in the breast; MELANOTIC C. malignant melanoma; see under MELANOMA; SCIRRHOUS C., C. with a hard structure owing to the formation of dense

connective tissue; SQUAMOUS CELL C. an invasive C. containing anaplastic squamous cells, arising in the squamous epithelium; often occurs on the lower lip; limited metastasis and curability; also called *epidermoid cyst*.

carcinosarcoma (kar' -si-nō-sar-kō' -ma): A tumour which has the cells and characteristics of both carcinoma and sarcoma; occurs most often in the uterus, oesophagus, or thyroid gland.

card-, cardia-, cardio-: Combining forms denoting: (1) the heart, or (2) heart action.

cardia (kar' -di-a): The oesophageal opening into the stomach.

cardiac (kar'di-ak): 1. Relating to the heart. 2. Relating to the cardia. 3. A person who has heart disease. 4. An agent or drug which acts especially on the heart. C. ARREST complete cessation of the heart's activity; C. ARRHYTHMIA abnormal rhythm of the heartbeat; C. ASTHMA see ASTHMA; C. ATROPHY fatty degeneration of the heart muscle; C. BED one which can be manipulated so that the patient is supported in a sitting position; C. BODY SURFACE MAPPING an electrocardiographic technique utilizing many electrodes producing signals that are fed into a computer which filters out the important readings; gives more information than the ordinary ECG about possible abnormalities; C. CATHETERIZATION see under CATHETERIZATION; C. COMPENSATION the maintenance of effective circulation in cases of cardiac disease or disorder, by some mechanism such as hypertrophy of the muscle; C. COMPRESSION (1) constriction of the heart which renders it unable to fill completely; may be due to pericardial fibrosis, or the accumulation of blood in the pericardial sac; (2) a procedure used in cardiopulmonary resuscitation; see C. MASSAGE; CONGESTIVE C. FAILURE a disorder where the heart loses its ability to pump blood efficiently; the body does not get as much oxygen and nutrients as it needs, leading to problems such as fatigue and shortness of breath; it is a chronic, long-term condition, managed with medications and lifestyle changes; C. CYCLE the period from the beginning of one heartbeat to the beginning of the next; includes systole, diastole, and rest period; C. DECOMPENSATION inability of the heart to maintain normal circulation; symptoms are dyspnoea, cyanosis, and oedema; C. FAILURE sudden fatal stoppage of the heart; C. INDEX the volume per minute of cardiac output per square metre of body surface; in the normal adult person the average output is approximately 2.2 litres per minute; C. INSUFFICIENCY inability of the heart to function normally; C. MASSAGE external or closed-chest massage consists of rhythmic compression of the lower end of the sternum every one and a half to two seconds; internal or open-chest massage consists of rhythmic compression of the heart after the chest has been opened surgically; C. MONITORING involves recording the activity of the heart; three methods are (1) hardware C.M. continuous monitoring of a patient on bed rest; (2) telemetry C.M. monitoring the heart of an ambulatory patient; and (3) Holter C.M. the use of a Holter monitor (*q.v.*) for 24 hours for a patient undergoing cardiac rehabilitation; C. MURMURS see MURMUR; C. NEUROSIS a form of anxiety neurosis characterized by chest pains, palpitation, dyspnoea, faintness; also called *neurocirculatory asthenia*; C. OEDEMA gravitational dropsy. C. ORIFICE the opening between the oesophagus and the stomach. C. OUTPUT the volume of blood expelled by either ventricle of the heart per unit of time, usually per minute; computed by multiplying the heart rate by the stroke volume; C. PACING regulating the rate of contraction of the heart muscle by means of an artificial cardiac pacemaker; C. RESERVE (1) the ability of the heart to increase its output to meet increased biological requirements; (2) the difference between C. output at rest and during maximum physical effort; C. STANDSTILL the sudden cessation of contraction of the myocardium; C. TAMPONADE compression of the heart; can occur in surgery or result from penetrating wounds of the heart which cause haemorrhage into the pericardium; may also result from rapid production of effusion, with the patient becoming pale with clammy extremities, engorgement of the neck veins, faint heart sounds, dependent oedema, and hepatomegaly.

cardiac care unit: A critical care unit for patients with myocardial infarcation; monitors are used to assess immediately changes in the status and functioning of the cardiac system.

cardialgia (kar-di-al'-ji-a): 1. Literally, pain in the heart. 2. A painful sensation in the 'pit of the stomach' often called *heartburn*.

cardiataxia (kar'-di-a-tak'-si-a): Irregularity of the heart action due to incoordination of the contractions.

cardiectasis (kar-di-ek'-ta-sis): Dilatation of the heart.

cardinal (kar'-di-nal): Primary or fundamental, as cardinal signs — temperature, pulse, respiration.

cardioaccelerator (kar'-di-ō-ak-sel'-e-rā-tor): An agent that speeds up the action of the heart.

cardiocatheterization (kar'-di-ō-kath-e-ter-ī-zā'-shun): Cardiac catheterization; see under CATHETERIZATION.

cardiocele (kar'-di-ō-sēl): The protrusion of the heart from its cavity through an opening in the diaphragm or a wound.

cardiocentesis (kar'-di-ō-sen-tē'-sis): Surgical puncture of the heart.

cardiochalasia (kar'-di-ō-ka-lā'-zi-a): Weakening or incompetence of the cardiac orifice of the stomach.

cardiodynamics (kar'-di-ō-dī-nam'-iks): The study of the forces involved in the functions and actions of the heart.

cardiogenesis (kar'-di-ō-jen'-e-sis): The development of the heart in the embryonic stage of life.

cardiogenic (kar'-di-ō-jen'-ik): 1. Relating to the development of the heart. 2. Developing or having its origin in the heart, *e.g.*, the shock in coronary thrombosis. C. SHOCK occurs when the cardiac output of blood is inadequate to meet body requirements.

cardiogram (kar'-di-ō-gram): A tracing, on special paper, showing the activity of the heart muscle; obtained by cardiography. Electrocardiogram.

cardiograph (kar'-di-ō-graf): An instrument for recording graphically the force and form of the heartbeat. — cardiographic, adj.; cardiographically, adv.

cardioinhibitor (kar'-di-ō-in-hib'-i-tor): An agent that slows or restrains the action of the heart. — cardioinhibitory, adj.

cardiokinetic (kar'-di-ō-kī-net'-ik): 1. Stimulating heart action. 2. An agent that influences heart action.

cardiology (kar-di-ol'-o-ji): That branch of medicine that deals with the heart, its functions and diseases.

cardiomegaly (kar'-di-ō-meg'-a-li): Enlargement of the heart.

cardiometry (kar-di-om'-e-tri): The procedure of measuring the size of the heart or the force exerted by its contractions.

cardiomyopathy (kar'-di-ō-mī-op'-a-thi): A disorder of heart muscle; acute, subacute, or chronic; cause may be obscure; may be associated with endocardial or pericardial pathology. — cardiomyopathic, adj.

cardiopathy (kar-di-op'-a-thi): Any heart disorder or disease. — cardiopathic, adj.

cardiopericarditis (kar′ -di-ō-per-i-kar-dī′ -tis): Inflammation of the heart muscle and pericardium.

cardioplegia (kar′ -di-ō-plē′ -ji-a): Cardiac arrest as may result from a direct blow or injury. May also be an elective procedure, utilizing drugs, during cardiac surgery.

cardioptosis (kar-di-op′ -to-sis): Downward displacement of the heart.

cardiopulmonary (kar′ -di-ō-pul′ -mō-ner-i): Pertaining to the heart and lungs. C. ARREST the absence of effective circulation or respiration, or both; C. BYPASS see BYPASS; C. RESUS-CITATION, see RESUSCITATION.

cardiorrhexis (kar-di-ō-rek′ -sis): Rupture of the heart wall.

cardiosclerosis (kar-di-ō-skle-rō′ -sis): Hardening of the heart muscle.

cardioscope (kar′ -di-ō-scōp): An instrument fitted with a lens and illumination, for examining the inside of the living heart — cardioscopic, adj.; cardioscopically, adv.

cardiospasm (kar′ -di-ō-spazm): Persistent spasm of the cardiac sphincter between the oesophagus and the stomach, causing secondary dilation of the upper part of the oesophagus and thus giving rise to substernal pain and sometimes regurgitation. Usually no pathological change is found but the pain is easily mistaken for cardiac pain.

cardiosphygmograph (kar′ -di-ō-sfig′ -mō-graf): An instrument for recording the heart movement and the pulse.

cardiotachometer (kar′ -di-ō-ta-kom′ -i-ter): An instrument for recording the heart rate continuously over days or longer.

cardiotherapy (kar′ -di-ō-ther′ -a-pi): Treatment of heart diseases and disorders.

cardiothoracic (kar′ -di-ō-tho-ras′ -ic): 1. Relating to the heart and thoracic cavity. 2. Pertaining to a specialized branch of surgery. C. RATIO the size of the heart as compared to the size of the thoracic cage.

cardiotocography (kar′ -di-ō-tō-kog′ -ra-fi): A combination of electrocardiography and tocography (q.v.). The fetal heart rate is obtained by a microphone placed on the mother's abdomen or by an electrode attached to the fetal scalp. At the same time the uterine contractions are measured by tocography. Both measurements are recorded on a monitoring device.

cardiotomy (kar-di-ot′ -o-mi): 1. Surgical incision of the heart. 2. An operation in which the cardiac sphincter is cut in order to reduce stricture of the oesophagus.

cardiotonic (kar′ -di-ō-ton′ -ik): Increasing the contractility of the heart muscle and slowing its rate, thus increasing efficiency of the cardiac pumping. Usually refers to agents that have this effect, especially drugs.

cardiotoxic (kar′ -di-ō-tok′ -sik): Having a toxic or harmful effect on the heart. — cardiotoxicity, adj.

cardiovalvulitis (kar′ -di-ō-val-vū-lī′ -tis): Inflammation of the heart valves.

cardiovascular (kar′ -di-ō-vas′ -kū-lar): Relating to the heart and blood vessels. C. SYSTEM the heart and blood vessels by which the blood is pumped and circulated throughout the body; it transports oxygen from the lungs to the tissues and returns carbon dioxide to the lungs to be removed.

cardioversion (kar′ -di-ō-ver′ -zhun): Restoration of the heart's normal rhythm by applying brief discharges of direct-current electricity across the intact chest and into the heart muscle to stop an arrhythmia or control fibrillation, and allow the normal heart to take over; usually an emergency measure. It is called defibrillation (q.v.) when used to correct ventricular fibrillation.

cardioverter (kar′ -di-ō-ver-ter): An instrument used to deliver a brief direct-current electric shock to the heart to terminate certain arrhythmias.

carditis (kar-dī′ -tis): Inflammation of the heart. A word seldom used without a descriptive prefix, e.g., endo-, myo-, pan-, peri-. RHEUM-ATIC C. associated with rheumatic fever; may be severe, causing congestive heart failure, pericarditis, and enlargement of the heart; STREPTOCOCCAL C. occurs as a result of a streptococcal infection.

care: See ACUTE CARE, CORONARY CARE UNIT, CO-OPERATIVE CARE, LONG-TERM CARE, MANAGED CARE, SELF-CARE.

care contracting: A procedure whereby the caregiver and the patient commit themselves to a precisely defined course of action and activities, usually in writing, stating specifically certain behaviours that are to occur and the conditions under which they are to occur, and establishing rewards and punishments appropriate to the outcomes.

caregiver: Any person who is involved in identifying, preventing, or treating patients, or in rehabilitating them; includes professionals, non-professionals, and community health workers.

care home: See NURSING HOME.

care manager: A person responsible for overseeing an individual's treatment and follow-up. See also MANAGED CARE.

care pathway: An integrated treatment plan using available evidence and guidelines, and agreed by the multi-disciplinary team (*q.v.*).

care plan: The document in which nursing information is recorded. It usually contains an assessment of the patient, details of actual and potential problems, goals, nursing interventions, implementation and an evaluation.

Care Programme Approach: A protocol for the delivery of community care services to people with mental health problems. The key elements are: a thorough and systematic assessment of health and social care needs; a detailed written care plan (*q.v.*); the appointment of a care coordinator; and regular reviews of health and social care needs. The care plan is agreed with members of the multidisciplinary team, GPs, service users and their carers. See KEY WORKER.

carer: Someone who provides substantial amounts of care or support on a regular basis to another person who, because of age, disability, or illness, cannot manage at home without help. A carer is not a care worker of any kind who is paid to provide care as part of a contract of employment. The Carers Recognition and Services Act (1995) aims to provide for assessment of the ability of carers to provide care and to ensure that carers receive services; it gives people who provide substantial care on a regular basis the right to ask for an assessment from social services, based on their ability to provide and continue to provide care; it applies only to informal carers, and the local authority does not have a duty to provide services to carers.

care rationing: The restriction of medical aid or services; usually a result of budgetary constraints.

Carer's Assessment of Management Index: A questionnaire for evaluating the person responsible for the care of someone with mental health problems. It assesses his or her strategies for managing and coping, and aims to develop these skills.

care standards: The quality of treatment expected in children's homes, independent hospitals, and care homes, as established by the Care Standards Act (2000).

caries (kā'-ri-ez): Inflammatory decay of bone or teeth, usually associated with pus formation. SPINAL C. Pott's disease (*q.v.*). — carious, adj.

caritas (kar'-i-tas): A term used to describe the aspects of the nurse–patient relationship, meaning love; charity; compassion.

carminative (kar-min'-a-tiv): 1. Having the power to relieve flatulence and associated colic. 2. An agent that helps to prevent the formation of gas and is capable of causing gas to be expelled from the gastrointestinal tract.

carneous (kar'-nē-us): Fleshy. C. MOLE see MOLE.

carnivorous (kar-niv'-o-rus): Subsisting entirely or chiefly on meat.

carotenaemia (kar-o-te-nē'-mi-a): The presence of an excessive amount of carotene in the blood; in large quantities it produces yellowing of the skin.

carotenase (kar'-ō-ti-nās): An enzyme that converts carotene into vitamin A.

carotene (kar'-ō-tēn): A yellow pigment, found in carrots, sweet potatoes and other yellow vegetables, leafy vegetables, milk fat and other fats, and egg yolk; is converted into vitamin A in the liver. A provitamin.

carotid (kar-ot'-id): The principal arteries on each side of the neck, which supply blood to the head and neck. They arise from the aortic arch on the left and the innominate artery on the right. At the bifurcation of each common carotid artery into the internal and external carotid arteries there are: (1) the C. BODIES a collection of chemoreceptors (*q.v.*) which, being sensitive to chemical changes in the blood, protect the body against lack of oxygen and aid in the reflex control of the blood pressure, heart rate, and respiration; and (2) the C. SINUS a slight dilatation of the common carotid artery at its bifurcation; it contains baroreceptors (*q.v.*) in its walls which are sensitive to pressure changes; pressure on the sinus causes vasodilation, slowing of the heart, and a drop in blood pressure.

carotid sinus syndrome: A condition characterized by bradycardia, severe hypotension, dizziness, faintness; caused by overactivity of the carotid sinus reflex.

carpal (kar'-pal): Relating to the wrist.

carpal tunnel: A deep cavity on the palm side of the carpus with a fibrous band across it forming a tunnel which accommodates the median nerves and some of the tendons of the hand. C.T. SYNDROME a fairly common symptom complex due to compression of the median nerve in the carpal tunnel; characterized by pain, paraesthesia, atrophy of the thenar muscles, oedema of the fingers, numbness, and tingling in the area of the hand innervated by the median nerve, with weakness, sometimes extending to the elbow; most severe at night. The compression may be caused by swelling of the structures in the tunnel and compression of the nerve as it passes through the fascial band. Most common in middle-aged women. Also called *carpotunnel syndrome.*

carpectomy (kar-pek′-to-mi): Excision of a carpal bone.

carpus (kar′-pus): The wrist. The eight small bones and surrounding structures between the hand and the forearm. The bones, arranged in two rows, are (1) the scaphoid, lunate, triquetral, pisiform; (2) the trapezium, trapezoid, capitate, hamate. — carpal, adj.

carrier (kar′-i-er): **1.** A healthy animal or human host who harbours a pathogenic or potentially pathogenic microorganism in the absence of discernible disease and serves as a possible source of infection. ACTIVE C. one who becomes a C. after recovering from the disease. **2.** An insect vector that transmits an infection. **3.** A heterozygote (*q.v.*) that carries a recessive gene together with its dominant allele.

car sickness: A form of motion sickness (*q.v.*).

cartilage (kar′-til-ij): Gristle; a tough connective tissue, characterized by firmness and having no neurovascular supply. There are three main varieties: (1) HYALINE C. a semi-transparent substance of a pearly bluish colour possessing considerable elasticity; (2) YELLOW ELASTIC C. possesses a network of yellow elastic fibres, branching and anastomosing in all directions; it is a true cartilage found, *e.g.,* in the external ear; and (3) white fibrocartilage, consists of dense white fibrous tissue of great strength and rigidity; it forms the intervertebral discs. AR-TICULAR C. the C. at the joint surfaces of bones; provides smooth surfaces for movement without friction; ARYTENOID C. one on either side forming the posterior wall of the upper rim of the larynx; their function is to regulate the opening and closing of the space between the vocal cords; COSTAL C. one of several cartilages that attach the first seven ribs to the sternum; CRICOID C. lies below the thyroid C.; shaped like a signet ring with the broad part at the back; forms the lateral and posterior walls of the larynx; lined with ciliated epithelium; EN-SIFORM C. the xiphoid process of the sternum; EPIPHYSEAL C. that present at the ends and shafts of the long bones in children; it allows for growth in length; THYROID C. the large cartilage of the larynx, in the front of the neck; 'Adam's apple'.

cartilaginous (kar-ti-laj′-i-nus): Composed of or relating to cartilage.

caruncle (kar′-ung-k′l): A red, fleshy projection. HYMENAL C. the tabs of skin that remain around the orifice of the vagina after rupture of the hymen. Also called *caruncula myrtiformes.* LACRIMAL C. a small reddish projection near the inner canthus of the eye; caruncula lacrimalis.

carus (kār′-rus): Stupor; coma.

cary-, caryo-: Combining forms denoting relationship to a nucleus; same as kary-, karyo-.

case: C. FINDING the process of identifying those at risk from a particular disease or illness, carried out within the National Service Frameworks (*q.v.*); also referred to as *screening*; C. HISTORY a biography of a patient's physical and pathological experiences, collected for scientific purposes; sometimes obtained by interview, sometimes collected over the years; includes the history of the present condition for which he or she is being treated; C. RECORD all of the data accumulated about a patient's history, disease, treatment, etc. during a hospital stay; it is placed in the permanent files of the hospital and is admissible as evidence in court; C. SERIES (1) collections of reports on the treatment of individual patients; (2) reports on a series of treatments of a single patient; also known as *case reports.* C. STUDY a method of learning about various diseases and their treatment; includes gathering, organizing, and recording all relevant data concerning a specific condition or status of an individual patient; C.S. RESEARCH the collection and analysis of data relating to a patient or group of patients.

caseation (kā-zē-ā′-shun): The precipitation of casein in milk to form cheese. C. NECROSIS necrosis of tissue whereby it is changed to a dry, crumbly consistency resembling cheese; characteristically associated with pulmonary tuberculosis.

casein (kā′-sē-in): A protein formed when milk enters the stomach. Coagulation occurs, due to the action of rennin on the caseinogen in the milk, splitting it into two proteins, one being casein. The casein combines with calcium and a clot is formed.

caseinogen (kā-sē-in′-ō-jen): The precursor of casein; a substance present in milk that is converted into casein by the action of rennin in the stomach.

cast: 1. Fibrous material and exudate that has been moulded to the form of the cavity or tube in which it has collected, *e.g.,* RENAL C. or URINARY C. it can be identified under the microscope and classified according to its constitution as bloody, epithelial, fatty, etc. **2.** A commonly used term for any abnormal turning of the eye. **3.** A stiff bandage or dressing impregnated with plaster of Paris or other hardening material; used to immobilize a part in cases of fracture or dislocation and in various orthopaedic conditions. AEROPLANE C. a spica cast that covers the upper torso as well as the affected arm and holds it in an abducted position; BANJO C. one with a large ring extension that holds the fingers in extension by the use of rubber bands; used mostly for finger fractures; BODY C. a c. that encloses the trunk; may extend from the neck to the groin; used for treating diseases and injuries of the vertebrae; CYLINDER C. a semi-rigid c., applied to the lower leg; extends from the thigh to the ankle; used for treating ankle and knee injuries; GAUNTLET C. encloses the wrist and extends to the palm; used for treating fractures of the metacarpus and phalanges; MINERVA JACKET a c. used in treatment of fractures of the cervical vertebrae; encloses the forehead, chin, occiput, and neck and extends down over the shoulders and trunk; SPICA C. used to immobilize an extremity by incorporating part of the body along with the injured extremity; the HIP SPICA is used in fractures of the femur, and in some hip, pelvic, and tibial fractures; the SHOULDER or ICA is used for treating fractures of the proximal humerus; the THUMB SPICA is used in fractures of the navicular bone in the wrist; the TOE SPICA is used after surgery for bunions and incorporates all or part of the foot; TURNBUCKLE JACKET a spica jacket c. which may include the head and arm; the side of the jacket is split and a turnbuckle inserted to allow for gradual opening of the two halves as correction progresses; used in treatment of scoliosis; WALKING C. a rubber walker is attached to a leg or foot cast to permit the patient to ambulate. See also UNNA'S BOOT.

cast brace: A device used with a walking cast to permit early ambulation following fracture of the tibia.

Castle's factor: A substance secreted by the stomach; necessary for the absorption of vitamin B_{12} (cyanocobalamin); deficiency or lack of this factor results in pernicious anaemia. Also called *Castle's intrinsic factor*.

castor oil: Obtained from the seed of the castor bean; used in medicine as a purgative; *oleum ricini*.

castration (kas-trā′-shun): The removal of testes or ovaries. C. ANXIETY or COMPLEX the unfounded fear of loss of one's genital organs; may be precipitated by some humiliating or worrisome life event or by feelings of guilt over forbidden sexual desires; in children it usually arises from guilt over oedipal feelings. See also OEDIPUS COMPLEX.

casualty (kaz′-ū-al-ti): An accidental or other type of injury, or a person who has suffered such an injury.

CAT: Abbreviation for computerized axial tomography (*q.v.*).

CATS: Abbreviation for Credit Accumulation Transfer System (*q.v.*).

cata-: Prefix denoting down, under, lower, away, against, through, concealed, along with.

catabolism (ka-tab′-ō-lizm): The series of chemical reactions in the living body in which complex substances, taken in as food, are broken down into simpler ones, accompanied by the release of energy. This energy is needed for anabolism (*q.v.*) and the other activities of the body. — catabolic, adj.

catagen (kat′-a-jen): The brief period in the hair growth cycle after the hair is formed and before the resting period that precedes shedding. See TELOGEN.

catagenesis (kat-a-jen′-e-sis): **1.** Involution. **2.** Retrogression.

catalase (kat′ a-lās): An enzyme found in many plant and animal tissues, and especially in anaerobic bacteria; catalyses the decomposition of hydrogen peroxide into water and oxygen.

catalepsy (kat′-a-lep-si): A conscious but trance-like state in which the muscles are rigid so that the subject remains in a fixed position over an indefinite period of time. — cataleptic; cataleptoid, adj.

catalyse (kat′-a-līz): To act as a catalyst or to influence a chemical reaction without taking part in it.

catalysis (ka-tal′-i-sis): A change in the rate at which a chemical action proceeds, produced by an agent which is not itself affected by the reaction. May be positive or negative. — catalytic, adj.

catalyst (kat′-a-list): An agent that produces catalysis (*q.v.*). It does not undergo any change during the process. Syn., *catalyser, enzyme*.

cataphoresis (kat′-a-fō-rē′-sis): Electrophoresis (*q.v.*).

cataphrenia (kat-a-frē′-ni-a): A mental state that resembles dementia and which tends to be temporary.

cataphylaxis (kat-a-fi-lak′-sis): The migration of leukocytes and antibodies to the site in the body that has been invaded by an infective organism.

cataplasia (kat-a-plā'-zi-a): Atrophy or degeneration of tissues in which they revert to an earlier, or embryonic state.

cataplexy (kat'-a-plek-si): A condition of sudden powerlessness due to muscular rigidity caused by intense emotional upheaval such as fear or shock, or hypnotic suggestion. The patient remains conscious; recovery is usually complete. — cataplectic, adj.

cataract (kat'-a-rakt): A progressive clouding of the crystalline lens of the eye or its capsule, or both, causing blurring of vision; may be due to senility, trauma, or diabetes mellitus or inherited factors; may also be congenital in infants who have a viral infection in utero. CONGENITAL C. may be due to the mother's having rubella during early pregnancy; HARD C. contains a hard nucleus, tends to be dark in colour, and occurs in older individuals; SENILE C. a hard C. that occurs as a result of the ageing process; SOFT C. one without a hard nucleus; occurs at any age but particularly in the young. Cataract usually develops slowly and when mature is called 'ripe'. — cataractous, adj.

catarrh (ka-tar'): Inflammation of mucous membrane with a constant flow of mucus; applied especially to the upper respiratory tract. POST-NASAL C. chronic rhinopharyngitis.

catastrophic (kat-a-strof'-ik): Sudden; disastrous; violent; life threatening.

catatonia (kat-a-tō'-ni-a): A type of behaviour that may occur in schizophrenia; the patient may assume certain odd postures for indefinite periods, have muscular spasms, refuse to speak, become negative, stuporous or indifferent to the environment. — catatonic, adj.

catchment area: A term used to describe the geographic area from which a health authority or health-care practice draws its patients.

catecholamine (kat-e-kōl'-a-mēn): Any one of a group of compounds that are secreted largely but not exclusively by the adrenal gland and which have the power to cause physiological changes resembling those caused by the action of the sympathetic nerves. Includes dopamine, noradrenaline, and adrenaline. Also produced synthetically as drugs for use as sympathomimetics (q.v.).

catgut (kat'-gut): A form of ligature and suture of varying thickness, strength and absorbability, prepared from sheep's intestines. After sterilization it is hermetically sealed in glass tubes according to size. The plain variety is usually absorbed in 5 to 10 days. Chromicized C. and iodized C. will hold for 20 to 40 days.

catharsis (ka-thar'-sis): 1. A cleansing or purging, said particularly of the intestine. 2. A method used in Freudian psychiatry; the analyst urges the patient to talk freely about things that come to mind during a train of thought and thus purge his mind of the memories of painful or unpleasant experiences that may be causing his psychological disturbance; syn., abreaction (q.v.).

cathartic (ka-thar'-tik): 1. Producing catharsis (q.v.). 2. An agent that promotes evacuation of the intestine. Cathartics are classed as laxatives or purgatives, according to the type and degree of evacuation they produce.

catheter (kath'-e-ter): A slender, hollow, flexible tube of varying lengths, bores and shapes, that is inserted into a structure (e.g., a vein or hollow organ); used to distend a hollow tube or passage, to distend or maintain an opening, or for injecting, instilling, or withdrawing fluid from a body cavity. Catheters are made of soft or hard rubber, gum elastic, glass, rubberized silk; silver and other metals; some are radiopaque. Catheters are often designated as French; sizes 16–18 French are usually used for adults. To convert from French scale to millimetres divide by 3; see FRENCH SCALE. BALLOON C. see FOLEY C. BROVIAC C. a C. designed for use in administering hyperalimentation; CARDIAC C. a long, slender C. designed for passage through a blood vessel into the heart; CHEST CATHETER a size 32 to 36 French catheter that is inserted in the 4th or 5th intercostal space at the midaxillary line of the affected side and connected to underwater seal and suction, to re-establish negative pressure in the pleural space for a patient with pneumothorax; in cases of haemothorax, the 36 French catheter is inserted in the second intercostal space; DEPEZZAR C. Malecot C.; FEMALE C. a short C. for catheterizing the urinary bladder of female patients; FOLEY C. a common type of indwelling C. held in place by an attached inflated balloon; HICKMAN C. used for administering hyperalimentation; it is designed to also allow for withdrawal of blood and administration of medications; INDWELLING C. one fastened in place for continuous drainage of the urinary bladder; INLYING C. one inserted for infusion after doing a cutdown; INTRACATHETER a C. inserted through a needle; used for intravenous infusions; the venepuncture is made with the needle and the C. is then inserted into the vein through the needle; JACQUES C. has a rounded end and an opening at the side; MALE C. a long catheter for use in catheterizing the male urinary bladder; MALECOT C. has a protuberance at the distal end; used to drain the bladder through a suprapubic opening; NASAL C. used to pass food into the stomach or to administer oxygen through the nose; NONRETENTION C. one used to empty the urinary bladder or to collect a clean urine specimen; is removed after use; RETENTION C. indwelling C. or self-retaining C., one fitted with a device to hold it in position when prolonged drainage of the urinary bladder is required; SUCTIONING C. one used to suction the upper respiratory tract; introduced through the nasotracheal route; SWAN–GANZ C. balloon-tipped, flow-directed, multilumen C. used for haemodynamic monitoring; has a transistorized thermistor that detects changes in blood temperatures which are used to compute cardiac output; it also measures right and left ventricular pressures and pulmonary capillary wedge pressure in the smallest pulmonary vessels accessible to the catheter. A transducer attached to the external end of the catheter translates pressure waves into electrical impulses; thus waves appear on an oscilloscope and the digital values are displayed on the monitor. Used in diagnosing and managing patients with heart failure from myocardial infarction or cardiogenic shock, those with pulmonary oedema or pulmonary embolus, those who have undergone cardiac bypass surgery; WHISTLE-TIPPED C. one with an opening on the end as well as the side.

catheterization (kath-e-ter-ī-zā′-shun): Insertion of a catheter into a body cavity or channel, often the urinary bladder. CARDIAC C. an invasive procedure consisting of the insertion of a fine polyethylene or radiopaque nylon tubing via the basilic, median cubital, basilar, or femoral vein into the heart to: (1) record pressures; (2) introduce a radiopaque substance prior to x-ray; (3) withdraw blood samples; and (4) determine blood flow in the heart. Either the right or left heart and one or more chambers may be catheterized; CONTINUOUS C. provides for continuous drainage of the bladder through an indwelling catheter; INTERMITTENT C. C. that is performed at intervals to remove accumulated urine from the bladder; SUPRAPUBIC C. is accomplished by surgically inserting an indwelling catheter through an opening just above the pubis.

catheterize (kath′-e-ter-īz): To introduce a catheter into a body cavity; often refers to the urinary bladder. See also CARDIAC CATHETERIZATION under CATHETERIZATION.

cathexis (ka-thek′-sis): In psychiatry, the conscious or unconscious fixing of one's psychic energy on some particular thing, person, or concept. — cathetic, adj.

cathode (kath′-ōd): The negatively charged terminal of an electrode or an electrolytic cell, as in a storage battery.

cation (kat′-ī-on): A positively charged ion; the opposite of anion (q.v.).

caul: A part or all of the amnion which sometimes covers or envelops the head of the fetus at birth. In olden days called 'Angel's veil' and thought to be a good omen.

cauliflower ear: A partially deformed auricle, usually due to injury; frequently seen in professional boxers.

cauloplegia (kaw-lō-plē′-ji-a): Paralysis of the penis.

causal (kaw′sal): Relating to a cause, as the agent causing a disease.

causalgia (kaw-sal′ji-a): Excruciating burning neuralgic pain, resulting from physical trauma to cutaneous nerve fibres.

causal hypothesis (kaw′-zal-hī-poth′-ē-sis): A theory that proposes a cause-and-effect relationship between two or more variables. See DEPENDENT VARIABLE; INDEPENDENT VARIABLE.

causality (kaw-zal′-i-ti): The relation between cause and effect.

caustic (kaw′-stik): 1. Corrosive or destructive to living tissue, or agents that produce this effect. Used therapeutically to destroy granulation tissue, warts, polyps. Carbolic acid, nitric acid, carbon dioxide snow, silver nitrate, and potassium hydroxide are most commonly employed. 2. Able to burn, corrode, or otherwise destroy by chemical action.

caustic soda: Sodium hydroxide; see under SODIUM.

cauterize (kaw′-ter-īz): 1. To apply a cautery. 2. To destroy tissue by heat, chemical action, or electricity. — cauterization, n.

cautery (kaw′-ter-i): A caustic agent or device such as a chemical, hot iron, electricity, or extreme cold to destroy living tissue. ACTUAL C. a hot iron used to apply direct heat; CHEMICAL C. a chemical substance used to burn or sear tissue; ELECTRIC C. a platinum wire maintained at red heat by an electric current; PAQUELIN'S C. a form of C. in which the hollow platinum point is kept at the required heat by a current of benzene which is constantly pumped into it. — cauterization, n.; cauterize, v.

cava (kā′-va): Plural of cavum. A vena cava.

cavamesenteric shunt (kā′-va-mes-en-ter′-ik): The upper end of the inferior vena cava is anastomosed to the superior mesentric vein; used in children when the portal vein is BLOCKED. SEE SHUNT.

Cavell, Edith L.: British nurse, matron of a Red Cross Hospital in Belgium during World War I; helped about 200 imprisoned English, French, and Belgian soldiers to escape; was arrested by the Germans, tried, and convicted, and was executed 12 October 1915. [1865–1915.]

cavernous (kav' -er-nus): Relating to a cavity or hollow. C. BODY see under BODY; c. respirations see under RESPIRATION; C. SINUS see under SINUS.

cavity (kav' -i-ti): A hollow; an enclosed area within the body. ABDOMINAL C. that area below the diaphragm and above the pelvis; the abdomen; BUCCAL C. the mouth; CEREBRAL C. the ventricles of the brain; CRANIAL C. the brain box formed by the bones of the cranium; DENTAL C. a hollow formed in a tooth as a result of decay of the organic matter following decalcification of the inorganic outer part of the tooth; syn., *caries (pl.)*; DORSAL C. the cavity enclosed by the vertebrae and the bones of the cranium.; GLENOID C. see under GLENOID; MEDULLARY C. the hollow centre of a long bone, containing yellow bone marrow or medulla; NASAL C. that in the nose, separated into right and left halves by the nasal septum; ORAL C. the buccal cavity; PELVIC C. that formed by the pelvic bones, more particularly the part below the iliopectineal line and containing primarily the rectum and reproductive organs; PERITONEAL C. a potential space between the parietal and visceral layers of the peritoneum. Similarly, the PLEURAL C. is the potential space between the pulmonary and parietal plurae which, in health, are in contact in all phases of respiration; SPINAL C. contains the spinal cord; SYNOVIAL C. the potential space in a synovial joint; THORACIC C. the part of the trunk lying above the diaphragm; TYMPANIC C. the cavity of the middle ear; see under EAR; UTERINE C. that of the uterus, in the form of a small triangle, the base extending between the orifices of the uterine tubes; VENTRAL C. the body C. in front of the spinal column, encloses the mouth, throat, thorax, abdomen and pelvis.

CBT: Abbreviation for cognitive behavioural therapy (*q.v.*).

cc: Abbreviation for cubic centimetre.

CCETSW: Abbreviation for Central Council for the Education and Training in Social Work.

CCF: Abbreviation for congestive cardiac failure, see under CARDIAC.

CCU: Abbreviation for: (1) coronary care unit (*q.v.*), (2) cardiac care unit (*q.v.*).

CD: Abbreviation for controlled drug, see under DRUG.

CDC: Abbreviation for Centers for Disease Control (USA) — (*q.v..*).

CD-ROM: Abbreviation for compact disk read-only memory (*q.v.*).

-cele: Combining form denoting: (1) tumour; (2) hernia.

cell (sel): A mass of protoplasm containing a nucleus. The basic physiological and structural unit of all living things. Consists of a central core, the nucleus, which is made up of nucleoplasm, enclosed in a membrane, and surrounded by cytoplasm, the whole being enclosed in a membrane which separates it from other cells. Certain cells are non-nucleated, *e.g.*, erythrocytes, and others are multinucleated, *e.g.*, the leukocytes. ARGYROPHILIC C. cells that are capable of being stained by silver salts. BAND C. a neutrophil with a nucleus in the form of a continuous band which may be coiled, twisted, or in the shape of a horseshoe; see NEUTROPHIL B C.S beta lymphatic cells that migrate directly into tissues without passing through the thymus; they mature into plasma cells and are responsible for the production of immunoglobulins; BETA C.S cells that make up most of the bulk of the islets of Langerhans in the pancreas; they secrete insulin; C. MEMBRANE the semipermeable membrane that bounds all animal cells; T C. a lymphocyte derived from the thymus and which participates in the body's immune defences; in the gate control theory T cells are assumed to respond to both excitatory and inhibitory impulses to cause or inhibit a response by the body to certain stimuli.

cell-mediated immunity: A specific type of immune reaction thought to be initiated by T lymphocytes. See T CELL under CELL.

cellular (sel' -ū-lar): Relating to or composed of cells.

cellulitis (sel-ū-lī' -tis): A diffuse inflammation of connective tissue, especially the loose subcutaneous tissue. When it involves the pelvic tissues in the female it is called parametritis. When it occurs in the floor of the mouth it is called Ludwig's angina.

cellulose (sel' -ū-lōs): A carbohydrate forming the outer walls of plant and vegetable cells. A polysaccharide which cannot be digested by humans but supplies roughage for stimulation of peristalsis (*q.v.*).

Celsius (sel' -si-us): A thermometric scale in which the boiling point of water at sea level is

100° and the melting point of ice is 0° (centigrade thermometer). [Anders Celsius, Swedish astronomer, 1701–1744.]

cement (sē-ment'): **1.** Any plastic material used to bind contiguous objects or materials together. **2.** Any material used for filling teeth or making other dental repairs. **3.** The hard, white, bone-like substance covering the roots of the teeth; cementum.

censor (sen'-sor): Term employed by Freud (*q.v.*) to define the resistance that prevents repressed material from readily re-entering the conscious mind from the subconscious (unconscious) mind unless it is disguised in some way.

census (sen'-sus): A complete enumeration of a population; specifically, a periodic survey of the population of a country by its government.

Centers for Disease Control: A federal agency in the Public Health Service in the USA, established to protect the health of the American nation by providing leadership and direction in the investigation, identification, prevention, control, and eradication of preventable and other diseases. Known internationally as *CDC*.

centesis (sen-tē'-sis): A puncture of a body cavity with a trocar, needle, or aspirator. Often used with other word elements to indicate the part of the body involved, *e.g.*, abdominocentesis.

centi-: Prefix used in the metric system to indicate one one-hundredth.

centigrade (sen'-ti-grād): Having one hundred divisions or degrees. Usually applied to the Celsius thermometric scale in which the freezing point of water is fixed at 0° and the boiling point at 100°.

centigram (sen'-ti-gram): A metric unit of weight; one one-hundredth part of a gram.

centilitre (sen'-ti-lē-ter): One one-hundredth of a litre.

centimetre (sen'-ti-mē-ter): In metric linear measurement, one one-hundredth of a metre.

centrad (sen'-trad): Towards a centre, or towards the median line of the body.

central nervous system: The part of the nervous system consisting of the brain, spinal cord, spinal nerves and their end organs.

central processing unit: the part of a computer (a microprocessor chip) that does most of the data processing; together with the memory, this forms the central part of a computer to which the peripherals are attached.

Central Sterile Supplies Department: A hospital sterilization and disinfection unit.

Central Sterile Supply Unit: A hospital sterilization and disinfection unit.

central venous pressure: See under BLOOD PRESSURE.

centre: 1. A group of neurons concerned with the control of a particular activity or function; usually named for the function they control, *e.g.*, respiratory centre, auditory centre, etc. **2.** The midpoint of a body.

centrifugal (sen-trif'-ū-gal): Efferent. Having a tendency to move away or outwards from a centre or from the cerebral cortex.

centrifuge (sen'-tri-fūj): An apparatus that rotates at high speed, thereby increasing the force of gravity so that substances of different densities are separated; usually used to separate particulate material from a suspending liquid. — centrifuge, v.

centriole (sen'-tri-ōl)· Either of two cylindrical granules in the cytoplasm of cells which migrate to opposite poles during cell division and determine the arrangement of the spindles in the dividing cell.

centripetal (sen-trip'-it-al): Afferent. Having a tendency to move towards a centre or towards the cerebral cortex.

centromere (sen'-trō-mēr): The part of the chromosome to which the spindle fibre is attached during mitosis (*q.v.*).

centrosome (sen'-trō-sōm): A minute spot in the cytoplasm of animal cells supposedly concerned with the division of the nucleus and which, in mitosis (*q.v.*), draws the divided chromosomes to opposite sides of the dividing cell.

centrosphere (sen'-trō-sfēr): A small body near the nucleus of an animal cell which contains the centrosome.

centrum (sen'-trum): A centre.

cephal-, cephalo-: Combining forms denoting head.

cephalalgia (kef'-al-al'-ji-a): Pain in the head; headache. Also spelled *cephalgia*.

cephalic (kef'-al'-ik): Relating to the head; near the head. C. INDEX the ratio of the width to the length of the head; C. VERSION an obstetric manoeuvre to change the fetal lie to a head presentation to facilitate delivery.

-cephalic, -cephalism, -cephaly: Combining forms denoting (1) the head; (2) headed or having a head.

cephalitis (kef'-a-lī'-tis): Encephalitis (*q.v.*).

cephalocele (kef'-a-lō-sēl): Hernia of the brain; protrusion of part of the cranial contents through the skull. ORBITAL C. protrusion of some of the cranial contents into the orbit of the eye; a birth defect usually accompanied by other eye defects.

cephalohaematoma (kef'-a-lō-hē-ma-tō'-ma): A collection of blood beneath the fibrous covering of the skull. Also spelled *cephalhaematoma*.

cephaloid (kef'-a-loyd): Resembling the head.

cephalometer (kef-a-lom'-i-ter): An instrument for measuring the head dimensions.

cephalometry (kef-a-lom'-i-tri): Measurement of the living human head.

cephalopelvic (kef'-a-lō-pel'-vik): Term used in referring to the size of the head of the fetus *in utero* in relation to the size of the mother's bony pelvis. C. DISPROPORTION a disparity between the size of an infant's head and that of the maternal pelvis or of the opening of the pelvis.

cephaloplegia (kef'-a-lō-plē'-ji-a): Paralysis of the muscles of the head and face.

cephalosporins (kef-a-lō-spōr'-ins): A group of broad-spectrum penicillinase-resistant antibiotics derived from *Cephalosporium*, a genus of fungi found in soil. Effective against Gram-negative and Gram-positive organisms, including *E. coli, Klebsiella, Haemophilus influenzae, Aerobacter*, and *Proteus*. Used in the treatment of certain severe infections of the respiratory and genitourinary tracts, bloodstream, bones and joints, and in staphylococcal and streptococcal infections of skin and soft tissues.

cephalotripsy (kef-a-lō-trip'-si): In obstetrics, the instrumental crushing of the fetal head when delivery is impossible.

cerat-, cerato-: Combining forms denoting: 1. The sclera. 2. Horny tissue. For words beginning thus see also words beginning kerato-.

cerate (sē'-rāt): A preparation for external use; has a wax or fat base; consistency is between that of an ointment and a plaster; does not melt at ordinary temperatures.

cerclage (ser-klazh'): 1. A technique used in reducing a fracture; a wire or other non-absorbable material is placed around the bone to hold it in the reduced position until the permanent fixation is accomplished. 2. The technique of stitching edges of an incompetent uterine cervix together with non-absorbable sutures to prevent spontaneous abortion; the sutures are removed at term.

cerebellar (ser-e-bel'-ar): Relating to or involving the cerebellum. C. ATAXIA a condition marked by muscular incoordination, due to a lesion or disease of the cerebellum; see also ATAXIA; C. GAIT a characteristic wide-based, unsteady, staggering, lurching gait; due to a lesion or disease of the cerebellum.

cerebellitis (ser'-e-bel-lī'-tis): Inflammation of the cerebellum.

cerebellospinal (ser'-e-bel-ō-spī'-nal): 1. Relating to the cerebellum and the spinal cord. 2. Proceeding from the cerebellum to the spinal cord, as a descending cerebellospinal tract.

cerebellum (ser-e-bel'-um): That part of the brain which lies behind and below the cerebrum and above the pons and medulla oblongata; consists of two lateral hemispheres with a narrow central portion; its chief functions are the coordination of fine voluntary movements and the maintenance of equilibrium. — cerebellar, adj.

cerebral (ser'-e-bral): Relating to or affecting the cerebrum. C. ACCIDENT or CEREBROVASCULAR ACCIDENT a common occurrence, caused by reduced blood supply to cerebral neurons; may result from haemorrhage, stenosis of cerebral arteries, embolism, or thrombosis; C. CORTEX the outermost cellular layer of grey matter covering the cerebrum; is responsible for higher mental activities during consciousness; CEREBRAL DEATH see BRAIN DEATH; C. CRY the high-pitched cry of an infant; may be indicative of meningitis; C. DIPLEGIA results from a birth injury to both hemispheres causing double hemiplegia and lack of development of limbs; C. HAEMORRHAGE haemorrhage into the cerebrum from a ruptured artery; may result from hypertension or arteriosclerosis; C. HERNIA a hernia in which some of the brain substance protrudes through an opening in one of the bones of the skull as may occur after surgery or injury; C. LOCALIZATION the specification of a certain area in the brain that controls a particular function such as speech, vision, etc.; C. MENINGITIS inflammation of the meninges of the brain. See MENINGITIS; C. PALSY a non-progressive, persistent disorder of motor power resulting from an impairment in the development of the nervous system, due to a birth injury of cerebral motor nerves; covers a large group of disabilities, the most common of which is lack of muscular control; symptoms appear in infancy or early childhood. Several types are recognized: (1) ataxic, in which many muscles are involved; (2) spastic, the most common form, in which attempts to use affected muscles results in incoordinated movements; (3) athetoid, in which severe muscular incoordination is uncontrolled and uncontrollable; and (4) flaccid, in which muscular incoordination is very severe; C. THROMBOSIS thrombosis occurring in a cerebral blood vessel.

cerebralgia (ser-e-bral′ -ji-a): Headache.

cerebrate (ser′ -e-brāt): To use the mind; to think.

cerebration (ser-e-brā′ -shun): Functional or mental activity of the cerebrum; thinking.

cerebritis (ser-e-brī′ -tis): Inflammation of the cerebrum.

cerebromalacia (ser′ -e-brō-ma-lā′ -shi-a): Softening of the substance of the cerebrum.

cerebromedullary (ser′ -e-brō-med-u′ lu-ri): Pertaining to the cerebrum and the spinal cord.

cerebrosclerosis (ser′ -ē-brō-sklē-rō′ -sis): Hardening of the substance of the cerebrum.

cerebroside (ser′ -e-brō-sīd): A lipid substance found in body tissues, particularly brain and nerve tissue.

cerebrospinal (ser′ -e-brō-spī′ -nal): Relating to the brain and spinal cord. C. FEVER an epidemic form of cerebrospinal meningitis (q.v.), C. FLUID the fluid filling the ventricles of the brain and the central canal of the spinal cord; also found in the cranial and subarachnoid spaces; it is colourless, odourless, and clear, with a specific gravity of 1.007; contains protein and a few white cells but no red cells; has a fluctuating glucose level; and a normal pressure of 80–180 millimetres of water when the patient is lying down; C. GANGLIA ganglia located on the dorsal root of each spinal nerve; see GANGLION; C. MENINGITIS inflammation of the meninges of the spinal cord; C. NERVE one that runs from or to the brain or spinal cord, i.e., a central nervous system nerve; C. PUNCTURE usually refers to a lumbar puncture, i.e., a puncture into the subarachnoid space between the third and fourth lumbar vertebrae; C. SYSTEM consists of the brain, spinal cord, and the nerves emanating from or running to them.

cerebrotonia (ser′ -e-brō-tō′ -ni-a): A temperamental trait manifested by restraint, inhibition in regard to physical enjoyment, apprehensiveness, and a tendency towards concealment.

cerebrovascular (ser′ -ē-brō-vas′ -ku-lar): Relating to the blood vessels of the brain, especially to pathological conditions or changes in these vessels. C. ACCIDENT the rupture of a blood vessel within or near the brain, as occurs in cerebral haemorrhage, a stroke, a transient ischaemic attack, or a change in the blood supply in the brain as a result of embolism or thrombosis that causes neurological dysfunction.

cerebrum (ser′ -e-brum, se-rē′ -brum): The largest and uppermost part of the brain; it does not include the cerebellum, pons, and medulla.

The longitudinal fissure divides it into two hemispheres, each containing a lateral ventricle. The internal substance is white, the outer convoluted cortex is grey. — cerebral, adj.

ceruloplasmin (sē-roo-lō-plaz′ -min): A protein found in plasma; contains most of the copper normally present in plasma; is markedly decreased in hepatolenticular degeneration (q.v.).

cerumen (se-roo′ -men): Ear wax. The soft, yellowish-brown, wax-like secretion of the ceruminous glands in the external auditory canal. — ceruminous, ceruminal, adj.

cervical (ser′ -vī-kal): Relating to the neck, or to the neck of an organ. C. ADENITIS inflammation of the lymph glands or nodes of the neck; C. CANAL the lumen of the cervix uteri which leads from the body of the uterus to the vagina; C. CAP a rubber contraceptive cap that fits over the end of the uterine cervix; C. COLLAR an appliance used to keep the head in neutral or slightly fixed position; C. HALTER a device used to increase vertebral separation and thus relieve pressure on cervical nerves; see C. TRACTION under TRACTION; C. INCOMPETENCE painless dilatation of the cervix of the pregnant uterus; usually causes termination of the pregnancy; C. RIB a rib-like process that sometimes appears on a cervical vertebra; may present no problems or it may press on the brachial plexus when it causes C. RIB syndrome; C. NERVES the first eight pairs of spinal nerves; C. VERTEBRAE the first (upper) seven bones of the spinal column.

cervicectomy (ser-vi-sek′ -to-mi): Amputation of the cervix of the uterus.

cervicitis (ser-vi-sī′ -tis): Acute or chronic inflammation of the uterine cervix.

cervicocolpitis (ser′ -vi-kō-kol-pī′ -tis): Inflammation of the uterine cervix and the vagina.

cervicovaginitis (ser′ -vi-kō-vaj-i-nī′ -tis): Inflammation of the uterine cervix and the vagina.

cervix (ser′ -viks): A neck or constricted part of an organ. C. UTERI the neck of the uterus; INCOMPETENT C. occurs usually at about the 16th to 20th week of pregnancy when the cervix dilates painlessly; a suturing procedure is sometimes utilized to avoid abortion; see CERCLAGE.

cestode (ses′ -tōd): Tapeworm. See TAENIA. — cestoid, adj.

CF: Abbreviation for cystic fibrosis, see under CYSTIC.

Chadwick's sign: See JACQUEMIER'S SIGN.

chafing (chāf′ -ing): Irritation of the skin due to: (1) irritants; or (2) two skin surfaces rubbing together.

CHAI: Abbreviation for Commission for Health-Care Audit and Inspection (*q.v.*).

chain reaction: A series of events each of which initiates or influences a following reaction.

chalasia (ka-lā′-zi-a): The relaxation of a body opening, particularly one that is normally guarded by a sphincter muscle. May be a cause of regurgitation or vomiting by infants when there is no other sign of distress.

chalazion (ka-lā′-zi-on): A cyst on the edge of the eyelid from retained secretion of the meibomian glands (*q.v.*). Similar to a stye, but painless. May disappear or may need to be surgically evacuated. — chalazia, pl.

chalicosis (kal-i-kō′-sis): A lung disease caused by inhalation of stone dust. Found chiefly among stonecutters. Pneumonoconiosis (*q.v.*).

challenging behaviour: Action(s) of such intensity, frequency or duration that the physical safety of the individual or others is likely to be placed in severe jeopardy; or conduct that is likely to seriously limit or deny access to the use of ordinary community facilities.

chalone (ka′-lon): Any one of several inhibitors of mitosis that is active within the tissue in which it is elaborated; inhibits proliferation of cells and thought to be reversible in action.

chalybeate (kal-ib′-ēt): 1. Containing iron, as occurs in the waters of various spas. 2. A pharmaceutical preparation containing iron.

chamber: In anatomy, an enclosed space or cavity, *e.g.*, the c.'s of the heart, or the anterior and posterior c.'s of the eye. See also HYPERBARIC OXYGEN CHAMBER under HYPERBARIC.

Chamberlen forceps: The original obstetric forceps, invented by Dr. Peter Chamberlen [English obstetrician, 1560–1631] but first described in the literature in 1773.

chamecephaly (kam-e-kef′-a-li, -sef′-a-li): The condition of having a flat head with a low cephalic index (*q.v.*). — chamecephalic, adj.

chancre (shang′-ker): A primary lesion, usually of syphilis or chancroid; formed at the site of infection two or three weeks after infection; usually on the lips, genitals, or fingers; consists of an ordinary round or oval red spot that may go unnoticed as it is usually painless; may develop into a papule, ulcer or erosion that is highly infectious. Associated with swelling of local lymph glands. Also called *hard chancre* and *Hunterian chancre*.

chancroid (shang′-kroyd): A type of non-syphilitic venereal infection caused by *Haemophilus ducreyi*; prevalent in warmer climates; associated with uncleanliness; transmitted by sexual contact; characterized by regional lymph node involvement, and multiple painful, ragged ulcers on the penis or vulva that have a purulent exudate.

Chandelier's sign: Tenderness of the cervix on digital examination and a feeling of fullness or masses at the sides of the pelvis; an indication of pelvic inflammatory disease.

change of life: The menopause (*q.v.*).

chaos theory (kā′-os): A mathematical philosophy used to explain apparent disorder in a very ordered way. Chaos theory states that things are not really random, just complex. Many apparently random events can be represented by a simple computations which, when iterated, produce complex results. Most natural processes, and many man-made ones, are chaotic systems which, although possible to predict generally, are hard to predict in detail.

chaplain (chap′-lin): 1. A clergyman in charge of a chapel. 2. A clergyman officially attached to an institution, such as a hospital, or to a family or court. 3. A person chosen to conduct religious exercises (as at a meeting of a club or society).

character (kar′-ak-ter): The sum total of the known and predictable mental characteristics of an individual, particularly his conduct. C. CHANGE denotes change in the form of conduct to one foreign to the patient's natural disposition, *e.g.*, indecent behaviour in a hitherto respectable person. Common in the psychoses; C. DISORDER term given to a pattern of behaviour that is disapproved or unacceptable in the person's social environment.

characteristic (kar′-ak-ter-is′-tik): 1. A specific, distinguishing attribute or trait. 2. A structural or functional feature of an organism.

charcoal (char′-kol): The residue after burning organic substances at a high temperature in an enclosed vessel. Used in medicine for its adsorptive and deodorant properties. ACTIVATED c., c. that has been treated to increase its adsorptive power; used in treating diarrhoea and as an antidote in some poisonings.

Charcot–Marie–Tooth disease: Progressive neuropathic muscular dystrophy. See MUSCULAR DYSTROPHY under DYSTROPHY.

Charcot's joint (shar′-kōs): Complete disorganization of a joint associated with syringomyelia or advanced cases of tabes dorsalis (locomotor ataxia). Condition is painless. Also called *neurogenic joint disease* and *Charcot's arthropathy*. C. TRIAD late manifestations of disseminated sclerosis — nystagmus, intention tremor, and staccato speech. [Jean Martin Charcot, French neurologist and clinician, 1825–1893.]

charge nurse: The title usually given to the nurse who is in charge of a particular ward or unit of a hospital.

charlatan (shar'-la-tan): One who pretends to have knowledge or skills that he or she does not possess; a quack.

Charles' law: States that, at constant pressure, the volume of a given mass of gas is directly proportional to the absolute temperature. Also called *Gay-Lussac's law*.

chart: A record of data; may be in tabular or graph form. GENEALOGICAL C. a design showing all descendents of a common ancestor; may be used to determine whether a disease is due to presence of a particular gene; PATIENT'S C. an individual record that is kept for each patient. Common usage refers to a collection of forms for recording various types of information, *e.g.*, laboratory and x-ray examination reports; patient's temperature, pulse and respirations; nurses' notes, including their observations of the patient's condition, food intake, etc. The chart becomes part of the hospital's permanent records; it is a legal document; SNELLEN'S C. a chart of block letters used in testing vision.

Chartered Society of Physiotherapists: The professional, educational and trade union body for chartered physiotherapists, physiotherapy students, and physiotherapy assistants in Britain.

charting: The recording on a patient's chart of the important data about a patient and his illness, his medical and nursing care, and the progress and outcome of his disorder.

CHC: Abbreviation for Community Health Council, see under COMMUNITY.

CHD: Abbreviation for coronary heart disease (*q.v.*).

cheek: The side wall of the oral cavity.

cheil-, cheilo-: Combining forms denoting relationship to the lips.

cheilosis (kī-lō'-sis): Fissuring and scaling of the lips, especially at the angles of the mouth, usually resulting from riboflavin deficiency.

cheir-, cheiro-: Combining forms denoting relationship to the hand.

cheiralgia (kī-ral'-ji-a): Pain in the hand. Also called *cheiragra*.

cheirarthritis (kī-rar-thrī'-tis): Inflammation of the joints of the fingers and hands.

cheiromegaly (kī-rō-meg'-a-li): Abnormal enlargement of the hands.

cheiropompholyx (kī-rō-pom'-fo-liks): Symmetrical eczematous eruption of the skin of the hands (especially fingers) characterized by the formation of tiny vesicles and associated with itching or burning. On the feet the condition is called podopompholyx.

cheirospasm, chirospasm (kī'-rō-spazm): Writer's cramp (*q.v.*).

chelating agents (kē' lā-ting): Soluble organic compounds that can fix metallic ions into their molecular structure; the chelates resulting from this action are used therapeutically in treatment of certain metal poisonings and the new compound formed in the body is excreted in the urine.

chemical (kem'-i-kal): 1. Of or relating to chemistry. 2. A substance produced by or used in a chemical process. C. CHANGE the transformation of a substance into a different substance through a chemical reaction; C. FORMULA the composition or structure of a substance as represented by chemical symbols; C. REACTION the interaction of two or more substances which results in chemical change; C. SYMBOL a single capital letter or a capital and small letter as an abbreviation for an atom of an element.

cheminosis (kem-i-nō'-sis): Any pathological condition caused by a chemical.

chemistry (kem'-is-tri): The science that deals with composition, structure, properties, behaviour, and reactions of substances and the changes they may undergo.

chemo-: Combining form denoting relationship to: (1) chemistry; (2) a chemical.

chemoceptor (kēm'-ō-sep-tor): Chemoreceptor (*q.v.*).

chemoprophylaxis (kē'-mō-prō-fi-lak'-sis): The prevention of a specific disease (or recurrent attack) by administration of chemotherapeutic agents — chemoprophylactic, adj.

chemopsychiatry (kē'-mō-si-kī-a-tri): Treatment of mental or emotional disorders by administration of drugs.

chemoreceptor (kē'-mō-rē-sep'-tor): 1. A chemical linkage in a living cell having an affinity for, and capable of combining with, certain other chemical substances. 2. A sensory end organ that responds to a chemical stimulus.

chemosis (kē-mō'-sis): Oedema or swelling of the bulbar conjunctiva. — chemotic, adj.

chemosurgery (kē-mō-sur'-jer-i): The destruction of diseased or unwanted tissue by the application of chemical agents.

chemosynthesis (kē-mō-sin'-the-sis): In physiology, the production of carbohydrates by use of energy derived from a chemical reaction rather than from light. See PHOTOSYNTHESIS.

chemotaxis, chemotaxy (kē-mō-tak′-sis): Response of organisms to chemical stimuli, attraction towards a chemical being positive C., and repulsion being negative C.

chemothalamectomy (kē′ mō-thal-a-mek′-to-mi): Destruction of part of the thalamus by the injection of a chemical. Done for the relief of tremor.

chemotherapy (kē-mō-ther′-a-pi): The oral, intramuscular, or intravenous administration of a specific chemical agent to arrest the progress of, or eradicate, a specific pathological condition in the body without causing irreversible injury to healthy tissue; widely used in the treatment of cancer.

chemtrode (kem′-trōd): A small hollow tube that can be implanted in the brain and used to deliver small amounts of chemicals to specific areas.

chenodeoxycholic acid (kē′-nō-dē-oks-i-kō′-lik as′-id): A normal constituent of bile; has been used in treatment of gall bladder disease since it allows the cholesterol in gallstones to dissolve.

cherry angioma: See under ANGIOMA.

chest: The thorax (*q.v.*). C. CAVITY the upper division of the body cavity, containing the heart, lungs, and related structures; C. TUBES tubes inserted into the second intercostal or fifth intercostal space for the removal of air or fluid from the pleural cavity; usually attached to a water-seal apparatus; FLAIL C an unstable thoracic cage due to fracture in which two or more ribs are detached; the segment is drawn inward on inspiration and pushed outward on exhalation; loss of rigidity of the chest wall may lead to inadequate ventilation and result in respiratory failure. C. X-RAY a radiogram of the C. See also BARREL CHEST; PIGEON BREAST.

Cheyne–Stokes respiration: A breathing pattern in which the respirations gradually increase in depth, then decrease in depth, and then stop altogether for a period, after which the pattern is repeated. See under RESPIRATION.

CHF: Abbreviation for congestive heart failure (*q.v.*).

CHI: Abbreviation for Commission for Health Improvement (*q.v.*).

chiasm (kī′-azm): An X-shaped crossing or decussation. OPTIC C. or CHIASMA OPTICUM the meeting of the optic nerves; where the fibres from the medial or nasal half of each retina cross the middle line on the ventral surface of the brain to join the optic tract of the opposite side.

chiasma (kī-az′-ma): Chiasm. — chiasmata, pl.

chiasmatic (kī-az-mat′-ik): Relating to a chiasm. Also called *chiasmal*.

chickenpox: A mild, specific, highly contagious disease of childhood, caused by a virus. Successive crops of vesicles appear first on the trunk; they scab and heal, sometimes causing scarring. Syn., *varicella*. See also under HERPES.

Chief Nursing Officer: One of the UK government's four most senior nursing advisors, who have responsibility for delivering the government's strategies for nursing, midwifery and health visiting in the four countries of the UK. They also play a key role in public health, social care, and the development of nursing internationally. Abbreviated CNO.

chilblain (chil′-blān): Congestion and swelling attended with severe itching and burning sensation in reaction to damp, cold weather; fingers, toes and ears are affected particularly. Erythema pernio.

child abuse: Beating, starving, neglecting, sexually or emotionally abusing, mistreating, or demeaning of a child by parents or other adult, often one who is emotionally disturbed. See also NON-ACCIDENTAL INJURY.

childbearing: Pregnancy and the delivery of a child. C. PERIOD the years of a woman's life during which she can normally bear children, *i.e.*, the years between puberty and menopause.

childbirth: Term applied to the normal outcome of pregnancy with the birth of an infant. FAMILY-CENTRED C. siblings and other family members are present during the birth process; birth takes place in the home or birthing room, etc.; incorporates the infant into the family unit immediately; NATURAL C. popular term for a form of C. that emphasizes reduction or elimination of the use of drugs; patient is prepared by courses in which she learns the anatomy and physiology involved, and practises a regimen of exercises during pregnancy.

childhood: The period of life between infancy and puberty. C. SCHIZOPHRENIA that which occurs before puberty; characterized by autism (*q.v.*) and immaturity.

child protection: The monitoring and care of children at risk from neglect or abuse.

Children Act: The Children Act 1989 became law in 1991. The main principles of this legislation are:

- the welfare of the child is the paramount consideration in court proceedings;
- wherever possible children should be brought up and cared for within their own families; children should be safe and protected by effec-

tive intervention if they are in danger but this should be open to challenge by parents in the courts;

- when dealing with children, courts should ensure that any delay is avoided, and may only make an order if to do so is better for the child than making no order at all;
- children should be kept informed about what happens to them, and should participate when decisions are made about their future;
- parents continue to have parental responsibility for their children, even when their children are no longer living with them. They should be kept informed about their children and participate when decisions are made about their children's future;
- parents with children in need should be helped by local authorities to bring up their children themselves;
- this help should be provided as a service to the child and their family and should be provided in partnership with the parents and meeting each child's identified needs. This service should be open to complaints and provide an effective partnership with other agencies.
- Local authorities are required to take children's racial origin, culture, linguistic background and religion into account when making decisions about them.

chill: A sudden sensation of cold, accompanied by shivering, often followed by rise in body temperature. Sometimes the initial symptom of an acute infection such as pneumonia; a characteristic symptom of malaria.

chimera (ki-mēr'-a): In genetics, refers to an individual whose body contains cells from two different cell lines that are derived from two different zygotes.

chin: The mentum; the lower anterior prominence of the mandible.

Chinese medicine: The collective term used for the holistic therapies originating in China, including herbalism, acupuncture (q.v.), and t'ai chi. Many of these therapies date back thousands of years and are based on ancient Chinese beliefs. Animal substances can be included in remedies, although most Western clinics use only plants.

chionablepsia (kī-ō-na-blep'-si-a): Snow-blindness.

chirology (kī-rol'-o-ji): A method of communicating with or between the deaf through hand signals. Also known as *dactylology* or *signing*. A specialist trained in the treatment of minor foot disorders. He or she will be qualified and registered with one of the professional bodies

that teach chiropody. Unlike a podiatrist (q.v.), a chiropodist does not perform foot surgery.

chiropodist (kī-rop'-o-dist):

chiropody (ki-rop'-o-di): The treatment of corns, callosities, bunions, and toenail conditions.

chiropractic (kī-rō-prak'-tik): A system of treatment based on the theory that disease is caused by impingement on the spinal nerves and that relief or cure can be effected through manual manipulation of the spinal column.

chiropractor: One who practises chiropractic (q.v.).

chiropsia (kī-rop'-si-a): Friction applied with the hands; massage.

chi-square test (ki): A statistical test to determine whether a significant difference exists between the observed data and the results expected according to a null hypothesis (q.v.).

Chlamydia (kla-mid'-i-a): A genus of parasitic Gram-negative organisms: two species are (1) *C. psittaci* which causes psittacosis and (2) *C. trachomatis*, a serious sexually transmitted pathogen which causes lymphogranuloma venereum (q.v.), inclusion conjunctivitis, blinding trachoma, epididymitis, pelvic inflammation, cervicitis, urethritis, salpingitis, prostatitis, Reiter's syndrome, infant pneumonia.

chloasma (klō-az'-ma): Painless yellowish or dark brown patches on the skin; melasma. C. GRAVIDARUM patches of brown discoloration on the forehead, cheeks, nipples and along the median line of the abdomen, occurring during pregnancy; sometimes called '*mask of pregnancy*'.

chlor-, chloro-: Combining forms denoting a green colour.

chloraemia (klō-rē'-mi-a): 1. Decrease in the haemoglobin and red cells; chlorosis (q.v.). 2. The presence of more than the normal amount of chlorides in the blood.

chloramines (klor'-a-mēns): Chlorine compounds used as topical antiseptics and disinfectants.

chlorate (klō'-rāt): Any salt of chloric acid.

chlordane (klor'-dān): An organic insecticide; may cause poisoning in humans if ingested, inhaled, or absorbed.

chlorhydria (klor-hī'-dri-a): An excess of hydrochloric acid in the gastric juice.

chloride (klō'-rīd): Any salt of hydrochloric acid; a compound composed of two substances, one of which is chlorine, that carries a negative charge.

chloride of lime: See under CHLORINATED.

chlorinated (klōr'-in-ā-ted): Said of a substance to which chlorine has been added, e.g., water,

C. LIME a substance made by passing chlorine over hydrated lime; formerly much used as a disinfectant, fumigant, and deodorant; also called *chloride of lime*.

chlorination (klōr-i-nā'-shun): The procedure of adding chlorine to a substance to disinfect it, *e.g.*, water, sewage.

chlorine (klor'-ēn): A yellowish-green gaseous element with an irritating, suffocating odour. Represented by the symbol Cl.

chloroform (klor'-ō-form): A clear, colourless, volatile, heavy liquid with a sweetish taste, once much used as a general anaesthetic.

chloroleukaemia (klō'-rō-lū-kē'-mi-a): A type of leukaemia in which no perceptible tumour masses occur, but the organs and body fluids have a definite green colour on autopsy.

chloroma (klō-rō'-ma): A condition in which multiple malignant greenish-yellow growths develop, especially on the periosteum of the facial and cranial bones and the vertebrae. Observed most frequently in children and young adults.

chlorophenothane (klō'-rō-fēn'-nō-thān): The insecticide, dichloro-diphenyl-trichloroethane; also called *DDT*. See DICOPHANE.

chlorophyll (klō'-rō-fil): The colouring matter of green plants; essential for photosynthesis (*q.v.*). Now prepared synthetically for use in medicine and as a deodorant.

chloroquine (klor'-ō-kwin): A chemical used as an antimalarial and antiamoebic.

chlorosarcoma (klō-rō-sar-kō'-ma): See CHLOROMA.

chlorosis (klō-rō'-sis): Simple iron-deficiency anaemia occurring especially in young women.

chloruretic (klor-ū-ret'-ik): 1. Promoting urinary excretion of chlorides. 2. An agent that promotes urinary excretion of chlorides.

chocolate cyst: See under CYST.

choke: To strangle or suffocate due to obstruction or compression of the trachea or larynx.

chol-, chole-, cholo-: Combining forms denoting bile, gall.

cholagogue (kō'-la-gog): A drug that causes an increased flow of bile into the intestine.

cholalic acid (kō-lal'-ik-as'-id): Cholic acid (*q.v.*).

cholangiocarcinoma (kō-lan'-ji-ō-kar-si-nō'-ma): An adenocarcinoma occurring usually within an intrahepatic bile duct.

cholangiogram (kō-lan'-ji-ō-gram): An x-ray film demonstrating the bile ducts. TRANSHEPATIC PERCUTANEOUS C. a procedure whereby a radiopaque dye is injected by needle through the abdominal wall into the biliary tree and the movement of the dye into the liver is observed on a fluoroscopic screen; used to differentiate between intrahepatic and extrahepatic jaundice.

cholangiography (kō-lan-ji-og'-ra-fi): Radiographic examination of hepatic, cystic, and bile ducts.

cholangiohepatitis (kō-lan'-ji-ō-hep-a-tī'-tis): Severe inflammation of the liver and small bile ducts in the liver; often associated with fluke infestation which causes obstructions in the ducts.

cholangiolitis (kō-lan'-ji-ō-lī'-tis): Inflammation of the bile ducts within the liver.

cholangioma (kō-lan'-ji-ō'-ma): A tumour in a bile duct, especially a duct within the liver.

cholangitis (kōl-an-jī'-tis): Inflammation of a bile duct; symptoms include pain in the upper right abdominal quadrant, fever, nausea, vomiting, jaundice.

cholecalciferol (kō-li-kal-sif'-er-ōl): Vitamin D$_3$, found in butter, egg yolk, and fish liver oils; also prepared synthetically. Prevents rickets.

cholecyst (kō'-li-sist): The gall bladder. — cholecystic, adj.

cholecystagogue (kō'-li-sis'-ta-gog): An agent that stimulates activity of the gall bladder and promotes the flow of bile from it.

cholecystalgia (kō'-li-sis-tal'-ji-a): Biliary colic; may be due to inflammation of the gall bladder or to the obstruction of a cystic duct by a gallstone.

cholecystangiogram (kō'-li-sis-tan'-ji-ō-gram): Film demonstrating gall bladder, cystic, and common bile ducts after administration of opaque medium.

cholecystectasia (kō-li-sis-tek-tā'-zi-a): Dilatation of the gall bladder.

cholecystectomy (kō-li-sis-tek'-to-mi): Surgical removal of the gall bladder.

cholecystenterostomy (kō'-li-sis-ten-ter-os'-to-mi): The surgical establishment of an anastomosis between the gall bladder and the small intestine.

cholecystic (kō-li-sis'-tik): Relating to the gall bladder.

cholecystitis (kō-li-sis-tī'-tis): Inflammation of the gall bladder; may be acute or chronic.

cholecystocholangiogram (kō'-li-sis-tō-kō-lan'-ji-ō-gram): X-ray of the gall bladder and the bile ducts.

cholecystocolostomy (kō'-li-sis-tō-ko-los'-to-mi): The surgical establishment of an anastomosis between the gall bladder and some portion of the colon, usually the upper part.

cholecystoduodenostomy (kō' -li-sis-tō-du-ō-dēn-os' -to-mi): The establishment of an anastomosis between the gall bladder and the duodenum. Usually necessary in cases of stricture of the common bile duct, which may be congenital or due to previous inflammation or operation.

cholecystogastrostomy (kō-li-sis-tō-gas-tros' -to-mi): The surgical establishment of an anastomosis between the gall bladder and the stomach; a palliative operation when the common bile duct is obstructed by an immovable growth.

cholecystogram (kō-li-sis' -tō-gram): An x-ray picture of the gall bladder obtained by cholecystography (q.v.).

cholecystography (kō-li-sis-tog' ra-fi): Radiographic examination of the gall bladder after it has been rendered opaque by the ingestion or intravenous injection of an opaque medium. — cholecystographic, adj.; cholecystographically, adv.; cholecystograph, n.

cholecystojejunostomy (ko-li-sis' tō-jē-ju-nos' -to-mi): The surgical establishment of an anastomosis between the gall bladder and the jejunum. Usually performed to relieve obstructive jaundice due to a growth in the head of the pancreas.

cholecystokinase (kō-li-sis-tō-kīn' -ās): An enzyme that promotes the breakdown of cholecystokinin.

cholecystokinin (kō-li-sis-tō-kīn' -in): A hormone secreted by the mucous membrane of the upper part of the small intestine; stimulates contraction of the gall bladder and the secretion of pancreatic enzymes. Also called *pancreozymin*.

cholecystolithiasis (kō-li-sis' -tō-li-thī' -a-sis): Cholelithiasis (q.v.).

cholecystolithotripsy (kō' -li-sis' -tō-lith' -ō-trip-si): The procedure of crushing gall stones within the gall bladder.

cholecystostomy (kō-li-sis-tos' -to-mi): A surgically established fistula between the gall bladder and the abdominal surface; used to provide drainage in empyema of the gall bladder or after removal of stones.

cholecystotomy (kō-li-sis-tot' -o-mi): A surgical incision in the abdominal wall for the purpose of removing gall stones or providing for drainage.

choledochectomy (kō-led-ō-kek' -to-mi): Surgical excision of part of the common bile duct.

choledochitis (kō-led-ō-kī' -tis): Inflammation of the common bile duct.

choledochoduodenostomy (kō-led' -ō-kō-dū' -ō-den-os' -to-mi): The formation of a passageway between the common bile duct and the duodenum.

choledochogastrostomy (kō-led' -ō-kō-gas-tros' -to-mi): The surgical establishment of an anastomosis between the common bile duct and the stomach.

choledochojejunostomy (kō led' -o-kō-je-jū-nos' -tō-mi): The surgical establishment of an anastomosis between the common bile duct and the jejunum.

choledocholith (kō-led' -o-ko-lith): A stone in the common bile duct.

choledocholithiasis (kō-led' -ō-kō-lith-ī' -a-sis): The presence of a stone or stones in the common bile duct.

choledocholithotomy (kō-led' -ō-kō-li-thot' -om-i): Surgical removal of a stone through an incision in the common bile duct.

choledocholithotripsy (kō-led' -o-kō-lith' -ō-trip-si): Crushing of a gall stone within the common bile duct.

choledochopancreatography (kō-led' -ō-kō-pan-kre-a-tog' -ra-fi): Visual examination of the common bile duct and the pancreatic duct with a fibre-optic endoscope.

choledochoscope (kō-led' -ō-ko-skōp): An instrument for viewing the interior of the common bile duct.

choledochostomy (kō-led-ō-kos' -to-mi): Drainage of the common bile duct through an incision in the abdominal wall, usually after exploration for a stone.

cholelith (kō' -lē-lith): A gall stone.

cholelithiasis (kō' -lē-li-thī' -a-sis): The presence of stones in the gall bladder or bile ducts.

cholelithotomy (kō' -lē-li-thot' -o-mi): Operation for the removal of gall stones through an incision in the gall bladder.

cholepoiesis (kō-lē-poy' -ē' -sis): The formation of bile in the liver.

cholera (kol' -er-a): An acute, infectious, enteric disease, endemic and epidemic in Asia; caused by the potent endotoxin produced by *Vibrio comma* (also called *Vibrio cholerae*); spread mainly by contaminated food and water, overcrowding, and generally unsanitary conditions. Symptoms include copious 'rice-water' stools, accompanied by agonizing cramp; severe, persistent vomiting; malaise; headache; muscular weakness; dehydration with depletion of minerals and electrolyte imbalance; rapid breathing; slow pulse rate; and circulatory collapse. The mortality rate is very high. Preventive measures include the use of cholera vaccine; boiling all drinking water; and cooking all foods; in addition, isolating and treating carriers.

choleresis (kol-er-ē'-sis): The production of bile by the liver.

cholesteatoma (kō-les-tē-a-tō'-ma): A benign, slow-growing encysted tumour, often containing cholesterol; occurs chiefly in the middle ear and mastoid region as a result of chronic otitis media, but also occurs in the meninges, skull, or brain.

cholesteraemia (kō-les-ter-ē'-mi-a): Excess cholesterol in the blood. Also called *cholesterolaemia*.

cholesterase (kō-les'-ter-ās): An enzyme that splits up the cholesterol.

cholesterol (kō-les'-ter-ol): A pale yellow crystalline substance occurring as granules or particles; of a fatty nature, occurring in foods of animal origin; found in brain, nerves, liver, kidneys, blood cells, and plasma, and is a major normal constituent of bile and bile acids. Not easily soluble and may crystallize in the gall bladder and form gallstones, and along arterial walls in atherosclerosis. When irradiated it forms vitamin D. Important in maintaining the permeability of cell membranes, and synthesis of steroid hormones, and in the functioning of certain body systems, *e.g.*, the nervous system. Normal values for human serum, 3.9–6.5 mmol per litre See also FATTY ACID. Cholesterol is an essential chemical for the efficient running of the human body. Only a small amount of cholesterol comes directly from food, the body makes most of it. Some individuals have high cholesterol levels, and the cause is hereditary; this requires monitoring and medical attention to correct because members of this group are prone to heart disease.

cholesterolopoiesis (kō-les'-ter-ol-ō-poy-ē'-sis): The synthesis of cholesterol by the liver.

cholesteroluria (kō-les'-ter-ol-ū'-ri-a): Cholesterol in the excreted urine.

cholesterosis (kō-les-ter-ō'-sis): Abnormal deposition of cholesterol, especially in the gall bladder; due to faulty metabolism of lipids. Also called *cholesterolosis*.

cholic acid (kō'-lik as'-id): One of the principal acids found in human bile, usually in conjunction with glycine and taurine; an important aid to digestion.

choline (kō'-lēn): A chemical found in most animal tissues as a constituent of lecithin and acetycholine. Part of the vitamin B complex, and known to be a growth factor. Appears to be necessary for fat transportation in the body. Useful in preventing fat deposition in the liver

in cirrhosis. Richest sources are dairy products, liver, kidney, brain, wheat germ, brewer's yeast, egg yolk.

choline acetyltransferase (kō'-lēn-a-set-il-trans'-fer-ās): An enzyme necessary for the formation of acetylcholine (*q.v.*).

cholinergic (kō-lin-er'-jik): Refers to parasympathetic nerves that liberate acetylcholine at their terminations when a nerve impulse passes. See ADRENERGIC. c. CRISIS severe muscular weakness and respiratory depression caused by an excess of acetylcholine in the body; likely to occur in patients with myasthenia gravis as a result of overdose of anticholinesterase drugs. c. FIBRES nerve fibres that liberate acetylcholine at the synapse.

cholinesterase (kō-lin-es'-ter-ās): An enzyme that hydrolyses acetycholine into choline and acetic acid, at nerve endings. Present in all body tissues.

choluria (kō-lū'-ri-a): The presence of bile in the urine. — choluric, adj.

chondral (kon'-dral): Cartilaginous; relating to cartilage.

chondralgia (kon-dral'-ji-a): Pain in a cartilage. Chondrodynia.

chondrectomy (con-drek'-to-mi): The surgical removal of a cartilage.

chondrification (kon-dri-fi-kā'-shun): Conversion into cartilage. — chondrify, v.

chondritis (kon-drī'-tis): Inflammation of the cartilage.

chondroblast (kon'-drō-blast): An embryonic cell that produces cartilage.

chondroblastoma (kon'-drō-blas-tō'-ma): A rare tumour, usually occurs in the epiphyses of long bones; generally benign; most often seen in young males.

chondrocostal (kon-drō-kos'-tal): Relating to the costal cartilages and ribs.

chondrocyte (kon'-drō-sīt): A cartilage cell.

chondrodynia (kon-drō-din'-i-a): Pain in a cartilage.

chondrodystrophy (kon-drō-dis'-tro-fi): A defect or disorder of cartilage formation. See ACHONDROPLASIA.

chondrogenesis (kon-drō-jen'-e-sis): The formation of cartilage. — chondrogenic, adj.

chondroid (kon'-droyd): Resembling cartilage.

chondroitin (kon-drō'-i-tin): A sulphur-rich compound that is a component of cartilage and is taken as a dietary supplement to relieve arthritis and other conditions.

chondrolipoma (kon-drō-li-pō'-ma): A benign tumour containing both cartilaginous and fatty tissue.

chondrolysis (kon-drol´-i-sis): Dissolution of cartilage. — chondrolytic, adj.

chondroma (kon-drō´-ma): A benign, slow-growing, painless tumour of cartilage. Tends to recur after removal. It causes no pain.

chondromalacia (kon-drō-mal-ā´-shi-a): Abnormal softness of cartilage, occurring most often in the knee. May be congenital, in which case the bones of the stillborn fetus are soft and pliable.

chondromatosis (kon-drō-ma-tō´-sis): A congenital condition, marked by the presence of many chondromata affecting chiefly the growing ends of long bones and bones of hands and feet; usually unilateral, resulting sometimes in shortening and deformity of the affected limb.

chondromucoid (kon´-drō-mū´-koyd): A glycoprotein; one of the main constituents of cartilage.

chondromyoma (kon´-drō-mī-ō´ ma): A myoma that contains cartilaginous elements.

chondro-osseous (kon-drō-os´-ē-us): Consisting of cartilage and bone.

chondroplasty (kon´-drō plas-ti): Plastic surgery on cartilage.

chondroprotein (kon-drō-prō´ tēn): One of several glucoproteins occurring naturally in cartilage.

chondrosis (kon-drō´-sis): The formation of cartilage.

chondrosteoma (kon´-dros-tē-ō´-ma): An osteoma that contains cartilaginous tissue. Also called *osteochondroma*.

chord (kord): Cord.

chorda (kor´-da): A collection of fibres forming a cord; a tendon. C. TYMPANI a branch of the facial nerve which passes through the tympanic cavity and joins the lingual branch of the trigeminal nerve; its fibres are distributed over the anterior two-thirds of the tongue; infection of the middle ear or mastoid may cause temporary or permanent loss of taste sensation for sweet, salt, and sour.

chordae (kor´-dē): Plural of chorda. C. TENDINAE fine, white, glistening cords stretching between the atrioventricular valves and the papillary muscles of the heart. When the muscles contract, the chordae are tightened, thus preventing the cusps of the atrioventricular valves from being swept back into the atria during ventricular contraction.

chordee (kor-dē´): Downward bending of the penile shaft; painful on erection; usually due to urethritis; common in gonorrhoea. CONGENITAL C. a cord-like anomaly extending from the scrotum up the penis, pulling it

downwards in an arc; congenital hypospadias is also present.

chorditis (kor-dī´-tis): Inflammation of a cord, usually refers to the spermatic or vocal cords.

chorea (ko-rē´-a): A nervous disorder of the extremities and face, sometimes the entire body; characterized by ceaseless, rapid, spasmodic, jerky, purposeless movements that are beyond the control of the individual. The childhood type is also called *rheumatic chorea* or *St. Vitus' dance*. HUNTINGTON'S C. an inherited, degenerative, and ultimately fatal chorea that is not usually evident until the fourth or fifth decade of life, characterized by insidious onset, loss of muscle tone, hand and body tremor, head nodding, mental deterioration and psychoses. Sometimes called *Woody Guthrie disease* after the folk singer who died of it in 1967; SENILE C. a benign chorea characterized by late onset and relatively few signs of mental deterioration; SYDENHAM'S C. occurs mainly in children; characterized by moderate convulsive movements; chorea minor.

choreiform (ko-rē´-i-form): Resembling chorea (*q.v.*), particularly the rapid, jerky, purposeless movements of chorea.

chorioadenoma (ko´-ri-ō-ad-e-nō´-ma): An adenomatous tumour of the chorion (*q.v.*). C. DESTRUENS a type of hydatidiform mole which may be transported to distant sites, particularly the lungs. Also called *metastasizing, malignant*, or *invasive mole*.

chorioamnionitis (ko´-ri-ō-am´-ni-ō-nī´-tis): Inflammation of the fetal membranes, associated with a bacterial infection.

chorioangioma (ko´-ri-ō-an-ji-ō´-ma): A vascular tumour of the chorion arising from placental capillaries.

choriocarcinoma (ko´-ri-ō-kar-si-nō´-ma): An extremely malignant tumour occurring most often in young women, starting in the uterus and less often in the ovary; spreads rapidly to the lungs, liver, brain, vagina, and pelvic organs. May follow abortion, ectopic pregnancy, or normal pregnancy, or may develop from hydatidiform mole, see MOLE.

choriogenesis (ko-ri-ō-jen´-e-sis): The development of the chorion (*q.v.*).

choriomeningitis (ko´-ri-ō-men-in-jī´-tis): Cerebral meningitis involving the choroid plexuses; see CHOROID PLEXUS, under PLEXUS. It is caused by a virus, affects chiefly young adults, and occurs most often during the autumn and winter months.

chorion (ko´-ri-on): The outermost of four fetal membranes that form the embryonic sac which surrounds the embryo; it secretes chorionic gonadotrophin during the first months of pregnancy and becomes an important part of the placenta. C. FRONDOSUM the part of the c. that bears the chorionic villi, see under CHORIONIC.

chorionepithelioma (ko'-ri-on-ep-i-thē-li-ō'-ma): A highly malignant tumour arising from chorionic cells, usually those of the uterus but also those of other female generative organs and the testes; may follow hydatidiform mole (*q.v.*) abortion, or even normal pregnancy; quickly metastasizes, especially to the lungs. Syn., *choriocarcinoma.* Also called *chorioepithelioma.*

chorionic (ko-ri-on'-ik): Relating to the chorion (*q.v.*). C. GONADOTROPHIN a hormone normally produced by the chorion of a fertilized ovum; C. VILLI many finger-like projections from the chorion through which the exchange of gases, nutrients, and waste products between the maternal and fetal blood takes place.

chorionic villus sampling: A test available to pregnant women, particularly those with a family history of inherited disorders or who are over the age of 35. It is an alternative to amniocentesis (*q.v.*), to test for serious fetal problems. It can be done earlier than amniocentesis, about 10 weeks after fertilization. These villi are formed by the division of the original fertilized egg and have exactly the same deoxyribonucleic acid (genetic codes) as the embryo, including any possible genetic abnormality. Any defect in one will be present in the other. This test is not without risk; in around 2% of cases the procedure results in spontaneous abortion.

chorionitis (ko-ri-on-ī'-tis): Inflammation of the chorion.

choroid (ko'-royd): The middle pigmented vascular coat of the posterior five-sixths of the eyeball, continuous with the iris in front. It lies between the sclera externally and the retina internally, and prevents the passage of light rays. C. PLEXUS see under PLEXUS. — choroidal, adj.

choroiditis (ko-royd-ī'-tis): Inflammation of the choroid. C. GUTTATA degenerative change affecting the retina around the macula lutea; believed to be caused by an atheromatous condition of the arteries; seen in older people; also called *Tay's choroiditis.*

choroidocyclitis (ko'-roy-dō-si-sklī'-tis): Inflammation of the choroid and ciliary body.

choroidoretinitis (ko-roy'-dō-ret-in-ī'-tis): Inflammation of both the choroid and the retina.

Christmas disease: Allied to haemophilia (*q.v.*). Caused by a hereditary deficiency of clotting factor IX (plasma thromboplastin component). Named for the patient in whom it was first described. Also called *haemophilia B.*

Christmas factor: Factor IX, a precoagulant factor normally present in plasma but deficient in patients with haemophilia B (Christmas disease, *q.v.*).

chrom-, chromat-, chromato-, chromo-: Combining forms denoting: (1) colour; (2) pigment.

chromaesthesis (krō-mes-thē'-zi-a): The association of a perception of colour with a sensation of hearing, taste, smell, or touch.

chromaffin (krō-maf'-in): Term used in reference to certain cells that take up and stain strongly yellow or brown with chromium salts; said of certain cells seen mostly in the adrenal medulla and less frequently along the sympathetic nerves and the abdominal aorta.

chromaffinoma (krō-maf-i-nō'-ma): 1. Any tumour containing chromaffin cells. 2. Phaeochromocytoma (*q.v.*).

chromatelopsia (krō-mat-e-lop'-si-a): Imperfect perception of colours; colour blindness.

chromatic (krō-mat'-ik): Relating to (1) colour; (2) chromatin (*q.v.*).

chromatid (krō'-ma-tid): Either of the two like subunits that result from the longitudinal splitting of a chromosome as a step in preparation for mitosis (*q.v.*); each chromatid eventually becomes a chromosome.

chromatin (krō'-ma-tin): The part of the cell nucleus that stains most readily with basic dyes; it consists of nucleic acid and proteins, the DNA-containing part of the nucleus; the physical basis of heredity.

chromatin (krō'-ma-tizm): 1. Abnormal pigmentation. 2. An abnormal condition characterized by hallucinatory perceptions of coloured light.

chromatodermatosis (krō'-ma-tō-der-ma-tō'-sis): Any disease of the skin accompanied by discoloration. Also called *chromodermatosis.*

chromatodysopia (krō'-ma-tō-dis-ō'-pi-a): Imperfect perception or differentiation of colours. Colour blindness.

chromatogenous (krō-ma-toj'-e-nus): Producing colour or pigmentation.

chromatogram (krō-mat'-ō-gram): The graphic record produced by chromatography (*q.v.*).

chromatography: A method used to separate the components of a mixture of closely related compounds. The mixture is applied to an adsorbent material and a solvent is added so that it moves over the mixture and through the adsorbent material. The different solutes are carried by the solvent at different speeds, resulting in bands of the separated compounds at different levels in the chromatogram. — chromatographic, adj.

chromatoid (krō´-ma-toyd): Relating to, resembling, or having the properties of chromatin (*q.v.*).

chromatometer (krō-ma-tom´-i-ter): An instrument for measuring the intensity of colour or colour perception.

chromatophil (krō-mat´-ō-fil): A cell or tissue that stains readily; chromophil.

chromatophore (krō-mat´-ō-for): **1.** A pigmented connective tissue cell. **2.** A pigmented phagocytic cell found chiefly in the skin, mucous membranes, and the choroid coat of the eye and, sometimes, in melanomas.

chromatopseudopsis (krō´-ma-tō-sū-dop´-sis): Colour blindness.

chromatopsia (krō-ma-top´-si-a): A visual defect in which objects that are normally seen as colourless are seen as having colour. May be due to optical or psychic disturbances or to the use of certain drugs.

chromatosis (krō-ma-tō´-sis): Abnormal pigmentation of the skin, as in Addison's disease (*q.v.*).

chromaturia (krō-ma-tū´-ri-a): The excretion of urine of an abnormal colour.

chromhydrosis (krōm-hī-drō´-sis): The secretion of coloured sweat.

chromium (krō´-mi-um): A hard, greyish metallic element. Chemical symbol, Cr.

chromoblastomycosis (krō´-mō-blas-tō-mī-kō´-sis): Any of a group of fungal skin infections characterized by itching and the appearance of nodules and papillomas which frequently progress to warty plaques or ulceration; seen on the feet, legs, and exposed areas.

chromocyte (krō´-mō-sīt): Any coloured or pigmented cell.

chromocytometer (krō-mō-sī-tom´-i-ter): An instrument for measuring colour, particularly one which measures the haemoglobin in red blood cells.

chromogen (krō´-mō-jen): Any substance that may give colour to another substance.

chromogenic (krō-mō-jen´-ik): Producing a pigment.

chromonychia (krō-mō-nik´-i-a): Any abnormal or unusual colouring of the nails.

chromophil (krō´-mō-fil): A cell, tissue, or structure that takes a deep stain easily. C. GRANULES see NISSL('S) BODIES; C. TUMOUR see PHAEO-CHROMOCYTOMA. — chromophilic, adj.

chromophobe (krō´-mō-fōb): Any cell or tissue that does not stain readily, especially the cells of the anterior hypophysis. C. ADENOMA the most common type of pituitary tumour with symptoms resembling those of a space-occupying lesion due to pressure on nervous system tissues; made up of chromophobe cells.

chromophytosis (krō-mō-fī-tō´-sis): **1.** Discoloration of the skin. **2.** Tinea versicolor (*q.v.*).

chromopsia (krō-mop-si-a): Chromatopsia (*q.v.*).

chromoptometer (krō-mop-tom´-i-ter): An instrument for measuring an individual's perception of colour.

chromosome (krō´-mo-sōm): Any one of the microscopic, dark-staining, thread-like bodies which develop from the nuclear material of the cell and which split longitudinally during cell division, one half going into the nucleus of each daughter cell. They carry the hereditary factors (genes), the number being constant for each species; they are also responsible for the determination of sex. The sex chromosomes are called X and Y; the female cell always contains two X chromosomes and the male cell contains one X and one Y chromosome.

chromotropic (krō-mō-trōp´-ik): Attracting colour or pigment.

chronaxia, chronaxie (krō-nak´-si-a, krō-nak´-sē): The length of time an electric current must flow in order to excite the tissue being tested. — chronaxic, adj.; chronaxy, n.

chronic (kron´-ik): Slowly developing, lingering, long-lasting. Opp. of acute. — chronically, adj.; chronicity, n.

chronic brain syndrome: An irreversible organic disorder; may be caused by viral or degenerative disease of the nervous system; often associated with brain trauma, encephalitis, meningitis, metabolic disorders, senility, cerebral arteriosclerosis; characterized by disorientation, faulty memory and comprehension.

chronic care: See LONG-TERM CARE.

chronic fatigue syndrome: A debilitating illness, usually following a viral infection, that may result in exhaustion, inability to concentrate, depression, and digestive problems. It is difficult to diagnose and can last for years. Also known as *ME, myalgic encephalomyelitis,* or *post-viral fatigue syndrome.*

chronicity (kro-nis´-i-ti): The quality or state of being chronic.

chronic obstructive airways disease: Term used in referring to pulmonary diseases of uncertain origins, characterized by persistent interference with air flow during expiration;

usually consists of emphysema with destruction of the distal air spaces, bronchitis, and bronchoconstriction, any one of which symptoms may predominate. Also called *chronic obstructive lung disease* and *chronic obstructive pulmonary disease*.

Chronic Sick and Disabled Persons Act 1970: Legislation in the UK, providing for the identification and care of those suffering from chronic or degenerative disease for which there is no cure and which can be only partially alleviated by treatment.

chronobiology (kron'-ō-bī-ol'-o-ji): The study of the mechanisms underlying predictable time-dependent biological rhythms that occur during human growth, development, and ageing, including the menstrual, sleep/wake, and rest/activity cycles, and the heartbeat.

chronogenesis (kron-ō-jen'-e-sis): The history and development of an organism or groups of organisms. — chronogenetic, adj.

chronognosis (kron-og-nō'-sis): Sensitivity to the passage of time.

chronograph (kron'-ō-graf): An instrument for measuring and recording small amounts of time in certain psychophysical experiments.

chronological age (kron-ō-loj'-i-kal): Age from birth; one's calendar age.

chronotropic (kron'-ō-trōp'-ik): Having an effect on the rate of rhythmic movements, *e.g.*, the heartbeat. C. DRUGS may increase or decrease the heart rate, depending on the drug.

chthonophagia (thon-ō-fā'-ji-a): The habit of eating dirt. Syn., *geophagia*. Also called *chthonophagy*.

chukka boot (chuk'-ka): An orthopaedic boot or shoe that has a three-quarter upper; it covers the malleolus.

Chvostek's sign (shvos'-teks): Excessive twitching of the facial muscles on tapping the facial nerve. A sign of tetany. [Franz Chvostek, Austrian surgeon, 1835–1884.]

chyle (kīl): Digested fats which, as an alkaline milky fluid, pass from the small intestine via the lymphatics to the bloodstream. — chylous, adj.

chylification (kī-lif-i-kā'-shun): The formation of chyle in the intestine and its absorption by the lacteals. — Syn., *chylopoiesis*.

chylopericardium (kī'-lō-per-i-kar'-di-um): The presence of a milky fluid in the pericardium; may result from trauma or from obstruction of the thoracic duct.

chylorrhoea (kī'-lō-rē'-a): 1. The production of an excessive amount of chyle. 2. Diarrhoea with stools that are milky in colour, due to rupture of lymphatics of the small intestine.

chylosis (kī-lō'-sis): The conversion of food into chyle in the intestine and its absorption by the tissues.

chylous (kī'-lus): Relating to or resembling chyle.

chymase (kī'-māz): An enzyme found in the gastric juice; it acts to hasten the action of pancreatic juice.

chyme (kīm): Partially digested food which as an acidic, creamy-yellow, thick fluid, passes from the stomach to the duodenum. Its acidity controls the pylorus so that c. is ejected at frequent intervals. — chymous, adj.

chymotrypsin (kī-mō-trip'-sin): Proteolytic enzyme of the pancreatic secretion; also prepared synthetically. Along with trypsin, c. acts to stimulate catabolism of proteins.

cicatrectomy (sik-a-trek'-to-mi): The surgical excision of a scar.

cicatricial (sik-a-trish'-al): Relating to or resembling a scar.

cicatrix (sik'-a-triks): A scar, formed from connective tissue in the healing of a wound. See KELOID. — cicatricial, adj.; cicatrization, n.

cicatrization (sik'-a-trī-zā'-shun): Scarring.

-cide: Combining form denoting kill, killing or to kill.

cilia (sil'-i-a): 1. The eyelashes. 2. Microscopic hair-like projections from certain epithelial cells. Membranes containing such cells are known as ciliated membranes, for example, those lining the respiratory tract and uterine tubes. — cilium, sing.; ciliary, ciliated, cilial, adj.

ciliary (sil'-i-a-ri): Hair-like. C. APPARATUS the nerves, muscles, and other structures of the eye that are concerned with adjusting the lens of the eye for vision at varying distances; C. BODY a specialized structure in the eye connecting the anterior part of the choroid to the circumference of the iris; it is composed of the ciliary muscles and processes; C. MUSCLES fine hair like muscle fibres arranged in a circular manner to form a greyish-white ring immediately behind the corneoscleral junction; C. PROCESSES 70 to 80 in number, are projections on the under surface of the choroid which are attached to the C. muscles; C. REFLEX see under REFLEX.

ciliospinal (sil'-i-ō-spī-nal): 1. Relating to the ciliary body (see under CILIARY) and the spinal cord. 2. Referring to the ciliary centre in the lower cervical and upper thoracic section of the spinal cord which governs the dilatation of the pupil. 3. C. REFLEX see under REFLEX.

cillosis (sil-lō'-sis): Spasmodic twitching of the muscles of the eyelid.

CINAHL: Abbreviation for Cumulative Index to Nursing and Allied Health Literature (*q.v.*).

Cinderella service: An area of healthcare that is not deemed to be mainstream and which may be less well funded than other departments; includes learning disabilities and older people.

cineangiocardiography (sin'-ē-an'-ji-ō-kar-diog'-ra-fi): Motion picture of the passage of contrast medium through the heart and blood vessels.

cineangiography (sin'-ē-an-ji-og'-ra-fi): Motion picture angiography (*q.v.*).

cinecystourethrography (sin'-ē-sist-ō-ū-rēthrog'-ra-fi): Radiographic demonstration of the lower urinary tract following the introduction of a radiopaque dye into the bladder; the organs are observed on a television monitor before, during, and after voiding.

cinefluorography (sin'-ē-floo-or-og'-ra-fi): Motion picture photography of images on a fluoroscopic screen.

cingulum (sin'-gū-lum): A collection of association fibres located in the cingulus gyrus of the brain; see CYRUS.

cion (sī-on): The uvula (*q.v.*).

cionectomy (sī-ō-nek'-to-mi): Excision of part or all of the uvula.

circadian (ser'-kā-di-an): Relating to a period of 24 hours. C. RHYTHM rhythm within a periodicity of 24 hours, especially in relation to biological variations.

circle of Willis: An anastomosis of arteries at the base of the brain, formed by the union of the branches of the internal carotids with the branches of the basilar artery. [Thomas Willis, physician to James II, 1621–1675].

circulating nurse: One who works in the operating theatre, usually a registered nurse, who is free to obtain needed supplies and deliver them to the operating team, to answer anaesthetists' requests for assistance, and perform other duties that the 'scrub' nurse and the operating team are not free to carry out.

circulation (ser-kū-lā'-shun): Passage in a circle. In anatomy, often refers to movement of blood in the body. C. OF BILE the passage of bile from the liver cells where it is formed to the gall bladder, then via the bile ducts to the duodenum and intestine where the bile salts and fats are reabsorbed into the blood; C. OF CEREBROSPINAL FLUID takes place from the ventricles of the brain to the cisterna magna, from whence the fluid bathes the surface of the brain, and cord, including its central canal. It is absorbed into the blood in the cerebral venous sinuses; COLLATERAL C. that established through anastomotic communicating channels, when there is interference with main blood supply; CORONARY C. that of blood through the heart walls; EXTRACORPOREAL C. blood is taken from the body, directed through a machine (heart–lung, artificial kidney) and returned to the general C.; FETAL C. that of blood through the fetus, umbilical cord and placenta; LYMPH C. that of lymph collected from the tissue spaces, which passes via capillaries, vessels, glands and ducts back into the bloodstream; PORTAL C. that of venous blood (collected from the intestines, pancreas, spleen and stomach) to the liver before return to the heart; PULMONARY C. deoxygenated blood leaves the right ventricle, flows through the lungs where it becomes oxygenated and returns to the left atrium of the heart; SYSTEMIC C. oxygenated blood leaves the left ventricle, and after flowing throughout the body, returns deoxygenated to the right atrium. — circulatory, adj.; circulate, v.

circulatory (ser'-kū-la-tor-i): Relating to circulation, particularly of the blood. C. ARREST cessation of circulation of the blood through the heart; may be due to hypoxia, pericardial effusion, arrhythmias due to drugs, electric current, often fatal; C. SYSTEM a system of channels through which nutrient fluids and oxygen are carried to the cells of the body; usually refers to vessels that carry blood.

circum-: Prefix denoting around; surrounding; on all sides.

circumcision (ser-kum-sizh'-un): Excision of the prepuce or foreskin of the penis. FEMALE C. excision of part or all of the prepuce, the clitoris, and the labia (*q.v.*).

circumduction (ser-kum-duk'-shun): **1.** The circular movements of an organ or part around a central axis; *e.g.*, the eye or a limb. **2.** The active or passive swinging of a limb in such a manner that it describes a cone-shaped figure with the apex of the cone being fixed at a joint and the distal end being moved to form a complete circle.

circumferential pneumatic compression: Treatment by application of a body garment (or trousers) which can be inflated sufficiently to produce pressure adequate to control internal haemorrhage from major arteries and veins; can also be used as an air splint for fractures of leg bones. Not to be used in the presence of pulmonary oedema, head, neck, or chest injuries, or haemorrhage from the upper extremities.

circumflex (ser'-kum-fleks): Winding round, designating particularly an artery or nerve that has a winding course. C. NERVE that supplying the deltoid muscle.

circumscribed (ser'-kum-scrībd): Limited; confined to a limited area.

circumstantiality (ser'-kum-stan-shi-al'-i-ti): A condition seen in schizophrenia and senile dementia; the patient is apparently aware of what he wants to express but cannot get beyond utterances that are beside the point.

circumvallate (ser-kum-val'-lāt): Surrounded by a raised ring or by a trench, as the papillae of the tongue.

circus movement: In electrocardiography, the term applies to a continuous movement of a wave that arises in an ectopic focus and travels in a circle around a ring of muscle within the atrial wall, with the result that only part of the impulse is conducted to the ventricle.

cirrhosis (si-rō'-sis): 1. Hardening of an organ. 2. Diffuse permanent damage to an organ. Applied almost exclusively to degenerative changes in the liver with resulting fibrosis; associated developments may include ascites (*q.v.*), obstruction of circulation through the portal vein, with haematemesis, jaundice, and enlargement of the spleen. ALCOHOLIC C. Laennec's C.; CRYPTOGENIC C., C. of unknown cause; often seen in patients with a history of hepatitis or alcoholism; LAENNEC'S C. the C. of the liver that develops in alcoholics; hobnail liver.

cirsectomy (ser-sek'-to-mi): The surgical excision of all or part of a varicose vein.

cirsoid (ser'-soyd): Resembling a tortuous dilated vein (varix, *q.v.*). C. ANEURYSM a tangled mass of pulsating blood vessels, usually seen as a subcutaneous tumour on the scalp.

cirsomphalos (sir-som'-fa-los): A varicose condition involving the navel. See CAPUT MEDUSAE under CAPUT.

cisplatin therapy: The use of cisplatin, an antineoplastic agent, in the treatment of metastatic ovarian and testicular cancer.

cissa (sis'-a): Pica (*q.v.*).

cistern (sis'-tern): A reservoir or large enclosed space for the storage of fluid, particularly the areas in the subarachnoid space where cerebrospinal fluid is stored. See also CISTERNA.

cisterna (sis-ter'-na): Any closed space serving as a reservoir for a body fluid. C. CHYLI the dilated part at the beginning of the thoracic duct which receives lymph from several lymph-collecting vessels; C. MAGNA a subarachnoid space in the cleft between the medulla oblongata and the cerebellum. — cisternal, adj.

cisternal puncture: See PUNCTURE.

cistoid (sis'toyd): 1. Like a bladder. 2. Like a cyst. 3. A tumour that resembles a cyst in that it contains fluid or pulpy material but which has no capsule.

citizen's juries: An approach to public participation designed to feed into the policy-making decisions of public bodies. A randomly selected group of citizens, the jury, is identified. The agenda for the jury focuses on the concerns of the policy makers but is structured in a way that is independent and open to the citizens' views. The jury is given time to examine evidence, discuss ideas and information, to reach a shared view and conclusion.

citrate (sī'-trāt): A compound of citric acid and a base.

citrated (sī'-trāt-ed): Containing a citrate; refers particularly to blood or milk to which a solution of potassium or sodium citrate, or both, has been added.

citrate–phosphate–dextrose–adenine: A preparation commonly used as an anticoagulant in whole blood (for transfusion) because it increases the maximal storage time. Abbreviated CPDA.

citric acid (sit'-rik): Occurs widely in fruits, especially in lemons and limes. Prevents scurvy; also has a diuretic action.

citrin (sit'rin): A mixture of bioflavonoids (*q.v.*) that act in the body to reduce permeability of the capillaries; useful in the treatment of certain purpuras. Also thought to enhance the action of vitamin C in prevention of scurvy. Found in rose hips, citrus fruits, and blackcurrants. Also known as *vitamin P complex*.

citta, cittosis (sit'-a, sit-tō'-sis): Pica (*q.v.*).

civil service: The administrative offices of a government or international agency exclusive of the armed forces.

CJD: Abbreviation for Creutzfeldt–Jakob disease (*q.v.*).

Cl: Chemical symbol for chlorine.

clairvoyance (klar-voy'-ans): The act or power of knowing about events without the use of the senses. Extrasensory perception; insight; divination.

clamp: Usually refers to an instrument used to compress vessels to prevent haemorrhage or to compress organs in order to prevent their contents from spilling into the operative field.

clap: A slang term for gonorrhoea.

clapping: A massage manoeuvre involving a type of percussion; the hands are either held flat or cupped and are brought down rapidly and repeatedly; often used on the chest to dislodge bronchial secretions.

Clark's rule: A formula for calculating the correct dose of medicine for a child:

$$\frac{\text{Weight of child in lbs}}{150} \times \text{adult dose} = \text{child's dose}$$

-clasis: A combining form meaning breaking up.

class: A group sharing the same economic or social status.

-clast: A combining form denoting something that breaks something else or causes separation of its parts.

claudicant (claw'-di-kant): 1. Relating to claudication (*q.v.*). 2. A person suffering from intermittent claudication.

claudication (klaw-di-kā'-shun): Limping, ataxic gait, or pain due to interference with the blood supply to the legs. The cause may be disease or spasm of the vessels themselves. INTERMITTENT C., C. characterized by severe pain in the calves when the person is walking; but after a short rest he is able to continue.

claustrophobia (klaws'trō-fō'-bi-a): Morbid fear of enclosed places, or of being locked in. — claustrophobic, adj.

clavicle (klav'-ik'l): The collarbone. It articulates with the sternum at one end and the acromion process of the scapula at the other. — clavicular, adj.

clavicular (kla-vik'-ū-lar): Relating to the clavicle. C. NOTCH a depression on either side of the upper end of the sternum for articulation of the medial ends of the clavicles.

clavus (klā'-vus): A corn or horny area on the skin. C. HYSTERICUS a pain described as feeling like having a nail driven into one's head.

clawfoot (klaw'-foot): Deformity in which the longitudinal arch of the foot is increased in height, and associated with clawing of the toes. It may be acquired or congenital in origin. Syn., *pes cavus*.

clawhand: A condition in which the hand is clawed and radially deviated due to paralysis of the flexor carpi ulnaris, ulnar half of the flexor digitorum longus, and the small muscles of the hand. Occurs in leprosy, syringomyelia, and in lesions of the ulnar and radial nerves.

clean: Uncontaminated; free of microorganisms. Frequently used to refer to objects that have had no contact with patients in isolation units, or to instruments, etc. that have been sterilized and kept free from contact with microorganisms.

clean-catch specimen: A urine specimen used in examination for the presence of bacteria.

The periurethral area is thoroughly cleansed and a sterile receptacle for the urine is held so it does not touch the body; the patient voids and discards a small amount of urine before collecting the specimen. Female patients are instructed to hold the labia apart while voiding.

cleavage (klēv'-ij): 1. Segmentation by mitosis of the fertilized ovum, with the resulting cells becoming smaller with each division. 2. The splitting of a molecule into two or more smaller molecules. 3. Linear clefts in the skin, most prominently in the skin of the palms and soles.

cleft: A long, narrow fissure, particularly one that develops in the embryo. C. LIP formerly known as harelip; C. PALATE congenital failure of fusion between the right and left palatal processes. If complete, it extends through both hard and soft palates, thus forming a single cavity for the nose and mouth; often associated with C. lip.

cleid-, cleido-: Combining forms denoting the clavicle.

cleidorrhexis (klī-dō-rek'-sis): The fracturing of the clavicle; usually refers to fracture of a fetus's clavicle during difficult labour.

click: A sharp brief sound. EJECTION C. a single high-pitched sound usually heard early in systole; arises from one of the great vessels or when the aortic or pulmonary valve opens forcefully; most often associated with septal defects, sometimes with hypertension; JOINT C. a sharp, high-pitched sound heard on joint movement; ORTOLANI'S C. a click that is felt in a congenitally dislocated hip when the thigh is abducted when in flexion and the head of the femur slides over the rim of the acetabulum; SYSTOLIC C. a sharp click heard during systole; often indicates a mitral valve defect. — clicking, adj.

client: In nursing, an individual who seeks and/or receives nursing care services, either from a health-care facility or from a health-care professional.

climateric (klī-mak'-ter-ik): The symptoms that accompany the cessation of ovarian function. It marks the end of the period of possible reproduction by the female, as evidenced by cessation of the menstrual periods; other bodily and emotional changes may occur. Cf. MENOPAUSE. In the male, it marks the beginning of the period of lessening sexual activity, usually between the ages of 40 and 60.

climacterium (klī-mak-tē'-ri-um): Climacteric (*q.v.*). C. PRAECOX premature appearance of the symptoms and physical changes associated with the climacteric.

climatology (klī-ma-tol'-o-ji): The study of climate and its effects on health and disease.

climax (klī'-maks): **1.** The period of greatest intensity of a disease; the crisis of a disease. **2.** The sexual orgasm. — climactic, adj.

clinic (klin'-ik): **1.** A centre for examination, study and treatment of outpatients. **2.** Medical instruction, with the examination of patients, before a group of students; usually conducted at the bedside. **3.** A type of medical practice wherein a group of medical specialists work cooperatively.

clinical (klin'-i-kal): **1.** Relating to a clinic. **2.** Relating to the actual observation and treatment of sick persons as distinguished from theoretical or experimental observations. C. DIAGNOSIS, see under DIAGNOSIS; C. NURSING see under NURSING; C. THERMOMETER a self-registering thermometer used to determine the temperature of the human body; its range is from 94° to 110° Fahrenheit and from 34.4° to 42° Centigrade (Celsius).

clinical audit: A cyclical measurement and evaluation process by health professionals of the clinical standards they are achieving, through which the quality of healthcare in general, and clinical quality in particular, can be improved.

clinical effectiveness: 1. The extent to which an intervention, when deployed in the field for a particular patient or population, maintains and improves health and secures the greatest possible health gain from the available sources. **2.** Demonstrable benefit from an intervention, measured in the relevant client group.

clinical governance: A framework through which NHS organizations are accountable for continually improving the quality of their services and safeguarding high standards of care by creating an environment in which excellence in clinical care will flourish. See also COMMISSION FOR HEALTHCARE AUDIT AND INSPECTION; COMMISSION FOR HEALTH IMPROVEMENT.

clinical guidelines: 1. A set of instructions to direct the management of a patient, developed by a group of experts using existing evidence. **2.** A suggested course of action, usually provided by an authoritative body, for the investigation and/or treatment of patients.

clinical indicators: Signs used to gauge the performance of the NHS. Directed at the outcomes of clinical care, these are not direct measures of quality but can be used to high-

light issues that may need further investigation or action.

clinical nurse specialist: A nurse in an area of healthcare who has undertaken advanced study and practices at a higher level; that is, a nurse who develops specific skills for an area of nursing, e.g., infection control, or a particular group of patients, e.g., those with diabetes or genitourinary disorders.

clinical reasoning: Examining the relevant factors before making decisions on a care or treatment. Includes consideration of the problem, the diagnosis and what to do, if anything. More experienced practitioners use shortcuts based on knowledge and previous experience. See also DIAGNOSE.

clinical supervision: The formal process of professional support, central to learning, where students and practitioners are called upon to deal with complex clinical situations under the supervision of a colleague. A range of clinical supervision models have been developed or refined to meet the needs of the many diverse groups of nurses.

clinical trials: Research studies conducted with patients, usually to evaluate a new treatment or drug. Each trial is designed to answer scientific questions and to find better ways to treat individuals with a specific condition.

clinician (kli-nish'-an): A medical practitioner who is engaged in clinical practice rather than research.

clinicopathology (klin'-i-kō-path-ol'-o-ji): The diagnosis of disease by observation of the patient's signs and symptoms, combined with a study of laboratory findings.

Clinitest (klin'-i-test): Trade name for a reagent tablet used in testing urine for sugar, particularly by patients at home; the administration kit contains the reagent tablets and the equipment needed for conducting the test.

clinodactylism (kli-no-dak'-til-izm): A congenital defect consisting of abnormal bending or deviation of the fingers and/or toes. Clinodactyly.

clip: A malleable metal staple that is fixed in the skin with special forceps to hold the edges of a surgical wound together.

clitoral (klit'-or-al): Relating to the clitoris. C. STAGE the stage in girls' psychosexual development that compares with the phallic phase in boys.

clitoridectomy (klit'-or-i-dek'-to-mi): Surgical removal of the clitoris; female circumcision.

clitoridotomy (klit'-or-i-dot'-o-mi): Incision into or excision of part of the clitoris.

clitoris (klit′-or-is): A small, erectile, highly erotogenic body situated just below the mons veneris at the junction anteriorially of the labia minora; the homologue of the penis in the male. — clitoral, clitoridean, adj.

clitorism (klit′-ō-rizm): Hypertrophy of the clitoris.

clofibrate (klō-fī′-brāt): A liquid chemical with a characteristic odour (chlorophenoxyisobutyrate); used in treatment of cholesterolaemia; it reduces the plasma levels of cholesterol, triglycerides, and uric acid.

clone (klōn): 1. One of a group of individuals with identical genetic make-up; produced by asexual reproduction of a single individual. 2. A group of cells produced from a single cell by the process of mitosis. — clonal, adj.; cloning, n. 3. An individual formed from a single somatic cell of another individual. The parent organism and clone are therefore genetically identical.

clonic (klon′-ik): Of the nature of clonus; pertains particularly to generalized seizures that are characterized by the rapid, alternating contraction and relaxation of the muscles.

clonic–tonic: See TONIC–CLONIC.

clonorchiasis (klō-nor-kī′-a-sis): An infection of the liver caused by the presence of the adult worms of the fluke. *Clonorchis sinensis*, in the biliary channels.

Clonorchis sinensis (klō-nor′-kis si-nen′-sis): A tapeworm (Chinese liver fluke) found in the Far East; infects both animals and humans. The latter become infected by eating raw or undercooked fish. Attacks primarily the biliary passages, producing symptoms of enlarged liver, oedema, and diarrhoea; often fatal.

clonus (klō′-nus): A series of regular, rapid, intermittent muscular contractions and relaxations following stimulation; usually indicates central nervous system disease and affects mostly the arms and legs.

closed: C. CHEST DRAINAGE continuous drainage of the pleural cavity by means of an intercostal drainage tube that is attached to an airtight collecting bottle to which suction is applied; C. HEART MASSAGE rhythmic compression of the chest by hand pressure applied over the sternum; C. HEART SURGERY that performed without making an incision into the chest cavity; C. REDUCTION OR FRACTURE reduction by manipulation of the bone without making an incision in the skin; C. TREATMENT OF BURNS the use of an occlusive dressing after cleansing the area and applying a topical medication.

Clostridium (klos-trid′-i-um): A bacterial genus; large Gram-positive anaerobic, variously shaped, pathogenic bacilli found as commensals of the gut of animals and humans, and as saprophytes in the soil. Produces endospores which are widely distributed. Many species are pathogenic for humans because of the endotoxins produced, *e.g.*, *C. botulinum* (botulism); *C. perfringens* (gas gangrene); *C. sporogenes*, a species of C. that frequently contaminates deep wounds; considered non-pathogenic, but causes a foul odour in wounds; *C. tetani* (tetanus); *C. welchii* (gas gangrene).

clot: 1. A semisolid mass. Usually refers to blood; fibrin forms a network that holds the formed elements in the blood in a mass. 2. To form into a clot; to coagulate.

clotting factor: Any of several substances in the blood that are concerned with the clotting process; principally fibrinogen, fibrin, prothrombin, thrombin, thromboplastin, and calcium ions.

clotting time: The time it takes for shed blood to clot. This is determined by test and differs from bleeding time in that it involves only the ability of the blood to clot, whereas bleeding time also involves the ability of the small capillaries to constrict.

Cloward procedure: A surgical procedure for immobilizing the cervical spine when external measures cannot maintain proper alignment; consists of fusion of the anterior spine of the cervical vertebra involved; utilizes a bone graft from another part of the body.

clubbed fingers: Fingers that are swollen with bulbous enlargement of the terminal phalanges, usually without any osseous change. See CLUBBING.

clubbing: Refers to the bulbous enlargement of the ends of the phalanges due to proliferation of the soft tissues without the same degree of change in the bones. May be familial and insignificant. Also sometimes seen in children with certain congenital heart defects and in adults with heart, lung, or gastrointestinal diseases.

clubfoot: A congenital malformation in which the foot is twisted out of shape or position; may be either unilateral or bilateral. See TALIPES.

clubhand: A congenital deformity analogous to clubfoot; type most commonly seen is the result of defective development of the radius.

clumping: See AGGLUTINATION.

Clutton's joints: Symmetrical swelling of joints, usually painless, the knees often being involved.

Associated with congenital syphilis. [Henry Hugh Clutton, English surgeon, 1850–1909.]

CMHT: Abbreviation for community mental health team, see under COMMUNITY.

CMV: Abbreviation for cytomegalovirus (*q.v.*).

CNO: Abbreviation for Chief Nursing Officer (*q.v.*).

CNS: Abbreviation for (1) central nervous system (*q.v.*) (2) clinical nurse specialist (*q.v.*)

Co: Chemical symbol for cobalt (*q.v.*)

CO: Chemical formula for carbon monoxide, see under CARBON.

CO₂: Chemical formula for carbon dioxide, see under CARBON.

COAD: Abbreviation for chronic obstructive airways disease (*q.v..*)

coagulant (kō-ag′-ū-lant): 1. An agent that causes or speeds clotting of the blood. 2. Having the effect of increasing the tendency of the blood to clot.

coagulase (kō-ag′-ū-lās): A clotting enzyme, *e.g.*, thrombin, rennin. Also produced by some bacteria (*e.g., Staph. aureus*), which clot plasma. Used to type bacteria into C. negative and positive.

coagulate (kō-ag′-ū-lāt): 1. To change from a fluid to a solid jelly-like mass, or to clot. 2. To cause clotting or curdling. — coagulation, coagulability, n.; coagulable, adj.

coagulation (kō-ag-ū -lā′-shun): 1. The process of changing a liquid to a solid or thickened state; the formation of a clot. 2. The process of changing fluid plasma of the blood to a solid gel by the conversion of fibrinogen to fibrin. C. FACTORS see under FACTOR; C. TIME see CLOT-TING TIME.

coagulometer (kō-ag-ū-lom′-i-ter): An instrument for determining the clotting time of blood.

coagulum (kō-ag′-ū-lum): Any coagulated mass. Scab.

coalesce (kō-a-les′): To grow together; to unite into a mass. Often used to describe the development of a skin eruption when discrete areas of affected skin coalesce to form sheets of a similar appearance, *e.g.*, in psoriasis (*q.v.*), pityriasis ruba pilaris. — coalescence, n.; co-alescent, adj.

coal tar: Thick black substance obtained from coal by distillation. Used in a variety of pharmaceutical preparations.

coal workers' pneumoconiosis: See under PNEU-MONOCONIOSIS.

coaptation (kō-ap-tā′-shun): The procedure of correctly aligning or placing displaced parts, as the ends of a fractured bone. C. SPLINT a

splint that prevents fragments of a bone from overriding.

coarctation (kō-ark-tā′-shun): Contraction, stricture, narrowing; applied to a vessel or canal. C. OF THE AORTA a pressing together or narrowing of the aorta or part of it; may be a congenital heart defect or may be due to pathological narrowing of the median coat of the artery.

coarctotomy (kō-ark-tot′-a-mi): Surgical division of a stricture.

coating: A covering; of pills, a covering to conceal an unpleasant taste. ENTERIC C. covering for a medicament which prevents its being absorbed from the stomach; the coating dissolves in the intestine only.

cobalamin (kō-bal′-a-min): Part of the vitamin B₁₂ group.

cobalt (kō′-balt): A mineral element considered nutritionally essential in minute traces; thought to be linked with iron and copper in prevention of anaemia. Cobalt-60, a radioisotope frequently used in radiotherapy for cancer.

coca (kō′-ka): The leaves of several varieties of the South American shrub, *Erythroxylon*, from which cocaine (*q.v.*) is obtained.

cocaine (kō-kān′): A crystalline alkaloid obtained from coca leaves; used as a narcotic; habituating; see also 'CRACK?' C. HYDRO-CHLORIDE a hydrochloride of cocaine, used as a topical anaesthetic.

coccobacillus (kok′-ō-ba-sil′-us): A short, thick, somewhat ovoid bacterial cell. — coc-cobacillary, adj.

coccogenous (kok-oj′-e-nus): Produced by cocci.

coccoid (kok′-oyd): Resembling a micrococcus.

coccus (kok′-us): A spherical or nearly spherical bacterium. Often classified according to the way it arranges itself, as can be seen under the microscope; diplococcus, when it occurs in pairs; streptococcus, when it occurs in chains; staphylococcus, when it occurs in bunches resembling bunches of grapes. — cocci, pl.; coccal, coccoid, adj.

-coccus: Combining form denoting berry-shaped. Used primarily in forming generic names for microorganisms.

coccy-: A combining form denoting coccyx.

coccygeal (kok-sij′-ē-al): Relating to or located in the region of the coccyx. C. NERVE one of the lowest pair of spinal nerves.

coccygeus (kok-sij′-ē-us): Relating to the coccyx. C. MUSCLE a muscle that extends from the pubis to the sacrum and coccyx; one of the two muscles that make up the pelvic diaphragm, the muscular floor that supports the pelvic organs.

coccyx (kok′-siks): The last bone at the base of the vertebral column. It is triangular in shape and curved slightly forward. It is composed of four rudimentary vertebrae, cartilaginous at birth, ossification being completed at about the 30th year. — coccygeal, adj.

cochlea (kok′-lē-a): A tightly coiled, fluid-filled, spiral canal resembling a snail shell, in the anterior part of the bony labyrinth of the inner ear; contains the essential organ of hearing, the organ of Corti, where the movement of special hair cells that are the receptors of sound waves stimulate the auditory nerve. — cochlear, adj.

cochleitis (kok-le-ī -tis): Inflammation of the cochlea. Also called *cochlitis.*

Cochrane Library (kok′-ran): A collection of seven separate databases. Five of these provide coverage of evidence-based medicine, and the other two provide information on research methodology. Also called *Cochrane database.* Available at http://www.cochrane.org/index0.htm

cocoa (ko′-kō): The seeds of *Theobroma cacao.* The powder is made into a nourishing pleasant beverage. Contains theobromine and caffeine. C. BUTTER the fat obtained from the roasted seeds; is used in suppositories, ointments and as an emollient (*q.v.*).

code (kō′d): **1.** A system of symbols, letters, or words given certain arbitrary meanings, used for transmitting messages requiring brevity. **2.** A systematic collection of regulations and rules of procedure or conduct, see CODE OF CONDUCT.

codeine (kō′-dēn): An alkaloid of opium; similar to morphine in action and habituating; used in medicine for its analgesic, sedative, hypnotic, antitussive, antidiarrhoeal and narcotic effects.

code of conduct: A set of rules that guide an individual's behaviour. See APPENDIX 4.

cod liver oil: Oleum morrhuae. The oil extracted from the liver of fresh codfish. Contains vitamins A and D and on that account is used as a dietary supplement in cases of mild deficiency. Also used as a preventive of rickets in children. Now often replaced by purer forms or concentrates of vitamins A and D.

codon (kō′-don): A basic informational unit of the genetic code, being a segment of the DNA molecule that specifies a certain amino acid.

coeliac (sē′-li-ak): Relating to the abdomen. C. DISEASE non-tropical sprue; occurs primarily in young children but also in adults; characterized by malabsorption of fats and inability to digest certain gluten grains, pain, vomiting, diarrhoea, distension, malnutrition, bulky foul-smelling stools; cause unknown; may be hereditary; C. CRISIS an acute attack of diarrhoea and vomiting resulting in dehydration and acidosis.

coelioma (sē-li-ō′-ma): A tumour of the peritoneum, particularly a mesothelioma (*q.v.*).

coelom (sē′-lom): The body cavity of the fetus; from it the principal cavities of the trunk arise.

coenzyme (kō-en′-zīm): An enzyme activator, *e.g.*, bile which facilitates the action of lipase in the digestion of fats.

cofactor: 1. Any factor functioning in cooperation with another factor. **2.** A coenzyme.

coffee-ground vomitus: Vomitus containing partly digested blood; has the appearance of coffee grounds.

cognition (kog-ni′-shun): The mental process involved in thinking, perceiving, knowing, comprehending, reasoning, judging, remembering, and being aware of one's thoughts and of objects. C. is one of three aspects of mind, the others being affection (feeling or emotion) and conation (willing or desiring); these aspects of mind work as a whole but any one of them may dominate any mental process. C. DEVELOPMENT refers to the development of the acquisition of conscious thought, intelligence, and problem-solving ability, an orderly process which begins in childhood; C. THERAPY refers to any of the several treatment methods that help an individual to alter the mental processes involved in perceiving, thinking, and reasoning that are maladaptive to his environment.

cognitive (kog′-ni-tiv): Related to or involving perception, including the elements of comprehension, judgement, memory, and reasoning. C. BEHAVIOURAL THERAPY a form of psychological treatment based on learning theory principles, used mostly for the treatment of depression but increasingly shown to be a useful component of treatment in schizophrenia (*q.v.*) and some personality disorders (*q.v.*); it involves improving thinking and social skills by teaching strategies to deal with problems and people more effectively; C. LEARNING THEORY the theory that it is the person's interpretation of the environment that determines which actions are or are not rewarding, which positive reinforcements are viewed as bribes, and which negative reinforcements are viewed as punishment. See also OPERANT LEARNING THEORY.

cogwheel rigidity: A type of movement in certain neurological conditions; when a hypertonic muscle is passively stretched it resists and responds with a rhythmic jerkiness of movement. Also called *cogwheel phenomenon, cogwheel resistance.*

cohabitation (kō-hab-i-tā′ -shun): The living together of a man and woman as man and wife; they may or may not be legally married.

cohort (kō′ -hort): A group of individuals having some common factor or objective; particularly used in statistics, *e.g.*, a birth cohort consists of people born within a specific period; a colleague, supporter, or associate.

coil: 1. A spiral or winding structure; helix. 2. An intrauterine contraceptive device. C. GLAND a sweat gland.

coitus (kō′ -i-tus): The act of sexual intercourse with a person of the opposite sex; copulation. C. INTERRUPTUS intercourse in which the penis is withdrawn before ejaculation occurs; C. RESERVATUS intercourse in which ejaculation is avoided, with the penis remaining in the vagina until flaccid.

col-, coli-, colo-: Combining forms denoting colon.

cola: See KOLA.

colchicine (kōl′ -chi-sēn): A pale yellow bitter alkaloid powder obtained from a European tree; poisonous; used in suppression and treatment of gout.

cold: 1. Opp. of heat. 2. A catarrhal inflammation of the upper respiratory tract; may be caused by infection or allergy.

cold abscess: An abscess that does not exhibit the usual signs, *i.e.*, redness, heat, swelling.

cold agglutination test: A test that demonstrates the cold agglutination phenomenon, that is, human erythrocytes of the group O type will agglutinate at 0° to 10°C, but not at normal body temperatures in cases of atypical pneumonia, trypanosomiasis, some viral infections, and several other disorders.

cold sore: A small vesicle or blister that appears, usually around or within the mouth, during a cold or a disease attended by fever. Often multiple. See HERPES. Also called *fever blister.*

cold-weather payment: Benefit for individuals receiving income support, aged over 60, disabled or with a long-term illness. It is paid automatically when the temperature drops below a certain level. The UK government decides what level the temperature must drop to before this money is received.

colectomy (kō-lek′ -to-mi): Excision of part or all of the colon.

coleitis (kōl-ē-ī′ -tis): Vaginitis.

coleocystitis (kol-ē-ō-sis-tī′ -tis): Inflammation of the vagina and the urinary bladder.

coleoptosis (kōl-ē-op′ -tō-sis): Prolapse of the vaginal wall.

coleotomy (kōl-ē-ot′ -ō-mi): Colpotomy (*q.v.*).

colibacillaemia (kō′ -li-bas-i-lē′ -mi-a): The presence of *Escherichia coli* in the blood.

colibacillosis (kō′ -li-bas-il-ō′ -sis): Infection caused by *Escherichia coli.*

colibacilluria (kō′ -li-ba-sil-ū′ -ri-a): The presence of the colon bacilli in the urine.

colibacillus (kō′ -li-ba-sil′ -us): The colon bacillus; found in the intestine of humans and many animals. *Escherichia coli.*

colic (kol′ -ik): 1. Abdominal pain that occurs in waves with relatively painless periods between the spasms of pain. 2. A complex syndrome seen in infants under three months of age, characterized by excessive crying, apparent severe abdominal pain, pulling up of the legs and clenching of the fists. BILIARY C. spasm of smooth muscle in a bile duct, caused by a gallstone; GALL BLADDER C. acute cholecystitis (*q.v.*); INTESTINAL C. abnormal peristaltic movement of an irritated intestine, causing abdominal pain; PAINTER'S C. spasm of the intestine and constrict of mesenteric vessels; associated with lead poisoning as may occur in painters; RENAL C. spasm of a ureter due to the presence of a stone; UTERINE C. dysmenorrhoea. — colicky, adj.

colic (kō′ -lik): Relating to or involving the colon.

colicin (kōl′ -i-sin): A protein secreted by certain strains of *Escherichia coli* that act to destroy other strains of the same species.

colicky (kol′ -i-ki): 1. Resembling or causing colic. 2. A person suffering from colic.

colicystitis (kō′ -li-sis-tī′ -tis): Cystitis caused by *Escherichia coli.*

coliform (kō′ -li-form): A word used to describe any bacterium of faecal origin which is morphologically similar to *Escherichia coli.*

colipyuria (kō′ -li-pī-ū′ -ri-a): Pus in the urine associated with infection caused by *Escherichia coli.*

colitis (ko-lī′ -tis): Inflammation of the colon; acute or chronic. ACUTE C. occurs suddenly as a result of infection or irritation; accompanied by pain and diarrhoea; AMOEBIC C. caused by an amoeba; GRANULOMATOUS C. inflammation of the colon characterized by formation of granulomas; MUCOUS C. see under IRRITABLE

BOWEL SYNDROME. PSEUDOMEMBRANOUS C. a relatively rare syndrome; may appear in postoperative patients who have received certain antibiotics; symptoms include diarrhoea, pain, cardiac collapse, and formation of a pseudomembrane over the mucosa of the bowel with necrosis; often fatal; SPASTIC C. irritable colon; see under COLON. ULCERATIVE C. an inflammatory and ulcerative condition of the mucosa of the colon; of unknown cause. Characteristically it affects young and early middle-aged adults, producing periodic bouts of diarrhoeal stools containing mucus and blood. Often chronic, it may vary in severity from a mild form with little constitutional upset to a severe, dangerous, and prostrating illness.

coliuria (kō-li-ū′-ri-a): See colibacilluria.

collaboration (kol-lab′-er-ā′-shun): **1.** Work done jointly with others, especially in an intellectual endeavour. **2.** Work with an agency or institution with which one is not immediately affiliated. **3.** Referring to multidisciplinary co-operation.

collagen (kol′-la-jen): An albuminoid substance, arranged in bundles, insoluble in water. It is the main protein constituent of the white fibres of connective tissue and cartilage and the organic substance of bone. The C. DISEASES are characterized by an inflammatory lesion of unknown origin with widespread pathology of the connective tissues and affecting the small blood vessels; they include dermatomyositis, lupus erythematosus, polyarteritis (periarteritis) nodosa, and scleroderma, rheumatoid arthritis, and rheumatic fever. — collagenic, collagenous, adj.

collagenase (kol′-aj′-in-ās): A proteolytic enzyme that hydrolyses collagen fibres and gelatin; an endotoxin produced by *Clostridium perfringens* (*q.v.*); attacks primarily subcutaneous tissues.

collapse: 1. Extreme physical or nervous prostration. **2.** The falling in of a hollow organ or vessel, *e.g.*, collapse of lung from change of air pressure inside or outside the organ. C. THERAPY artificial pneumothorax (*q.v.*), induced to collapse and immobilize a lung. Also called *collapsotherapy*.

collarbone: The clavicle (*q.v.*).

collateral (ko-lat′-er-al): Accessory, secondary. C. CIRCULATION established by blood flowing in nearby anastomosing small vessels when a main vessel has become blocked.

collectivism (kol-lek′-ti-vizm): A political or economic theory advocating common control, especially over production and distribution.

Colles fracture: See under FRACTURE.

colliquative (kol-lik′-wa-tiv): **1.** Profuse; excessive. **2.** Characterized by excessive fluid discharge.

collodion (ko-lō′-di-on): A flammable, viscous solution of pyroxylin, ether and alcohol. It forms a flexible film on the skin and is used mainly as a protective dressing. FLEXIBLE C. collodion mixed with camphor and castor oil.

colloid (kol′-loyd): A glue-like non-crystalline substance; diffusible but not soluble in water and unable to pass through an animal membrane. Some drugs can be prepared in their colloidal form. C. GOITRE abnormal enlargement of the thyroid gland, due to the accumulation in it of viscid, iodine-containing colloid. — colloidal, adj.

collopexia (kol-ō-pek′-si-a): The surgical fixation of the neck of the uterus.

collum (kol′-um): **1.** The neck. **2.** A neck-like part.

collyrium (kol-lir′-i-um): **1.** Eyewash. **2.** Eye drops.

colocentesis (kō′-lō-sen-tē′-sis): Surgical puncture of the colon, usually to relieve distension.

colocolostomy (kō′-lō-ko-los′-to-mi): An anastomosis between two parts of the colon not formerly contiguous.

colocystoplasty (kōl-ō-sis′-tō-plas-ti): Operation to increase the capacity of the urinary bladder by using part of the colon. — colocystoplastic, adj.

colon (kō′-lon): The large bowel extending from the caecum to the rectum. In its various parts it has appropriate names. — ASCENDING C., TRANSVERSE C., DESCENDING C., SIGMOID C.; IRRITABLE C. one in which there is a tendency to hyperperistalsis, colic, and sometimes diarrhoea; emotional stress is thought to be a contributing factor. See also IRRITABLE BOWEL SYNDROME. — colonic, adj.

colonic (ko-lon′-ik): Relating to the colon. C. LAVAGE or IRRIGATION the introduction of a large amount of fluid into the colon to cleanse and flush it out.

colonization (kol′-on-ī-zā′-shun): **1.** The formation of compact groups of microorganisms as occurs when bacteria begin to reproduce on the surface of or within a culture medium, or in a location to which they have metastasized. **2.** Innidiation (*q.v.*).

colonoscope (kō-lon′-o-skōp): An instrument for examining the lower part of the colon. — colonoscopy, n.

colonoscopy (kō-lon-os′ -kō-pi): Examination of the colon, usually with a flexible fibre-optic endoscope.

colony (kol′ -on-i): A mass of bacteria, growing on a culture, which is the result of multiplication of one or more organisms. A colony may contain many millions of individual organisms and become macroscopic (q.v.); its physical features are often characteristic of the species. C. COUNT bacterial count; a method of estimating the number of bacteria in a unit of sample; C. COUNTER a device for counting colonies of bacteria growing in culture medium.

coloproctectomy (ko-lō-prok-tek′ -to-mi): Surgical removal of the colon and the rectum.

coloproctitis (ko-lō-prok-tī′ -tis): Inflammation of the colon and the rectum.

coloproctostomy (ko-lō-prok-tos′ -to-mi): An anastomosis between the colon and the rectum.

coloptosis (ko-lop′ -tō-sis): The downwards displacement of the colon.

colorectal (ko-lō-rek′tal): Relating to the colon and the rectum.

colorectitis (ko-lō-rek-tī′ -tis): Inflammation of the colon and the rectum.

colorectum (ko-lō-rek′ -tum): The lower 28 cm of the bowel including the distal part of the colon and the rectum considered together, regarded as an organic entity.

colorrhagia (ko-lō-rā′ -ji-a): An abnormal discharge from the rectum.

colosigmoidostomy (ko′ -lō-sig-moy-dos′ -tō-mi): An anastomosis between the sigmoid and another part of the colon.

colostomy (ko-los′ -to-mi): A surgically established fistula between the colon and the surface of the abdomen; this acts as an artificial anus and may be temporary or permanent. TRANSVERSE C. a surgical anastomosis between the ileum and the transverse colon.

colostrum (ko-los′ -trum): The thin pale yellow serous fluid secreted in the breasts during the first few days after parturition, before the formation of the true milk is established. It contains white blood cells, protein, water, and carbohydrates, and is immunologically active, rich in lactalbumin; also acts as a laxative for the infant, promoting the excretion of meconium. C. CORPUSCLE or BODY one of many round bodies containing fat droplets found in colostrum early in lactation and again when milk is diminishing; thought to be modified leukocytes; a galactoblast.

colotomy (ko-lot′ -o-mi): Incision into the colon.

colour blindness: Achromatopsia (q.v.). See also under BLINDNESS.

colour index: A term used to indicate the relative amount of haemoglobin in red blood cells of a patient. It is the ratio of the percentage of haemoglobin (100% = 14.6 g of haemoglobin per 100 ml) to the percentage of red blood cells (100% = 5 million per cu mm). The normal index ranges from 0.85 to 1.1.

colour scotoma: Colour blindness in only a part of the visual field.

colp-, colpo-: Combining forms denoting: 1. A fold or hollow. 2. The vagina.

colpectomy (kol-pek′ -to-mi): Surgical excision of the vagina, or part of it.

colpeurysis (kōl-pū-ris′ -is): Surgical dilatation of the vagina.

colpocele (kol′ -pō-sēl): A hernia into the vagina.

colpocystitis (kol′ -pō-sis-tī-tis): Inflammation of the vagina and the urinary bladder.

colpohysterectomy (kol′ -pō-his-ter-ek′ -to-mi): Surgical removal of the uterus through the vagina.

colpoperineoplasty (kol′ -pō-per-i-nē′ -ō-plas-ti): Plastic repair of the vagina and perineum.

colpoperineorrhaphy (kol′ -pō-per-in-ē-or′ -a-fi): The surgical repair of an injured vagina and perineum.

colpoplasty (kol′ -pō-plas-ti): Plastic surgery of the vagina.

colpoptosis (kol-pop-tō′ -sis): Prolapse of the vagina.

colporrhaphy (kol-por′ -a-fi): 1. Surgical repair of a tear in the vagina. 2. Suturing of the vaginal wall to narrow the vaginal canal.

colporrhexis (kol-pō-rek′ -sis): 1. Rupture or laceration of the vaginal vault. 2. The forcible tearing away of the uterine cervix from the vaginal walls; a rare occurrence during childbirth.

colposcope (kol′ -pō-skōp): An endoscope for viewing the vagina and cervix. — colposcopic, adj.; colposcopically, adv.; colposcopy, n.

colposcopy (kol-pos′ -ko-pi): Examination of the vagina and cervix by means of a colposcope.

colpostenosis (kol-po-ste-nō′ -sis): Constriction or narrowing of the vaginal canal.

colpotomy (kol-pot′ -o-mi): Incision of the vaginal wall. POSTERIOR C. performed to drain an abscess in the pouch of Douglas through the vagina.

colpoxerosis (kol-pō-zē-rō′ -sis): Abnormal dryness of the vaginal mucous membrane.

column (kol′ -um): In anatomy, a structure of the body resembling a column or pillar, e.g., the spinal column. RENAL C. one of the structures that lie between the pyramids in the cortex of the kidney (*q.v.*); VERTEBRAL C. see under VERTEBRAL.

coma (kō′-ma): A prolonged state of complete loss of consciousness, from which the patient cannot be awakened; insensibility. Seen in alcoholism and other poisonings, diabetes, epilepsy, encephalitis, brain tumour, haematoma, vascular diseases. DIABETIC C. occurs suddenly in patients with diabetes mellitus; due to excess of insulin in the blood and the resulting severe acidosis; HEPATITIS C., C. that accompanies hepatic encephalopathy; see under ENCEPHALOPATHY; HYPERGLYCAEMIC C., C. due to an excess of glucose in the circulating blood; HYPOGLYCAEMIC C., C. due to an excess of insulin in relation to the glucose content of the circulating blood; INSULIN C., C. due to an excess of insulin in the blood; see also INSULIN THERAPY under THERAPY.

comatose (kō′-ma-tōs): In a state of coma.

combat fatigue: A state of physical and emotional fatigue experienced by soldiers in military combat. Also called *combat neurosis, battle neurosis,* and *shell shock.* See also GULF WAR SYNDROME.

combustion (kum-bust′-shun): In chemistry, rapid oxidation accompanied by heat and sometimes light.

comedo (kom′-ē-dō): Blackhead. A worm-like cast of sebum which occupies the outlet of a sebaceous gland in the skin. Comedones have a black colour because of oxidation; a feature of acne vulgaris. — comedones, pl.

comma bacillus (kom′-ma bas-il′-us): VIBRIO COMMA the comma-shaped organism that causes cholera. Also called *Vibrio cholerae.*

commensal (ko-men′-sal): One of two organisms living in a state of commensalism (*q.v.*) without invading tissues or causing infection; however, when transferred to an abnormal site, some commensals are potentially pathogenic.

commensalism (ko-men′-sal-izm): The harmonious living together of two organisms, one of which obtains food, protection or other benefit from the other without either damaging or benefiting the other.

comminuted (kom′-i-nū-ed): Broken or shattered into a number of small pieces; term often used to denote a shattering fracture of a bone. — comminution, n.

Commission for Health-care Audit and Inspection: An organization created, in draft form in 2003, to take on the functions of: the Commission for Health Improvement (*q.v.*);

the National Care Standards Commission (*q.v.*) (in respect of private and voluntary healthcare); and the Audit Commission (*q.v.*) (in respect of national studies of the efficiency, effectiveness, and economy of healthcare). It succeeded the Commission for Health Improvement in April 2004. It aims to improve the quality of healthcare by providing an independent assessment of the standards of services provided to patients, whether by the NHS or privately.

Commission for Health Improvement: A regulatory body established to improve the quality of patient care in the NHS. It does this by reviewing the care provided by the NHS in England and Wales, examining three key areas: strategic capacity; resources and processes; and information. (Scotland has its own equivalent regulatory body, the Clinical Standards Board.) It aims to address unacceptable variations in NHS patient care in the UK by identifying both notable practice and areas where care could be improved. See also COMMISSION FOR HEALTH-CARE AUDIT AND INSPECTION.

Commission for Patient and Public Involvement in Health: An independent, non-departmental public body, sponsored by the Department of Health, set up in January 2003, with a remit to ensure that the public is involved in decision-making about health and provision of health services. It aims to promote the involvement in health of all sections of the community, but especially of those whose views are not usually heard. A Patient and Public Involvement Forum has been set up for every NHS Trust and Primary Care Trust in England. These are made up of local people who play an active role in health-related decision-making within their communities.

Commission for Social Care Inspection: Body proposed to replace the Social Services Inspectorate and National Care Standards Commission. It will monitor standards of care by social services and in private nursing homes.

commissure (kom′-mi-shūr): 1. The point or line of union between two parts, *e.g.*, the angle or corner of the eyelids or lips. 2. A band of nerve fibres that cross from one side of the brain or spinal cord to the other.

Committee on the Safety of Medicines: An advisory board responsible for informing the UK licensing authority of the quality, efficacy, and safety of medicines. It maintains the high standards that the public and health professionals expect.

common bile duct: The duct formed by the union of the hepatic and pancreatic ducts; empties into the duodenum.

common cold: See COLD.

communicable (ko-mū′-ni-ka-b′l): Transmissible from one source to another or from one person to another, either directly or indirectly. C. DISEASE an infectious disease that is transmitted from one person to another, directly or by an animal or insect vector, or a carrier. See also NOTIFIABLE.

Communicable Disease Center: See CENTERS FOR DISEASE CONTROL.

communication (kuh-mū′-ni-kā′-shun): The process of exchanging thoughts or information in a reciprocal relationship; may be carried on verbally or non-verbally as, *e.g.*, by writing, gestures, facial expression, or body behaviour.

communism: 1. A theory advocating elimination of private property. 2. A system in which goods are owned in common and are available to all as needed.

community (ko-mū′-ni-ti): A group of people living in the same geographic area and under the same government. C. CARE the provision of help and treatment for people in their home environment; these services can be provided by unpaid carers, such as family or friends, and some health- and social-care professionals; see PRIMARY HEALTHCARE. C. CHILDREN'S NURSE a nurse concerned with the health and well-being of children and their families in the home and other settings outside of the hospital; C. DEVELOPMENT the process by which all members of a neighbourhood are encouraged to influence the decisions that affect their lives, through education concerning local issues; C. HEALTH the discipline concerned with preventing disease and prolonging life through organized effort to control communicable disease, provide services for early diagnosis and treatment of disease, and provide health maintenance education for individuals, families, and the community at large; C. HEALTH COUNCIL a group of local residents appointed to voice the patient's point of view in relation to district Health Service provision; C. MEDICINE the branch of medicine concerned with the health status of populations rather than individuals, and with conditions that affect health and the purity of food, milk, water, etc. C. MENTAL HEALTH TEAM a group of health-care professionals having the common aim of providing people having severe and enduring mental health problems with a single point of access to a range of specialist services; such groups consist of a consultant psychiatrist and junior medical staff, a specialist occupational therapist, community psychiatric nurses, social workers specializing in mental health, and psychologists; some may have a support worker; C. NURSES, nurses working with people and their families in their own homes. They may be health visitors, midwives, community learning disability nurses, children's nurses, district nurses, and community psychiatric nurses; C. PSYCHIATRIC NURSE, a qualified nurse, based outside a hospital, who has specialist training in mental health; he or she usually works as part of a community mental health team (*q.v.*) and may also work closely with doctors' surgeries, administering medication and providing advice and long-term support; such help is normally arranged through a doctor (GP), psychiatrist, or community mental health team.

compact (kom-pakt′,kom′-pakt): Dense or solid in structure. C. BONE the hard outer layer of bones, especially the long bones.

compact disk read-only memory: A storage devise for data that can be read by personal computers.

compartment (kom-part′-ment): 1. A small enclosure within a larger space, *e.g.*, the areas between the muscle groups in the leg. 2. One of the two main fluid-containing areas in the body: (a) the INTRACELLULAR C. the space occupied by the fluid within the cell membranes; makes up about 40% of total body weight; and (b) the EXTRACELLULAR C. the space occupied by the plasma and interstitial fluid; makes up about 30% of total body weight.

compartmental syndrome (com-part-men′-tal): A condition in which increased pressure within a compartment interferes with the circulation of blood to the contents of that space.

compatibility (kom-pat-i-bil′-i-ti): Suitability; congruity. The property of a substance that enables it to mix with another without ill effects, *e.g.*, two medicines, blood plasma and cells. See BLOOD GROUPS. — compatible, adj.

compensate (kom′-pen-sāt): To counterbalance a lack or defect in a bodily or physiological function.

compensation (kom-pen-sā′-shun): 1. A form of compromise. 2. A psychic mechanism employed by a person to cover up a weakness by exaggerating a more socially acceptable quality. 3. The state of counterbalancing or making up for a structural or functional defect or deficiency through overgrowth of another organ or increased function of unimpaired parts of the same organ. CARDIAC C. a condition in which adequate circulation is maintained in patients with cardiac disease.

competence (kom'-pe-tens): 1. The quality or state of being capable of an act. 2. The knowledge that enables a person to understand and speak about something. See APPENDIX 8; see also INCAPACITY.

competencies: Clusters of skills, abilities, and knowledge necessary for the performance of certain jobs. See APPENDICES 4 and 8.

complaint (kom-plānt'): A lay term used to describe a disease, ailment, or group of symptoms which cause the individual to seek medical advice.

complement (kom'-ple-ment): Any of a group of several factors normally present in plasma that are of importance in the mechanism of immunity. Thermolabile and non-specific, they are absorbed into antigen–antibody complexes and this leads to the completion of reactions such as bacteriolysis and the killing of bacteria. C. FIXATION TEST a test that measures the amount of complement fixed by any given antigen–antibody complex.

complemental (kom-ple-men'-tal): Complementary (q.v.). C. AIR, see AIR.

complementary (kom-ple-men'-ta-ri): Supplying a deficiency. C. MEDICINE a broad term covering a range of unorthodox therapies based on the holistic treatment of physical disorders; these treatments generally address the perceived causes of illness rather than the symptoms, and are also used for disease prevention; they are used as adjuncts to conventional medicine; the term embraces therapies such as acupuncture (q.v.), herbalism (q.v.), and homeopathy (q.v.); see C. THERAPIES; C. THERAPIES unorthodox techniques or approaches often used in addition to standard medical and nursing treatments; for example, acupuncture (q.v.), homeopathy (q.v.), aromatherapy (q.v.); see C. MEDICINE.

complete blood count: Includes, in addition to numerical and differential count of white blood cells, a count of red blood cells and estimates of platelets, haemoglobin and haematocrit.

complex (kom'-pleks): A Freudian term for a series of emotionally charged ideas, repressed because they conflict with ideas acceptable to the individual, but which significantly influence attitudes and behaviours. CAIN C. rivalry and destructive impulses between brothers; CASTRATION C. fear of loss or damage of one's sexual organs as punishment for forbidden sexual desires; ELECTRA C. a syndrome attributed to sup-

pressed sexual desire of a daughter for her father; also called *father* C.; INFERIORITY C. an abnormal feeling of being inferior which causes an individual to behave in an overly assertive, aggressive manner; may stem from organic inferiority, low social status, or from an emotional disturbance resulting from not being able to attain one's goals; INVERTED OEDIPUS C. refers to a girl who feels hopeful love for her mother and an ambivalent love–hatred for her father, with whom she identifies and who she copies in her personality, developing masculine behaviours, the result being that she may become homosexual; LEAR C. lustful desire of a father for his daughter; MOTHER C. OEDIPUS C.; OEDIPUS C. a syndrome attributed to suppressed sexual desire of a son for his mother; PERSECUTION C. paranoia (q.v.); SUPERIORITY C. (1) an exaggerated feeling of being superior; (2) intense striving for superiority as compensation for supposed inferiority.

complex needs: Multiple and complex presenting problems, where the demands of the case are not met or sustained by existing health or social services. Individuals may have challenging behaviours that place them at high risk to themselves, service staff and/or the community. There can be additional issues that increase their social isolation and lack of support.

complexity theory (kom-pleks'-i-ti): A hypothesis concerned with the behaviour over time of certain kinds of complicated systems. Under certain conditions, some things perform in regular, predictable ways; under other conditions they exhibit behaviour in which regularity and predictability are lost. Almost undetectable differences in initial conditions lead to gradually diverging system reactions and the eventual evolution of quite dissimilar behaviours.

compliance (kom-plī'-ans): 1. The quality or behaviour of yielding to pressure, suggestion, or force. 2. In physiology, an expression of the ability of an air- or fluid-filled organ such as the lung or bladder to yield to pressure or force. 3. In respiratory conditions, the elasticity of the lung or the ease with which it is inflated. 4. In healthcare, the extent to which a patient agrees with and carries out the prescribed activities of a therapeutic regimen in terms of agreeing with and accepting the specific requirements, taking the recommended medications, keeping appointments, and making changes in his lifestyle required by the regimen. See also NON-COMPLIANCE.

complication (kom-pli-kā'-shun): In medicine, a concurrent condition or disease, or an accident or second disease arising in the course of primary disease and adding to its severity.

compos mentis (kom'-pos men'-tis): A Latin term meaning 'of sound mind'.

compound (kom'-pownd): A substance composed of two or more elements, chemically combined in a definable proportion to form a new substance with new properties. C. FRACTURE see FRACTURE.

comprehension (kom-pre-hen'-shun): The act of grasping, with the mind, meaning and relationships or the knowledge that results from this action.

compress (kom'-pres): A pad or folded piece of cloth applied firmly to a part to cover a wound, exert pressure or control haemorrhage, or to relieve pain, swelling or inflammation. May be dry or wet, hot or cold.

compression (kom-presh'-un): 1. The state of being compressed. 2. The act of pressing or squeezing together. CEREBRAL C. arises from any space-occupying intracranial tumour, haemorrhage, or other lesion; C. BANDAGE see under BANDAGE; DIGITAL C. pressure applied by the fingers, usually to an artery to stop bleeding.

compromise (kom'-pro-mīz): A mental mechanism whereby a conflict (q.v.) is evaded by disguising the repressed wish to make it acceptable in consciousness.

compulsion (kom-pul'-shun): An irresistible, repetitive urge to engage in some act that the individual knows is irrational, or against his or her best judgement or his or her usual standards of behaviour. The term is also descriptive of thoughts, fears, and use of words over which the individual has no control.

compulsive (kom-pul'-siv): 1. Having the power of compulsion (q.v.). 2. Relating to acts performed under compulsion. C. PERSONALITY one characterized by an irresistible impulse to perform, under compulsion, acts that have to do with such qualities as orderliness or cleanliness.

compulsiveness (kom-pul'-siv-ness): An uncontrollable urge to perform certain physical actions or rituals; in psychiatry, considered a defence mechanism.

compulsory powers (kom-puls'-o-ri): The legal rights that empower the clinical supervisor to provide care and treatment for a person with a mental disorder in the absence of his or her consent.

compulsory treatment: The mandatory care given to mentally ill individuals who fail to comply with medical treatment, either in the community or in hospitals. The power to do this is being introduced under the proposed mental health legislation and review of the 1983 Mental Health Act.

computer-assisted learning: The use of computers to provide flexible approaches to learning and an aid to more traditional forms of learning.

computerized axial tomography: Painless diagnostic procedure for examining soft tissues; consists of a radiographic scan in which hundreds of x-ray pictures are taken as a camera revolves through 180°; the pictures are fed into a computer which integrates them and a cross-section picture is displayed on a computer screen. The procedure, called CAT scan, allows for visualization of grey matter, necrotic tissue, and tumours, is utilized in determining the location and size of brain tumour and such conditions as cancer of the pancreas, and in injuries of the liver, spleen, pancreas, or kidney.

computerized tomography: Computerized axial tomography (q.v.).

conarium (kō-na'-ri-um): The pineal gland.

conation (kō-nā'-shun): The act of willing, desiring, striving. The conscious tendency to action. One of the three aspects of mind, the others being cognition (awareness, understanding) and affection (feeling or emotion).

conative (kon'-a-tiv): Relates to (1) the act of making an effort or of striving; (2) the exertive power of the mind; the will power.

concave (kon'-kāv'): Having a somewhat depressed or hollowed surface like the inner surface of a bowl. Opp. to convex.

concavity (kon-kav'-i-ti): A hollowed-out space or depression on the surface of an organ or structure.

conceive (kon-sēv'): 1. To become pregnant. 2. To form a conception of.

concentrate (kon'-sen-trāt): 1. To bring together at a common point. 2. To increase the strength or bulk of a substance by condensing it. 3. A pharmaceutical preparation that has been strengthened by evaporation of some of its liquid content. — concentration, adj.

concentration (kon-sen-trā'-shun): 1. Close or fixed attention. 2. Strength or density. 3. The ratio of the solute to the volume of a solution.

concept (kon'-sept): C. ANALYSIS a statistical theory that identifies conceptual structures among data sets; its method of formal data analysis has been applied successfully to many fields, such as medicine and psychology.

1. Something conceived in the mind. **2.** An abstract or generic idea inferred from particular instances.

conception (kon-sep´-shun): **1.** The union of an ovum and a spermatozoon to begin a new life. **2.** The act of becoming pregnant. **3.** An abstract mental image or idea, or the act of forming such an image or idea.

conceptus (kon-sep´-tus): That which is conceived; a fetus; an embryo.

concha (kon´-ka): A shell or shell-like structure. AURICULAR C. the external ear; NASAL CONCHAE three long thin bony projections from the lateral walls of the nasal cavity; identified according to position as superior, medial, and inferior. — conchae, pl.

concomitant (kon-kom´-i-tant): Occurring at the same time or together.

concretion (kon-krē´-shun): A deposit of hard material in the tissues or in a natural cavity of the body; a calculus.

concurrent (kon-kur´-ent): Occurring at the same time or acting together. C. INFECTION two or more infections occurring in an individual at the same time; C. DISINFECTION the immediate disinfection of discharges from the body of an infected person or of materials that have been contaminated by such discharges or by the patient.

concussion (kon-kush´-un): A violent shaking or jarring of the body or a part of it as may result from a fall, a hard blow, or an explosion, or the condition resulting from such an action. BRAIN C. a morbid condition resulting from a violent impact to the head; characterized by partial or complete transient loss of consciousness, dizziness, pallor, coldness, visual disturbances, unequal pupils, and sometimes an increase in pulse rate and incontinence of urine and faeces; recovery is usually swift and complete except when injury is severe, or is repeated, as occurs in boxers, for example.

condensation (kon-den-sā´-shun): **1.** The process of becoming thicker, or more dense or compact. **2.** The process of changing a gas into a liquid or a liquid into a solid. **3.** A psychological process whereby two or more concepts or events are fused into a single symbol; often occurs in dreams.

condition: **1.** A state of being, as of health or disease. **2.** To produce, through training or repeated application, a particular response to a particular stimulus. — conditioned, adj.

conditioned: C. REFLEX see under REFLEX; C. RESPONSE a response aroused by some stimulus other than that which naturally produces it; c.

STIMULUS one to which a conditioned reflex has been developed.

conditioning: Term sometimes used synonymously with learning. Specifically, a process whereby a person learns to modify or adapt his behaviour when certain stimuli are applied. In group therapy, a technique used to help the patient learn to cope with discomfort and to carry on with his daily activities. NEGATIVE C. learning in which a neutral stimulus produces a desired response after repeated application of the stimulus, along with the stimulus that originally produced the desired response; OPERANT C., C. that is the result of rewarding (or not punishing) the individual who, having once responded to a stimulus in a desired manner, is likely to respond similarly to the same stimulus in the future.

condom (kon´-dom): A flexible rubber or plastic sheath worn over the penis as a contraceptive or as protection against sexually transmitted disease.

conduction (kon-duk´-shun): **1.** The transmission of heat, light, or sound waves through suitable media. **2.** The passage of electrical currents and nerve impulses through body tissues. C. SYSTEM in cardiology, consists of the S-A node, the A-V juntion, the bundle of His, right and left bundle branches, and the Purkinje fibres; it conducts impulses through the heart to produce the heartbeat; C. TEST an electrical test to determine whether a nerve is capable of transmitting nerve impulses; C. TIME the time it takes for a nerve to react to stimulation, measured by a recording device such as an electromyograph; C. VELOCITY the speed with which a nerve impulse is transmitted; expressed in metres per second.

conductive (kon-duk´tiv): Relating to conduction. C. HEARING LOSS a defect in the external or middle ear causing an impedance to sound-wave conduction, without loss of interpretation of sounds; various appliances that compensate for this loss are available.

conductivity (kon-duk-tiv´-i-ti): In physiology, the ability to transmit an impulse from one point to another in the body; said of nerves and the heart.

conductor (kon-duk´-tor): A substance or medium which transmits heat, light, sound, electric current, etc. POOR, GOOD, or NON-CONDUCTOR designate degrees of conductivity.

condylar (kon´-di-lar): Relating to a condyle.

condylarthrosis (kon´-di-lar-thrō´-sis): A joint in which an ovoid surface or condyle fits into an elliptical articular surface.

condyle (kon'-dīl,-dil): A rounded, knuckle-like projection at the articular end of a bone, such as occur on the humerus and tibia; they articulate with adjacent bones and provide anchorage for ligaments.

condylectomy (kon-di-lek-to-mi): Excision of a condyle.

condyloid (kon'-di-loyd): Resembling a condyle.

condyloma (kon-di-lō'-ma): Papilloma. C. ACUMINATUM a pointed dry wart found under the prepuce in the male and on the vulva and vestibule of the female, or on the skin of the perineal area; not necessarily venereal; C. LATUM a flat, highly contagious, moist, venereal wart with a greyish yellow discharge; found on the vulva, penis, anus, and axillae in late secondary syphilis. — condylomata, pl.; condylomatous, adj.

cone: A solid figure that has a circular base and tapers to a point. In anatomy, usually refers to one of the cone-like bodies found along with the rods of the layers of neurons in the retina; together the rods and cones are the receptors for light stimuli. C. BIOPSY see under BIOPSY.

confabulation (kon-fab-ū-lā'-shun): A symptom common in confusional states when there is impairment of memory for recent events. The gaps in the patient's memory are filled in with fabrication of his own invention. Occurs in senile and toxic confusional states, cerebral trauma and Korsakoff's syndrome (q.v.).

confidence interval (kon'-fi-dens): A statistical term referring to a range of values from a sample. The range has a specific probability of containing any value from the sample population. For the 95% confidence interval, the probability that the true population value will fall outside the range will be 5%.

confidential information: Privileged communication. A statement made to a doctor or certain other people in positions of trust which, by law, may not be revealed, even in court.

confidentiality (kon'-fi-den-shē-al'-i-ti): The ethical principle that a care giver may not disclose information to others about a patient without first gaining consent and that such information will be used only in connection with treatment or in the planning of healthcare.

confinement (kon-fin'-ment): 1. Restraint of an individual within a designated area. 2. The natural termination of pregnancy, with labour, and the delivery of an infant; lying-in.

conflict (kon'-flikt): A mental struggle caused by the simultaneous presence of two incompatible contrasting impulses, desires, or drives which are of equal or comparable intensity. The conflict is termed intrapsychic when it occurs between urges within the personality, and extrapsychic when it occurs between urges within the self and the environment. When the conflict becomes intolerable, one of the urges may be suppressed and result in some form of neurosis.

confluent (kon'-floo-ent): Becoming merged; flowing together. In medicine, a uniting as of neighbouring pustules, e.g., C. SMALLPOX a variety of which the pustules coalesced. Opp. to discrete. — confluence, n.

confounding variable (kon-fownd'-ing): A variable, other than those under investigation, which is not controlled for and which may distort the results of experimental research.

confusion (kon-fū'-shun): Term used to describe a mental state which is out of touch with reality and associated with clouding of consciousness and impairment of the patient's ability to think clearly, perceive, and respond decisively; often accompanied by disorientation as to time, place, and person. May be due to decreased cerebral blood flow, damage to brain tissue, or mental disturbance; may also be present following epileptic fits, and in cerebral arteriosclerosis, trauma, or severe toxaemia.

confusional state (kon-fu'-zhun-al): Mental confusion manifested in either chronic brain syndrome (q.v.) or as a symptom of some general disease; SYMPTOMATIC C.S temporary disruption of cerebral function, often reversible if the underlying disease is recognized and treated.

congenital (kon-jen'-it-al): Referring to mental or physical conditions that are present at birth; they are acquired during the development in the uterus and are to be differentiated from conditions that are hereditary (q.v.). C. ANOMALY an abnormality present at birth; C. DISLOCATION OF THE HIP an anomaly due to faulty formation of the acetabulum; C. HEART DISEASE developmental anomalies of the heart, resulting postnatally in imperfect oxygenation of the blood, manifested by cyanosis and breathlessness; later there is clubbing of the fingers. See CLUBBING, BLUE BABY; C. MEGACOLON Hirschsprung's disease (q.v.); C. SYPHILIS acquired by the fetus from the mother during intrauterine life.

congestion (kon-jes'-chun): Hyperaemia; abnormal accumulation of blood in a part or an organ. ACTIVE C. due to increased flow of blood to the part due to dilatation of the vessels;

HYPOSTATIC C. occurs in the lowest part of an organ or part; due to gravity and impaired circulation; PASSIVE C. results from slowing down of venous return, as in the lower limbs or the lungs. — congest, v.; congestive, adj.

congestive heart failure: Inability of the heart to maintain an adequate output of blood from one or both ventricles, resulting in manifest congestion and overdistension of certain veins and organs with blood, an inadequate blood supply to the body tissues, and excessive retention of water and salt; usually chronic. Clinical manifestations include arteriosclerotic or hypertensive heart disease, dyspnoea, nocturia, tachycardia, gallop rhythm, splenomegaly.

conglutinate (kon-gloo'-ti-nāt): To adhere or stick together as if by a glutinous substance. — conglutination, n.; conglutinant, adj.

conglutination (kon-gloo-ti-nā' shun): The abnormal joining together of two contiguous bodies or surfaces.

congruence (kon' groo-ens): 1. Agreement. 2. A coinciding, agreeing or being in harmony.

coniosis (kō-ni-ō' sis): A pulmonary disease caused by the inhalation of dust. See PNEUMONOCONIOSIS.

conization (kon-i-zā'-shun): Removal of a cone-shaped part of the cervix by the knife or cautery.

conjoint (kon-joynt'): 1. Joined together. 2. Relating to two things that are done together.

conjugal (kon'-jū-gal): Relating to marriage or to a husband and wife.

conjugate (kon'-jū-gāt): 1. Paired; working together. 2. OBSTETRIC C. the true conjugate diameter, an important diameter of the pelvis. See DIAMETER. C. OCULAR MOVEMENTS close coordination of eye movements to keep them both looking at the same object.

conjugation (kon-jū-ga'-shun): The joining together of two substances to form another substance. The joining together of two compounds, *e.g.*, a toxic substance and a substance from the body, to form a compound that the body can eliminate. — conjugated, adj.

conjunctiva (kon-jungk-tī'-va): The delicate transparent mucous membrane that lines the inner surface of the eyelids and reflects over the exposed anterior surface of the eyeball. BULBAR C. that which covers the anterior third of the eyeball; PALPEBRAL C. that which lines the eyelids.

conjunctival (kon-jungkt-tī'val): Relating to or affecting the conjunctiva. C. REFLEX see under REFLEX; C. SAC or CUL-DE-SAC the potential space, lined with conjunctiva, between the eyelids and the eyeball, particularly that between the lower lid and the eyeball.

conjunctivitis (kon-jungkt-ti-vī'-tis): Inflammation of the conjunctiva; may be bacterial, viral, or allergic in origin. CATARRHAL C. pinkeye; may be due to *Haemophilus* or staphylococcal organisms, or to pollutants in the atmosphere; marked by burning of the eyes, photophobia, and mucous or purulent discharge; FOLLICULAR C. dense infiltration of the connective tissue of the conjunctiva; due to irritation or virus; GONORRHOEAL C. an acute, severe form of c.; caused by the *Neisseria gonorrhoeae* organism; may progress to panophthalmitis; INCLUSION C., C. of the newborn; acquired during passage through the birth canal; caused by *Chlamydia trachomatis*; PURULENT C. characterized by discharge of pus; 'SWIMMING POOL' C,, C, often acquired in swimming pools; acute and purulent.

conjunctivoma (kon-junkt-ti-vō'-ma): A tumour involving the conjunctival tissue.

connective tissue: The binding and supportive tissues of the body, the principal varieties of which are (1) aerolar, (2) fibrous, and (3) elastic. Adipose and lymphoid tissue, bone, and cartilage belong to the same group of bodily structures.

Connexions (kon-nek'-shunz): An advice, guidance, and support service for all 13- to 19-year-olds in England. Connexions can help with information and advice on issues relating to health, housing, relationships with family and friends, career and learning options, money, and leisure activities. See www.connexions.gov.uk

consanguinity (kon-san-gwin'-i-ti): Blood relationship. — consanguineous, adj.

conscious (kon'-shus): 1. Being aware; capable of voluntary perception in response to stimuli and of having subjective experiences. 2.. Refers to all mental phenomena of which one is aware. 3. Being awake and in full possession of one's faculties.

consciousness (kon'-shus-ness): 1. Being conscious (*q.v.*). 2. Awareness of self and of one's environment at any given time, with each instance of awareness being experienced as a thought, perception, idea, sensation, or emotion. In psychoanalysis, that part of one's psychic or mental life of which one is aware and that is accessible to others through verbal report or by inference from one's behaviour. See also DROWSINESS, STUPOR, COMA.

consensual (kon-sen'sū-al): 1. Relating to involuntary movements that occur simultaneously with voluntary movements. 2. Relating to excitation that occurs involuntarily in response to stimulation of another part. 3. A similar reaction of both pupils to a stimulus applied to only one eye.

consent: The voluntary consent of a patient (or of someone authorized to give consent) that is required prior to any surgical, diagnostic, or special therapeutic procedure, except in emergency situations requiring immediate surgery to preserve life. INFORMED C. based on full disclosure of the whole truth before the patient submits to any surgery or invasive tests; the consent form states the diagnosis; treatment planned, drugs or procedures to be employed; prognosis; the risks involved; alternative therapies; and whether it is intended to conduct research or experimental studies on the patient. The form must be signed by the patient, unless he or she is mentally incompetent or a minor (when a surrogate assumes this responsibility), and must be witnessed. It is the responsibility of the doctor to obtain informed consent. The Gillik competence (officially known as the Fraser Guidelines) establishes the framework for assessing the competence of a child or adolescent to give informed consent to treatment.

conservatism (kon-serv'-a-tizm): 1. Conservative political principles and policies. 2. The principles and practice of Conservative politicians or supporters, for example, in the UK or Canada.

consolidation (kon-sol-i-dā'-shun): Becoming solid, as, for instance, the state of the lung due to exudation and organization in lobar pneumonia.

constipation (kon-sti-pā'-shun): An implied chronic condition of infrequent and often difficult evacuation of the faeces; may be due to lack of normal tone of the intestine, insufficient food or fluid intake, obstruction, the presence of tumour or diverticuli, or to habitual failure to empty the rectum. ACUTE C. signifies obstruction or paralysis of the gut; of sudden onset; HYPERTONIC C., C. in which there is increased contraction of the bowel but the stool is not evacuated and becomes hard and dry from reabsorption of water; HYPOTONIC C. due to lack of motility of the colon; the stool remains soft but becomes impacted in the rectum.

constitution (kon-sti-tū'-shun): 1. The general state of someone's health. 2. The system of fundamental laws and principles that prescribes the nature, functions, and limits of a

government or another institution. 3. The composition or structure of something; make-up.

constrict (kon-strikt'): To contract or draw together.

constriction (kon-strik'-shun): 1. A morbid sensation of being tightly squeezed or bound. 2. A narrowing or binding of a tissue or part as occurs in syndactyly (*q.v.*). 3. The narrowing of a blood vessel or of an opening such as the pupil.

constructivism: An approach in social science based on the assumption that human beings make their own social reality, and that the social world cannot exist independently of human beings. In research terms this means that both participants and researcher construct meaning together.

consultant nurse: A specialized health-care professional responsible for developing personal practice, being involved in research and evaluation, and contributing to education, training, and development of the multidisciplinary team. In the UK they are expected to spend a minimum of 50% of their time working directly with patients, ensuring ·that people using the NHS continue to benefit from the very best nursing and midwifery skills. See HIGHER-LEVEL PRACTICE; NURSE CONSULTANT.

consultation (kon-sul-tā'-shun): A discussion by two or more health professionals concerning the aspects of a condition in a particular patient.

consumer groups: Organizations that represent the interests of purchasers of goods and services by lobbying on behalf of their members, in consultative and advisory bodies at local, regional, or national level. *E.g.* Age Concern.

consumers: People who access services; also referred to as customers, clients, or patients. In healthcare there has been a shift from people being passive recipients to a more expectant and demanding group.

consumption (kon-sump'-shun): 1. The act of consuming or using up. 2. A wasting of body tissues; in this sense, the term was formerly much used for pulmonary tuberculosis (which 'consumed' the body). — consumptive, adj.

contact (kon'-takt): 1. A mutual touching or connection. 2. Direct or indirect exposure to infection. 3. A person who has been so exposed. C. DERMATITIS a type of eczema due to irritants, friction, sensitivity; C. LENS of glass or plastic, worn under the eyelids in direct contact with conjunctiva (in place of spectacles) for therapeutic or cosmetic purposes.

contagion (kon-tā'jun): **1.** Communication of disease from person to person. **2.** A contagious disease. **3.** The living organism by which a disease is transferred from person to person. — contagious, adj.; contagiousness, n.

contagious (kon-tā'-jus): **1.** Capable of transmission from one person to another, by direct or indirect contact. **2.** Highly communicable, referring to a disease that is easily transmitted from one person to another.

contagium (kon-tā'-ji-um): Any infective matter that may spread a disease.

contaminant (kon-tam'-i-nant): A substance or object that contaminates (*q.v.*).

contaminate (kon-tam'-i-nāt): **1.** To soil or infect with extraneous matter, particularly pathogenic bacteria. **2.** To render unfit for human use by pollution with unhealthful or disease-producing elements, *e.g.*, pollution of drinking water. — contamination, n.

content analysis: A systematic, replicable technique used in the qualitative analysis for compressing many words of text, transcripts, and images into fewer content categories, based on explicit rules of coding. It allows researchers to discover and describe data from an individual, group, or institution. It can be undertaken by hand, or using computer programs such as NVivo, ATLAS, or Ethnograph.

continence (kon'-ti-nens): **1.** Self-restraint; refusal to yield to an impulse or desire, *e.g.*, voluntary refrainment from sexual intercourse. **2.** The ability to retain a bodily discharge until the conditions are proper for evacuation, *e.g.*, urine or faeces.

continent (kon'-ti-nent): In medicine, the state of being able to control such normal bodily functions as defecation or urination until conditions are proper for carrying them out.

continuing care: A general term used to describe the care that people need over an extended period of time, as a result of accident, illness, or disability. It can cover physical and mental health needs. It may require health and social care input, and can be provided in hospital, nursing or residential homes, or in the individual's own home. See INTERMEDIATE CARE.

continuing education: For professional nurses, courses of instruction for practising nurses for the purpose of updating professional knowledge and skills, developing professionalism in nursing, and assisting nurses in advancing their careers. The Nursing and Midwifery Council (*q.v.*) in its code of professional conduct (2002) recognizes that registered nurses,

midwives, and health visitors are personally accountable for professional practice, and that in the exercise of professional accountability must maintain and improve professional knowledge and competence.

continuing professional development: A requirement for paid workers in a dynamic sector (e.g. healthcare) to keep up to date with changes and innovations within their line of work. See APPENDIX 8.

continuous: Extending without interruption or cessation. C. BATH, one in which the patient is kept immersed in water at 32° to 37°C; a therapeutic measure for quieting agitated psychiatric patients; C. POSITIVE AIRWAY PRESSURE a technique of respiratory assistance involving the use of a respirator when it is necessary to increase the functional capacity of the lung, expand atelectic areas within the lung, and to diminish the tendency of alveoli to collapse on expiration; especially useful in treating infants with hyaline membrane disease. Also called *positive pressure breathing*.

contraception (kon-tra-sep'-shun): The voluntary and artificial prevention of conception or impregnation.

contraceptive (kon-tra-sep'-tiv): An agent or device used to prevent conception, *e.g.*, condom, spermicidal vaginal cream, soft diaphragm to cover the mouth of the uterus, intrauterine contraceptive device, or pills that are taken orally. — contraception, n.

contract (kon-tract'): **1.** To draw together; shorten; decrease in size. **2.** To acquire by contagion or infection.

contract (kon'-trakt): **1.** An agreement, usually written, between two individuals with different interests and concerns, to describe their future actions; specifies conditions under which behaviour is to occur, and usually includes the consequences of not following the conditions as outlined. **2.** In clinical psychology, written CONTINGENCY. C.'s between therapist and patient are utilized as instruments for achieving certain agreed upon behaviours; the contingencies are specified, and the patient agrees to treatment which includes the behaviours agreed upon.

contractile (kon-trak'-til): Possessing the ability to shorten — usually occurs as a response to a stimulus; a particular characteristic of muscle tissue.

contraction (kon-trak'-shun): Shortening, especially applied to muscle fibres. ISOMETRIC C., c. of a muscle in which there is no change in its length because there is no movement of a joint; also called *static contraction*; ISOTONIC C., C. of a muscle that results in motion and, consequently, a change in its length.

contracture (kon-trak'-chur): Permanent shortening of a muscle, tendon, or scar tissue, or fibrosis of tissue supporting a joint, producing a deformity and limiting movement of the joint; may result from disuse or improper position. DUPUYTREN'S C. painless, chronic flexion of the fingers, especially the third and fourth, towards the palm; aetiology uncertain. [Guillaume Dupuytren, French surgeon, 1777–1835.] VOLKMANN'S C. a rapidly developing flexion deformity of the wrist and fingers, with loss of power, resulting from fixed contracture of the flexor muscles of the forearm. The cause is ischaemia of the muscles by injury or obstruction to the brachial artery near the elbow. Sometimes follows improper use of a tourniquet. [Richard von Volkmann, German surgeon, 1830–1889.]

contraindication (kon'-tra-in-di-kā'-shun): A sign, symptom, or condition suggesting that a certain line of treatment (usually used for that disease) should be discontinued or avoided.

contralateral (kon-tra-lat'-er-al): Relating to, located on, or occurring in or on the opposite side. — contralaterally, adv.

contrast medium: A substance that is radiopaque and which helps to outline an organ or space on x-ray films; may be swallowed, injected intravenously, or introduced by enema.

contrecoup (kon'-tre-koo): Injury or damage at a point opposite the impact, resulting from transmitted force. More likely to occur in an organ or part containing fluid, as the skull.

control: 1. To maintain influence over the conduct of a situation, function, or activity. **2.** A standard against which to measure an experiment or test.

control and restraint: 1. Techniques applied to control violent, aggressive, or abusive behaviour. The Nursing and Midwifery Council has produced guidance in therapeutic management of violence and aggressive behaviour. **2.** (prison) A series of physical locks and holds used to restrain and move a resisting prisoner in a controlled manner from one location to another.

control group: In research, the sample under observation that is not exposed to the independent variable (*q.v.*).

Control of Substances Hazardous to Health: A set of regulations (published in 1988, amended in 1998) covering the concept of risk assessment in the workplace. Health hazards are categorized and employers are obliged to assess substances against these criteria, and to have the systems in place to control these risks. This is an ongoing activity and accurate records must be maintained.

contusion (kon-tū'-shun): A bruise; slight bleeding into tissues while the skin remains unbroken. — contuse, v.

conus (kō'-nus): C. ARTERIOSUS the cone-shaped eminence of the right ventricle of the heart; the pulmonary artery trunk arises from it; C. MEDULLARIS the cone-shaped lower end of the spinal cord; also called *conus terminalis*.

convalescence (kon-va-les'-ens): The period of recovery following an illness, operation, or accident. — convalescent, adj. and n.

convalescent (kon-va-les'ent): Relating to convalescence. C. CARRIER a person who continues to carry the pathogenic organisms within his or her body during recovery from a disease; C. SERUM blood serum of a patient recently recovered from a specific disease, sometimes given by injection to another person to prevent the occurrence of the disease.

convection (kon-vek'-shun): Transfer of heat from the hotter to the colder part; the heated substance (air or fluid), being less dense, tends to rise. The colder portion, flowing in to be heated, rises in its turn, thus C. currents are set in motion.

converge (kon-verj'): To come to a point, as light rays do when passing through a lens. — convergence, n.; convergent, adj.

convergence (kon-ver'-jens): Moving together towards a common point, as occurs when the two eyes move in coordination towards fixation on the same point or object.

conversion (kon-ver'-zhun): **1.** Correction of the position of a fetus, or part of it, during labour. **2.** In psychiatry, a Freudian term for the defence mechanism whereby intrapsychic conflicts are expressed in a variety of sensory or motor symptoms such as pain, blindness, deafness, paralysis, or other loss of function. C. DISORDERS see HYSTERICAL NEUROSIS, CONVERSION TYPE, under NEUROSIS. C. APHONIA see under APHONIA.

convex (kon-veks'): Having an evenly rounded external surface that bulges outwards. Opp. to concave.

convoluted (kon'-vō-loo-ted): Folded, curved, contorted, twisted, or winding.

convolutions (kon-vō-loo'-shunz): Folds, twists, or coils as found in the intestine, renal tubules, and surface of brain. — convoluted, adj.

convulsant (kon-vul′-sant): An agent that causes convulsions.

convulsion (kon-vul′-shun): Violent, uncontrolled, involuntary contractions of groups of muscles, resulting from abnormal stimulation from many causes. Occurs with or without loss of consciousness. CLONIC C. alternating contraction and relaxation of muscle groups; FEBRILE C. usually a generalized C. occurring in children with fever; TONIC C. sustained muscular rigidity. Also called *fit, seizure.* — convulsive, adj.

convulsive (kon-vul′-siv): Related to, producing, or characterized by convulsions. C. DISORDER any condition characterized by convulsions, particularly the various types of epilepsy; C. THERAPY one of the physical methods of treatment for mental disorders, notably depressive states, mania, stupor; before introduction of electroshock therapy, drugs were widely used to produce the convulsions that are basic to this kind of therapy. Also known as *electroplexy, electrotherapy, electroconvulsive therapy.* See INSULIN THERAPY under THERAPY.

Cooley's anaemia: Thalassaemia (*q.v.*). [Thomas Benton Cooley, American paediatrician, 1871–1945.]

Coombs′ test: DIRECT C. TEST used in early diagnosis of erythroblastosis fetalis (*q.v.*) and in cross-matching blood for high-risk recipients. INDIRECT C. TEST used to detect various minor blood type factors, including the Rh factor.

cooperative care: A care programme in the USA in which a family member or close friend lives in the hospital with an adult patient, assists in routine duties and learns how to care for the patient at home. Parents stay with their children, thus reducing the child's fears and loneliness.

Cooper's ligaments: 1. A band of fascia attached to the iliopectineal spine and the pubic spine. **2.** A group of fibres that connect the olecranon with the coronoid process at the elbow joint. **3.** The suspensory ligaments of the breast.

coordination (kō-or′-di-nā′-shun): Moving or functioning in harmony. MUSCULAR C. the harmonious action of muscles, permitting free, smooth, and efficient movements under perfect control.

co-ossify (kō-os′-i-fi): To grow or become joined together by ossification (*q.v.*).

COPD: Abbreviation for chronic obstructive pulmonary disease, see CHRONIC OBSTRUCTIVE AIRWAYS DISEASE.

cope (kōp): The ability to deal with problems and stresses.

coping (kō′-ping): **1.** Behaviour that protects a person from feelings of anxiety; includes such unconscious mechanisms as denial, rationalization, repression, etc. **2.** The problem-solving efforts employed by an individual in making a choice among possible alternatives for adapting to a crisis event. C. STRATEGIES planned techniques whereby the individual under stress attempts to regain emotional equilibrium and freedom from the stress-inducing situation.

copiopia (kop′-i-o-pē′-a, ko′-pi): Eye strain; asthenopia (*q.v.*).

copious (kōp′-i-us): Profuse; abundant.

copr-, copra-, copro-: Combining forms denoting faeces, dung, filth.

copremesis (kop-rem′-e-sis): The vomiting of material containing faeces.

coprolith (kop′-rō-lith): A stony concretion or hard mass of faecal material in the intestine.

coprostasis (kop-ros′-ta-sis): Faecal impaction in the intestine. Also called *coprostasia.*

copulation (kop-ū-lā′-shun): Sexual intercourse.

cor (kor): The muscular organ that keeps the blood circulating in the body; the heart. C. PULMONALE chronic or acute right ventricular hypertrophy or acute strain of the right heart following disorders of the lungs; sometimes accompanied by heart failure; usually persistent. Signs and symptoms include oedema, liver congestion, hepatomegaly, ascites, high venous blood pressure, substernal pain, cough, dyspnoea, syncope on exertion; C. TRIATRIUM a congenital cardiac anomaly which may be of several types; most commonly, the heart has three instead of two atria.

coracoid (kor′-a-koid): **1.** Beak-shaped. **2.** Denoting a process of the upper part of the scapula.

cord: A long, rounded, flexible, thread-like structure. SPERMATIC C. that which suspends the testes in the scrotum; SPINAL C. a cord-like structure which lies in the spinal column, reaching from the foramen magnum to the first or second lumbar vertebra; consists of an inner core of grey matter surrounded by a layer of white matter that is composed mostly of myelinated nerve fibres. It is a direct continuation of the medulla oblongata and is about 45 cm long in the adult. UMBILICAL C. attaches the fetus to the placenta; gives passage to the umbilical vein and arteries; it is about 60 cm long and 1 cm in diameter; VOCAL C.'s membranous bands in the larynx, the vibrations of which are responsible for the production of voice.

cordate (kor′-dāt): Heart-shaped.

cordial (kord'-yal): **1.** An invigorating preparation used for its stimulating effect on the heart and circulation. **2.** An alcoholic preparation with a pleasant taste, used for its stimulating effect on the digestion.

corditis (kor-dī'-tis): Inflammation of the spermatic cord.

core: Central portion, often applied to the mass of necrotic material in the centre of a boil. C. TEMPERATURE, see BODY TEMPERATURE under TEMPERATURE.

corectasis (kō-rek'-ta-sis): Dilatation of the pupil; usually refers to dilatation caused by some pathological condition.

corediastasis (kō-rē-dī-as'-ta-sis): Dilatation of the pupil or a state of dilatation of the pupil of the eye.

Cori cycle: An energy cycle occurring in carbohydrate metabolism in which muscle glycogen is broken down in the peripheral tissues, producing lactic acid which is carried to the liver, where it is converted into liver glycogen. This is converted into glucose which is then carried to the muscles, where it is reconverted into muscle glycogen.

corium (kō'-ri-um): The internal layer of the skin lying immediately beneath the epidermis, composed of a dense bed of connective tissue with many blood vessels; also contains the hair follicles, the sweat glands and their ducts, and the sebaceous glands and their ducts, as well as smooth muscle tissue. Also called *the dermis, true skin, cutis vera.*

corn: A cone-shaped overgrowth and hardening of epidermis, with the point of the cone in the deeper layers, as on a toe; produced by friction or pressure. HARD C. usually occurs over a toe joint. SOFT C. occurs between the toes.

cornea (kor'-nē-a): The outwardly convex transparent membrane forming part of the anterior outer coat of the eye. It covers the iris and the pupil and admits light, occupies about one-sixth of the circumference of the eyeball, and merges backwards into the sclera. C. GUTTATA degeneration of the cornea; may progress to dystrophy of the epithelial cells; C. PLANA congenital flatness of the cornea.

corneal (kor'-nē-al): Relating to the cornea. C. GRAFT the replacement of opaque corneal tissue with healthy, transparent human cornea from a donor; C. REFLEX see under REFLEX; C. TRANSPLANT see KERATOPLASTY.

corneitis (kor-nē-ī'-tis): Inflammation of the cornea.

corneoplasty (kor'-nē-ō-plas-ti): Syn., *keratoplasty.* See CORNEAL GRAFT.

corneous (kor'-nē-us): Horny.

corneum (kor'-nē-um): The horny outer layer of the skin; the stratum corneum.

cornified (kor'-ni-fid): Relates to tissue that has been converted into a horny state. — cornification, n.

cornu (kor'-nū): Any horn-shaped structure. — cornua, pl.; cornual, cornuate, adj.

corona (ko-rō'-na): A crown. In anatomy, refers to a crown-like eminence or a surrounding structure. C. DENTIS the crown of a tooth. C. RADIATA (1) a mass of white nerve fibres that pass from the internal capsule to every part of the cerebral cortex; (2) a mass of granulosa cells derived from the Graafian follicles that surround the zona pellucida (*q.v.*); persists for some time after ovulation.

coronal (kor-ō'-nal): **1.** Relating to any crown-like structure. **2.** Relating to the crown of the head. C. SUTURE the jagged transverse line of union between the parietal and frontal bones of the cranium.

coronary (kor'-o-nar-i): Crown-like; encircling in the manner of a crown; said of a blood vessel or nerve that encircles a part or organ. C. ARTERIES the right and left arteries that supply blood to the heart itself; the first pair to be given off by the aorta as it leaves the left ventricle. Spasm or narrowing of these vessels produces angina pectoris; C. OCCLUSION stoppage of flow through the coronary arteries by an obstruction; C. SINUS the channel receiving most cardiac veins and opening into the right atrium; C. THROMBOSIS occlusion of a coronary vessel by a clot of blood.

coronary artery bypass: Open-heart surgery, done to improve circulation to the heart muscle. With the patient established on the heart–lung machine, one end of a section of healthy blood vessel (often taken from the saphenous vein of the leg) is affixed to a coronary artery and the other end to the ascending aorta, thus bypassing an obstructed or narrowed coronary artery. The graft may be 15 to 20 cm in length. Double, triple, or quadruple grafts are done to relieve blockage in several areas of the coronary arteries; these areas are predetermined by coronary arteriography before surgery. Bypassing is also sometimes done to relieve the pain of angina pectoris. See CORONARY ARTERY under CORONARY, ARTERIOGRAPHY, HEART–LUNG MACHINE, and BYPASS.

coronary artery disease: Any of the pathological conditions that affect the arteries of the heart, particularly those that lessen the flow of oxygen and other nutrients to the heart muscle.

Atherosclerosis is the most common cause of CAD, and angina is the most common symptom. Causes include cigarette smoking, hypertension, high blood cholesterol, fats, salt, and coffee, and deficiencies in certain vitamins.

coronary care unit: A specially equipped and staffed area in a hospital that provides concentrated, specialized care for the treatment of patients who have suffered a coronary (*q.v.*) thrombosis and for observation of those with signs and symptoms of impending heart attack.

coronary heart disease: A condition caused by a deficiency of oxygen in the myocardium; usually due to narrowing of the lumen of the coronary arteries and or the presence of coronary atheromas; may be temporary or permanent; the outstanding symptom is pain; may be associated with coronary thrombosis and myocardial infarction, and may result in sudden death. Also called *ischaemic heart disease*.

coronavirus (kō-rō-na-vī'-rus): One of a large group of viruses that are capable of causing acute disease of the upper respiratory tract. So called because when viewed with the electron microscope, the virion appears to be surrounded by a crown with projections that are bulbous at the tip. Also written *corona virus*.

coroner (kor'-o-ner): A public official, often a solicitor, barrister or a physician, whose main duty is to investigate any death not obviously due to natural causes. The coroner must be notified if a patient dies within 24 hours of being admitted to hospital. All anaesthetic/theatre deaths must also be reported.

corotomy (kō-rot'-o-mi): Iridotomy (*q.v.*).

corporeal (kor-po-rē'-al): Relating to the physical, material body; not spiritual.

corpse (korps): A dead body. Cadaver.

corpulence (kor'-pū-lens): Obesity; fatness. — corpulent, n. Also called *corpulency*.

corpus (kor'-pus): 1. A discrete mass of material, *e.g.*, specialized tissue. 2. The body of an animal or human, especially a dead body. 3. The main part of an organ or structure. C. ALBICANS the degenerated corpus luteum which atrophies and remains on the surface of the ovary as a white scar; C. CALLOSUM a band of white nerve fibres passing beneath the longitudinal fissure and connecting the two cerebral hemispheres; C. CAVERNOSUM two cylinders of erectile tissue that make up the greater part of the penis; C. LUTEUM the yellow, progesterone-secreting body formed in the ovary after rupture of a Graafian follicle; if pregnancy supervenes, it persists and enlarges; FALSE C.L. is formed in the non-pregnant state and

persists for approximately one month, when it is reabsorbed, TRUE C.L. occurs in pregnancy, persists for six months, and has almost disappeared by the end of the 9th month; C. SPONGIOSUM PENIS the cylinder of the erectile tissue surrounding the penile urethra; C. STRIATIUM a stalk-like arrangement of grey and white matter at the base of the brain, thought to have a steadying effect on voluntary movement, but no power of initiation of same. — corpora, pl.

corpuscle (kor'-pus'l): A microscopic mass of protoplasm. There are many named varieties but the term generally refers to the red and white blood cells. See ERYTHROCYTE and LEUKOCYTE. — corpuscular, adj.

corrective (ko-rek'-tiv): 1. Changes, counteracts or modifies something harmful. 2. A drug that modifies the action of another drug.

corrosion (ko-rō'-shun): The slow wearing away or destruction of a part or tissue.

corrosive (ko-rō'-siv): 1. A caustic; a substance that weakens or destroys the surface or substance of a tissue or other material. 2. Having the power to weaken or destroy the surface or substance of tissue or other material.

corset (kor'-set): An orthopaedic appliance that encircles the trunk or part of it, or a part of a limb. MILWAUKEE C. see MILWAUKEE BRACE.

cortex (kor'-teks): 1. The outer bark or covering of a plant. 2. The outer layer of an organ beneath its capsule or membrane. ADRENAL C. the thick outer portion of the adrenal gland which encloses the medulla of the gland; CEREBELLAR C. the superficial layer of grey matter covering the cerebellum; CEREBRAL C. the thin layer of convoluted grey matter on the surface of the cerebral hemispheres; it controls most of the complex sensory-motor reactions and is the seat of memory, thought, and language; RENAL C. the smooth-textured outer layer of the kidney; it extends in columns between the pyramids of the medulla; is composed chiefly of glomeruli and secretory cells. — cortices, pl.; cortical, adj.

Corti: ORGAN OF C. the elongated spiral structure lying on the basilar membrane of the cochlea and containing the hair cells where the fibres of the auditory nerve begin; the actual receptor for hearing. [Alfonso Corti, Italian anatomist, 1822–1888.]

cortical (kor'-ti-kal): Relating to or referring to a cortex.

corticifugal (kor-ti-sif'-ū-gal): Moving or conducting away from the cortex; said particularly of nerve fibres. Also called *corticofugal*.

corticoafferent (kor′ -ti-kō-af′ -er-rent): Relating to nerves that carry impulses towards the cerebral cortex.

corticoefferent (kor-ti-kō-ef′ -er-rent): Relating to nerves that carry impulses away from the cerebral cortex.

corticoid (kor′ -ti-koyd): A name for the several groups of steroid substances produced by the adrenal cortex and for synthetic compounds with similar actions. Examples of the three main groups are: hydrocortisone, cortisone, prednisolone and prednisone in the first; deoxycorticosterone acetate (DOCA) in the second; and the sex hormones in the third.

corticospinal (kor′ -ti-kō-spī′ -nal): Relating to the cortex of the brain and the spinal cord. C. TRACTS tracts of motor nerve fibres that descend from the cerebral cortex, pons, and medulla where they cross to form lateral and anterior tracts of fibres that descend the spinal cord; they are concerned with fine motor movements.

corticosteroid (kor′ -ti-kō-stē′ -royd): Any of the hormones produced by the adrenal cortex, or any synthetic substitute.

corticosterone (kor-ti-kos′ -ter-ōn): A secretion of the adrenal cortex; influences the metabolism of carbohydrates, potassiums and sodium.

corticotrophin (kor′ -ti-kō-trō′ -pin): The hormone of the anterior pituitary gland which specifically stimulates the adrenal cortex to produce steroid hormones. Available commercially as a purified extract of animal anterior pituitary glands (ACTH); only active by injection. Also called *corticotrophin*.

corticotrophin releasing factor: A factor produced in the hypothalamus which stimulates the release of corticotrophin by the anterior pituitary gland.

cortisol (kor′ -ti-sōl): A glucocorticoid (*q.v.*); steroid hormone secreted by the adrenal cortex. Hydrocortisone (*q.v.*). Also called *17-hydrocorticosterone*.

cortisone (kor′ -ti-sōn): A hormone produced in the adrenal cortex; also produced synthetically; important in carbohydrate metabolism and in body response to stress; converted into cortisol before use by the body. An excess of C. occurs in Cushing's syndrome (*q.v.*). It has powerful anti-inflammatory properties, and is used in ophthalmic conditions, rheumatoid arthritis, pemphigus and Addison's disease. Side-effects, such as salt and water retention, may limit its therapeutic use.

coruscation (kor-us-kā′ -shun): The subjective sensation of light flashes before the eyes.

Corynebacterium (kō-rī-nē-bak-tē′ -ri-um): A bacterial genus: Gram-positive, rod-shaped bacteria, averaging 3 microns in length, showing irregular staining in segments (metachromatic granules). Many strains are parasitic; some are pathogenic, *e.g.*, C. *diphtheriae*, which produces a powerful exotoxin and is the cause of diphtheria. C. *VAGINALIS*, see GARDNERELLA VAGINITIS under *GARDNERELLA*.

coryza (kō-rī′ -za): An acute upper respiratory infection of short duration, usually due to a filterable virus; highly contagious; attacks produce only temporary immunity. Also called *acute rhinitis*.

COSHH: Abbreviation for Control of Substances Hazardous to Health (*q.v.*).

cosmetic (koz-met′ -ik): 1. Relating to that which is done to improve the appearance, *e.g.*, C. surgery. 2. A preparation used to improve the appearance.

cost-, costi-, costo-: Combining forms denoting rib(s).

costa (kos′ -ta): A rib. — costae, pl.; costal, adj.

costal (kos′ -tal): Of or relating to a rib or ribs. C. ANGLE the angle formed by the right and left costal cartilages at the xiphoid process; C. BREATHING breathing that involves primarily the chest structures; occurs in patients with gastric or abdominal pain or distension, and in paralytics. See also COSTAL CARTILAGE and under CARTILAGE

cost–benefit analysis: A method of gauging the expense of the provision of health intervention versus the returns in terms of money.

costectomy (kos-tek′ -to-mi): Surgical removal of one or more ribs or part of one or more ribs.

cost effective: Refers to the least costly plan for meeting specific objectives, or to a service that is less costly than one to which it is being compared; often a factor when considering health services.

cost effectiveness: A measure of how well an intervention performs under cost–benefit analysis (*q.v.*).

costicartilage (kos-ti-kar′ -ti-lij): The cartilage of a rib.

costochondritis (kos′ -tō-kon-drī′ -tis): Inflammation of a costal cartilage; characterized by anterior chest wall pain, swelling, redness, tenderness to touch. See also TIETZE'S SYNDROME.

costosternal syndrome (kos-tō-ster′ -nal): A condition in which the patient experiences intermittent pain in the entire anterior chest wall that is intensified by deep inspiration; may last for months.

costotomy (kos-tot'-o-mi): Excision of all or part of a rib.

cot: C. DEATH sudden infant death syndrome (*q.v.*); FINGER C. a rubber or plastic covering for the finger; used when examining a body passage as the rectum or vagina, or as a protective covering over a bandage. Also called *finger stall*.

cotyledon (kot-i-lē' don): One of the subdivisions of the uterine surface of the placenta.

cotyloid (kot'-i-loid): Cup-shaped; pertaining to the acetabular cavity.

cough (kawf): **1.** A sudden forcible noisy expulsion of air from the lungs in an effort to expel mucus or other extraneous matter from the air passages; may be productive or unproductive. **2.** A chronic or transient condition characterized by frequent coughing due to irritation of the respiratory mucosa. **3.** To expel air forcefully after a deep inspiration and closure of the glottis. C. REFLEX an involuntary protective nervous response to irritation of the mucosa of the larynx, trachea, or bronchi, which causes coughing; C. SYNCOPE fainting following a severe coughing spell; WHOOPING C. see PERTUSSIS.

Council for Health Regulators: An emerging council that will have responsibility for the regulation of a wide range of health-care professions. It is being introduced as part of the regulatory restructuring of the health-care professions central to the modernization of the health service. The new regulatory body will be accountable, open and transparent, responsive to change, with consistency of approach and integration and co-ordination between the regulatory bodies. See NHS PLAN: www.doh. gov.uk/hrinthenhsplan/

Council for the Regulation of Health-care Professionals: An organization working in conjunction with regulatory bodies, such as the Nursing and Midwifery Council (*q.v.*) and the General Medical Council (*q.v.*), to build and manage a strong system of self-regulation that puts patients' interests first.

counselling (kown'-sel-ing): A process of consultation and discussion between two individuals, one of whom (the counsellor) offers advice or guidance to the other (the client), helping to identify and clarify problems while providing support as the client makes adjustments to overcome or come to terms with them. PASTORAL C. a form of counselling undertaken by ministers and priests.

Counselling, Assessment, Referral, Advice and Throughcare Scheme: A service for prisoners with drug and alcohol problems.

counteraction (kown-ter-ak'-shun): The action of a drug or other therapeutic agent which opposes that of some other drug or agent.

counterconditioning (kown'-ter-kon-dish'-un-ing): The application of a stimulus which ordinarily produces a certain emotional response, simultaneously with another stimulus that produces an opposite response, with the purpose of changing the affective value of the first stimulus.

counterextension (kown'-ter-eks-ten'-shun): Traction upon the proximal extremity of a fractured limb, opposing the pull of the extension apparatus on the distal extremity.

counterphobia (kown'-ter-fō'-bi-a): A reaction in which the individual attempts to overcome a fear by seeking out situations that are consciously feared.

countershock (kown'-ter-shok): Usually refers to an electric shock given via two electrodes placed on the chest to convert atrial or ventricular fibrillation to normal rhythm.

counterstain (kown'-ter-stān): A second stain of a different colour applied to a smear to make the organisms that are to be viewed microscopically more distinct.

countertraction (kown-ter-trak'-shun): In orthopaedics, a traction that affects another type of traction; sometimes used in reducing fractures.

countertransference (kown'-ter-trans-fer'-ens): **1.** The psychiatrist's conscious or unconscious emotional reactions to the patient; see TRANSFERENCE. **2.** An emotional response of the nurse to the patient that is inappropriate to the therapeutic relationship.

coup (koo): Stroke. COUP DE SOLEIL sunstroke.

coup–contrecoup injury (koo-kon'-tre-koo): Injury, usually to the brain, beneath the point of impact and more extensive injury to the opposite side of the brain.

coupling (kup'-ling): In cardiology, a term used to describe a pulse in which two beats occur in rapid succession followed by a slight pause; often a sign of digitalis poisoning.

couvade syndrome (koo'-vād): The psychophysiological response of a pregnant woman's husband who experiences the same symptoms as his wife, including nausea, vomiting, abdominal pains.

Couvelaire uterus: (koo-ve-lair'): See under UTERUS.

coverglass (kuv'-er-glas): A small piece of special optical glass that is placed over a specimen on a slide for microscopic study.

covert video surveillance: The use of hidden cameras, usually to prevent theft or other illegal activities occurring on the premises. It has been used in the diagnosis of Münchausen syndrome by proxy (*q.v*).

Cowling's rule: A rule for determining the correct dosage of medicines for children:

$$\frac{\text{age in years at nearest birthday}}{24} \times \text{adult dose} = \text{child's dose}$$

Cowper's glands (kow'-perz): Bulbourethral glands. Two in number, lying lateral to the membranous urethra, below the prostate gland, and deep to the perineal membrane. They open via short ducts into the anterior (penile) urethra. [William Cowper, English surgeon, 1666–1709.]

cowpox (kow'-poks): Vacccinia. Viral disease in cows. Lymph from infected animals was used in vaccination of humans against smallpox (variola).

coxsackievirus (kok-sak'-e-vī-'-rus): One of a large group of enteroviruses that produce symptoms resembling those of poliomyelitis but without the paralysis; associated with cardiac conditions, pneumonia, hepatitis, acute haemorrhagic conjunctivitis, aseptic meningitis, encephalitis, and an influenza-like fever. First isolated in Coxsackie, New York. Also written *Coxsackie virus*.

CPA: Abbreviation for Care Programme Approach (q.v.).

CPAP: Abbreviation for continuous positive airway pressure, see under CONTINUOUS.

CPD: Abbreviation for continuing professional development (*q.v*).

CPK: Abbreviation for creatinine phosphokinase, see under CREATININE.

CPN: Abbreviation for community psychiatric nurse, see under COMMUNITY.

CPPIH: Abbreviation for Commission for Patient and Public Involvement in Health (*q.v*).

CPR: Abbreviation for cardiopulmonary resuscitation, see RESUSCITATION.

CPU: Abbreviation for central processing unit (*q.v*.)

crab louse (krab lows): *Phthirus pubis* (*q.v*.).

'crack': A highly concentrated, highly addictive, chemically reconstituted, and relatively inexpensive preparation of cocaine that is sold in the form of small rocks or pebbles and is smoked rather than snorted. Produces more intense 'highs' and 'lows' than the powdered form of cocaine and leads more quickly to addiction. Also known as *rock*.

crackling (krak'-ling): Fine, moist crepitant-like sound heard on auscultation of the lungs; lower in pitch than crepitant sounds;

also called subcrepitant sounds. See CREPITUS.

cradle: A frame, usually of wood or wire, used to keep the bed clothes from contact with an injured or fractured limb; also used when dry heat is being applied to an extremity. C. CAP an accumulation of greyish-yellow crust-like material on the crown of the scalp of an infant with eczema.

cramp: Spasmodic, involuntary, painful contraction of a muscle or group of muscles. Occurs in tetany, food poisoning, and cholera. In gynaecology, a colloquial term for dysmenorrhoea. HEAT C. muscular spasm attended by weak pulse, dilated pupils and prostration, seen in those who work in intense heat and who lose much salt and water through perspiration, *e.g*., stokers, miners; MUSCLE C. sudden painful involuntary contraction of a skeletal muscle; WRITERS' C. an occupational disease characterized by spasmodic contraction of muscles of fingers, hand and forearm; a similar condition occurs in others whose occupations involve use of fine muscles.

cranial (krā'-ni-al): Relating to the cranium (*q.v*.). C. CAVITY the cavity of the skull which contains the brain; C. DECOMPRESSION reduction of excessive pressure on the brain by means of surgery; C. FOSSA any one of the three shallow depressions on the upper surface of the base of the skull; C. NERVE any one of the twelve pairs of nerves given off by the brain rather than the spinal cord; they are named and numbered in the following order: 1, olfactory; 2, optic; 3, oculomotor; 4, trochlear; 5, trigeminal; 6, abducens; 7, facial; 8, acoustic; 9, glossopharyngeal; 10, vagus; 11, accessory; 12, hypoglossal.

craniectomy (krā-ni-ek'-to-mi): Surgical removal of a portion of skull.

craniocele (krā'-ni-ō-sēl): Protrusion of part of the cranial contents through a defect in the bones of the cranium.

craniomalacia (krā'-ni-ō-ma-lā'-shi-a): Abnormal softness of the skull bones.

craniomegaly (krā-ni-ō-meg'-a-li): Enlargement of the head.

craniopharyngioma (krā'-ni-ō-fa-rin-jē-ō'-ma): A solid or cystic benign congenital brain tumour in the area of the pituitary; associated with intracranial pressure on the hypothalamus and optic chiasm; causes visual impairment and hormone disturbances; seen in children and young adults.

cranioplasty (krā'-ni-ō-plas-ti): Surgical repair of a skull defect. — cranioplastic, adj.

craniostenosis (krā'-ni-ō-ste-nō'-sis): Premature fusion of the cranial sutures with consequent cessation of growth, resulting in deformity and a small skull.

craniosynostosis (krā'-ni-ō-sin-os-tō'-sis): Premature closure of the cranial sutures before or shortly after birth; due to hypercalcaemia; the resulting abnormal shape of the head depends on the sutures involved. Brain growth is restricted and learning disability often follows. Also called *craniostosis*.

craniotabes (krā'-ni-ō-tā'-bēz): A softening and wasting of the cranial bones, and widening of the sutures and fontanels (*q.v.*) occurring in infancy, due to lack of normal mineralization of the bones. — craniotabetic, adj.

craniotomy (krā-ni-ot'-o-mi): A surgical opening of the skull in order to remove a growth, relieve pressure, evacuate a blood clot, arrest haemorrhage, or to reduce the size of the head of an unborn dead infant to facilitate its delivery.

cranium (krā'-ni-um): The part of the skull enclosing the brain. It is composed of eight bones: the occipital, two parietals, frontal, two temporals, sphenoid and ethmoid. — cranial, adj.

crash team: An organized team in a hospital trained to be available in any emergency; includes nurses, physicians, anaesthetists. A crash trolley is kept ready for their use; it is equipped with drugs and equipment needed to handle emergency situations in patients with cardiac, respiratory, circulatory, or central nervous system conditions.

crash trolley: An emergency trolley containing supplies, equipment, instruments and drugs needed for cardiopulmonary resuscitation or other life-saving procedures. Items that have been used are immediately replaced and the trolley is returned to a designated location where it is readily available.

-crasia: A combining form denoting combination, mixing, constitution.

craving (krā'-ving): A persistent hunger or need for a drug or other substance; may be the result of either physical or psychological factors.

C-reactive protein: A globulin found in the serum of persons with inflammation or necrosis; tests for the presence of this protein are used in diagnosing rheumatic fever.

creatinaemia (krē-a-ti-ne'-mi-a): The presence of an excess of creatine in the blood.

creatinase (krē-at'-i-nās): An enzyme that acts as a catalyst in the decomposition of creatine.

creatine (krē'-a-tin): In biochemistry, a crystalline substance synthesized in the body; found chiefly in vertebrate muscle tissue; combines with phosphate to form phosphocreatine, a source of quickly available energy for the muscles; is increased in pregnancy and decreased in hypothyroidism. C. CLEARANCE TEST a test for renal function; C. KINASE an enzyme found in cardiac and skeletal muscle; is active in the conversion of phosphocreatine and adenosine diphosphate to creatinine and adenosine triphosphate; used in several diagnostic tests including those for muscle disorders; C. PHOSPHOKINASE C. kinase.

creatinine (krē-at'-i-nin): A waste substance that is an end product of protein metabolism and is found in muscle, blood, and urine; it is liberated from muscle and secreted in the urine at a constant rate. C. CLEARANCE TEST a test for measuring glomerular filtration, a major function of the kidney that decreases in renal disease; C. PHOSPHOKINASE an enzyme found in cardiac muscle, skeletal muscle, and brain tissue; helps control the amount of energy available for use in the body; is elevated in disorders involving cardiac muscle, cardiac surgery, and cardiac defibrillation.

creatinuria (krē-a-ti-nū'-ri-a): Increased or abnormal amounts of creatinine in the urine. Occurs in metabolic disorders and conditions in which muscle is rapidly broken down, *e.g.*, acute fevers, starvation. — creatinuric, adj.

Credé's method (krē-dāz'): 1. A method of delivering the placenta by gently rubbing the fundus of the uterus until it contracts, and then by squeezing the fundus, expressing the placenta into the vagina whence it is expelled. 2. Periodically pressing on the urinary bladder to expel urine; also called *Credé's manoeuvre*. [Karl Sigmund Franz Credé, German obstetrician, 1819–1892.]

Credit Accumulation Transfer System: A points system recognized by all UK higher education institutions as a method of quantifying credit for a particular course. To attain an undergraduate degree you would need to accumulate 120 points at level 1, 120 points at level 2, and 120 points at level 3. Abbreviated CATS.

cremation (krē-mā'-shun): The burning or incineration of the body of a deceased person.

crenate (krē'-nāt): Scalloped, indented or notched. In physiology, descriptive of the indented edges of red blood cells that have shrunken from exposure to air or to a hypertonic solution. Also called *crenated*. — crenation, n.

crepitation (krep-i-tā'-shun): 1. Grating of bone ends in fracture. Also crepitus. 2. Crackling sound heard via stethoscope in lung infections.

3. Crackling sound elicited by pressure on emphysematous tissue.

crepitus (krep'-i-tus): 1. A dry, crackling sound such as might be produced by the grating ends of a broken bone, or as heard by stethoscope in some pneumonias. 2. The noisy discharge of flatus from the bowel.

cresol (krē'-sol): Colourless to brownish aromatic liquid obtained from wood tar; disinfectant. *Lysol* is a proprietary name for a compound solution of C.

crest: A projection or ridge, especially at the border of a bone.

cretinism (kre-'-tin-ism): A condition originating in fetal life or early infancy; due to congenital thyroid deficiency; characterized by stunted mental and physical development, dwarfism, large head, thick legs, pug nose, dry skin, scanty hair, swollen eyelids, short neck, protruding abdomen, clumsy uncoordinated gait. — cretinistic, cretinoid, cretinous, adj.

Creutzfeldt–Jakob disease (kroyts'-feld-yak' 'ob): Three forms occur: sporadic cases, which have an unknown cause; familial cases associated with a gene mutation; and iatrogenic cases resulting from the accidental transmission of the causative agent via contaminated surgical equipment or as a result of cornea or dura mater transplants or the administration of human-derived pituitary growth hormones. See VARIANT CREUTZFELDT–JAKOB DISEASE.

cribriform (krib'-ri-form): Perforated, like a sieve. C. PLATE that portion of ethmoid bone that forms the roof of the nasal cavity; has many perforations for the passage of fibres of the olfactory nerve.

cricoid (krī'-koyd): Ring-shaped. Applied to the cartilage forming the inferior posterior part of the larynx.

cricothyroid membrane or ligament (krī-kō-thī'-royd): A sheet of fibroelastic connective tissue which is attached at its lower edge to the cricoid cartilage, at its upper edge to the thyroid cartilage, with the lateral parts of its upper margin forming the vocal ligaments.

cricothyrotomy (krī'-kō-thī-rot'-o-mi): An incision through the skin and the cricoid and thyroid cartilages, required in some instances to create and maintain a patent airway; may be preliminary to emergency tracheostomy.

cricotracheotomy (krī'-kō-tra-kē-ot'-mi): The procedure of making an incision into the trachea through the cricoid cartilage.

cri-du-chat (krē-du-shah'): A syndrome consisting of a group of congenital anomalies including brachycephaly, low forehead, wide-spaced eyes, strabismus, micrognathia, and mental handicap characterized by a catlike cry in infants.

Criminal Records Bureau: A body set up to improve and widen access to police checks on people intending to work with children or vulnerable people.

-crine: A suffix denoting secretion, or secreting.

crisis (krī'-sis): 1. The turning point or an abrupt change in the course of a disease, as the point of defervescence in fever. 2. Muscular spasm in tabes dorsalis referred to as visceral crisis (gastric, vesical, rectal, etc.). 3. A period of stress or an episode that interferes with normal functioning activities. ADDISONIAN C. a sudden onset or worsening of the signs and symptoms of Addison's disease; ANAPLASTIC C. a transient condition caused by disappearance of red blood cells from the bone marrow; may develop during serious infections or in certain haemolytic disorders; ASTHMATIC C. status asthmaticus; see under STATUS; CHOLINERGIC C. respiratory failure resulting from overtreatment with anticholinesterase drugs; DIETL'S C. a complication of ptosis of the kidney; the chief symptom is severe sudden pain in the kidney that may follow the intake of large amounts of water but is usually due to kinking of the ureter; other symptoms are nausea, vomiting, hypotension, tachycardia, scanty blood-stained urine; possibly collapse; MATURATIONAL C. one that occurs during life periods marked by social, physical, or psychological change; MYASTHENIC C. sudden deterioration with weakness of respiratory muscles due to an increase of myasthenia; OCULOGYRIC C. see OCULOGYRIC; SITUATIONAL C. one that arises as a result of a stressful event; THYROTOXIC C. sudden return of symptoms of thyrotoxicosis, due to a shock, injury, or thyroidectomy.

crisis intervention: A term used to describe a brief type of treatment in which a psychotherapist or a team intervenes in a situation in order to assist the family and the patient to secure help in solving an immediate problem; may include medications, referral to a community agency, changing the patient's environment, etc.

criteria (krī-tēr'-i-a): Standards on which a judgment or decision may be based. — criterion, sing.

critical (krit'-i-kal): 1. Arising from or characterized by crisis. 2. Implying serious risk or uncertainty as to outcome. 3. Crucial.

critical care unit: A special unit in a hospital where patients with critical disorders or diseases of the vital physiological systems (cardiovascular, respiratory, renal, electrolytic, neurological) are provided with the care required to sustain life. May be combined with an intensive care unit (*q.v.*).

critical incident: A compressed case study that poses a problem but offers no preferred solution; usually where an event has the potential to lead to an undesirable outcome. Often used in clinical supervision. See CRITICAL INCIDENT TECHNIQUE; CLINICAL SUPERVISION.

critical incident technique: A technique that involves the collection of detailed reports of incidents in which an individual did something that was especially effective or especially ineffective in achieving the purpose of an activity. The incidents must be collected from individuals who personally observed the actions of the individual. These incidents are used to discern whether the outcome of the action was beneficial or otherwise, and whether it was the individual's action, rather than other factors, that was in fact critical to the outcome. See CRITICAL INCIDENT; CLINICAL SUPERVISION.

critical reflection: The process of reflecting back on prior learning to determine whether what we have learned is justified under present circumstances; seen as a major objective of higher education. To engage in critical reflection requires moving beyond the acquisition of new knowledge and understanding, into questioning of existing assumptions, values, and perspectives.

critical theory: The view that people can critically evaluate social phenomena and change society.

critical thinking: A sociological theory that aims to dig beneath the surface of social life and uncover the assumptions that keep us from a full understanding of how the world works.

Crohn's disease: Regional ileitis; a chronic intestinal disorder in which segments of the intestine become inflamed and swollen; cause unknown. May be acute or chronic; onset usually before age 35; symptoms include nausea, vomiting, diarrhoea, abdominal pain, fever, weight loss, malaise. Chief complications are perforation and haemorrhage. Also called *regional colitis, regional enteritis, granulomatous colitis*. [Burrill N. Crohn, American gastroenterologist, 1884–1983.]

cross-contamination: The introduction of infectious material from one source to another.

cross-dependence: A condition in which one drug can prevent withdrawal symptoms in an addict who is withdrawing from use of another drug.

crossed: C. EXTENSOR RESPONSE a normal response in the newborn; when the infant is in the supine position and the sole of one foot is stroked, it responds by flexing the other leg and then adducting and extending it to try to push the stimulus away; C. LATERALITY a combination of right-handedness and left-eyedness or vice versa.

cross-eyed: Convergent strabismus. A squint in which one or both eyes turn inward towards the nose. Esotropia. — cross-eyed, adj.

crossmatching: A procedure for determining the compatibility of bloods before transfusion. See BLOOD GROUPS, BLOOD CROSSMATCHING.

cross-section: A cut or slice made through an object at right angles to the long axis.

cross-tolerance: A condition in which tolerance to one drug produces a reduced response to another drug in the same general class.

crotch (krotch): The angle formed by the parting of two leg-like parts or branches. In anatomy, the angle formed by the inner side of the thigh and the trunk.

croup (kroop): A condition resulting from acute spasmodic laryngitis, occurring in infants and children, most often at night; characterized by harsh, brassy cough, crowing inspirations, dyspnoea, and with or without membrane formation. Croupy breathing in a child is often called stridulous, meaning noisy or harsh-sounding. Narrowing of the airway gives rise to the typical attack with crowing inspiration; may result from oedema, allergy, inflammation of the larynx, spasm. C. KETTLE a kettle for producing steam or medicated vapour which is either directed into a C. tent or allowed to escape into the air to humidify it; used in croup and bronchial conditions; C. TENT a covering for the head and shoulders into which a stream of steam or medicated vapour is directed; used to relieve croup and some other respiratory conditions. — croupous, croupy, adj.

crown: The highest or topmost part of anything. In anatomy, the topmost part of an organ or structure, *e.g.*, the top of the head.

Crown II Report: The final report of the *Review of prescribing, supply and administration of medicines* (Department of Health 1999). The report recommends the introduction of two new groups of prescribers: independent prescribers who make the initial clinical assessment, usually making a diagnosis and then prescribes, as appropriate; and dependent prescribers, who do not diagnose, but once the diagnosis is made, would follow clinical guidelines and prescribe.

crowning (krown'-ing): The phase in the second stage of labour when part of the fetal scalp can be seen at the vaginal orifice.

crow's feet: Wrinkles emanating from the outer canthus of the eye in a fan-like pattern.

CRP: Abbreviation for c-reactive protein (*q.v.*).

crucial (kroo'-shal): 1. Cross-shaped. 2. Severe; essential, as being decisive.

cruciate (krū'-shi-āt): Shaped like a cross c. LIGAMENTS OF THE KNEE strong, thick ligaments that run from the intercondylar of the tibia to the femur and cross within the knee joint; they provide stability to the joint and prevent dislocation of the tibia.

crush injury: An injury in which the physical force caused by crushing, pressure, or by blast is transmitted to the soft tissues, bones, or viscera. Often refers to injuries of the chest when there may or may not be fractured ribs; symptoms include severe breathing difficulty immediately after the injury; later the person may develop oedema of the lungs, dyspnoea, cyanosis; sometimes fatal.

crush syndrome: Traumatic uraemia. A condition resulting from damage to the renal tubules because their blood supply has been interfered with. Following an extensive trauma to muscle, there is a period of delay before the effects of renal damage manifest themselves. There is an increase of non-protein nitrogen of the blood, with oliguria, proteinuria and urinary excretion of myohaemoglobin. Loss of blood plasma to damaged area is marked. Symptoms include thirst, nausea, somnolence, hypertension, features of severe shock, pulmonary oedema, and cardiac involvement.

crust: A hardened covering formed on a lesion on the surface of the skin from the accumulation of dried exudate and other debris. A scab.

crutch: Artificial support used by those who require aid in walking due to injury, disease or a birth defect. Made in different sizes to accommodate people of various heights, and may be adjustable in handgrip-to-ground length. ELBOW C. a c. which consists of an adjustable aluminium tube with a horizontal handgrip and a plastic forearm grip. C. PALSY paralysis or weakness of one or both of the upper extremities caused by compression of the brachial plexus or of the radial nerve.

crutchwalking: Walking with the aid of crutches when normal weight bearing is not possible. Several gaits are utilized, depending on the particular orthopaedic problem involved. In the TWO-POINT GAIT the person advances the right foot and the left crutch together, then the left foot and right crutch together. In the THREE-POINT GAIT the person advances both crutches and the affected leg together, then the unaffected leg. In the FOUR-POINT GAIT the person puts one crutch forward, then the opposite leg, then the other crutch, and then the other leg. In the SWING-THROUGH GAIT both crutches are advanced, the legs are swung through to a point past the crutches, then the crutches are brought to the legs. In the SWING-TO GAIT the crutches are advanced and then the legs are brought to the crutches.

crux (cruks): A cross or structure shaped like a cross. C. OF THE HEART the area around the junction of the walls of the four chambers of the heart.

cry-, cryo-: Combining forms denoting relationship to (1) cold; (2) freezing.

cryaesthesia (krī-es-thē'-zi-a): Unusual sensitivity to cold.

crymodynia (krī-mō-din'-i-a): Rheumatic pain brought on by damp or cold weather.

crymotherapy (krī-mō-ther'-a-pi): Cryotherapy (*q.v.*).

cryocautery (krī-ō-kaw'-ter-i): The destruction of living tissue by the application of extreme cold, *e.g.*, using solid carbon dioxide.

cryogenic (krī-ō-jen'ik): 1. Relating to or causing very low temperatures. 2. Describing any means or apparatus involved in the production of low temperatures.

cryogenics (krī-ō-jen'-iks): Low-temperature physics; concerned with the production of very low temperatures and the phenomena that occur at those temperatures.

cryonics (krī-on'-iks): The practice of using intense cold therapeutically for such purposes as producing local anaesthesia, or removing superficial skin lesions, and including the freezing of dead bodies and maintaining them at temperatures of −196°C in a sealed capsule suspended in liquid nitrogen.

cryoprecipitate (krī'-ō-pre-sip'-i-tāt): A precipitant substance containing factor VIII; derived from rapidly freezing fresh human plasma from a single donor, then slowly thawing, which removes all factors not related to clotting; used to help prevent or control haemorrhage and in treating haemophilia.

cryosurgery (krī'-ō-sur'-jer-i): The destruction of tissue by the application of extreme cold, *e.g.*, the destruction of an area in the thalamus for treatment of parkinsonism, or the treatment with cold of malignant tumours of the skin. Also called *chryosurgery, crymosurgery*.

cryotherapy (krī-ō-ther′-a-pi): Therapeutic use of extreme cold, either local or general.

crypt (kript): In anatomy, a small sac, follicle, or pit-like depression opening on a free surface of an organ or of the body. ANAL C. one of the depressions between the folds of the mucous membrane in the anal canal; CRYPTS OF LIEBER-KÜHN, intestinal glands; simple tubular glands in the mucous membrane of the intestine, thought to be concerned with secretion of intestinal enzymes; TONSILLAR C. one of several crypts in the palatine tonsils.

crypt-, crypto-: Combining forms denoting (1) hidden, covered, invisible; (2) latent.

Cryptococcaceae (krip′-tō′-kok-kā′-sē-a): A family of yeast-like fungi including several that are pathogenic to man, e.g., *Cryptococcus, Candida, Trichosporum*, and *Pityrosporon*.

cryptococcosis (krip′-tō-kok-ō′-sis): A sub-acute or chronic infection involving the lungs, bones or skin, but especially the brain and meninges; caused by *Cryptococcus neoformans* (q.v.).

Cryptococcus (krip-to-kok′-us): A genus of fungi. C. NEOFORMANS is pathogenic to humans; it has a marked predilection for the central nervous system, causing symptoms similar to those of tuberculosis, cancer, brain tumour, even insanity; it may also affect the skin, liver, spleen, or joints.

cryptoinfection (krip-tō-in-fek′-shun): A hidden or latent infection.

cryptolith (krip′-tō-lith): A concretion or stone formed within a gland follicle or a crypt; the tonsil is a frequent site.

cryptomenorrhoea (krip′-tō-men-ō-rē′-a): Retention of the menses although other symptoms of menstruation may be present. Due to a congenital obstruction such as an imperforate hymen or atresia of the vagina. Syn., *haematocolpos*.

cryptomnesia (krip-tom-nē′-zi-a): Subconscious memory; the recall of a forgotten episode or event which seems new to the individual.

cryptorchidopexy (krip′-tor-ki-dō-pek′-si): Surgical fixation of an undescended testis in the scrotum.

cryptorchism (krip-tor′-kizm): A development defect whereby the testes do not descend into the scrotum; in TRUE C. they remain in the abdominal cavity; in ECTOPIC C. they remain within the inguinal canal. Also *cryptorchidism*. — cryptorchid, n. and adj.

crystallin (kris′-ta-lin): Either of two globulins; the principal constituents of the lens of the eye.

crystalline (kris′-ta-līn): Like a crystal; transparent. Applied to various structures. C. LENS a transparent biconvex body, oval in shape, which is suspended just behind the pupil and the iris of the eye, and separates the aqueous from the vitreous humour. It is slightly less convex on its anterior surface and it refracts the light rays so that they focus directly on the retina.

crystalloid (kris′-ta-loid): 1. Resembling a crystal. 2. A substance that forms a true solution; the opposite of a colloid (q.v.).

CSF: Abbreviation for cerebrospinal fluid, see under CEREBROSPINAL.

CSP: Abbreviation for Chartered Society of Physiotherapists (q.v.).

CSSD: Abbreviation for Central Sterile Supplies Department (q.v.).

CSSU: Abbreviation for Central Sterile Supply Unit (q.v.).

CT: Abbreviation for computed tomography, see COMPUTERIZED AXIAL TOMOGRAPHY.

Cu: Chemical symbol for copper.

cubic centimetre (kū′-bik sen′-ti-mē-ter): 1. A mass of material that, in cube form, measures 1 centimetre on each side. Abbreviated cu cm or cc. 2. In liquid capacity it is equal to one one-thousandth of a litre or 0.27 fluidrams; called millilitre and abbreviated ml.

cubital tunnel syndrome: Pain, tenderness, weakness, paraesthesia, and atrophy occurring along the ulnar nerve distribution in the hand and forearm; caused by an injury to the ulnar nerve at the elbow.

cubitus (kū′-bi-tus): 1. The forearm. 2. The bend between the arm and forearm. C. VALGUS a greater than normal degree of valgus at the elbow joint; in severe cases the ulnar nerve may be affected; C. VARUS the carrying angle of the elbow is decreased; may be due to previous surgery, injury, or infection.

cuboid (kū′-boid): 1. Shaped like a cube; 2. One of the tarsal bones.

cul-de-sac (kul′-de-sak): A blind pouch or a cavity closed at one end. C. OF DOUGLAS see RECTO-UTERINE POUCH under POUCH.

culdocentesis (kul-dō-sen-tē′-sis): The aspiration of pus or any other fluid from Douglas' puch through a retrovaginal puncture or incision.

culdoscope (kul′-do-skōp): An endoscope used via the vaginal route. See CULDOSCOPY.

culdoscopy (kul-dos′-kō-pi): Passage of a culdoscope through the posterior vaginal fornix, behind the uterus, to enter the peritoneal cavity, for viewing internal genitalia. A form of peritoneoscopy, laparoscopy. — culdoscopic, adj.; culdoscopically, adv.

culdotomy (kul-dot'-o-mi): An incision into the cul-de-sac called Douglas' pouch; see RECTO-UTERINE POUCH under POUCH.

Cullen's sign: A bluish-red discoloration around the umbilicus; may be indicative of intra-abdominal haemorrhage, or ruptured ectopic pregnancy; sometimes also seen in acute pancreatitis.

cultural competence: The integration and transformation of knowledge about individuals and groups of people into specific standards, policies, practices, and attitudes used in appropriate cultural settings to increase the quality of services and produce better outcomes.

culture (kul'-chur): 1. The beliefs, customs, practices and social behaviour of a particular nation or people. 2. A group of people whose shared beliefs and practices identify the particular place, class or time to which they belong. 3. The development of microorganisms on artificial media under ideal conditions for growth. 4. A growth of microorganisms on a culture medium. 5. The act of cultivating microorganisms on an artificial medium. C. MEDIUM a sterile preparation suitable for cultivation and growth of microorganisms; may have a meat infusion as a base; MIXED C. growth of two or more organisms in the same culture, PURE C. specific growth of only one species of organism in a culture.

cu mm: Abbreviation for cubic millimetre.

cumulative action (kū'-mū-lā-tiv): Occurs when the dose of a slowly secreted drug is repeated too frequently. This can be dangerous as, if the drug accumulates in the system, toxic symptoms may occur, sometimes quite suddenly. Long-acting barbiturates, thyroid extract, strychnine, mercurial salts, and digitalis are examples of drugs with a cumulative action.

Cumulative Index to Nursing and Allied Health Literature: A computerized database of literature relevant to nursing and allied health professionals. Abbreviated CINAHL.

cumulus (kū'-mū-lus): A small heap or mound. C. OOPHORUS a small solid mass of follicular cells surrounding the ovum and protruding into the fluid in the cavity of the Graafian follicle.

cuneate (kū'-nē-āt): Wedge-shaped.

cunnilingus (kun-i-lin'-gus): Oral stimulation of the female genitalia.

cunnus (kun'-us): The female genitalia; the vulva.

cup: In anatomy, a cup-shaped part or structure. C. ARTHROPLASTY a surgical procedure where-

by the acetabulum is reshaped and the head of the femur is replaced with a metallic prosthesis.

cupping (kup'-ing): 1. A once-popular method of counterirritation. A small bell-shaped glass (in which the air is expanded by heating, or exhausted by compression of an attached rubber bulb) is applied to the skin, resultant suction producing hyperaemia — dry C. When the skin is scarified before application of the cup it is termed wet C. 2. Rapid, rhythmic tapping over the lungs with the cupped hands; often performed along with vibration produced by placing the fingertips firmly on the area over the lungs and shaking the arms; done to loosen tenacious mucus in the bronchial tree.

curare (kū-rar'ē): A bitter poison, sometimes used as a drug; prepared as an abstract of a variety of South American plants. Inert when given orally but a powerful muscle relaxant when given by intravenous or intramuscular routes. Sometimes used to promote muscle relaxation in convulsions, spasms, shock, and as an adjunct of anaesthesia. Has been known to cause death from paralysis of respiratory muscles. Syn., *Indian arrow poison*.

curative (kūr'-a-tiv): 1. Having a tendency to heal or cure. 2. Related to or useful in curing disease and restoring health.

cure (kūr): 1. To heal or restore to health. 2. A restoration to health. 3. A system or special course of treatment. 4. A medicine or agent used in treating a disease.

curet, curette (kū'-ret): 1. A spoon-shaped instrument or metal loop for scraping the walls of a cavity or other surface (curetting) to remove growths or other abnormal or diseased tissue, or to obtain material for biopsy. 2. To remove growths or other abnormal tissue from a surface such as bone or from the walls of a cavity, as the uterus, by scraping with a spoon-shaped instrument.

curettage (kū-re-tazh'): The scraping of unhealthy or exuberant tissue from a cavity or from a surface such as bone, using a spoon-shaped instrument. SUCTION C. or VACUUM C., C. using a suction device, often to produce abortion during the first trimester of pregnancy. — cuert, v.

curettings (kū-ret'-ingz): The material obtained by scraping or curetting and usually sent for examination in the pathology laboratory.

curie (kū'-rē): A unit of measurement of radioactivity it is that quantity of any radioactive nuclide that has 3700×10^{10} disintegrations per second.

Curie, Pierre and Marie: French chemist (1859–1919) and his Polish-born scientist wife, Marie Curie (1867–1934); known for their discovery of radium in 1898.

current (kur'-rent): Something which flows. AL-TERNATING C. an electric current that periodically reverses its flow; DIRECT C. an electric current that always flows in the same direction.

curriculum vitae: 1. Latin for 'course of life'. **2.** A summary of academic and professional history and achievements.

curvature of the spine: An abnormal curve in the spinal column; may be to the front (lordosis), to the back (kyphosis) or to the side (scoliosis).

cushingoid (kush'-ing-oyd): **1.** Having the appearance of a person with Cushing's disease or syndrome; said of the appearance resulting from the administration of corticosteroid drugs. **2.** Having the appearance of one with Cushing's disease or syndrome, but none of the other features of that disorder.

Cushing's disease: A rare disorder, mainly of females, characterized by symptoms of Cushing's syndrome, principally virilism, obesity of trunk and face, hyperglycaemia, glycosuria, and hypertension. Due to intrinsic and excessive hormone stimulation of the adrenal cortex by tumour or by hyperplasia of the anterior pituitary gland.

Cushing's syndrome: A disorder similar to Cushing's disease, but commoner, in which excessive hormonal excretion of adrenocorticotropic hormone is caused by intrinsic hyperplasia or, most often, by tumour of the adrenal cortex *per se*, or by prolonged administration of glucocorticoids. Occurring most often in females, the symptoms include fatness of the face ('moon' face), neck and trunk, abnormal distribution of the hair and hypertrichosis, florid complexion, hypertension, kyphosis due to softness of the vertebrae, muscular weakness, polycythaemia, atrophy of the genital organs, impotence, and amenorrhoea. Also called *hyperadrenocorticism, basophilism; pituitary basophilism.* [Harvey Williams Cushing, American surgeon, 1869–1939.]

cusp (kusp): A projecting point such as that of the edge of a tooth or a leaflet of a valve, such as the heart valves that control the flow of blood between the atria and ventricles; the tricuspid valve in the right heart has three cusps, the mitral (bicuspid) valve in the left heart has two.

cuspid (kus'-pid): A tooth having only one cusp; the third tooth on either side from the midline of the jaws; a canine tooth.

cutaneous (kū-tā'-nē-us): Relating to the skin. C. LEISHMANIASIS see under LEISHMANIASIS; C. URETEROSTOMY transplantation of the ureters so that they open on to the skin of the abdominal wall.

cutdown (kut'-down): A small surgical incision to expose a vein into which a needle, cannula, or catheter is inserted for the administration of intravenous fluids or medications.

cuticle (kū'-ti-k'l): The epidermis (*q.v.*); dead epidermis, as that which surrounds a nail. See EPONYCHIUM. — cuticular, adj.

cutis (kū'-tis): The corium or deeper layer of the skin; the derma; true skin. C. ANSERINA erection of the papillae of the skin due to contraction of the arrectores pilorum; produced by fear, cold, excitement or other stimulus. Often called *gooseflesh* or *goose pimples*; C. MARMORATA transient pinkish or purplish mottling of the skin, seen chiefly in children on exposure to the cold; C. RHOMBOIDALIS NUCHAE thickening and furrowing of the skin, especially of the neck, from years of exposure to sun and weather; C. VERA the dermis.

CV: Abbreviation for curriculum vitae (*q.v.*).

CVA: Abbreviation for cerebrovascular accident, see under CEREBROVASCULAR.

CVP: Abbreviation for central venous pressure, see under BLOOD PRESSURE.

CVS: Abbreviation for (1) cardiovascular system, see under CARDIOVASCULAR; (2) chorionic villus sampling (*q.v.*).

CXR: Abbreviation for chest x-ray, see under CHEST.

cyan-, cyano-: Combining forms denoting dark blue.

cyanaemia (sī-a-nē'-mi-a): Bluishness of the blood; as in cyanosis; due to insufficient oxygen.

cyanide (sī'-a-nīd): Any compound containing cyanogen with the –CN radical; all are deadly poisons.

cyanocobalamin (sī-an-ō-kō-bal'-a-min): Vitamin B_{12}, a member of the vitamin B complex; essential to life. C. is a red crystalline water-soluble substance containing cobalt; essential for the metabolism of fats, proteins, and carbohydrates, and for normal formation of blood cells; deficiency results in pernicious anaemia and brain damage. Found in liver, kidney, eggs, fish, meats, dairy products. Used prophylactically and as a specific in treatment of pernicious anaemia; also useful in treatment of several other anaemias, sprue, polyneuritis, and herpes zoster. Also called *cobalamin*, and *intrinsic factor*.

cyanosis (sī-a-nō′-sis): A bluish tinge manifested by hypoxic tissue, observed most frequently under the nails, lips, and skin. It is always due to lack of oxygen, and the causes of this are legion. CENTRAL C. blueness seen on warm surfaces such as the oral mucosa and tongue, due to impaired gas exchange between the alveoli and the pulmonary capillaries; PERIPHERAL C. blueness of the hands, feet, tip of the nose; disappears on massage of the part; due to low cardiac output; occurs after chilling, smoking, ingestion of certain drugs. — cyanotic, cyanosed, adj.

cyanotic (sī-a-not′-ik): Refers to the bluish-purple discoloration of the mucous membranes and skin due to insufficient oxygen in the capillaries.

cyasma (sī-az′-ma): The peculiar freckle-like discoloration of the skin sometimes occurring in pregnant women.

cybernetics (sī-ber-net′-iks): The comparative study of electronic communication systems which combines the disciplines of neurophysiology, mathematics, and electrical engineering; it is concerned with the processes of information flow through which the brain controls the body and through which computers control machines. It supports the hypothesis that the functioning of the human brain is similar to that of electronic control devices.

cyclarthrosis (sik-lar-thrō′-sis): A pivot joint; one which allows for rotation.

cycle (sī-k′l): A regular series of movements or events; a sequence which recurs regularly. CARDIAC C. the series of movements through which the heart passes in performing one heartbeat which corresponds to one pulse beat and takes about one second. See DIASTOLE and SYSTOLE; MENSTRUAL C. the periodically recurring series of changes in breasts, ovaries, and uterus, culminating in menstruation. See also KREBS CYCLE. — cyclic, cyclical, adj.

cyclical (sī-klik-al): Relating to or occurring in a cycle or cycles. C. SYNDROME term used currently for premenstrual symptom complex, to emphasize that these symptoms are due to normal physiological interaction between several endocrine glands under the cyclical control of the hypothalamus and pituitary; C. VOMITING periodic attacks of vomiting, associated with ketosis; no demonstrable pathological cause; occurs in nervous persons, children in particular.

cyclitis (sīk-lī′-tis): Inflammation of the ciliary body of the eye, often coexistent with inflammation of the iris.

cycloid (sī′-kloyd): In psychiatry, descriptive of behaviour characterized by alternating periods of well-being and happiness with mild depression.

cyclophosphamide (sī-klō-fos′-fa-mīd): A preparation of nitrogen mustard with cytotoxic effects; used in medicine as an antineoplastic agent.

cyclopropane (sī-klō-prō′-pān): A highly flammable and explosive anaesthetic gas; of low toxicity and produces anaesthesia rapidly; now largely replaced by non-flammable substances.

cyclops (sī′-klops): A congenital anomaly in which the individual has only one eye or in whom the two eye sockets are fused.

cyclosporin A (sī-klō-spōr′-in): An immunosuppressant derived from a fungus and used prophylactically to prevent graft-versus-host disease (*q.v.*) in organ and tissue transplantation.

cyclothymia (sī-klō-thī′-mi-a): An affective disorder characterized by a tendency to alternation between moods of elation and depression that are not caused by external circumstances. — cyclothymic, adj. CYCLOTHYMIC DISORDER: see AFFECTIVE DISORDERS.

cyclotron (sī′-klō-tron): An apparatus that gives high energy to certain particles by means of an alternating electric field and a powerful magnet; these particles can produce neutrons or can impart artificial radioactivity to various substances.

cyesis (sī-ē′-sis): Pregnancy. See also PSEUDOCYESIS.

cylindruria (sil-in-drū′-ri-a): The presence of an increased number of cylindroid casts in urine; they are formed in the nephron and are diagnostic of renal rather than urinary tract disease.

cyllosis (sil-ō′-sis): Clubfoot.

cynophobia (sī-nō-fō′-bi-a): A morbid or unreasonable fear of dogs.

cynorexia (sī-nō-rek′-si-a): Morbidly excessive hunger or appetite. See also BULIMIA.

cypridophobia (sip-ri-dō-fō′-bi-a): **1.** A morbid fear of contracting a veneral disease. **2.** Morbid fear of sexual intercourse.

cyst (sist): **1.** The encapsulated stage in the life cycle of certain protozoa. **2.** An encapsulated area, filled with fluid or semi-fluid material, in the dermis or subcutaneous tissue. ADVENTITIOUS C. one formed about a foreign body or exudate; BRANCHIAL C. one in the neck region arising from anomalous development of the embryonal branchial cleft(s); CHOCOLATE C. a c. filled with degenerated blood; the ovaries are the most usual site; CHOLEDOCHAL C. a congenital dilatation of the common bile duct which is usually manifested early in life; characterized by pain, enlarged liver, jaundice, cirrhosis, tumour; also called choledochous C. and bile C.; COLLOID C. contains jelly-like material; occurs particularly in the third ventricle; DERMOID C. congenital in origin, usually occurring in the ovary, containing elements of hair, nails, skin, teeth, etc. EXTERNAL ANGULAR DERMOID C. a C. usually occurring above the eye on the lateral aspect of the eyebrow; an anomaly occurring in a neonate or infant; FOLLICULAR C. occurs in the ovary when the Graafian follicle fails to rupture; menstrual irregularities and menorrhagia may result; HYDATID C. the envelope in which *Taenia echinococcus* (tapeworm) produces its larvae — usually in the liver; INCLUSION C. a C. that develops from the implantation of epidermal tissue into another structure of the body; may occur in embryonic development or following trauma; MEIBOMIAN C. see CHALAZION. NABOTHIAN C. cyst-like formations in the Nabothian glands of the cervix; caused by occlusion of the outlets for the secretion of the glands; OVARIAN C. ovarian new growth, usually cystic but may be solid, such as fibroma. To be differentiated from a cystic ovary, see under OVARY; O.C. is enucleated from the ovary which is conserved; PAPILLARY C. an ovarian C., in which there are nipple-like (papillary) outgrowths from the wall. May be benign or malignant; PILONIDAL C. a sacrococcygeal dermoid C. containing hairs; RETENTION C. caused by blocking of a duct, as a ranula (*q.v.*); SEBACEOUS C. retention C. of a sebaceous gland, a wen; THYROGLOSSAL C. a cystic distension of the thyroglossal duct near the hyoid bone in the neck region.

cyst-, cysti-, cysto-: Combining forms denoting a fluid-filled sac, as the gall bladder or urinary bladder.

-cyst-: Suffix denoting a bladder.

cystectomy (sis-tek′-to-mi): 1. Usually refers to the surgical removal of part or the whole of the urinary bladder, this may involve transplantation of one or both ureters cutaneously or into the bowel. 2. Surgical removal of the cystic duct or of the cystic duct and the gall bladder. 3. The excision of a cyst. 4. Removal of part of the capsule of the crystalline lens, a procedure in the operation for removal of a cataract. OVARIAN C. excision of a cyst from an ovary with conservation of the remaining ovarian tissue.

cysteine (sis′-tē-in): A sulphur-containing amino acid found in most proteins.

cystic (sis′-tik): 1. Relating to the urinary bladder or the gall bladder. 2. Relating to or resembling a cyst. C. BREAST DISEASE fibrocystic disease of the breast; see under FIBFBROCYSTIC; C. DEGENERATION degeneration of tissue with formation of cysts; C. DUCT the duct that leads from the gall bladder and joins the hepatic duct from the liver to form the common bile duct; C. FIBROSIS an inherited condition characterized by accumulation of thick tenacious mucus which obstructs tubular structures, particularly the bronchioles; symptoms include a high level of electrolytes in the sweat, deficient pancreatic functioning, dyspnoea, productive cough, voracious appetite, abdominal cramps, bulky malodorous stools, impaired growth; affects about one in every 2500 children; occurs most often in Caucasian children; prognosis beyond adolescence is poor; survival depends on avoidance of pulmonary infections; see MUCOVISCIDOSIS; FIBROCYSTIC; C. MASTITIS cystic breast disease.

cystine (sis′-tēn): A sulphur-containing amino acid, produced by the breaking down of proteins during the digestive process. C. STONES sometimes occur as a deposit in urine or forming stones in the bladder.

cystinuria (sis-ti-nū′ri-a): A hereditary disorder in which cystine appears in the urine; often associated with liver disease or jaundice. A cause of renal stones. — cystinuric, adj.

cystitis (sis-tī′-tis): Inflammation of a bladder, the urinary bladder in particular. May be acute or chronic, primary or secondary to stones, etc., but the exciting cause is usually bacterial; may be associated with pathological conditions of the kidney, prostate, or ureters; more common in women than men because the urethra is short. Symptoms include pain on urination, frequency, haematuria. CYSTIC C., C. characterized by formation of multiple cysts in the bladder wall; INTERSTITIAL C. chronic C. which extends into the deeper tissues of the bladder, often accompanied by ulcer formation. See also TRIGONITIS.

cystocele (sis′-tō-sēl): Prolapse or pouching of the posterior wall of the urinary bladder into the anterior vaginal wall.

cystogram (sis′-tō-gram): An x-ray film demonstrating the urinary bladder. MICTURATING C. taken during the act of passing urine.

cystography (sis-tog′-ra-fi): Radiography of the urinary bladder after it has been rendered radiopaque. — cystographic, adj.; cystographically, adv.

cystoid (sis′-toyd): 1. Like a bladder. 2. Like a cyst. 3. A tumour that resembles a cyst in that it contains fluid or pulpy material but which has no capsule.

cystolith (sis′-tō-lith): A stone in the urinary bladder.

cystolithectomy (sis′-tō-li-thek′-to-mi): Removal of a stone or stones from the urinary bladder by cutting into the bladder.

cystometrogram (sis-tō-met′-rō-gram): A graphic record, made with a cystometer, of the changes in pressure within the urinary bladder under various conditions; used in the study of certain disorders of bladder function.

cystoplasty (sis′-tō-plas-ti): Surgical repair of the bladder. — cystoplastic, adj.

cystopyelitis (sis-tō-pī-e-lī′-tis): Inflammation of the urinary bladder and the pelvis of the kidney.

cystopyelonephritis (sis-tō-pī′-e-lo-ne-frī′-tis): Inflammation of the urinary bladder associated with pyelonephritis.

cystorectocele (sis-tō-rek′-tō-sēl): Herniation of the urinary bladder and the rectum into the vagina.

cystorrhoea (sis-tō-rē′-a): Mucous discharge from the urinary bladder.

cystoscope (sis′-to-skōp): An endoscope equipped with a light and viewing lenses for examining the urinary tract. — cystoscopic, adj.

cystoscopy (sis-tos′-kō-pi): Observation of the bladder by means of a fibre-optic cystoscope (q.v.), for diagnostic purposes.

cystostomy (sis-tos′-to-mi): The operation whereby a fistulous opening is made into the bladder via the abdominal wall.

cystotomy (sis-tot′-o-mi): 1. Incision into the urinary bladder or gall bladder; may be done to remove calculi or a tumour; PERINEAL C. one in which the opening into the urinary bladder is made through the perineum; SUPRAPUBIC C. one in which the opening into the urinary bladder is made just above the symphysis pubis. 2. Incision into the capsule of the crystalline lens.

cystoureterogram (sis′-tō-ū-rē′-ter-ō-gram): An x-ray of the urinary bladder and ureters.

cystourethrogram (sis-tō-ū-ri′-thrō-gram): A x-ray film demonstrating the urinary bladder and the urethra.

cystourethrography (sis′-tō-ū-ri-throg′-ra-fi): Radiographic examination of the urinary bladder and the urethra after they have been rendered radiopaque. — cystourethrographic, adj.; cystourethrographically, adv.

cyte-, cyto-: Combining forms denoting (1) cells; (2) cytoplasm.

cythaemolysis (sī-thēm-ol′-i-sis): Dissolution of blood cells, erythrocytes and leukocytes.

cytobiology (sī-tō-bī-ol′-o-ji): The study of cell biology.

cytoblast (sī′-tō-blast): The nucleus of a cell.

cytoclasis (sī-tok′-la-sis): The destruction or necrosis of cells.

cytodendrite (sī-tō-den′-drīt): Dendrite.

cytodiagnosis (sī′-tō-dī-ag-nō′-sis): Diagnosis by microscopic study of cells. EXPOLIATIVE C. diagnosis by the examination of cells from the external or internal surfaces of the body. See CYTOLOGY.

cytogenetics (sī-tō-je-net′-iks): That branch of biology concerned with the origin, development, structure, functions, etc. of cells, particularly of the chromosomes and genes.

Cytoglomerator (sī-tō-glom′-e-rā-tor): A machine that is used for freezing donated blood for long-time storage after the plasma has been extracted and the red cells coated with glycerol; the freezing temperature is −85°C; this process has increased the storage life of blood.

cytoid (sī′-toyd): Resembling a cell.

cytokinesis (sī-tō-kin-ē′-sis): The changes that take place in the cytoplasm of a cell during cell division.

cytology (sī-tol′-ō-ji): Subdivision of biology, consisting of the study of the structure, function, and pathology of the body cells. EXFOLIATIVE C. microscopic study of cells from the surface of an organ or lesion after suitable staining. — cytological, adj.

cytolysin (sī-tol′-i-sin): A substance or antibody that is capable of causing cells to dissolve. When a C. acts upon a specific type of cell, it is named accordingly, e.g., haemolysin.

cytolysis (sī-tol′-i-sis): The degeneration, destruction, disintegration or dissolution of living cells. — cytolytic, adj.

cytomegalic inclusion disease: A disease especially of the newborn; due to infection with a cytomegalovirus (q.v.) which often occurs before birth; in the neonate is characterized by enlarged spleen and liver, small head, diarrhoea, haematemesis, haematuria, cerebral haemorrhage, anaemia, mental and motor retardation. Diagnostic cells that contain large acidophil intranuclear inclusions are found in the ducts or acini of the salivary glands, also sometimes in other organs, e.g., liver, kidney. Congenital form is the most severe; formerly thought to be rare in adults; but it has been reported in that age group as an illness resembling infectious mononucleosis (*q.v.*).

cytomegalovirus (sī-tō-meg'-a-lō-vī'-rus): One of a group of several DNA viruses, closely related to the herpes virus, that infect monkeys and rodents as well as humans, causing mononucleosis, (*q.v.*), cytomegalic inclusion disease (*q.v.*), and various pulmonary disorders. Although it is not highly contagious, studies show that by age 35 most adults have been infected with it. When it is acquired *in utero* it sometimes causes deafness or hearing loss, and mental retardation. It causes serious illness in the newborn and in those on immunosuppressive therapy, especially those who have had a transplant. The virus is spread by saliva, breast milk, blood, and semen.

cytomegaly (sī-tō-mcg'-a-li): Marked enlargement of cells. — cytomegalic, adj.

cytomorphosis (sī-tō-mor-fō'-sis): The changes occurring in cells in the course of their development.

cytomycosis (sī-tō-mī-kō'-sis): A fungal infection characterized by enlargement of the spleen, leukopenia, fever; attacks the phagocytes in the blood; often fatal. Also called *histoplasmosis*.

cyton (sī'-ton): The cell body of a neuron.

cytopathology (sī-tō-pa-thol'-o-ji): The branch of pathology that deals with alterations within cells.

cytopenia (sī-tō-pē'-ni-a): A deficiency of blood cells or in the cellular elements in blood.

cytophagy (sī-tof'-a-ji): The engulfing of cells by other cells. See PHAGOCYTOSIS.

cytopheresis (sī-tō-fer-ē'-sis): The removal of cells, especially white blood cells, from whole blood and returning the remaining blood to the donor.

cytophysiology (sī-tō-fiz-ē-ol'-o-ji): The physiology of cells.

cytoplasm (sī'-tō-plazm): The material (protoplasm) of the cell other than that of the nucleus.

cytoscopy (sī-tos'-ko-pi): The microscopic examination of cells.

cytosome (sī'-tō-sōm): The cell body exclusive of the nucleus.

cytotoxic (sī'-tō-tok'-sik): 1. Relating to any substance that is toxic to cells. 2. An agent that damages or deranges cellular organization. Applied to a group of drugs used for treatment of carcinomas and reticuloses.

cytotoxin (sī'-tō-tok'sin): A toxin or antibody that is destructive to specific cells of certain organs, or which inhibits their functioning. See ANTIBODIES, CYTOTOXIC.

cytozoic (sī-tō-zō'-ik): Living on or within cells; parasitic.

cytozyme (sī-tō-zim): Thromboplastin (*q.v.*).

D

Dacron (dak′-ron): Trade name for a synthetic textile fibre; resistant to stretching and wrinkling. Sometimes used in replacement surgery.

dacry-, dacryo-: Combining forms denoting (1) lacrimal, or (2) tears.

dacryoblennorrhoea (dak′-ri-ō-blen-ō-rē′-a): Mucous discharge from the lacrimal gland through the lacrimal duct; often chronic.

dacryocystotomy (dak′-ri-ō-sis-tot′-o-mi): Surgical incision of the lacrimal duct; usually done to facilitate drainage.

dacryorrhoea (dak-ri-ō-rē′-a): Excessive secretion and flow of tears.

dactyl (dak′-til): A digit, finger, or toe. — dactyli, pl.; dactylar, dactylate, adj.

dactyl-, dactylo-: Combining forms denoting relationship to a digit, finger, or toe.

-dactylia, dactyl-: Combining forms denoting digit, finger, or toe.

dactylion (dak-til′-i-on): Webbing or adhesion of the fingers. See SYNDACTYLY.

dactylogram (dak-til′-ō-gram): A fingerprint.

dactylology (dak-til-ol′-o-ji): Communication between individuals by signs made with the hands and fingers. See also SIGN LANGUAGE.

dactylus (dak′-til-us): A finger or toe.

Dakin's solution: A neutral antiseptic solution formerly much used for cleansing wounds; contains 0.5% solution of sodium hypochlorite. [Henry D. Dakin, English chemist working in the USA, 1880–1952.]

Daltonism (dawl′-ton-izm): 1. Colour blindness; named after John Dalton, English chemist and physicist [1766–1844], who was afflicted with it. 2. Red–green colour blindness.

damp: 1. Humid or moist. 2. Relating to noxious or foul gases found in mines and caves. BLACK D. noxious atmosphere that collects in a mine from the absorption of oxygen and the giving off of carbon dioxide by coal.

dance: D. THERAPY see under THERAPY. D. REFLEX see under REFLEX; ST. VITUS' D. see under CHOREA.

D and C: Abbreviation for dilatation and curettage (q.v.).

dandruff (dan′-druf): 1. The dried, scaly material normally shed by the scalp. 2. Seborrhoeic dermatitis of the scalp; see under DERMATITIS.

Dandy–Walker syndrome: A condition characterized by hydrocephalus due to distension of the fourth ventricle of the brain; thought to be caused by constriction of the foramina of Luschka and Magendi.

dangerous and severe personality disorder: A term used to describe the condition of individuals who pose a significant risk of serious harm to others as a result of their psychological problems.

dark adaptation: The adjustment of the retina and iris for seeing in a dim light or in darkness.

dartos (dar′-tos): A thin layer of smooth muscle tissue that makes up part of the superficial fascia of the scrotum; it envelops the testes. Cold causes it to contract, thus bringing the testes closer to the abdomen for warmth; warmth causes it to relax, thus the testes are kept at a fairly even temperature. Also called *tunica dartos*.

Darwinian tubercle: A blunt-pointed tubercle that projects from the upper part of the helix of the external ear; when it is abnormally enlarged it is referred to as Darwinian ear.

Darwinism (dar′-wi-nizm): The theory of evolution proposed by Darwin that organisms have evolved from earlier forms in response to natural and environmental influences. [Charles Darwin, English naturalist, 1809–1882.]

DASE: Abbreviation for Denver Articulation Screening Examination (q.v.).

data (dā′-ta, da′-ta): Information collected for a specific purpose, e.g., clinical nursing data collected at the initial interview with a patient or client. See DATA COLLECTION.

data analysis: The interpretation of collected information. For example, following an initial interview with a patient or client, the information is examined closely to identify problems or issues. Also used in research for the interpretation of qualitative or quantitative results. See APPENDIX 6; CONTENT ANALYSIS.

database (dā′-ta-bās, da′-): An organized collection of data. In clinical care the term may be used to describe only data collected at the initial interview with a patient. Alternatively it may refer to all the information regarding a patient or to the collected data for a group of patients to be analysed retrospectively.

data collection: The gathering of information, usually in a structured format. Information can be obtained verbally, in the form of an interview that is recorded, or by measurement, *e.g.*, 24-hour fluid balance. See DATA; DATA PROTECTION ACT 1998.

data processing: The processing of raw data to produce ordered, meaningful information.

Data Protection Act (1998): A law that implements EC Directive 95/46/EC on the protection of individuals with regard to the processing of personal data and on the free movement of such data. One of its purposes is to safeguard the fundamental rights of individuals.

daughter cell: A cell resulting from subdivision of a mature mother cell.

Dawson's encephalitis: Subacute sclerosing panencephalitis; see under PANENCEPHALITIS.

day blindness: Inability to see well in bright daylight; hemeralopia.

day care centre: A facility that provides a programme of rehabilitation and occupation usually for mental health and older people for part of the day.

daydream: A pleasant reverie indulged in while awake; an imagining usually involving pleasant visions or wishful thinking. — daydream, v.

day hospital: A centre where non-hospitalized patients, particularly older persons who do not require surgical intervention or 24-hour nursing care, may spend time and may be provided with needed diagnostic, medical, nursing, and rehabilitative services.

day treatment: Treatment given in a care facility during the day only, sometimes in a hospital, as a substitute for inpatient care. Patients spend the day at the facility receiving surgery, medical interventions, pharmacotherapy, and nursing care.

db, DB: Abbreviations for decibel(s) (*q.v.*).

DBT: Abbreviation for dialectical behavioural therapy (*q.v.*).

DC: Abbreviation for direct current, see under DIRECT.

DDA: Abbreviation for Disability Discrimination Act (*q.v.*).

deacidification (dē'-a-sid-i-fi-kā'-shun): The neutralization of an acid or correction of a condition of acidity.

dead space: 1. In the respiratory tract, the ANATOMICAL D.S. consists of those parts of the nose, mouth, and terminal bronchioles that do not take part in the exchange of oxygen and carbon dioxide; the PHYSIOLOGICAL D.S. consists of the anatomical D.S. plus that in the alveoli which does not take part in exchange of gases. **2.** In a hypodermic syringe, the space at the tip of the syringe and in the hub of the needle after an injection.

deaf (def): Partially or completely unable to hear. May be due to anatomical defect, dysfunction or disease of the ear or part of it, brain disorder, or dysfunction of the vestibulocochlear nerve. — deafened, adj.; deafness, n.

deafferentation (dē'-af-fer-en-tā'-shun): Eliminating or interrupting afferent impulses, usually by destroying the afferent nerve pathway.

deafness (def'-nes): Lack, loss, or impairment of usable hearing; may be acute or chronic; congenital or acquired. ACOUSTIC, BOILERMAKER'S or OCCUPATIONAL D., D. that occurs in individuals who work in extremely noisy places; AVIATORS'D. an occupational disease of aviators; may be temporary or permanent; caused by prolonged exposure to loud noise; CENTRAL D., D. caused by alterations in the auditory pathways and/or the auditory centre of the brain; CONDUCTION D., D. that results from interference with conduction of sound waves within the ear; due possibly to the presence of hardened wax or to infection of the outer or middle ear; HYSTERICAL D., D. that appears and disappears in hysterical people without discernible physical cause; NERVE D., D. that results from damage to the auditory nerve; ORGANIC D., D. due to a defect in the ear or auditory apparatus; PRESBYCUSIC D. see PRESBYCUSIS; profound D., no usable hearing; PSYCHIC D. hearing sounds without comprehension; SENSORIMOTOR D. the D. that occurs in old age; usually due to presbycusia; may also be due to a lesion in the cochlear division of the 8th cranial nerve; also called perceptive D.; SENSORINEURAL D., D. due to a lesion in the acoustic nerve or the central neural pathways, or both; SIMULATED D. feigned D.; TONE D. inability to distinguish musical sounds; TOXIC D., D. due to the effect of toxins on the auditory nerve; WORD D., D. in which sounds are heard, but interpretation of words is impossible.

deaf without speech: A person without the sense of hearing whose normal method of communication is by signs, finger spelling or writing.

deaf with speech: A person who, even with a hearing aid, has little or no useful hearing but whose normal method of communication is by speech and lipreading.

deaminase (dē-am'-i-nās): An enzyme that catalyzes the splitting off of an amino group from an organic compound.

dearticulation (de'-ar-tik-ū-lā'-shun): The dislocation of a joint.

death: The permanent cessation or end of life. In the past death was said to occur when the heart ceased to beat and the respiration stopped. CLINICAL D. occurs at the time of cardiac or respiratory arrest, and BIOLOGICAL D., which is irreversible, 3 to 8 minutes later when the body cells have become anoxic. The tendency today is to include BRAIN D., the irreversible cessation of brain function, in determining the time of death. Criteria for determining brain death are governed in the UK by a set of guidelines ratified by the Medical Royal Colleges. These criteria include: (1) unreceptivity and unresponsivity to external stimuli; (2) no movement or breathing for at least one hour; (3) no reflexes can be elicited. Two independent medical opinions are required before brain death is agreed. D. CERTIFICATE certificate issued by the registrar for deaths after the receipt of a preliminary signed notification from the attending doctor indicating the probable cause of death. It is only after the issue of this certificate registering the death that the body can be disposed of; D. INSTINCT an unconscious tendency towards self-destruction which may be expressed in a variety of aggressive acts usually aimed at oneself; thought by Freud to co-exist with the 'life' instinct; D. MASK a mould, usually of the face of a person, made after death; D. RATE the ratio of deaths over a certain period of time among 1000 of the population in a certain area; D. RATTLE sound sometimes heard in dying patients; caused by the loss of the cough reflex and the breathing of air through mucus that has collected in the trachea; D. STRUGGLE, AGONY, THROE a final twitching or convulsion sometimes seen in a dying person.

debilitant (de-bil'-i-tant): 1. An agent that weakens or enfeebles. 2. Causing debility.

debilitate (de-bil'-i-tāt): To make weak or to enfeeble. — debilitating, adj.

debility (de-bil'-i-ti): A state of weakness, feebleness or infirmity. See also ASTHENIA.

débridement (dā-brēd'-mon): In surgery, thorough cleansing of a wound with removal of all foreign matter and devitalized, injured or infected tissue. — debride, adj.

debris (de-brē'): Accumulated devitalized tissue or foreign matter.

dec-, deca-: Prefixes denoting (1) ten; (2) multiplied by ten.

decacurie (dek-a-kū'-rē): A unit of radioactivity; ten curies.

decadence (dek'-a-dens): A process or condition of deterioration, decline, or decay.

decagram (dek'-a-gram): In the metric system, ten grams.

decalcification (dē'-kal-si-fik-ā'-shun): Removal of calcium or calcium salts, as from teeth in dental caries, bone in disorders of metabolism.

decalcify (dē-kal'-si-fi): To deprive of calcium, as in decalcification of bones.

decalitre (dek'-a-lē-ter): In the metric system, liquid volume equal to ten litres.

decameter (dek'-a-mē-ter): In the metric system, a measure of length equal to ten metres.

decannulation (dē-kan-ū-lā'-shun): The removal of a cannula (q.v.), especially a tracheostomy cannula.

decant (dē-kant'): To pour off liquid without disturbing the sediment or precipitate in it.

decapeptide (dek-a-pep'-tīd): A polypeptide that contains ten amino acid groups.

decapitation (dē-kap-i-tā'-shun): 1. The removal of the head from the body. 2. The removal of the head of a bone from its shaft.

decay rate (di-kā'): In radiobiology, the rate at which a radioactive substance decays; radioactive disintegration.

decedent (dē-sē'-dent): A dead person.

decerebrate (dē-ser'-e-brāt): 1. To remove the cerebrum. 2. To eliminate cerebral function by transecting the brain stem. 3. Without cerebral function; a state of deep unconsciousness. D. POSTURE or POSITION a condition of the unconscious patient in which all four limbs are spastic; the legs are hyperextended at the hip and knee, the shoulders are rotated inward, and the arms are flexed; indicates severe damage to the cerebrum; D. RIGIDITY flexion of the arms, wrists, and fingers, and extension of the legs; indicates interruption in the corticospinal tracts in the cerebral hemisphere. — decerebrate, n.; adj.

decibel (des'-i-bel): A standard unit that has been adopted for measuring the amount of sound perceptible to the normal ear; it is the smallest change in sound intensity that the normal ear can detect; one-tenth of a bel (q.v.).

decidua (dē-sid'-ū-a): The endometrial lining of the uterus thickened and altered for reception of the fertilized ovum, and which is shed when pregnancy terminates and during menstruation. D. BASALIS the part of the D. that lies under the embedded ovum and forms the maternal part of the placenta; D. CAPSULARIS that part of the D. that lies over the developing fetus; it surrounds the chorionic sac; D. MENSTRUALIS that part of the outer layer of the endometrium that is shed during menstruation; D. VERA the part of the decidua lining the rest of the uterus; also called the D. PARIETALIS. — decidual, deciduate, adj.

deciduation (dē-sid-ū-ā'-shun): The shedding of the decidua (*q.v.*).

deciduous (dē-sid'-ū-us): Not permanent; said of something that is shed or falls out, at maturity. Term often applied to the teeth of the primary dentition; see under DENTITION.

decigram (des'-i-gram): One-tenth of a gram.

decilitre (des'-i-lē-ter): One-tenth of a litre.

decimetre (des'-i-mē-ter): One-tenth of a metre.

decision-making: The process of choosing courses of action or reaching conclusions regarding important matters. In nursing this usually involves the patient/client and other health-care professionals. Seven steps to better decision-making are: Stop and think; Clarify goals; Determine facts; Develop options; Consider consequences; Choose; and Monitor and modify.

decoagulent (dē-kō-ag'-ū-lant): An agent or substance that reduces the coagulability of the blood by reducing the amount of coagulants or procoagulants in it.

decompensation (dē'-kom-pen-sā'-shun): 1. A failure of compensation, particularly in heart disease; inability of the heart to maintain adequate circulation. 2. In psychiatry, the deterioration of existing defences, resulting in exacerbation of pathological behaviour.

decompose (dē'-kom-pōz'): To decay or rot.

decomposition (dē'-kom-pō-zish'-un): 1. The separation of a substance into simpler compounds or its constituent elements. 2. The chemical breakdown of a substance. 3. Rot; decay; putrefaction.

decompression (dē'kom-presh'-un): Removal of pressure or of a compressing force. ABDOMINAL D. removal of pressure from the abdomen during the first stage of labour; improves blood supply and results in shorter and less painful labour; CARDIAC D. removal of fluid from the pericardial sac by means of an incision into the sac; D. OF THE BRAIN achieved by trephining the skull; D. OF THE BLADDER achieved in cases of chronic urinary retention by continuous or intermittent drainage via a catheter inserted into the urethra; D. CHAMBER a compressed air chamber for gradual reduction of barometric pressure; used when returning deep-sea divers and caisson workers to the surface, to avoid decompression sickness; D. SICKNESS caisson disease (*q.v.*).

deconditioning (dē-kon-dish'-un-ing): A type of therapy used in patients with neurotic phobias; after discussing with the patient his/her particular fear, the therapist gradually exposes the patient to the fear itself with further discussion following each exposure.

decongestant (dē-kon-jes'-tant): An agent that reduces congestion.

decongestion (dē-kon-jest'-yun): Relief or reduction of congestion (*q. v*). — decongestive, adj.

deconstruction (dē-kon-struk'-shun): A method of analysing texts based on the ideas that language is inherently unstable and shifting, and that the reader, rather than the author, is central in determining meaning. It was introduced by the French philosopher Jacques Derrida in the late 1960s.

decontamination (dē'-kon-tam-in-ā'-shun): The process of destroying, removing, or neutralizing potentially harmful agents, *e.g.*, bacteria, war gas, or radioactive material, from persons, objects, or an area. — decontaminate, v.

decrudescence (dē'-krōo-des'-ens): The lessening of intensity of symptoms of a disease.

decubation (dē-kū-ba'-shun): The period in the course of an infectious disease after the symptoms have subsided and lasting until complete recovery.

decubitus (dē-kū-bi-tus): The recumbent position; lying down. D. ULCER an ulceration or pressure sore, usually ocurring in a patient long confined to bed, arising from continual pressure of the flesh over a bony prominence or from friction, obesity, emaciation, impaired circulation to the part, paralysis, old age, lowered vitality, lack of cleanliness, failure to keep the bed dry, smooth and free of irritating particles. The usual sites are the buttock, hip, shoulder, heel, elbow. The first warning is redness of the area, which becomes hot and tender, later smarting. Discoloration ensues and is followed by breaking of the skin, thus producing an open sore which may or may not become infected and which sloughs before healing takes place by granulation. Skin grafting may be necessary. See PRESSURE AREAS; WATERFLOW PRESSURE SORE PREVENSION/TREATMENT POLICY. — decubiti, pl.; decubital, adj.

dedentition (dē-den-tish'-un): The loss or shedding of teeth.

deduction (dē-duk'-shun): The process of drawing a conclusion from available information.

deductive reasoning: The logical thinking process that proceeds from general to specific. Opp. of inductive reasoning.

defecation (def-e-kā'-shun): Discharge of faecal matter from the rectum; evacuation of the bowels. — defecate, v.

defect (dē'-fekt): 1. An imperfection or flaw. 2. The malformation or absence of a body part or organ.

defeminization (dē'-fem-i-nī-zā'-shun): The loss or diminishment of feminine sexual characteristics, *e.g.*, increased muscle mass and decreased breast size; often the result of dysfunction or removal of the ovaries. VOLUNTARY D. the voluntary giving up of feminine characteristics and assumption of those of males.

defence mechanism: In psychiatry, an unconscious manoeuvre that helps to prevent, and to obtain relief from, anxiety or emotional distress. Among the many mechanisms employed are conversion, denial, disassociation, identification, rationalization, repression, substitution, and sublimation.

defensive medicine: Medical practice characterized by the reliance of the physician on objective tests rather than on personal judgement alone in making decisions as to diagnosis and treatment; usually the purpose is to provide protection against possible legal action being brought by patients.

deferens (def'-er-ens): Vas deferens (*q.v.*).

defibrillation (dē-fib-ri-lā'-shun): The arrest of fibrillation of the cardiac muscle (atrial or ventricular), and restoration of normal rhythm. Usually refers to treatment by application of electric shock (cardioversion). — defibrillate, v.

defibrillator (dē-fib'-ri-lā-tor): 1. Any agent (*e.g.*, an electric shock) that interrupts ventricular fibrillation and restores normal rhythm. 2. An apparatus that administers electric shock used for defibrillation.

defibrinate (dē-fi'-brin-āt): To remove fibrin, particularly from blood or serum. — defibrinated, adj.; defibrination, n.

deficiency disease: Any disease resulting from a deficiency of essential nutrients, vitamins, or minerals in the diet, or an inability of the body to utilize any of these substances. Dehydration, diabetes mellitus, specific vitamin deficiencies, and deficiencies in potassium, calcium, magnesium, and iron intake are the most common of these disorders.

deflection (dē-flek'-shun): A turning aside or a state of being turned aside. D. OF THE NASAL SEPTUM displacement of one side of the bone separating the two nasal cavities, leading to discomfort; often corrected by surgery.

defluvium (dē-floo'-vi-um): 1. Falling out of the hair. 2. Falling out of the nails.

deformity (dē-form'-i-ti): Congenital or acquired malformation, disfigurement or distortion of the body or a part of it when the deviation from normal is apparent. GUNSTOCK D. deformity of the elbow caused by fracture of either condyle of the humerus; the forearm is displaced to one side; LOBSTER-CLAW D. congenital absence of all fingers except the first and fifth; bidactyly; MADELUNG'S D. congenital, accidental, or pathological dislocation of the lower end of the ulna with radial deviation of the hand; SPRENGEL'S D. a D. consisting of a congenitally high scapula and permanent elevation of the shoulder; often association with other deformities. [Otto G.K. Sprengel, German surgeon, 1852–1915.]

degeneracy (dē-jen'-er-a-si): A state of deterioration of physical and mental functioning, or of social behaviour, sexual behaviour in particular.

degeneration (dē-jen-er-ā'-shun): 1. Deterioration in quality or function. 2. Regression from more to less specialized type of tissue. AFFERENT D. degeneration spreading upwards along sensory nerves; AMYLOID D. a wax-like change in tissues; CASEOUS D. cheese-like tissue resulting from atrophy in a tuberculoma or gumma; COLLOID D. mucoid degeneration of tumours; CYSTOID D. OF THE RETINA a condition characterized by the formation of cystic spaces in the retina; FATTY D. characterized by the presence of droplets of fat in atrophic tissue, as in the myocardium; HYALINE D. said of connective tissue, especially of blood vessels, in which the tissue takes on a homogeneous or formless appearance; MACULAR D. pathological changes in the macula lutea that results in loss of central but not peripheral vision; may be hereditary or be caused by atherosclerosis, trauma, or senility; a leading cause of blindness in people over 60 years of age; SENILE D. the clinical picture of old age in which acuity of thought is blunted; SUBACUTE COMBINED D. a complication of untreated pernicious anaemia, starting with paraesthesia; WALLERIAN D., D. of a motor or sensory nerve fibre that has been cut off from its source of nutrition and is ultimately destroyed. — degenerative, adj.; degenerate, v.

degenerative (dē-jen'-er-a-tiv): Referring to progressive deterioration of cells, tissue, or a body part. D. DISEASE one in which loss of efficiency or function of an organ, structure, or tissue is gradual and progressive and usually non-reversible, *e.g.*, arteriosclerosis; D. JOINT DISEASE a chronic disorder of the joint cartilage, enlargement of the bone, and pain on activity; affects primarily the weight-bearing joints and the distal interphalangeal joints of the fingers, occurs chiefly in older people.

degradation (deg-ra-dā′-shun): The reduction of a chemical compound to a simpler one that has fewer carbon atoms.

degustation (dē-gus-tā′-shun): The act of tasting.

dehumanize (dē-hū′-man-īz): To deprive one of individuality, human qualities, and attributes.

dehydrate (dē-hī-drāt): To remove water from any substance, including the body.

dehydration (dē-hī-drā′-shun): Loss or removal of fluid. In the body, this condition arises when the fluid intake fails to replace fluid loss. This is liable to occur where there is bleeding, diarrhoea, excessive sweating, fever, polyuria, or vomiting, and usually upsets the body's electrolyte balance; may also cause tachycardia, impaired sensorium, and decreased intraocular pressure. If suitable fluid replacement cannot be achieved orally, parenteral administration is usually prescribed. HYPOTONIC D., D. in which, proportionally, the loss of electrolytes exceeds the loss of water; ISOTONIC D., D. in which there is a proportionate loss of water and electrolytes.

7-dehydrocholesterol (dē-hī-drō-ko-les′ ter-ol): A sterol found in the skin which forms vitamin D_3 when properly irradiated.

dehydrocorticosterone (de hī′-drō-kor-ti-kos′-ter-ōn): 11-dehydrocorticosterone, the chemical name for a steroid from the adrenal cortex; it has an effect on protein and carbohydrate metabolism.

dehydroepiandrosterone (dē-hī′-drō-ep-i-an-dros′-ter-ōn): An androgen (*q.v.*) occurring in normal urine; may also be synthesized from cholesterol.

dehydrogenase (dē-hī-droj′-en-ās): Any of a class of enzymes that activates or mobilizes a substance so that it gives up its hydrogen and transfers it to an acceptor other than oxygen.

dehydrogenate (dē-hī-droj′-en-āt): To remove hydrogen from a compound.

deinstitutionalization (dē-in-sti-tū′-shi-nal-ī-zā′-shun): Refers to the movement to place institutionalized persons in the community and provide the necessary supportive services; the goal is rehabilitation; the persons are usually disabled in some way.

deionize (dē-ī′-ō-nīz): The removal of ions from a fluid to produce a mineral-free substance.

déjà vu phenomenon (dā-zha voo′ fe-nom′-e-non): Intense feeling of familiarity as if something had been seen, or had happened, before.

dejection (dē-jek′-shun): **1.** Mental depression. **2.** Defecation (*q.v.*).

delactation (dē-lak-tā′-shun): **1.** Weaning. **2.** Cessation of the secretion of milk.

deLange's syndrome: See AMSTERDAM DWARFISM under DWARFISM.

delayed discharge: The postponement of a patient's release from hospital until a package of care or resources is available in the community or residential care sector to meet the patient's needs.

delegation (del-i-gā′-shun): **1.** A group of people chosen to represent or act on behalf of others. **2.** The act of giving of some power, responsibility or work to somebody else.

deleterious (del-e-tē′-ri-us): Hurtful, injurious, destructive, noxious, pernicious.

deliberate self-harm: Intentional damage to one's own body. Often (but not always) associated with mental illnesses, such as bipolar disorder or anorexia, and with a history of trauma and abuse, and with mental traits such as perfectionism. People who self-harm are not usually attempting suicide, but are trying to relieve emotional pressure. Self-harm is also very rarely attention-seeking behaviour. A common form of self-harm presents as shallow cuts to the skin of the arms or legs.

delimitation (dē-lim-i-tā′-shun): **1.** Setting limits or bounds. **2.** Preventing the spread of disease in an individual or in the community.

delinquency (dē-lin′-kwen-si): Unacceptable, anti-social behaviour which is sometimes in violation of the law, including such offences as theft, vandalism, and truancy. Used especially with reference to children or adolescents.

delinquent (dē-lin′-qwent): **1.** Failing or neglecting to do what the law and society require, committing offences, and behaving in an unacceptable manner; often refers to an adolescent. **2.** A person who behaves in an unacceptable anti-social, and, sometimes, illegal manner.

delipidation (dē-lip-i-dā′-shun): The removal of lipid by the use of fat solvents.

delirium (dē-lir′-i-um): A state of frenzy or uncontrollable excitement, characterized by disorientation, mental confusion, impulsive behaviour, incoherent speech; often accompanied by delusions and hallucinations. May be present in various forms of mental disease but more frequently seen in patients with high fever, a toxic condition, or injury; usually of short duration. D. TREMENS a violent form of delirium resulting from prolonged use of alcohol; the patient is confused, terrified, and restless; has a marked tremor and hallucinates; also called *mania à potu*. In psychiatry, a condition occurring in primary degenerative dementia of senile onset. — delirious, adj.

delouse (dē-lows'): To remove lice from or to destroy lice.

Delphi technique (del'-fī, del'-fi): A research method where the consensus of a group of experts is obtained by asking the contributors to rate a number of items in order of importance.

delta: The fourth of a series. D. WAVES see under WAVE.

deltoid (del'-toyd): Triangular. D. MUSCLE large shoulder muscle, the apex of which is inserted into the midshaft of the humerus; D. LIGAMENT the large ligament on the medial side of the ankle.

delusion (dē-lū'-zhun): A false fixed belief held only by the affected person, which cannot be altered by argument or appeal to reason; found as a psychotic symptom in several types of psychopathy, notably schizophrenia, paranoia, senile psychosis, mania, and the depressive states, including involutional melancholia. D. OF GRANDEUR megalomania (*q. v.*); D. OF GUILT, D. occurring in psychotic depressed persons; HYPOCHONDRIACAL D. D. of bodily disease in spite of no evidence; occurs in schizophrenic persons; NIHILISTIC D., D. Relating to nothingness; the person believes the world and everything in it, including himself, has ceased to exist; PARANOID D. the person wrongfully believes that someone or something wishes to do him harm; D. OF PERSECUTION the false notion that one is being wilfully persecuted by a particular person or group of persons; the patient is hostile, aggressive, suspicious; RELIGIOUS D. the patient thinks he hears voices that give direct commands from God; SOMATIC D. the fixed belief that one has an imaginary lesion or supposedly abnormally functioning organ; SYSTEMATIZED D. a D. in which the patient distorts the truth to justify his actions or reasoning.

delusional (dē-lū'-zhun-al): Relating to or characteristic of delusions. D. SPEECH excessive verbalization of delusions of grandeur or of persecution.

demand: 1. A clear and firm request that is difficult to ignore or deny. **2.** A customer interest in acquiring something; the level of desire or need that exists for particular goods or services. **3.** A need for resources or action; an urgent requirement for time, facilities, resources, or action.

demarcation (dē-mar-kā'-shun): **1.** A separation or distinction. **2.** An outlining of the junction of diseased and healthy tissue; often refers to the line formed at the edge of a gangrenous area.

demasculinization (dē-mas'-kū-lin-ī-zā'-shun): The loss or diminishment of normal masculine characteristics.

demedicalization (dē-med'-i-kal-ī-zā'-shun): **1.** The tendency in health-care programmes and activities to lessen the autonomy of the doctor–patient relationship by emphasizing the importance of a healthy lifestyle, elaborating codes of patients' rights, utilizing nurse practitioners, and de-emphasizing the sick role by referring to patients as clients or consumers. **2.** A trend in rehabilitation to remove disabled people from medical supervision after stabilization and to provide opportunities for them to be responsible for managing their own lives.

demented (di-ment'-ed): Insane; deprived of reason.

dementia (di-men'-shi-a): An organic mental disorder severe enough to prevent normal social and occupational functioning; deterioration of one's intellectual abilities along with alterations in one's memory, judgement, and personality. ARTERIOSCLEROTIC D., D. characterized by headache, dizziness, and confusion; runs a fluctuating course with steady intellectual decline; ATHEROSCLEROTIC D., D. resulting from changes in the blood supply to the brain cells; often accompanied by physical and neurologic disorders, impairment of the intellect, memory, and personality; D. PARALYTICA general paresis; see PARESIS; D. PRAECOX obsolete term for schizophrenia that develops during adolescence or early adult life; PRIMARY DEGENERATIVE D. SENILE ONSET (after age 65 and at or before age 65, formerly referred to as senile or presenile dementia); mental deterioration marked by loss of memory, disturbed sleep patterns, disorientation, delusions, preoccupation with death, and false notions of persecution; progresses to total lack of ability to deal with the environment; D. PUGILISTICA cerebral concussion resulting from repeated blows to the head as happens to professional boxers; MULTI-INFARCT D. a common form of D., resulting from a series of small strokes in the brain that destroy brain tissue. TOXIC D., D due to use of some toxic substance.

demineralization (dē-min'-er-al-ī-zā'-shun): The loss of mineral salts from the body, the bones in particular. See DECALCIFICATION.

demise (dē-mīs'): Death.

democracy (de-mok'-ra-si): A form of government in which the people, either directly or indirectly, take part in the running of their country. The word democracy originates from Greek, *demos* meaning 'the people', and *kratein* meaning 'to rule'.

demographic (dem-o-graf'-ik): **1.** A statistic characterizing human populations, or segments

demographic 173 dentinogenesis

of human populations broken down by age, sex or income, etc. 2. In marketing, a demographic comprises a market segment. Demographics often relate to age-bands, though social class and other categories may contribute towards the definition.

demography (dē-mog'-ra-fi): The study of mankind or of human populations, especially their size, density, geographic distribution, physical environments, and vital statistics, including birth and mortality rates, and sometimes morbidity rates. — demographic, adj.

demonomania (dē'-mon-ō-mā'-ni-a): The psychotic belief that one is possessed by devils.

demulcent (dē-mul'-sent): 1. Soothing; softening. 2. A slippery mucilaginous fluid that allays and soothes inflammation, especially of the mucous membranes.

demyelinate (dē-mi'-e-lin-āt): To remove or destroy the myelin sheath of a nerve or nerves. — demyelination, n , demyelinize, v.

dendriform (den'-dri-form): Tree-shaped or branch-like.

dendrite or dendron (den'-drit, den'-dron): One of the branched filaments that are given off from the body of a nerve cell; it is the part of the neuron that transmits impulses from the terminations of other neurons to the nerve cell body. — dendritic, adj.

dendritic (den-drit'-ik): Relating to or resembling a dendrite. D. ULCER a linear corneal ulcer that sends out tree-like branches; usually caused by herpes simplex.

denervation (dē-ner-vā'-shun): The act of depriving an area of its nerve supply. Usually refers to incision, excision, or blocking of a nerve. — denervate, adj.

dengue (den'-gā): An acute, epidemic, febrile disease that occurs sporadically in the tropical and subtropical parts of the world. The cause is an arbovirus transmitted by the *Aédes* mosquito. Characterized by headache, fever, rheumatic pains, sore throat, a spotty skin eruption. HAEMORRHAGIC D. a serious form of D. which affects primarily children; symptoms include prostration, respiratory distress, haemorrhage, circulatory collapse, and shock.

denial: 1. In psychology, a defence mechanism, usually unconscious, whereby a person does not admit that certain facts exist, or he avoids disagreeable realities in order to avoid pain, anxiety, or guilt feelings. 2. Refusal to perceive; often part of a normal phenomenon such as occurs in the fantasies of children at play.

denitrogenation (dē-nī'-trō-je-nā'-shun): The removal of dissolved nitrogen from the body,

by breathing nitrogen-free gas, a treatment to prevent the development of caisson disease (*q.v.*) or aeroembolism (*q.v.*).

de novo (de-nō'-vō): A Latin term meaning over again or anew.

dens: 1. A tooth. 2. The odontoid process of the axis that provides a pivot on which the atlas can rotate, thereby allowing for rotary movements of the head. — dentes, pl.

density (den'-si-ti): 1. The closeness of the particles in a substance. 2. The mass of a given substance per unit volume. 3. The number of inhabitants per unit of a given area.

dent-; denta-; dento-: Combining forms denoting relationship to a tooth or teeth.

dental (den'-tal): Relating to the teeth. D. ANAESTHESIA anaesthesia for dental operations; D. CARIES or CAVITIES disintegration of the substance of teeth; D. CALCULUS the deposit of mineral matter on the teeth; tartar; D. PLAQUE a thin deposit of mucoid material on the teeth; D. PROSTHESIS a substitute for natural teeth; D. PULP the vascular tissue in the pulp cavity and root canals of the teeth.

dental hygienist: A person educated and specially trained to provide such dental services as cleaning teeth, assisting dentists, and promoting dental health. The dental hygienist's training course lasts 9 to 12 months followed by an examination for the Certificate of Proficiency in Dental Hygiene. To practise the hygienist must register on the Roll of Dental. Hygienists maintained by the General Dental Council.

dental technician: A person who has had special training in the making of such dental appliances as bridges, dentures, crowns, etc.; may have taken an educational course or learned on the job.

dentate (den'-tāt): Having teeth or pointed, tooth-like projections.

dentia (den'-shi-a): 1. A condition relating to teeth and their development. 2. A word element relating to teeth. D. PRAECOX the presence of erupted teeth at birth, or the premature eruption of teeth; D. TARDA delay in eruption of teeth beyond the normal time for their appearance.

dentin, dentine (den'-tēn): The hard material, similar to bone, that makes up the chief substance of the teeth. It encloses the pulp cavity, is covered with enamel on the crown and cementum on the root of a tooth.

dentinogenesis (den'-ti-nō-jen'-e-sis): The formation of dentin. D. IMPERFECTA a hereditary condition in which teeth are small, the pulp cavity is lacking, and early wearing away of the crown and enamel destroys the teeth.

dentist (den´ -tist): A person trained for the practice of dentistry.

dentistry (den´ -tis-tri): The branch of medicine that is concerned with the prevention, diagnosis, and treatment of diseases of the teeth and surrounding tissues, and with restoring missing natural dental structures.

dentition (den-tish´ -un): 1. The process of teething. 2. The character and arrangement of an individual's teeth. PRIMARY D. eruption of the deciduous, milk or temporary teeth; SECONDARY D. eruption of the adult or permanent teeth.

dentoalveolar (den´ -tō-al-vē´ -ō-lar): Relating to the alveolus of a tooth or alveoli of the teeth. D. ABSCESS the formulation of an abscess around the root of a tooth.

denture (den´ -chur): A set of teeth. Term usually designates an artificial replacement of one, several or all of the natural teeth.

denude (di-nūd´): To remove a covering or to lay bare. — denudation, n.

Denver Articulation Screening Examination: An examination to discriminate between normal development in the acquisition of speech sounds and developmental delay; used for children 2½ to 6 years of age.

Denver Developmental Screening Test: A popular, reliable test for evaluating a child's development and for identifying delayed development in such areas as social adaptation, fine motor activities, and use of language; most useful in children between ages of one month and six years.

deodorant (de-ō´ -dōr-ant): Any substance that destroys or masks an (unpleasant) odour. — deodorize, v.

deodorizer (de-ō´ -dor-ī-zer): An agent that absorbs or neutralizes an odour. — deodorize, v.

deossification (dē-os-i-fi-kā´ -shun): Removal or reduction in the amount of mineral content of a bone or bones.

deoxidation (dē-ok-si-dā´ -shun): The removal of all or part of the oxygen from a compound. — deoxidize, v.

deoxy-; desoxy-: Prefixes denoting (1) loss or removal of oxygen from a compound, or (2) replacement of the OH group by a hydrogen atom.

deoxycorticosterone (dē-ok´ -si-kor-ti-kos´ -ter-ōn): A steroid substance produced in the adrenal cortex, concerned chiefly with metabolism and retention of salt and water, and with excretion of potassium; used in the treatment of adrenal insufficiency; also called *desoxycorticosterone* and *deoxycortone*.

deoxygenate (dē-ok´ -si-jen´ -āt): To deprive an organism of oxygen. To remove all or part of the oxygen from a compound. — deoxygenation, n.

deoxyhaemoglobin (dē-ok´ -si-hēm-ō-glō´ -bin): Haemoglobin that is not associated with oxygen.

deoxyribonuclease (dē-ok´ -si-rī-bō-nū´ -klē-ās): An enzyme that serves as a catalyst for the hydrolysis of deoxyribonucleic acid (DNA).

deoxyribonucleic acid (DNA) (dē-ok´ -si-rī-bō-nū-klē´ -ik as´ -id): A derivative of nucleic acid, DNA is found in the nuclei and protoplasm of animal cells, many plant cells, most bacterial cells, and many viruses; is the carrier of genetic information in living cells and considered to be the autoreproducing component of chromosomes; is required for the production of proteins and for cell reproduction. Genes are segments of the DNA molecules, which consist of two long chains of alternate sugar and phosphate groups joined together by bases and twisted into a double helix; see WATSON–CRICK HELIX under HELIX. Also spelled *desoxyribonucleic*.

Department of Health: A government department that is responsible for commissioning, managing, monitoring, and evaluating healthcare in England. Similar government departments perform this role in Scotland, Northern Ireland, and Wales .

Department of Social Security: A UK department of central government that supports the Secretary of State for Social Security in meeting the Minister's accountability to Parliament for social and welfare matters.

Department of Work and Pensions: A governmental organization in the UK, responsible for delivering support and advice through a network of services to people of working age, employers, pensioners, families and children, and disabled people. This is achieved through: Jobcentre Plus, helping people of working age to find work and get any benefits they are entitled to, and a service to employers to fill their vacancies; the Pension Service, providing services and support for pensioners and people looking into pensions and retirement; the Child Support Agency, administering the Child Support scheme; the Disability and Carers Service, delivering a range of benefits to disabled people and carers; the Appeals Service, providing an independent tribunal body for hearing appeals; and Debt Management, delivering debt management and recovery systems.

depend: 1. To hang or hang down. **2.** To rely, as for support. **3.** To be contingent to. — depend-ence, n.; dependent, adj.

dependence: CHEMICAL D. the need of body tissues for the continued use of any abused chemical substance, including drugs and alco-hol; if not satisfied regularly, withdrawal symptoms occur; CROSS D. a condition in which one drug causes dependence but its use can prevent the development of withdrawal symptoms from another, possibly more harm-ful drug; PHYSICAL D. chemical D.; PSYCHO-LOGICAL D. a condition marked by intense desire for the pleasurable effects of a drug which invariably leads to use of that drug.

dependency (dē-pen'-den-si): The state of being abnormally reliant on something that is psychologically or physically habit-forming; e.g., alcohol or narcotic drugs.

dependent variable: In a study of the cause and effect of one factor on another, the dependent variable is the effect, or outcome, being caused by a change in the other causal (inde-pendent) variable (q.v.).

depersonalization (dē-per'-sun-al-ĭ-zā'-shun): A subjective state in which the person loses his sense of reality and of his own personality, and may feel that he no longer exists; caused by partial or total disruption of the ego and self-concept; occurs in schizophrenia and sometimes in depressive states.

depigmentation (dē-pig-men-tā'-shun): Partial or complete loss of pigment. — depigmented, adj.

depilate (dep'-i-lāt): To remove hair from. — depilatory, adj.; depilation, n.

depilatories (di-pil'-a-tor-iz): Substances, usu-ally made in pastes (e.g., barium sulphide), which remove excess hair temporarily; they do not act on the papillae, consequently the hair grows again. See EPILATION.

deplete (dī-plēt'): **1.** To empty or deprive of a principal substance. **2.** To reduce the strength of a person or substance.

depletion (dī-plē'-shun): **1.** Withdrawal or re-moval of a body constituent, especially blood. **2.** An exhausted state, often referring to results of loss of blood. D. SYNDROME a condition resulting from loss of essential body constituents or from inadequate intake of protein and calories.

depolarization (dē-pō'-lar-ĭ-zā'-shun): The re-moval, destruction, or neutralization of the electrical polarity of a substance. In neuro-physiology, the tendency of the cell to become positively charged in relation to the substances surrounding the cell. — depolarize, adj.

deposit (di-poz'-it): **1.** Sediment; dregs; a pre-cipitate. **2.** Morbid particles of matter that have collected in a body tissue or cavity.

depot (de-pō'): A place in the body where a sub-stance, e.g., fat or drugs, can be stored and from which it can be released and distributed. D. INJECTION a deep muscular injection of a substance in a vehicle that tends to keep it at the site of injection, so that absorption occurs over a prolonged period; may be used, for example, in the administration of some psy-chotrophic drugs when clients fail to take their medication.

depraved (dē-prāvd): **1.** Deteriorated. **2.** Abnor-mal. — depravity, n.

depressant (di-pres'-ant): An agent that reduces or slows down the functional activity of an organ or system of the body; often refers to certain drugs.

depressed (di-prest'): **1.** Below the normal level. **2.** Refers to the condition of depression; see DE-PRESSION. D. FRACTURE a skull fracture in which the fractured part of the bone is depressed below the level of the other cranial bones.

depression (dē-presh'-un): **1.** A hollow place or an indentation, e.g., a fossa in a bone. **2.** Dimin-ution of power or activity, either mental or physical. **3.** A mood or feeling state character-ized by sadness, discouragement, and self-doubt that may occur at the loss, or possible loss of, a loved one or something valued; may be brought about by the actions or criticisms of others or failure to meet self-set goals. **4.** In psychiatry, depression states are now classified as neurotic disorders and categorized as major affective disorders, and further categorized as bipolar disorders that are identified as mixed, manic, or depressed, and as major depression, single episode or recurrent. Depression is con-sidered neurotic when the condition follows an event or situation that the individual can iden-tify, and psychotic when it is due to a traumatic situation that the individual can identify and is accompanied by severe functional impairment, including insomnia, anorexia, weight loss, im-potence, and often delusions. ANACLITIC D. occurs in young children often due to neglect; characterized by apathy, anorexia, frequent stools, progressive marasmus; sometimes fatal; INVOLUTIONAL D., D. occurring during menopause; ORGANIC D., D. associated with a physical disorder, usually one of the nervous system; REACTIVE D., see under REACTIVE.

depressive (dē-pres'-iv): **1.** Relating to depres-sion. **2.** Causing depression. D. NEUROSIS a dis-order in which the individual seeks relief, or partial relief, through depression and self-depreciation; D. PERSONALITY a type of personality characterized by low spirits, subservience, and vulnerability to disappointment D. STATE a mental disorder characterized by severe depression; D. STUPOR a condition characterized by muteness, unresponsiveness, retention of both urine and faeces for long periods, and possibly death from starvation.

depressor (dē-pres′-or): Anything that depresses a bodily activity or function. Applies to muscles, drugs, nerves, as well as instruments. TONGUE D. a spatula-like blade, usually of wood, used to hold the tongue down during examination of mouth and throat.

deprivation (dep-ri-vā′-shun): The loss, absence, removal or withholding of powers, or things that are needed. D. SYNDROME usually the result of parental rejection of offspring; may include malnutrition, dwarfism, pot-belly, gluttonous appetite, superficial attachment to any adult.

der-: A combining form denoting relationship to the neck.

derangement (dē-rānj′-ment): 1. Mental disorder. 2. A disturbance in the normal order or arrangement of a part or an organ.

derealization (dē-rē′-al-ī-zā′-shun): Feelings of unreality and detachment from one's surroundings, may occur simultaneously with depersonalization; a symptom often found in schizophrenic and depressive states.

derivative (dē-riv′-a-tiv): In chemistry, a chemical substance that is not original or fundamental, but which is derived from another substance.

derived (dē-rīvd′): Developed or formed from something else.

-derm: Combining form denoting (1) skin; (2) cutaneous.

derm-, derma-, dermat-, dermato-, dermo-: Combining forms denoting skin.

derma: The skin; specifically, the corium (*q.v.*). — dermic, dermal, adj.

-derma: Combining forms denoting: 1. Skin; integument. 2. An abnormal or pathological condition of the skin.

dermabrasion (der-ma-brā′-zhun): A surgical procedure for the removal of acne scars, tattoos, or naevi. Wire brushes, sandpaper or other abrasives are used.

dermafat (der′-ma-fat): The adipose content of the skin.

dermal (der′-mal): Relating to the skin, especially the true skin. D. GRAFT a skin graft utilizing a split or full thickness of dermis; D. SENSE recognition of the sensations of heat,

cold, pain, or pressure through stimulation of receptors in the skin.

dermatalgia (der-ma-tal′-ji-a): Localized pain in the skin with no lesion at the site of the pain; sometimes due to a nervous disorder. Syn., *dermatodynia, dermalgia.*

dermatitis (der-ma-tī′-tis): Inflammation of the skin, acute or chronic, and by custom limited to conditions that present with one or more of the following symptoms at some stage: itching, redness, blisters, crusting, scaling, oozing, fissuring, thickening, hardening, or abnormal pigmentation. ACTINIC D. caused by sunlight; not a sunburn; ATOPIC D. chronic eczematous D., usually affecting the face, antecubital, and popliteal areas; CONTACT D. caused by touching a substance to which the person is sensitive, *e.g.*, a chemical, cosmetic, or plant such as spurge or rue; Syn., *irritant D.* D. ARTEFACTA self-induced D., produced by heat, chemicals, or other means; D. DYSMENORRHOEICA, D. that occurs during the menstrual period, usually on the face; D. VENENATA contact D.; EXFOLIATIVE D., D. characterized by pink to deep red sin colour, intense itching, and desquamation; EXFOLIATIVE D. OF INFANCY a type of pemphigus; starts with a red patch or blister; D. HEIMALIS a recurrent eczema occurring in cold weather; winter itch; D. HERPETIFORMIS an intensely itchy skin eruption of unknown cause, most commonly characterized by vesicles, bullae, and pustules on urticarial plaques, which remit and relapse; when occurring in pregnancy it is known as *hydros gravida*; D. MEDICAMENTOSA skin eruption due to drugs taken internally; NUMMULAR D. a vesicular D. with coin-shaped patches, usually seen on the forearms and legs; OCCUPATIONAL D. occurs as a result of handling some sensitizing agent while at work; SEBORRHOEIC D. occurring in the areas where oil glands abound, *e.g.*, the face, scalp, pubis, around the anus; characterized by yellowish-grey oily scales; SECONDARY EXFOLIATIVE D., D. that may arise during treatment with certain drugs, *e.g.*, arsenic, gold, etc.; STASIS D. chronic inflammation of the skin of the legs; associated with vascular stasis in the lower extremities; TRAUMATIC D. due to exposure to irritating substances or physical agents; VARICOSE D. usually seen in the lower part of the leg; due to varicosities of the smaller veins; WEEPING D. an oozing D. that results from scratching to relieve itching; X-RAY D. due to exposure to x-rays. — dermatitides, pl.

dermato-autoplasty (der′-ma-tō-aw′-tō-plas-ti): The grafting to a denuded area of skin taken from some other part of the patient's own body.

dermatoglyphics (der-ma-tō-glif′-iks): The skin patterns or surface markings, especially those found on the palms of the hands and soles of the feet. They have been classified and are used as identification since they are unique to each individual and never change.

dermatoheteroplasty (der′-ma-tō-het′-er-ō-plas-ti): The grafting of skin taken from the body of another.

dermatologist (der′-ma-tol′-o-jist): A doctor who studies skin diseases and is skilled in their treatment. A skin specialist.

dermatology (der-ma-tol′-o-ji): The medical specialty which deals with the skin, its structure, functions, diseases and their treatment. — dermatological, adj.; dermatologically, adv.

dermatolysis (der-ma-tol′-i-sis): Abnormal looseness of the skin, usually congenital, causing it and the subcutaneous tissues to hang in folds. Also called *dermatomegaly*.

dermatome (der′-ma-tōm): 1. An instrument used in cutting a thin slice of skin, particularly for use in skin grafting. 2. An area of skin that is enervated by sensory fibres from a single spinal nerve. There is considerable overlapping of the contiguous dermatomes.

dermatopathy (der-ma-top′-a-thi): Any disease or disorder of the skin.

Dermatophagoides farinae: (der′-mat-ō-fag-oy′-dēz-fa′-ri-nē): The common household dust mite, which causes allergic reactions in sensitive individuals.

dermatophylaxis (der′-ma-tō-fi-lak′-sis): Protection of the skin against infection.

dermatophyte (der′-ma-tō-fīt): One of a group of fungi that invade the superficial skin causing such skin diseases as tinea pedis, eczema, and ringworm.

dermatophytosis (der′-ma-tō-fi-tō′-sis): An eruption caused by one of the dermatophytes (*q.v.*). Most commonly seen on the feet (athlete's foot). Characterized by itching, small vesicles, fissures and scaling. See TINEA PEDIS.

dermatoplasty (der′-ma-tō-plas′-ti): Plastic repair of the skin; skin grafting.

dermatosis (der′-ma-tō′-sis): Generic term for skin disease. — dermatoses, pl.

dermatrophia (der-ma-trō′-fi-a): Atrophy of the skin.

-dermia: Combining form denoting a skin condition.

dermis (der′-mis): The true skin; the cutis vera; the layer below the epidermis. — Syn., *corium*.

dermitis (der-mī′-tis): Dermatitis (*q.v.*).

dermoid (der′-moyd): Relating to or resembling skin and/or its related tissues. D. CYST a benign teratoma (*q.v.*); when it occurs in the ovary it may contain sebaceous fluid, hair, and sometimes, teeth and bone; is usually unilateral and seen mostly in women between 20 and 35 years of age.

DES: Abbreviation for diethylstilboestrol (*q.v.*).

desalination (dē′-sal-i-nā′-shun): The process of removing salt from a substance.

desaturation (dē-sat′-ū-rā′-shun): The process of converting a saturated substance into an unsaturated one by the removal of hydrogen.

descending (di-sen′ ding): Directed or extending downward. D. AORTA the part of the aorta between the distal end of the arch and the bifurcation into the iliac arteries; D. COLON the part of the colon between the splenic flexure and the sigmoid colon; D. NEURITIS weakness or paralysis of muscles, beginning at the shoulder and spreading downwards towards the hands and feet; D. TRACT a collection of nerve fibres that conduct impulses down the spinal cord.

desensitization (dē-sen′-si-tī-zā′-shun): The neutralization or lessening of acquired hypersensitiveness to some agent acting on the skin or internally. Used in asthma and for treatment of people who have become allergic to drugs such as penicillin and streptomycin. The process usually consists of giving small, repeated doses of the protein to which the person is sensitive. SYSTEMATIC D. in psychiatry, a procedure in behavioural therapy whereby the patient is repeatedly exposed to scenes depicting an anxiety-causing situation while relaxing the deep muscles, with the expectation that the real-life situation will no longer produce an anxiety reaction.

desensitize (dē-sen′-si-tīz): 1. To render a person insensitive to an antigen by the administration of a series of small, steadily increasing doses of a particular allergen. 2. To deprive a person of sensation by nerve block with an anaesthetic drug or by sectioning a particular nerve. 3. In psychiatry, to relieve or remove a person's phobia by frequent exposure to the stressful situation or by repeated discussions of it. — desensitization, n.

desexualize (dē-seks′-ū-a-līz): To castrate.

desiccant (des′-i-kant): Promoting dryness of a substance by absorbing or expelling water from it, or an agent that does this.

desiccate (des' -i-kāt): To dry out thoroughly. — desiccation, n.

-desis: Combining form denoting binding or fusing.

desoxycorticosterone (des-ok' -si-kor-ti-kos' -ter-ōn): deoxycorticosterone (q.v.).

desoxyribonucleic acid: Deoxyribonucleic acid (q.v.).

desquamation (des-kwa-mā' -shun): Shedding or flaking off, usually referring to the normal shedding of the superficial layer of the skin. Commonly increased after diseases attended by a rash, e.g., scarlet fever, measles. — desquamate, v.; desquamative, adj.

detachment (dē-tach' -ment): D. OF THE RETINA the separation of the inner, neural layer of the retina from the pigment layer. Retinal detachment.

detergent (di-ter' -jent): A purifying or cleansing agent resembling soaps in its ability to emulsify oils and hold them in suspension, but differing in chemical composition.

deteriorioration (di-ter-i-ō-rā' -shun): The state of being worse or process of becoming worse. — deteriorate, v.

determinant of health (di-ter' -mi-nant): A factor that has a direct relationship with the well-being of an individual or population; e.g., age, sex, gender, culture, social class, access to health services, unemployment, work conditions, level of education, living conditions, genetic inheritance, economics, and personal lifestyle.

determinism (di-ter' -min-izm): In psychiatry, the concept that all emotional and mental life is determined by pre-existing conditions or forces outside of one's control, that one has no freedom of choice, and that the individual is incapable of purposeful, self-generated action.

detoxication (dē-tok-si-kā' -shun): The process of removing the poisonous property of a substance. — detoxicant, adj., n.; detoxicate, v.

detoxification (dē-toks' -i-fi-kā' -shun): A major mode of medical treatment by which the effects of a drug are lessened in victims of overdosage or in addicts. D. UNIT a unit in a healthcare facility that provides for medically supervised withdrawal from addiction to alcohol or other drugs. — detoxify, v.

detrition (dē-trish' -un): A wearing off or away by friction, rubbing, or use.

detritus (dē-trī' -tus): Organic or non-organic matter produced by detrition, or waste matter resulting from disintegration or wearing away of tissues.

detrusor (dē-troo' -ser): Term applied to any part of the body that pushes downward. D. URINAE the external longitudinal layer of muscle of the urinary bladder that contracts to empty the bladder.

detubation (dē-tū-bā' -shun): The withdrawal of a tube. — detubate, v.

deuteranopia (dū' -ter-a-nō' -pi-a): Colour blindness in which red and green are incorrectly perceived, green in particular. — deuteranopic, adj.

deutero-: Combining form denoting second.

devascularize (dē-vas' -kū-lar-īz): To remove the blood supply to an area by destroying, obstructing, or removing the blood vessel(s). — devascularization, n.

development: In human biology, the gradual growth and maturation of the body systems, of adaptability to the environment, and of creative expression — developmental, adj.

developmental: Relating to development. D. AGE an individual's age as estimated from the degree of anatomical development; D. AGRAPHIA delayed development in learning to write; D. ALEXIA delayed development in learning to read; D. APHASIA delayed development in learning to speak; D. DYSLEXIA greater than normal difficulty of the school-age child in learning to read; D. QUOTIENT the score derived by dividing the child's mental age (as measured by the Gesell Development Schedule) by his chronological age, and multiplying by 100, abbreviated DQ.; D. TASKS the knowledge and skills that an individual needs to learn at different stages throughout the ageing process.

deviancy (dēv' -i-an-si): Variation from the norm in quality, state, or behaviour.

deviant (dē-vi-ant): 1. Varying from an accepted normal standard. 2. Something that differs from what is considered normal, especially a person whose behaviour or characteristics vary from what is acceptable in the group to which he or she belongs.

deviate (dē' -vi-āt): 1. To vary from the norm or from the accepted standard. 2. A person whose attitude and behaviour differ from the norm or from the accepted social and moral standard. 3. A sexual pervert.

deviation (dē-vi-ā' -shun): 1. A departure from normal. 2. Failure to conform to normal standards. In optics, strabismus (q.v.).

device (di-vīs'): Something contrived or constructed for a particular purpose or use. CONTRACEPTIVE D. one used to prevent conception; INTRAUTERINE D. a D. that is inserted into the uterus to prevent conception by preventing implantation of a fertilized ovum.

devitalize (de-vī' -tal-īz): To destroy or deprive of life, vitality, force, effectiveness. In dentistry, to destroy the pulp and nerve supply of a tooth. — devitalization, n.

devolution (dev' -ō-lū' -shun): 1. Catabolism; degeneration; the opposite of evolution. 2. Transfer or delegation of authority from central to regional government; for example, the devolution of power from the central government in Westminster to assemblies in Wales, Scotland, and Northern Ireland.

dexamethasone (dek-sa-meth' -a-sōn): A synthetic substance resembling cortisol in biological action; used in medicine as an anti-inflammatory agent.

dexter (deks' -ter): Related to or situated on the right. In anatomy, on the right-hand side.

dextr-, dextro-: Combining forms denoting the right, or towards the right side.

dextrad (deks' -trad): Toward the right.

dextrality (deks-tral' -i-ti): The voluntary preferential use of the right one of the paired organs of the body, as the eye or hand.

dextran (deks' -tran): A blood plasma substitute or expander obtained from the action of a specific bacterium (*Leuconostoc mesenteroides*) on sucrose; available in several preparations. Used in treatment of shock, severe burns, haemorrhage, hypovolaemia, hydration, and certain kidney diseases.

dextrimaltose (deks' -tri-mal' -tōs): A sugar preparation used in infant formulas; contains maltose and dextrin.

dextrin (deks' -trin): A soluble polysaccharide formed during the hydrolysis of starch.

dextropedal (deks-trop' -e-dal): Preferential use of the right leg and foot.

dextroposition (deks' -trō-pō-zish' -un): Displacement to the right. D. OF THE HEART displacement of the heart into the right half of the thorax.

dextrose (deks' -trōs): 1. Glucose (*q.v.*); a soluble, readily absorbed and utilized carbohydrate (monosaccharide); may be given by almost any route; widely used by intravenous infusion in dehydration, shock, and postoperatively. Also given orally as a readily absorbed sugar in acidosis and other nutritional disturbances. 2. The end product of carbohydrate digestion.

dextrosinistral (deks' -trō-sin' -is-tral): Extending from right to left. Also descriptive of a person who is left-handed but has trained himself to use the right hand for certain performances, *e.g.*, writing.

dextroversion (deks' -trō-ver' -zhun): A moving or turning to the right, as of the eyes.

dhobie itch (dō'bi): *Tinea cruris*; a fungal infection of the skin of the groin and inner thigh, seen most often in the obese and in warm climates; a type found in the laundrymen of India is thought to be caused by a laundry-marking ink made from the cashew nut. See TINEA.

di-: A prefix denoting two; twice; double.

DI: Abbreviation for donor insemination (*q.v.*).

dia-: A prefix denoting between, apart, across, through, completely.

diabetes (dī-a-bē' -tēz): Any of a group of metabolic disorders marked by the excessive secretion and excretion of urine and excessive thirst; when used without qualification it means D. MELLITUS. BRITTLE D., D. that is difficult to control because of alternating episodes of hyperglycaemia and hypoglycaemia; also called *unstable D.* or *labile D.*; BRONZE D., D. that also involves the liver; the skin is deeply pigmented D. INNOCENS a condition marked by glycosuria that is not associated with pancreatic disease; D. INSIPIDUS a disease caused by inadequate secretion of antidiuretic hormone by the pituitary gland; may be congenital or follow injury or infection; characterized by dehydration, polydipsia, and polyuria; D. MELLITUS a chronic disorder characterized by faulty carbohydrate metabolism, due mainly to a relative or absolute lack of effective insulin, which results in alterations in the metabolism of fats and proteins; the urine is pale and of high specific gravity because of its sugar content. Other features include dehydration, polydipsia, polyuria, weight loss, lassitude, retinopathy, neuropathy, nephropathy, lowered resistance to infection, decreased ability of wounds to heal and vascular abnormalities; in more advanced cases there is coma and ketosis. Sometimes leads to accelerated atherosclerosis affecting particularly the blood vessels of the eye, kidneys, and nerves see Type 1 D., Type 2 D.; DRUG-INDUCED D., D. caused by certain chemicals that may have a cytotoxic effect on the beta cells of the pancreas or may antagonize insulin and thus increase hyperglycaemia; GESTATIONAL D., D. that occurs during pregnancy; LIPOTROPHIC D., D. characterized by deficient storage of fat in the body; NEUROGENOUS D. D. that occurs in association with certain brain lesions; SECONDARY D. D. that is secondary to disease of the pancreas, liver, or any of several other organs; STARVATION D. glycosuria following ingestion of glucose after prolonged fasting; attributed to a reduced ability to form glycogen; SUBCLINICAL D., D. in which the glucose tolerance test is abnormal but the patient has no other clinical signs of diabetes; TYPE I (INSULIN-DEPEND-ENT, KETOSIS-PRONE) D., D. that develops before the age of 16 (formerly called juvenile-onset D.); symptoms are more severe than in D.; TYPE 2 NON-INSULIN-DEPENDENT, KETONE RESIST-ANT D., D. that usually occurs in obese individuals over 40 years of age; they have a variable but less than normal amount of plasma insulin, and their D. can often be controlled by diet alone or by an oral hypoglycaemic drug; formerly called *adult-onset D.*

diabetic (dī-a-bet′ -ik): 1. Relating to diabetes. 2. An individual suffering from diabetes. D. ACID-OSIS caused by an excess of ketone bodies in the blood; signs include thirst, air hunger, weakness, headache, coma. D. CATARACT see CATARACT; D. COMA see COMA; D. DIET a diet that consists of calculated amounts of protein, carbohydrates, and fats, with sugar restricted; D. GANGRENE that occurring in diabetic patients, often following an injury. See GAN-GRENE; D. IDENTIFICATION CARD one carried by diabetics; lists patient's and doctor's names, addresses, and telephone numbers, states the kind and amount of insulin the patient is receiving, and directions for treatment should the person become ill when in a public place; D. KETOACIDOSIS see KETOACIDOSIS; D. RETINO-PATHY see RETINOPATHY.

diabetogenic (dī-a-bet′ -ō-jen′ -ik): Causing diabetes.

diabetogenous (dī-a-be-toj′ -e-nus): Caused by diabetes.

diaceturia (dī-as-e-tū′ -ī-a): The presence of diacetic (acetoacetic) acid in the urine.

diacetylmorphine (dī-a-se′ -til-mor′ -fen): Heroin.

diagnose (dī′ -ag-nōs): To recognize the distinctive signs and symptoms of a disease or disorder. Experienced practitioners use three main methods, or a combination, in making a diagnosis; these are the hypothetico-deductive approach, pattern recognition, and signs and symptoms.

diagnosis (dī-ag-nō′ -sis): The name of a disease or condition that distinguishes it from other diseases or conditions. CLINICAL D., D. based on physical examination, and the patient's history; does not include laboratory tests; DIFFER-ENTIAL D., D. made after comparing the symptoms with two or more diseases; LABORA-TORY D., D. arrived at after laboratory study of specimens taken from the patient; POST-MOR-TEM D., D. based on findings at autopsy; SERO-LOGICAL D., D. based on laboratory study of the patient's blood serum; TENTATIVE D. one

judged by apparent symptoms and facts pending further study and examination. — diagnoses, pl.; diagnose, v.; diagnostic, adj.

Diagnosis and Treatment Centres: Institutions in the UK where routine hospital operations are dealt with separately from emergency treatment, to ensure that non-emergency patients are provided rapidly with the diagnostic procedures and operations that they need. These centres, financed in partnership with the private sector, are contributing to the large-scale capacity increase required in the NHS.

Diagnosis Related Groups: A cost control system used in the USA in which patients are categorized as to age and diagnosis or surgical procedure, according to 467 different groupings; used in estimating how much each patient in a DRG may be expected to cost the hospital in service by anticipating the amount of service the patient may require and the length of hospital stay. It allows hospitals that are reimbursed by Medicare insurance to collect in advance for services and improves their cash flow. If the length of the hospital stay is shorter than the DRG estimate, the hospital makes a profit; if the stay is longer than the DRG estimate, the hospital suffers a loss.

diagnostic (dī-ag-nos′ -tik): 1. Relating to diagnosis. 2. Serving as evidence in diagnosis. — diagnostician, n.

dialectical behavioural therapy (dī-a-lek′ -ti-kal): A specific type of cognitive behavioural therapy (*q.v.*) which includes skills training and exposure to emotional cues, found to be particularly effective in treating those with self-harming behaviour. It is delivered according to a manual to ensure adherence to effective interventions.

dialysance (dī-al′ -i-sans): A measure of the rate of exchange that takes place between the blood and the bath fluid in haemodialysis or peritoneal dialysis, in a certain time period, usually one minute.

dialysate (dī-al′ -i-sāt): 1. The fluid used in dialysis. 2. The part of the liquid that passes through a dialysing membrane in dialysis. D. BATH the isotonic solution used in dialysis; contains almost all of the ions found in the blood and that diffuse across the semi-permeable membrane and are needed to establish normal blood levels.

dialysis (dī-al′ -i-sis): The separation of certain substances in solution by taking advantage of their differing diffusibility through a porous membrane to remove metabolic waste products, poisons, toxins, drugs taken in overdose, or to correct electrolyte imbalance. CONTINUOUS AMBULATORY PERITONEAL D. takes place inside the body using the peritoneum, which acts as the D. membrane; this allows the procedure to be done at home, usually 4 times every day, taking less than 30 minutes each time, enabling the individual to take responsibility for his or her own care; EXTRACORPOREAL D., D. that utilizes the artificial kidney; see HAEMODIALYSIS; PERITONEAL D. a method of irrigating the peritoneum by continuously or intermittently infusing dialysing fluid into the peritoneal cavity by a soft peritoneal catheter, where it remains for a preset period of time, during which an exchange takes place between the dialysing fluid and the body fluids containing waste products of metabolism; the fluid is then withdrawn into a collecting bag.

dialysis disequilibrium syndrome: A condition occurring usually one to two hours after the start of dialysis; characterized by nausea, vomiting, mental confusion including hallucinations, and sometimes convulsions.

dialyser (dī′-a-līz-ɐr): The apparatus used in performing dialysis, or the membrane in the apparatus.

diameter (dī-am′-e-ter): In anatomy, a straight line between two opposite points of a structure that is more or less spherical or cylindrical in shape, e.g., the cranium and the bony pelvis.

Diana children's community nursing team: Groups of health-care professions who support parents and children with life threatening or severely disabling conditions, such as cancer, cystic fibrosis, AIDS and progressive, degenerative conditions, at home. The teams include children's nurses experienced in community care, GPs, paediatricians, psychologists, trained counsellors and other support staff. Set up in memory of Diana, Princess of Wales.

diapedesis (dī′-a-pe-dē′-sis): The passage of blood cells through the unbroken vessel walls into the tissues, usually refers to passage of white cells through capillary walls in response to infection or injury. — diapedetic, adj.

diaphoresis (dī′-a-fo-rē′-sis): Perspiration, particularly that which is excessive; may be associated with muscular activity, stress, use of certain drugs, exposure to heat, fever.

diaphoretic (dī′-a-fo-ret′-ik): **1.** An agent that induces diaphoresis; a sudorific. **2.** Relating to diaphoresis.

diaphragm (dī′-a-fram): **1.** The dome-shaped musculomembranous partition between the thorax above and the abdomen below; the chief muscle of respiration. **2.** Any partitioning membrane, such as that used in dialysis. **3.** A saucer-like contraceptive rubber cap with a spring that fits over and occludes the cervix.

diaphragmatic (dī′-a-frag-mat′-ik): Relating to the diaphragm. D. BREATHING see under BREATHING; D. FLUTTER rapid rhythmic contractions of the diaphragm which may simulate cardiac pain, D. HERNIA see under HERNIA.

diaphragmatocele (dī′-a-frag-mat′-ō-sēl): Hernia through the diaphragm.

diaphysis (dī-af′-i-sis): The shaft of a long bone. — diaphyses, pl.; diaphyseal, adj.

diarrhoea (dī-a-rē′-a): Loose or watery and frequent evacuation of stools, with or without discomfort. BACTERIAL D. caused by contaminated food; CHRONIC D. often associated with diverticulosis, colitis, and cancer of the colon; DIETETIC D. due to overindulgence in laxative foods; EPIDEMIC D., D. of the newborn, a highly contagious infection seen in maternity hospitals; FOOD POISONING D. a serious condition caused by food contaminated with bacterial toxins, especially those of the *Salmonella* group; SUMMER D. occurs chiefly in children in exceptionally hot weather; TRAVELLERS' D. occurs commonly in travellers in tropical or subtropical areas particularly; often thought to be due to imperfect sanitation and caused by *Escherichia coli*.

diarthric (dī-ar′-thrik): Relating to two joints or affecting two joints at the same time.

diarthrosis (dī-ar-thrō′-sis): A synovial, freely movable joint, such as the hip joint. — diarthrodial, adj.; diarthroses, pl.

diastalsis (dī-a-stal′-sis): The downwards moving wave of contraction in the small intestine during digestion. — diastaltic, adj.

diastasis (dī-as′-ta-sis): **1.** A separation of bones without fracture; dislocation. **2.** The separation of epiphysis from the body of a bone. D. RECTI ABDOMINIS separation of the rectus abdominalis at the midline; results from weakening of the supporting tissues, usually as a result of pregnancy or surgery.

diastematomyelia (dī-a-stē′-ma-tō-mī-ē′-li-a): A congenital condition in which the spinal cord is split into halves separated by a fibrous band; each half has its own dural sac; occurs most often in spina bifida (*q.v.*).

diastole (dī-as′-tō-li): The normal relaxation period of the cardiac cycle, when the heart rests, the muscle fibres lengthen, and the respective chambers fill with blood. Alternates with systole (*q.v.*).

diastolic (dī-a-stol'-ik): Relating to the diastole. D. MURMUR an abnormal sound heard during diastole; occurs in valvular diseases of the heart; D. PRESSURE the blood pressure during the relaxation phase of the cardiac cycle; it is the lowest pressure reached during any ventricular cycle.

diathermy (dī'-a-ther-mi): The passage of a high-frequency electric current through the tissues whereby heat is produced. When both electrodes are large, the heat is diffused over a wide area according to the electrical resistance of the tissues. In this form it is widely used in the treatment of inflammation, especially when deeply seated (e.g., sinusitis, pelvic cellulitis). When one electrode is very small the heat is concentrated in this area and becomes great enough to destroy tissue. In this form (surgical diathermy) it is used to stop bleeding during surgery by coagulation of blood, or to cut through tissue in operations for malignant disease.

diathesis (dī-ath'-e-sis): An inherited predisposition or combination of attributes that makes a person susceptible to certain diseases or classes of diseases. HAEMORRHAGIC D. bleeding D.; a predisposition to spontaneous haemorrhage.

DIC: Abbreviation for disseminated intravascular coagulation, see under DISSEMINATED.

dichorionic (dī-kō-ri-on'-ik): Having two chorions (q.v.). D. TWINS twins having separate chorions.

dichotomy (dī-kot'-o-mi): A division into two parts, classes, or groups that are normally mutually contradictory or exclusive. — dichotomization, n.; dichotomous, adj.

dichromatopsia (dī'-krō-ma-top'-si-a): Colour blindness in which the individual is able to recognize and distinguish only two of the three primary colours red, blue, and green; either the red–green or the blue–yellow system is lacking, the first type being relatively common and the second being the rarest of all types of colour blindness.

dichromophil (dī-krō'-mō-fil): Relating to a cell or tissue that takes both a basic and acidic stain.

dicophane (dī'-kō-fān): Chlorophenothane, a well-known highly toxic insecticide formerly sometimes used against pediculosis capitis and other body parasites as a lotion or dusting powder.

dicrotic (dī-krot'-ik): Relating to, or having a double beat, as indicated by a second expansion of the artery during diastole. D. PULSE a small wave of distension of the blood vessel after the normal beat; D. WAVE the second rise in the tracing of a dicrotic pulse.

didactylism (dī-dak'-til-izm): The congenital condition of having only two fingers on one hand or two toes on one foot; bidactyly.

didymitis (did-i-mī'-tis): Inflammation of a testis; orchitis.

didymous (did'-i-mus): Growing or arranged in a pair or pairs.

-didymus (did'-i-mus): A combining form meaning (1) a testis, or (2) a conjoined pair of twins with the first element of the word designating the part of the bodies that is not fused.

diencephalon (dī-en-kef'-a-lon, sef'-): That part of the forebrain or cerebrum lying between the telencephalon and the mesencephalon; contains the thalamus, hypothalamus, and the greater part of the third ventricle.

diesterase (dī-es'-ter-ās): An enzyme such as nuclease which acts to split the bonds binding the nucleotides (q.v.) in nucleic acid.

diet: 1. The food normally consumed in the course of living. 2. A prescription of food that is required by or permitted for a patient. 3. To eat only simple, easily digested food in limited quantities. ACID-ASH D. a D. that yields an acidic residue; may be prescribed to help prevent the formation of urinary calculi; consists of cereals, fish, eggs, and meat, with restrictions on fruit and vegetables and the elimination of milk and cheese; BALANCED D. one that contains all the elements in the correct quantities needed for growth and repair of body tissues; BLAND D. one that contains no stimulating or irritating foods; DIABETIC D. one adapted to the needs of a diabetic patient; contains weighed amounts of fats, carbohydrates, and proteins; FULL LIQUID DIET consists of only liquids, but includes ice cream and cream soups; HIGH CALORIC D. one that provides 4000 or more calories per day; KETOGENIC D. one high in fat, low in protein and carbohydrate; LIGHT D. one suitable for a person taking little exercise, e.g., a bed patient or convalescent; includes foods from the Basic Four group (q.v.), but excludes foods that are difficult to digest and those that are fried, highly seasoned, or spicy; LOW CALORIE D. one that provides 1000 calories or less per day; LOW FAT DIET, one low in fat; antiketogenic D.; LOW PROTEIN D., one containing the minimum amount of protein; LOW RESIDUE D., one low in cellulose and fibre; prescribed in certain bowel disorders; LOW SALT D., one low in sodium, often used in treatment of oedema, hypertension, congestive heart disease; MACROBIOTIC D. see under MACROBIOTIC; NEPHRITIC D. one low in nitrogen content and eliminating spices, alcohol, and condiments; RICE D. a low fat, low salt, low cholesterol D. consisting of rice and fruit supplemented with vitamins and iron; used in treatment of arterial hypertension and chronic kidney disease; SIPPY D. a dietary regimen for treatment of peptic ulcer. The objective is to neutralize the hydrochloric acid in the stomach by frequent feedings; starting with milk and cream only and gradually adding bland foods as the symptoms subside until finally the patient is able to take a normal diet; SOFT DIET one consisting of milk, eggs, custard, mashed potatoes, ice cream, or other non-irritating easily digested foods; VEGETARIAN D. one in which all flesh foods are eliminated in favour of vegetables, cereals and dairy products. — dietary, dietetic, adj.

dietetics (die-tet´-iks): The interpretation and application of the scientific principles of nutrition to feeding in health and disease.

diethylstilboestrol (di-eth´-il-stil-bes´-trol): A synthetic oestrogenic substance used therapeutically as a substitute for natural oestrogenic hormones. Should not be used during pregnancy since there have been instances of daughters of women who took DES during pregnancy developing cancer of the cervix.

dietitian (di-e-tish´-un): One who applies the principles of nutrition to the feeding of an individual, or a group of individuals in various settings, *e.g.*, hospitals, institutions, schools, restaurants, hotels, etc. STATE REGISTERED D. a dietitian who has undertaken a recognized form of training leading to a degree in nutrition or a graduate in a relevant subject who has undertaken a postgraduate course in dietetics. State Registration is obtained by application to the Council for Professions Supplementary to Medicine; THERAPEUTIC D. one involved in treatment of patients through modification of their diet.

Dietl's crisis: Acute obstruction of a kidney causing severe pain in the loins. The obstruction usually occurs in the region of the renal pelvis causing the kidney to become distended with urine.

differential (dif-fer-en´-shul): Related to or constituting a difference. D. BLOOD COUNT the estimation of the relative proportions of the different leukocyte cells in the blood, with the normal differential count being (1) granular leukocytes; eosinophils, 1–4%, basophils, 1–4%, and neutrophils, 51–67%; and (2) non-

granular leukocytes; lymphocytes, 25–33%, monocytes, 2–6%; D. DIAGNOSIS diagnosis based on comparison of the symptoms of diseases that have similar manifestations, and evaluating the signs and symptoms that are dissimilar; D. FORGETTING selective forgetting, especially the faster forgetting of erroneous responses than of correct ones; D. STAIN a stain used to differentiate bacteria; see GRAM'S STAIN.

diffusate (di-fu´-zat): Material that passes through or has passed through a membrane; dialysate (*q.v.*).

diffuse (di-fuz): 1. To pour out, extend, or scatter. 2. To spread out or disperse. 3. (di-fus) Scattered or spread throughout a substance or an area; not localized or limited.

diffusion (di-fu´-zhun): The process of homogenization whereby liquids, solutions, gases, and some solids intermingle when brought into contact, with the molecules from an area of higher concentration moving to an area of lower concentration until the two substances are of equal density. — diffuse, v. See DIALYSIS.

digest (di-jest´): In physiology, to change food by mechanical and chemical processes, in the mouth, stomach and intestines, so that it can be absorbed by the body.

digesta (di-jes´-ta): The contents of the stomach and intestine in the process of being digested.

digestant (di-jest´-ant): An agent that aids in digestion of food.

digestion (di-jest´-yun): The mechanical and chemical process by which food is broken down in the gastrointestinal tract and rendered absorbable. — digestible, digestive, adj.; digestibility, n.; digest, v.

digestive (di-jes´-tiv): Relating to digestion. D. SYSTEM the organs associated with the ingestion and digestion of food; includes the mouth and associated structures, pharynx, oesophagus, stomach, small and large intestine, and associated glands; also called *alimentary system; digestive canal*, or *tract*. D. TUBE alimentary T., see under ALIMENTARY.

digit (dij´-it): In anatomy, a finger or toe. — digital, adj.

digital (dij´-i-tal): 1. Using the fingers, or operated by a finger or fingers. 2. Processing, operating on, storing, transmitting, representing, or displaying data in the form of numerical digits, as in a computer; most commonly, this means binary data represented using electronic or electromagnetic signals.

digitalis (dij-i-tal´-is): A drug prepared from the leaf of the common foxglove plant, which is the source of a large group of drugs used exclusively in cardiac conditions to strengthen and slow the heartbeat. Especially useful in auricular fibrillation and congestive heart failure. *Digitalis purpurea* furnishes the glycosides digitalin and digitoxin while *Digitalis lanata* furnishes digoxin. These drugs have a cumulative effect.

digitoplantar (dij-i-tō-plan′-tar): Relating to the toes and the sole of the foot.

digitoxin (dij-i-toks′-in): A cardiotonic glucoside that comes from several species of *Digitalis*; has an action similar to that of digitalis; useful in treatment of congestive heart failure.

digitus (dij′-i-tus): Digit; a finger or toe. D. FLEXUS hammertoe (*q.v.*). — digiti, pl.

dilatation (dil-a-tā′-shun): The condition of being stretched or enlarged. May occur physiologically, pathologically, or be induced artificially. — dilate, v.; dilation, n.

dilatation and curettage: Dilatation of the cervix and scraping of the lining of the uterus. Done to remove any remaining contents of the uterus after abortion, to obtain material for histological examination or diagnosis, for treatment, or when radon or radium seeds are to be implanted.

dilatation and evacuation: An operation to remove the products of conception; the cervix is dilated and the uterus curetted by suction or other method of curettage.

dilate (dī′-lāt): To expand or enlarge.

dilation (dī-lā′-shun): The act of dilating or stretching of an orifice or cavity of the body.

dilator (dī′-lā-tor): Anything that dilates or stretches an opening or canal or a part of the body, *e.g.*, a muscle, drug or instrument, or other device.

diluent (dil-ū′-ent): A diluting or dissolving agent.

dilute (dī-lūt′): 1. To make weaker or thinner by the addition of liquid. 2. Descriptive of a solution that has been weakened or thinned, thereby lessening its potency.

dilution (dī-lū′-shun): 1. The state of being diluted. 2. A solution that has been made weaker or thinner.

dimorphism (dī-mor′-fizm): The condition of having, or of existing in, two different forms. SEXUAL D. the condition of having some of the characteristics of both sexes.

dimorphous (dī-morf′-us): Having the quality of existing in two distinct forms.

dimple (dim′-p′l): A slight depression in bone or other body tissue. — dimpling, n.

dimpling (dim′-pling): A depression in the skin caused by retraction; occurs in subcutaneous tumours, especially in those of the breast. May also occur at sites of repeated insulin injection.

Diogenes syndrome (dī-oj′-i-nēz): A condition characterized by a grossly abnormal lifestyle; the person, usually elderly, lives in filthy surroundings, sometimes with many animals as pets, but is intellectually normal, often very bright, and resists any attempts to change his or her way of life.

diopsimeter (dī-op-sim′-i-ter): An instrument used to measure the field of vision.

diopter, dioptre (dī-op′-ter): A unit of measurement in refraction. A lens of one dioptre has a focal length of 1 metre.

dioptometer (dī-op-tom′i-ter): An instrument used for measuring the refractive ability of the eye.

diorthosis (dī-or-thō′-sis): The surgical correction or straightening of a deformed or injured extremity.

diotic (dī-ō′-tik): Relating to or affecting both ears.

dioxide (dī-ok′-sīd): An oxide in which the molecules contain two oxygen atoms.

DipEd: Abbreviation for Diploma in Education.

dipeptidase (dī-pep′-ti-dās): An enzyme that catalyses the splitting of dipeptides into amino acids.

dipeptide (dī-pep′-tīd): A peptide that yields two amino acids on hydrolysis.

diphasic (dī-fā′-zik): Occurring in two stages or phases.

diphenylhydantoin (dī′-fen-il-hī-dan′-tō-in): A white, odourless, powdery substance, soluble in water; used for its anticonvulsant action in the treatment of grand mal epilepsy. Also called *phenytoin*.

diphtheria (dif-thē′-ri-a): An acute, specific, highly infectious, epidemic and endemic disease caused by the *Corynebacterium diphtheriae* [Klebs–Loeffler bacillus]; transmitted by direct and indirect contact and carriers. A notifiable disease. Primarily a disease of children, formerly occurring in the autumn and winter months; protection is obtained by immunization, usually combined with immunization for pertussis (*q.v.*) and tetanus (*q.v.*). Characterized by the formation of a greyish, leathery, adherent membrane growing on an epithelial surface which bleeds on removal, and the development of a potent systemic toxin that may attack the heart muscle and nerves. CUTANEOUS D. a form that affects the skin, characterized by deep ulcerating lesions; associated with poor hygiene; D. ANTITOXIN a serum containing antibodies that neutralize the D. TOXIN; obtained from horses that have been immunized to the toxin produced by *Corynebacterium diphtheriae*; D. TOXIN a protein exotoxin produced by the *Corynebacterium diphtheriae*; is responsible for the development of symptoms of diphtheria; D. TOXIN–ANTITOXIN a mixture used to produce active immunity against the disease; now largely replaced by diphtheria toxoid; D. TOXOID, D. toxin that has been detoxified; used to produce active immunity to diphtheria; LARYNGEAL D. membranous croup; a serious condition seen primarily in infants; NASAL D., D. confined to the nose; usually mild; but may spread to surrounding structures and tissues; PHARYNGEAL D. that which affects primarily the pharynx; WOUND D. name given to a false membrane that forms on the surface of a wound.

diplegia (dī-plē'-ji-a): Symmetrical paralysis of the same parts on both sides of the body. CONGENITAL or INFANTILE D. birth palsy, FACIAL D., D. affecting both sides of the face. SPASTIC D. see LITTLE'S DISEASE. Cf. PARAPLEGIA. — diplegic, adj.

diplo-: A combining form denoting double, twice, twofold.

diplobacillus (dip'-lō-ba-sil'-us): A pair of short rod-shaped organisms joined end to end as a result of incomplete fission.

diplocardia (dip-lō-kar'-di-a): A condition in which the right and left sides of the heart are partially separated by a deep fissure.

diplococcus (dip'-lō-kok-'-us): A coccal bacterium characteristically occurring in pairs, *e.g.*, the pneumococcus.

diploë (dip'-lō-ē): The cancellous tissue between the outer and inner layers of compact bone, *e.g.*, the flat bones of the skull. — diploetic, adj.

diploic (dip-lō'-ik): 1. Diploetic. 2. Double. 3. Pertaining to the diploë. D. VEINS the large, thin-walled veins situated in the diploë of the cranial bones.

diploid (dip'-loyd): 1. Having two sets of chromosomes; a normal occurrence in the somatic cells of humans. 2. An individual having two full sets of chromosomes that are homologous. — diploidy, n.

diplomatic (dip'-lō-mat-ik): Being tactful; dealing well with people.

diploneural (dip-lō-nū'-ral): Being supplied with two nerves; said of certain muscles.

diplopia (dip-lō'-pi-a): Double vision; the perception of two images of only one object.

diplosomatia (dip-lō-sō-mā'-shi-a): The condition of being completely formed twins that are joined at some part of their bodies.

DipN: Abbreviation for Diploma in Nursing.

DipNEd: Abbreviation for Diploma in Nursing Education.

dipsesis (dip-sē'-sis): Thirst. — dipsetic, adj.

dipsogen (dip'-sō-jen): An agent that induces thirst and intake of fluids.

dipsomania (dip-sō-mā'-ni-a): Alcoholism in which uncontrollable drinking occurs in bouts, often with long periods of sobriety inbetween. — dipsomaniac, adj., n.

dipsosis (dip-sō'-sis): Abnormal thirst, or a craving for unusual drinks.

dipstick (dip'-stik): A strip of cellulose impregnated with chemicals that will react with certain substances in the urine and discolour the strip.

direct (di-rekt'): 1. Straight. 2. Without anything between or intervening. D. CONTACT referring to the passing of a disease directly from one person to another; D. CURRENT an electric current that flows continuously; opp. to alternating current; D. PAYMENT a method of benefit issue whereby the money is transferred straight into the recipient's account at a bank, building society, or Post Office. It is the way all benefits, state pensions and war pensions will be paid in the UK. D. TRANSFUSION transfusion of blood directly from person to another. See also NHS DIRECT.

director (di-rek'-tor): 1. A grooved instrument used for guiding the knife in surgical operations. 2. A person in a position involving guiding or directing.

dirt-eating: Geophagia or chthonophagia (*q.v.*).

dis-: Prefix denoting: 1. To do the opposite of; reverse; deprive of; exclude. 2. Absence of; opposite of. 3. Not.

disability: As a medical term, refers to any lasting impairment of physiological, anatomical, or psychological functioning caused by an injury, illness, or birth defect, with resultant loss of learning power, or limitation of one's capacity to perform some key life functions or activities. While disability usually stems from a physical or mental medical condition, you can distinguish between impairment caused by actual defect and disability caused by the attitude of society. Someone who is unable to walk and needs a wheelchair has an impairment; however, environmental factors such as lack of access to transport, public toilets and buildings cause his or her disability.

Disability Discrimination Act 1995: An Act of Parliament that aims to end the discrimination faced by many disabled people. This Act gives disabled people rights in the areas of: employment; access to goods, facilities, and services; and buying or renting land or property. The employment rights and first rights of access came into force on 2 December 1996; further rights of access came into force on 1 October 1999; and the final rights of access come into force in October 2004.

Disability Rights Commission: An independent body set up by the UK government to help secure civil rights for disabled people. Its statutory duties are: to work to eliminate discrimination against disabled people; to promote equal opportunities for disabled people; to encourage good practice in the treatment of disabled people; and to advise the government on the working of disability legislation.

Disability Rights Commission Act 1999: An Act of Parliament that led to the establishment of the Disability Rights Commission (*q.v.*) in April 2000. It sets out its statutory duties.

Disabled Living Centres Council: The lead organization for a national network of centres giving free advice on disability equipment and related matters.

disaccharidase (dī-sak′-a-ri-dās): An enzyme that acts to hydrolyse a disaccharide into two monosaccharides.

disaccharide (dī-sak′-a-rīd): Any one of a class of carbohydrates ($C_{12}H_2O_{11}$) that yields two molecules of monosaccharide on hydrolysis, *e.g.*, lactose, maltose, sucrose.

disarticulation (dis-ar-tik-ū-lā′-shun): A disjointing, or separation at a joint.

disc: A circular or rounded, flattened organ or structure. ARTICULAR D. a fibrocartilage or fibrous tissue pad found in some synovial joints; INTERVERTEBRAL D. a layer of fibrocartilage between the bodies of the vertebrae; consists of a fibrous ring with a pulpy centre; OPTIC D. the intraocular portion of the optic nerve formed by the fibres converging from the retina and appearing as a white disc; SLIPPED D., herniated D., see under HERNIATED. Also called *discus*.

discectomy (dis-kek′-to-mi): The surgical removal of an intervertebral disc.

discharge (dis-charj′): 1. To liberate or set free. 2. To release a patient from a healthcare facility; (dis'charj). 3. The flowing away of a secretion or excretion. 4. Material that is expelled, evacuated, or flows away from a body cavity or wound, *e.g.*, faeces, urine, pus.

dischronation (dis-krō-nā′-shun): A disturbance in one's consciousness of time.

discission (di-sizh′-un): A cutting out or division; specifically, the rupturing of the lens capsule in surgery for soft cataract.

discography (dis-kog′-ra-fi): X-ray of an intervertebral disc after it has been rendered radiopaque. — discographic, adj.; discographically, adv.; discograph, n.

discoid (dis′-koyd): Having the shape of a disc.

discopathy (dis-kop′-a-thi): Any disease or disorder involving an intervertebral disc.

discrete (dis-krēt′): Separate; not continuous. Often said of skin lesions that do not blend or join others. Opp. to confluent (*q.v.*).

discrimination (dis-krim-i-nā′-shun): 1. The ability to perceive distinctions. D. IN HEARING the ability to discriminate between words having the same or very similiar sounds. 2. Allowing personal opinions on race, religion, sex, national origin, sexual orientation, disability, etc. to create a bias that affects actions concerning specific people.

discus (dis′-kus): A disc.

disease (di-zēz′): Sickness, illness. A departure from a state of health caused by an interruption or modification of any of the vital functions, and characterized by a definite train of symptoms. ACUTE D. an abnormal condition of the body characterized by sudden onset of symptoms of a violent nature, and by a short course terminating in either recovery or death; CHRONIC D. an abnormal condition of the body; of long continuance, marked by lack of violent symptoms, sometimes ending in recovery; COMMUNICABLE D. one that is transferable from one person to another by means of the causative organism; CONGENITAL D. one that is present at birth; may or may not be due to hereditary factors; DEGENERATIVE D. that is the result of cellular and tissue changes that occur naturally in old age; FUNCTIONAL D. dysfunction of some part of the body with no obvious pathology to account for it; HEREDITARY D., D. that is transferred from parent to offspring genetically; IATROGENIC D. induced by a physician or by a treatment being utilized for some other condition; IDIOPATHIC D., D. for which the cause is not known; INFECTIOUS D., D. that may be transmitted; NOTIFIABLE D. a disease, the occurrence of which must by law be reported to the public health authorities; OCCUPATIONAL D. a disease arising from various factors associated with the patient's occupation; PSYCHOSOMATIC D., D. that originates in the person's mind or emotions; SUBCLINICAL D., D. in which the symptoms have not yet appeared; TERMINAL D., D. from which the person cannot be expected to recover. See also under SEXUALLY TRANSMITTED DISEASES.

disengagement (dis-en-gāj' -ment): 1. The emergence from a confined space, in particular the emergence of the infant's head from the vagina during childbirth. 2. A process in which the individual withdraws from society, disregards personal obligations and ties, and is in turn disregarded by society; happens chiefly in the elderly. D. THEORY implies that both society and the aged prepare for death by withdrawal and by gradually reducing their life contacts, a process that leads to poor relationships, egocentricity, and, sometimes, depression; often the result of physiological deficits such as deafness.

disequilibrium (dis-ē' -qwi-lib' -ri-um): Lack or loss of balance; may be physical or mental. D. SYNDROME a condition seen in persons who are severely catabolic; marked by restlessness, twitching, jerking, mental confusion.

disinfect (dis-in-fekt'): To kill pathogenic organisms by physical or chemical means or to cause them to become inert; refers particularly to cleansing of inanimate objects. — disinfection, n.

disinfectant (dis-in-fek' -tant): An agent that is used to destroy pathogenic organisms or to cause them to be inert. — disinfectant, adj.

disinfection (dis-in-fek' -shun): A vague term, implying the destruction of pathogenic microorganisms, except spores, by physical or chemical means; can refer to the action of antiseptics (q.v.) as well as disinfectants.

disinhibition (dis' -in-hi-bish' -un): The abolition or removal of an inhibition.

disintegrate (dis-in' -te-grāt): To decompose or break up. — disintegration, n.

disintoxication (dis' -in-tok-si-kā' -shun): 1. Detoxication (q.v.). 2. Treatment to assist an addict to overcome his or her drug habit.

disjoint (dis-joynt'): To separate at a joint or to disarticulate; said of separating bones from their natural relationship at joints.

dislocation (dis-lō-kā' -shun): A displacement of organs or articular surfaces, more especially of a bone at a joint; accompanied by pain and deformity. Syn., *luxation.* — dislocated, adj.; dislocate, v.

dismemberment (dis-mem' -ber-ment): Amputation of an extremity or part of it. — dismember, v.

disorder (dis-or' -der): A disturbance or abnormality of physical or mental health or function.

disorientation (dis' -ō-ri-en-tā' -shun): Permanent or temporary loss of orientation or of the ability to identify oneself in relation to time, place, and person. May occur as a result of trauma, severe illness, the use of alcohol or certain drugs, or psychiatric disturbance. When it is a result of organic brain disease, D. for time and place occurs before D. for person.

disparate (dis' -pa-rat): Unequal; not alike; unmatched.

dispensary (dis-pen' -sa-ri): A pharmacy in a hospital or clinic where medications are dispensed.

dispense (dis-pens'): In pharmaceutical practice, to prepare and deliver medicines.

dispersion (dis-per' -zhun): 1. The act of separating or scattering. 2. The incorporation of particles of one substance into another, as occurs in solutions and suspensions. — disperse, v.

displacement (dis-plās' -ment): 1. Removal from the normal position; dislocation. 2. In psychiatry, a defence mechanism whereby an emotion provoked by one person or situation is transferred to another less threatening person or situation. 3. In chemistry, the action whereby one substance in a compound is displaced by another. — displaceability, adj.

disposition (dis-po-zish' -un): A prevailing tendency, mood, attitude.

disproportion (dis-prō-por' -shun): In anatomy, lack of normal relationship between two body areas or parts. CEPHALO-PELVIC D. in obstetrics, the head of the fetus is too large or the pelvis is too small to allow the head to engage. See ENGAGEMENT.

dissect (dis-sekt'): 1. To cut apart or separate; applied particularly to tissues of a cadaver for anatomical study. 2. In surgery, to separate a structure by cutting or tearing along the natural lines rather than by making a wide incision.

dissection (di-sek' -shun): 1. The act or process of dissecting. 2. An anatomical specimen obtained by dissection. BLUNT D. a method of separating tissues along natural lines by using a finger or blunt instrument instead of cutting; SHARP D. the separation of tissues by cutting with a scalpel, scissors, or other sharp instrument.

disseminated (dis-sem' -i-nā-ted): Widely extended, scattered, or distributed. D. INTRAVASCULAR COAGULATION an acute or chronic disorder of clotting in which platelets and clotting factors are depleted by haemorrhage or some other circumstance; sometimes occurs as a secondary condition in trauma or following the administration of large amounts of thromboplastic substances.

dissemination (dis-sem' -i-nā' -shun): The act of distributing or spreading something, especially information, or causing it to become widespread, *e.g.*, research findings.

dissimilate (dis-sim′-i-lāt): To break a substance down into its component parts; to produce energy or to separate out materials to be eliminated. The reverse of assimilate. — dissimilation, n.

dissociation (dis-sō′-shi-ā′-shun): 1. The separation or breakdown of a complex substance into simpler parts. 2. The release of ions in solution by electrovalent compounds; also called ionization. 3. In psychiatry, a defence mechanism in which the mind achieves non-recognition and isolation of certain unpalatable facts. This involves the actual splitting off from consciousness of all the unpalatable ideas so that the individual is no longer aware of them. D. is commonly observed in such involuntary states as hysteria, schizophrenia, fugue, somnambulism, and dual personality, but is seen in its most exaggerated form in delusional psychosis.

dissociative disorders: See under DISSOCIATION.

dissolution (dis-sō-lū′-shun): 1. The chemical separation of a compound into its component elements. 2. The liquefaction of a solid substance. 3. Death.

dissolve (di-zolv′): 1. To cause a substance to pass into solution by placing it in a solvent.

dissonance (dis′-sō-nans): A combination of tones that produce harsh or disagreeable sounds.

distal ((dis′-tal): Farthest from the head, centre, or any point of reference. Located away from the centre of the body and towards the extremities. — distally, adv.; distad, adj. Cf. PROXIMAL.

distance learning: Learning that takes place outside of a dedicated learning environment such as a university or training department, *e.g.*, courses run by the Open University. It can refer to correspondence courses and e-learning (*q.v.*). See FLEXIBLE LEARNING; OPEN LEARNING.

distensible (dis-ten′-si-b'l): Capable of being distended.

distension (dis-ten′-shun): The state of being enlarged or distended. ABDOMINAL D. that which occurs after some operations when there is an abnormal accumulation of gas in the intestines.

distichia (dis-tik′-i-a): The presence of an extra row of eyelashes at the inner border of the eyelid, which turn in and rub on the cornea; a congenital anomaly.

distil (dis-til′): To change a liquid to vapour by the application of heat and then, by cooling, to change the vapour to a liquid.

distillation (dis-til-ā′-shun): The process of driving off gas or vapour by heating solids or liquids, and then condensing the resulting products. — distil, v.

distocclusion (dis′-tō-kloo′-zhun): Malocclusion of the teeth in which the teeth and lower jaw are in a distal or recessive position in relation to the upper jaw and teeth.

distortion (dis-tor′-shun): The state of being twisted out of the natural position or shape. In psychiatry, a mechanism through which the individual disguises or denies material that he or she cannot accept and substitutes material that is less offensive to his or her self-concept.

distraction (dis-trak′-shun): 1. The dislocation of joint surfaces caused by extension but without injury to the parts involved. 2. Anything that diverts the attention. 3. Great mental or emotional distress, confusion, or disturbance.

distress (dis-tres′): Anguish or suffering, physical or mental.

district nurse: A registered nurse who also holds a District Nursing Certificate and provides skilled nursing care for patients in their own homes.

diurese (dī-ū-res′): The act of causing or producing diuresis.

diuresis (dī-ū-rē′-sis): Increased secretion and excretion of urine.

diuretic (dī-ū-ret′-ik): 1. Having the effect of increasing the flow of urine. 2. An agent that increases the flow of urine.

diuria (dī-ū′-ri-a): Frequency of urination during the waking hours.

diurnal (dī-er′-nal): 1. Occurring or recurring during the daytime. 2. Recurring every day.

divergence (dī-ver′-jens): A spreading out or drawing apart from a common point. In ophthalmology, the abduction of one eye or of both eyes at the same time. — divergent, adj.

divers' ear: Middle ear inflammation caused by sudden changes in atmospheric pressure; often a symptom in decompression sickness.

diversion (dī-ver′-zhun): A turning aside or the act of diverting from a course. URINARY D. the surgical procedure of creating an alternate route for the elimination of urine; following removal of all or part of the urinary bladder, the ureters are severed from the bladder and attached to the ileum or sigmoid, or they may be brought out to the surface of the abdominal wall. See ILEAL CONDUIT under ILEAL.

diversional (dī-ver′-shun-al): Tending to produce relaxation or diversion. D. THERAPY a pastime that causes a person to turn his thoughts away from himself and his problems.

diverticulectomy (dī'-ver-tik-ū-lek'-to-mi): Surgical excision of a diverticulum (*q.v.*).

diverticulitis (dī'-ver-tik-ū-lī'-tis): Inflammation of one or more diverticula.

diverticulosis (dī'-ver-tik-ū-lō'-sis): A condition in which there are many diverticula, especially in the sigmoid colon.

diverticulum (dī'-ver-tik-ū-lum): A circumscribed pouch or sac of variable size protruding from the wall of a tube or hollow organ; occurs chiefly in the intestine, but also in the rest of the alimentary tract, including the oesophagus, and in the urinary tract; may be congenital or acquired. MECKEL'S D. a blind tube that arises from the ileum at some distance from the ileocaecal valve; it represents a persistent end of the embryonic yolk stalk; ZENKER'S D. a pharyngoesophageal d. — diverticula, pl.; diverticular, adj.

divulse (di-vuls'): To separate or pull apart forcibly. — divulsion, n.

dizygotic (dī'-zī-got'-ik): Referring to twins that develop from two fertilized ova; termed fraternal twins.

dizziness (diz'-i-nes): A disturbed, unpleasant sense of one's relationship to space, in which objects seem to whirl about; giddiness. May be due to disturbance in any of the body systems that normally keep a person aware of his or her position in space.

DLCC: Abbreviation for Disabled Living Centres Council (*q.v.*).

DN: Abbreviation for district nurse (*q.v.*).

DNA: Abbreviation for deoxyribonucleic acid (*q.v.*).

DNA viruses: A group of viruses that includes the herpesviruses, adenoviruses, papoviruses, poxviruses, and the bacteriophages, all of which have a core of deoxyribonucleic acid.

DOA: Abbreviation for death on arrival.

doctor: 1. A person registered with the General Medical Council to practise medicine. 2. To treat the sick or injured. 3. To dilute, tamper with, or falsify.

Döderlein's bacillus: A large, Gram-positive, non-pathogenic rod bacterium commonly found in the vagina; also found in the intestine when the diet is rich in milk or milk products; said to be identical with *Lactobacillus acidophilus*. [Albert Döderlein, German obstetrician and gynaecologist. 1860–1941]

DOH: Abbreviation for Department of Health (*q.v.*).

domiciliary care (dom-i-sil'-i-a-ri): Social care provided for people in their own homes.

domiciliary services (dom-i-sil'-i-a-ri): Health and social services provided in the home for the elderly and those who are not quite able to manage living independently.

dominance (dom'-in-ans): 1. In genetics, the ability of one of a pair of genes to suppress the other (recessive) gene. 2. In neurology, the tendency of one side of the brain to be more important than the other in controlling certain functions, *e.g.*, speech, handedness. 3. In psychiatry, a predisposition to play an important or controlling role in interpersonal relationships.

dominant (dom'-in-ant): In genetics, refers to a character possessed by one parent, which in the offspring masks the corresponding alternative character derived from the other parent. Opp. to recessive. See MENDEL'S LAW. D. HAND the hand of greater skill, *e.g.*, in writing; D. HEMISPHERE the cerebral hemisphere that appears to be more important in the control of body movements; it is contralateral to the D. hand.

donor (dō'-nor). One who supplies living tissue or material to be used by another. D. INSEMINATION insemination of a woman with donor sperm; either by direct insertion into the cervical canal or combined with *in vitro* fertilization (*q.v.*) techniques; UNIVERSAL D. a person who has group O blood which, in an emergency, can safely be given to patients with blood of any type.

dopa (dō'-pa): An amino acid produced by the oxidation of tyrosine; a precursor of dopamine and an intermediate product in the synthesis of noradrenaline, adrenaline, and melanin. The naturally occurring form, L-dopa, and the synthetic form, levodopa, are used in the treatment of Parkinson's disease.

dopamine (dō'-pa-mēn): A neurotransmitter found in the brain; an intermediate product in the synthesis of adrenaline and noradrenaline, which increases cardiac output and renal blood flow but does not produce peripheral vasoconstriction. In Parkinson's disease there is a depletion of dopamine in the caudate nucleus of the brain.

dope (dōp): 1. Any drug taken habitually for other than medical purposes. 2. To administer or take a habit-forming drug. D. ADDICT a person who is physically and psychologically dependent on a drug, due to habitual use.

Doppler: 1. D. DEVICE a highly sensitive ultrasonic device for measuring the blood pressure of infants and children. 2. D. EFFECT the observable change in the frequency of an acoustic or electromagnetic wave; due to the relative movement of the source of the wave and the observer away from or towards each other. D. FLOWMETER an ultrasonic device for measuring the circulation of blood in the extremities; D. PHENOMENON or PRINCIPLE see D. EFFECT; D. SHIFT the amount of change in the frequency of light, sound, or frequency waves that occurs as the wave source and the observer move towards or away from each other; D. ULTRASONIC TEST a test that utilizes an ultrasonic probe and transducer for detecting shifts in sound that are reflected from a blood vessel and augmented by an audio speaker. [Christian Johann Doppler, Austrian physicist and mathematician, 1803–1853].

dorsal (dor'-sal): Relating to the back, or the posterior part of an organ. Opp. to ventral. D. surface of the foot refers to the top of the foot; D. surface of the hand refers to the back of the hand. D. RECUMBENT POSITION see under POSITION.

dorsi-, dorso-: Combining forms denoting relationship to the back or back part of the body.

dorsiduct (dor'-si-dukt): To draw towards the dorsum or back.

dorsiflexion (dor-si-flek'-shun): Bending backwards, as of the hand or foot. In the case of the great toe, upwards. See BABINSKI'S REFLEX.

dorsum (dor'-sum): The back or the surface that corresponds to the back. — dorsa, pl.

dosage (dō'-sij): 1. The determination of the proper amount of a medicinal agent to be given. 2. The giving of prescribed amounts of a medicinal agent. 3. The amount of a medication to be given at one time.

dose (dōs): A quantity of any therapeutic agent to be given at any one time, or at stated intervals, as an amount of medicine or a quantity of radiation. BOOSTER D. one given some time after a primary immunization to maintain protection of the individual; DIVIDED D. one given in fractional amounts at specific intervals; ERYTHEMA D. the smallest amount of radiation that will produce reddening of the skin within ten days to two weeks after application; LETHAL D. one likely to cause death; MAINTENANCE D. one given in protracted illness to keep the patient under an influence achieved by an initial dose of a drug; MAXIMUM D. the largest amount of a drug that can be given with safety; MINIMUM D. the smallest amount of a drug that will produce the desired effect; MINIMUM LETHAL DOSE the smallest amount of toxin that will kill a laboratory animal; OPTIMAL D. the amount of an agent that will produce the desired effect without any

undesirable effects; SENSITIZING D. the initial D. of an allergen; the patient has no antibodies to it.

dosimeter (dō-sim'-i-ter): A device that measures the amount of exposure to x-rays or other radioactive emanations; worn by health-care personnel who are in frequent contact with radioactive substances or emanations.

dosimetry (dō-sim'-i-tri): The determination of dosages. In radiography, the measurement of doses of x-ray or radioactive emanations.

dossier (dōs'-ē-ā): The file that contains the accumulated case history of a patient.

double: D. DECOMPOSITION a chemical reaction in which the ions of two compounds exchange places and two new compounds are formed; D. PNEUMONIA pneumonia in both lungs; D. VISION diplopia (q.v.).

double-blind: Refers to a manner of conducting experiments with neither experimenter nor subjects knowing the controlling elements; the objective is to secure statistically reliable results.

douche (doosh): A stream of water, gas or vapour directed against the body or into a body cavity for cleansing or therapeutic purposes.

Douglas' pouch: Rectouterine pouch; see under POUCH.

downer or **downs:** Slang for a drug or drugs having a depressive action.

Downey cells: Atypical lymphocytes, which may be seen on a peripheral blood smear from a patient with infectious mononucleosis and certain other viral infections.

Down's syndrome: A congenital anomaly caused by one of two types of abnormality of chromosome 21: (1) failure of the chromosome to divide; infants with this anomaly are usually born to older mothers; (2) an abnormality within the chromosome itself with the total number of chromosomes being normal; infants with this anomaly are usually born of younger mothers, and there is a high risk of recurrence in subsequent pregnancies. This syndrome is characterized by learning disability and such physical features as oval tilted eyes, short flat-bridged nose, thickened tongue, flattened occiput, pallor, smaller than normal brain, broad hands and feet with widened space between first and second digits, stubby fingers, hyperflexibility of joints. Also called *Trisomy 21 syndrome* and formerly called *mongolism*.

doxogenic (dok-sō-jen'-ic): Caused by or resulting from one's own mental processes and conceptions, said of certain diseases.

DPhil: Abbreviation for Doctor of Philosophy.

DPT: Abbreviation for diphtheria–pertussis–tetanus (vaccine).

DQ: Abbreviation for developmental quotient, see under DEVELOPMENTAL; GESSELL DEVELOPMENT SCHEDULE.

drain (drān): 1. To draw off by degrees an accumulation of such material as pus, lymph, or secretion. 2. A device or substance that provides a channel or means of exit for the discharge from a wound or cavity.

drainage (drān'-ij): The withdrawal, or flow, of fluid from a wound or cavity. D. TUBE a hollow tube inserted into a cavity or wound to allow fluids to escape; POSTURAL D. that achieved by putting the patient in a position in which gravity aids the process; TIDAL D. drainage of a paralysed urinary bladder utilizing an apparatus that allows for filling the bladder to a certain level and then emptying it either by siphonage or gravity; UNDER-WATER SEAL D. a chest drainage system that prevents air from re-entering the chest.

drape (drāp): A sheet of fabric or other material used to cover parts of the body that do not need to be exposed for examination or carrying out a procedure — drape, v.

drastic (dras'-tik): Term applied to a treatment or medication that has a powerful or thorough effect.

draught (draft): 1. A current of air circulating in a limited space. 2. A large dose of liquid medicine to be taken at a single swallow.

draw sheet: A narrow sheet placed crosswise on the bed to protect the lower sheet. It can be removed when soiled by pulling to the side.

DRC: Abbreviation for Disability Rights Commission (q.v.).

drepanocytaemia (drep'-nō-sī-tē'-mi-a): Sickle cell anaemia; see under ANAEMIA.

drepanocyte (drep'-a-nō-sīt): A sickle cell (q.v.).

dressing (dres'-ing): 1. Any material or substance applied to a wound or lesion to cover it, to prevent infection, to aid in healing, or to absorb drainage. 2. The application of any one of various materials to protect or cover a wound or lesion. DRY D., a D. consisting of dry material such as absorbent gauze; WET D., a D. that has been moistened with plain water or a fluid containing a medication. — dressings, pl.

Dressler beat: A fusion beat heard in digitalis toxicity; indicates that an ectopic impulse is originating in the ventricle.

Dressler's syndrome: Postmyocardial infarction syndrome (q.v.).

DRG: Abbreviation for Diagnosis Related Groups (q.v.).

dribble (drib'-'l): 1. To drool. 2. To fall in drops, as urine from the bladder of patients with distended or paralysed bladder.

drift: 1. A condition caused by muscle weakness following mild hemiparesis; the hand pronates when the patient stands with arms outstretched and the palms facing each other; the foot becomes everted when the patient sits with legs extended, feet together, and eyes closed. 2. Movement of teeth from their normal position, due to loss of other teeth.

drip: 1. To instill a medication drop by drop, e.g., eye drops. 2. The slow continuous drop-by-drop administration of a solution into a body cavity. INTRAVENOUS D. continuous drop-by-drop instillation of a solution into a vein; nutrients or drugs may be added to the solution; POSTNASAL D. dripping of irritating material from the posterior nares into the pharynx, often a feature of sinusitis.

drive: 1. An urgent, instinctive need that causes one to press for its satisfaction, e.g., the sex drive. 2. A powerful concern or interest that motivates one to consistent and continual effort.

dromotropic (drō-mō-tro-pik): Having an effect on the conductivity of nerves. D. DRUGS drugs that may speed up or slow conductivity of nerve impulses, depending on the drug.

drool: 1. To let saliva or other liquid run from the mouth. 2. To flow from the mouth, as saliva.

drooling (droo'-ling): Uncontrolled salivation.

drop: D. ATTACK loss of equilibrium and falling, without vertigo or loss of consciousness, followed by rapid recovery; D. FOOT an abnormal downwards position of the foot due to paralysis of the flexors of the foot; often due to pressure of bedclothes on the foot or to poorly fitted casts or splints. Also called foot-drop; EAR D. medication to be dropped into the ear; EYE D. medication to be dropped into the conjunctival sac; NOSE D. medication to be dropped into the nose; WRIST D. flaccid paralysis of the wrist as a result of injury to a nerve by fracture or trauma.

droplet (drop'-let): A very small drop. D. INFECTION one transmitted by small droplets expelled when talking, sneezing or coughing; D. NUCLEI microscopic particles that, when surrounded by moisture, become airborne.

dropsy (drop'-si): A common term used to describe an abnormal accumulation of fluid in cellular tissue or a cavity. See ASCITES,

HYDROCEPHALUS, HYDROTHORAX. — dropsical, adj.

drowsiness (drowz'-i-nes): A state of semi-wakefulness characterized by lethargy, sleepiness, lessened sensibility, sometimes confusion.

drug: 1. A substance used in the diagnosis, prevention, or treatment of disease; often of vegetable or chemical origin. **2.** A medicine or substance that is capable of modifying one or more functions of the body or mind. D. ABUSE use of any drug for other than medical treatment; D. ADDICTION a state in which habitual use of a drug has (1) created a strong physical and/or psychological dependence that cannot be controlled; (2) causes the individual to concentrate their activities on securing the required drug to the exclusion of other forms of socially acceptable activity; and (3) has resulted in a condition wherein withdrawal of the substance causes severe distress symptoms; CONTROLLED D. the distribution of such a drug is limited and monitored according to government regulations; D. DEPENDENCE the physical or psychological desire for continuous use of a drug over a period of time and the compulsion to take it continuously to experience its pleasurable effects and to prevent withdrawal symptoms, pertains to both drug abuse and drug addiction, including dependence on alcohol, the hallucinogens, narcotics, analgesics, tranquillizers, or marijuana; D. REACTION an unexpected or undesirable effect produced by a drug and which may or may not be harmful, ranging from nausea, skin rash, nervousness, and gastrointestinal upset to anaphylactic shock; see ANAPHYLACTIC; D. RESISTANCE the ability to develop resistance to the bacteriostatic action of certain drugs; D. TOLERANCE the decreasing effect of a drug with continued administration so that larger and larger doses are required to produce the same effect.

drug fever: Fever, with chills, urticaria, myalgia, angiodema, arthralgia; usually due to a hypersensitivity to certain drugs; may occur in a few days or up to two weeks after starting certain drug therapies.

drug trials: Tests of efficacy and safety undertaken during the development of a new drug. There are four different stages: Phase I trials involve a small number of healthy volunteers; only small doses of the drug are given and the volunteers are monitored carefully for adverse reactions; Phase II trials involve patients and the efficiency of the drug is compared with that of other therapies; Phase III trials are larger, multicentre studies prior to the drug being approved and licensed; Phase IV trials take place after the drug is in clinical use; reactions and adverse reactions are monitored and recorded.

drum: In anatomy, the ear drum or tympanic membrane. Also called *drumhead*.

drunkenness: Intoxication, particularly that produced by alcoholic beverages.

drusen (droo'-sen): Small colloid or hyaline bodies seen in the retinal pigment cells in degeneration of Bruch's membrane.

dry: Not wet; free from and not associated with moisture. D. COUGH one not productive of mucus or phlegm; D. GANGRENE death of tissue due to interference with the blood supply to the part; D. ICE solid carbon dioxide, see CARBON DIOXIDE SNOW; D. LABOUR labour following premature rupture of the amniotic sac; D. SOCKET alveolitis following extraction of a tooth.

dry eye syndrome: Lack of adequate secretion of tears; a common condition that may be due to irritation from any cause; is increased in persons taking diuretics and following cataract surgery. Symptoms include dryness of the conjunctiva, burning, sensation of a foreign body in the eye. Symptoms are increased in persons taking antihistamines or following cataract surgery. Treatment includes use of artificial tears or of a humidifier or vaporizer.

DSM IV: Abbreviation for *Diagnostic and Statistical Manual of Mental Disorders*, 4th edition.

DSPD: Abbreviation for Dangerous and Severe Personality Disorder (*q.v.*).

DTP: Diphtheria and tetanus toxoids combined with pertussis vaccine, used for active immunization of normal infants and children.

DTs: Abbreviation for delirium tremens. See DELIRIUM.

dual (dū'-al): Consisting of two parts. D. DIAGNOSIS the identification of two associated illnesses contributing to a single set of symptoms; e.g., a person who has both an alcohol or drug problem and an emotional or mental health problem; to recover fully, the person needs treatment for both problems; D. PERSONALITY see under PERSONALITY DISORDER.

Duchenne: D.'S DISEASE tabes dorsalis,; see under TABES; D.'s muscular dystrophy, pseudohypertrophic infantile muscular dystrophy; see under DYSTROPHY; D.'S PARALYSIS progressive bulbar paralysis; see ERB–DUCHENNE PARALYSIS under PALSY. [G. B. A. Duchenne, French neurologist, 1807–1875.]

Duchenne–Griesinger disease (doo-shen'-grē'-sing-er): An inherited disorder, marked by wasting and weakness of calf and shoulder muscles, waddling gait, sclerosis. Symptoms appear in childhood and increase until the individual is unable to walk; death usually occurs in early teens from respiratory infection. Also called *pseudohypertrophic muscular dystrophy*.

Ducrey's bacillus (*Haemophilis ducreyi*) (dū'krāz'): Small Gram-negative rod. The causative organism of soft chancre (chancroid), a venereal disease. [Augosto Ducrey, Italian dermatologist, 1860–1940.]

duct (dukt): A passageway or tube, especially one for the passage of secretions or excretions. EJACULATORY D.S, two fine tubes, one on either side, commencing at the union of the seminal vesicle with the vas deferens, and terminating at their union with the prostatic urethra.

duction (duk'-shun): 1. The act of leading, conducting, or bringing. 2. Movements of the eyes into positions upward, downward, towards the nose, and towards the temples.

ductless (dukt'-les): Having no duct, as the ductless glands. See ENDOCRINE GLANDS.

ductule (dukt'-ūl): A small duct.

ductus (duk'-tus): Duct. D. ARTERIOSUS a fetal blood vessel connecting the left pulmonary artery to the aorta, to bypass the lungs in the fetal circulation; it normally closes at birth and may cause serious heart problems if it persists; D. VENOSUS a fetal blood vessel connecting the umbilical vein to the inferior vena cava, thus the venous blood bypasses the liver; it ceases to function at birth but remains in the liver as a ligament. See also COMMON BILE DUCT (ductus choledochus); EJACULATORY DUCTS (ductus ejaculatorius) under DUCT; LACTIFEROUS DUCTS (ductus lactiferi); NASOLACRIMAL DUCT (ductus nasolacrimalis); STENSEN'S DUCT; SUDORIFERUS DUCT (ductus sudoriferus); THORACIC DUCT (ductus thoracacius); VAS DEFERENS (ductus deferens).

dull: 1. Lacking mental alertness. 2. Not sharp. 3. Not resonant, said of sounds heard on examination by percussion.

dumb (dum): 1. Mute; unable to speak. 2. Stupid (slang).

dum-dum fever: Kala-azar (*q.v.*).

dummy: 1. Term sometimes used synonymously with placebo (*q.v.*); 2. Pacifier (*q.v.*).

dumping syndrome: The name given to the symptoms which often follow a partial gastrectomy — bilious vomiting, nausea, sweating, palpitation, and a feeling of faintness and weakness after meals.

Dunant, Henri: Swiss philanthropist whose work with the wounded at the battle of Solfer-

ino in 1859 inspired him to work for an organization to aid wounded soldiers and eventually led to the establishment of the International Red Cross in 1864. [1828–1920].

duodenal (dū-ō-dē'-nal): Relating to or affecting the duodenum.

duodenectomy (dū-ō-de-nek'-tō-mi): Surgical excision of all or part of the duodenum.

duodenocholecystostomy (dū-ō-dē'-nō-kō-lē-sis-tos'-to-mi): Surgical creation of a passage between the gall bladder and the duodenum.

duodenoduodenostomy (dū-ō-dē'-nō-dū-ō-dē-nos'-to-mi): An anastomosis of two sections of the duodenum, done to correct an abnormality that prevents duodenal contents from passing through the lumen.

duodenostomy (dū-od-e-nos'-to-mi): Surgical creation of an opening into the duodenum with the establishment of a fistula between it and another cavity or the outside.

duodenotomy (dū-od-e-not'-o-mi): Incision into the duodenum.

duodenum (dū ō-dē'-num): The fixed curved, first portion of the small intestine, 20–25 cm long, connecting the stomach above to the jejunum below. — duodenal, adj.

dupp (dup): A syllable used to describe the second sound heard at the apex of the heart in auscultation. It is higher pitched and shorter than the first sound, lupp.

Dupuytren's contracture: See under CONTRACTURE.

dura mater (dū'-ra mā'-ter): The outermost, fibrous, and toughest of the three meninges that surround the brain and spinal cord. — dural, adj.

duritis (dū-rī'-tis): Inflammation of the dura; also called *pachymeningitis*.

Dutch cap: A contraceptive device that covers the cervix.

duty of care: A requirement that a person acts towards others with the watchfulness, attention, caution and prudence that a reasonable person in the same circumstances would use. If a person's actions do not meet this standard of care, then the acts are considered negligent, and any damages resulting may be claimed in a lawsuit for negligence.

duty of partnership: A requirement placed on NHS bodies and local government to develop joint plans of local care delivery involving other parts of the NHS, local voluntary organizations and businesses.

DVT: Abbreviation for deep vein thrombosis, see under THROMBOSIS.

dwarf (dwawf): 1. An abnormally short or undersized person, especially one whose body proportions are abnormal. 2. To prevent, or preventing normal growth and development.

dwarfism (dwawf'-izm): Abnormal smallness or development of the body; AMSTERDAM D. a congenital syndrome in which severe mental handicap is associated with many anatomical abnormalities including short stature with short tapering fingers, short wide head, low-set ears, bushy eyebrows, fish-like mouth, excessive hairiness; 10% of the afflicted have epilepsy; deLange's syndrome. PITUITARY D., D. due usually to hypofunction of the hypophyseal or anterior lobe of the pituitary gland, but may also result from pituitary lesions or trauma, or from deficiency of thyrotrophic and adrenocorticotrophic hormones; in young persons characterized by stunted growth and development, childish appearance, and delayed sexual maturation; in older persons the outstanding characteristic is premature senility; THANATOPHORIC D. severe congenital dwarfism with very small limbs, narrow chest, long head, flattened vertebral bodies; death occurs early due to pulmonary difficulties.

dyad (dī'-ad): A pair. A couple, *e.g.*, mother and father, mother and baby. In cytology, either of two spiral filaments that are joined by the centrosome and constitute a chromosome; they separate during cell division and each becomes a chromosome in the daughter cells. — dyadic, adj.

dynamic (dī-nam-ik): Pertinent to or having physical energy or force. D. PSYCHOLOGY a psychological approach that stresses the element of energy in mental processes.

dynamics (dī-nam'-iks): 1. The branch of mechanics that deals with forces and the laws governing them. 2. The various forces operating in a field. 3. The implementation of the mechanics of a situation or procedure. 4. In psychiatry, the determination of how individuals develop emotional reactions and patterns of behaviour.

dys-: Prefix denoting painful, difficult, abnormal, diseased, impaired, faulty, poorly.

dysaesthesia (dis-es-thē'-zi-a): Impairment of the sense of touch.

dysaphia (dis-ā'-fi-a): Impairment in the sense of touch (pressure).

dysarthia (dis-ar'-thri-a): Difficulty in articulating words; may be due to a cerebellar disturbance, spasticity of the tongue and muscles of speech, or emotional stress. — dysarthric, adj.

dysarthrosis (dis-ar-thro'-sis): Any joint deformity, disease or other condition limiting movement.

dysbasia (dis-bā'-zi-a): Difficulty in walking, particularly when it is due to a nervous system lesion.

dyschesia (dis-kē'-zi-a): A form of constipation with accumulation of faeces in the rectum and difficult or painful defecation. Also dyschezia.

dyschondroplasia (dis-kon-drō-plā'-zi-a): A disease affecting the growth of long bones, metacarpals and phalanges; the cartilage develops regularly but ossifies very slowly, thus arresting the growth of the long bones while the head and trunk develop normally. This produces a condition of stocky dwarfism.

dyschromia (dis-krō'-mi-a): Any discoloration of the skin or hair.

dysdipsia (dis-dip'-si-a): Difficulty in swallowing liquids.

dysendocriniasis (dis'-en-dō-krin-ī'-a-sis): Any functional disorder of the hormone-secreting glands.

dysentery (dis'-en-ter-i,-tri): A term for a variety of disorders that may be epidemic or endemic and that are characterized by inflammation and sometimes ulceration of the intestines accompanied by evacuation of watery stools containing blood and mucus and attended by colic and tenesmus. Causative agent is usually a bacterium, protozoon or parasitic worm that is spread chiefly through contaminated food or water. AMOEBIC D., D. caused by the *Entamoeba histolytica*; BACILLARY D., D. caused by a bacillus of the genus *Shigella*. See AMOEBIASIS. — dysenteric, adj.

dysfunction (dis-funk'-shun): Abnormal functioning of any body organ or part. COLONIC D. sluggish muscular action of the colon resulting in distension and constipation; MINIMAL BRAIN D. that which may be caused by an inherited metabolic defect or damage or destruction of brain cells before birth; or it may follow infection with high fever, trauma, or lack of oxygen. Affected children may be hyperactive, have a short attention span, and be poor learners; UTERINE D. the slowing down or cessation of uterine contractions during labour; *inertia uteri*.

dysgeusia (dis-gū'-si-a): Impairment in the sense of taste, or perversion of taste; those affected often say that all foods have a vile taste.

dyshaematopoiesis (dis-hē'-ma-tō-poy-ē'-si-a): Imperfect blood formation.

dyshidrosis (dis-hid-rō'-sis): 1. Any abnormality in the production of sweat. 2. A vesicular skin eruption, occurring chiefly on the hands and feet; thought to be caused by a blockage of the sweat glands at their orifices; pompholyx (*q.v.*).

dyskinesia (dis-kī-nē′-si-a): Impairment of the ability to perform voluntary movements. TARDIVE D. aetiology not always known; may occur as a side effect of certain psychotropic drugs; characterized by facial tics and grimaces; blinking, chewing, sucking, and lip-smacking movements; choreoathetotic movements of the trunk may occur as well as torticollis, pelvic thrusting, foot-tapping; resembles parkinsonism in many ways.

dyslexia (dis-lek′-si-a): Impairment of the ability to read with comprehension; the child usually has difficulty with groups of letters, but the intelligence is unimpaired; often associated with poor instruction in reading, impaired hearing, or emotional stress.

dyslogia (dis-lō′-ji a): 1. Delay or interference in the development of the power of speech; often due to a central nervous system lesion. 2. Inability to think logically or to reason.

dysmelia (dis-mē′-li u): A congenital malformation characterized by shortening or complete absence of one or more limbs.

dysmenorrhoea (dis-men-ō-rē′-a): Painful or difficult menstruation. CONGESTIVE D. that which occurs during the premenstrual period; may be due to ischaemia and water retention; characterized by dull aching pain in the lower abdomen accompanied by feelings of depression and irritability; PRIMARY D. seen mostly in girls in their mid- and late teens; arises 24 hours before menstruation starts and is worse during the first 12 hours; causes a muscle incoordination, changes in hormonal secretion; may be accompanied by nausea and diarrhoea; SECONDARY D. seen mostly in women in their late 20s; pain starts before menstruation begins and continues through the flow; may be due to retroversion of the uterus, to pelvic inflammation, or endometritis; may be accompanied by anxiety and depression; SPASMODIC D. pain limited to the lower abdomen and back, accompanied by nausea and faintness; starts on the first day of the menses; due to muscle contractions.

dysmetria (dis-mē′-tri-a): Impairment of the sense of distance in controlling muscular action, *e.g.*, hand movements that overshoot the mark, as in the finger–nose test; seen in persons with cerebellar lesions.

dysmorphia (dis-mor′-fi-a): Deformity; abnormality in shape.

dysopia (dis-ō′-pi-a): Impaired vision.

dysorexia (dis-o-rek′-si-a): A diminished or unnatural appetite.

dysostosis (dis-os-tō′-sis): Defective formation of a bone or bones. CLEIDOCRANIAL D. defective ossification of cranial bones and of the clavicle. CRANIOFACIAL D. a rare birth defect consisting of a premature closure of the skull sutures, underdevelopment of the maxillae, exophthalmos, strabismus, nystagmus; MANDIBULOFACIAL D. see under MANDIBULOFACIAL; METHAPHYSEAL D. a form of D. in which the metaphases of long bones are spottily calcified and remain largely cartilaginous.

dyspareunia (dis-pa-roo′-ni-a): Painful or difficult coitus in women.

dyspepsia (dis-pep′-si-a): Disturbed digestion, characterized by heartburn, gas, nausea and a sense of over-fullness; indigestion. May be due to morbid condition of some organ or part of the digestive system or to the psychic effects of emotional tension, anxiety, fits of temper, etc. — dyspeptic, adj.

dysphagia (dis-fā′-ji-a): Painful or difficult swallowing; may result from local mouth or throat disorders, anxiety, or certain central nervous system disorders.

dysphasia (dis-fā′-zi-a): Loss or impairment of power to use or understand language due to injury or damage to the brain. — dysphasic, adj.

dysphemia (dis-fē′-mi-a): Stammering.

dysphonia (dis-fō′-ni-a): Unnatural sound of the voice, hoarseness, or difficulty in pronouncing sounds; due to organic, functional, or psychic causes.

dysphoria (dis-fo′-ri-a): Unpleasant mood; malaise; restlessness. Opp. of euphoria.

dysplasia (dis-plā′-zi-a): Abnormal development of organs, tissues or cells. CERVICAL D. a progressive D. of the cervix; seen most often in young women; may lead to carcinoma; FIBROMUSCULAR D. idiopathic D. leading to stenosis of the arteries, especially the renal artery, causing hypertension; usually seen in young women; MONOSTOTIC D., D. in which only one bone becomes deformed due to displacement by fibrous tissue; POLYOSTOTIC D. same as monostotic D. except that more than one bone is involved, usually on only one side of the body.

dyspnoea (dis′-nē-a): Difficult or painful breathing. EXERTIONAL D. that which occurs during even moderate exercise and is relieved when the exercise is discontinued; EXPIRATORY D., D. in which the expiratory time is prolonged, caused by obstruction in the bronchioles or small bronchi; may be associated with asthma, bronchitis, or obstructive emphysema; INSPIRATORY D., D. caused by some hindrance to the intake of air; may be due to presence of a foreign body, laryngitis, tumour, or compression of the trachea; often stridulous; NOCTURNAL D., D. that increases steadily during the day until by night it is very distressing; ORTHOSTATIC D., D. that occurs when one is in the erect position; PAROXYSMAL D., D. that occurs when one is lying down, particularly at night; associated with congestive heart failure.

dyspraxia (dis-prak'-si-a): Difficulty in performing, or partial loss of ability to perform, coordinated movements.

dysrhythmia (dis-rith'-mi-a): Disordered or abnormal rhythm. CEREBRAL D. disturbance or irregularity of brain waves as recorded by electroencephalography.

dyssocial (dis-sō'-shul): Relating to the behaviour of an individual who disregards the social and moral codes of the community and engages in predatory, illegal, sometimes criminal, activities.

dyssynergia (dis-sin-er'-ji-a): A disturbance in muscular coordination; due to lack of cooperation between agonist and antagonist muscles that usually act in unison. Ataxia.

dystaxia (dis-tak'-si-a): Difficulty in controlling voluntary movements. Mild ataxia (*q.v.*).

dysthesia (dis-thē'-zi-a): Impatience, ill temper, fretfulness.

dystocia (dis-tō'-si-a): Difficult, slow, or abnormal labour or delivery.

dystonia (dis-tō-ni-a): Disordered or defective muscle tone. D. MUSCULORUM DEFORMANS a relatively rare hereditary disease characterized by involuntary contractions of muscles, particularly those of the trunk, arms, and legs, which occur chiefly when walking. — dystonic, adj.

dystopia (dis-tō'-pi-a): Displacement or malposition of an organ. — dystopic, adj.

dystrophy (dis'-trō-fi): Term applied to many disorders, musculoskeletal disorders in particular, that arise from faulty nutrition. FUCH'S D., D. characterized by erosion of the epithelium of the cornea; LANDOUZY–DEJERINE D. a form of muscular D. in which there is atrophy of the face, shoulder girdle and arm; characterized by inexpressive face, drooping shoulders, inability to raise the arms; also called *facioscapulohumeral D.* LIMB-GIRDLE D. a hereditary, slowly progressive type of muscular D.; begins in childhood; may involve either the shoulder or pelvic girdle; MUSCULAR D. a group of familial, progressive, primary degenerative muscle disorders characterized by atrophy and wasting away of muscles, affecting primarily children and young adults; of unknown cause. Several types are recognized with the DUCHENNE type being the most severe; onset begins before five years of age; characterized by pseudohypertrophy of muscles followed by atrophy, skeletal deformities, lordosis, protruding abdomen, congestive heart failure, and frequent respiratory infections; MYOTONIC D., D. characterized by progressive weakness and atrophy of muscles of the face and limbs especially, early baldness, cataracts, often mental deficiency; SYMPATHETIC REFLEX D., D. characterized by superficial or deep pain in an upper or lower extremity, with throbbing, burning, aching, local oedema and erythema; occurs after some physical disturbance in that extremity; VITELLIFORM D. congenital degeneration of the macula; occurs in childhood; characterized by yellow or reddish lesions that eventually form pigmented areas on the macula, causing loss of central vision; syn.

dysuria (dis-ū'-ri-a): Difficult or painful urination.

E

ear: The organ of hearing. EXTERNAL E. consists of the semicircular flap on the side of the head called the auricle or pinna and the external auditory meatus or canal that extends to the middle ear from which it is separated by the tympanum or ear drum. MIDDLE E. consists of an air-containing cavity, bounded laterally by the tympanum; anteriorly it communicates with the Eustachian tube and thus with the throat. Stretched across this cavity are the tiny bones, the malleus, incus and stapes; these bones are in contact with the tympanic membrane and with one of the openings into the inner ear; their function is to transmit sound waves from the tympanum to the inner ear. INTERNAL or INNER E. the deepest part of the ear; consists of a bony labyrinth in which a similar membranous labyrinth is suspended in a fluid called perilymph. It is divided into the vestibule cochlea and three semicircular canals and contains a fluid called endolymph. Its walls hold the endings of the nerve of hearing. E. DRUM the membrane that separates the external from the middle ear; also called *tympanic membrane, tympanum;* E. LOBE the lower, usually fleshy part of the pinna; E. PLUG a small device of wax, rubber, or plastic worn in the external auditory canal to keep out noise, water when swimming, etc. E. WAX cerumen (*q.v.*).

earache (ēr′-āk): Pain in the ear. Syn., *otalgia, otodynia.*

ear drops: Liquid medication to be instilled into the external canal of the ear, drop by drop.

Early Sign Scale: A 34-item assessment scale used to predict deterioration in people with schizophrenia. Each item is rated on a 0 to 3 scale (0 = no problem; 3 = marked problem).

EBL: Abbreviation for enquiry-based learning (*q.v.*).

EBM: Abbreviation for evidence-based medicine (*q.v.*).

Ebola virus disease (eb′-o-la): A rare central African viral fever with acute onset. Involves cutaneous lymph nodes; symptoms include headache, muscle and abdominal pain, diarrhoea, intravascular clotting; often fatal. Incubation period is 2–21 days.

ebonation (ē-bō-nā′-shun): Removal of bone fragments from a wound after an injury.

EBP: Abbreviation for evidence-based practice (*q.v.*).

EC: Abbreviation for European Community, see EUROPEAN UNION.

eccentric (ek-sen′-trik): 1. Abnormal or peculiar in manner, speech, or ideas. 2. Proceeding outward from a centre.

ecchymoma (ek-i-mō′-ma): A slight haematoma or swelling due to a bruise and resulting from subcutaneous extravasation of blood.

ecchymosis (ek-i-mō′-sis): An extravasation of blood under the skin; marked by purple discoloration gradually changing to brown, green, yellow. Syn., *bruise.* — ecchymoses, pl.; ecchymosed, ecchymotic, adj.

eccrinology (ek-ri-nol′-ō-ji): The branch of anatomy and physiology that deals with the secretions and excretions of the exocrine glands. See EXOCRINE.

eccyesis (ek-sī-ē′-sis): Ectopic pregnancy; See under ECTOPIC.

ecdemic (ek-dem′-ik): Neither epidemic nor endemic, ecdemic refers to a disease that is carried to an area from a distant source.

ECG: Abbreviation for electrocardiogram (*q.v.*) Also *EKG* (USA).

echocardiography (ek′-kō-kar-di-og′-ra-fi): A painless procedure for recording the echo produced by directing ultrasound waves through the chest wall; shows the position and motion of the heart walls and great vessels; particularly useful in evaluating certain heart structures and abnormalities and in diagnosing and treating valvular heart disease.

echoencephalography (ek′-ō-en-kef-a-log′-ra-fi,-sef-): A non-invasive technique in which ultrasonic waves are beamed at both sides of the head; the echoes from the central part of the brain, which are recorded on a graphic tracing, may indicate the presence of a central mass in the brain; useful in detecting abscesses, blood clots, injury, or tumour within the brain. — echoencephalogram, n.

echogram (ek′-ō-gram): The pictorial representation of body structures and activity obtained by recording the echo produced by a technique utilizing ultrasound.

echopony (ek-of′-o-ni): The echo of a vocal sound heard during auscultation of the chest.

echovirus (ek-ō-vī′-rus): *E*nteric *C*ytopathic *H*uman *O*rphan, name given to a group of viruses originally found in stools of diseaseless children; most of them appear to be harmless but several have been known to cause various respiratory infections; enteritis, and non-bacterial meningitis.

eclampsia (ek-lamp′-si-a): **1.** A severe manifestation of toxaemia of pregnancy, often accompanied by convulsions and sometimes coma; associated with hypertension, oedema, proteinuria, oliguria; other symptoms include headache, blurred vision, gastric pain; complications include cerebral haemorrhage, retinal haemorrhage, sometimes with blindness, pulmonary oedema, renal failure, premature detachment of the placenta. May also occur during the puerperium. **2.** A sudden convulsive attack. — eclamptic, adj.

eclectic (ek-lek′-tik): Refers to the practice of selecting what seems to be the best from diverse systems, sources, etc. In medicine, refers to the use of biological, psychological, sociological, and cultural factors by physicians in constructing the framework within which they practice. — eclecticism, n.

ecography (ē-kog′-ra-fi): The use of ultrasound as a diagnostic aid in differentiating between solid and cystic structures within the body. The technique involves measuring the variations in echoes reflected by ultrasonic vibration of bodies of varying density. Ultrasonography (*q.v.*).

E. coli (kō ′-li): See *ESCHERICHIA COLI*, under *escherichia*.

ecology (ē-kol′-o-ji): The branch of biology that deals with the interactions of organisms with their environments and with each other.

ecosystem (ē′kō-sis-tem): A community and its environment functioning as a unit in nature; ecological system.

ecstasy (ek′-sta-sē): **1.** A state of exaltation, exhilaration or delight; a trance. **2.** Popular name for 3,4-methylenedioxymethamphetamine (MDMA for short), an illegal stimulant associated with rave parties. Also known as *E.* — ecstatic, adj.

ecstasia (ek′-tā′-zi-a): An overstretching or dilatation of a tubular organ or vessel. MAMMARY DUCT E. inflammation of the collecting ducts of the mammary gland with a sticky multicoloured discharge from the nipple, accompanied

by pain, itching, and redness around the nipple; SENILE E. dilated tufts of capillaries appearing as red or purplish spots on the skin of the upper chest and trunk of older persons.

ECT: Abbreviation for electroconvulsive therapy. See ELECTROTHERAPY.

ectad (ek′-tad): Outward; without.

-ecstasia, -ectasis: Combining forms denoting dilatation, stretching.

ecthyma (ek-thī′-ma): A pyogenic skin infection occurring chiefly on the thighs and legs, most often seen in tramps, filthy persons, and neglected children and characterized by large flat papules, with hardened bases and thick brownish crusts, that ulcerate and heal with pigmented scars. A similar condition may occur in syphilis.

ecto-: Combining form denoting external, outer, outside, situated on, out of place.

ectoblast (ek′-tō-blast): The ectoderm (*q.v.*).

ectocardia (ek-tō-kar′-di-a): A congenital condition in which the heart is misplaced, either within or outside the thoracic cavity.

ectocinerea (ek-tō-si-nē′-rē-a): The cortical part of the grey matter of the brain.

ectoderm (ek′-tō-derm): The external primitive germ layer of the embryo. From it are developed the skin structures, the nervous system, organs of special sense, mucous membrane of the mouth and anus, pineal gland and part of the pituitary and adrenal glands. — ectodermal, adj.

ectomorph (ek′-tō-morf): An individual whose body build tends to be lean and fragile, with thin muscles and slightly underdeveloped digestive organs. Compare with ENDOMORPH and MESOMORPH. — endomorphic, adj.

-ectomy: Combining form denoting a cutting out; surgical removal.

ectopia (ek-tō′-pi-a): Displacement of an organ or structure, especially if congenital. E. CORDIS displacement of the heart; may be in the abdomen or outside the chest wall; E. LENTIS displacement of the crystalline lens of the eye; E. VESICAE a congenital anomaly in which the urinary bladder protrudes through or opens onto the abdominal wall. — ectopic, adj.

-ectopia: Combining form denoting a condition in which an organ or part is out of place.

ectopic (ek-top′-ik): **1.** Occurring at an abnormal time, in an abnormal place, or in an abnormal position. **2.** Situated outside a normal position, said of an organ or part; may be congenital or acquired. E. BEAT a heartbeat caused by an impulse that originates in an area other than the sinoatrial node; E. FOCUS a group of cells in the heart which may or may not be able to control the heartbeat when the natural pacemaker fails to function normally; E. GESTATION or PREGNANCY extrauterine pregnancy; the fertilized ovum fails to reach the uterus but becomes implanted elsewhere; in most cases the site is the uterine tube but sometimes it is the peritoneal cavity. At about the 6th week of pregnancy, the tube ruptures, causing a surgical emergency. This is a serious condition and may be accompanied by severe pain, shock, and intra-abdominal haemorrhage. Prognosis is good if diagnosis and treatment are early, poor if treatment is omitted or unduly delayed.

ectoplasm (ek′-tō-plazm): The outer layer of protoplasm of a cell.

ectopy (ek′-to-pi): Displacement or malposition.

ectozoa (ek-tō-zō′-a): Animal parasites living on the outside of the body of the host. ectozoon, sing.

ectrogeny (ek-troj′-e-ni): The congenital absence of any organ or part of the body.

ectropion (ek-trō′-pi-on): An abnormal turning of a part, as of an eyelid, when it is due to laxity of the structures that support it; this causes eversion with resulting exposure of the lid conjunctiva. CERVICAL E. outward turning of the edges of the endocervix; usually results from chronic cervicitis or laceration of the external os; SENILE E., E. due to atrophy of the eyelid or flaccidity of the lid muscles.

ECV: Abbreviation for external cephalic version, see under CEPHALIC.

eczema (ek′-ze-ma): An all-inclusive term used to describe a non-contagious condition of the skin; may be chronic. Characterized by redness, inflammation, itching, formation of vesicles, papules or pustules that discharge and later become scaly and crusted. Cause is unknown but the condition is usually associated with allergies, drug sensitivity, fungus infection, nutritional deficiency, uncleanliness. CRAQUELE E., E. characterized by round erythematous lesions; E. VACCINATUM generalized vaccinia resulting from inoculation with vaccinia virus when there is an existing topical eczema; symptoms include crops of vesicles over the entire body, high fever, malaise, enlargement of lymph nodes; has a high mortality. INFANTILE E. an allergic E. of infants from about two months to two years, often limited to forehead and cheeks; very irritating; due to an allergy to foods, baby oil, or powder, etc.; NUMMULAR E., E., characterized by coin-

shaped scaly lesions; STASIS E. stasis dermatitis (q.v.). — eczematous, adj.

EDD: Abbreviation for expected date of delivery (q.v.).

edema, edematogenic: See OEDEMA, OEDEMATOGENIC.

edentulous (ē-den′-tū-lus): Without teeth.

EDTA: Abbreviation for ethylenediamine-tetraacetic acid, a substance that is mixed with blood specimens to prevent them from clotting.

Edwards syndrome: Trisomy 18 syndrome (See under TRISOMY).

EEG: Abbreviation for electroencephalogram (q.v.).

effacement (i-fās′-ment): 1. A change or obliteration of form or features. 2. The shortening of the cervical canal during labour until it becomes a circular orific continuous with the lower part of the uterus.

effect (i-fekt′); A condition or result produced by some agent, force, or action.

effectiveness (i-fek′-tiv-ness): 1. A measure of the accuracy or success of a diagnostic or therapeutic technique when carried out in an average clinical environment. 2. The extent to which a treatment achieves its intended purpose.

effector (i-fek′-tor): 1. A motor or secretory nerve ending in a muscle, gland, or organ. 2. A muscle that contracts or gland that secretes in response to a nerve impulse.

effemination (i-fem-i-nā′-shun): The development of feminine attributes in a male.

efferent (ef′-er-ent): Carrying, conveying, or conducting away from a centre. Opp. to afferent. E. NERVE one that conveys impulses away from the central nervous system to a part of the body such as a muscle or gland.

effervescent (ef-er-ves′-ent): Bubbling, foaming, giving off gas bubbles.

efficiency: 1.The production of the desired effects or results with minimum waste of time, money, effort or skill. 2. A measure of effectiveness; specifically, the useful work output divided by the energy input.

effleurage (ef-loo-razh′): A long, deep or superficial stroking movement used in massage.

efflorescence (ef-lō-res′-ens): In medicine, a rash or skin eruption in which the lesions are numerous and conspicuous.

effluvium (ef-floo′-vi-um): 1. An exhalation or emanation, especially one that is foul smelling. 2. A shedding, especially of hair.

effusion (i-fū′-zhun): Extravasation or escape of fluid into a tissue or cavity; may be serous, bloody, purulent. ENCYSTED E. the effused fluid is enclosed in a cyst, sac, or bladder; PERICARDIAL E. the accumulation of fluid exudate in the pericardial sac following pericarditis, most commonly associated with pyogenic infections, acute fibrinous pericarditis, rheumatic fever, or tuberculosis; PLEURAL E. effused fluid in the space between the lungs and pleura; may be bloody, purulent, or chylous; see EMPYEMA, HAEMOTHORAX; PULMONARY E. the presence of fluid in the air sacs and interstitial tissue of the lungs.

Egan Three Stage Mode (ē'-gan): A skills model of counselling. The initial stage is a review of the present situation; followed by development of a new or preferred scenario; finally the action phase, where the client puts the scenario into practice.

egest (ē-jest'): To discharge unabsorbed food residue from the digestive tract. — egestion, n.

ego (ē' -gō): 1. Self-esteem. 2. In psychoanalytic theory, the unconscious self, the 'I', that part of personality that deals with reality and is influenced by social forces. It modifies behaviour by unconscious compromise between the primitive instinctual urges (the id), internalized parental and social prohibitions (the superego), and reality.

egocentric (ē-go-sen' -trik): Self-centred; selfish; limited in outlook to one's own wishes and desires. Syn., *egotropism.* — egocentrism, n.

egomania (ē-gō-mā' -ni-a): Morbid preoccupation with self and self-esteem.

egotism (ē' -gō-tizm): Overvaluation of oneself; self-conceit. — egotistic, adj.

Ehrlich (air' -lik): E.'s side-chain theory, postulated that body cells consist of a stable nucleus and unstable side chains or chemoreceptors which, under certain conditions, are overproduced and released into body fluids; these free receptor groups become antibodies and are capable of combining specifically with certain antigen molecules; E.'s 606, arsphenamine (Salvarsan), discovered in 1909 as a result of his 606th experiment; the first specific treatment known for syphilis, yaws, and related infections. [Paul Ehrlich, German bacteriologist, 1854–1915.]

Eisenmenger's syndrome (ī-sen-meng-er): A condition in which a congenital septal defect allows for shunting of blood from the right side of the heart to the left side, with the result that some oxygen-poor blood gets pumped into the circulation and some oxygen-rich blood gets pumped into the lungs; symptoms include pulmonary hypertension and cyanosis; E.'s TETRALOGY a congenital anomaly consisting

of ventricular septal defect, dextroposition of the aorta, dilatation of the pulmonary artery, and right ventricular hypertrophy. [Victor Eisenmenger, German physician, 1864–1932.]

ejaculation (i-jak-u-lā' -shun): A sudden emission or expulsion, said particularly of semen. PREMATURE E., E. at the beginning of or prior to coitus; RETARDED E. occurs when the individual cannot effect E. when desired; RETROGRADE E. occurs when semen is ejaculated into the bladder; may occur in diabetic males.

ejaculatory (i-jak' -ū-la-tor-i): Relating to ejaculation. E. DUCT see under DUCT.

ejection click: A sound produced by the heart; caused by the sudden dilatation of the pulmonic artery and the aorta or to the forceful opening of the aortic valve; may indicate some pathologic condition but also heard in many normal, healthy persons.

EKG: Abbreviation for electrocardiogram (*q.v.*) (US). Also called *ECG.*

elastance (ē-las' -tans): A measure of the ability of an organ or structure to return to its original form when its contents are removed; refers often to an air-filled lung or fluid-filled urinary bladder.

elastic (i-las' -tik): Capable of being stretched, twisted, or distorted and then resuming its natural shape; E. BANDAGE a bandage of rubber or woven elastic material used to exert continuous pressure on oedematous or swollen limbs, broken ribs, or varicose veins; E. STOCKING a stocking made of woven elastic material; used to exert pressure on veins in the lower limbs; E. TISSUE connective tissue made up of yellow elastic fibres.

elasticity (ē-las-tis' -i-ti): The ability of a material to undergo distortion and return to its original size, shape, and condition.

elastin (i-las' -tin): The protein substance that forms the base of yellow elastic tissue.

elastinase (ē-las' -tin-ās): An enzyme that acts to dissolve elastic tissue by its action on elastin. Also called *elastase.*

elastofibroma (i-las' -tō-fī-brō' -ma): A tumour consisting of both elastic and fibrous tissue; usually occurs in the subscapular area, particularly of the elderly.

Elastoplast: Trademark for a type of elastic bandage made of cotton cloth without rubber, has porous, adhesive, non-fray edges.

elation (i-lā' -shun): Joyfulness; excitement that is marked by increased physical and mental activity. It becomes pathological when not consistent with the patient's circumstances.

elbow: The joint between the arm and forearm. E. CRUTCH see under CRUTCH; E. JERK involuntary bending of the elbow when the triceps muscle is struck suddenly; MINER'S E., STUDENT'S E. inflammation and enlargement of the bursa over the tip of the elbow caused by leaning on the elbow while digging or writing. NURSE-MAID'S E. subluxation of the head of the humerus; TENNIS E. radiohumeral bursitis; inflammation of the epicondyle of the humerus; occurs in those who engage in certain sports including tennis, but also occurs as a result of some unusual strain; due to repeated, sudden, jerky, vigorous movement of the extended forearm.

elder abuse: Actions that harm an older person, either through violence or neglect. There are three basic categories of elder abuse: (1) domestic elder abuse; (2) institutional elder abuse; and (3) self-neglect or self-abuse.

elderly (el'-der-li): Relating to individuals who are beyond middle age but not yet considered old. See OLD.

e-learning: Education achieved through the use of electronic multimedia such as interactive CD-ROMs and the World Wide Web (q.v.). It allows people to access learning opportunities at times and places that best fit their lifestyles.

elective (i-lek'-tiv): Term applied to procedures, usually surgical, that may be advantageous to the patient but not necessary to save his life; either the doctor or the patient may make the choice as to whether to perform the procedure at all or to schedule it for some convenient future date.

Electra complex (e-lek'-tra kom'-pleks): Term derived from Greek mythology. Refers to excessive fondness of a daughter for her father. The female counterpart of the Oedipus complex (q.v.).

electrical silence: Absence of the electrical activity of the brain as shown on the electroencephalogram; brain death.

electricity (ē-lek-tris'-i-ti): A fundamental physical entity of nature, now believed to be caused by the motion of negatively charged particles (electrons); it is observable in its attraction and repulsion of electrified bodies and the phenomena of luminescence and heating effects.

electric shock therapy: See ELECTROCONVULSIVE.

electrocardiogram (ilek-trō-kar'-di-ō-gram): A graphic recording of the electrical changes in the heart muscle during the cardiac cycle; obtained with an electrocardiograph (q.v.).

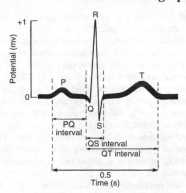

Standard electrocardiogram (ECG) record for resting heart rate.

electrocardiograph (i-lek-trō-kar'-di-ō-graf): An instrument containing a string galvanometer through which passes the electrical current produced by the heart's contraction. The electric impulses arising in the heart are picked up by several electrodes placed on the patient's body and amplified, and a permanent record (electrocardiogram) (q.v.) of these oscillations is made on a moving drum of graph paper.

electrocardiography (i-lek'-trō-kar-di-og'-ra-fi): The process and technique of recording and interpreting the electrical activity of the heart.

electrocardiophonograph (i-lek'-trō-kar'-di-ō-fō'-nō-graf): An instrument that records electrical potentials simultaneously with heart sounds produced during contraction of the heart muscle.

electrocardioscope (i-lek-trō-kar'-di-o-skōp): An instrument for visualizing the interior of the chambers of the heart.

electrocauterization (i-lek'-trō-kaw-ter-ī-zā'-shun): Cauterization by means of a wire heated by direct or alternating current of electricity.

electrocoagulation (i-lek'-trō-kō-ag-ū-lā-shun): A technique of surgical diathermy. Coagulation of bleeding points, or hardening of tumours or diseased tissue by the application of electricity.

electroconvulsive (i-lek'-trō-kon-vul-siv): Usually refers to therapy for some mental disorder; consists of passing an electric current through the patient's brain, producing a convulsion and coma.

electrocorticography (i-lek'-trō-kor-ti-kog'-ra-fi): An electroencephalogram in which the electrodes are attached directly to the cortex of the brain. — electrocorticographic, adj.; electrocorticographically, adv.

electrode (i-lek´-trōd): In electrotherapy, a conductor in the form of a pad or plate whereby electricity enters or leaves the body.

electrodesiccation (i-lek´-trō-des-i-kā´-shun): A technique of surgical diathermy in which a high-frequency current is applied to tissue with a needle electrode; there is drying and subsequent removal of the tissue.

electrodiagnosis (i-lek´-trō-dī-ag-nō´-sis): The use of graphic recordings of electrical irritability of tissues in diagnosis. — electrodiagnostic, adj.

electroencephalogram (i-lek´-trō-en-kef´-a-lō-gram, -sef´-): A graphic record made with the electroencephalograph (q.v.)

electroencephalograph (i-lek´-trō-en-kef´-a-lō-graf, -sef-): An instrument for obtaining a recording of the electric currents developed in the brain by means of electrodes that may be attached to the scalp or the surface of the brain, or placed within the substance of the brain. The electrodes pick up electric changes produced by activity in the brain and amplify them for recording. The record is an electroencephalogram (EEG), useful in localizing brain lesions or tumours and in studying some forms of mental disorder and brain function. — electroencephalographic, adj., electroencephalographically, adv.

electroencephalography (i-lek´-trō-en-kef-a-log´-ra-fi, -sef-): The recording of electric currents developed in the brain. See ELECTROENCEPHALOGRAPH.

electroexcision (i-lek´-trō-ek-siz´-zhun): The excision of tissue or a body part by electrosurgical means.

electrogram (i-lek´-tro-gram): A recording, on paper or film, of an electrical event, as occurs, e.g., in an electrocardiogram.

electrolarynx (i-lek-trō-lar´-inks): Any of several types of electronic devices that enable laryngectomees who can use oesophageal speech to communicate. See OESOPHAGEAL SPEECH under OESOPHAGEAL.

electrolysis (i-lek-trol´-i-sis): 1. Chemical decomposition of a substance by passage of an electric current through it. 2. Destruction and permanent removal of hairs (epilation), moles, spider naevi, etc. by means of electricity.

electrolyte (i-lek´-trō-līt): 1. A liquid or solution of a substance that is capable of conducting electricity and is decomposed by the passage of it; see ELECTROLYSIS. 2. In physical chemistry, any substance that dissociates into positive

and negative ions when in solution; in physiology, refers to body anions and cations. E. BALANCE (1) the normal state when there is the correct balance between positive and negative ions in body fluids, tissues, and blood; (2) the state of the body in relation to intake and output of electrolytes.

electrolyte and fluid balance: See FLUID and ELECTROLYTE BALANCE and BALANCE.

electromyogram (i-lek-trō-mī´-ō-gram): 1. An electrophysiological recording of the electrical activity of a muscle, either that which occurs spontaneously or that which is produced by an electric current. 2. A graphic recording of movements of the eye during reading. Abbreviated EMG.

electromyograph (i-lek-trō-mī´-ō-graf): An instrument used for measuring the electrical currents generated in muscle tissue activity.

electromyography (i-lek´-trō-mī-og´-ra-fi): 1. A graphic recording of electrical currents generated when a muscle contracts as a result of the application of an electric stimulus. 2. The science and study of the recordings made by an electromyograph.

electron (i-lek´-tron): A negatively charged subatomic particle that revolves around the positively charged nucleus of an atom. E. MICROSCOPE a modern M. that differs from the ordinary M. in several ways; in particular, instead of using ordinary light it utilizes electron beams that have a much shorter wavelength than that of ordinary visible light and this allows for much greater magnification; E. THEORY the theory that all bodies are complex structures made up of atoms together with still smaller particles — electrons, protons, and neutrons.

electronic (i-lek´-tron´-ik): 1. Relating to or carrying electrons (q.v.). 2. Relating devices that operate on the principles of electronics (q.v.).

electronic health record: A computerized longitudinal log of a patient's health and healthcare which combines information from primary health-care with periodic input from other institutions.

electronic patient record: Computer-based information on the care provided for a client, mainly by one organization, such as an acute hospital or mental health trust

electronics (i-lek´tron-iks): The branch of physics that deals with the emission and effects of electrons and with the use of electronic devices. The pure study of such devices is considered as a branch of physics, while the design and construction of electronic circuits to solve practical problems belong to the fields of electrical and computer engineering. The main uses of electronic circuits are the controlling, processing and distribution of information, and the conversion and distribution of electromagnetic power. Both of these uses involve the creation or detection of electromagnetic fields and electric currents. Electronic systems are divided into: inputs – electrical or mechanical sensors (also known as *transducers*); signal processing circuits – components connected together to manipulate, interpret and transform the signals; and outputs – actuators or other devices (also called *transducers*).

electronic tagging: Use of a transmitter, tracking device on the body that uses a global positioning satellite to identify and check an individual's exact location. Most commonly used for criminal offenders released early from prison.

electronystagmography (i lek′-trō-nī-stag-mŏg′-ra-fi): The electroencephalographic recording of eye movements for use in assessing nystagmus (*q.v.*).

electrophoresis (i-lek-trō-fo-rē′-sis): Migration of charged particles in solution to the positive or negative electrode when an electric current is passed through the solution.

electropuncture (i-lek-trō-punk′-chur): The use of needles as electrodes for applying electric current to a nerve or muscle.

electroscission (i-lek′-trō-sizh-un): The division of tissues using an electrocautery knife.

electroshock (i-lek′-trō-shok): Shock produced by applying an electric current to the brain. E. THERAPY see ELECTROCONVULSIVE.

electrospectrography (i-lek′-trō-spek-tog′-ra-fi): A recording of electroencephalographic wave patterns, and their study and interpretation. See ELECTROENCEPHALOGRAPH.

electrotherapy (i-lek-trō-ther′-a-pi): Treatment of disease by means of electricity, *e.g.*, diathermy, electroshock therapy. Also *electrotherapeutics, electroshock, electroplexy.*

element (el′-e-ment): One of the constituents of a compound. The elements are primary substances which, alone or combined with other elements in compounds, constitute all matter. The basic unit of an element is an atom. – elementary, adj.

-eleo: Combining form denoting oil.

elephantiasis (el-e-fan-tī′-a-sis): A chronic disease, usually of the tropics, caused by an obstruction in the lymphatics. Often due to *Filaria* but in non-tropical areas may occur as a result

of syphilis or recurrent streptococcal infections. Characterized by thickening and hardening of the skin and subcutaneous tissues and hypertrophy of the affected areas; legs and external genitalia most often affected. Also called *Barbados leg, pachydermia.* – elephantoid, elephantiasic, adj.

elevator (el′-e-vā-tor): 1. An instrument for lifting or separating parts, *e.g.*, periosteum from bone. 2. An instrument for extracting roots of teeth. 3. One of the extraocular muscles.

eliminant (e-lim′-in-ant): An agent that increases excretion of waste materials.

elimination (e-lim-i-nā′-shun): The removal of wastes from the body.

ELISA: Abbreviation for enzyme-linked immunosorbent assay (*q.v.*).

elixir (ē-lik′-ser): A clear, sweetened, flavoured, often alcoholic, solution containing a medicinal agent; administered by mouth.

elliptocytosis (e-lip′-tō-sī-tō′-sis): A rare hereditary type of anaemia in which many of the red blood cells are oval in shape; seen in certain blood dyscrasias, thalassaemia, and in pernicious, sickle cell, and iron-deficiency anaemias.

emaciation (i-mā-shi-a′-shun): Excessive leanness, or wasting of body tissue. – emaciate, v.

e-mail: Messages sent from computer to computer via the Internet (*q.v.*). Also known as *electronic mail.*

emanation (em-a-nā′-shun): 1. Exhalation. 2. That which is given off, such as the gaseous disintegration products of radioactive substances.

emasculation (e-mas-kū-lā′-shun): Castration.

embalm (em-balm′): To treat a dead body with preservatives to prevent its decay.

embolectomy (em-bō-lek′-to-mi): Surgical removal of an embolus (*q.v.*).

embolic (em-bol′-ik): Relating to an embolus (*q.v.*) or an embolism (*q.v.*).

embolism (em-bō-lizm): The sudden obstruction of a blood vessel by a bit of foreign matter, *e.g.*, a clot, air bubble, fat particle, or clump of bacteria that is brought to the site by the blood current. AIR E., E. caused by a bubble of air; usually occurs following surgery or injury to a blood vessel, but may also be a serious complication of intravenous therapy; ARTERIAL E., E. that is usually characterized by sudden onset of pain, ischaemia, coldness of the part supplied by the artery, absent or diminished pulses; FAT E., E. caused by a tiny drop of fat in the bloodstream; most commonly occurring in association with diabetes, pancreatitis, fatty liver disease, skeletal trauma, PULMONARY E., E. that occurs when a bubble of air or fat, but most often a free-flowing clot in the circulation, becomes lodged in the pulmonary artery or a branch of it, causing an impedance of pulmonary circulation characterized by sudden respiratory distress, pleural pain, restlessness; may be a serious complication of intravenous therapy.

embolization (em-bō-lī-zā´-shun): The therapeutic occlusion of a blood vessel, usually by introducing into the circulation any of several substances that will occlude the vessel.

embolus (em´-bō-lus): A body such as a clot or an air bubble transported in the blood until it causes obstruction by blocking a blood vessel. Besides clots and air bubbles, emboli may consist of masses of bacteria, tumour cells, parasites, tissue fragments, or fat globules. — emboli, pl.

embrocation (em-bro-kā´-shun): The application of a liquid to the body, especially by rubbing.

embryo (em´-brē-ō): The early stage in the development of an organism. Fertilization of an egg following fusion of the gametes (q.v.) result in a zygote which undergoes progressive cell division (q.v.), producing an embryo. In human anatomy, the term is applied to the conceptus from the time of generation until all of the internal and external organs are present and undergoing further development, which occurs at approximately the end of the seventh week of pregnancy, after which it is called a fetus.

embryoctomy (em-bri-ok´-to-mi): Feticide; the intentional destruction of the embryo or the fetus *in utero* for abortion or when delivery is impossible.

embryogenesis (em´-brē-ō-jen´-e-sis): 1. The period in prenatal development when the characteristics of the embryonic body are established; usually considered to extend from the second through the eighth week, after which the conceptus is called a fetus. 2. The development of a new individual by the process of sexual reproduction.

embryology (em-brē-ol´-o-ji): Study of the development of an organism from fertilization to extrauterine life. — embryological, adj., embryologically, adv.

embryonic (em-brē-on´-ik): 1. Relating to an embryo. 2. Rudimentary.

embryopathy (em-brē-op´-a-thi): A disease or abnormal condition resulting from interference with the normal development of the embryo or fetus. More serious if it occurs during the first three months. Includes the rubella syndrome, anomalies that occur in the fetus as a result of the mother's having had German measles (rubella) in early pregnancy.

emergency (ē-mer´-jen-si): 1. A pathological condition that develops suddenly and requires immediate medical therapy or surgical intervention. 2. A suddenly occurring threat to life or health, such as an epidemic or a disaster, that calls for immediate attention to seriously ill or injured victims.

emergency contraception: A form of birth control to be taken by a woman when other contraceptive precautions fail or are not taken. Usually in the form of a pill that induces a hormonal imbalance, resulting in rejection of the embryo. Its efficacy is increased the earlier it is taken after unprotected sexual intercourse. In the UK, it can be purchased through direct pharmacy supply, providing an additional point of access to birth control. This is advantageous at weekends and evenings when other services might not be available. Hormonal emergency contraception will remain available for women, including under the 16s, free of charge on prescription from GPs and Family Planning clinics.

emergency trolley: See CRASH TROLLEY.

emesis (em´-e-sis): Vomiting.

emetic (ē-met´-ik): 1. Causing the act of vomiting. 2. Any agent used to produce vomiting.

EMG: Abbreviation for electromyogram (q.v.).

EMI scanner: Name given to the first computerized axial tomography (q.v.) (manufactured in England by Electrical and Musical Instruments). The machine permits safe, painless serial viewing of organs or parts of the body that do not show up on x-ray photographs; used especially for viewing the brain.

-emia: Combining form denoting (1) blood, (2) a condition of blood.

eminence (em´-i-nens): A prominence or projection, especially on the surface of a bone.

emiocytosis (ē´-mi-ō-sī-tō´-sis): The passage of the granular cell material through the cell membrane; said particularly of the insulin granules in the cells of the islets of Langerhans, which migrate to the cell membrane where they fuse, the membrane ruptures, and the insulin passes out of the cell into the circulation.

emission (i-mish'-un): An ejaculation or sending forth, specifically an involuntary ejaculation of semen. NOCTURNAL E. involuntary emission of semen during sleep, occurring in normal males beginning with puberty.

emmenia (e-mē'-ni-a): The menses (*q.v.*).

emmetropia (em-e-trō'-pi-a): Normal or perfect vision — emmetropic, adj.

emollient (ē-mol'-i-ent): An agent that softens and soothes skin or mucous membrane.

emotion (i-mō'-shun): A strong feeling such as fear, anger, grief, joy, or love, or an aroused mental state recognized in ourselves by certain bodily changes, and in others by certain characteristic behaviour.

emotional (i-mō'-shun-al): Characteristic of or caused by emotion. E. BIAS tendency to allow one's E. attitude to affect logical judgment; E. ILLNESS a mental disorder; E. INSTABILITY a condition characterized by hysterical behaviour; E. INTELLIGENCE a term describing the ability to perceive, assess, and positively influence your own and other people's emotions; E. LABILITY fluctuations in emotional expression that are beyond the person's control; may shift from crying to laughing, from anger to fear, and so on; often due to a frontal lobe lesion; E. LABOUR the stresses inherent in the conduct of work activities involving strong feelings, where effective performance may require individuals to express attitudes that they do not feel and may consider false or personally distressing; E. MATURITY the state of having achieved maximum emotional control; E. REACTION reaction based on emotion rather than logic; E. STATE effect of emotions on normal mood, *e.g.*, agitation. — emotionality, n.

empathy (em'-pa-thi): The ability to identify with the emotions, feelings and reactions that another person is experiencing, and to communicate that understanding effectively to the individual.

emphysema (em-fi-sē'-ma, -fi-): A non-reversible chronic pulmonary disorder, often secondary to smoking or the hazards of certain occupations; characterized by the breakdown of the septal walls between the alveoli, destruction of the connective tissue that is responsible for the elastic recoil of the lung, and the resulting gaseous distension of the tissues or organs with air. CENTRIACINAR E. affects chiefly the bronchioles rather than the alveoli; there is focal dilatation of air spaces which are scattered throughout normal tissue of the entire lung; also called centrilobular E.; INTERSTITIAL E. a condition in which air is trapped in the lung tissue instead of moving into the alveoli; occurs in respiratory distress syndrome of infants; OBSTRUCTIVE E. overdistension of the lung resulting from partial obstruction of the air passages, which allows air to enter the alveoli but interferes with expiration; PANACINAR E. panlobular E., affects all lung segments; the alveoli atrophy and the vascular bed is destroyed; PULMONARY E. alveolar distension, which may be (1) generalized; often accompanying chronic bronchitis, or (2) localized, occurring distally to partial obstruction of a bronchus or in alveoli adjacent to a segment of collapsed lung; SUBCUTANEOUS E. air or gas in subcutaneous tissues; when it occurs in the connective tissue under the skin it is called *cutaneous E.*; SURGICAL E. air or gas in subcutaneous tissues following surgery or trauma. — emphysematous, adj.

empirical (em-pir'-i-kal): Based on careful observational testing of a hypothesis; rational.

empiricism(em-pir'-i-sizm): 1. The belief, in philosophy or psychology, that all knowledge is the result of our experiences. Empiricism is closely allied with philosophical materialism and positivism and opposed to rationalism or intuitionism. 2. Using experience as a guide to practice or to the therapeutic use of any remedy.

empower: To give someone official authority or the freedom to do something.

emptysis (emp'-ti-sis): Haemoptysis (*q.v.*).

empyema (em-pī-ē'-ma): A collection of pus in a cavity, hollow, organ, or space; if unspecified, refers to pus in the pleural cavity. — empyemic, adj.

emulsify (i-mul'-si-fi): To convert a substance into an emulsion by combining two solutions that do not normally mix, so that the result is a liquid containing particles in suspension.

emulsion (i-mul'-shun): A fluid containing fat or oil particles in the state of subdivision and suspension, so that a smooth, milky white fluid results.

enamel (en-am'-el): The hard external covering of the crown of a tooth.

enarthrosis (en-ar-thrō'-sis): A ball and socket joint such as a hip joint.

encapsulation (en-kap-sū-lā'-shun): Enclosure within a capsule.

encelitis (en-si-li'-tis): Inflammation in any of the abdominal organs.

encephal-, encephala-, encephalo-: Combining forms denoting the brain.

encephalasthenia (en-kef-el-as-thē'-ni-a, -sef-): Mental fatigue, particularly when of emotional origin.

encephalic (en-ke-fal' -ik, -sef-): Relating to the structures within the cranium or to the brain alone.

encephalitis (en-kef-a-lī' -tis, -sef-): Inflammation of the brain; may be a specific disease entity or occur as a sequel to another disease. Characterized by headache, malaise, fever, slowed mental and motor responses, and stuporous sleep. ACUTE DISSEMINATED E. postinfection E.; ARBOVIRUS E. caused by an arborvirus such as Eastern equine or St Louis equine; E. AXIALIS DIFFUSA a form of E. occurring in children and adults, and characterized by destruction of the white matter of the brain; symptoms include progressive mental deterioration, bilateral spasticity, deafness, and blindness; also called *Schilder's disease*; HERPES E., E. caused by the herpes simplex virus; usually fatal; E. LETHARGICA a sporadic and occasionally epidemic form of virus infection. Profound cerebral damage with cranial nerve palsies; stupor and delirium can occur. May be followed by alteration of personality or Parkinson's disease; POSTINFECTION E. an acute infection of the central nervous system in persons recovering from an infectious disease, usually one caused by a virus; POST-RUBEOLA E., E. that usually develops within four to six days following the skin eruption; marked by sudden rise in temperature and drowsiness, stupor, neurological signs; often fatal; POST-VACCINIAL E. acute E. sometimes follows vaccination. — encephalitides, pl.; encephalitic, adj.

encephalocele (en-kef' -a-lō-sēl, -sef-): Hernia of the brain with protrusion of the brain substance through an opening in the skull. Often associated with hydrocephalus when the protrusion occurs at a suture line.

encephalogram (en-kef' -a-lō-gram, -sef-): An x-ray picture of the contents of the skull. See PNEUMOENCEPHALOGRAM.

encephalography (en-kef-a-lōg' -ra-fi, -sef-): Roentgenology of the skull contents, particularly of the brain. See PNEUMOENCEPHALOGRAPHY.

encephaloid (en-kef' -a-loyd, -sef-): Resembling the substance of the cerebrum. E. CANCER encephaloma, a malignant tumour of the brain.

encephalolith (en-kef' -a-lō-lith,-sef-): A concretion in the brain tissue or in one of the ventricles.

encephalomeningitis (en-kef' -a-lō-men-in-jī' -tis, -sef-): Inflammation of the brain and its meninges.

encephalomeningocele (en-kef' -a-lō-me-ning' -gō-sēl, -sef-): Protrusion of the cerebral membranes and brain substance through a defect in the bones of the skull.

encephalomyelitis (en-kef' -a-lō-mī-e-lī' -tis, -sef-): Inflammation of the brain and spinal cord. EQUINE E. a viral disease transmitted by ticks and mosquitoes to horses and man.

encephalomyelopathy (en-kef' -a-lo-mī-e-lop' -a-thi, -sef-): Disease affecting both the brain and spinal cord. POSTINFECTION E., E. that occurs secondarily to such common diseases as mumps, measles, chickenpox, influenza.

encephalopathy (en-kef' -a-lop' -a-thi, -sef-): Any disease or dysfunction of the brain. ALCOHOLIC E. see WERNICKE'S E.; HEPATIC E., E. that occurs in patients with advanced liver disease; marked by nervous system disturbances, changes in behaviour and consciousness which may proceed to confusion, lethargy, tremor, disorientation, stupor, coma; may also occur in patients having a porta-caval shunt; HYPERTENSIVE E., E. marked by convulsions, coma; associated with malignant hypertension; HYPOGLYCAEMIC E., E. induced by severe hypoglycaemia as in overstorage of glycogen or disturbances in insulin secretion; TRAUMATIC E., E. that occurs in boxers and others subject to persistent trauma to the head; marked by headache, confusion, slowing of mental activity, and memory loss; WERNICKE'S E. a condition caused by deficiency of vitamin B_1 (thiamine); commonly seen in chronic alcoholics, and characterized by delirium, various eye signs, paralysis of some of the eye muscles causing a squint or rhythmic jerking of the head when the patient tries to look to one side. See also BOVINE SPONGIFORM ENCEPHALOPATHY; CREUTZFELDT-JAKOB DISEASE; VARIANT CREUTZFELDT-JAKOB DISEASE

encephalopyosis (en-kef' -a-lō-pī-ō' -sis, -sef-): A purulent inflammation or abscess of the brain.

encephalorrhagia (en-kef' -a-lō-rā' -ji-a, -sef-): Haemorrhage from the brain or within it.

encephalosclerosis (en-kef' -a-lō-sklē-rō' -sis, -sef-): Hardening of the brain.

encephalosepsis (en-kef' -a-lō-sep' -sis, -sef-): Septic inflammation of the brain.

encephalosis (en-kef-a-lō' -sis, -sef-): Any organic disease of the brain.

enchondroma (en-kon-drō' -ma): A benign cartilaginous tumour occurring in a part where cartilage is not normally found or within a bone near the epiphyseal line. — enchondromata, pl.; enchondromatous, adj.

encopresis (en-kō-prē' -sis): Involuntary passage of faeces not due to disease or organic defect. In children, often due to emotional problems. — encopretic, adj.

encounter group therapy: A type of therapy whereby patients meet in groups, designed to improve their orientation to reality and their relations with others. See also SENSITIVITY TRAINING.

Endamoeba: See ENTAMOEBA.

endarterectomy (end-ar-ter-ek′-tō-mi): Surgical removal of the innermost lining of an artery when it has become thickened by atheromatous plaque. CAROTID E. surgical removal of atheromatous plaque from the intima of a carotid artery; may be done when transient ischaemic attacks are thought to be due to such plaque; may involve both internal and external carotids; CORONARY E. surgical removal of occluding material from the coronary artery.

endarterial (end-ar-tē′-ri-al): 1. Within an artery. 2. Pertinent to the intima of an artery.

end bulb: A term used to describe certain sensory nerve endings in some areas of the skin or mucous membrane.

end-diastolic (dī-as-tol′-ik): Refers to the time period following diastole (end-diastole) just before the systolic contraction begins. E. PRESSURE the pressure of the blood in the ventricles at end-diastole; E. VOLUME the volume of blood in the ventricles just before the beginning of systole.

endemic (en-dem′-ik): Peculiar to a certain area; said of diseases that are habitually present within a given locality. — endemically, adv.; endemicity, n.

endemiology (en-dē-mi-ol′-ō-ji): The special study of endemic diseases.

endo-: Combining form denoting within; inner.

endobronchial (en-dō-brong′-ki-al): Within a bronchus. E. TUBE a double lumen tube that can be inserted into the bronchus of one lung to permit deflation of the other lung for thoracic surgery; also may be used in administration of inhalation anaesthetic.

endobronchitis (en-dō-bron-kī′-tis): Inflammation of the lining of the bronchi.

endocardial (en-dō-kar′-di-al): Relating to the endocardium. E. FIBROELASTOSIS a heart disease of unknown cause; occurs mostly in infants; the lining of the heart chambers becomes thickened with elastic tissue, especially in the left ventricle, which impairs cardiac function.

endocarditis (en-dō-kar′-dī′-tis): Inflammation of the inner lining of the heart and/or the covering of the valves of the heart; most commonly due to rheumatic fever. ABACTERIAL E., E. that

is not due to an invading organism; sometimes associated with lupus erythematosus; ACUTE BACTERIAL E., E. caused by pyogenic organisms, usually streptococcus, gonococcus, pneumococcus, or meningococcus; rapidly progressive; often fatal; ACUTE E. the nonbacterial E. that is often due to rheumatic fever; INFECTIVE E. infection of the endocardium; usually caused by a streptococcic, staphylococcic, or enterococcic organism; may occur in patients with congenital heart malformations or, more often, following valvular heart surgery. Also frequently occurs in patients having dental surgery and in those with infection of the periodontal membranes. Prophylaxis consists chiefly of preoperative administration of antibiotics; MALIGNANT E. acute fulminating E.; usually associated with suppuration elsewhere in the body; MARANTIC E. non bacterial E., usually associated with a neoplasm or other debilitating condition; RHEUMATIC E. the E. of rheumatic fever, often involving the heart valves; SUBACUTE BACTERIAL E. usually due to *Streptococcus viridans*; usually confined to the valves; of gradual onset; seen most often in young adults; VALVULAR E., E. that affects one or more of the heart valves; VERRUCOUS E. vegetative E.; associated with formation of fibrinous clots on the endocardium and forming ulceration on the valves; often associated with lupus erythematosus.

endocardium (en-dō-kar′-di-um): The thin serous membrane lining the chambers of the heart and covering the surfaces of the heart valves. It is continuous with the lining of the vessels entering and leaving the heart.

endocervix (en-dō-ser′-vix): The mucous membrane lining of the cervix of the uterus. — endocervical, adj.

endochondral (en-dō-kon′-dral): Situated or occurring within cartilage; usually refers to the formation of bone within cartilage by the process of replacement.

endocranial (en-dō-krā′-ni-al): Within the cranium.

endocrine (en-dō-krin, krīn): Secreting within; term applied to the ductless glands of the body whose secretions pass directly from the gland into the interstitial tissues, from which they are diffused into the blood or lymph to be carried to other parts of the body where they affect the functioning of other organs or parts. The opposite of exocrine (*q.v.*). E. GLANDS include the pineal, pituitary, thyroid, parathyroid, thymus, adrenals, ovaries, testes, and islands of Langerhans in the pancreas. E. SECRETIONS those produced by the E. glands; they have important influences on the metabolic processes; E. SYSTEM consists of all glands that deliver their secretions directly into the bloodstream; E. THERAPY treatment with E. preparations.

endocrinology (en-dō-kri-nol'-o-ji): The study of the ductless glands and their internal secretions.

endocrinotherapy (en-dō-krin-ō-ther'-a-pi): Treatment of disease by administration of endocrine substances.

endocytosis (en'-dō-sī-tō'-sis): The engulfing by a cell of particles that are too large to diffuse through the cell membrane, as occurs in phagocytosis (q.v.).

endoderm (en'-dō-derm): The innermost of three layers of cells that form during the early development of the embryo; it gives rise to the epithelium of the digestive tract, liver, pancreas, urinary bladder and urethra, pharynx, auditory tube, larynx, trachea, bronchi, lungs, and the thyroid, parathyroid, and thymus glands, and the adenohypophysis. Also called *entoderm.*

endodontium (en-dō-don'-shi-um): The pulp of a tooth.

endogamy (en-dog'-a-mi): 1. In biology, sexual reproduction by conjugation of two gametes descended from the same ancestor cell. 2. In anthropology, the restriction of marriage to members of the same tribe, social group, or community.

endogenic (en-dō-jen'-ic): Of inside origin; endogenous.

endogenous (en-doj'-e-nus): Originating within a structure, organ, or organism, as contrasted with exogenous.

endolymph (en'-dō-limf): The fluid contained in the membranous labyrinth of the internal ear.

endometrial (en-dō-mē'-tri-al): Relating to or affecting the endometrium. E. ASPIRATION use of a low-pressure suction apparatus to remove the endometrium and the products of conception; E. CANCER a fairly common type of uterine cancer; usually an adenocarcinoma; E. LAVAGE a procedure for obtaining endometrial cells for examination by injecting a solution of normal saline into the uterus as a lavage.

endometrioma (en'-dō-mē-tri-ō'-ma): A tumour containing shreds of misplaced endometrium; found most frequently in the ovary. Adenomyoma (q.v.). See CHOCOLATE CYST under CYST. — endometriomata, pl.

endometriosis (en'-dō-mē-tri-ō'-sis): The presence of functioning endometrium in abnormal places both within and without the uterus;

often the cause of abdominal and/or pelvic pain which becomes more severe at menstruation, and of unusually heavy menstrual flow. Adhesions may form around these deposits and cause distortion of the pelvic organs and their functions. See CHOCOLATE CYST under CYST.

endometrium (en-dō-mē'-tri-um): The lining mucosa of the uterus. — endometrial, adj.

endomorph (en-dō-morf): An individual whose body build differs from the normal in that the digestive viscera are large, there are accumulations of fat about the abdomen, the trunk and thighs are large and the extremities are tapering. Compare with ECTOMORPH and MESOMORPH. — endomorphic, adj.

endomysium (en-dō-mis'-i-um): The delicate connective tissue sheath that surrounds individual muscle fibres within a fasciculus and serves to support blood vessels and nerves that branch between the fibres.

endoneurium (en-dō-nū'-ri-um): The delicate, inner connective tissue surrounding the nerve fibres.

endoparasite (en-dō-par'-a-sīt): Any parasite living within its host. — endoparasitic, adj.

endophytic (en-dō-fit'-ik): Having a tendency to grow inward and proliferate within an organ or structure; often refers to tumours of the skin.

endoplasm (en'-dō-plazm): The central, more fluid portion of a unicellular organism, as distinguished from the ectoplasm (q.v.).

end organ: An encapsulated structure containing the terminal part of a sensory nerve fibril in muscle tissue, skin, mucous membrane or a gland.

endorphin (en-dor'-fin): Any of several neuropeptides produced by the pituitary gland and widely distributed in the central nervous system; alpha, beta, and gamma E.'s have been isolated. E.'s have a molecular structure similar to that of morphine; they act as neurotransmitters and neuromodulators and have the effect of reducing pain. See also ENKEPHALIN.

endorrhachis (en-dō-rā'-kis): The spinal cord dura mater.

endosalpinx (en-dō-sal'-pinks): The mucous membrane lining of the uterine tubes; it is continuous with the lining of the uterus.

endoscope (en'-dō-skōp): A tubular, lighted instrument for visualization of the interior of body cavities or organs. — endoscopic, adj.; endoscopy, n.

endospore (en'-dō-spōr): A bacterial spore that has a purely vegetative function. It is formed by the loss of water and probable rearrangement of the protein of the cell, so that metabolism is minimal and resistance to environmental conditions, especially high temperature, desiccation and anti-bacterial drugs, is high; two genera that include pathogenic species that form spores are *Bacillus* and *Clostridium*.

endosteal (en-dos'-tē-al): 1. Relating to the endosteum. 2. Located or occurring within a bone.

endosteum (en-dos'-tē-um): The thin vascular connective tissue lining the medullary canal of a long bone. — endosteal, adj.

endothelial (en-dō-thē'-li-al): Relating to or resembling epithelium.

endotheliocyte (en-dō-thē'-li-ō-sīt): A macrophage (*q.v.*).

endotheliocytosis (en-dō-thē'-li-ō-sī-tō'-sis): An abnormal increase in the production of endotheliocytes.

endothelioma (en'-dō-thē-li-ō'-ma): A tumour derived from the epithellal cells that make up the lining of blood or lymph vessels or serous cavities; may be benign or malignant.

endothelium (en-dō-thē'-li-um): The very thin smooth vascular membrane lining of serous cavities, heart, blood and lymph vessels. — endothelial, adj.

endotoxaemia (en-dō-tok-sē'-mi-a): A condition in which endotoxins are present in the bloodstream; may be a sign of impending shock.

endotoxin (en-do-tok'-sin): A toxin present in the cell wall of certain bacteria, caused chiefly by Gram-negative organisms, which is freed only when the microorganism is broken down in the body; has a pyrogenic action and increases capillary permeability; associated with shock, thrombopenia, leukopenia. Opp. to exotoxin. — endotoxic, adj.

endotracheal (en-dō-tra'-kē-al): Within the trachea. E. TUBE an airway catheter inserted through the nose or mouth into the trachea in tracheal intubation. See INTUBATION.

end plate: The ending of a motor nerve fibre in relation to skeletal muscle fibres. MOTOR E. P. a complex myoneural junction where the axon of a motor nerve fibre makes contact with striated muscle fibres by way of a synapse.

enema (en'-e-ma): The injection of a liquid into the rectum, to be returned or retained. It can be further designated according to the function of the fluid; to promote evacuation of faeces; to provide nutrients or medicinal substances; to introduce opaque material in x-ray examination of the lower intestinal tract. — enemata, pl.

energy (en'-er-ji): The capacity to do work; manifested in various forms such as motion, light, heat.

enervation (en-er-vā'-shun): 1. General weakness; loss of strength; lack of vigour or nervous energy. 2. Removal of a nerve or part of one.

engagement (en-gāj'-ment): In obstetrics, the entrance of the presenting part of the fetus into the superior pelvic strait. The beginning of the descent through the pelvic canal. Usually occurs about the fourth week before delivery and often accompanied by a sensation called lightening.

engorged (en-gorjd'): Distended or swollen with blood or other fluid; term is applied to a tissue, an organ, or a vessel. — engorgement, adj.

engorgement (en-gorj'-ment): Congestion and distension of a tissue, organ, or vessel with fluid or other material.

engram (en'-gram): An enduring mark or trace. In psychology, a lasting impression made by an experience.

enhaematospore (en-hēm'-a-tō-spor): A spore of the malarial parasite that forms within the bloodstream. Also called *haematophore*.

enkephalin (en-kef'-a-lin): Either of two pentapeptides normally found in the body, the brain in particular but also in the gastrointestinal tract and the pituitary gland; composed of five amino acids. The effect of enkephalins of the central nervous system derives from their combining with certain receptors to reduce the individual's perception of pain. See also ENDORPHIN.

enophthalmos (en-of-thal'-mus): Retraction of the eyeball within its orbit. Opp. to exophthalmos.

enquiry-based learning: The process of learning through asking questions. This usually involves a deep engagement with a complex problem and incorporates forms of support to guide students in their enquiries. See PROBLEM-BASED LEARNING.

ensiform (en'-si-form): Sword-shaped. Term applied to the process at the lower end of the breast bone. Syn., *xiphoid*.

ENT: Abbreviation for ear, nose, and throat.

ental (en'-tal): Internal; inner; central.

Entamoeba (ent-a-mē'ba): A genus of protozoon parasites, some species of which affect man. *E. COLI* nonpathogenic, infests the human intestinal tract; *E. GINGIVALIS* infests the mouth about the gums and found in tartar on teeth; nonpathogenic; *E. HYSTOLYTICA* pathogenic; causes amoebic dysentery, see under DYSENTERY.

enter-, entero-: Combining forms denoting intestine.

enteral (en'-ter-al): 1. Within the gastrointestinal tract. 2. Relating to the small intestine. E. NUTRITION provides nutrition for those who are not able to ingest adequate nutrients orally but who are able to utilize them in the body; given through nasoduodenal, gastric or jejunostomy tubes.

enteric (en-ter'-ik): Relating to the intestine. E. BACTERIA bacteria living in or isolated from the intestine; E.-COATED, refers to a pill or other medicaton that is coated with a substance that will not dissolve until it reaches the intestine; E. FEVER includes typhoid fever (*q.v.*) and paratyphoid fever (*q.v.*).

enteritis (en-ter-ī'-tis): Inflammation of the intestine, the small intestine in particular.

enteroanastomosis (en'-ter-ō-a-nas-tō-mō'-sis): The surgical union of two parts of the intestine; term usually refers to the small intestine.

Enterobacter (en'-ter-ō-bak'-ter): A genus of the family Enterobacteriaceae; widely distributed in nature; *E. AEROGENES* a species found in soil, sewage, water, dairy products, and intestinal canal of humans and other animals; often acts as an opportunistic pathogen.

Enterobacteriaceae (en'-ter-ō-bak-tēr-i-ā'-sē-ē): A large family of motile and non-motile Gram-negative bacteria which act on glucose to produce acid and gas; includes the *Escherichia coli*, *Salmonella*, *Shigella*, *Proteus*, and *Klebsiella* organisms.

Enterobius vermicularis (en-ter-ō'bi-us ver-mik-ū-lar'is): A nematode which infests the small and large intestine. Threadworm; pinworm; seatworm. Found more often in children than adults. Presence in the rectum causes intense itching. Transmitted in the ova of the worm which is found in faeces of infected persons. Prevalent among those whose environmental and personal hygiene are poor. Distribution is worldwide.

enterocele (en'-ter-ō-sēl): 1. Hernia of the intestine. 2. Prolapse of the intestine, sometimes into the upper posterior part of the vagina.

enterococcus (en-ter-ō-kok'-us): A Gram-positive encapsulated streptococcus that occurs in short chains and is relatively resistant to heat. It is found in the human intestine; sometimes is the causative organism in infections of the urinary tract, ear, and wounds and, more rarely, in endocarditis (*q.v.*).

enterocolitis (en'-ter-ō-ko-lī'-tis): Inflammation of the mucous membrane lining of the intestines and the colon. HAEMORRHAGIC E., E. characterized by haemorrhage breakdown of the mucous lining of the intestinal mucosa; NECROTIZING E. severe inflammation of the gastrointestinal tract; when it occurs in high-risk neonates it may be fatal; REGIONAL E. see CROHN'S DISEASE; PSEUDOMEMBRANOUS E. see PSEUDO-MEMBRANOUS COLITIS under COLITIS.

enterocystocele (en-ter-ō-sis'-tō-sēl): A hernia involving both the urinary bladder and the intestine.

enteroenterostomy (en'-ter-ō-en-ter-os'-to-mi): The surgical anastomosis of two parts of the intestine that do not normally adjoin each other.

enterogastritis: (en'-ter-ō-gas-trī'-tis): Inflammation of the small intestine and the stomach.

enterolysis (en-ter-ol'-i-sis): The surgical freeing of the intestine from adhesions.

enteron (en'-te-ron): The gut, the small intestine in particular.

enteropeptidase: An enzyme in intestinal juice. It converts inactive trypsinogen into active trypsin.

enteroptosis (en-ter-op-tō'-sis): Descent or downwards displacement of the intestines, usually associated with the downwards displacement of other abdominal organs. Also called *enteropsia, abdominal ptosis, visceroptosis.* — enteroptotic, adj.

enterostenosis (en'-ter-ō-ste-nō'-sis): A stricture or narrowing of a portion of the intestine.

enterostomy (en-ter-os'-to-mi): The surgical establishment of an artificial anus or opening into the intestine through the abdominal wall.

enterotomy (en-ter-ot'-o-mi): An incision into the intestine, the small intestine in particular.

enterotoxin (en-ter-ō-tok'-sin): A toxin produced in the intestine by certain species of bacteria and which produce symptoms associated with food poisoning. — enterotoxigenic, adj.

enterovirus (en-ter-ō-vī'-rus): One of a group of more than 70 related viruses that were formerly classified as echovirus, coxsackievirus, and poliovirus, which enter the body through the alimentary tract and tend to invade the central nervous system.

enterozoon (en-ter-ō-zō'-on): Any animal parasite that infects or inhabits the intestine. — enterozoa, pl.

entity (en'-ti-tē): The existence of a thing or condition separate from its attributes and in contrast to them. In medicine, a distinct and separate disorder or disease.

entochondrostosis (en'-tō-kon-dros-tō'-sis): The development of bone within cartilage.

entomology (en-tō-mol'-o-ji): The branch of biology that deals with the study of insects. MEDICAL E. the branch of medicine that deals with the study of insects that cause disease in humans or serve as vectors of disease.

entopic (en-top'-ik): Occurring in the correct place; opp. of ectopic (q.v.).

entrails (en'-trāls): Intestines, or viscera; most often referring to those of animals.

entropion (en-trō'-pē-on): The turning inward of a margin or edge, particularly the inversion of an eyelid so that the lashes are in contact with the globe of the eye, occurring as a result of laxity of the structures supporting the eyelid.

enucleation (e-nū-klē-ā'-shun): The removal of an organ or tumor in its entirety, as of an eyeball from its socket. — enucleate, v.

enuresis (en-ū-rē'-sis): Involuntary urination, especially bedwetting, when it is not due to any organic disease of the urinary organs. Can be treated by psychotherapy, behaviour therapy or tricyclic anti-depressant drugs.

environment (en-vī-ron-ment): External surroundings. The total of all the conditions and forces that surround and act upon an organism or any of its parts.

environmental (en-vī-ron-men'-tal): Relating to the environment. E. MANIPULATION in psychiatry, an attempt to help an individual by changing his environment so as to make it less stressful.

Environmental Health Officer: A specially qualified person in the field of environmental health and related issues employed by a local authority to safeguard, maintain and improve public health. Responsibilities include monitoring housing, sanitation, food, clean air, noise and water supplies to ensure that standards set by legislation are met.

enzygotic (en-zī-got'-ik): Development from one zygote. E. TWINS identical twins.

enzyme (en'-zīm): A protein, produced by living cells, that acts specifically to accelerate or produce some chemical change without itself being changed. Each E. is specific for one particular chemical transformation only. — enzymic, enzymatic, adj.

enzyme-linked immunosorbent assay: A serological assay in which the bound antigen or antibody is detected by a linked enzyme that converts a colourless substrate to a coloured product.

enzymolysis (en-zī-mol'-i-sis): Lysis that is activated by or caused by the action of an enzyme.

eosinophil(e) (ē-ō-sin'-ō-fil): A cell having an affinity for the stain eosin. A type of white blood cell that constitutes about 1 to 4% of the total leukocytes in the blood and increases in number during allergic states and infestation with worms.

eosinophilia (ē-ō-sin-ō-fil'-i-a): An increase above normal in the number of eosinophils per unit volume in peripheral blood. PULMONARY E. a transient condition, usually due to worm infestation, but may also be produced by certain drugs; SPUTUM E. the presence of an abnormal number of eosinophils in the sputum, a characteristic of asthma; TROPICAL E. pulmonary E., a type of E. occurring mainly in the tropics; may be associated with polyarteritis or asthma.

ep-, epi-: Prefix denoting upon, above, over; beside; anterior; on the outside.

ependyma (ep-en'-di-ma): The membrane lining of the ventricles of the brain and the central canal of the spinal cord. — ependymal, adj.

ephebic (e-fē'-bik): Pertaining to puberty or adolescence.

ephelis (ef-ē'-lis): A freckle. — ephelides, pl.

ephemeral (e-fem'-er-al): Fleeting; transient.

epiblepharon (ep-i-blef'-a-ron): A congenital anomaly in which an excess fold of skin on the lower eyelid causes the lashes to turn inward; seen in Down's syndrome and certain other abnormalities; to be differentiated from the epicanthal folds normal to people from the Far East.

epicardia (ep-i-kar'-di-a): The lower end of the oesophagus between the diaphragm and the opening into the stomach. — epicardial, adj.

epicardium (ep-i-kar'-di-um): The thin visceral or inner layer of the pericardium that immediately invests the heart. — epicardial, adj.

epicondyle (ep-i-kon'-dīl): A bony projection situated above a condyle on a bone. — epicondylar, adj.

epicritic (ep-i-krit'-ik): Term applied to a set of nerve fibres in the skin and oral mucosa that enable one to discriminate fine variations in the sensations of touch, temperature, or pain, and to localize these sensations. The opposite of protopathic (q.v.).

epicureanism (ep-i-kūr-ē'-an-izm): A philosophy of life that emphasizes pleasure, the happiness of the moment, and instant gratification.

epidemic (ep-i-dem'-ik): **1.** Simultaneously affecting many people in an area. Cf. ENDEMIC **2.** The occurrence in a community or region of a group of illnesses of a similar nature, in excess of normal expectancy, and derived from a common source. **3.** Of, or pertaining to epidemics.

epidemicity (ep-i-de-mis'-i-ti): The characteristic of being a community-wide and rapidly proliferating occurrence of disease.

epidemiologist (ep-i-dē-mi-ol' -o-jist): A person who specializes in epidemiology.

epidemiology (ep-i-dē-mi-ol' -o-ji): The study of the effect of the physical and social environment on the frequency, distribution, and cause of an infectious or non-infectious disease in a population. — epidemiological, adj., epidemiologically, adv.

epidermal (ep-i-der' -mal): Relating to or involving the epidermis.

epidermis (ep-i-der' -mis): The external, non-vascular layer of the skin; composed of several individual layers; the cuticle. Also known as the *scarf skin.* — epidermal, adj.

epidermodysplasia (ep-i-der' -mō-dis-plā' -zi-a): Faulty or incomplete development of the epidermis. E. VERRUCIFORMIS a congenital defect characterized by verrucous lesions on the hands, feet, neck, or face; caused by a virus.

epidermoid (ep-i-der' -moyd): Resembling epidermis or epidermal cells. E. CARCINOMA malignant epithelioma occurring in the skin; E. CYST a cyst arising from aberrant epithelial cells, commonly occurring in subcutaneous areas as a steatoma or wen, but may also be seen in the skull, meninges, or brain.

Epidermophyton (ep-i-der-mof' -i-ton): A genus of fungi that affects the skin and nails. E. FLOCCOSUM the causative agent of several types of ringworm, including ringworm of the scalp and athlete's foot.

epidermosis (e-pi-der-mō' -sis): A skin disease which affects only the epidermis; characterized by decreased glandular secretion, water loss, degeneration of cells of the dermis, thinning and wrinkling.

epididymectomy (ep-i-did-i-mek' -to-mi): Surgical removal of the epididymis.

epididymis (ep-i-did' -i-mis): A small oblong body attached to the posterior surface of the testis. Consists of the first convoluted portion of the excretory duct of the testis; conveys the spermatozoa from the testis to the vas deferens.

epididymo-orchidectomy (ep-i-did-ī' -mō-or-kid-ek' -tō-mi): The surgical removal of a testis or epididymis.

epidural (ep-i-dū' -ral): Upon or external to the dura mater. E. BLOCK injection of local anaesthetic, usually in the lumbar or caudal region prior to rectal examination and surgery; also in childbirth, especially, a forceps delivery, or Caesarean section. Also used for crush injuries to the chest; the analgesia can be maintained for a week or more; E. SPACE the space outside the dura mater of the brain and spinal cord.

epigastric (ep-i-gas' -trik): Relating to the epigastrium. E. ANGLE the angle made by the xiphoid process and the body of the sternum.

epigastrium (ep-i-gas' -tri-um): The abdominal region lying directly over the stomach; the 'pit' of the stomach. — epigastric, adj.

epiglottitis (ep-i-glot-tī' -tis): Inflammation of the epiglottis. The acute form, which occurs mainly in children, may cause respiratory difficulty due to swelling of the epiglottis; other symptoms include croupy cough, stridulous breathing, cyanosis, and prostration.

epilation (ep-il-ā' -shun): Extraction or destruction of hair roots, *e.g.*, by coagulation necrosis, electrolysis, or forceps. — epilate, v.

epilemma (ep-i-lem' -ma): The outer sheath of very small nerves.

epilepsy (ep' -i-lep-si): A recurrent paroxysmal disorder of cerebral function characterized always by variable clouding of consciousness, often associated with generalized convulsions, and due to an abnormal discharge of nerve impulses in the brain. E. can be classified on causation: (1) SYMPTOMATIC E., E. due to a recognized cause or agent, *e.g.*, cerebral tumour, trauma, or vascular abnormality; or (2) IDIOPATHIC E., E. of unknown cause; or of clinical features: (1) GRAND MAL E. loss of consciousness with generalized convulsions; (2) PETIT MAL E. clouding of consciousness with no generalized convulsions; or (3) JACK-SONIAN E. convulsions beginning in one muscle group and either remaining localized or else spreading in an orderly march to involve wider muscle groups, and which may then involve loss of consciousness; or according to age at onset: (1) PRIMARY E., E. with onset of seizures usually occurring in the first two weeks of life or later in adolescence; heredity is a factor in the aetiology; (2) SEC-ONDARY E. which begins in childhood or after age 30; with many causative factors including brain tumour, trauma, infection, meningitis, encephalitis, exposure to toxic substances. AB-DOMINAL E. a rare form characterized by recurrent episodes of abdominal pain without the usual convulsions of epilepsy; AKINETIC E. epileptic manifestations without movement and usually no loss of consciousness; FOCAL E. minor recurrent seizures limited to one side of the body; MYOCLONIC E. a hereditary E. which begins in childhood; characterized by sudden attacks of muscle clonus and shock-like jerks of a limb or the body; often occurs in the morning; PSYCHOMOTOR E. convulsions follow soon after a head injury and may not recur, or convulsive attacks start a month or more after injury and are then likely to recur; REFLEX E. a form of E. characterized by attacks that are brought on by an external stimulus; SENILE E. includes several disorders that occur in the elderly; the person may not have seizures but usually has drop attacks; TEMPORAL LOBE E. psychomotor E., characterized by impaired consciousness, semi-purposeful movements of arms or legs, hallucinations. See STATUS EPILEPTICUS under STATUS.

epileptic (ep-i-lep'-tik): 1. A person affected with epilepsy. 2. Relating to epilepsy. E. AURA premonitory subjective phenomena (tingling in the hand or visual or auditory sensations) that precede an attack of grand mal; E. CRY the croak or shout heard from the epileptic person as they fall unconscious.

epimenorrhagia (ep-i-men-ō-rā'-ji-a): Too frequent and too excessive menstruation.

epimenorrhoea (ep-i-men-ō-rē' a): Reduction in the length of the menstrual cycle resulting in too frequent menstruation.

epimysium (ep-i-miz'-i-um): The external fibrous sheath of a skeletal muscle.

epineurium (ep-i-nū'-ri-um): The connective tissue covering of a nerve trunk.

epiphenomenon (ep-i-fe-nom'-e-non): An unexpected, or accidental event or condition occurring during the course of a disease; may or may not be related to the disease itself.

epiphora (ē-pif'-o-ra): Pathological overflow of tears onto the cheek. May be due to excessive secretion, obstruction, or narrowing of the lacrimal passages.

epiphysial, epiphyseal (ep-i-fiz'-i-al): Referring to or related to an epiphysis (q.v.). E. FRACTURE the separation of the epiphysis from a long bone; results from injury; E. PLATE the thin plate of cartilage between the shaft of a long bone and its epiphysis in children and young adults; it is the site of growth in bone length and when growth is completed it is replaced by bone, the resulting area being called the E. LINE.

epiphysiodesis (ep'-i-fiz-i-od'-e-sis): Premature ossification of an epiphysis, resulting in cessation of bone growth. In surgery, the procedure of fixing a separated epiphysis to the diaphysis of the bone; done especially on children when the bones are of uneven length.

epiphysis (ē-pif'-i-sis): The growing part of a bone, especially a long bone, that is separated from the end of the main shaft by a plate of

cartilage; the latter disappears and becomes part of the bone when growth ceases. SLIPPED E. displacement of an E., especially the upper femoral; also called epiphysiolisthesis. — epiphyses, pl.; epiphysial, epiphyseal, adj.

epiploon (ē-pip'-lō-on): The greater omentum; see under OMENTUM. — epiploic, adj.

episioperineoplasty (ē-piz'-i-ō-per-i-nē'-ō-plas-ti): Repair of a lacerated vulva and perineum by plastic surgery.

episiorrhaphy (ē-piz-i-or'-ra-fi): The surgical repair of a lacerated vulva or of an episiotomy after childbirth.

episiotomy (ē-piz-i-ot'-o-mi): Incision of the vulva made during the birth of a child when the vaginal orifice does not stretch enough and laceration of the perineum seems imminent.

epispadias (ep-i-spā'-di-as): A congenital anomaly in the male in which the urethral opening in the penis is on the dorsal side; occurs rarely in the female, when the opening is above the clitoris.

epispastic (ep-i-spas'-tik): 1. Causing blistering. 2. A blistering agent or vesicant.

epistasis (e-pis'-ta-sis): 1. In genetics, the suppressive effect of one gene on another as occurs, e.g., in albinism, in which the determining gene for pigmentation patterns is suppressed. 2. The control or stoppage of haemorrhage.

epistaxis (ep-i-stak'-sis): Bleeding from the nose. — epistaxes, pl.

epistemology (ep-is-te-mol'-o-ji): The branch of philosophy that deals with the nature of knowledge and truth. It encompasses the study of the origin, nature, and limits of human knowledge.

episternum (ep-i-ster'-num): The manubrium or upper part of the sternum.

epitendineum (ep'-i-ten-din'-ē-um): The fibrous sheath that covers tendons.

epithelial (ep-i-thē'-li-al): Relating to the epithelium. E. PEARLS or NESTS multiple rounded or oval, variously sized, aggregates of neoplastic epidermal material, frequently found in squamous cell carcinomata.

epithelialization (ep-i-thē'-li-al-ī-zā'-shun): The growth of epithelium over a raw area; the final stage of healing. Also called epithelization.

epitheliolysin (ep'-i-thē-li-ol'-i-sin): A specific lysin in the blood serum that causes dissolution of epithelial cells. — epitheliolytic, adj.

epithelioma (ep-i-thē-li-ō'-ma): A malignant growth arising in epithelial tissue, usually the skin; a squamous cell carcinoma. BASAL CELL E. skin cancer which often follows exposure to radium, radiation, or sunlight; starts as slow-growing nodules, sometimes pigmented with later ulceration that penetrates into the deep tissues; may be fatal; SCROTAL E. also called *chimney-sweep's cancer*; caused by irritation due to coal soot.

epithelium (ep-i-thē'-li-um): The surface layer of cells covering cutaneous, mucous, and serous surfaces. It is classified according to the arrangement of the cells it contains as (1) simple squamous; (2) simple cuboidal; (3) simple columnar; and (4) pseudo-stratified columnar. E. protects underlying tissues from wear and tear and must be continually renewed; some epithelial cells are able to absorb certain substances; others have secretory or excretory functions.

epitrochlea (ep-i-trok'-lē-a): The medial epicondyle (*q.v.*) of the humerus. — epitrochlear, adj.

epizoon (ep-i-zō-on): An animal parasite living on the outside of the host's body. — epizoa, pl. epizoic, adj.

eponychia (ep-ō-nik'-i-a): An infection of the fold of skin around the nail.

eponychium (ep-ō-nik'-i-um): The horny layer of skin attached to the margin of the nails.

eponym (ep'-o-nim): 1. One for whom something is named. 2. The name of something formed from or including a person's name, such as Cushing's syndrome.

Epsom salt: Magnesium sulphate; formerly in wide use as a cathartic.

Epstein–Barr virus: Virus particles that resemble herpesvirus; associated with infectious mononucleosis; also thought to be a possible cause of Burkitt's lymphoma and nasopharyngeal carcinoma. Also called *Barr–Epstein virus*.

Epstein's pearls: Small, yellowish white, slightly elevated cysts or masses seen on each side of the hard palate and sometimes on the gums in many newborns. [A. Epstein, Prague paediatrician, 1880–1965.]

equation (ē-kwā'-shun): An expression of equality of two things, or quantities; often involves the use of mathematical and/or chemical symbols.

equilibrium (ē'-kwi-lib'-ri-um): 1. A state of balance between forces or processes. 2. The normal, oriented state of the body in respect to its position in space, maintained through the labyrinthine sense. ACID–BASE E. the state of the body when the acids and bases in body fluids are present in their normal ratio; NITROGENOUS E. the condition of the body when the amount of nitrogen excreted is in the normal ratio to that taken in.

equinovalgus (ē-kwī-nō-val'-gus): Talipes equinovalgus; elevation and outward rotation of the heel.

equinovarus (ē-kwī'-nō-var'-us): Talipes equinovarus; elevation and inward rotation of the heel; the most common form of clubfoot.

equinus (ē-kwī'-nus): Talipes equinus. See under TALIPES.

equity (ek'-wi-ti): 1. Actions, treatment of others, or a general condition characterized by justice, fairness, and impartiality. 2. Justice applied in conformity with the law, but influenced at the same time by principles of ethics and fair play. 3. The system of jurisprudence that supplements common and statutory law, when those bodies of law are inadequate in the attainment of justice. 4. A claim that is judged to be just and fair.

erasion (ē-rā'-zhun): Surgical removal of tissue by scraping. E. OF A JOINT arthrectomy (*q.v.*).

Erb's paralysis, palsy, Erb–Duchenne palsy: See under PALSY. E.'S POINT a point 2 or 3 cm above the clavicle at the side of the neck where pressure on the brachial plexus gives rise to Erb's paralysis; E.'S SIGN, (1) loss of the patellar reflex, an early sign of tabes dorsalis; or (2) increased excitability to faradic or galvanic current; seen in tetany. [William H. Erb, German neurologist, 1840–1921.]

erectile (ē-rek'-tīl): Upright; capable of being elevated. E. TISSUE highly vascular tissue, which, under stimulus, becomes rigid and erect from hyperaemia.

erection (ē-rek'-shun): The condition achieved when erectile tissue is made rigid or elevated due to hyperaemia. The enlarged, rigid penis of the male (or clitoris of the female) under stimulus of sexual excitement is said to be in a state of erection.

erector (ē-rek'-tor): A muscle that achieves erection of, or raises, a part.

erethism (er'-e-thizm): Heightened responsiveness of the nervous system.

erethisophrenia (er'-e-thiz-ō-frē'-ni-a): Abnormally heightened mental activity.

ERG: Abbreviation for electroretinogram.

ergogram (er'-gō-gram): The graphic recording made by an ergograph.

ergograph (er'-gō-graf): An instrument that measures the amount of movement a muscle is capable of performing or the amount of work it is able to do; utilizes a weight or spring against which the muscle contracts.

ergometer (er-gom'-i'-ter): An instrument for measuring the work done by muscular activity.

BICYCLE E. one used for measuring the energy expended while using a stationary bicycle.

ergometry (er-gom'-et-ri): Measurement of work done by muscles. — ergometric, adj.

ergonomics (er-gō-nom'-iks): The application of various biological disciplines in relation to humans and their working environment.

ergosterol (er-gos'-ter-ol): A provitamin present in the subcutaneous fat of humans; also found in plants and foodstuffs. On irradiation with sunlight or ultraviolet light it is converted into vitamin D_2 which has antirachitic properties.

ergot (er'-got): A fungus that is parasitic on rye. It is the source of several valuable alkaloids used in medicine; causes contraction of muscular coat of the arteries, raises blood pressure and contracts uterine muscle; widely used in control of post-partum haemorrhage. Also useful in treatment of certain vascular disorders, including migraine headache.

Erlenmeyer flask: A flask with a cone-shaped body, a broad base, and a narrow neck; especially suitable for certain chemical procedures. [Emil Erlenmeyer, German chemist, 1825–1909.]

erode (ē-rōd): To diminish or destroy gradually; to wear away.

erogenous (ē-roj'-e-nus): Descriptive of body areas or skin that are capable of arousing sexual excitement when stimulated, e.g., the oral, anal, and genital areas. Also called *erotogenic*.

eros (ē'-ros): 1. Physical love; sexual desire. 2. The Greek god of love. 3. In psychiatry, the life instinct, i.e., the instinctive tendency towards self-preservation.

erosion (ē-rō'-zhun): 1. The superficial wearing away of tissue or a surface. 2. Loss of superficial epidermis. CERVICAL E. ulceration of the superficial tissues at the squamocolumnar junction in the vaginal portion of the cervix.

erotic (ē-rot'-ik): Relating to sexual passion or interest; lustful.

erotica (ē-rot'-i-ka): Artistic or literary work that has an erotic theme or quality.

eroticism (ē-rot'-i-sizm): Sexual desire. In psychoanalysis any manifestation of the sexual instinct, specifically the heightened sexual response derived from stimulation of mucous membranes or special sense organs.

ERPC: Abbreviation for evacuation of retained products of conception, see EVACUATION.

erratic (e-rat'-tik): 1. Wandering, said of pain or other symptoms. 2. Eccentric.

error: 1. A defect in structure or function. 2. In biostatistics: (a) a mistaken decision, as in hypothesis testing; (b) the difference between the true value and the observed value of a variate, ascribed to randomness or misreading by an observer. 3. False positive and false negative results in a dichotomous trial. 4. A false or mistaken belief; in biomedical and other sciences; there are many varieties of error, for example due to bias, inaccurate measurements or faulty instruments.

erubescence (er-ū-hes'-ens): A reddening of the skin; a blush. — erubescent, adj.

eructation (e-ruk-tā'-shun): Noisy, oral expulsion of gas from the stomach. The act of belching.

eruption (i-rup'-shun): 1. The act of becoming visible or breaking out. 2. The appearance of a rash or visible lesion on the skin due to disease; characterized by redness, prominence, or both. — erupt, v.

eruptive (i-rup'-tiv): Relating to or characterized by eruption; appearing suddenly.

erysipelas (er-i-sip'-e-las): An acute, contagious inflammatory cellulitis involving the skin and subcutaneous tissues; caused by a haemolytic streptococcus. The inflammation begins around a wound often too small to be noticed. The characteristic eruption is painful, red with small blebs, and has a raised edge. The disease is accompanied by fever and other severe constitutional symptoms. Sometimes called *Saint Anthony's fire* (q.v.).

erythema (er-i-thē'-ma): Inflammatory redness of the skin. E. ABIGNE a reddish mottling and macular eruption of the skin over the shins, as occurs in stokers, bakers, and others whose work exposes them to radiant heat, or those who sit too close to a fire or electric heater; E. INFECTIOSUM a mild, non-febrile infection, probably viral, characterized by macropapular erythematous eruption, also called *fifth disease* and *Sticker's disease*. E. MULTIFORME successive painless, toxic or allergic skin eruptions of short duration, appearing chiefly on the extremities; the lesions are violet-pink or dark red papules; E. NODOSUM an eruption of painful red nodules on the front of the legs; occurs in young women and is often accompanied by rheumatic pains; may be a symptom of many diseases including tuberculosis, acute rheumatism, gonococcal septicaemia; also caused by certain drugs or food poisoning; E. PERNIO chilblain (q.v.); E. TOXICUM E. caused by allergic reaction to some substance, e.g., a drug or a bacterial toxin; characterized by a generalized macular erythematous eruption; E. TOXICUM NEONATORUM a self-limited condition occurring during the first few days of life; characterized by a temporary blotchy erythematous rash, sometimes papules or pustules; due to some allergy, often to mother's or cow's milk. — erythematous, adj.

erythr-, erythro-: Combining forms denoting: **1.** Erythrocyte. **2.** Red or redness.

erythroblast (ē-rith′-rō-blast): An immature, nucleated red blood cell found in the red bone marrow and from which the erythrocytes are derived. — erythroblastic, adj.

erythroblastaemia (ē-rith′-rō-blas-tē′-mi-a): The presence of abnormally large numbers of erythroblasts (*q.v.*) in the peripheral blood.

erythroblastosis (ē-rith′-rō-blas-tō′-sis): The presence of erythroblasts in the circulating blood. E. FETALIS or NEONATORUM is a haemolytic disease of the fetus or the newborn; occurs when the mother's blood is Rh-negative, causing the development of antibodies against the fetus whose blood is Rh-positive. Red blood cell destruction occurs with anaemia, jaundice, hepatomegaly, splenomegaly, an excess of erythrocytes in the blood, and often generalized oedema.

erythrochloropia (ē-rith′-rō-klō-rō′-pi-a): A form of colour blindness in which only the colours red and green can be distinguished correctly.

erythroclasis (er-ē-throk′-la-sis): The fragmentation of red blood cells.

erythrocyte (ē-rith′-rō-sīt): A non-nucleated, bi-concave, disc-shaped blood cell containing an oxygen-carrying pigment, haemoglobin, which gives blood its red colour. Produced in the marrow of spongy bone, at the ends of long bones, and in flat, irregular bones. Chief function is to carry oxygen to the cells of all the tissues of the body. Adult blood contains about five million erythrocytes per cubic millimetre; the average life of erythrocytes is about 120 days.

erythrocyte sedimentation rate: The rate at which red blood cells settle to the bottom of a glass tube within a given amount of time. The rate is increased in infections and conditions in which cell destruction occurs and decreased in abnormal morphology of red blood cells, as occurs in certain anaemias, especially sickle cell anaemia, and in bleeding, congestive heart failure, and diseases of the bone marrow. Useful in diagnosing and following up on such illnesses as rheumatic fever, arthritis, and myocardial infarcation.

erythrocythaemia (e-rith′rō-sī-thē′-mi-a): Overproduction of red blood cells. This may be (1) a physiological response to the need for greater oxygenation of the tissues (congenital heart disease), and is referred to as erythrocytosis or

secondary polycythaemia; or (2) idiopathic, when the condition is called polycythaemia vera; see POLYCYTHAEMIA. — erythrocythaemic, adj.

erythrocytolysis (e-rith′-rō-sī-tol′-i-sis): Destruction or dissolution of red blood cells with escape of haemoglobin into the plasma.

erythrocytopenia (e-rith′-rō-sī-tō-pē′-ni-a): Deficiency in the number of red blood cells. — erythrocytopenic, adj.

erythrocytosis (e-rith′-rō-sī-tō′-sis): An increase in the red blood cells in the circulating blood resulting from a known cause; see ERYTHROCYTHAEMIA. STRESS E. a condition occurring in tense, anxiety-prone individuals; there is no increase in the red blood cell mass but a diminished plasma volume leads to an increase in peripheral haematocrit.

erythrocyturia (e-rith-rō-sī-tū′-ri-a): The presence of red blood cells in the urine.

erythroderma (e-rith′-rō-der′-ma): Excessive redness of the skin. Also called *erythrodermia*.

erythrodermatitis (e-rith′-rō-der-ma-tī′-tis): Reddening and inflammation of the skin.

erythroedema (er-ith-ro-dē′-ma): A disease of infancy characterized by bluish-red swollen extremities, tachycardia, photophobia; cause unknown. Nervous irritability is extreme, leading to anorexia and disordered digestion, followed by multiple arthritis and muscular weakness. Syn., *pink disease, Swift's disease, infantile acrodynia*.

erythrogenic (e-rith-rō-jen′-ik): **1.** Producing or causing a rash. **2.** Producing red blood cells, or relating to their formation.

erythroid (er′-i-throyd): Of a red colour.

erythroleukaemia (e-rith′-rō-lū-kē′-mi-a): A malignant blood disorder characterized by the proliferation of erythroblasts and leukoblasts.

erythrolysis (er-i-throl′-i-sis): The dissolution or destruction of erythrocytes.

erythropenia (e-rith-rō-pē-ni-a): Deficiency in the number of red blood cells in the blood.

erythrophage (e-rith′-rō-fāj): A phagocyte that engulfs and destroys red blood cells.

erythroplasia (e-rith-rō-plā′-zi-a): A condition characterized by the formation of erythematous papules with ill-defined borders, at the junction of mucous membrane and epithelium, chiefly at the anus, vulva, and mouth; when it occurs on oral mucous membrane it may be a sign of early cancer.

erythropoiesis (e-rith′-rō-poy-ē′-sis): The production of red blood cells. See HAEMOPOIESIS.

erythropoietin (e-rith′-rō-poy-ē′-tin): A substance found in many animals and humans; secreted by the kidney, it circulates in the blood and is concerned with the stimulation and regulation of the production of erythrocytes.

erythrorrhexis (e-rith-rō-rek'-sis): Fragmentation of red blood cells.

erythrostasis (e-rith-rō-stā'-sis): A condition due to stasis of the blood in the capillaries and hence stasis of the erythrocytes, which are then denied access to fresh plasma from which they would normally receive oxygen.

eschar (es-kar): A dry slough, as results from application of caustics, or from burns, especially second- or third-degree burns. See SLOUGH. — escharotic, adj.

Escherichia (esh-e-rik'-i-a): A genus of bacteria of the tribe Eschericheae; short Gram-negative rods, non-motile, widely distributed in nature. *E. COLI* a natural inhabitant of the intestinal tract in humans; usually non-pathogenic, but pathogenic strains frequently cause urinary tract infections, enteritis, peritonitis, cystitis, wound infections; also called *colon bacillus*.

Esmarch's bandage: A rubberized roller bandage used to temporarily arrest the flow of blood in an extremity to create a bloodless field for surgery. [Johann Friedrich August von Esmarch, German military surgeon, 1823–1908.]

eso-: A combining form denoting within.

esocataphoria (ēs-ō-kat-a-fō'-ri-a): A convergent squint with the eye turning downwards and inward.

esotropia (ēs-ō-trō'-pi-a): Convergent strabismus (*q.v.*); occurs when one eye fixes on an object and the other eye deviates inward. Opp. of exotropia. — Syn., *esophoria*.

ESR: Abbreviation for erythrocyte sedimentation rate (*q.v.*).

essence (es'-sens): 1. That which is the real nature of a thing and so the source of its particular qualities. 2. A solution of a volatile oil in alcohol.

essence of care: A term referring to the fundamental and essential aspects of nursing, which include: principles of self-care; food and nutrition; personal and oral hygiene; continence and bladder and bowel care; pressure ulcers; record keeping; safety of clients/patients with mental health needs in acute mental health and general hospital settings; and privacy and dignity. The term arose from a commitment in *Making a Difference* (*q.v.*) to explore the benefits of benchmarking (*q.v.*) in the NHS. See NHS PLAN; www.doh.gov.uk/essenceofcare/

essential (ē-sen'-shal): Of prime importance; indispensable. In medicine the term is often used to describe conditions of unknown origin, *e.g.*, essential hypertension. E. OIL an undiluted, volatile oil extracted from plants, having the odour or flavour of the plant from which it comes; used in perfume, flavourings, and in aromatherapy (*q.v.*).

ester (es'-ter): Any organic compound formed by the combination of an acid and an alcohol with the elimination of water.

esterase (es'-ter-ās): An enzyme that acts as a catalyst in the hydrolysis of an ester (*q.v.*).

estrogen, estrus: For these and related words see OESTROGEN, OESTRUS, etc.

ethacrynic acid (eth-a-krin'-ik): A diuretic drug.

ethanol (eth'-a-nōl): Ethyl alcohol.

ether (ē'-ther): Thin, colourless, volatile, inflammable liquid; one of the oldest volatile general anaesthetics. — Syn., *diethyl ether*, *diethyl oxide, sulphuric ether*

ethical decision-making: The protocol for solving ethical dilemmas. It includes consideration of the barriers to and the consequences of doing the right thing, and what to do when unethical situations arise. See DECISION-MAKING.

ethics (eth'-iks): A branch of philosophy which studies questions relating to right and wrong, good and bad.

ethisterone (ē-this'-ter-ōn): A steroid that resembles both progesterone and testosterone; used as a progestational agent. See PROGESTATIONAL.

ethmoid (eth'-moid): 1. Sieve-like; cribriform. 2. The sieve-like bone that separates the nasal cavity from the brain; the olfactory nerves pass through perforations in it; contains small cavities called ethmoid sinuses.

ethnic (eth'-nik): Relating to a social group whose members share certain common qualities, especially cultural or physical characteristics, have common national origin, and speak a common language.

ethnicity (eth-nis'-i-ti): The cultural characteristics that connect a particular group or groups of people to each other. While ethnicity and race are related concepts, the concept of ethnicity is rooted in the idea of societal groups, marked especially by shared nationality, tribal affiliation, religious faith, shared language, or cultural origins or traditional backgrounds.

ethnic monitoring: The process used to collect, store and analyse data about the ethnic background of individuals. Ethnic monitoring can be used to highlight possible inequalities and investigate their underlying causes.

ethnocentrism (eth-nō-sen'-trizm): Assessing all other cultures through the values of your own.

ethnography (eth-nog' -ra-fi): 1. The practice of writing an anthropological description of an individual human society or of a situation within a society. 2. An anthropological description of a society or situation. See also ETHNOLOGY.

ethnology (eth-nol' -o-ji): A branch of anthropology that uses ethnographies (*q.v.*) and other sources to compare systematically the beliefs and practices of different societies.

ethnomethodology (eth'-nō-meth-o-dol' -ō-ji): Systematic study of the ways in which people use social interaction to make sense of their situation and their everyday activities. See also SOCIOLOGY.

ethyl (eth'-il): C_2H_5; derived from ethane.

ethyl chloride (eth'-il klaw'-rīd): A volatile general anaesthetic for short operations, and a local anaesthetic as a result of the intense cold produced when applied to the skin.

ethylene (eth' -i-lēn): A colourless, highly flammable, explosive gas formerly used as an inhalation anaesthetic.

E trisomy: See under TRISOMY.

eu-: Combining form denoting (1) well, good; (2) well being.

EU: Abbreviation for European Union (*q.v.*).

EUA: Abbreviation for examination under anaesthetic.

eugenics (ū-jen' -iks): The study of methods for controlling the characteristics of future generations through selective breeding. — eugenic, adj.

eunoia (ū-noy' -a): A normal mental state.

eunuch (ū' -nuk): A human male from whom the testes have been removed; a castrated male.

eunuchoidism (ū' -nuk-oyd-izm): Lack of masculine sex characteristics and sexual desire; due to a deficiency of androgen secretion which may, in turn, be due to lack of development or inadequate functioning of the testes.

euphoria (ū-fo' -ri-a): A state of bodily comfort; well-being. In psychology, an exaggerated feeling of well-being, usually not justified by the circumstances. — euphoric, euphoretic, euphoriant, adj.

euphorigenic (ū-for-i-jen' -ik): Tending to produce a state of euphoria.

eupnoea (ūp-nē' -a): Normal easy respiration.

eupraxia (ū-prak' -si-a): The ability to perform perfectly movements involving coordination of muscles.

eurhythmic (ū-rith' -mik): 1. Harmonious development and relationship of the body parts. 2. Descriptive of a pulse beat that is regular.

eurhythmics (ū-rith' -miks): Harmonious body movements performed to music.

European Community: see EUROPEAN UNION.

European Medicine Evaluation Agency: The organization responsible for the safety of medicines. It authorizes the use of medicinal products within the European Union and works with the drug regulatory bodies of the member nations.

European Union: A political alliance between some European countries, where there exists a common market with unified external tariffs. It was originally called the European Economic Community (EEC), then the European Community (EC).

European Working Time Directive: International law stipulating a working limit of an average of 48 hours per week. It applies to all directly employed NHS workers. An NHS derogation concerning career-grade doctors provides some flexibility in complying with regulations while enabling 24-hour service cover to be provided.

eurysomatic (ū' -ri-sō-mat' -ik): Having a thickset body.

eusol (ū' -sol): An antiseptic solution prepared from chloride of lime and boric acid. The name is derived from the initials of Edinburgh University Solution of Lime.

Eustachian (ū-stā' -shi-an): A canal, partly bony, partly cartilaginous, measuring 2.5 to 5 cm in length, connecting the pharynx with the tympanic cavity. It allows air to pass into the middle ear, so that the air pressure is kept even on both sides of the eardrum. E. CATHETER an instrument used for dilating the Eustachian (auditory) tube when it becomes blocked; E. TUBE auditory tube; see under AUDITORY; E. VALVE the valve guarding the entrance of the inferior vena cava into the right atrium of the heart. [Bartholomeo Eustachius, Italian anatomist, 1520–1574.]

euthanasia (ū' -tha-nā' -zi-a): 1. An easy painless death. 2. The act of killing, or helping to kill, painlessly a hopelessly ill or injured individual, as an act of mercy. ACTIVE E. involves doing something that results in a person's death; DIRECT E. involves an act intended to result in the death of an individual; INDIRECT E. involves an act in which death is not the main intention; INVOLUNTARY E. refers to E. carried out for patients who are comatose or otherwise unable to make decisions; PASSIVE E. involves not doing something that might prevent death; VOLUNTARY E. refers to E. produced with the person's knowledge and consent. See LIVING WILL.

evacuation (i-vak' ū-ā' shun): 1. The act of emptying a cavity; generally refers to the discharge of faecal matter. 2. The material discharged from the rectum. 3. SUCTION E. a procedure used to produce abortion of a fetus of less than 14 weeks' gestation. 4. The production of a vacuum by removing the air from a closed container.

evagination (ē-vaj-i-nā′-shun): An outpouching or protrusion of a layer or a part of an organ or of a tissue.

evaluation (i-val-ū-ā′-shun): A process that attempts to determine, as systematically and objectively as possible, the relevance, effectiveness and impact of activities in the light of their objectives.

evanescent (ev-a-nes′-ent): Fleeting, unstable, unfixed, vanishing.

Evans' formula: A solution consisting of 50% colloids and 50% lactated Ringer's solution.

evaporate (i-vap′-o-rāt): To convert from the liquid or solid state to the gaseous state by conversion to vapour. — evaporation, n.

eventration (ē-ven-trā′shun): 1. Protrusion of some of the contents of the abdomen through the abdominal wall. 2. Surgical removal of the contents of the abdominal cavity. E. OF THE DIAPHRAGM a condition in which the muscular action of the diaphragm is defective, the left part being abnormally high and not moving during normal excursion; UMBILICAL E. omphalocele (*q.v.*).

eversion (ē-ver′-zhun): 1. A turning inside out or back upon itself, as the eversion of an eyelid to expose the conjunctival sac. 2. Turning inward of the ankle. 3. The position of a part when it is turned away from the midline of the body. — evert, v.

evidence-based medicine: Medical practice using the best external clinical evidence, obtained from a review of research literature, combined with the expertise of the clinician, to help make informed decisions about the care of an individual patient.

evidence-based nursing: The process by which nurses make clinical decisions using the best available research evidence, their clinical expertise and patient preferences, in the context of available resources.

evidence-based practice: A systematic analysis of information on the effectiveness and use of treatments in providing the best health outcomes.

evisceration (i-vis-e-rā′-shun): 1. Removal of the thoracic or abdominal organs. 2. Post-operative protrusion of viscera through a ruptured abdominal incision.

evolution (ēv-o-lū′-shun): 1. The process of continual, gradual and orderly growth and development or advance. 2. The theory that the variety and complexity of life on Earth has developed from earlier forms. See also DARWINISM; NEO-DARWINISM.

Ewing's tumour: Sarcoma involving the shaft of long bone before the 20th year; arises in the medullary tissue; characterized by pain, fever, leukocytosis. Also called *Ewing's sarcoma* and *endothelial myeloma*. [James Ewing, New York pathologist, 1866–1943.]

ex-: Prefix denoting out, outside, outside of, outward, away from, lacking. Opp. to end-, endo-. Variants are e-, ef-.

exacerbation (eks-as-cr-bā′-shun): Increased severity as of symptoms, or a flareup of symptoms that have subsided.

examination (eks-am-i-nā′-shun): 1. The procedure of inspecting a patient to determine his physical condition and to aid in diagnosing his ailment. PELVIC E. usually refers to examination of the female internal genitalia; see 2. under BIMANUAL; PHYSICAL E. examining the physical state of a person by inspection, palpitation, percussion, and auscultation.

exania (ek-sā′-ni-a): Prolapse of the rectum.

exanthema (eks-an-thē′-ma): 1. Any eruptive disease such as measles. 2. A skin eruption. — exanthematous, adj.

exarticulation (eks-ar-tik-ū-la′-shun): 1. The amputation of a limb at a joint. 2. The removal of part of a joint.

exchange list: See FOOD EXCHANGE LIST.

exchange transfusion: See TRANSFUSION.

excise (ek′-sīz): To remove by cutting out or off.

excision (ek-sizh′-un): The act of removing a part by cutting out or off.

excitability (ek-sīt-a-bil′-i-ti): 1. The state of readiness of cells or an organism to respond to stimuli. 2. A state of being easily irritated.

excitation (ek-sī-tā′-shun): The act of stimulating an organ or tissue.

excitatory (ek-sīt′-a-tor-i): Tending to or able to excite or stimulate.

excoriation (eks-ko-ri-ā′-shun): Loss or removal of skin such as that produced by heat, moisture, scratching, scraping, burns, chemicals, or similar means. See ABRASION. — excoriate, v.

excrement (eks-kre-ment): Waste matter cast off by the body; usually refers to faeces.

excrescence (eks-kres′-ens): Any abnormal protuberance or growth of the tissues; usually refers to surface outgrowths.

excreta (eks-krē´-ta): The waste matter which is normally discharged from the body, particularly urine and faeces.

excrete (eks-krēt): To separate and throw off from the body as waste matter.

excretion (eks-krē´-shun): The elimination of waste material from the body, and also the matter so discharged. — excretory, adj.; excrete, n; v.

excretory (eks´-kre-tō-ri): Relating to excretion. E. SYSTEM term used to describe groups of organs that eliminate waste products from the body; urinary, digestive, and respiratory systems, and the skin.

excruciating (eks-krū´ shi-āt-ing): 1. Agonizing or torturing, as pain. 2. Causing severe suffering.

excursion (eks-kur´-zhun): Any movement of a part of the body with the expectation that it will return to the original position, as the movement of the mandible from side to side or the movement of the diaphragm during respiration.

exdwelling drainage system: A system for collecting drainage material or a bodily excretion, such as urine, without inserting a tube into the organ or cavity; involves the use of a specially constructed apparatus that is attached to the skin and provides for collection in an appropriate container, such as a conveen.

exencephaly (eks-en-kef´-a-li, -sef-): A congenital anomaly marked by deficient formation of the cranium; the brain is exposed or extrudes through the skull.

exenteration (eks-en-te-rā´-shun): Evisceration. Removal of the viscera. PELVIC E. The removal of the pelvic organs, a radical operation for removal of malignant growths.

exercise (ek´-ser-sīz): Performance of physical exertion for the purposes of improving one's health, correcting a deformity, or developing a particular skill. ACTIVE E. voluntary muscular activity performed by one's own efforts; ACTIVE ASSISTED E. performed partly by a mechanical device or by a therapist, to increase range of motion or strength; AEROBIC E., E. performed while breathing continuously, as in dancing, walking, jogging, bicycling, swimming, playing tennis; advocated to promote cardiac fitness; ANAEROBIC E., E. or sport that requires short bursts of energy during which the person may 'hold' his breath until the exercise is completed, the needed oxygen being released from various oxygen compounds in the body; such E. is limited to short periods of vigorous activity; E.

ELECTROCARDIOGRAM see BRUCE TREADMILL TEST; E. TOLERANCE TEST a test to determine the oxygen requirement of the myocardium during exercise; helps in estimating the extent of coronary disease that may be present and to measure the person's capacity for exercise; may utilize the treadmill or the Master's two-step test; ISOMETRICE E. exercises involving contraction of the muscle that has both ends fixed so that the muscle is tensed without its length being changed; ISOTONIC E. in which one end of the muscle is attached to a light weight which is lifted when the muscle shortens; the tone of the muscle does not change; opp. to isometric; PASSIVE E. massage, manipulation, or movement of the body or parts of it, performed by another person, a machine, or other outside force without any effort on the part of the patient; RANGE OF MOTION E. see RANGE OF MOTION; RESISTIVE E. exercises against resistance of the therapist or a fixed object; TCDB E. turning, coughing, deep breathing exercises; UNDERWATER E., E. carried out under water where the movements of weakened muscles are facilitated by buoyancy. See also BUERGER'S EXERCISE; BUERGER-ALLEN EXERCISE; YOGA.

exfoliation (eks-fō-li-ā´-shun): The scaling off of tissue in layers, particularly of dead cells from the epidermis. — exfoliative, adj.

exhalation (eks-ha-lā´-shun): The giving forth of a gas or vapour. In physiology, the breathing out of air from the lungs.

exhale (eks-hāl´): To breathe out; to force or let air out of the lungs.

exhaustion (eg-zaws´-chun): 1. Extreme weariness or fatigue. 2. Inability to respond to stimuli. 3. The using up of a supply of anything. HEAT E. a condition caused by excessive heat, either from exposure to the sun or from working in hot places; characterized by prostration, subnormal temperatures, weakness, dehydration, and collapse.

exhibitionism (ek´-si-bish´-un-izm): Any kind of 'showing off' or extravagant behaviour to attract attention, including such perverted behaviour as exposure of their genitalia, by males, for the purpose of obtaining sexual excitement and the desire to shock the victim who is usually female. — exhibitionist, n.

exhibitionist (ek´-si-bish´-un-ist): One who derives sexual stimulation or gratification from exposing parts of the body that are conventionally covered, the genitalia in particular, to someone of the opposite sex.

exo-: Prefix demoting external, exterior, outside, outer, outer part.

exocrine (ek'-sō-krēn): Term applied to glands that deliver their secretions to an epithelial surface either directly or through a duct, or to the secretions such glands produce. Opp. to endocrine (*q.v.*). — exocrinal, adj.

exogenous (eks-oj'-en-us): Of external origin.

exomphalos (eks-om'-fa-los): A congenital condition due to failure of the abdominal wall to develop properly; the abdominal viscera herniate through a gap in the umbilical region. Umbilical hernia.

exophthalmic goitre (eks-of-thal'-mik goy'-ter): See EXOPHTHALMOS and GOITRE.

exophthalmos (ek-sof-thal'-mos): Abnormal protrusion of the eyeballs; most frequently occurs in hyperthyroidism. Opp. to enophthalmos. See GOITRE.

exoserosis (ek-sō-ser-ō'-sis): The exudation or oozing of serum from the skin surface.

exosmosis (eks-os-mo'-sis): Osmosis. The outward diffusion of a liquid through a membrane.

exotoxin (ek-sō-tok'-sin): A toxic product of living bacteria that is passed into the environment of the cell, becomes diffused and attacks specific tissues. The organisms causing diphtheria and typhoid fever produce exotoxins. Opp. to endotoxin. — exotoxic, adj.

exotropia (ek-sō-trō'-pi-a): Outward deviation of the visual axis of one eye. Opp. to esotropia. Also called *divergent strabismus, divergent squint, 'walleye'*.

expansiveness (ek-span'-siv-nes): In psychiatry, behaviour marked by euphoria, talkativeness, and an exaggerated sense of one's own importance.

expected date of delivery: The predicted date of a pregnant woman's delivery. Usually calculated from the first day of the last normal period even though fertilization takes place midpoint in the menstrual cycle. Pregnancy lasts approximately 280 days or 40 weeks. The expectant mother is advised that the expected date of delivery is only an estimate and will usually give birth within 2 weeks before or more commonly 2 weeks after the given date.

expected outcome: A statement in the patient's care plan of what a planned nursing intervention is intended to achieve.

expectorant (eks-pek'-to-rant): An agent that promotes or increases the expectoration of mucus or other exudate from the lungs, bronchi and trachea.

expectoration (ek-spek-to-rā-shun): 1. The elimination of secretion from the respiratory tract by coughing and spitting. 2. Sputum (*q.v.*). — expectorate, v.

expel (eks-pel'): To force out.

experiential learning (ek-spe-ri-en'-shul): The process of learning through participation; learning by doing.

experiment (ek-sper'-i-ment): A procedure undertaken to (1) discover a fact, principle, or effect; (2) test a hypothesis; (3) illustrate a principle or point. A test or trial.

expert (eks'-pert): A person with special knowledge or abilities who performs skilfully. See CLINICAL NURSE SPECIALIST; CONSULTANT NURSE; EXPERT PATIENT.

expertise (eks-pert-ēz'): The skill, knowledge, or opinion of somebody who is an expert.

expert patient: An informed patient taking greater responsibility for his or her own care. The idea to encourage this emerged from the NHS plan (*q.v.*) www.ohn.gov.uk/ohn/people/expert.htm

expiration (eks-pi-rā'-shun): 1. The act of breathing out air from the lungs. 2. Death. — expire, v.; expiratory, adj.

expiratory (eks-pī'-ra-tō-ri): Relating to expiration. E. GRUNT grunting sound heard on expiration in comatose adults; may be a neurological reflex or caused by partial obstruction of the airway. In infants it is a sign of impending respiratory distress; E. RESERVE VOLUME the amount of air that remains in the lungs after a maximum exhalation; for the normal adult, about 1200 ml; E. RETARD a device that provides expiratory resistance sufficient to slow expiration.

expire (eks-pīr'): 1. To exhale or breathe out. 2. To die.

explant (eks-plant'): To transfer tissue from the body to an artificial medium for growth, or the material so transferred.

exploration (eks-plo-rā'-shun): The act of exploring for diagnostic purposes, usually involving surgery or endoscopy.

expression (eks-presh'-un): 1. Expulsion by force, squeezing, or pressing out, as the placenta from the uterus, milk from the breasts. 2. Facial reflection of feeling, mood, etc.

expulsion (eks-pul'-shun): The act of forcing out, as faeces from the rectum or urine from the bladder. — expel, v.; expulsive, adj.

exsanguinate (ek-sang'-win-āt): To drain off blood. — exsanguination, n.; exsanguine, adj.

exsanguine (ek-sang'-win): Bloodless; anaemic.

extended family: One that includes aunts, uncles, grandparents, and other relatives in addition to the nuclear family.

extended role: Responsibility above and beyond that generally given to nurses, including tasks normally undertaken by a doctor. Appropriate training beyond that of the initial nursing qualification and assessment of competency are prerequisites.

extension (ek-sten'-shun): **1.** Traction upon a fractured or dislocated limb. **2.** The act of straightening a flexed limb or part.

extensor (ek-sten'-sor): A muscle which on contraction extends or straightens a part. Opp. to flexor.

exterior (eks-tēr'-i-or): The outside or outer part, or situated on or near the outside.

external: On the outside or surface of the body; in anatomy, situated towards or near the outside of the body. E. CARDIAC MASSAGE see under CARDIAC; E. HAEMORRHAGE that in which blood escapes to the outside of the body; opposite to internal haemorrhage; E. MALLEOLUS the prominence on the lateral side of the ankle formed by the rounded eminence on the lateral side of the fibula; E. RESPIRATION the transport of oxygen from the atmosphere through the lungs to the alveoli, and of carbon dioxide from the lungs to the atmosphere; E. ROTATION turning of the anterior surface of a limb outwards or laterally.

external acoustic meatus: The tubular structure leading from the pinna of the external ear to the tympanic membrane. Also called *external auditory canal.*

external verifier: An individual appointed by the Awarding Body (*q.v.*) to monitor the operation of the National Vocational Qualification (*q.v.*) scheme and to ensure that all appropriate procedures are adhered to. The external verifier will carry out regular spot checks of approved centres.

exteroceptive (eks-ter-ō-sep'-tiv): Relating to or activated by a stimulus to a sense receptor located at the surface of the body.

exteroceptor (eks'-ter-ō-sep'-tor): A sensory nerve terminal located in the skin or mucous membrane and that receives such external stimuli as heat, cold, pain, touch, taste, and smell.

extinction (ek-sting'-shun): In psychiatry, the weakening or cessation of a behaviour pattern as a result of negative reinforcement. In neurophysiology, the loss of excitability by a nerve or by nervous tissue.

extortion (eks-tor'-shun): **1.** Rotation of the eye away from the midline of the face. **2.** Outward rotation of a limb or organ.

extra-: Prefix denoting outside of, beyond, without, or in addition to.

extra-articular (eks-tra-ar-tik'-ū-lar): Outside a joint.

extracapsular (eks'-tra-kap'-sū-lar): Outside a capsule, usually referring to the capsule of a joint.

extracellular (eks-tra-sel'-ū-lar): Occurring outside a cell or cells. E. FLUID found outside of cells; includes interstitial fluid, cerebrospinal fluid, and plasma; also called *E. compartment.*

extracorporeal (eks'-tra-kor-po-rē'-al): Relates to something existing or taking place outside the body or unrelated to it. E. CIRCULATION circulation of the blood outside the body as by a mechanical pump or pump-oxygenator, often done while surgery is being performed on the heart.

extract (eks'-trakt): A preparation obtained by evaporating a solution of a drug until it contains a predetermined portion of the drug; the resulting preparation is several times stronger than the crude drug.

extraction (eks-trak'-shun): **1.** The preparation of an extract. **2.** The act or process of drawing or pulling out. E. OF LENS surgical removal of the lens of the eye. EXTRACAPSULAR E. being removal of the lens after rupturing its capsule, and INTRACAPSULAR E. being removal of the lens within its capsule; VACUUM E. the delivery of a fetus or extraction of uterine contents by application of a vacuum.

extractor (eks-trak'-tor): A surgical instrument used for removing a tooth, foreign object, or stone from the body.

extradural (eks-tra-dū'-ral): External to the dura mater (*q.v.*), or on the outer side of it.

extramural (eks-tra-mū'-ral): Refers to something situated or occurring outside the walls of an organ. — extramurally, adj.

extraneous (eks-trā'-nē-us): **1.** Originating, existing, or coming from outside of the organism. **2.** Inessential; not vital.

extrapyramidal (eks-tra-pi-ram'-i-dal): Outside of or independent of the pyramidal tracts; refers to other descending motor pathways. See PYRAMIDAL, MOTOR FIBRES. E. DISEASE characterized by disorders of movement such as tremor, rigidity, contractures, slowness, gait changes, flailing movements as seen in Parkinson's disease and Huntington's chorea.

extrasensory perception (eks-tra-sen'-so-ri per-sep'-shun): Thought transference. Relates to capacities or forms of perception of the thoughts or actions of others that are not dependent upon the five senses or explainable in relation to the senses.

extrasystole (eks'-tra-sis'-to-li): A premature beat that is independent of the regular pulse rhythm; the beat follows closely the preceding beat and is followed by a long pause before the next beat.

extravasation (eks-trav'-a-sā'-shun): An inadvertent escape of blood, lymph, intravenous infusions or medications from a vessel, or other natural enclosure into the surrounding subcutaneous tissues. — extravasate, v.

extraversion (eks-tra-ver'-zhun): Extroversion (q.v.).

extravert (eks'-tra-vert): Extrovert (q.v.).

extremitas (eks-trem'-i-tas): In anatomy, a term used to designate a distal or terminal part of an organ or structure.

extremity (eks-trem'-i-ti): The terminal end of an elongated structure or thing. In anatomy, term refers to a distal or terminal position and is used to designate such parts as arm, leg, hand, foot.

extrinsic (eks-trin'-sik): Developing or having its origin at a site outside of the location where it is found or upon which it acts; often referring to muscle. E. FACTOR Vitamin B_{12} (cyanocobalamin), which is normally present in the diet and absorbed from the gut, it is essential for normal haemopoiesis.

extro-: Prefix denoting outward, outside. Opp. to intro-.

extroversion (eks-trō-ver'-zhun): Turning outward; turning inside out; exstrophy. In psychology, the turning of one's thoughts to the external world and the focusing of one's interest on things outside oneself. Opp. of introversion.

extrovert (eks-trō-vert): Used by Jung (q.v.) to describe one extreme of personality dimension. Those described as E. regulate their behaviour in response to other people's attitude, they are sociable, good mixers and interested chiefly in external things and the actions of others. Opp. of introvert.

extrude (eks-trood'): To force or push out of the position normally occupied, or to occupy such a position. — extrusion, n.

extubation (eks'tū-bā'shun): The removal of a tube that has been inserted into an organ or orifice, e.g., a tracheostomy tube.

exudate (eks'-ū-dat): The matter that has passed through a vessel wall or membrane into surrounding space or tissue, or is deposited in the tissues; occurs in inflammation.

exuviae (eks-ū'-vi-a): Something cast off from the body, as desquamated skin or slough.

eye: The organ of vision, located in the eye socket of the skull.

eyeball: The globe of the eye without any appendages such as the extrinsic muscles.

eyebrow: The area at the upper edge of the bony orbit that contains the eye, particularly the hairs covering it.

eyelash: One of the hairs that project from the edge of the eyelid.

eyelid: One of two movable folds of skin (upper and lower) that is continuous with the skin of the face, lined with conjunctiva (q.v.), and has a row of stiff hairs at the edge. See MEIBOMIAN GLAND, CANTHUS.

eyepiece: Usually refers to the part of a microscope that the viewer looks into.

eyestrain: Fatigue of the eye from overuse, poor lighting, or an uncorrected defect in focusing.

F

F: Abbreviation for fahrenheit.

F2052SH: An active document used to highlight and identify prisoners who are, or may be, at risk of suicide or self-harm.

Faber's anaemia: Iron-deficiency anaemia, often seen in association with achlorhydria (*q.v.*); seen most often in women 30 to 50 years of age. Also called *achlorhydric anaemia*.

face: The anterior aspect of the human head, including the mouth, cheeks, nose and forehead. F. LIFTING plastic surgery to restore youthful contours; F. MASK (1) a mask made of several layers of folded gauze, worn over the nose and mouth by operating room and certain other healthcare personnel; (2) a device that fits over the nose and mouth, used in oxygen therapy to allow for variations in the concentration of oxygen in the inspired air; PARKINSON'S F. the characteristic facies seen in persons with Parkinson's disease; see under FACIES; F. PRESENTATION the position of the fetus when the face presents first in labour and delivery.

facet (fas′ et): A small, smooth, flat surface on a bone. ARTICULAR F. a small plane surface on a bone at a place where it articulates with another.

facial (fā′ -shul): Relating to the face. F. NERVE one of the seventh pair of cranial nerves; supplies motor fibres to muscles used in facial expression, and to the salivary and lacrimal glands; supplies sensory fibres to the front two-thirds of the tongue; F. NEURALGIA neuralgia (*q.v.*) in that part of the face supplied by the trigeminal (fifth cranial) nerve; F. PALSY Bell's palsy (*q.v.*); F. PARALYSIS paralysis of the muscles supplied by the facial nerve; F. SPASM muscular spasm on one side of the face or around the eye, irregular and not under conscious control.

-facient: Suffix denoting: **1.** A person or agent that brings something about or initiates an action. **2.** Making; causing.

facies (fā′ -shi-ēz): An anatomical term used to designate a surface of a body structure or part, the expression on the face, or the face itself. ABDOMINAL F. the expression seen in peritonitis; the skin is livid, the eyes sunken, and the lips dry; ADENOID F. open-mouthed, vacant expression seen in children with enlarged adenoids; F. HIPPOCRATICA the drawn, pale, pinched expression indicative of extreme prostration and approaching death; MOON F. the round, full face seen in persons with Cushing's syndrome (*q.v.*); may also occur in those receiving corticosteroid therapy; PARKINSON'S F. the mask-like appearance seen in persons with Parkinson's disease; saliva may trickle from the corner of the mouth.

facilitation (fa-sil′ -i-tā-shun): The act of increasing the ease with which an action or function is carried out, *e.g.*, the reinforcement of a reflex action by impulses from some source other than a reflex centre.

facio-: Combining form denoting face or relationship to the face.

factitious (fak-tish′ -us): Artificial. F. DISORDERS SEE MÜNCHAUSEN'S SYNDROME.

factor (fak′ -tor): Something that contributes to the production of a result, *e.g.*, an agent, constituent, ingredient. In heredity, a gene; in nutrition, a desirable ingredient or essential element, *e.g.*, a vitamin. ANTIANAEMIC F. vitamin B_{12} (cyanocobalamin); ANTIHAEMOPHILIC F. factor VIII; ANTIHAEMORRHAGIC F. vitamin K (*q.v.*); ANTIRACHITIC F. Vitamin D (*q.v.*); ANTISTERILITY F. vitamin E, see under TOCOPHEROL; clotting factors, 13 are identified and numbered I to XIII; essential for clotting or coagulation of blood; EXTRINSIC F. vitamin B_{12} (cyanocobalamin); FACTOR I fibrinogen (*q.v.*); FACTOR II prothrombin (*q.v.*); FACTOR III tissue thromboplastin; important in relation to activity of thromboplastin in clotting; FACTOR IV calcium; required in many phases of coagulation. FACTOR V proaccelerin, also called *accelerator globulin*, the clotting factor essential for converting prothrombin to thrombin; found in plasma but not serum; heat and storage-labile; also called *Labile F.*; FACTOR VI function indefinite; FACTOR VII prothrombinogen or serum prothrombin conversion accelerator is concerned with a coagulation deficiency which results in a tendency to haemorrhage due to prolonged prothrombin time; FACTOR VIII called antihaemophilic factor or antihaemophilic globulin present in plasma, but not serum; participates in formation of thromboplastin; a deficiency is associated with haemophilia A, a hereditary haemorrhagic tendency; see VON WILLEBRAND'S DISEASE. FACTOR IX a precoagulant called *Christmas factor*, found in normal plasma; deficiency is associated with classic haemophilia B, a hereditary haemorrhagic tendency. FACTOR X present in plasma and serum; deficiency may be inherited or be the result of anticoagulant therapy with certain drugs; also called *Stuart–Prower F.*; FACTOR XI an antecedent to plasma prothrombin and important in the functioning of the intrinsic factor; FACTOR XII, found in normal serum but deficient in individuals with hereditary bleeding disorders; necessary for rapid coagulation; FACTOR XIII a fibrin stabilizing factor; necessary to fibrin in the formation of a firm clot; HAGEMAN FACTOR factor XII; INTRINSIC F. a mucoprotein secreted by the gastric glands; essential for the absorption of vitamin B_{12}; absent in pernicious anaemia; RH FACTOR see under RHESUS; RHEUMATIC F. an immunoglobulin found in the blood serum of many individuals with rheumatic arthritis; TRANSFER F. a F. occurring in some leukocytes that have been sensitized in one individual and that can apparently transfer the hypersensitivity to another individual in whom the leukocytes have not been sensitized.

faculty (fak'-ul-ti): **1.** An inherent normal power, capability, function, or attitude; pertains chiefly to the human body or its parts, particularly in reference to mental endowments. **2.** The teaching staff of an educational institution.

faecal (fē'-kal): Relating to faeces. F. IMPACTION an accumulation of hardened faeces in the rectum or sigmoid colon, resulting from prolonged constipation and which is immovable by normal intestinal activity; F. VOMITING the vomiting of faecal matter; often a sign of intestinal obstruction.

faeces (fē'-sēz): The waste matter excreted from the bowel, consisting of indigestible cellulose, unabsorbed food, mucus, intestinal secretions, water, and bacteria. Also called *stool* or *defecation.* — faecal, adj.

Fahrenheit (far'-en-hīt): A thermometric scale; the freezing point of water is 32° and its boiling point 212°, the normal body temperature is 98.4°–98.6°. [Gabriel Fahrenheit, German physicist, 1686–1736.]

failure: Inability to perform a normal duty or expected action. HEART F. sudden cessation of the heart's action.

failure-to-thrive syndrome: A condition of infants and young children characterized by malnutrition, faulty physical and emotional development, apathy, irritability, anorexia, sometimes vomiting and diarrhoea; may be the result of underfeeding, congenital anomalies, infection, or disturbed mother–child relationship.

faint: 1. Weak; lacking in strength or in courage. **2.** A swoon; a state of temporary unconsciousness. Syn., *synscope.*

fainting: Loss of consciousness due to lack of adequate blood to the brain.

falciform (fal'-si-form): Sickle-shaped. F. LIGAMENT a fold of peritoneum that separates the two main lobes of the liver.

Fallopian (fal-lō'-pi-an): F. LIGAMENT the round ligament of the uterus; F. TUBE one of two ducts that open out of the upper part of the uterus. Each measures about 10 cm. The distal ends lie near the ovary, are funnel-shaped and fimbriated, with one of the fimbriae reaching the ovary. The function is to carry the ova from the ovary to the uterus. Also called *uterine tubes, oviducts.* [Gabriele Fallopius, 16th C. Italian anatomist.]

Fallot's tetralogy (fa-lōz'): Tetralogy of Fallot (*q.v.*).

fallout: Radioactive particles that result from a nuclear explosion and descend through the atmosphere.

false: Not true; not genuine. F. LABOUR painful contractions of the uterus that resemble those of true labour but without dilatation of the cervix; F. NEGATIVE an incorrect result of a diagnostic or other test that indicates the absence of a finding or of a pathological condition; F. PAINS abdominal pains during pregnancy that are not true labour pains; F. PELVIS that part of the pelvis above the pelvic brim; F. POSITIVE an incorrect result of a diagnostic or other test that indicates the presence of a pathological condition that does not exist; F. PREGNANCY unfounded preoccupation with thoughts of pregnancy and motherhood, intense desire to have a baby, sometimes accompanied by morning sickness, amenorrhoea, and even enlarged breasts; F. RIBS the lower five pairs of ribs, so called because they attach to the sternum by means of a cartilage rather than directly; F. VOCAL CORDS see under VOCAL.

falx (falks): A sickle-shaped structure. F. CEREBELLI the short process of the dura mater that extends from the occipital bone into the posterior notch between the two hemispheres of the cerebellum; F. CEREBRI the fold of dura mater that separates the two cerebral hemispheres.

familial (fa-mil' -i-al): Relating to the family, as of a disease affecting several members of the same family, or one that occurs in members of the same family in successive generations.

family: Any group of persons closely related by blood and certain other ties; may or may not be living under the same roof. EXTENDED F. a nuclear F. plus blood-related others, *e.g.*, aunts, uncles, cousins, grandparents; F. HEALTH PLAN (public health), an assessment tool that reviews the family in the context of its life cycle. MATRIARCHAL F. one headed by a woman; NUCLEAR F. consisting of only parents and their children living together; ONE-PARENT F. one in which only one parent remains with the children; PATRIARCHAL F. one headed by a man; F. PLANNING is concerned with the avoidance of or spacing of pregnancies, with infertility, and with methods of effecting conception; F. THERAPY see under THERAPY.

Family Planning Certificate: A qualification awarded on completion of a course that covers contraception, screening, menopause, sexual history taking, clinical governance, and applying national directives to local practice.

Fanconi's syndrome: A rare hereditary condition of two types: (1) characterized by various anomalies of the musculoskeletal and genitourinary systems, hypoplasia of the bone marrow and pancytopenia, and uneven brown skin discoloration; also called *Fanconi's anaemia* and (2) characterized by short stature, osteomalacia and rickets, glycosuria, aminoaciduria, and the deposit of cystine in various parts of the body, including the liver, spleen, cornea, and bone marrow. Both types are known by several other names that are descriptive of the anomalies involved.

fantasy (fan' -ta-si): Imagination in which images or chains of images are directed by the desire or pleasure of the thinker, normally accompanied by a feeling of unreality; a normal process in childhood when learning to distinguish between wish and reality. Occurs pathologically in schizophrenia. Also spelled *phantasy*. — fantasize, v.

farad (far' -ad): A unit of electrical capacity. — faradic, adj.

Farber's disease: Disseminated lipogranulomatosis. See LIPOGRANULOMATOSIS. [S. Farber, American pathologist, 1903–1973.]

far-sightedness: Hyperopia (*q.v.*).

fascia (fash-i-a): A connective sheath consisting of fibrous tissue and fat, which unites the skin to the underlying tissues. DEEP F. forms a sheath for muscles, either separating them or

holding them together; also invests such other deep structures as nerves and blood vessels; F. LATA the strong, tough F. that envelops the muscles of the thigh; SUPERFICIAL F. formed by the subcutaneous tissue; contains fat, small arteries and branches of nerves; is loosely attached to the deep F. — fasciae, pl.; fascial, adj.

fascial (fash' -i-al): Relating to a fascia.

fascicle (fas'i-k'l): A small bundle, as of nerve or muscle fibres. Also called *fascicule*.

fascicular (fa-sik' -ū-lar): 1. Relating to a fascicle. 2. Arranged in a bundle.

fasciculation (fa-sik-ū-lā' -shun): 1. The formation of fascicles. 2. The uncoordinated contraction or twitching of several groups of muscle fibres that are all supplied by the same motor neuron; may be indicative of any one of several nutritional or neurological disorders; also occurs as a side effect of certain drugs. When it occurs in heart muscle it is called fibrillation.

fasciectomy (fash-i-ek' -tō-mi): Excision of a fascia or of strips of fascia.

fasciitis (fash-i-ī' -tis): Inflammation of fascia.

fascioscapulohumeral (fas' -i-ō-scap' -ū-lō-hūm' -er-al): Pertinent to the face, scapula, and upper arm. F. MUSCULAR DYSTROPHY also called *Landouzy–Déjerine dystrophy*; see under DYSTROPHY.

fast: 1. To abstain from eating. 2. To be resistant to destruction or to staining, said of bacteria.

fastidious (fas-tid' -i-us): In microbiology, pertains to an organism that is difficult to grow under ordinary laboratory conditions.

fastidium (fas-tid' -i-um): Repugnance or aversion to food or to eating. Squeamishness.

fastigium (fas-tij' -i-um): 1. The highest point of a fever; the period of full development of a disease. 2. The highest point in the roof of the fourth ventricle of the brain.

fasting blood sugar test: A test for diagnosis of a glucose metabolism disorder; requires the patient to fast for 12 hours before the test.

fat: 1. Plump, stout, obese. 2. The oily substance that makes up most of the cell content of adipose tissue. 3. An oil of animal or vegetable origin, either solid or liquid. POLYUNSATURATED F. refers to fats that have many unsaturated chemical bonds and which tend to be liquid at room temperature; these fats are found in corn, cottonseed, soybean, and safflower oils, and in fish and poultry. SATURATED FATS tend to be solid at room temperature; they are found in meats, chocolate, butter, cheese, cream, whole milk. — fatty, adj.

fatal (fā′-tal): Causing death; deadly.

fat embolism syndrome: A condition caused by the lodgement of a fat embolism in the pulmonary circulation; symptoms resemble those of adult respiratory distress syndrome; an emergency situation requiring immediate correction.

fatigue (fa-tēg′): The feeling of weariness and of reduced capacity for mental or physical work, usually resulting from prolonged or excessive labour or exertion. In physiological experiments on muscle the term is used to denote diminishing reaction to stimuli. — fatigability, n.; fatigable, adj.

fat soluble: Usually refers to the vitamins A, D, E, and K, which are soluble in fat but not in water.

fatty: Relating to or characterized by fat. F. DE-GENERATION degeneration (q.v.) of tissues which results in appearance of fatty droplets in the cytoplasm, found especially in diseases of the liver, kidney and heart.

fatty acid: Any organic acid that will combine with glycerine to form fat, especially oleic, palmitic, and stearic acids. Obtainable from most plants and animals. Used by the tissues as a major source of energy. ESSENTIAL F.A. an unsaturated F.A. that cannot be formed in the body; must be supplied by the diet; SATURATED F.A. not capable of absorbing any more hydrogen; palmitic and stearic are the most common of this group; found in products of both animal and vegetable origin including dairy products; beef, lamb, veal, and pork; coconut and palm oils; and chocolate. Diets heavy in these products have been found to be associated with high serum cholesterol levels; UNSATURATED F.A. (essential F.A.) capable of absorbing more hydrogen; linoleic and arachidonic are the most common of this group; found in fowl and fish; olive and safflower oils; sunflower seeds and cottonseeds; soybeans; walnuts, peanuts, cashew nuts, almonds, and pecans. Diets high in unsaturated F.A. have been found to be associated with low serum cholesterol levels.

fauces (faw′-sēz): The space between the mouth and the pharynx, bounded above by the soft palate, below by the tongue. PILLARS OF THE F. anterior and posterior, lie laterally and enclose the tonsil. — faucial, adj.

FBC: Abbreviation for full blood count (q.v.).

FBS: Abbreviation for fasting blood sugar (q.v.).

Fe: Chemical symbol for iron. (q.v.).

fear: An unpleasant, strong emotion occurring in response to recognition of danger or a threat; apprehension, dread, alarm. When carried to morbid excess it is called a phobia (q.v.).

febri-: Combining form denoting fever.

febrile (feb′-ril): Feverish; accompanied by fever, or having a fever. F. ALBUMINURIA albiminuria that is due to fever; F. SEIZURE a generalized convulsive seizure induced by sudden elevation in temperature; usually occurring in children between six months and five years of age; thought to be due to underdevelopment of the body's capacity to adjust to sudden changes in the body temperature.

fecal, feces: For these and other related words SEE FAECAL, FAECES, etc.

feculent (fek′-ū-lent): 1. Foul. 2. Having sediment. 3. Relating to, containing, or of the nature of faeces.

fecundate (fē′-kun-dāt): 1. To fertilize; to impregnate. 2. To render fertile.

fecundation (fē′-kun-dā′-shun): Impregnation. Fertilization.

fecundity (fē-kun′-di-ti): 1. Pronounced fertility; the power to reproduce offspring in large numbers. 2. The innate physiological ability of an individual to produce offspring, as opposed to fertility.

feedback: In general, all information resulting from a process. In nursing, the results of planned nursing interventions in the form of information that can be applied to the control and improvement of patient care. See also BIOFEEDBACK.

feeding: The giving or taking of food. DEMAND F. feeding an infant when hungry rather than on a set schedule; F. TUBE a tube for introducing food into the stomach; FORCED F. giving food by force when the patient refuses to eat; INTRAVENOUS F. feeding by introducing liquid nourishment (nutrient fluids) into a vein; NASOGASTRIC F. gavage; introduced feedings into the stomach via the nose, pharynx, and oesophagus; TRANSPYLORIC F. feeding of a special formula through a tube positioned through the nares into the stomach, then into the duodenum or jejunum; used for feeding neonates or small infants when necessary, or sometimes adults after surgery; TUBE F. introducing food via a tube into the stomach, or duodenum. See HYPERALIMENTATION.

feeling: 1. The sense of touch. 2. The awareness of the sensations produced by the special sense organs. 3. An emotion or mental state that is recognized as pleasurable or unpleasurable.

fellatio (fe-lā′-shi-ō): Insertion of the penis into the mouth of another person, male or female. Oral coitus.

felon (fel′-un): A purulent infection involving the end of a finger, usually near the nail, usually follows a minor penetrating wound. WHITLOW.

Felty's syndrome: A combination of adult rheumatoid arthritis and hypersplenism, often accompanied by pigmented spots on the skin of the legs, by anaemia, thrombocytopenia, and granulocytopenia, leukopenia, splenomegaly.

female (fē′-mal): 1. Pertinent to the sex that produces the ovum and becomes pregnant. 2. A person of the female sex. F. PSEUDOHERMAPHRODITISM a condition in which the external genitalia are male but the internal genitalia are entirely female.

femaleness (fē′-māl-nes): The anatomical and physiological features of a female that are concerned with procreation and nurturing of offspring.

feminine (fem′-i-nin): Relating to the qualities and role behaviour of a female apart from her procreative and nurturing capacities.

feminism (fem′-i-nizm): 1. Femaleness. 2. The possession of feminine traits and characteristics by the male. 3. The social movement for equality of women. 4. A set of social theories and political practices that are critical of past and current social relations and primarily motivated and informed by the experience of women. It involves a critique of gender inequality and the promotion of women's rights and interests.

feminization (fem′-i-nī-zā′-shun): 1. The normal development of female traits and characteristics. 2. The development of female characteristics in a male, *e.g.*, high-pitched voice, female type of breast.

femoral (fem′-or-al): Relating to the femur or to the thigh as a whole. F. ARTERY the main blood vessel supplying blood to the leg; F. CANAL a conical canal, about 1.25 cm in length, situated in the region between the anterior superior spine of the ilium and the symphysis pubis; a frequent site of hernia; F. HERNIA see under HERNIA; F. NERVE originates in the lumbar plexus; enervates the muscles of the front of the thigh, and the leg, hip, and knee joints; F. PULSE the pulse of the femoral artery which may be felt in the groin; F. VEIN the large vein in the upper two-thirds of the thigh.

femoropopliteal (fem′-or-ō-pop-li-tē′-al): Relating to the femur and the popliteal space, or to the femoral and popliteal arteries. F. BYPASS the insertion of a vascular prosthesis between the femoral and politeal arteries to bypass an obstructed segment.

femur (fē′-mur): The thigh bone; the longest and strongest bone in the body extending from the hip to the thigh. — femora, pl.; femoral, adj.

fenestra (fe-nes′-tra): 1. A window-like opening. 2. An aperture or opening cut into a plaster of Paris bandage or cast to give access for inspection, relieve pressure, or give skin care. F. OVALIS the oval window, an oval opening between the middle and inner ear. Below it lies the F. ROTUNDA, round window, a round opening in the wall between the middle and inner ear.

fenestration (fen-es-trā′-shun): 1. Perforation. 2. The surgical procedure of creating a new opening in the labyrinth of the inner ear to restore hearing in persons with otosclerosis. (*q.v.*).

ferment: 1. (fer-ment′): To undergo fermentation (*q.v.*). 2. (fer′-ment): Any substance that causes other substances to undergo fermentation.

fermentation (fer-men-tā′-shun): The chemical changes brought about by the action of enzymes or ferments on complex carbohydrates, usually accompanied by the liberation of heat and gas. Excellent examples are the making of cheese and wine.

fern test: A test for ovulation. Mucus from the cervix during the preovulatory phase will show a fern-like pattern when dried and examined under a microscope. After ovulation this pattern disappears.

ferr-, ferri-, ferro-: Combining forms denoting or relating to iron.

ferric (fer′-ik): Relating to iron. F. AMMONIUM CITRATE an iron preparation sometimes used in treatment of anaemia; F. CHLORIDE a water or tincture preparation of iron that is sometimes used as a styptic or as an astringent in treatment of skin disorders.

ferritin (fer′-i-tin): An iron–protein complex formed in the intestinal mucosa and stored in the liver, spleen, and bone marrow; essential for haematopoiesis.

ferrous (fer′-rus): Relating to divalent iron, as of its salts and compounds.

fertile (fer′-tīl): Fruitful; not sterile or barren; capable of conceiving and bearing young. — fertility, n.

fertility (fer-til′-i-ti): The ability of a man to impregnate a woman or of a woman to conceive and give birth to a live infant. F. PLANNING see FAMILY PLANNING; F. RATE the number of live births per 1000 women of child-bearing age in a specific population.

fertilization (fer′ti-lī-zā′shun): The impregnation of an ovum by a spermatozoon. Conception.

fester (fes'-ter): To ulcerate, generate pus, or suppurate superficially.

festination (fes-ti-nā'-shun): An involuntary hastening in gait as seen in paralysis agitans and some other nervous system disorders.

fetal (fē'-tal): Relating to a fetus (*q.v.*). F. ALCO-HOL SYNDROME a group of features seen in new-borns whose mothers are alcoholics; consists of low birth weight, poor growth pattern, failure to thrive, and mental handicap; F. AS-SESSMENT determination of the well-being of the fetus using a combination of several techniques and procedures, including family and medical history, physical examination, ultrasonography, assessment of fetal activity, chemical assessment of placental functioning, and amniocentesis. F. CIRCULATION see under CIR-CULATION; F. MONITORING the continuous and simultaneous recording of uterine contractions together with the fetal heart rate. Often recorded during labour so that any potential problems related to fetal distress can be detected early in order to prevent perinatal morbidity and death.

fetation (fe-tā'-shun): 1. Pregnancy 2. The formation and development of the fetus

fetid (fet -id): Having an offensive odour; stinking.

fetish (fet'-ish): An inanimate object that is believed to have magical or supernatural power, or that is worshipped or regarded with unreasonable devotion.

fetishism (fet'-ish-izm): 1. The worship of an inanimate object as a substitute for, or symbol of, a loved person. 2. The displacement of the natural erotic interest from a human to an inanimate object. In psychiatry, a form of sexual deviation in which the person feels a strong attachment for an inanimate object usually associated with the other sex, or uses a non-human object for sexual arousal.

fetoprotein (fē-tō-prō'-tē-in): A fetal antigen that may also be found in adults. ALPHA-F. when increased in the fetus, as shown by amniocentesis or maternal blood sampling, may be diagnostic of neural tube defects; may also appear in the serum of persons with certain liver diseases, including malignancies. BETA-F. a protein found in fetal liver; may also be found in the liver of adults with some liver diseases; is identical with ferritin (*q.v.*).

fetor (fē'-tor): Offensive odour; stench. F. EXORE bad breath; halitosis. F. HEPATICUS the peculiar breath odour noticed in patients with terminal liver disease; due to exhalation of sulphur-containing substances formed in the intestine by bacterial action on sulphur-containing amino acids.

fetoscope (fē'-to-skōp): A stethoscope for auscultating the fetal heartbeat.

fetus (fē'-tus): An unborn child. In the human, the term usually refers to the unborn child from the end of the seventh week after gestation when all of the internal and external organs are present and are undergoing development, until birth. CALCIFIED F. a. F. that has died but remained in the uterus and become calcified; MUMMIFIED F. a dead F. that has taken on the characteristics of a mummy; F. PAPYRACEUS a mummified dead F. pressed flat by the presence of a growing twin.

FEV: Abbreviation for forced expiratory volume (*q.v.*).

fever (fē'-ver): 1. An elevation of body temperature above normal (37°C; 98.6°F) Syn., *pyrexia*. 2. Designates some infectious condition, *e.g.*, paratyphoid fever, scarlet fever, etc. F. BLISTER herpes simplex of the lip; F. OF UN-DETERMINED ORIGIN, F. that persists for weeks or months, often exceeding 101°F.; of obscure origin, more commonly known as pyrexia of undetermined origin, (*q.v.*); HECTIC F., F. that occurs daily and tends to rise in the afternoon; seen in tuberculosis and septicaemia.

fibr-, fibro-: Combining forms denoting (1) fibre; (2) fibrous tissue; (3) fibrin.

fibraemia (fi-brē'-mi-a): The presence of fibrin in the blood.

fibre (fi'-ber): A slender, elongated, threadlike structure. — fibrous, adj. NERVE F. a slender process of a neuron, particularly from an axon; may vary in length up to several feet; see GANGLION, NEURON, PLEXUS.

fibreoptic (fī-ber-op'-tik): Refers to the fine, flexible, coated glass or plastic tubes of the fibrescope that have special refractive properties, making it possible to visualize body parts not previously visible, such as the oesophagus, stomach, bronchus, bladder and rectum. Combined with the laser beam, the F. endoscope is useful in controlling gastrointestinal bleeding.

fibrescope (fi'-ber-skōp): An instrument made of flexible glass, embodying light, an eyepiece and a photographic device; it provides a valuable diagnostic tool, as it permits close examination of the bronchial tree, stomach, oesophagus, duodenum, and part of the jejunum as well as parts of the large bowel. Also used for doing biopsies. — fibreoscopy, adj.

fibril (fi'-bril): A component filament of a fibre, as of a muscle or nerve. A small fibre. — fibrillar, fibrillary, adj.

fibrillation (fi-bri-lā´-shun): Uncoordinated, rapid, quivering contraction of muscle, referring usually to ATRIAL F. in the myocardium wherein the atria beat very rapidly and not in synchronization with the ventricular beat. The result is a total irregularity in the pulse rhythm; VENTRICULAR F. similar to atrial F. and resulting in rapid, wavering, and ineffectual contraction from the ventricle, seen most often in association with organic heart disease, such as hypertension, thyrotoxicosis, mitral valve disorder, rheumatic heart disease.

fibrin (fi´-brin): An elastic, thread-like, insoluble protein that forms the matrix on which a blood clot is formed. Derived from soluble fibrinogen of the blood by the catalytic (enzymatic) action of thrombin. — fibrinous, adj.

fibrinase (fi´-brin-ās): factor XIII; see under FACTOR.

fibrinogen (fi-brin´-ō-jen): A soluble protein of the blood from which is produced the insoluble protein called fibrin (q.v.) essential to blood coagulation. Also called *plasminogen*. See FACTOR I under FACTOR.

fibrinogenopenia (fi-brin´-ō-jen-ō-pē´-ni-a): Lack of blood plasma fibrinogen. May be congenital or due to liver disease. Fibrinopenia. Also called *Hypofibrinogenaemia*.

fibrinolysin (fi´-bri-nol´-i-sin): An enzyme which causes the destruction of fibrin, thereby aiding in the dissolution of blood clots. Thought to dissolve the fibrin that occurs in tissues after minor injuries. Also called *plasmin*.

fibrinolysis (fi--bri-nol´-i-sis): The digestion or dissolution of fibrin by various enzymes and mechanisms. — fibrinolytic, adj.

fibrinolytic (fi´-bri-nō-lit´-ik): 1. Relating to fibrinolysis. 2. A drug that dissolves blood clots.

fibroadenoma (fi´-brō-ad-e-nō´-ma): A benign tumour containing fibrous and glandular tissue. Often occurs as a breast tumour in women under 30; the mass is firm, movable, well defined; appears suddenly and may become very large; biopsy confirms the diagnosis.

fibroblast (fi´-brō-blast): A large stellate cell from which connective tissue arises, including fibrous tissues, tendons, aponeuroses, and other supporting connective tissues; also commonly seen in developing tissues and tissue that is undergoing repair. Syn., *fibrocyte*. — fibroblastic, adj.

fibroblastoma (fi´-brō-blas-tō´-ma): A tumour arising from the ordinary connective tissue cells or from fibroblasts.

fibrocarcinoma (fi´-brō-kar-si-nō´-ma): A carcinoma that contains fibrous elements.

fibrocartilage (fi´-brō-kar´-ti-lij): Cartilage containing fibrous tissue, found especially in the intervertebral discs.

fibrochondroma (fi´-brō-kon-drō´-ma): A benign tumour of cartilaginous tissue which contains a considerable amount of fibrous tissue.

fibrocyst (fi´-brō-sist): A fibroma that has undergone cystic degeneration with the cyst becoming the predominant component of the lesion.

fibrocystic (fī-brō-sis´-tik): Relating to a fibrocyst. F. DISEASE OF BONE, cysts may be solitary or generalized. The latter condition, when accompanied by decalcification of bone, is due to hyperparathyroidism; F. DISEASE OF THE BREAST mastitis characterized by the formation in the female breast of cysts that contain straw-coloured fluid; usually occurs at or near menopause; F. DISEASE OF THE PANCREAS see MUCOVISIDOSIS.

fibrocyte (fī-brō-sīt): See FIBROBLAST. — fibrocytic, adj.

fibroelastic (fī-brō-i-las´-tik): Containing both fibrous and elastic elements.

fibroepithelioma (fi´-brō-ep-i-thē-li-ō´-ma): A skin tumour consisting of fibrous tissue and basal cells of the epidermis; may develop into basal cell carcinoma.

fibroid (fī´-broyd): 1. Being fibrous in nature. 2. A benign tumour originating in smooth muscle tissue often found in the endometrium in multiparous women between 30 and 50 years of age, and which tends to regress at menopause; may occur singly or as multiple firm, round, encapsulated tumours. Most common symptoms are a feeling of dragging in the pelvis; pain and irregular spotting and/or excessive bleeding may occur. Also called *fibroma uteri* and *leiomyoma uteri*.

fibroidectomy (fī´-broid-ek´-tō-mi): Surgical removal of a uterine fibroid.

fibrolymphoangioblastoma (fī´-brō-lim´-fō-an´-ji-ō-blas-tō´-ma): A fibrous tumour of the breast; it is hard and freely movable although somewhat adherent to the skin.

fibroma (fī-brō´-ma): An irregularly shaped, firm, slow growing, benign tumour composed chiefly of fibrous or fully developed connective tissue; usually painless; a fibroid. JUVENILE NASOPHARYNGEAL F. a benign neoplasm of the nasopharynx; most often seen in young males.

fibromatosis (fī-brō-ma-tō´-sis): A condition in which several fibromata develop at the same time; they may be quite widely distributed throughout the body.

fibromyitis (fī´-brō-mī-ī´-tis): Inflammation of the muscles, followed by degeneration of the muscle fibres.

fibromyoma (fī´-brō-mī-ō´-ma): A benign tumour consisting of fibrous and muscle tissue. — fibromyomata, pl.; fibromyomatous, adj.

fibromyositis (fī´-brō-mī-ō-sī´-tis): Any of a large group of acute or chronic disorders characterized by inflammation of muscles, overgrowth of connective tissues, and stiffness of the joints.

fibroneuroma (fī´-brō-nū-rō´-ma): A tumour that has elements of both a fibroma and a neuroma.

fibro-osteoma (fī´-brō-os-tē-ō´-ma): A tumour that has the characteristics of both a fibroma and an osteoma.

fibroplasia (fī-brō-plā´-zi-a): The formation of fibrous tissue; occurs in the healing of wounds; usually implies an abnormal increase of fibrous tissue. RETROLENTAL F. the presence of fibrous tissue in the vitreous, from the retina to the lens, causing blindness. Noticed shortly after birth, more commonly in premature babies who have had continuous oxygen therapy. — fibroplastic, adj.

fibrosarcoma (fī´-brō-sar-kō´-ma): A sarcoma that develops from fibroblasts; begins with small skin nodules and metastasizes early.

fibrose (fī´-brōs): 1. The forming of fibrous tissue. 2. Fibrous.

fibrosis (fī-brō´-sis): The formation of fibrous tissue in an organ or part; usually refers to excessive formation as part of a reparative process. It is the cause of adhesions of the peritoneum and other serous tissues. CYSTIC F. OF THE PANCREAS see CYSTIC, FIBROCYSTIC; F. OF THE LUNGS the formation of scar tissue in the stroma of the lungs following an infection or inflammation. PERIGLOMULAR F. the deposition of collagen in Bowman's capsule, (*q.v.*), see under NEPHRON; PULMONARY F. progressive F. of the walls of the alveoli resulting in severe dyspnoea; the acute form may be rapidly fatal.

fibrositis (fī´-brō-sī´-tis): Inflammation of the white fibrous tissue, especially that of some of the muscles. Syn., *muscular rheumatism*. See BORNHOLM DISEASE, LUMBAGO, PLEURODYNIA.

fibrotic (fī-brot´-ik): Characterized by or pertinent to fibrosis.

fibrous (fī´-brus): Consisting of, containing, or like fibres. F. TISSUE a type of connective tissue that is made up of strong, tough, white fibres; forms tendons, ligaments and fascia.

fibula (fib´-ū-la): One of the longest and thinnest bones of the body; situated on the outer side of the leg and articulating at the upper end with the lateral condyle of the tibia and at the lower end with the lateral surface of the talus (astragalus) and tibia. — fibular, adj.

Fick principle: States that an indirect measure of cardiac output per minute can be obtained by comparing the amount of oxygen consumed per minute to the amount of oxygen absorbed by each millilitre of blood as it passes through the capillaries of the lungs. See also CARDIAC OUTPUT under CARDIAC.

field (fēld): A limited area; an open space. F. OF HEARING the space within which sounds are audible. Also called *auditory field*; F. OF VISION the entire area in which objects can be seen by the fixed eye.

fight-or-flight reaction: 1. In physiology, the response of the sympathetic nervous system and the adrenal medulla to stress, which results in alterations in metabolism and blood flow that, in turn, promote preservation of the individual in emergency situations. 2. In psychiatry, the response of the individual to stress; he or she may fight by striving to adjust, or flee by taking refuge in psychosis, which allows him or her to ignore the stressful circumstance.

filament (fil´-a-ment): A delicate fibre or thread-like structure. — filamenta, filaments, pl.; filar, filamentous, adj.

filial (fil´-i-al): Relating to a son or daughter.

film badge: A small packet device containing x-ray sensitive film, worn by individuals exposed to ionizing radiation in their work, for estimating the amount of radiation to which they have been exposed.

filter (fil´-ter): 1. To screen out or strain the solids from a substance by passing it through a device that will hold back the solids larger than a certain size while letting the liquid pass. 2. Any substance or device that screens or strains out certain suspended particles. In radiotherapy the term applies to a sheet of metal that lets certain rays pass through while holding others back. F. PAPER a coarse-grained paper used for filtering solutions; F. PASSING VIRUS see VIRUS.

filterable (fil´-ter-a-b'l): Capable of passing through a filter. F. VIRUS a pathogenic agent that is so small it passes through the pores of the finest filter available.

filtrate (fil´-trāt): That part of a solution that has passed through a filter.

filtration (fil-trā´-shun): The process of straining through a filter. The act of passing fluid through a porous medium. F. UNDER PRESSURE occurs in the kidneys, due to pressure of the blood in the glomeruli.

filum (fī´-lum): Any filamentous or thread-like structure. F. TERMINALE a strong, fine cord blending with the spinal cord above, and the periosteum of the sacral canal below; the terminal end of the spinal cord.

fimbria (fim´-bri-a): A fringe or frond resembling a frond of a fern, especially one of the frond-like processes at the end of a uterine tube. — fimbriae, pl.; fimbriate, fimbriated, adj.

finger: A digit of the hand. CLUBBED F. swelling of the terminal phalanx of digits that occurs in many persons with heart or lung disease; F. COT see under COT; INDEX F. that nearest the thumb; F. READING Braille reading; see BRAILLE; F. SPELLING a method of communication between deaf people; the letters of the alphabet are formed by various positions of the hands and fingers; F. STALL, F. cot; TRIGGER F. one that locks when flexed so it can be opened only with difficulty, making a snapping noise; due to chronic tenosynovitis; WEBBED F. one that is joined to another by a fold of skin.

finger–finger test: A test for cerebellar function; the patient is asked to stretch his arms out to the sides and then bring the tips of the index fingers together; normally the motion is carried out smoothly and accurately.

finger–nose test: A test for cerebellar function; the patient extends his arm to one side and then slowly tries to touch the end of his nose. Test is conducted in several ways, all involving touching the end of the nose.

fingerprint: The impression made when the ends of the fingers are inked and then pressed on a piece of paper. Used for identification purposes as no two persons have the same pattern of ridges in the skin at the ends of the fingers.

fingersweep: A technique utilized before administering the abdominal thrust manoeuvre to a choking or unconscious patient; the curved index finger of one hand is inserted at the side of the cheek and quickly passed over the back of the throat and sides of the cheek to remove any food or other object that may be obstructing the airway.

finished consultant episode: The point at which a patient has completed a period of care under a specialist, and is either discharged or transferred to another consultant.

first aid: The immediate treatment given to a person who is injured or who becomes suddenly ill, before the doctor arrives or medical treatment can be obtained.

first intention healing: See under HEALING.

fish-skin test: Ichthyosis (*q.v.*).

fission (fish´-un): The action of splitting. In biology, the reproduction of a cell by simple division into two approximately equal parts. In nuclear physics, the splitting of the nucleus of the atom, causing the release of great quantities of energy.

fissure (fish´-ur): A split, crack, or groove in tissue; may be structured and normal or abnormal. ANAL F. or F. IN ANO a crack or linear ulcer on the margin of the anus; causes severe pain on defecation; usually treated surgically; LONGITUDINAL F. separates the right and left hemispheres of the cerebrum; PALPEBRAL F. the opening between the eyelids; F. OF ROLANDO see ROLANDIC; F. OF SYLVIUS see SYLVIUS.

fistula (fis´-tū-la): An abnormal tube-like communication between two body surfaces or cavities, or between an internal organ and the surface of the body, *e.g.*, a gastrocolic F. between the stomach and the colon, or a colostomy between the colon and the abdominal surface. ABDOMINAL F. one leading from an abdominal viscus to the exterior; ANAL F. fistula in ano; ARTERIOVENOUS F. an abnormal communication between an artery and a vein; CIMINO-BRESCIA F. a F. created between a cephalic vein and the radial artery; made to provide a mode of entry to the circulation for dialysis; COLONIC F. a F. between the intestine and the skin of the abdomen or between the colon and another hollow organ; FAECAL F. a F. that opens onto the surface of the body; it discharges faeces; F. IN ANO a deep slit in the skin around the anus; often a sequela to perineal abscess; INTESTINAL F. an abnormal passage into the intestine; may refer to one surgically created; PANCREATIC F. (1) an opening from the pancreas to the surface of the body; may be created in certain gastric or duodenal operations; or (2) a surgically created internal passage from the pancreas to the small intestine or gallbladder; RECTOVAGINAL F. a fistulous opening between the rectum and vagina; TRACHEAL F. an abnormal passage opening into the trachea; TRACHEOESOPHAGEAL F. a communication channel between the trachea and the oesophagus; a serious congenital anomaly requiring immediate surgey; VESICOINTESTINAL F. a fistulous communication between the urinary bladder and the intestine; VESICOVAGINAL F. a fistulous opening between the urinary bladder and the vagina. — fistular, fistulous, adj.; fistulae, pl.

fit: Convulsion (*q.v.*). Inappropriate, sudden attack of motor or psychic activity, or both. Typical episode involves patient in involuntary and paroxysmal muscular movements (writhing) associated with loss of consciousness. See EPILEPSY.

Fitness for Practice: A UKCC report published in 1999, which reviewed the pre-registration nurse education programme and made recommendations for change. Also known as the *Peach Report.*

fix: To fasten firmly. See FIXATION.

fixation (fik-sā'-shun): 1. The act of fastening something into a fixed position, often by suturing. 2. The condition or state of being fixed in a certain position. 3. In microscopy, a method of treating material to be examined so as to preserve it or to make possible a more thorough examination. 4. In personality development, the arrest of development at a level short of maturity; may result in unnatural behaviour, *e.g.*, excessive emotional attachment for a parent. 5. In optics, the direct focusing of one or both eyes so that the image falls on the *fovea centralis.* COMPLEMENT F. when antigen and homologous antibody unite to form a complex, complement may unite with such a complex, and this is referred to as F.; SKELETAL F. a method of treating fractures that are difficult to treat by traditional means; utilizes a rigid metal plate or apparatus that holds the bones in alignment; when applied to the surface of the body it is called EXTERNAL F., when surgically applied directly to the bone it is called INTERNAL F.

fixative (fik'-sa-tiv): An agent that hardens and preserves specimens for laboratory study.

fixator (fiks-ā'-ter): Name given to the apparatus used to immobilize fractures without casting when there is skin loss or injury, or in compound fractures.

flaccid (flak'-sid, flas'-id): Soft, flabby, not firm; term is often used to describe muscles that have lost all or part of their tone. Also sometimes used to describe a certain type of personality. See PARALYSIS. — flaccidity, n.

flagella (fla-jel'-a): Plural of flagellum (*q.v.*).

flagellant (flaj'-e-lent): 1. Relating to flagella. 2. One who practises flagellation. 3. Relating to a stroking manoeuvre in massage.

flagellate (flaj'-e-lāt): Having flagella. See FLAGELLUM.

flagellation (flaj-e-lā'-shun): 1. A massage manoeuvre consisting of whipping the skin with the fingers. 2. A sadistic or masochistic act in which one or both partners derive pleasure from whipping.

flagellum (fla-jel'-um): A fine hair-like appendage capable of lashing movement. Characteristic of spermatozoa, certain bacteria and protozoa; used for locomotion. — flagella, pl.

flail (flāl): Refers to flaccidity or lack of normal control over a part. F. CHEST see under CHEST; F. JOINT one that is excessively mobile and cannot be controlled due to paralysis of the muscles that control its movements.

flank: That part of the trunk of the body that lies between the lowest ribs and the ilia.

flap: A piece of skin or soft tissue of varying size, shape, and thickness that has been detached from the underlying tissue but left attached at some point to retain its own circulation; used in various plastic operations and to cover the end of bone after amputation of a part. SKIN F. refers to a true flap of skin created by a curved incision, leaving a portion attached.

flare (flār): Diffuse reddening of an area around an injury or an infected area.

flask: A bottle with a narrow neck; has many laboratory uses.

flatfoot: A congenital or acquired condition in which the arch of the instep is depressed so that the entire sole of the foot touches the ground when one is standing or walking. See TALIPES.

flatulence (flat'-u-lens): Gastric and intestinal distension with air or gas. — flatulent, adj.

flatus (flā'-tus): Gas or air in the stomach or intestines. F. BAG a bag attached to a rectal tube which may drain into a vented container that may or may not contain water; F. TUBE a rectal tube; see under RECTAL.

flatworm: Any worm belonging to the phylum Platyhelminthes, including tapeworms and flukes.

flea (flē): A blood-sucking wingless parasitic insect of the order Siphonaptera; it may act as host and transmit such diseases as typhus and plague. Its bite leaves a portal of entry for infection. HUMAN F. *Pulex irritans*; RAT F. *Xenopsylla cheopis*, transmitter of plague (*q.v.*).

flesh: The soft tissues of an animal or human body, especially the muscle tissue. GOOSE F. cutis anserina (*q.v.*); PROUD F. the excessive growth of granular tissue in a wound.

flex (fleks): 1. Bend. 2. To move a joint so that the two parts it connects are brought closer together.

flexibility (flek-si-bil'-i-ti): The ability to change, bend, or conform.

flexible learning: A term used for a versatile approach to learning, where the student is central to the process and teaching occurs on the student's terms with respect to his or her needs, time and available resources. See COMPUTER-ASSISTED LEARNING.

flexion (flek'-shun): 1. The act of bending. 2. The condition of being bent. 3. The movement of certain joints so as to decrease the angle between the two parts it connects, as in bending the elbow. Opp. of extension.

Flexner's bacillus (*Shigella flexneri*): A pathogenic Gram-negative rod bacterium which is the most common cause of bacillary dysentery epidemics, and sometimes infantile gastroenteritis. It is found in the faeces of cases of dysentery and carriers, from whence it may pollute food and water supplies, or be transferred by contact. [Simon Flexner, American pathologist, 1863–1946.]

flexor (flek'-sor): A muscle which on contraction flexes or bends a part. Opp. to extensor.

flexure (flek'-shur): A bend. HEPATIC F. the bend between the ascending and transverse colon on the right side near the liver; SIGMOID F. the S-shaped bend at the lower end of the descending colon, at its juncture with the rectum below; SPLENIC F. the bend at the junction of the transverse and descending parts of the colon on the left side near the spleen. — flexural, adj.

flight of ideas: Sometimes seen in acute mania when a patient talks continually and repeatedly changes his line of thought.

floaters (flō'-ters): Opaque specks in the vitreous space that float across the visual field and cast moving shadows on the retina; may be congenital or due to degenerative changes in the vitreous or retina.

floating: In anatomy, an organ that is out of, or has become detached from, its normal position in the body. F. KIDNEY see NEPHROPTOSIS. F. RIBS a name sometimes given to the 11th and 12th pairs of ribs because they are not attached to the sternum.

flooding: 1. In psychiatry, behaviour therapy in which treatment of phobias consists of repeated exposure to the worst possible phobic situations, progressing from fantastic to real-life situations. Also called *implosion*. 2. Bleeding profusely as from the uterus following childbirth.

'floppy baby': Descriptive of an infant with respiratory distress syndrome (*q.v.*); rapid respirations, grunting expirations, retraction of the sternum and ribs are prominent signs.

floppy mitral valve syndrome: A structural alteration of the mitral valve leading to stretching and weakness of the cusps of the valve which allows some of the blood to leak back into the left atrium when the heart pumps instead of being pushed through the aorta. Also called *Barlow's syndrome*.

flora (flaw'-ra): The collective plant life of a certain area. In human physiology, the bacterial and fungal life that normally inhabits an area. INTESTINAL F. the bacteria normally found in the intestinal canal; NORMAL F. refers to flora that normally inhabit certain areas of the body without causing infection.

Florence Nightingale Foundation: A charity that raises funds to provide scholarships for nurses, midwives and health visitors, to allow them to study at home and abroad, to promote innovation in practice, and to extend knowledge and skills to meet changing needs.

florid (flor'-id): 1. Having a bright red colour. 2. A flushed appearance of the skin, especially of the face.

flow chart: A chronological record in graph or tabular form that reflects ongoing observations; used to follow a patient's progress when rapid changes in condition are occurring. Observations usually recorded are temperature, pulse rate, blood pressure, respirations, reflexes. Also called *flow sheet*.

flowmeter (flō'-mē-ter): A device that monitors the flow of oxygen and other gases and liquids.

fluctuate (fluk'-tū-āt): 1. To change from time to time or to vary irregularly. 2. To move with wave-like motion or to undulate.

fluctuation (fluk-tū-ā'-shun): A wave-like motion felt on digital examination of an organ or structure containing fluid. — fluctuant, adj.

fluid (floo'-id): A substance composed of particles that may change their relative positions but do not separate from the mass, and which is capable of flowing. AMNIOTIC F. see under AMNIOTIC; EXTRACELLULAR F. the interstitial F. plus the blood plasma; constitutes about 20% of body weight; EXTRAVASCULAR F. all body fluid that is outside the blood vessels; constitutes about 50% of body weight; F. BALANCE see under BALANCE; INTERSTITIAL F. that which is in the spaces between the cells; constitutes about 16% of body weight; INTRACELLULAR F. that which is inside the cells; PLEURAL F. the minute amount of F. between the visceral and parietal pleura; PROSTATIC F. the whitish F. secreted by the prostate gland; a constituent of semen; SEMINAL F. semen; SYNOVIAL F. the clear fluid that serves as a lubricant for joints and bursae.

fluidextract (floo-id-eks'-trakt): A concentrated alcoholic solution of a drug of such strength that each millilitre contains the equivalent of one gram of the dry form of the drug.

fluke 235 follicle

fluke (flook): A small, flat, unsegmented trematode worm that may be parasitic to animals and to man, particularly in tropical countries.

fluorescence (floo-ō-res'-ens): The property of emitting radiation, usually visible light, as a result of having absorbed energy derived from radiation of another, usually shorter, wavelength.

fluorescent (floo-ō-res'-ent): Having the property of emitting electromagnetic radiation following absorption of radiation from some other source. F. ANTIBODY TEST a rapid sensitive laboratory test which, among other uses, can be used to detect the presence of streptococci that cause rheumatic fever. F. SCREEN one that gives temporary visualization of a structure when it is interposed between the subject and a source of x-rays; F. TREPONEMAL ANTIBODY ABSORPTION TEST a test performed on cerebrospinal fluid to confirm the diagnosis of neurosyphilis.

fluoridate (floo-or'-i-dāt): To add fluorine salts to a community water supply to aid in control of dental caries.

fluoridation (floo or-i-dā'-shun): The addition of fluorine salts to water; term usually refers to treatment of the water supply of a community as a public health measure to reduce the incidence of dental caries; the dilution is usually 1:1,000,000. See FLUORINE.

fluoride (floo'-or-īd): A compound of fluorine and another element; the form of fluorine used as an additive to drinking water to prevent caries. Also applied directly to the teeth.

fluoridize (floo-or'-i-diz): 1. To add fluoride to the drinking water. 2. To apply fluoride to the teeth as a preventive measure against the formation of caries.

fluorine (floo'-or-rēn): A non-metallic gaseous element; in the human body it is found chiefly in bones and teeth. When present in natural water supply, it tends to reduce dental decay; in excess it gives a mottled appearance to the teeth. See FLUORIDATION.

flush: A sudden reddening of the skin, especially the face and neck. HECTIC F. redness of the cheeks seen as a characteristic of certain chronic infections, e.g., pulmonary tuberculosis; HOT F. lay term for sudden reddening of the face and a subjective feeling of heat experienced by women during menopause.

flutter: A rapid pulsation or vibration tremulousness; said especially of the heart. ATRIAL F. a type of cardiac arrhythmia in which the atrial contractions may reach 250–400 per minute, but remains rhythmic and of uniform strength; the ventricular rate is usually about 150; this pattern produces saw-tooth waves in the ECG; it is a manifestation of underlying heart disease involving particularly the coronary arteries; OCULAR F. spontaneous horizontal oscillations of the eye during fixation; often associated with cerebellar pathology; VENTRICULAR F. rapid ventricular tachycardia with the ECG showing no distinct QRS or T waves.

flux: 1. An excessive flow of any of the body secretions. 2. Diarrhoea. BLOODY F. dysentery.

focal (fō'-kal): Limited to one area; localized, F. INFECTION one localized more or less in one site, from which it spreads to other parts of the body; F. SEIZURE an epileptic seizure due to irritation of a localized area of the brain; usually there is no loss of consciousness.

focus (fō'-kus): 1. A point at which rays converge; said of light and sound waves. 2. The area of the body where disease or a morbid process is localized. — foci, pl., focal, adj.

focus group research: A form of qualitative investigation in which a sample of people are asked about their attitude towards a product, concept, advertisement, idea or packaging. Questions are asked in an interactive setting where participants are free to talk amongst themselves.

foetal, foetus: For these and related words see FETAL, FETUS, etc.

folacin (fō'-la-sin): Folic acid (q.v.).

folate (fō'-lāt): A salt of folic acid. Folates are present in natural foods; they act as coenzymes (q.v.).

fold: A thin margin or doubling of tissue, or a plica.

Foley catheter: See under CATHETER.

folic acid (fō'-lik): A water-soluble constituent of the vitamin B complex; found in certain nuts, leafy plants, yeast, liver, kidney. Has anti-anaemic properties, and in conjunction with vitamin B_{12} is important in formation of red blood cells in the bone marrow. Effective in preventing sprue, and pernicious and megaloblastic anaemia; is commonly deficient in the average diet. Folic acid is prescribed in pregnancy for the prevention of neural tube defects.

follicle (fol'-ik'l): 1. A small secreting sac. 2. A simple tubular gland. GRAAFIAN F. a minute vesicle in the stroma of the ovary containing a single ovum; HAIR F. the tubular oil-secreting invagination of epithelium in which the hair grows; OVARIAN F. Graafian F.; PILOSEBACEOUS F. the hair follicle with its attached oil gland.

follicle-stimulating hormone: A hormone of the anterior pituitary lobe which stimulates the Graafian follicles of the ovary, promotes maturation of the follicle and liberation of oestrogen (*q.v.*). In the male it stimulates the production of spermatozoa through stimulation of the epithelium of the seminiferous tubules.

follicular (fo-lik′-ū-lar): Relating to a follicle, or follicles. F. CYST a cyst developing in a follicular space, as in the ovary; F. HORMONE oestrogen produced in the ovarian follicle; F. TONSILLITIS see under TONSILLITIS.

folliculitis (fo-lik-ū-lī′tis): Inflammation of a follicle; usually refers to infection around the hair follicles. F. BARBAE infection of the hair follicles of the beard with formation of papules and pustules; also called *ringworm of the beard* and *barber's itch*; F. DECALVANS an alopecia (*q.v.*) of the scalp characterized by pustulation and scars.

fomentation (fō′ -men-tā′ -shun): A hot, wet application used to reduce pain or inflammation. When the skin is intact, strict cleanliness is observed (medical F.); when the skin is broken, aseptic technique is observed (surgical F.).

fomite (fō′ -mīt): Any article that has been in contact with infection and is capable of transmitting same. Also called *fomes*. — fomites, pl.

fontanel, fontanelle (fon′ -ta-nel′): Any one of the six spaces ('soft spots') between the converging cranial bones in which ossification is not complete at birth. The diamond-shaped ANTERIOR F. lies at the junction of the frontal and parietal bones; it usually closes at about the eighteenth month of life. The triangular-shaped POSTERIOR F. lies at the junction of the occipital and parietal bones; it usually closes at about the second month of life. The two ANTEROLATERAL F.S. lie at the junction of the frontal, parietal, temporal, and sphenoid bones; they usually close at about the third month of life. The two POSTEROLATERAL F.S. lie at the junction of the parietal, occipital, and temporal bones; they do not usually close until the second year of life.

food exchange list: Any of several lists of foods and the quantities of each that will provide the same number of calories and the same amount of nutritive value. Useful in planning regular diets as well as those for persons requiring special diets. The main groups on the list are milk, vegetables, bread, meat and fats.

food groups: A reference to food lists that have been called the Basic Four, (*q.v.*): meats, milk, fruits and vegetables, breads and cereals; well-planned meals will contain foods from each classification.

food intolerance: Inability of the body to digest certain foods due to lack of an enzyme necessary to their digestion and metabolism; to be differentiated from food allergy. See also COELIAC DISEASE.

food poisoning: Characterized by vomiting, with or without diarrhoea, resulting from eating food contaminated with chemical poison, preformed bacterial toxin, or live bacteria.

foot: That portion of the lower leg that is below the ankle, consisting of the tarsus, the metatarsus and the phalanges. The sole or bottom is called the plantar surface; the top side is called the dorsal surface. ATHLETE'S F. tinea pedis (*q.v.*); DROP F. or FOOTDROP inability to dorsiflex the foot, as in severe sciatica and nervous conditions affecting lower lumbar regions of the cord; sometimes resulting from failure to protect feet from pressure of bedclothing; MADURA F. see MYCETOMA; TRENCH F. immersion F., so called because it occurred among soldiers in trenches; also occurs in frostbite and other conditions of exposure when there is local deprivation of blood supply.

foot-and-mouth disease: An acute, highly infectious viral disease of cattle, transmissible to causing a vesicular eruption of the mucous membranes of the mouth and nose and of the skin of the interdigital spaces; other symptoms include headache, fever, malaise. — Syn., *aphthous fever*.

footling breech: An intrauterine position of the fetus in which one or both feet are folded under the buttocks at the inlet of the maternal pelvis, one foot presenting in a single footling breech, both feet in a doubling footling breech.

footprint: An ink impression of the sole of the foot. Used in the USA as a means of identification of newborn infants.

foramen (fō-rā′ -men): A natural hole or opening. Generally used with reference to a bone or a membranous structure. F. MAGNUM the opening in the occipital bone through which the spinal cord passes and becomes continuous with the medulla oblongata; F. OF MAGENDIE an opening in the roof of the fourth ventricle of the brain for the passage of cerebrospinal fluid into the subarachnoid space; F. OF MORGAGNI a small gap on either side of the diaphragm between the sternal and costal portions through which the superior epigastric blood vessels and some lymphatics pass; F. OF MUNRO a communication between the lateral and third ventricles of the brain; also called *intraventricular f.*; F. OVALE the fetal communication between the left and right atria; closes at birth; F. SPINOSUM an opening in the great wing of the sphenoid to accommodate the middle meningeal artery; NUTRIENT F. any of the channels through which nutrient-carrying vessels enter the medullary cavity of long bones; OBTURATOR F. an aperture situated in the anterior portion of the innominate bone; VERTEBRAL F. the space in the vertebrae through which the spinal cord passes.

forced expiratory volume: The volume of gas exhaled over a given time period while performing forced vital capacity determination.

forced vital capacity: The maximal amount of gas that can be expelled from the lungs following a maximal inspiration with an expiration as forceful and rapid as possible.

force-field analysis: A method of weighing pros and cons. This can be done by listing all forces for change in one column, and all forces against change in another column; assigning a score to each force, from 1 (weak) to 5 (strong); drawing a diagram showing the forces for and against change, and showing the size of each force as a number next to it.

forceps (for'-seps): Surgical instruments with two opposing blades which are used to grasp or compress tissues, swabs, needles, and many other surgical appliances. The two blades are controlled by direct pressure (tong-like), or by handles (scissor-like). KELLY F. a surgical instrument used to clamp large blood vessels; OBSTETRIC F. used in the second stage of labour to help extract the infant's head from the birth canal, in cases where this mode of delivery is safer for the mother or infant.

forearm (for'-arm): That part of the arm that is between the elbow and the wrist. Antebrachium.

forebrain (for'-brān): The part of the embryonic brain that develops into the telencephalon and diencephalon.

foreconscious (for-kōn'-shus): Information not usually within consciousness but which can be recalled voluntarily; preconscious.

forefinger: The index finger, *i.e.*, the one next to the thumb.

forefoot (for'-foot): The front or fore part of the foot.

foregut (for'-gut): The embryonic structure from which most of the small intestine, stomach, liver, oesophagus, lung, and pharynx develop.

forehead (for'-hed): The anterior part of the cranium that is above the eyes; the brow.

foreign body: Any substance or object lodged in a place in the body where it does not belong.

forensic medicine (for-en'-sik): 1. The relationship and influence of law on the practice of medicine. 2. The use of autopsy findings and medical facts in trials for murder or deaths from suspicious causes. See MEDICAL JURISPRUDENCE.

forensic mental health services: Mental health services provided for offenders.

foreplay (for'-plā): Sexual stimulation preceding and leading to sexual intercourse.

foreskin (for'-skin): The prepuce or skin covering the glans penis.

forewaters (for'-wat-erz): In pregnancy, the liquor amnii found in the membranes lying below the presenting part of the fetus.

formaldehyde (fu-mal'-de-hīd)· A colourless, pungent, irritating gas that has disinfectant and germicidal properties. Used in the gas form and also in solution. See FORMALIN.

formalin (for'-ma-lin): Approximately a 40% solution of formaldehyde. Used mainly for room disinfection and for fixing and preserving pathological specimens.

formic acid (for'-mik as'-id): An organic acid found naturally in ants and other insects as well as in some plants, *e.g.*, nettles.

formicant (for'-mi-kant): Producing a sensation resembling that of ants crawling on the skin. F. PULSE a feeble small pulse resembling the movements of ants.

formula (for'-mū-la): 1. A prescription. 2. Recipe for an infant's feeding. 3. A simplified statement of a general fact or rule expressed in figures, symbols, or simple language. 4. A rule or method of doing something, especially something done regularly and automatically. 5. An expression of the composition of a compound by symbols and figures that show the proportions of the various constituents.

formulary (for'-mū-lar-i): A collection of formulas, recipes, prescriptions. BRITISH NATIONAL F. a book issued twice a year by the British Medical Association and the Pharmaceutical Society of Great Britain containing details of nearly all drugs currently available on prescription in the UK.

fornicate (for'-ni-kāt): To have sexual intercourse with a person to whom one is not married. — fornication, n.

fornix (for'-niks): An arch-shaped structure or space, often referring to the space between the vaginal wall and the cervix of the uterus. CONJUNCTIVAL F. the line of reflection of the conjunctiva from the eyelids into the eyeball. — fornices, pl.

fortified (for'-ti-fid): In nutrition, refers to the addition of substances intended to make food more nutritious.

fossa (fors'a): In anatomy, a depression, hollow, pit, or furrow. ANTECUBITAL F. the hollow at the front of the elbow; also called *cubital F.*; CORONOID F. the hollow at the distal end of the humerus; it accommodates the coronoid process of the ulna in flexion; HYPOPHYSEAL F. a deep depression in the middle of the sella turcica; it contains the pituitary gland; ILIAC F. the large smooth concave area occupying most of the inner surface of the wing of the ilium; INTERCONDYLAR F. lies between the medial and lateral condyles of the lower end of the femur; OLECRANON F. a depression on the posterior surface of the humerus into which the olecranon of the ulna fits when the arm is extended; F. OVALIS CORDIS a depression on the right side of the interatrial septum of the heart; it represents the remains of the fetal foramen ovale; POPLITEAL F. the space at the back of the knee; contains blood vessels and nerves; SUPRACLAVICULAR F. a depression on the surface of the body just above and behind the clavicle and lateral to the tendon of the sternocleidomastoid muscle. — fossae, pl.

fossette (fos-set'): 1. A small deep ulcer of the cornea. 2. A small depression.

Fothergill's operation: An operation to correct prolapse of the uterus by fixation of the uterine ligaments. [William Fothergill, English gynaecologist, 1865–1926.]

foulage (foo-lazh'): A movement in massage consisting of kneading and pressing the muscles; also called *petrissage*.

Foundation of Nursing Studies: A UK-based charity, the sole purpose of which is to help nurses, midwives and health visitors improve patient care by encouraging them to use the most up-to-date methods.

fourchette (foor-shet'): A membranous fold connecting the posterior ends of the labia minora.

Fournier's disease: Gangrene of the genitalia, the scrotum in particular.

fovea (fo'-ve-a): A small depression or fossa, particularly the fovea centralis retinae in the macula lutea of the retina, the site of most distinct vision.

foxglove (foks'-glov): See DIGITALIS.

FPCert: Abbreviation for Family Planning Certificate (*q.v.*).

fractional sterilization: Sterilizing material by submitting it to temperatures of 100°C on three or four successive days to kill the spores that may develop in the periods between heatings. Also called *intermittent sterilization*.

fracture (frak'cher): A break in the continuity of a bone, epiphyseal plate, or joint surface. AVULSION F. results from forceful contraction of a muscle, which causes a fragment of bone to be torn loose at the tendinous insertion of the muscle; BARTON'S F. dorsal dislocation of the carpus on the radium, with fracture of the dorsal articular surface of the radius; BASOCERVICAL F., F. at the base of the femoral neck; BENNETT'S F., F. of the first metacarpal, often the result of a fall or a fight; BLOWOUT F., F. of the floor of the bony orbit of the eye, caused by direct blunt trauma to the eyeball, which causes increase in intraorbital pressure; BOXER'S F. impacted F. of the necks of the fourth and fifth metacarpals, caused by striking the knuckles on a hard object; BURSTING F. a F. with many fragments occurring most often in the first cervical vertebra; BUTTERFLY F. a F. in which wedge-shaped segments split off laterally so that the fracture looks like a butterfly with outspread wings; CHAUFFEUR'S F., F. of the distal radial styloid, caused by twisting or snapping type of injury; these were formerly caused by cranking a car; CHIP F. a F. in which a chip of bone is separated from a bony process; CLOSED F. a F. with no break in the skin; COLLES'F., F. of the lower end of the radius giving a typical dinner-fork deformity; COMMINUTED F. one which has multiple fracture lines; COMPLETE F. the bone is broken completely; COMPLICATED F. in addition to the F. there is injury to the surrounding organs and/or structures; COMPOUND F., the skin is broken, allowing communication of the broken ends of bone with the atmosphere; also called *open f.*; COMPRESSION F. usually occurs in the lumbar region, due to hyperflexion of the spine; the anterior vertebral bodies are crushed together; COTTON'S F., F. of the ankle involving the medial, lateral, and posterior malleoli; DEPRESSED F. the fragmented bone presses on and may penetrate an underlying structure, as the lung; usually refers to skull or rib F.; DISPLACED F. the bone fragments are no longer in anatomical alignment; DOUBLE F. segmented F. of a bone in two places; EPIPHYSEAL F. a F. that involves the cartilaginous growth plate of a bone; FATIGUE F. a stress F. resulting from strenuous physical activity over a short period of time; FISSURE F. a crack in the surface of a long bone; GALLEAZZI'S F., F. in the lower part of the shaft of the radius, with dislocation of the distal end of the ulna; GOSSELIN'S F. a V-shaped F. of the distal end of the tibia; GREEN-STICK F., an incomplete F., occurring in children; the periosteum on one side of the bone remains intact; IMPACTED F. one end of the bone is driven into the other; INCOMPLETE F. the bone is only cracked and fissured; INTER-TROCHANTERIC F. a F. between the greater and lesser trochanters of the femur; LEFORT'S F. bilateral horizontal F. of the maxilla; classified as Type I, II, or III according to the location and extent of the F. and what other facial bones are involved; LINEAR F. a lengthwise F., usually of a long bone; it implies no displacement; MARCH F., F. in the shaft of the second or third metatarsal; caused by excessive marching; MONTEGGIA F., F. in the upper shaft of the ulna with dislocation of the head of the radius; MUL-TIPLE F. two or more lines of fracture in the same bone; NIGHT-STICK F, an undisplaced F. of the shaft of the ulna caused by a direct blow; OBLIQUE F. a slanted F. of the shaft of a long bone; OCCULT F. one that is not detected by x ray; hidden; PARATROOPER'S F., F. of the malleolus and/or the margin of the posterior tibia; PATHOLOGICAL F. one caused by osteoporosis or other local disease of the bone or where there is bony metastasis in cancer sufferers; POTT'S F., F. of the distal end of the fibula and the tibial malleolus, often accompanied by dislocation of the tarsal bones and injury to ligaments with lateral displacement of the foot; SECONDARY F. occurs in a bone weakened by disease; SIMPLE F. closed F., not compound, with the ends of the bone in proper alignment; SMITH'S F., F. of the lower end of the radius near the joint, with displacement of the lower fragment; SPIRAL F. one in which the fracture line is spiral in shape.; also called *torsion f.* when it is caused by a twisting force; SPONTAN-EOUS F. one occurring without force; SPRIN-TER'S F., F. of the antero-inferior spine of the ilium, with a fragment of the bone being pulled by muscular violence as at the start of a sprint; STABLE F. one that can be reduced and can be maintained with a cast or splint; STELLATE F., a F. with a central point of injury from which several fracture lines radiate; STIEDA'S F., F. of the internal condyle of the femur; STRESS F. caused by repeated or prolonged stress on a bone; T-F. intercondylar F., shaped like a T; TEARDROP F. a F. of the anterior lip of a cervical vertebra; shaped like a teardrop; TRANSVERSE F. the line of fracture goes across a long bone at right angles to its length; UNSTABLE F. a F. that cannot be held in reduction by splinting or traction without internal fixation; UNUNITED F. failure to form a bridge of callus at the end of a fractured bone; the ends become fragmented and a false joint results; Y-F., an intercondylar F. shaped like a Y; WEDGE F., a compression F. of a vertebra.

fracture–dislocation: Fracture of a bone accompanied by dislocation of the bone from its normal position in a joint.

fragile X syndrome: A genetic condition caused by a defective X chromosome, one of the sex chromosomes; it results in a form of learning disability.

fragilitas (fra-jil′-i-tas): Brittleness. F. CRINIUM brittleness of the hair; F. OSSIUM congenital disease characterized by abnormal fragility of bone, multiple fractures and a china-blue discoloration of the sclera; F. SANGUINIS fragility of the red blood cells; F. UNGUIUM abnormal brittleness of the nails.

fragility (fra-jil′-i-ti): Brittleness; the tendency to break down or disintegrate. F. OF THE BLOOD refers to the increased tendency of the red blood cells to break down under certain conditions.

fragmentation (frag-men-tā′shun): The division or breaking into small pieces or parts.

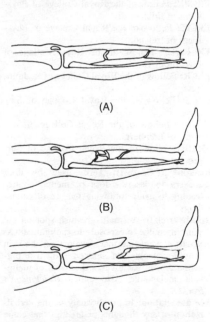

Classification of fractures: (a) simple: (b) comminuted: (c) compound

frame: See BRADFORD, STRYKER.

Francisella: A genus of nutritionally fastidious Gram-negative rods; belongs to the family Brucellacaea. *F. tularensis,* the causative organism of tularaemia in wild animals; may be transmitted to humans by contaminated water, by blood-sucking insects, or through handling infected animals. See TULARAEMIA.

frank: Obvious or clinically evident, such as the unequivocal presence of a condition or a disease.

fraternal twins: Twins that have developed from the fertilization of two ova; may or may not be of the same sex or identical in appearance. Dizygotic twins.

FRC: Abbreviation for functional residual capacity; see under FUNCTIONAL.

FRCGP: Fellow of the Royal Collge of General Practitioners.

FRCN: Fellow of the Royal College of Nursing.

FRCOG: Fellow of the Royal College of Obstetricians and Gynaecologists.

FRCP: Fellow of the Royal College of Physicians.

FRCPath: Fellow of The Royal College of Pathologists.

FRCPE: Fellow of the Royal College of Physicians of Edinburgh.

FRCPI: Fellow of the Royal College of Physicians of Ireland.

FRCPsych: Fellow of the Royal College of Psychologists.

FRCR: Fellow of the Royal College of Radiologists.

FRCS: Fellow of the Royal College of Surgeons.

FRCSE: Fellow of the Royal College of Surgeons of Edinburgh.

FRCSI: Fellow of the Royal College of Surgeons of Ireland.

freakout (frēk'-owt): Term used by drug abusers to describe loss of mental control leading to panic following the use of certain drugs.

freckle (frek'l): A small brownish spot on the skin, often due to exposure to sunlight. MELANOTIC F. a macule that develops on the skin of older people; of uneven brownish pigmentation. In some cases the focus of malignant melanoma. Also called *Hutchinson's freckle.*

free association: In psychoanalysis, the verbalization of any thoughts or feelings that come to mind without selection or repression of any kind.

Freedom of Information Act 2000: A law that requires all NHS bodies to have a publication scheme in place. This scheme must set out the type of information the body publishes or intends to publish, its format and details of any changes. The Act will be fully in force by January 2005.

free market: An idealized market economy (*q.v.*) in which buyers and sellers are permitted to carry out transactions without government intervention.

freezing: 1. Frostbite. 2. The use of freezing temperatures to produce temporary anaesthesia, *e.g.,* spraying the skin with liquid carbon dioxide snow or the use of ice bags. When used for therapeutic purposes, it is called CRYOTHERAPY.

fremitus (frem'-i-tus): A vibration that can be felt by resting the fingers on the chest or certain other parts of the body. It is diminished in some respiratory diseases and increased in certain other pathological conditions such as tumour or consolidation. TACTILE F. vibration that can be felt by palpitation on the chest wall over the trachea and bronchi; produced by the spoken voice; VOCAL F. vibration of vocal sounds heard on auscultation of the chest; is decreased in emphysema, pulmonary oedema and other pathological conditions marked by pleural effusion.

French chalk: Talc (*q.v.*).

French scale: Scale used in sizing catheters and certain other tubular instruments. It is a measure of the outside diameter, each unit being roughly equivalent to 0.33 millimetres; can be converted by dividing by 3. French sized catheters 16 to 18 are commonly used for adults.

frenetic (fre-net'-ik): Wild, excited, frantic, frenzied. — frenetically, adv.

Frenkel's exercises: Exercises for persons with tabes dorsalis, to teach muscle and joint sense in order to restore lost coordination. [Heinrich Frenkel, Swiss neurologist. 1860–1931.]

frenulum (fren'-ū-lum): A small frenum (*q.v.*). F. CLITORIDIS a F. formed by the union of the folds of the labia minora on the under surface of the glans clitoris; F. LINGUAE the vertical fold of mucous membrane under the tongue; F. PREPUTII PENIS the fold of tissue on the underside of the penis that connects with the prepuce.

frenum (frē'-num): A small fold of mucous membrane from a more or less fixed part extending to two movable parts which checks or limits their movement. See FRENULUM.

frenzy (fren'-zē): Violent, abnormal, compulsive excitement or agitation.

frequency: 1. The rate of regular recurrences in a given time, *e.g.*, the heartbeat. 2. In electricity, the number of alternations per second in an alternating current. 3. In vital statistics, the number of occurrences of a recognized entity per unit of time in a specific population. 4. The number of vibrations per minute made by a sound wave; expressed in cycles per second (cps) or Hertz. 5. The felt need to urinate more often than normally.

Freud, Sigmund (froyd): Physiologist, medical doctor, psychologist, and father of psychoanalysis. The basic structure of psychoanalysis as the study of unconscious mental processes is still Freudian. Freud used a variety of techniques, including hypnosis and free association. His collaborations with others (including Bleuler, Jung, and Adler) ended with their protest against Freud's emphasis on infantile sexuality and the Oedipus complex (*q.v.*). Freudian theory has had a wide impact, influencing fields as diverse as anthropology, education, art, and literary criticism. [1856–1939.]

freudian (froyd'-ē-an): Relating to Freud (*q.v.*) or his doctrines.

friable (frī'-a-b'l): Easily crumbled; readily pulverized. – friability, n.

fricatives (frik-a-tivs): Sounds produced when breath is forced through a constricted passageway, as are the sounds of *f, v, z, ch, t*.

friction (frik'-shun): Rubbing. F. BURN a wound caused by strenuous rubbing or friction; also called *brush burn*; F. MURMUR heard through the stethoscope when two rough or dry surfaces rub together, as occurs in pleurisy and pericarditis; PERICARDIAL F. RUB PLEURAL F. RUB see under RUB.

Friedländer's bacillus (frēd'-lend-erz, frēd'-land-erz): *Klebsiella pneumoniae*; see under KLEBSIELLA.

Friedreich's ataxia (frēd'-rīks): A rare progressive familial disease with symptoms beginning in childhood, in which there develops a sclerosis of the sensory and motor columns in the spinal cord, with consequent muscular weakness and staggering (ataxia), impairment of speech and lateral curvature of the spine. Also called *hereditary cerebellar ataxia*. [Nikolas Friedreich, German neurologist, 1825–1882.]

frolement: (frōl-mon'): 1. A rustling sound heard on auscultation in pericardial disease. 2. A massage manoeuvre consisting of very light friction with the hands.

frontal (frun'-tal): 1. Relating to the front or anterior part of an organ of the body. 2. The bone of the forehead. F. SINUS a cavity at the inner aspect of each orbital ridge on the F. bone; F. SUTURE the line of union between two halves of the frontal bone.

frontal lobe syndrome: A syndrome occurring after lobotomy or injury to the frontal area of the brain; symptoms include behavioural changes, lessened self-control, emotional dullness, lack of energy, mental deterioration with loss of ability to concentrate, impulsiveness, and aggression.

frost: A deposit resembling frozen vapour. UREA F. the deposit of salt crystals on the skin following the evaporation of sweat in urhidrosis (*q.v.*). Also called *uraemic frost*.

frostbite (frost-bīt): Freezing of the skin and superficial tissues resulting from exposure to extreme cold. The fingers, toe, nose and ears are most frequently affected. The lesion is similar to a burn and may become blistered, with deep-seated destruction of tissue and possible development of gangrene.

frottage (fro-tahzh'): 1. A rubbing movement in massage. 2. Obtaining sexual satisfaction by rubbing or pressing against another person; may occur in crowded situations.

frozen: F. SECTION section cut from frozen tissue for histological examination, *e.g.*, that removed from the body during surgery and examined immediately for possible malignancy; F. SHOULDER disability of the shoulder joint in which there is limited abduction and rotation of the arm; results from a fibrositis (*q.v.*) of unknown origin; initial pain is followed by stiffness which lasts several months; as the pain subsides exercises are intensified until full recovery is gained.

fructose (fruk'-tōs): A monosaccharide found with glucose in plants. It is the sugar in honey and is a constituent of cane sugar. Also called *levulose*.

frustration (frus-trā'-shun): The condition of emotional tension resulting when forces outside oneself block or thwart the performance of acts which, if carried out, would result in satisfaction or gratification of specific needs or desires.

FSH: Abbreviation for follicle-stimulating hormone (*q.v.*).

-fugal: Combining form denoting (1) passing from, driving away; (2) relieving or dispelling.

fugitive (fū'-ji-tiv): Wandering; transient. Descriptive of certain inconstant symptoms.

fugue (fūg): An attempt to escape from reality. A period of loss of memory as to identity but with retention of habits, skills, and mental faculties; sometimes involving flight from familiar surroundings. During the fugue, the patient may appear to act in a purposeful manner, but after recovery he has no memory of what occurred during the state although earlier events are remembered. Occurs in schizophrenia, hysteria; sometimes after an epileptic seizure.

full term: Mature — when pregnancy has lasted 40 weeks.

fulminating (ful'-mi-nā-ting): Developing quickly with severity, characterized by a severe course and an abrupt termination. In obstetrics, such conditions include severe pre-eclampsia and eclampsia, when they arise very suddenly. Also called *fulminant*. — fulminate, v.

fumes (fūmz): Vapours, particularly those that are irritating.

fumigation (fū-mi-gā'-shun): Disinfection by exposure to the fumes of a vaporized disinfectant.

fuming (fū'-ming): Smoking; emitting a visible vapour, usually unpleasant.

function: 1. The special action or physiological property of an organ or other part of the body. 2. The general properties of any substance, depending on its chemical character and relation to other substances. 3. A quality, trait or fact that is so related to another as to be dependent upon and to vary with it. 4. A role or action for which an object was created or adapted.

functional: 1. Relating to function. 2. Describing a disorder of the function but not the structure of an organ or system. 3. In psychiatry, a disorder of neurotic origin, *i.e.*, psychogenic, without primary organic disease. F. ASSESSMENT an assessment of a person's ability to function physically, mentally, emotionally, and socially, within his or her environment, and to carry out the activities of self-maintenance; F. DISEASE a disorder in which the function of an organ or part is disturbed but there is no evidence of structural disease; F. RESIDUAL CAPACITY the volume of air in the lungs at rest, i.e., the amount remaining in the lungs at the end of a normal quiet respiration; it equals the sum of respiratory reserve volume and residual volume. Abbreviated FRC.

functionalism (funk'-shun-a-lizm): 1. The branch of psychology that deals with the function of mental processes, particularly the role played by the intellect, emotions, and behaviour of a person in his adaptation to his environment. Opp. of structuralism (*q.v.*). 2. A social theory based on the premise that all societies have certain basic needs i.e., func-

tional requirements that must be met if a society is to survive. Functionalists are concerned with the contribution that the various parts of a society make towards its needs, and the necessity for social order and stability to prevail in society.

fundus (fun'-dus): The basal portion of a hollow structure; the part that is farthest from the opening. F. OF THE EYE the inside of the back part of the eye seen by looking through the pupil; F. OF THE UTERUS that part which is above the points of insertion of the uterine tubes. — fundal, adj.; fundi, pl.

funduscope (fun'-dus-scōp): An instrument for examining the fundus of the eye, an ophthalmoscope.

fungaemia (fun-jē'-mi-a): 1. The presence of fungi in the circulating blood. 2. A fungal infection that is carried by the bloodstream.

fungal (fung'-gal): Relating to or caused by a fungus; fungous.

fungate (fung'-gāt): 1. To grow rapidly or to granulate rapidly. 2. To assume a fungus-like form. 3. To produce fungus-like growths.

fungicide (fun'-ji-sīd): An agent that is lethal to fungi. — fungicidal, adj.

fungiform (fun'ji-form): Resembling a mushroom in shape.

fungistat (fun'ji-stat): An agent that inhibits the growth of fungi. Also fungistatic.

fungoid (fung'-goid): Resembling a fungus; usually referring to a heavy growth on the surface of the body.

fungus (fung'-gus): A low form of vegetable life including mushrooms, toadstools, moulds, and many microscopic organisms that live on organic matter; a few are capable of producing disease in humans. — fungi, pl.; fungoid, fungous, adj. See also RINGWORM, TINEA PEDIS.

funicular (fū-nik'-ū-lar): Relating to the spermatic or to the umbilical cord. F. PROCESS the part of the tunica vaginalis that covers the spermatic cord.

funiculus (fū-nik'ū-lus): A cord-like structure. F. UMBILICALIS the umbilical cord.

funis (fū'-nis): A cord; the umbilical cord in particular.

funny bone: Lay term for a place at the back of the elbow that responds with a tingling sensation when struck; it is the place where the ulnar nerve passes over the medial condyle of the humerus.

furcal (fur'-kal): Forked.

furor (fū'-ror): Fury; madness; rage. Violent angry outbursts.

furrow: In anatomy, a groove or crease.

furuncle (fū' -rung-k'l): An acute, painful, circumscribed inflammatory lesion of the skin and subcutaneous tissue, usually caused by infection of a hair follicle with *Staphylococcus aureus*; suppuration occurs with the formation of a central core that is eventually discharged. It has but one opening for drainage in contrast to a carbuncle (*q.v.*). A boil.

fusiform (fū' -zi-form): Resembling a spindle; round in the middle and tapering at both ends. F. BACILLI found in the mouth, gums, and fauces in cases of Vincent's angina (*q.v.*).

fusion (fū' -zhun): In surgery, the introduction of bony ankylosis in joints when it is desirable to immobilize them. BINOCULAR F. the fusion of two separate images of an object into one clear image, as occurs in binocular vision; SPINAL F. the surgical procedure of joining two or more of the vertebrae by bone grafts to immobilize part of the spinal column; used in cases of arthritis, severe trauma, herniated disc, or tuberculosis of the spine.

Fusobacterium fusiformis (fū-zō-bak-tēr-i-um fū-zi-fōr' -mis): A genus of anaerobic Gram-negative bacteria found in the normal mouth, intestine, and genitalia, and in necrotic lesions. Also the causative organism in Vincent's angina.

FVC: Abbreviation for forced vital capacity.

G

g: Abbreviation for gram(s).

Ga: Chemical symbol for gallium (*q.v.*).

GABA: Abbreviation for gamma-aminobutyric acid (*q.v.*).

gag: 1. A device that is placed between the teeth to keep the mouth open. 2. To prevent one from speaking. 3. The reflex action which occurs when the back of the throat is stimulated. G. REFLEX, the contraction of the constrictor muscle of the pharynx when the back of the pharynx or the soft palate is touched; also called *pharyngeal reflex*.

gait: A manner of walking. ATAXIC G., G. in which the foot is raised high, then brought down suddenly; CEREBELLAR G. reeling, staggering, lurching G. FESTINATING G. seen in patients with paralysis agitans and other nervous disorders; the person takes short, increasingly rapid steps, often on tiptoe; PARKINSONIAN G. seen in Parkinsonian patients; the body is held rigid with the head bent forward while the person takes short, mincing steps interrupted by sudden uncontrolled propulsive movements; SCISSOR G., G. in which the legs cross each other in progression; SLAPPING G. a G. in which the feet are wide apart, raised high and slapped down while the person's gaze is fixed on the floor to guide placement of the feet; SPASTIC G. a stiff, shuffling G. with the legs held closely together; STAGGERING G. a reeling, uncertain G. resembling that of an intoxicated person; TABETIC G. ataxic G.; TANDEM G., G. with one heel placed directly in front of the toes of the other foot in walking; used as a test of the person's ability to control motor activity; TRENDELENBURG G. see under TRENDELENBURG; WADDLING G. exaggerated alternation of lateral trunk movements with a marked elevation of the hip.

galact-, galacto-: Combining forms denoting: 1. Milk. 2. Galactose.

galactic (ga-lak′-tik): 1. Relating to or resembling milk. 2. An agent that increases the flow of milk.

galactocele (ga-lak′-tō-sēl): 1. A cyst in the mammary gland containing milk; due to occlusion of a milk duct. 2. A hydrocele that contains a milky fluid.

galactokinase (ga-lak′-tō-kī′-nās): An enzyme that is involved in the metabolism of galactose.

galactopoiesis (ga-lak′-tō-poy-ē′-sis): The production and secretion of milk. — galactopoietic, adj.

galactorrhoea (ga-lak-tō-rē′-a): 1. Excessive flow of milk. 2. Continued flow of milk after a child has been weaned. 3. Spontaneous, excessive flow of milk in the absence of a recent pregnancy.

galactose (ga-lak′-tōs): A monosaccharide found with glucose in lactose or milk sugar; it is converted into glycogen in the liver.

galactose tolerance test: A test of the carbohydrate tolerance of the liver to determine whether the liver is functioning normally.

gall (gawl): Bile.

gallbladder, gall bladder (gawl′-blad-der): A pear-shaped bag on the right underside of the liver. Between meals it concentrates and stores bile; during digestion it releases the bile into the duodenum where it acts on fats. G. SERIES x-ray examination of the gall bladder for diagnostic purposes.

gallipot (gal′-i-pot): A small pot for storing ointments or lotions.

gallium (gal′-i-um): A rare metallic chemical element; has been used in scanning to evaluate presence of active infection in the kidney, in localizing neoplasms, and in detecting perinephritic and psoas abscesses. RADIOACTIVE G. an isotope of G., used in treatment of neoplasms of bone.

gallop: See under RHYTHM.

gall stone (gawl′-stōn): A stone or concretion consisting of crystalline cholesterol that forms within the gall bladder or bile ducts, often multiple and faceted. *Cholelith.*

galvanic (gal-van′-ik): Relating to a direct current of electricity, particularly that produced by a battery. G. SKIN RESPONSE easily measured skin changes in response to various stimuli; used in many experimental studies.

galvanism (gal′-van-izm): Treatment by galvanic electric current. DENTAL G. a phenomenon experienced when dissimilar metals have been used in dental fillings or to replace missing teeth; an electric current is created, causing sharp painful shocks to the involved teeth; may cause inflammation of the tooth pulp.

gam-, gamo-: Combining forms denoting relationship to marriage or sexual contact.

gamete (gam'-ēt): 1. A mature male or female reproductive cell; see OVUM, SPERMATOZOON. 2. The sexual form of the malarial parasite during its existence in the stomach of the mosquito.

gambe intrafallopian transfer (in'-ter-to'-pi-an): An assisted conception technique. Oocytes and spermatozoa are mixed together and transferred to a patent uterine tube. The fertilization takes place *in vivo*

gametocyte (ga-mē'-tō-sīt): An undifferentiated cell from which gametes are produced. Often refers to the sexual stage of the malarial parasite in blood, which may produce gametes after being taken in by the mosquito host.

gametogenesis (gam'-e-tō-jen'-e-sis): The formation and development of gametes.

Gamgee (gam'-jē): A surgical dressing of absorbent cotton enclosed in a fine gauze mesh.

gamma: The third letter of the Greek alphabet; sometimes used in scientific nomenclature to designate the third in a series. G. RADIATION radiation from radioactive cobalt; has been used to replace x-rays in treatment of malignancies; large doses are used to sterilize instruments and dressings; G. RAYS electromagnetic radiation similar to x-rays but with greater penetrating power.

gamma-aminobutyric acid (gam'-ma-am'-i-nō-bū-tir'-ik): An amino acid found in brain tissue; found also in yeast, green plants, and certain bacteria. Considered a neurotransmitter and thought to be implicated in several psychiatric and neurological conditions, chiefly Huntington's chorea.

gamma globulin (gam'-ma glob'-ū-lin): A broad general term for the chemically extracted fraction of human plasma, made up of proteins, that contains immunoglobulins having specific antibody activity against a variety of viruses, specifically the immunoglobulins A, D, E, G, and M. May be used in temporary protection against various infections including measles and hepatitis. GAMMA-A GLOBULIN an immunoglobulin that comprises about 10% of the antibodies in human plasma; the chief immunoglobulin in tears, saliva, colostrum, and intestinal fluid.

gamma-glutamyl transpeptidase (gam'-ma-glū-tam'-il trans-pep'-ti-dās): An enzyme found chiefly in the kidney, liver, and pancreas, but also in lesser amounts in the prostate, salivary glands, brain, and heart. Elevated levels are seen in liver damage; laboratory determinations are useful in diagnosis. Also of medicolegal significance in investigations of rape, because seminal fluid contains high concentrations of it.

gammopathy (gam-mop'-a-thi): A disorder characterized by abnormally increased levels of gamma globulins in the blood; may be seen in myeloma, macroglobulinaemia, Hodgkin's disease, and lymphatic leukaemia. Also called *gammaglobulinopathy, immunoglobulinopathy*.

Gamna's disease: Slow progressive enlargement of the spleen; splenomegaly.

gamogenesis (gam-ō-jen'-e-sis): Sexual reproduction.

gangli-, ganglio-: Combining forms denoting ganglion.

ganglial (gang'-gli-al): Relating to a ganglion.

gangliectomy (gang-gli-ek'-to-mi): The excision of a ganglion. Also called *ganglionectomy*.

ganglioblast (gang'-gli-ō-blast): An embryonic cell from which the cerebrospinal ganglia develop.

gangliocyte (gang'-gli-ō-sīt): A ganglion cell; a neuron in which the body of the cell lies outside of the brain and spinal cord.

ganglion (gang'-gli-on): 1. A semi-independent, organized mass of nerve cell bodies outside the brain and spinal cord, forming a subsidiary nerve centre that receives and sends out nerve fibres, *e.g.*, the ganglionic masses forming the sympathetic system. 2. A cystic tumour on a tendon or aponeurosis; sometimes on the back of the wrist due to strain, such as excessive piano practice. 3. An enlargement of the course of a nerve such as is found on the receptor nerves before they enter the spinal cord. 4. An enlarged lymphatic gland. GASSERIAN G. is deeply situated within the skull, on the sensory root of the fifth cranial nerve. It is involved in trigeminal neuralgia. — ganglia, pl.; ganglionic, adj.

ganglionectomy (gang'-gli-ō-nek'-to-mi): Surgical excision of a ganglion; usually of a dorsal root ganglion, to control intractable pain; also called gangliectomy.

ganglioneuroma (gang'-gli-ō-nū-rō'-ma): A firm encapsulated benign neoplasm made up of nerve fibres and ganglionic cells, often with foci of calcification.

ganglioside (gang'-gli-ō-sīd): General term for a number of galactose-containing cerebrosides (*q.v.*) found in the tissues of the central nervous system.

gangrene (gang'-grēn): Death of part of the tissues of the body. Usually the result of inadequate blood supply, but occasionally due to direct injury (traumatic G.) or infection (gas G., for example). Deficient blood supply may result from pressure on blood vessels (*e.g.*, tourniquets, thigh bandages, or swelling of a limb); from obstruction within healthy vessels; from frostbite when the capillaries become blocked; from spasm of a vessel wall; or from thrombosis due to disease of the vessel. ARTERIOSCLEROTIC G. dry G. of the extremities due to failure of the terminal circulation in patients with arteriosclerosis; DIABETIC G., G. that occurs in the course of diabetes mellitus, usually as a result of a slight injury; may be of the dry or moist variety; DRY G. occurs when circulation of the blood through the affected part is inadequate; usually starts in the toes; tissues become shrunken and black; EMBOLIC G. follows the cutting off of blood supply by an embolism; GAS G. results from infection of a dirty lacerated wound by anaerobic organisms, usually *Clostridium welchii*; the gas that forms spreads through the muscles, so they give a crackling sound when touched; formerly a serious problem in wartime wounds; MOIST G. a form of G. in which the necrosed tissue is soft and moist due to decomposition caused by putrefactive bacteria; SENILE G. arteriosclerotic g.

gangrenous (gang′ -gre-nus): Relating to or of the nature of gangrene.

Gardnerella vaginitis: A vaginal infection, often caused by *Gardnerella vaginale*; characterized by a thin, frothy, greyish discharge with a foul odour; usual treatment includes use of antibiotics and treatment of the sexual partner. Formerly called *Haemophilus vaginalis*.

Gardner's syndrome: Familial intestinal polyposis (*q.v.*) of the colon, which may become malignant, with the presence of supernumerary teeth, tumour formations in bone, sebaceous cysts, and deformities of the skull.

gargle: 1. The act of washing the throat by tipping back the head and holding liquid at the back of the throat while forcing expired air through it. **2.** The liquid material used to gargle, usually medicated.

gargoylism (gar′ -goyl-izm): Rare congenital mucopolysaccharide disorder of metabolism with recessive or sex-linked inheritance. Characterized by skeletal abnormalities, dwarfism, coarse features, heavy ugly facies, enlarged liver and spleen, mental handicap. Also called *lipochondrodystrophy, Hunter syndrome, Hurler syndrome*, and *Hunter–Hurler syndrome*.

Gártner's bacillus: *Salmonella enteritidis*. A motile Gram-negative rod bacterium, widely distributed in domestic and wild animals, particularly rodents, and sporadic in humans as a cause of food poisoning. [August Gártner, German bacteriologist, 1848–1934.]

gas: 1. One of the three states of matter. It retains neither shape nor volume when released but expands so that it is evenly distributed in whatever container or area it is released into. **2.** Any gas that is utilized for lighting or heating an area. BLOOD G.S a term used to express the clinical determination of the partial pressures of oxygen and carbon dioxide exchange in the circulating blood; G. EMBOLUS the presence of small bubbles of gas in the blood which occlude the smaller vessels; a disorder frequently affecting deep-sea divers; aeroembolism; G. GANGRENE see under GANGRENE; G. POISONING see ASPHYXIA and CARBON MONOXIDE. LAUGHING G. nitrous oxide, a gas anaesthetic which sometimes causes a patient to experience an amusing delirium before the anaesthetic has become fully effective; MARSH G. methane (*q.v.*); METHANE G. a gas that develops in marshy places and mines; it results from the decay of organic matter; it is colourless, odourless and inflammable; MUSTARD G. a poisonous gas developed for use in warfare; TEAR G. a gas that irritates the mucous membranes, particularly the conjunctiva, causing a heavy flow of tears.

gasp: 1. To catch one's breath audibly in response to shock or emotion. **2.** To breathe with difficulty through the open mouth.

gasserectomy (gas-er-ek′ -to-mi): Surgical excision of the Gasserian ganglion (*q.v.*).

Gasserian ganglion (gas-sē′ -ri-an): A large flattened ganglion of the sensory root of the 5th cranial nerve (trigeminal); located in a cleft in the dura mater over the anterior part of the temporal bone; gives off the ophthalmic and maxillary nerves and part of the mandibular nerve.

gastr-, gastri-, gastro-: Combining forms denoting: **1.** The stomach. **2.** The ventral area.

gastrectomy (gas-trek′ -to-mi): Removal of a part or the whole of the stomach. PARTIAL G. the most common operation carried out for peptic ulcer; also referred to as SUBTOTAL G.; TOTAL G. carried out only for cancer of the stomach.

gastric (gas′ -trik): Relating to the stomach. G. ANALYSIS analysis of gastric contents for diagnostic purposes; patient is given a meal and specimens are withdrawn at intervals during digestion in the stomach; G. GAVAGE introduction of food through a tube that is passed from the mouth into the stomach; G. HORMONE see GASTRIN; G. INFLUENZA a term used when gastrointestinal symptoms predominate; G. JUICE juice secreted by the glands in the mucous lining of the stomach; the two main ingredients are pepsin and hydrochloric acid; G. LAVAGE a washing out of the stomach; G. PARTITIONING the surgical creation of a smaller pouch and a smaller stoma; sometimes done in treatment of morbid obesity; G. SUCTION intermittent or continuous suction to keep the stomach empty after abdominal operations; G. TUBE a tube for introducing food into the stomach or for washing out the stomach; G. ULCER, see under ULCER.

gastrin (gas'-trin): A hormone secreted by the gastric mucosa on entry of food, which causes a further flow of gastric juice, and helps to stimulate the secretion of bile and pancreatic enzymes.

gastritis (gas-trī'-tis): Inflammation of the mucous membrane lining the stomach; may be acute or chronic. The acute form is usually due to viral or bacterial infection, ingestion of alcohol or certain drugs including aspirin; symptoms include nausea, vomiting, and gastric pain. The chronic form usually indicates the presence of some pathological condition, e.g., peptic ulcer or cancer. ATROPHIC G., G. that is characterized by atrophy of parts of the gastric mucosa; likely to be associated with gastric achlorhydria (q.v.).

gastroanastomosis (gas'-trō-a-nas-to-mō'-sis): The surgical creation of a passageway between two pouches of stomach for the relief of a condition described as hourglass stomach.

gastrocele (gas'-trō-sēl): Hernia of part of the stomach.

gastrocnemius (gas-trok-nē'-mi-us): The large two-headed muscle of the calf of the leg.

gastroduodenostomy (gas'-trō-dū'-ō-de-nos'-to-mi): A surgical anastomosis between the stomach and the duodenum.

gastroenteritis (gas'-trō-en-ter-ī'-tis): Inflammation of mucous membranes of stomach and small intestine; although sometimes the result of dietetic error, the cause is usually a bacterial or viral infection, or food poisoning. EPIDEMIC NEONATAL G. of insidious onset; usually caused by various strains of Escherichia coli, and usually develops after first week of life; symptoms include listlessness, pallor, watery yellow stools, and dehydration.

gastroenterology (gas'-trō-en-ter-ol'-o-ji): The branch of medicine concerned with the physiology and pathological conditions of the stomach, intestines, and accessory organs of digestion. — gastroenterological, adj.

gastroenterostomy (gas'-trō-en-ter-os'-to-mi): The surgical creation of an anastomosis between the stomach and the small intestine, most often the jejunum.

gastroesophageal (gas'-trō-ē-sof'-a-jē'-al): Relating to the stomach and oesophagus. G. REFLUX see under REFLUX. G. VARICES enlarged and tortuous blood vessels of the stomach and oesophagus.

gastrogavage (gas-trō-ga-vazh'): The introduction of food directly into the stomach via a tube through an opening in the wall of the stomach.

gastroileostomy (gas'-trō-il-ē-os'-to-mi): The surgical creation of an anastomosis between the stomach and the ileum.

gastrointestinal (gas'-trō-in-tes'-ti-nal): Relating to the stomach and intestine. G. TRACT the stomach and intestine considered as a continuous structure.

gastrojejunostomy (gas'-trō-je-joo-nos'-to-mi): A surgical anastomosis between the stomach and the jejunum.

gastrolavage (gas'-trō-la-vazh'): Washing out of the stomach.

gastrolith (gas'-trō-lith): A calculus or stone formed in the stomach.

gastroplasty (gas'-trō-plas-ti): Any plastic operation on the stomach; may refer to surgery to reduce the size of the gastric pouch.

gastroscope (gas'-tro-skōp): An endoscope for viewing the interior of the stomach. See ENDOSCOPE. — gastroscopic, adj.

gastroscopy (gas-tros'-kō-pi): Examination of the interior surface of the stomach with a fibreoptic endoscope.

gastrostomy (gas-tros'-to-mi): A surgically established fistula between the stomach and the exterior abdominal wall; usually for artificial feeding.

gastrula (gas'-troo-la): The double-walled stage of the embryo succeeding the blastula (q.v.); the outer layer of cells becomes the ectoderm and the inner layer differentiates into the mesoderm and endoderm.

gate control theory: The theory, first proposed in 1965 by psychologist Melzack and anatomist Wall, that there is a 'gating system' in the central nervous system that opens and closes to let pain messages through to the brain or to block them. The basis for this theory is that psychological as well as physical factors guide the brain's interpretation of painful sensations and the subsequent response. For example, many athletes do not experience pain during intense activity, yet after the activity, when they turn their attention to their injuries, the pain suddenly appears.

gauge (gāj): An instrument with a graduated scale for measuring a dimension of a structure.

gauze (gawz): A thin open-mesh material used in all surgical procedures and for making surgical and other dressings. TUBULAR G., G. prepared in tubular form and applied with a special applicator; particularly useful for finger dressings.

gavage (ga-vazh'): Forced feeding through a tube that is passed into the stomach through the nose, pharynx, and oesophagus.

gay: Popular term for a male person who is a homosexual.

gegenhalten (gā'-gen-hal-ten): Paratonic rigidity see PARATONIA. A form of passive involuntary resistance to movement; the patient is unable to relax his muscles evenly when the arms or legs are being held by another person, and his walking may be characterized by going and stopping; occurs in persons with certain cerebral cortical disorders.

Geiger counter: A device for detecting and registering radioactivity. Also called *Geiger Müller counter*.

gel (jel): A substance consisting of a liquid and a colloid, the mixture being more solid than liquid in form. See COLLOID.

gelatin (jel'-a-tin): The protein-containing, gluelike substance obtained by boiling bones, skin and other animal tissues. Used in various ways in pharmaceutical preparations, as a bacteriological culture medium, and as a food. — gelatinoid, gelatinous, adj.

gelatinase (je-lat'-i-nās): An enzyme found in bacteria, moulds, yeasts; acts to liquefy gelatin.

Gelle's test: A hearing test to determine whether a person has a conductive hearing loss. It tests the mobility of the stapes.

gelose (jel'-ōs): Agar (*q.v.*).

geminate (jem'-i-nāt): Occurring in pairs.

geminus (jem'-i-nus): A twin.

-gen: Combining form denoting an agent that produces or generates.

gen-; geno-: Combining forms denoting production.

gender (update) The socially determined category describing femininity/masculinity. The number of categories and their associated roles vary within and between cultures, although some aspects are more widespread than others.

gender (jen'-der): The socially determined category describing femininity/masculinity. The number of categories and their associated roles vary within and between cultures, although some aspects are more widespread than

others. G. ROLE DISORDER problem associated with the individual's sense of masculinity or feminity. Marked by a sense of inappropriateness regarding sexual behaviour and sexual anatomy, includes transvestism and transsexuality.

gene (jēn): The factor in the chromosome that is responsible for the determination and transmission of hereditary characteristics. Genes are capable of self-reproduction and occur typically in pairs, occupying definite places on the chromosomes, one being found on the chromosome received from the father and one on that received from the mother. Genes are composed, in general, of deoxyribonucleic acid (DNA) and protein, and are the smallest unit of heredity. DOMINANT G. one that is capable of transmitting its characteristics regardless of whether it is present in the chromosome from the other parent; RECESSIVE G. one that will transmit its characteristics only if it is present in the chromosomes from both parents. — genetic, genic, adj.

genera (jen'-e-ra): Plural of genus (*q.v.*).

general: Said of a disease that affects all or many parts of the body. G. ANAESTHETIC see ANAESTHETIC; G. PARESIS see PARESIS; G. PRACTICE the system of medical care in the UK which is the first point of contact for a patient with a new illness, or for follow-up of chronic disease which does not require the expertise of a hospital consultant; the care is provided by general practitioners and other health workers, such as nurses, midwifes, and health visitors, making up primary health-care teams within the community; may also be referred to as primary care (*q.v.*); G. PRACTITIONER a qualified medical practitioner working in the community as part of a primary care team, involving nurses, health visitors, and other staff, addressing the physical and psychosocial needs of the local population; he or she may work alone or in partnership at a medical centre.

generalizability (jen'-e-ra-līz-a-bil'-i-ti): The degree to which the results of a study or systematic review can be extrapolated to other circumstances, in particular to routine health-care situations.

General Medical Council: The statutory regulatory body for doctors in the UK, responsible for licensing doctors to practise medicine. Abbreviated GMC.

General Social Care Council: The regulatory board responsible for registering social care workers and regulating their training and conduct. Abbreviated GSCC.

generation (jen-er-ā'-shun): **1.** A group of individuals who came into being at approximately the same time and who have some experience, attitude, or belief in common. 2. The time period, usually about 30 years, between the genesis of one generation and the next. 3. The process of producing offspring; procreation.

generic (je-ner′-ik): 1. Relating to a genus (*q.v.*). 2. Distinctive. 3. Not protected by patent or trademark; said of drugs. G. MEDICINES drugs marketed without a brand name; in the UK, they account for nearly 52% by volume of all prescriptions dispensed in the primary health-care sector; G. WORKER an individual who incorporates a combination of work from different traditions in a single post; such a worker is trained to provide both health and social care; this system of work is linked to role substitution but is not identical.

genesis (jen′-e-sis): The production, generation, or origin of a substance, organism, or other entity.

genetic (je-net′-ik): 1. Relating to origin or reproduction. 2. Inherited or produced by a gene. 3. Relating to the science of genetics. G. CODE the form in which genetic information is transmitted; the characteristics in genes that are passed from one generation to the next; G. COUNSELLING counselling of prospective parents in regard to risks, diagnostic procedures available, and possible recurrence of congenital or inherited disorders in a family; involves chromosomal studies of both prospective parents.

genetically modified: Organisms into which new genetic characteristics have been introduced to increase their usefulness; *e.g.*, modified bacteria that produce human insulin, and crop plants with increased yields or resistance to pests or disease.

geneticist (je-net′-i-sist): A scientist who specializes in genetics.

genetics (je-net-iks): The study of heredity. BEHAVIOURAL G. the branch of psychology that deals with the influence of heredity on behaviour.

Geneva Convention: An agreement between European nations signed in Geneva, Switzerland, in 1864, and later adopted by other nations, specifying that prisoners of war, the sick, wounded and dead, as well as those caring for them, would be humanely treated. The founding of the International Red Cross Society was a direct outcome of this meeting.

-genic: Combining form denoting: (1) forming, producing, produced by, formed from; (2) of or relating to a gene; or (3) suitable for production or reproduction.

genital (jen′-it-al): Relating to the organs of regeneration. G. HERPES see HERPES GENITALIS under HERPES; G. STAGE according to Freud, the stage in human psychosexual development, from about the second to the sixth year, when the child is interested in his genitals and when infantile masturbation is common.

genitalia (jen-i-tā′-li-a): The organs of reproduction. EXTERNAL G. the reproductive organs that are not located within the pelvic cavity; INTERNAL G. the reproductive organs that are contained within the pelvic cavity. See PENIS, VAGINA.

genito-: Combining form denoting the genital organs.

genitourinary medicine: A branch of medicine involving the investigation and management of sexually transmitted diseases (*q.v.*) and human immunodeficiency virus (*q.v.*). Mostly outpatient based, this can include more specialized services such as young people's clinics; genital dermatosis, sexual dysfunction, and psychosexual medicine; and outreach services for sex workers and drug users. Abbreviated GUM.

genoblast (jē′-nō-blast): The nucleus of a fertilized ovum.

genocide (jen′-ō-sīd): The systematic killing or destruction of an entire population, ethnic group, or tribe.

genogram (jen′-ō-gram): An outline of family history in which each member of a group gives his or her own family history; helps both the individual and the social investigator to visualize the family structure and to gain perspective on an individual in light of successive events in his background.

genome (jē′-nōm): 1. The genetic make-up of a species. 2. The human genetic complement of 23 pairs of chromosomes, 22 of which appear in both sexes; the 23rd pair is the sex chromosomes, which are identified as XX in the female and XY in the male. G. PROJECTS research and technology development efforts aimed at mapping and sequencing the genetic code of human beings and certain model organisms. See HUMAN GENOME PROJECT.

genotype (jen′-ō-tīp): 1. The entire inherent genetic endowment of an individual. 2. A group of organisms in which all members have the same genetic constitution. — genotypically, adj.

-genous: A suffix denoting produced by, resulting from, or arising in.

gentian violet: A dye derived from coal tar; widely used as a stain in biological and histological laboratories and as a topical anti-infective, antifungal and anthelmintic agent.

genus (jē′-nus): A classification ranking between family (higher) and species (lower).

geopathic stress (jē-ō-path′-ik): Harm done to the human body by radiation from the Earth.

geophagia (jē-ō-fā′-ji-a): The habit of eating earth, clay, or similar unsuitable substance. Also called *geophagism* and *geophagy*.

geotrichosis (jē′-ō-tri-kō′-sis): Infection by a fungus; sites most frequently affected are the lungs, mouth, and intestine.

ger-; gerat-: Combining forms denoting old age.

geratology (jer-a-tol′-ō-ji): Gerontology (*q.v.*).

geriactivist (jer-i-ak′-tiv-ist): A recently coined term used to describe an older person who is himself active in the causes of the elderly.

geriatric (jer-ē-at′-rik): Relating to advanced age or to the elderly. G. NURSING specialist nursing care, treatment and support provided for elderly patients.

geriatrics (jer-i-at′-riks): The branch of medical science that deals with the application of the knowledge of ageing in providing care for the elderly with all kinds of physical and mental illnesses.

germ (jurm): **1.** A small bit of living substance capable of developing into a new individual. **2.** Any microorganism, particularly a pathogenic bacterium. **3.** The part of a cereal grain that is separated from the starchy part in the milling process, *e.g.*, wheat germ. **4.** A beginning. **5.** One of three layers of cells in the embryo from which the organs and structures of the body develop (ectoderm, mesoderm, endoderm).

German measles: See RUBELLA.

germ cell: A sexual reproductive cell; an ovum or spermatozoon in any stage of its development.

germicide (jer′-mi-sīd): An agent that kills germs (pathogenic bacteria). — germicidal, adj.

germination (jer-min-ā′-shun): In physiology, the development of a fertilized ovum into an embryo.

germ plasm: The protoplasm of the germ cell (*q.v.*); it contains the hereditary material of the cell.

gero-, geront-, geronto-: Combining forms denoting old age or ageing.

gerontological (jer′-on-tō-loj′-ik): Of or relating to the study of gerontology. G. MEDICINE the branch of medicine dealing with the medical treatment of age-related diseases and disorders occurring in the elderly; G. NURSING nursing practice that is concerned with the study of the ageing process, geriatric nursing, and nursing research in healthcare of the elderly.

gerontology (jer-on-tol′-ō-ji): The scientific study of the ageing processes and the problems of the ageing; a multidisciplinary field that draws its content and methods from biology, medical science, psychology, sociology, philosophy, political science, economics, education, and social services. BIOLOGICAL G. the biology of longevity, ageing, and death.

gerontoxon (jer-on-tok′-son): An area of degeneration around the outer circumference of the cornea creating a greyish or white ring. Also called *arcus senilis* and *arcus cornealis*.

Gesell Development Schedule: A test for assessing child development, used with children between four weeks and six years of age. The areas emphasized include motor and language development, adaptive behaviour, and personal — social behaviour. The test measures responses to standardized materials and situations, both qualitatively and quantitatively; the results are expressed first as developmental age, which is then converted into developmental quotient, see under DEVELOPMENTAL.

gestalt (ge-stalt): A school of psychology founded in Germany by Dr. Frederick Perls; holds that objects that come to mind are perceived as total configurations arising from the interrelations of their component parts and cannot be split into separate parts; and that the word gestalt means 'integrated unit', hence individuals are treated as complete functional units in their particular setting and condition.

gestation (jes-tā′-shun): **1.** Pregnancy. **2.** The development of an individual from conception to birth.

gestational age (jes-tā′-shun-al): The age of a conceptus, computed from the first day of the mother's last menstrual period, expressed in weeks.

gestosis (jes-tō′-sis): Any toxic disorder of pregnancy.

-geusia: Combining form denoting taste, or the sense of taste.

GFR: Abbreviation for glomerular filtration rate, see under GLOMERULAR.

GGTP: Abbreviation for gamma-glutamyl transpeptidase (*q.v.*).

GH: Abbreviation for growth hormone, see under GROWTH.

GHIH: Abbreviation for growth hormone inhibiting hormone, see under GROWTH.

GHRH: Abbreviation for growth hormone releasing hormone, see under GROWTH.

GI: Abbreviation for gastrointestinal (*q.v.*).

giant-cell tumor: See OSTEOCLASTOMA.

Giardia lamblia (ji-ar′-di-a): A flagellated organism that attaches itself to the intestinal wall; usually does not cause pathology but may cause giardiasis (*q.v.*). Also called *Lamblia intestinalis*.

giardiasis (ji-ar-dī′-a-sis): Infection with the protozoan *Giardia lamblia*; usually there are no definite symptoms, but occasionally the organism gives rise to diarrhoea and dysentery. Transmitted by foods, water, and lack of handwashing among caregivers and others. Incubation period may be as short as 5 days or as long as 25 days. Symptoms include sudden onset of violent diarrhoea, abdominal cramps; nausea and vomiting, low grade fever, chills. Attacks may be of short duration or may last as long as several weeks.

giddiness (gid′-i-nes): An unpleasant sensation resembling dizziness.

GIFT: Abbreviation for gamete intrafallopian transfer (*q.v.*).

gigantism (jī′-gan-tizm): An abnormal overgrowth, especially in height. May be associated with anterior pituitary tumour if the tumour develops before fusion of the epiphyses. ACROMEGALIC G. pituitary G.; FETAL G. excessive size of the fetus or newborn; may be seen in offspring of diabetic mothers, when it is called *fetoprotein diabetica*; PITUITARY G. that due to excessive pituitary secretion; occurs before puberty.

Gilles de la Tourette syndrome (zhēl′ de la tooret′): A relatively rare condition characterized by progressively violent tics or jerks of muscles of the face, shoulder, and extremities; by compulsive acts, echolalia, explosive obscene utterances, grunting, barking, or hissing. Usually begins between ages of 2 and 14 years. [Gilles de la Tourette, French neurologist, 1857–1904.]

ginger (jin′-jer): The dried rhizome of a tropical plant; sometimes used in medicine in treatment of colic and flatulence. POWDERED G. ROOT prepared in capsules for use by travellers to avoid air, car, or other motion sickness.

gingiva (jin′-ji-va, jin-jī′-va): The gum; the dense fibrous tissue covered with mucous membrane into which the teeth are set. — gingivae, pl.; gingival, adj.

gingivitis (jin-ji-vī′-tis): Inflammation of the gingivae; often the result of poor oral hygiene with the formation of bacterial plaque. DESQUAMATIVE G. a condition sometimes seen in menopausal women and older people; a grey necrotic membrane forms on the gingivae and eventually sloughs off; usually chronic.

ginglymus (jin′-gli-mus): A hinge joint (*q.v.*). — ginglimoid, adj.

girdle (ger′-dl): 1. A belt. 2. An encircling structure or part, G. PAIN a constricting pain around the waist region, occurring in tabetic persons; PELVIC G. comprises the two innominate bones, sacrum, and coccyx; SHOULDER G. comprises the two clavicles and scapulae.

Girdlestone: G.'S ARTHROPATHY the insertion of a partial or total artificial hip joint. G.'S OPERATION a surgical procedure for draining a seriously infected hip joint. [G. R. Girdlestone, English surgeon, 1881–1950.]

Glasgow Coma Scale.

Test	Response	Score
Eye opening	Spontaneous	4
	To speech	3
	To pain	2
	None	1
Best verbal response	Oriented	5
	Confused	4
	Inappropriate	3
	Incomprehensible	2
	None	1
Best motor response (arm)	Obedience to commands	6
	Localization of pain	5
	Withdrawal response to pain	4
	Flexion response to pain	3
	Extension response to pain	2
	None	1

girth (gerth): Circumference, particularly of the abdomen.

gland: An organ, structure or group of cells capable of manufacturing a fluid substance (1) to be eliminated from the body, or (2) to be used in some part of the body other than the place it is made. LYMPHATIC G. (node) does not secrete but is concerned with filtration of the lymph. See ENDOCRINE, EXOCRINE. — glandular, adj.

glandular (glan'-dū-la): 1. Relating to or resembling a gland. 2. Relating to the glans penis. G. FEVER see INFECTIOUS MONONUCLEOSIS under MONONUCLEOSIS.

glans (glanz): The bulbous termination of the clitoris and penis.

Glasgow Coma Scale: A neurological evaluation tool based on eye, motor, and verbal responses; the various responses are given a number value on the scale, and the patient's state of responsiveness is expressed in the total of the number values; the lowest possible score is 3 and the highest is 15.

glaucoma (glaw-kō'-ma): A condition of the eye in which vision is lost due to increased intraocular pressure when the rate of absorption of the fluid within the eye is slower than the rate of production; may be acute or chronic, causing damage to the retina and optic nerve, hardening of the globe of the eye, and blindness if undetected or untreated; the classic symptom is seeing halos around lights. The cause may not be known, but the disorder may follow a blow on the head, emotional stress, diabetes, sudden dilatation of the pupil; heredity may also be involved. G. occurs most often in people over 40 years of age, but is also seen in young children. Not considered curable but can be kept from progressing through treatment. HAEMORRHAGIC G. caused by retinal haemorrhage. NARROW-ANGLE or CLOSED-ANGLE G. increased intraocular pressure due to blocking of the angle of the anterior chamber by fibrous bands; of sudden onset; characterized by intense pain, blurring or loss of vision, redness of the conjunctiva; may become chronic with permanent closure of the angle; surgical treatment is necessary to drain off the rapidly building pressure and prevent damage to the optic nerve; WIDE-ANGLE or OPEN-ANGLE G. increased intraocular pressure of insidious onset; the angle remains open but the filtration of intraocular fluid is diminished, leading to increased pressure, often with eventual loss of vision; treated with eye drops and oral medication.

glenoid (glē'-noyd): Resembling a pit or socket, particularly the cavity on the scapula into which the head of the humerus fits to form the shoulder joint. G. FOSSA the depression in the temporal bone in which the condyle of the lower jaw rests.

glia (glī'-a): The non-nervous supporting tissue of the brain and spinal cord; the neuroglia.

-glia: Combining form denoting neuroglia in which the elements are of a particular kind or size, *e.g.*, microglia.

gliadin (glī'-a-din): A protein derived from the gluten of grains such as wheat, rye, and oats.

gliding: A smooth, continuous movement. G. JOINT a synovial joint in which the movement is limited as to plane, as occurs in the wrist or ankle joints.

glioma (glī-ō'-ma): An infiltrative neoplasm, usually malignant, that arises in the neuroglia, often in the cerebral hemispheres or spinal cord of adults. The tumour has no well-defined border; it blends into the surrounding tissues, making complete excision almost impossible. One form occurring in the retina is hereditary. ASTROCYTIC G. see ASTROCYTOMA; GANGLIONIC G. see NEUROBLASTOMA; OPTIC NERVE G. a slow-growing neoplasm of the optic nerve or chiasm, beginning with visual loss; later symptoms include bulging of the eyeball, strabismus, and loss of eye movement. — gliomatous, adj.

gliosis (glī'-ō-sis): A condition marked by the presence of tumours or overgrowth in the neuroglia.

glitter cells: Leukocytes that, when viewed under the microscope, appear to have granules that move about and have a sparkling appearance.

globalization (glō-bal-ī-zā'-shun): 1. The process by which social institutions become adopted on a worldwide scale. 2. The process by which a business or company starts operating at an international level.

globin (glō'-bin): A protein that combines with haematin to form haemoglobin.

globule (glob'-ūl): A small spherical mass. — globoid, globular, adj.

globulin (glob'-ū-lin): A fraction of serum or plasma protein. ANTIHAEMOPHILIC G. FACTOR VIII; see under FACTOR; ANTILYMPHOCYTIC G. a purified serum produced in animals; used in combatting rejection reaction in organ transplantation; GAMMA G. see GAMMA GLOBULIN; HYPERIMMUNE G., G. prepared from serum of patients recently recovered from certain viral diseases, including those caused by herpesviruses and hepatitis B, and by certain encephalitides and zoonoses.

globulolysis (glob-ū-lol´-i-sis): Destruction of red blood cells. — globulolytic, adj.

glomerular (glō-mer´-ū-lar): Relating to a glomerulus (q.v.). G. FILTRATE the non-protein filtrate of plasma produced by Malpighian corpuscles of the kidney and that passes into the lumen of Bowman's capsule (q.v.); G. FILTRATION RATE the rate at which the kidney filters fluid from the circulating blood; measured in volume per unit of time, either minutes or hours.

glomerulonephritis (glō-mer´-ū-lō-nē-frī-tis): A term used in non-suppurative acute or chronic disease of the kidney, primarily of the glomeruli. In children and young persons. ACUTE G. often follows streptococcal infections, marked by haematuria, hypertension, oedema, and proteinuria; the prognosis is good. In older persons, the disease is marked by malaise, nausea, joint pain, proteinuria, hypertension, and pulmonary complications; all symptoms are more severe than in children and the prognosis is somewhat less favourable; POSTINFECTIOUS G. acute G., often follows streptococcal infections but may also follow infections caused by staphylococcal and pneumococcal organisms.

glomerulosclerosis (glō-mer´-ū-lō-skle-rō-sis): Fibrosis of the glomeruli of the kidney, the result of inflammation. INTERCAPILLARY G. is a common pathological finding in persons with diabetes mellitus. — glomerulosclerotic, adj.

glomerulus (glō-mer´-ū-lus): A coil of minute arterial capillaries held together by scanty connective tissue. It invaginates the entrance of a uriniferous tubule in the kidney cortex. — glomerular, adj. glomeruli, pl.

glomus (glō´-mus): In anatomy, a small encapsulated globular body containing many arterioles that are connected to veins, and having a rich nerve supply, especially sensory receptors, e.g., the G. CAROTICUM, situated behind the carotid artery at its bifurcation; G. TUMOUR, a neoplasm of unknown cause; consists of a slightly elevated, rounded, firm, nodular mass, occurring chiefly in the skin; generally seen on distal ends of fingers and toes and in the nailbed; treatment is surgical removal.

glos-, glosso-: Combining forms denoting: (1) the tongue, (2) language.

glossa (glos´-a): The tongue. — glossal, adj.

glossitis (glos-ī´-tis): 1. Inflammation of the tongue, 2. Cellulitis of the tongue. MOELLER'S G. see PAPILLITIS.

glossocele (glos´-ō-sēl): Oedema and swelling of the tongue; resulting in its protrusion from the mouth.

glossopharyngeal (glos´-ō-fa-rin´-jē-al): Relating to the tongue and pharynx. G. NERVE one of the 9th pair of cranial nerves; has motor fibres that go to the parotid gland and sensory fibres for the sensations of touch, temperature, and pain from the back of the tongue, tonsils, and pharynx; and taste from the back one-third of the tongue; G. NEURALGIA a condition marked by pain in the tongue and throat; seen most often in the elderly.

glossophytia (glos-ō-fit´-i-a): Black tongue. Blackish to yellow, fur-like, painless patches at the back of the tongue; often due to a fungal infection.

glossoplegia (glos-ō-plē´-ji-a): Paralysis of the tongue.

glottis (glot´-is): The part of the larynx that is concerned with voice production. See VOCAL CORDS, — glottides, pl; glottic, adj.

gluc-, gluco-: Combining forms denoting glucose.

glucagon (gloo´-ka-gon): Hormone produced in alpha cells of pancreatic islets of Langerhans. Causes breakdown of glycogen into glucose, thus preventing blood sugar from falling too low during fasting.

glucocorticoid (gloo´-kō-kor´-ti-koyd): Any steroid hormone that promotes gluconeogenesis (i.e., the formation of glucose and glycogen from protein) and antagonizes the action of insulin. Occurs naturally in the adrenal cortex as cortisone and hydrocortisone; also produced synthetically. G. INSUFFICIENCY see ADDISON'S DISEASE.

glucogenesis (gloo-kō-jen´-e-sis): The formation in the body of glycogen from the breakdown of glucose. — glucogenic, adj.

gluconeogenesis (gloo´-kō-nē´-ō-jen´-e-sis): Glyconeogenesis (q.v.).

glucose (gloo´-kōs): Dextrose or grape sugar. A common and important monosaccharide, present in most fruits. The chief end product of the digestion of carbohydrates and the form in which they are absorbed from the gastrointestinal tract. A normal constituent of blood and other fluids of the body. The chief source of energy in the body. Excess over what is needed or utilized by the body is stored in the form of glycogen or in body tissues as fat.

glucose tolerance test: Useful in the diagnosis of diabetes mellitus and other causes of glycosuria. Serial collections of blood are estimated for blood glucose following the oral or intravenous administration of glucose, and urine samples are simultaneously tested for glucose.

glucoside (gloo'-kō-sīd): Any of a group of natural vegetable substances that decomposes into glucose and another substance; many have medicinal properties with specific uses in medicine.

glucuronidase (gloo-kū-ron'-i-dās): An enzyme that acts as a catalyst in the hydrolysis of glucuronides; occurs in the liver, spleen, and endocrine glands.

glue ear: An accumulation of a tenacious, sticky, glue-like substance in the middle ear which causes distension of the ear drum, producing impaired hearing.

glue-sniffing: The inhalation of fumes from epoxy glue; initial stimulation of the central nervous system is followed by depression. The effect of the inhalation is enhanced when the glue is poured into a plastic bag that is placed over the nose and mouth.

glutamic acid decarboxylase (gloo-tam'-ik as'-id dē-kar-boks'-i-lās): An enzyme affecting regulation of the neurotransmitter, gamma-aminobutyric acid (q.v.), which is markedly reduced in Huntington's chorea.

glutamine (gloo'-ta-mēn): An amino acid found in certain proteins, blood, and other tissues; on hydrolysis it yields glutamic acid and ammonia.

glutaraldehyde (gloo-ta-ral'-de-hīd): A compound used for fixing a tissue specimen for examination by electron microscopy; it preserves very fine details.

glutathione (gloo-ta-thī'-ōn): A tripeptide that has been isolated from yeast, liver, and muscle; thought to be important in cellular respiration.

gluteal (gloo'-tē-al): Relating to the buttocks. G. FOLD the crease between the posterior thigh and the buttock; G. REFLEX contraction of the gluteal muscles from stimulation of the skin over them.

gluten (gloo'-ten): A protein constituent of wheat and several other grains; used commercially for making adhesives. G. ENTEROPATHY adult coeliac disease; see under COELIAC.

gluteus (gloo'-tē-us): G. MAXIMUS the largest and most superficial of the three large muscles that form the buttock; G. MEDIUS the middle of the muscles that form the buttock; G. MINIMUS the innermost of the muscles that form the buttock.

glutinous (gloo'-ti-nus): Viscid; adhesive; sticky.

glyc-, glyco-, gluco-: Combining forms denoting glycogen.

glycaemia (glī-sē'-mi-a): The presence of glucose in the blood.

glycase (glī'-kās): An enzyme that converts maltose to maltodextrin and dextrose.

glycerin(e) (glis'-er-in): A clear, syrupy liquid prepared synthetically or obtained as a by-product in soap manufacture. It has a hygroscopic action. Widely used in pharmaceutical preparations as a solvent or vehicle for drugs in syrups, lozenges, suppositories. Useful as an emollient (q.v.).

glycerol (glis'-er-ol): An alcohol that is a component of fats. Glycerol is soluble in ethyl alcohol and water. Pharmaceutical preparations are called glycerin (q.v.).

glyceryl trinitrate: Nitroglycerin. Glyceryl trinitrate is a vasodilator and is used to relieve certain types of pain, especially in the prophylaxis and treatment of angina pectoris (q.v.). It is administered sublingually or by transdermal patch or gel.

glycine (glī'-sēn): A non-essential amino acid; the simplest of the amino acids; found widely distributed in animal and plant proteins; also prepared synthetically; has some uses in medicine. Also called *aminoacetic acid.*

glycocholic acid (glī'-kō-kol-ik): An acid found in bile.

glycogen (gli'-kō-jen): The form into which glucose is converted by insulin for storage in the body; when it is needed it is converted to monosaccharides, providing an immediate source of energy.

glycogenase (glī'-kō-jen-ās): An enzyme necessary for the conversion of glycogen into glucose.

glycogenesis (glī-kō-jen'-e-sis): The synthesis or formation of glycogen from glucose or other monosaccharides. — glycogenetic, adj.

glycogenolysis (glī-kō-je-nol'-i-sis): The conversion of glycogen into glucose.

glycogeusia (glī-kō-gū'-si-a): A sweet taste in the mouth.

glycokinase (glī-kō-kī'-nās): An enzyme that, in the presence of ATP (q.v.), catalyzes the conversion of glucose to glucose-6-phosphatate.

glycolysis (glī-kol'-i-sis): The enzymatic, anaerobic breakdown of glucose or other carbohydrate in the body, with the formation of lactic acid or pyruvic acid and the release of energy.

glycometabolism (glī'-kō-me-tab'-ō-lizm): The utilization of sugar in the body. — glycometabolic, adj.

glyconeogenesis (glī'-kō-nē-ō-jen'-e-sis): The formation of sugar from protein or fat when there is lack of available carbohydrate.

glycopenia (glī-kō-pē'-ni-a): A deficiency of sugar in the body tissues.

glycopexis (glī-kō-pek'-sis): The fixation and storage of glycogen in the liver. — glycopexic, adj.

glycophilia (glī-kō-fil'-i-a): A condition characterized by the production of hyperglycaemia following the ingestion of a small amount of sugar.

glycoprotein (glī-kō-prō'-tē-in): Refers to a class of proteins that contain a carbohydrate group (conjugated proteins); they include the mucins, the mucoids, and the chondroproteins.

glycoside (gli'-kō-sīd): A complex natural substance composed of a sugar with another compound, particularly as found in some plants, e.g., digitalis, strophanthus, and others. The non-sugar fragment is sometimes of therapeutic value.

glycostatic (glī-kō-stat'-ik): Tending to maintain a constant level of glycogen in the body tissues.

glycosuria (glī-kō-sū'-ri-a): The presence of an abnormal amount of sugar in the urine.

glycuronic acid (glī-kū-ron'-ik): An acid formed by oxidation during animal metabolism; found in urine in combination with several other substances.

GM: Abbreviation for genetically modified (q.v.).

GMC: Abbreviation for General Medical Council (q.v.).

gnathoschisis (nath-os'-ki-sis): Congenital cleft in the upper jaw, as occurs in cleft palate.

-gnosis: Combining form denoting recognition; knowledge.

goblet cells: Special secreting cells, shaped like a goblet, found in the mucous membranes, particularly in the stomach, intestines, and respiratory tract; they secrete mucus.

Goeckerman method (ger'-ke-man): A method of treating psoriasis whereby tar is applied to the entire body, which is then irradiated with ultraviolet light and later bathed to remove scales; takes 21 days to complete.

Goffman, Irving: A sociologist who used microsociological analysis and unconventional subject matter to explore the details of individual identity, group relations, the impact of environment, and the movement and interactive meaning of information. A product of the Chicago school, his symbolic, interactionist perspective provided new insight into the nature of social interaction and the psychology of the individual.

goitre (goy'-ter): A chronic enlargement of the thyroid gland, causing a swelling in front of the neck; may be due to iodine deficiency in the diet, tumour, inflammation, or hyper- or hypo-function of the thyroid gland. ADENOMATOUS G. one in which the gland becomes firm and enlarges more on one side than the other; it may grow slowly and then enlarge greatly during middle age; may become toxic or not; COLLOID G. the gland enlarges and becomes soft due to collection of gelatinous matter in the follicles; ENDEMIC G. occurs in certain areas of the world where the food and water do not contain the normal amount of iodine, but the goitres are usually of the simple type. Also called *Derbyshire neck*. EXOPHTHALMIC G. gland may or may not enlarge; excess of thyroid hormone is secreted, leading to physical symptoms such as nervousness, loss of weight, profuse sweats, accelerated pulse, psychic disturbances, increased basal metabolism, fine muscle tremor, and exophthalmos (q.v.). Also called *Graves' disease*; LYMPHADENOID G diffuse enlargement of the thyroid; of unknown cause, marked by epithelial changes and lymphoid hyperplasia. Also called *struma lymphomatosa*; MULTINODAL G., G. in which there are several enlarged colloid lobules; occurs most often in women; NON-TOXIC G. simple G., not accompanied by any of the symptoms seen in exophthalmic goitre, due to an enlargement of the gland in response to iodine insufficiency in the diet; may disappear spontaneously; SUBSTERNAL G. enlargement chiefly of the lower part of the isthmus of the thyroid, only slightly palpable or not at all; TOXIC G. exophthalmic G.

gold: A solid yellow metallic element; its salts are used therapeutically in treatment of rheumatoid arthritis. RADIOACTIVE G. used in treatment of certain types of cancer and as a diagnostic scinti-scanning agent.

Goldthwaite: G.'S BELT a wide belt with a metal support; for treating back injuries; G.'S SIGN pain occurring in the sacroiliac region when the leg is held straight and flexed at the hip; a sign of sprain of the sacroiliac ligaments; G.'S STRAP a support strap used in treating an injured foot. [Joel Goldthwaite, American orthopaedic surgeon, 1866–1961.]

golfer's elbow: A condition comparable to tennis elbow (q.v.), with the affected area being the medial condylar region of the humerus; treatment is as for tennis elbow.

Golgi bodies, also **Golgi apparatus** (gol'-jē): An anastomosing network of delicate fibrils found near the nucleus in the cytoplasm of nearly all cells. [Camillo Golgi, Italian histologist, 1843–1926.]

gomphosis (gom-fō'-sis): An immovable joint, where a conical eminence fits into a socket, *e.g.*, a tooth, or the styloid process of the temporal bone.

gonad (gō´-nad): One of the essential sex glands of the male or female. See OVARY, TESTIS. — gonadal, adj.

gonad-, gonado-: Combining forms denoting a gonad (*q.v.*).

gonadotrophic (gon´-ad-ō-trō´-fin): Having an affinity for influencing or stimulating the gonads; often refers to the two secretions of the anterior pituitary, *i.e.*, the follicle-stimulating hormone and the luteinizing hormone.

gonadotrophin (gon´-ad-ō-trō´-fin): Any gonad-stimulating hormone. HUMAN CHORIONIC G. produced in the placenta during the first trimester of pregnancy, reaching a peak in 15 to 18 days following the first missed menses, then declining; its function is to stimulate growth and secretion of the corpus luteum and thus help to maintain the pregnancy; may be demonstrated in the urine and blood; tests for its presence are reliable tests for pregnancy. Also may be used in treatment for underdevelopment of the sex glands.

gonepoiesis (gon-e-poy-ē´-sis): The formation of semen.

goniopuncture (gō´-ni-ō-punk´-tur): An operation for glaucoma in which a knife is inserted through the cornea, across the anterior chamber, and through the opposite corneoscleral wall.

goniotomy (gō-ni-ot´-o-mi): Operation for glaucoma. Incision is through the anterior chamber angle to the canal of Schlemm.

gonococcal complement fixation test: A specific serological test for the diagnosis of gonorrhoea.

gonococcus (gon-ō-kok´-us): *Neisseria gonorrhoeae*; a Gram-negative, encapsulated diplococcus, usually occurring in pairs; the causative organism of gonorrhoea. — gonococci, adj.

gonorrhoea (gon-ō-rē´-ah): An infectious disease of venereal origin caused by the *Neisseria gonorrhoeae* organism; the incubation period is two to five days. Chief manifestations in the adult male are purulent urethritis and dysuria; in the adult female urethritis and endocervicitis; often spreads to the uterine tubes and the periotoneum. In rare cases the infection is carried by the bloodstream to the heart, joints, or other structures. In children the infection is usually accidental and may occur as (1) ophthalmia neonatorium, (notifiable disease) acquired during passage through the birth canal, or (2) gonococcal valvovaginitis in girls before puberty and acquired through contact with an infected adult.

gonorrhoeal (gon-ō-rē´-al): Resulting from or caused by gonorrhoea. G. ARTHRITIS a manifestation of gonorrhoeal infection; G. CONJUNCTIVITIS severe purulent conjunctivitis that causes scarring of the cornea and possible blindness. G. OPHTHALMIA one form of ophthalmia neonatorum; G. SALPINGITIS see PELVIC INFLAMMATORY DISEASE under PELVIC.

Goodell's sign: Softening of the cervix of the uterus; considered evidence of pregnancy. [W. Goodell, American gynaecologist, 1829–1894.] See HEGAR'S SIGN.

Goodenough's Draw-a-Person Test: A test for assessing the intelligence of children 3 to 10 years of age.

Goodpasture's syndrome: A serious glomerulonephritis affecting mostly young men; associated with or preceded by pulmonary problems, haemoptysis, anaemia, haematuria, proteinuria, and hypertension; rapidly progressive and often fatal. Haemodialysis is used in treatment and, sometimes, kidney transplant.

gooseflesh: Cutis anserina. Roughness of the skin produced by the erection of papillae when the arrectores pilorum muscles attached to the sides of the hair follicles contract under stimulation, usually cold or fear. Also called *goose bumps, goose pimples.*

gouge (gowj): A chisel with a grooved blade for removing bone.

gout (gowt): A metabolic disorder stemming from biochemical defects in purine metabolism; uric acid is overproduced and retained in the body, and sodium urate crystals are deposited around the joints and other places in the body. Characterized by redness, swelling, pain, and inflammation of the joints, particularly in the great toe; and by hyperuricaemia and the formation of stones in the urinary collecting system and tract. Frequently said to be due to heavy eating of rich foods and consumption of alcohol, but may also be familial in origin. TOPHACEOUS G., G. involving an increasing number of joints, including the ankle, knee, and elbow; tophaceous deposits of sodium urate form in subcutaneous and periarticular tissues, the pinna of the ear, along the tendons of fingers and toes, and in bursae. — gouty, adj.

GP: Abbreviation for general practitioner, see under GENERAL.

Graafian follicle: See under FOLLICLE.

gracilis (gras´-il-is): G. MUSCLE the long slender muscle at the inner side of the thigh.

graduate (grad´-ū-āt): A pitcher-shaped vessel marked with lines at different levels; used for measuring liquids.

graduate primary care mental health worker: A new kind of health-care employee, trained specifically to improve access to psychiatric support in primary care. This post was created in order to help meet the NHS Plan (*q.v.*) and National Service Framework (*q.v.*) requirements for mental health. These workers will be recruited from a wide graduate entry background, see www.doh.gov.uk/mental-health/ fastforwardguidancejan03.pdf

graft: A tissue or organ that is transplanted to another part of the body of the same animal (autograft), or to another animal of the same species (homograft), or to another animal of a different species (heterograft). AUTOGENOUS G. an autograft; BONE G. a piece of bone, usually taken from the tibia (or supplied by a bone bank), and used elsewhere in the body of the individual or another recipient; BYPASS G. a G. utilizing a synthetic tube to create a diversion in the bloodstream to bypass an obstructed or weakened blood vessel; CORNEAL G. the transplantation of healthy corneal tissue to a defective cornea; FULL-THICKNESS G. a G. utilizing a full thickness of skin and the subcutaneous tissue; ISOGRAFT tissue or an organ transplanted from one identical twin to the other; NERVE G. replacement of a segment of a defective nerve with a section from a sound one; PATCH G. a G. of living tissue used to close an incision made in a vein to enlarge its lumen; PEDICLE G. a flap of skin and subcutaneous tissue attached to a pedicle; PINCH G. a small thin piece of skin obtained by lifting it with a needle and slicing it off; SPLIT-THICKNESS G. a skin G. utilizing only part of the skin thickness; THIERSCH G. utilizes small thin, split strips of epidermis with part of the dermis; also called *Ollier–Thiersch* G. and *Ollier* G..

graft-versus-host disease/reaction: A condition occurring in an immunologically incompetent host or recipient following a graft of tissue or of an organ. The liver, skin, and gut are the systems most severely affected resulting in erythema, ulceration, oedema, heart and joint lesions, etc. Drugs that suppress the immune reaction, such as steroids and cyclosporin A, may be given to reduce the severity of the reaction.

grain: 1. A seed, normally of a cereal plant.

-gram: Combining form denoting (1) something written down, (2) something drawn, (3) a recording.

gram, gramme: The unit of weight in the metric system. Equal to one thousandth of a kilogram.

gram molecular weight: The molecular weight of a compound expressed in grams.

gram molecule: The weight of a substance expressed in grams, the number of grams being equivalent to the molecular weight of the substance, *e.g.*, the molecular weight of hydrogen is 2, therefore a gram molecule of hydrogen weighs 2 grams. Also called *gram mole*.

Gram-negative: See under GRAM'S STAIN.

Gram-positive: See under GRAM'S STAIN.

Gram's stain: A bacteriological stain for differentiation of microorganisms. First, a violet stain is applied, followed by an application of iodine solution; then the material is decolorized by alcohol or an acetone solution, and a counter-stain, safranin, is applied. Organisms that retain the violet colour are called Gram-positive and those that appear as rose-pink due to discoloration of the first stain are called Gram-negative. Also called *Gram's method*. [Hans Christian Gram, Danish physician, 1853–1938.]

grand mal (grahn mal): Major epilepsy; see EPILEPSY. G. M. SEIZURE characterized by loss of consciousness, generalized convulsions, frothing at the mouth, cyanosis of the face; usually preceded by an aura.

granular (gran'-ū-lar): Made up of, marked by the presence of, or resembling granules.

granulation (gran-ū-lā'-shun): The outgrowth of new capillaries and connective tissue cells from the surface of an open wound that is not healing by first intention; see under HEALING. G. TISSUE the young, soft tissue formed by granulation.

granule (gran-ūl): A grain, or a very small distinct mass.

granuloblast (gran'-ū-lō-blast): An immature granulocyte.

granulocyte (gran'-ū-lō-sīt): Any cell containing granules; refers particularly to neutrophils, eosinophils, or basophils that contain granules in their protoplasm; constitutes 60% of all leukocytes; their function is to engulf and kill invading bacteria by means of a chemical substance formed in the granules.

granulocytopenia (gran'-ū-lō-sī-tō-pē'-ni-a): Decrease of granulocytes in the blood but not to a degree sufficient to warrant the term agranulocytosis (*q.v.*).

granulocytopoiesis (gran'-ū-lō-sī-tō-poy-ē'-sis): The formation or production of granulocytes.

granulocytosis (gran'-ū-lō-sī-tō'-sis): The presence of an abnormally large number of granulocytes in the circulating blood.

granuloma (gran-ū-lō′-ma): A tumour formed of granulation tissue. G. ANNULARE a G. characterized by hard reddish nodules that enlarge progressively until a ring is formed; chronic and self-limited; usually seen on the extremities; EOSINOPHILIC G. a benign chronic proliferative process in bone with many eosinophilic cells present, producing one or more bone lesions; G. INGUINALE one of the venereal diseases in which lesions form on the genitals and in the inguinal region; PYOGENIC G., G. characterized by a fungating growth, with the granulations consisting of masses of pyogenic organisms; also called *septic g.*; SWIMMING POOL G. a granulomatous lesion that may develop in abrasions sustained in swimming pools; usually heals spontaneously but slowly; thought to be caused by *Mycobacterium balnei*; WEGENER'S G. a rare serious variant of polyarteritis nodosa, marked by the formation of granulomata in the nose and mouth, which ulcerate causing pain, erosion of bone, renal problems, and development of pulmonary nodules.

granulomatosis (gran′-ū-lō-ma-tō′-sis): A condition characterized by the formation of multiple granulomas in bones and elsewhere. LYMPHOMATOID G. a type of G. that resembles leprosy; the lesions have the features of both lymphoma and granuloma; WEGENER'S G. a form of G. marked by progression and lesions in the respiratory tract, arteriolitis, and inflammation of most of the body organs.

granulopenia (gran′-ū-lō-pē′-ni-a): A decreased number of granulocytes in the circulating blood.

granulosa cells (gran-ū-lō′-sa): Modified epithelial cells that surround the ovum in a follicle; after ovulation they are transformed into granular cells of the corpus luteum.

graph (graf): A diagram or curve presenting clinical or experimental data in pictorial form that shows relationships between sets of data.

-graph: Combining form denoting (1) something written; (2) an instrument for writing, recording, or transmitting.

graphology (graf-ol′-o-ji): The scientific study of handwriting for clues as to an individual's character, aptitudes, and temperament.

graphospasm (graf′-ō-spazm): Writer's cramp; cramping and pain around the muscles of the hand and forearm caused by writing for long periods of time.

-graphy: Combining form denoting (1) writing; (2) a writing on a particular subject.

grasp reflex: The grasping motion exhibited by the fingers or toes in response to stimulation by stroking the palm or sole.

grass: Street term for cannabis or marijuana.

grattage (gra-tazh′): The scraping or brushing of a surface to stimulate healing, or to remove granulations as in treatment of glaucoma.

grave (grāv): Severe; serious; life-threatening.

gravel: Minute stones or sandy deposit occurring in the gall bladder or urinary bladder.

Graves′ disease: Hyperthyroidism; see THYROTOXICOSIS. [Robert James Graves, Irish physician, 1797–1853.]

gravida (grav′-i-da): A pregnant woman. Gravida I designates the first pregnancy, gravida II the second, and so on.

gravidarum (grav-id-ar′-um): Literal translation is 'of the pregnant'. G. STRIAE the purplish longitudinal marks that occur on the skin of the lower abdomen during the later weeks or months of pregnancy.

gravitational (grav-i-tā′-shun-al): Subject to the force of gravity. G. ULCER varicose ulcer, see under ULCER.

gravity (grav′-i-ti): Weight. SPECIFIC G. the weight of a substance compared with that of an equal volume of water.

greater: 1. GREATER MULTANGULAR synonym for the trapezium, one of the bones of the wrist. 2. GREATER OMENTUM see under OMENTUM. 3. GREATER TROCHANTER the larger of the two processes of the femur at the point where the neck joins the shaft; it projects medially and laterally and serves as a site for the attachment of muscles including the gluteal muscles. 4. GREATER VESTIBULAR GLANDS see BARTHOLIN'S GLANDS.

greenhouse effect: The theory that industrial 'greenhouse gas' emissions are connected with the observed heating of the Earth's atmosphere. See GLOBAL WARMING.

Green Paper: A government report containing proposals for discussion and consultation, *e.g., Our Healthier Nation*, Department of Health (1998). Green Papers are frequently followed by White Papers (*q.v.*).

greenstick fracture: See FRACTURE.

grey matter: Nervous system tissue consisting mostly of cell bodies of neurons and unmyelinated nerve fibres; of greyish colour. Occurs in the cortex of the brain, the basal ganglia, and the central H-shaped portion of the spinal cord.

grid: A chart with horizontal and perpendicular lines on which curves may be plotted. WETZEL G. a chart on which weight, height, and other factors of growth and development are plotted; used for evaluating physical fitness of young and adolescent children.

grief (grēf): The normal emotional reaction of deep distress, caused by the loss of a loved one or of a treasured object, usually self-limited. Phases of the grief process have been described as (1) numbness or shock, accompanied by disbelief in the grievous event; (2) protest and yearning, accompanied by anger and longing; (3) disorganization, accompanied by chaos, despair, and depression; and (4) reorganization, characterized by acceptance of the event and making plans to resolve the crisis it created. ANTICIPATORY G. grieving that occurs prior to an actual loss either by death or separation from a loved person or object.

Griffiths Report: A government-chartered appraisal of management in the NHS, intended to consider ways of strengthening the management function within the NHS in order to improve accountability and value for money. The report by Sir Roy Griffiths, the Chief Executive of J. Sainsbury's supermarkets, recommended a new system of general management by specialist administrators rather than by health professionals, entrusting accountability to nonclinicians. This report, by a retail-based individual, was key to the introduction of the internal market in healthcare; its implementation greatly changed the way hospitals were run and administered.

grinders (grīn'-derz): The molars or 'double' teeth.

grinders' asthma: See under ASTHMA.

gripe (grīp): **1.** Colic. **2.** A sharp, spasmodic intestinal pain.

gristle: Cartilage (*q.v.*).

groin: The junction, or the area of the junction, of the thigh with the abdomen.

grommet (gro'-met): A small plastic tube inserted into the tympanic membrane of the ear to act as an artificial auditory tube, thus preventing the accumulation of fluid in the middle ear. Used in the treatment of 'glue ear' (*q.v.*). It is extruded spontaneously after a period of time.

groove: In anatomy, a long narrow depression, especially one in a bone or tooth substance.

gross (grōs): **1.** Large or coarse. **2.** Seen as a whole, without fine details. **3.** Visible without the use of a microscope.

grounded theory: A qualitative (*q.v.*) research approach where the theory is generated from the data. The theory is emergent – discovered in the data obtained.

group: A number of persons or things gathered closely together and forming a recognizable unit. G. PRACTICE a partnership of two or more general practitioners sharing premises and often secretarial help; the advantages include ease of consultation and the convenience of covering for each other. G. PSYCHOTHERAPY see GROUP THERAPY under THERAPY.

grouping: Blood grouping. See BLOOD GROUPS.

growing pains: Pains in the musculoskeletal system, the limbs particularly, during youth; thought by some to be rheumatic in origin; other causes that have been suggested are postural defects, emotional problems, muscle fatigue.

growth: 1. Normal progressive development or normal increase in size of any organism. **2.** An abnormal increase in size of cells or of tissue, as in a tumour. G. FACTOR any substance such as hormones that promote growth; G. HORMONE a secretion of the anterior part of the pituitary gland that promotes growth and helps to regulate the metabolism of proteins, fats, and carbohydrates; G. HORMONE INHIBITING HORMONE a peptide hormone that inhibits the release of growth hormone from the hypothalamus; G. HORMONE RELEASING HORMONE a peptide hormone related to the glucagon family, released from the pituitary, acts on the adenohypophysis to release growth hormone.

grunt: A deep gutteral sound in the chest; usually signifies chest pain, as in pneumonic conditions, rib fracture, and neonatal respiratory distress syndrome.

gryposis (grī-pō'-sis): An abnormal curvature. G. PENIS chordee (*q.v.*); G. UNGUIUM abnormal curvature of the nails.

GSCC: Abbreviation for General Social Care Council (*q.v.*).

GTN: Abbreviation for glyceryl trinitrate (*q.v.*).

guaiac test: (gwī'-ak): A test for the presence of occult blood in the faeces.

guarana (gwa-ra'-na): An astringent prepared from the seeds of a Brazilian tree (*Paullinia cupana*); used as treatment for diarrhoea.

guidelines: Directions or principles presenting current or future rules of policy. Guidelines may be developed by government agencies at any level, institutions, professional societies, governing boards, or by the convening of expert panels. The text is generally a comprehensive guide to problems and approaches in any field of activity.

Guillain–Barré syndrome (gē-yan´ -bar-rā´): A neurological syndrome; cause unknown but thought to be due to a virus; symptoms include pain, tenderness, and progressive weakness and flaccidity of muscles, ascending paralysis; chief laboratory finding is an increase in protein in the cerebrospinal fluid without accompanying increase in the cell count. Also called *idiopathic polyneuritis, acute febrile polyneuritis, infectious polyneuritis.*

guillotine (gil´ -o-tēn): A surgical instrument for excision of the tonsils.

guilt (gilt): In psychiatry, unconscious G. consists of mental reactions that are initiated by unconscious punishment fantasies; suffering that results from gratification of, or drive toward, gratification of a repressed wish.

Guinea worm: A genus of nematodes parasitic to humans, found especially in Africa and India; transmitted through infected water; the long thread-like worm burrows through the skin and into the subcutaneous and muscular tissues. Also called *Dracunculus medinensis.*

Gulf War syndrome: A group of medical symptoms, including fatigue, skin disorders, and muscle pains, experienced by some soldiers who fought in the Gulf War of 1991. These conditions are believed by some people to have been caused by exposure to pesticides, vaccines, and chemical and biological warfare agents.

gullet (gul´ -let): The tube by which food passes from the mouth to the stomach; includes the pharynx and oesophagus.

gum: 1. The dried sap from certain trees and shrubs, insoluble in ether or alcohol, but mixes with water to form a viscid mass. 2. The gingiva, the fleshy tissue that covers the alveolar processes of the jaw.

GUM: Abbreviation for genitourinary medicine (*q.v.*).

gumboil: An abscess on a gum (gingiva); may be due to infection of a tooth, injury, or tooth decay; may rupture spontaneously or require incision.

gumma (gum´ -a): A localized area of soft, gummy, vascular, granulation tissue, such as is seen in the later stages (tertiary) of syphilis; may occur in almost any tissue. Obstruction to the blood supply results in necrosis, and gummata near the surface of the body tend to break

down, forming chronic ulcers in such places as the nose, lower leg, and palate which heal slowly and probably are not infectious. — gummata, gummas, pl.; gummatous, adj.

gurgling (gur´ -gling): A coarse sound heard when auscultating over a large cavity or when there is a large amount of secretion in the trachea.

gustation (gus-tā´ -shun): 1. The act of tasting. 2. The sense of taste.

gut: 1. The intestines. (informal). 2. Suture material made from the intestine of sheep.

Guthrie test: A test for the presence of phenylketonuria in newborns. A drop of blood is obtained by heel prick and examined for the presence of phenylalanine; carried out on the 6th day of life. It is necessary to confirm the diagnosis in those infants with a positive test. [Robert Guthrie, American paediatrician, 1916–1995.]

GVHD: Abbreviation for graft-versus-host disease (*q.v.*).

gymnastics (jim-nas´ -tiks): Physical exercises that may be simple or complicated, ranging from callisthenics to acrobatics and performed with or without special equipment; may be done for prophylactic, curative, or corrective purposes.

gyn-, gynae-, gynaec-, gynaeco-, gyno-: Combining forms denoting (1) woman; (2) female reproductive organs.

gynaecological (gīn-e-kō-loj´ -ik, jī-ne): 1. Affecting or relating to the female reproductive tract. 2. Related to gynaecology.

gynaecology (gīn-e-kol´ -ō-ji, jī-ne): The branch of medicine that deals with disorders of the female genital tract.

gynaecomastia (gīn-e-kō-mas´ -ti-a, jī-ne): Excessive enlargement of the male mammary glands.

gynandrism (gǐ-nan´ -drizm, ji-nan): Female pseudohermaphroditism. See PSEUDOHERMAPHRODITISM.

gynandromorphism (gǐ-nan-drō-mor´ -fizm, ji-): An abnormality in which certain parts of an individual have both female and male characteristics. — gynandromorphous, adj.

gynatresia (gǐ-na-trē´ -zi-a, ji-): The occlusion of part of the female genital tract, particularly the vagina.

gypsum (jip´ -sum): Plaster of Paris (calcium sulphate).

gyrate (ji´ -rāt): 1. To revolve. 2. Twisted into a spiral or ring shape.

gyrus (jī-rus): Convolution. Term is used specifically to describe the tortuous elevations on the surface of the cortex of the brain; these elevations are separated from each other by shallow grooves called sulci and deep grooves called fissures.

H

H: Symbol for hydrogen.

habilitate (ha-bil′-i-tāt): To clothe, equip, educate or train those with disabilities to function better in their environment. — habilitation, n.

habit: 1. A constant automatic response to a given situation, acquired by frequent repetition; when applied to thoughts, thinking habits become attitudes that influence behaviour patterns. 2. The repeated, steady use of addictive drugs or narcotics. H. SPASM sudden, rapid, twitching, coordinated movement of muscles of a certain area, habitually repeated, voluntary at first, becoming involuntary; H. TRAINING teaching a child to acquire certain habits that will enable the child to adjust to their environment as they grow, primarily habits related to eating, dressing, sleeping, and elimination.

habitual (ha-bit′-ū-al): 1. Formed or established, by frequent repetition. 2. Usual, frequent, steady, much seen or done, or used. H. ABORTION abortion occurring spontaneously three or more times, always before the 20th week of a pregnancy.

habituation (ha-bit-ū-ā′-shun): The act or process of becoming accustomed to a stimulus or environment. DRUG H. psychological dependence on a drug when there is no physical need for it; the craving for the pleasurable or desirable effects of a drug is usually followed by its compulsive use. Usually there is no tendency to increase the dose and, on this basis, H. is often differentiated from drug addiction.

habitus (hab′-i-tus): The physical characteristics of a person, particularly the tendency to develop some disease or such fault as an inborn error of metabolism.

hacking (hak′-ing): 1. Short, chopping blows; a manoeuvre used in massage. 2. Short, dry, interrupted coughing.

haem-, haema-, haemat-, haemo-: Combining forms denoting blood.

haemafaecia (hēm-a-fē′-si-a, he-ma-): Blood in the faeces.

haemagglutination (hē′-ma-gloo′-ti-nā′-shun, hem′-a-): Clumping of red blood cells; may be caused by antibodies or viruses.

haemagglutinin (hē′-ma-gloo′-ti-nin, hem′-a-): A substance that agglutinates (clumps) red blood cells.

haemagogue (hēm′-a-gog, he′-ma-): An agent that promotes the flow of blood, especially the menstrual flow.

haemangioblastoma (hē-man′-ji-ō-blas-tō′-ma): A tumour of immature blood vessels, especially of the capillaries of the cerebellum; may be associated with polycythaemia (*q.v.*).

haemangioma (hē-man′-ji-ō′-ma): A benign lesion of blood vessels that may occur in any part of the body. When it occurs in the skin it may be called *birthmark, port wine stain*, or *strawberry mark*. CAVERNOUS H. a benign tumour made up of large thin-walled blood vessels. — haemangiomatoma, pl.; haemangiomatous, adj.

haemangiosarcoma (hē-man′-ji-ō-sar-kō′-ma): A malignant neoplasm composed of anaplastic cells derived from the blood vessels; highly progressive and infiltrative.

haemarthrosis (hēm-ar-thrō′-sis): The extravasation of blood into a joint or the synovial cavity of a joint.

haematemesis (hē′-ma-tem′-e-sis, hem′-a-): Vomiting of blood; vomitus has bright red colour when the haemorrhage is recent; 'coffee ground' colour indicates blood has been in the stomach long enough to be acted on by the gastric juice.

haematin (hēm′-a-tin, he′-ma-): An iron-containing constituent of haemoglobin.

haematinic (hēm-a-tin′-ik, he′-ma-): 1. Relating to haematin. 2. Any substance required for the production of red blood cells and their constituents. 3. An agent that improves the quality of red blood cells and haemoglobin.

haematoblast (hē′-ma-tō-blast, hem′-a-): 1. A primitive cell from which a blood cell develops. 2. An immature erythrocyte.

haematocele (hē′ma-tō-sēl, hem′-a-): 1. A swelling filled with blood. 2. An effusion of blood into a body cavity or a sac, particularly into the sac that covers the testes.

haematochromatosis (hē′-ma-tō-krō-ma-tō′-sis,hem′-a-): Staining of tissues with blood pigment.

haematocrit (hē-mat′-ō-krit, he′m-a-tō): **1.** The term commonly used to express the percentage of the volume of red blood cells in the blood. **2.** The calibrated tube, the centrifuge, or the procedure used to determine the percentage volume of red cells in the blood.

haematocyst (hē-mat′-ō-sist, hem′a-tō): **1.** A cyst containing blood. **2.** Effusion of blood into the urinary bladder.

haematocyte (hē-mat′-ō-sīt, hem′-a-tō): A blood corpuscle; haemocyte.

haematocytopenia (hē′-ma-tō-sī-tō-pē′-ni-a): A deficiency or decrease in the cellular content of the blood.

haematocytosis (hē′-ma-tō-sī-tō′-sis, hem′-a-): An increase in the cellular content of the blood.

haematocyturia (hē′-ma-tō-sī-tū-ri-a, hem′-a-): The presence of red blood cells in the urine.

haematogenesis (hē′-ma-tō-jen′-e-sis, hem′-a-): The formation of blood or red blood cells.

haematology (hē-ma-tol′-o-ji, hem′-a-): The science dealing with the formation, composition, functions, and diseases of the blood and the morphology of the blood-forming organs. — haematological, adj.; haematologically, adv.

haematoma (hē-ma-tō′-ma, hem′-a-): A localized mass of blood, usually clotted, within a tissue or body part; caused by a break in a blood vessel. EPIDURAL H. a collection of blood between the dura mater and the skull; may also be referred to as EXTRADURAL H.; INTRACRANIAL H. one within the cranium; usually due to loss of venous integrity; H. OF THE BREAST occurs as a result of trauma; may be mistaken for malignant tumour; SUBDURAL H. occurs between the dura mater and the arachnoid; may involve one or both hemispheres of the brain; usually due to trauma but may also be seen in certain blood dyscrasias; signs and symptoms may vary with the patient's age, but usually include depressed consciousness; severe headache, possibly hemiplegia.

haematosepsis (hē-ma-tō-sep′-sis, hem′-a-): Septicaemia (q.v.).

haematotoxin (hē′-ma-tō-toks′-in, hem′-a-): Any substance that causes the destruction of red blood cells. Also called haemotoxin.

haematozoa (hē′-ma-tō-zō′-a, hem′-a-): Animal parasites living in the bloodstream. — haematozoon, sing.

haematuria (hē-ma-tū′-ri-a, hem′-a-): The presence of red blood cells in the urine; caused by bleeding in any part of the urinary tract. GROSS H. that which can be observed without the use of microscopy. MICROSCOPIC H. that which can be demonstrated only by the use of the microscope.

haem (hēm): The pigment-carrying non-protein portion of haemoglobin. Formerly called haematin.

haemoblast (hē′-mō-blast): An immature blood cell; a blood platelet.

haemocidal (hē-mō-sī′-dal): **1.** Destructive to red blood cells. **2.** An agent that destroys red blood cells.

haemoconcentration (hē′-mō-kon-sen-trā′-shun): Relative increase of volume of red blood cells to volume of plasma, usually due to loss of the latter. May occur in such conditions as shock, burns, diabetes mellitus. The degree of concentration is determined by a haematocrit (q.v.).

haemocyte (hē′ mō-sīt): **1.** A blood corpuscle. **2.** Any blood cell.

haemocytolysis (hē′-mō-sī-tol′-i-sis): Destruction of blood cells.

haemodialyser (hē-mō-dī′ a-lī-zer): A machine for haemodialysis (q.v.). Artificial kidney.

haemodialysis (hē′-mō dī al′ i sis): A process of removing metabolic waste products, other poisons, and excess fluids from the blood and replacing essential blood constituents by a process of diffusion through a semi-permeable membrane. Such a technique is used in the artificial kidney. The patient's blood is diverted from a blood vessel by cannula and tubing into a dialysis machine where it is treated and then returned to the patient's circulation by another cannula inserted into a different vessel. May be used in treatment of acute or chronic renal failure, drug overdosage, hepatic coma, or other situations in which the natural kidney function is inadequate.

haemodilution (hē′-mō-dī-lū′-shun): A condition in the blood in which the ratio of blood cells to plasma is reduced. It is the first step in the reconstitution of the blood after severe blood loss. Also a natural occurrence during pregnancy.

haemodynamics (hē′-mō-dī-nam′-iks): Study of the movement of blood in the body and of the forces and mechanisms involved.

haemoglobin (hē-mō-glō′-bin): The oxygen-carrying colouring matter in the red blood cells. It is composed of an iron-containing substance called haem (q.v.) combined with globin. Has the reversible function of combining with and releasing oxygen. See OXYHAEMOGLOBIN. SICKLE CELL H. the haemoglobin found in sickle cell anaemia; see under ANAEMIA.

haemoglobinaemia (hē'-mō-glō-bi-nē'-mi-a): Free haemoglobin in the blood plasma. PAR-OXYSMAL H. haemolysis occurring during sleep; usually associated with intramuscular thrombosis, a rare condition.

haemoglobinopathy (hē'-mō-glō-bi-nop'-a-thi): Any disease caused by an abnormality of the haemoglobin; many are caused by inherited erythrocytic deficits, *e.g.*, sickle cell anaemia.

haemolysin (hē-mol'-i-sin): Any agent or condition that causes disintegration of red blood cells by liberating their haemoglobin.

haemolysis (hē-mol'-i-sis): Laking; disintegration of red blood cells with liberation of contained haemoglobin. May be caused by bacterial toxins, antibodies, immune bodies, various chemical agents, freezing or heating, venom of various snakes, hypotonic salt solution. Causes reddish discoloration of urine. See ANAEMIA, HAEMOGLOBINAEMIA. — haemolytic, adj.; haemolyse, v.

haemolytic (hē-mō-lit'-ik): 1. Relating to haemolysis. 2. Being able to cause haemolysis. H. ANAEMIA see under ANAEMIA. H. DISEASE OF THE NEWBORN see ERYTHROBLASTOSIS FETALIS. H. STREPTOCOCCI see LANCEFIELD'S GROUPS.

haemolytic uraemic syndrome: An acute condition occurring chiefly in infants, characterized by bloody diarrhoea, haemolytic anaemia, thrombocytopenia, and azotaemia; cause unknown; sometimes follows respiratory infection. Most frequent cause of renal failure in children.

haemoperfusion (hē'-mō-per-fū'-zhun): The passing of blood over an absorbent material to remove a toxic substance; activated charcoal is often used.

haemophagia (hē-mō-fa'-ji-a): Phagocytosis (*q.v.*) of red blood cells.

haemophilia (hē-mō-fil'-i-a): An inherited bleeding disease found mainly in males and transmitted through carrier females. Under special genetic circumstances, females with H. may be produced. Patient is subject to prolonged bleeding following minor injuries. CLASSIC H., HAEMOPHILIA A. due to deficiency in activity of factor VIII. HAEMOPHILIA B. Christmas disease, is due to deficiency of activity of factor IX. See also VON WILLEBRAND'S DISEASE.

haemophiliac (hē-mō-fil'-i-ak): 1. Relating to haemophilia. 2. A person afflicted with haemophilia.

haemophilic (hē-mō-fil'-ik): 1. Relating to haemophilia. 2. Blood-loving; said of microorganisms.

Haemophilus (hē-mof'-i-lus): A genus of bacteria; small Gram-negative rods that vary greatly in shape; strict parasites that require the presence of certain accessory substances in the blood for their growth; found in the respiratory tracts of vertebrates and often associated with acute and chronic diseases such as influenza, whooping cough, pink-eye. See DUCREY'S BACILLUS. H. AEGYPTIUS the causative agent of catarrhal conjunctivities (pink-eye); H. INFLUENZAE TYPE B. the causative agent of such serious pyogenic infections as meningitis, pneumonia, otitis media, croup, and bacteraemia, particularly in children; early symptoms may be mistaken for those of a common cold; sequelae may include deafness, partial paralysis, and mental handicap. H. VAGINITIS see under GARDNERELLA VAGINITIS.

haemopneumothorax (hē'-mō-nū-mō-thor'-aks): The presence of blood and air in the pleural cavity causing compression of lung tissue.

haemopoiesis (hē'-mō-poy-ē'-sis): The formation and development of the various types of blood cells.

haemopoietic (hē'-mō-poy-et'-ik): 1. Relating to the formation of blood cells. 2. An agent that affects the production of blood cells. H. SYSTEM the tissues concerned with the production of blood, including the lymphatic tissues and bone marrow.

haemoproctia (hē-mō-prok'-shi-a): Haemorrhage from the rectum.

haemoptysis (hē-mop'-tis-is): The coughing up of blood or blood-stained sputum. — haemoptyses, pl.

haemorrhage (hem'-or-rij): The escape of copious amounts of blood from a vessel by diapedesis through a vessel wall or by direct outflow through a break in the vessel walls. The terms ARTERIAL H., VENOUS H., and CAPILLARY H. designate the type of vessel from which it escapes. PRIMARY H. occurs at the time of surgery or injury. SECONDARY H. may also occur after surgery or injury but after a considerable time has elapsed. ACCIDENTAL ANTEPARTUM H. bleeding from separation of a normally situated placenta after the 28th week of pregnancy. The term *placental abruption* is now preferred. ANTEPARTAL H. vaginal bleeding before the onset of labour; BRONCHIAL H. haemoptysis; CEREBRAL H., H. into the substance of the cerebrum; CONCEALED H. internal H.; EXTRADURAL H. extravasation of blood into the space between the skull and the dura mater.; GASTRIC H., H. into the stomach; INTERNAL H., H. with the extravasated blood remaining in one of the organs or cavities of the body; INTRACEREBRAL H., H. within the substance of the brain; INTRAPARTAL H. occurs during labour; MASSIVE H. loss of a large amount of blood in a short time; NASAL H. epistaxis; PETECHIAL H. bleeding from small capillaries into the skin, forming petechiae; POSTMENOPAUSAL H. vaginal blood loss after menopause; requires immediate attention; may indicate presence of a malignancy; POSTPARTUM H. excessive bleeding within 24 hours after giving birth; PULMONARY H. haemoptysis; REACTIONARY H. a surgical complication that may occur in the first 12 to 24 hours after surgery; caused by dislodgement of an insecure or loose suture; SUBARACHNOID H. bleeding into the space between the arachnoid and the pia mater; SUBDURAL H. bleeding into the space between the dura mater and the arachnoid. — haemorrhage, v.; haemorrhagic, adj.

haemorrhagic (hem-ŏ-raj'-ik): Relating to or marked by haemorrhage. H. DISEASE OF THE NEWBORN a tendency to bleeding in the neonatal period; results from deficiency of vitamin K-dependent blood clotting factors II, VII, IX and X and prolonged prothrombin time; erythroblastosis fetalis (q.v.). H. PURPURA purpura haemorrhagica (q.v.).

haemorrhoid (hem'-o-royd): Varicosity of a vein in the rectal area. EXTERNAL H. one outside of the anal sphincter covered with skin. INTERNAL H. one inside the anal sphincter covered with mucous membrane.

haemorrhoidal (hem-o-royd'-al): 1. Relating to haemorrhoids. 2. Applied to nerves and blood vessels in the anal region.

haemorrhoidectomy (hem'-o-royd-ek'-to-mi): Surgical removal of the haemorrhoids.

haemosiderosis (hē'-mō-sid-er-ō'-sis): A condition in which haemosiderin accumulates in the tissues; occurs in diseases in which there is marked destruction of red blood cells; may be associated with several types of anaemia, chronic infection, malnutrition; often affects the kidney and lung.

haemostasis (hē-mō-stā'-sis, hē-mos'ta-sis): 1. Arrest of bleeding. 2. Stagnation of blood within its vessel, due to interruption of its flow.

haemostat (hē'-mō-stat): 1. An agent that arrests bleeding. 2. An instrument for constricting a blood vessel to stop or control the flow of blood.

haemostatic (hē-mō-stat'-ik): 1. An agent that arrests bleeding. 2. Having the effect of arresting bleeding.

haemothorax (hē-mō-thō'-raks): The presence of bloody fluid in the pleural cavity.

Hageman factor: Factor XII. See under FACTOR.

Hagie pin: A pin used in surgical treatment of fracture of the hip.

Hahnemannian (hah-ne-man'-i-an): Relating to Hahnemann or to the doctrine of homeopathy which he taught. See HOMEOPATHY. — Hahnemannism, n.

hair: Thread-like filament present on all parts of the human skin except the palms, soles, lips, glans penis and that surrounding the terminal phalanges. Also the aggregation of such filaments, especially on the scalp. Consists of a shaft and a bulb-like root. EXCLAMATION-MARK H. the broken off stump found at the periphery of spreading bald patches in alopecia areata; atrophic thinning of the hair shaft gives this characteristic shape — hence its name; H. CELLS usually pertains to the hairs in the organ of Corti in the inner ear, they function as receptors for the sensation of sound. H. FOLLICLE see under FOLLICLE. H. PULLING trichotillomania. H. TRANSPLANTATION the surgical process of transplanting hair follicles from one part of the scalp to another, a time-consuming technique that is sometimes used to correct baldness.

hairball: Trichobezoar (q.v.).

hairy tongue: A condition in which the filiform papillae of the tongue become enlarged and discoloured, due to the presence of bacteria and food pigments. May also occur as a side effect of certain antibiotics.

halal ((ha-lal'): Used to describe meat from animals that have been slaughtered in the ritual way prescribed by Islamic law, or relating to such meat.

Haldane effect: The amount of carbon dioxide that can be carried by the blood as carbamino-haemoglobin decreases when the pO_2 of the blood increases. [John S. Haldane, British physiologist, 1860–1936.]

half-life: 1. The time it takes the radioactivity of a substance to decay to one-half its original value. 2. In pharmacology, the time it takes for the concentration of a drug to decrease by one-half in the blood serum; used to determine the optimum dosing interval to provide the person with therapeutic but non-toxic dosage.

halfway house: A special residence for individuals who do not need full-time hospital care but are not yet ready to return to independent community living, or who are not able to behave in a manner acceptable to the community at large.

halibut liver oil: A very rich source of vitamins A and D. The smaller dose required makes it more acceptable than cod liver oil.

halitosis (hal-i-tō′ -sis): Bad breath. Often due to poor oral hygiene, but may also be caused by oral infections, dental problems, certain foods, alcohol, smoking, systemic disease.

hallucination (ha-lū′ -si-nā′ -shun): A sensory experience of something that does not exist; unique to the individual; occurs without any true sensory stimulus but regarded by the person as real. May be auditory, gustatory, olfactory, kinetic, tactile, or visual. A common symptom in severe schizophrenia and confusional states; may be induced by drugs, alcohol, or stress. COMMAND H., H. in which the person is 'commanded' by imaginery voices to perform certain acts; HYPNAGOGIC H. occurs at a time between sleep and wakefulness; KINAESTHETIC H. involves a false perception of the sensation of movement; LILLIPUTIAN H., H. of small objects or animals, often rapidly moving; SENSORY H. involves a mental impression of sensory vividness without any external stimulation; includes H.s of taste, smell, hearing, vision; VISCERAL H. involves visceral sensations. — hallucinatory, adj.

hallucinogen (ha-lū′ -si-nō-jen): An agent, drug, or specifically, a chemical such as mescaline or LSD, that is capable of altering the perception of sensations such as sight, sound, and touch, and of producing hallucinations.

hallucinogenic (ha-lū′ -si-nō-jen′ -ik): 1. Relating to a stimulus that creates the impression that one is having a hallucination. 2. Relating to hallucinogens.

hallucinosis (ha-lū-si-nō′ -sis): A psychosis in which the patient is grossly hallucinated, although in a state of clear consciousness. Usually a subacute state of delirium; the predominant symptoms are auditory, gustatory, or visual illusions and hallucinations. ALCOHOLIC H. that occurring in chronic alcoholism.

hallux (hal′ -uks): The great toe. H. DOLOROSUS pain in the great toe, especially when walking, often associated with flatfoot; H. FLEXUS hammertoe involving the great toe; H. RIGIDUS ankylosis and progressive loss of motion in the great toe joint, may be due to arthritis, trauma, or deformity; H. VALGUS lateral deviation of the great toe, as in a bunion; H. VARUS inward deviation of the great toe.

halo (hā′ -lō): A circle of light, particularly the flashing coloured circles seen around lights by patients with glaucoma. H. TRACTION see under TRACTION.

halogen (hal′ -ō-jen): Any one of a family of elements that includes bromine, chlorine, fluorine, and iodine.

halothane (hal′ -ō-thān): A clear, colourless, non-explosive liquid used as an inhalation anaesthetic.

Halsted's operation: 1. Radical mastectomy including removal of the supraclavicular lymph nodes; done for cancer of the breast, see also MASTECTOMY. 2. Radical surgery for correction of inguinal hernia.

hamartoma (ham-ar-tō′ -ma): A malformation that resembles a neoplasm but is caused by faulty development of an organ. There is an abnormal arrangement or proportion of the elements normally found in the particular location; the malformation grows at the same rate as normal tissues grow. — harmartomatous, adj.

hamate (ham′ -āt): The medial bone in the second row of wrist bones. Also called *hamatum*.

hammer: The hammer-shaped bone of the middle ear; the malleus. PERCUSSION H. a rubber-headed hammer used to tap various parts of the body to produce sounds for diagnostic purposes; REFLEX H. rubber-headed hammer for tapping tendons, muscles or nerves to elicit reflexes during physical examination.

hammertoe: A claw-like deformity of the foot in which there is permanent hyperextension of the first phalanx and plantar flexion of the second and third phalanges. May be congenital or the result of hallux valgus (*q.v.*) or too tight shoes.

hamstring: Name given to (1) the tendons on either side of the popliteal space; (2) the three muscles on the posterior aspect of the thigh; their function is to flex the leg at the knee and to adduct and extend the thigh; they are the semimembranous, semitendinous, and biceps femoris muscles.

handedness: A tendency to prefer to use one or the other hand in all voluntary motor acts, depending on cerebral dominance, *i.e.*, in a right-handed person the left side of the cerebrum is dominant, and vice versa.

hand–foot syndrome: A condition seen in patients with sickle cell haemoglobinopathy. There is painful swelling of the hands and feet, occurring at about two years of age; in older persons other joints are affected; caused by an impairment in circulation to the metacarpal and metatarsal bones.

hand roll: A roll of cloth or cylinder-shape object held in the hand to counteract the tendency to remain contracted and closed or loosely open and flaccid. The objective is to prevent contractures by keeping the hand in a functional position.

hangnail (hang'-nāl): A narrow strip of skin, partly detached from the nail fold.

hangover: Popular term for the headache, nausea, thirst, fatigue, irritability, and other unpleasant after-effects, usually occurring in the morning, after overindulgence in alcoholic beverages or other central nervous system depressants.

haploid (hap'-loid): Having half the number of chromosomes normally carried by the particular cell or cells.

hapten (hap'-ten): A low molecular weight chemical that does not itself induce antibody formation but enhances the antibody response to a carrier molecule to which it binds.

haptoglobins (hap-tō-glō'-binz): Globulins that bind any free haemoglobin in the blood plasma and then allow it to be excreted in the urine; increased in any inflammatory disease and in patients on steroid therapy; decreased in haemolysis, severe liver disease, and infectious mononucleosis.

hard drug: An illegal substance, such as heroin, that is physiologically addictive and causes long-term harmful effects. A term used in relation to drug misuse.

harlequin colour change: A condition sometimes seen in normal newborns, especially the immature. A transient redness of the skin that develops on the side on which the baby is lying; the coloration stops abruptly at the midline.

Harrington rod: Part of the Harrington distraction system for correcting scoliosis; consists of a rigid rod that is wedged beneath the lamina of the vertebrae at either end of the curve on the concave side and then forcibly opened to the degree possible during a fusion operation; the rod remains *in situ*.

Hartmann's solution: A saline solution containing sodium lactate; used in treating acidosis. Lactated Ringer's solution (*q.v.*).

Hartnup disease: A disease believed to be due to an inborn error of protein metabolism. Associated with a learning disability. Characterized by red scaly rash following exposure to sunlight, cerebellar ataxia, emotional instability.

Harvey, William: Noted English physician [1578–1657]; discovered how the blood circu-lates in the body; expounded his theory of circulation in 1628.

Harvey–Rand–Rittler plates: Any one of several polychromatic plates used in assessing colour vision.

Hashimoto's disease: An autoimmune thyroid disorder characterized by the production of antibodies in response to thyroid antigens and the replacement of normal thyroid structures with lymphocytes and lymphoid germinal centres. The thyroid, typically enlarged and lumpy on the surface, shows dense lymphatic infiltration, and the remaining thyroid tissue frequently contains small empty follicles. The goitre is usually asymptomatic, but symptoms occasionally include dysphagia and a feeling of local pressure. Also called *Hashimoto's thyroiditis, struma lymphomatosa* and *lymphadenoid goitre*. See AUTOIMMUNIZATION. [H. Hashimoto, Japanese surgeon, 1881–1934.]

hashish, hasheesh (hash'-ēsh): A resinous product of *Cannabis sativa*, see CANNABIS.

Hassall's corpuscle: A characteristic, rounded body in the medulla of the thymus gland; it is considered to be the source of thymosin, which has some of the properties of a hormone. Also called *Hassall's body*.

haunch: The hip and buttock.

haustration (haws-trā'-shun): 1. Haustrum (*q.v.*). 2. The formation of a haustrum.

haustrum (haw'-strum): One of the sacculations in the colon; these sacculations or pouches are caused by the longitudinal bands along the colon that are slightly shorter than the gut itself. — haustra, pl.; haustral, adj.

Haversian (ha-ver'-shan): H. SYSTEM the make-up of the compact bone. Consists of a central canal that contains blood vessels, lymphatics, nerves; lamellae (*q.v.*) arranged around the canal; spaces between the lamellae are called lacunae; and the fine channels are called canaliculi, which bring nutrients and oxygen to the osteocytes. H. CANALS see above. [Clopton Havers, English physician, 1650–1702.]

Hawthorne effect: An increase in worker productivity produced by the psychological stimulus of being singled out and made to feel important.

hay fever: A seasonal form of allergic rhinitis in which the release of histamine in response to exposure to a pollen, or other antigen to which the individual is sensitive, results in irritation of the conjunctiva and the mucous membranes of the upper respiratory tract.

Haygarth's nodes: Swelling of joints (exostoses) sometimes seen in the fingers of patients suffering from arthritis. [John Haygarth, English physician, 1740–1827.]

HAZ: Abbreviation for Health Action Zone (*q.v.*).

Hb: Abbreviation for haemoglobin. (*q.v.*).

HBcAg: Abbreviation for hepatitis B core antigen.

HBeAg: Abbreviation for hepatitis B e antigen.

HBIG: Abbreviation for hepatitis B immunoglobulin.

HBsAg: Abbreviation for hepatitis B surface antigen (*q.v.*).

HBV: Abbreviation for hepatitis B virus, see HEPATITIS.

HC: Abbreviation for head circumference (*q.v.*).

HCA: Abbreviation for health-care assistant (*q.v.*).

hCG: Abbreviation for human chorionic gonadotrophin, obtained from the placenta. HCG TEST a serology test using anti-hCG, which will show the presence or absence of hCG in the serum; a positive test result is a reliable indicator of pregnancy.

HCO: Abbreviation for health-care officer (*q.v.*)

HCV: Abbreviation for hepatitis C virus.

HDL: Abbreviation for high-density lipoprotein.

HDU: Abbreviation for high-dependency unit.

head: 1. The uppermost structure of the body, containing the brain and organs of hearing, speech, smell, and taste. 2. The superior or uppermost part of an organ or structure. 3. A rounded eminence on a bone that articulates with another bone at a joint. H. NOISES see TINNITUS.

headache: Pain or ache in the head. Often accompanied by nausea, as in migraine H. Of many types; described both as to location and quality of the pain; frontal, one-sided, top-of-the-head, sharp, dull, pulsating or throbbing, steady, intermittent, depressing. May be hereditary or familial, and of sudden or gradual onset. Causes include worry, lack of sleep, fatigue, hunger, tension, anxiety, high blood pressure, epilepsy, indigestion, constipation, liver and kidney disorders, allergy, eye disorders, sinusitis, fever, onset of a communicable disease, intake of certain foods, *e.g.*, chocolate, or premenstrual tension. CLUSTER H. migrainous neuralgia; occurs in clusters, with attacks several times a day for days or weeks, followed by long headache-free periods; the intense pain is unilateral, located in the eye region, and accompanied by coryza, tearing, flush, and constricted pupil; MIGRAINE H. see MIGRAINE; OCULAR H. results from a pathological or functional disorder of one or more ocular structures; SICK H. migraine H.; SINUS H. caused by congestion and oedema of the nasal and paranasal mucous membranes; may be related to allergens, infection, or some anatomical anomaly; TENSION H. due to habitual overwork or emotional strain; TRACTION H. caused by stretching of intracranial structures by a space-occupying lesion; VASCULAR H. migraine H.

head box: A device that fits loosely around the head; used in oxygen therapy for pre-term infants and small babies to confine oxygen-rich atmosphere.

head circumference: The measurement of a child's head along its largest dimension (above the eyebrows and ears and around the back of the head). During routine check-ups, the distance is measured in centimetres and compared to previous measurements; normal ranges are based on sex and age (weeks, months). Values for normal growth rates of infants' and young children's heads have been incorporated into standardized graphs for girls and boys from birth to 18 months of age. A deviation from the expected normal head growth may alert the nurse to a developing problem.

head halter: See HALTER TRACTION, under TRACTION.

headward acceleration: In aerospace travel, the acceleration of the body forward following the direction of the head; this causes the blood to rush from the head downwards in the body.

Heaf multiple puncture test: A test for tuberculosis that utilizes a stainless-steel disc with four prongs or tines, precoated with tuberculin, a purified protein derivative of tubercle bacilli; when the tines are pressed against the volar surface of the forearm; they penetrate the outer layer of skin. The test is said to be positive if a hard raised red spot develops around the puncture area. Also called *tine test*.

healing (hē'-ling): Curing. The natural process of getting well or of repair of disordered body parts or tissues. H. BY FIRST INTENTION occurs when the edges of a clean wound are accurately held together and heal with the minimum of scarring and deformity; H. BY SECOND INTENTION occurs when the edges of a wound unite after the formation of granular tissue; H. BY THIRD INTENTION occurs when granular tissue fills the wound cavity, followed by the formation of scar tissue.

health: 1. The state in which an organism is in homeostatic balance, with inputs and outputs of energy and mass in approximate equilibrium, and positive prospects for continued survival. It is a subjective experience and includes emotional well-being. **2.** The WHO definition: a state of complete physical, mental and social well-being and not merely the absence of disease or infirmity (WHO, 1946: 100).

Health Action Zone: Designated areas of deprivation and ill-health in England and Northern Ireland established by the government to tackle health inequalities and modernize services through local innovation. These communities vary significantly in their local characteristics, yet they face common problems of ill-health and disadvantage.

Health and Safety Commission: A body that, along with the Health and Safety Executive, regulates most of the risks to health and safety in the UK. Together they protect people's health and safety by ensuring that risks in the workplace are properly controlled. http://www.hse.gov.uk

Health and Safety Executive: See HEALTH AND SAFETY COMMISSION.

health assessment: An evaluation of a person's state of health based on data obtained from the health history and the physical examination.

health behaviour: Any health maintenance activity that is undertaken by an individual who believes himself to be healthy, as opposed to illness behaviour, which refers to activities undertaken by one who has symptoms of illness.

health care: A service sought by people who need help for physical or emotional problems. H.C. INSTITUTIONS institutions devoted to the care of the sick, aged, or infirm; includes hospitals, hospices, health clinics, nursing homes and convalescent homes. PRIMARY H.C. includes ambulatory care, treatment of acute illnesses and disabilities, management of common chronic disorders, guidance and counselling to individuals and families, preventive measures.

health-care assistant: A worker who supports health-care professionals in the delivery of care. Abbreviated HCA.

health-care officer: A registered nurse within the prison service; a specialist prison officer who has undertaken relevant training. Abbreviated HCO.

health-care system: The World Health Organization uses this term to describe the means by which a government organizes the administration of healthcare policies and services. In the UK, healthcare is provided primarily through the National Health Service and is the respon-

sibility of the Department of Health headed by a Secretary of State and a team of Ministers accountable to Parliament. Private healthcare also exists outside government control and is paid for by the consumer.

health-care team: A group of health-care professionals working both independently and collaboratively in providing healthcare to patients; may include physicians, nurses, social workers, various therapists.

health centre: A community provision centred around the general practitioner's services linking local health agencies in providing healthcare to clients and patients within their own homes and communities.

Health Committee: A board appointed by the House of Commons to examine the expenditure, administration, and policy of the Department of Health and its associated bodies.

health economics: A social system that studies the supply and demand of health-care resources and the impact of health services on a population.

health education: Informing people of health issues, to increase awareness and influence the attitudes and knowledge relating to the improvement of health. It can work on a number of levels, from the individual to the entire community. Its success depends upon acknowledging both health beliefs and individuals' perceptions about their susceptibility and the seriousness of disease. See HEALTH PROMOTION.

health history: Data obtained from the patient, family, and other sources regarding present and past physical and psychological health; used in diagnosing present illness and in planning care and follow-up.

Health Improvement Programme: A document produced by each health authority in England, setting out the strategic framework for improving health, reducing inequalities, and delivering faster, more responsive services of a consistently high standard.

health informatics (in-for-mat'-iks): The knowledge, skills, and tools which enable information to be collected, managed, used, and shared to support the delivery of healthcare and to promote health. See also Appendix 7.

Health of the Nation Outcome Scale: A measure of the health and social functioning of people with severe mental illness. It consists of a 12-item instrument that measures behaviour, impairment, symptoms, and social functioning.

Health Professions Council: An independent, UK-wide regulatory body responsible for setting and maintaining standards of professional training, performance, and conduct of the 12 health-care professions that it regulates; *e.g.,* art therapists, paramedics, and dieticians. www.hpc-uk.org

health promotion: A term used to describe any measure aimed at health improvement for individuals, communities, or the population. The World Health Organization (WHO) identified health promotion strategy as: building public policy; creating supportive environments for health; developing personal skills; strengthening community action; and reorientation of health services from treatment to preventative approaches. See HEALTH EDUCATION.

Health Service Ombudsman/Commissioner (om' -buds-man, kom-mish' -un-er): An official appointed to protect the interest of patients in the administration and provision of healthcare provided by the NHS. He or she undertakes independent investigations and is responsible directly to Parliament.

health services evaluation: An investigation into the success of programmes such as drug rehabilitation. See HEALTH SERVICES RESEARCH.

health services research: Applied research that examines the practical problems and decisions associated with healthcare. See HEALTH SERVICES EVALUATION.

health statistics: Summated data on any aspect of the health of populations.

Health Technology Assessment Programme: A national syllabus of research established and funded by the Department of Health. Its purpose is to ensure that high-quality information on costs, effectiveness, and the impact of health technologies is produced for those who manage and provide care in the NHS.

health visitor: In the UK, a registered nurse who has undertaken an approved course leading to a qualification in health visiting and is registered to practise as a health visitor. The health visitor works within the community promoting good health and providing preventive care primarily to mothers with children under five years, although some health visitors work within the school health service and in preventive care for the elderly. Abbreviated HV.

hearing: 1. The special sense that enables one to perceive sound. **2.** The ability to perceive the sensation of sound. H. LOSS impairment in ability to hear, sometimes within only certain frequencies. May be (1) CONDUCTIVE LOSS due to damage to the conducting mechanism of the ear, usually by a congenital malformation or an obstruction, or may be the result of

infection; (2) MIXED LOSS consisting of both conductive and sensorineural loss; or (3) SENSORINEURAL LOSS due to damage to the organ of Corti (*q.v.*), the cochlear nerve, or the auditory branch of the acoustic nerve. H. TEST any test of one's ability to hear, usually by means of an audiometer or tuning fork; RESIDUAL H. the amount of hearing that a hard-of-hearing person has retained.

hearing aid: Any of several types of devices worn in or near the external auditory canal to improve hearing. The type which is worn on the body has a receiver that is worn in the external auditory canal and is connected by an electric cord to a case containing a microphone, amplifier, transmitter, and battery. Many all-in-the-ear types are available.

Hearing Voices Network: An organization offering information, support, and understanding to people who hear voices and those who support them. Its aims are: to raise awareness of voice hearing, visions, tactile sensations, and other sensory experiences; give those who have these experiences an opportunity to talk freely about them; and support anyone with these experiences seeking to deal with them in their own way.

heart: The hollow muscular organ that pumps blood through the body; situated behind the sternum, lying obliquely between the two lungs. It weighs 227 to 340 grams in the female and 283 to 340 grams in the male. The heart is made up of four chambers, the right and left atria and the right and left ventricles. The muscular heart wall has three layers; the outer serous layer, the epicardium; the middle muscular layer, the myocardium; and the inner membranous layer, the endocardium. The flow of blood into, out of, and through the heart is controlled by valves. The heart is enclosed in a fibroserous sac, the epicardium, and the space between it and the pericardium is called the pericardial cavity. H. ARREST cardiac arrest, see under CARDIAC; HEART ATTACK see MYOCARDIAL INFARCTION under INFARCTION; H. CATHETERIZATION cardiac catheterization, see under CATHETERIZATION; H. FAILURE sudden fatal stoppage of the heartbeat as may occur in coronary thrombosis; when it is the result of failure to maintain adequate circulation in all parts of the body there is congestion of blood in the portal and pulmonary circulations, and then it is called congestive heart failure; H. MASSAGE cardiac massage, see under CARDIAC; H. MURMUR see MURMUR; H. RATE the number of times the heartbeats per minute; H. SOUNDS four sounds heard over the heart area are recognized; the first sound (lub), S_1, is dull and prolonged; it coincides with the closing of the mitral and tricuspid valves and the beginning of ventricular systole. The second sound (dup), S_2, coincides with the closing of the aortic and pulmonary valves and the beginning of the filling of the atria. The third sound is dull, weak, and low-pitched; may be heard most clearly over the apex; is often compared to the sound of Ken-tuk´-kē; is caused by the rapid filling of the ventricles and may be normal in children and adults; may also indicate some cardiac pathology, hypertension or congestive heart failure. The fourth sound is heard best at the apex during atrial contraction and may or may not be considered pathological. When the third and fourth sounds are considered pathological they are referred to as gallop. See also GALLOP, CLICK, MURMUR, THRILL; HEART STROKE VOLUME see under VOLUME; H. VALVES the valves that control and regulate the flow of blood through and from the heart; they are the atrioventricular (mitral and tricuspid), aortic, and pulmonary valves.

heart block: Partial or complete inhibition of the conduction of the electrical impulse from the atrium to the ventricle of the heart. The cause may be an organic lesion or a functional disturbance. In its mildest form it can only be detected electrocardiographically, while in its complete form the ventricles beat at their own intrinsic rate uninfluenced by the atria. Usually described according to degree: first-degree block, all impulses from the atria reach the ventricles but only after lengthy delay at the A-V node; second-degree block, some but not all of the impulses from the atria reach the ventricles; third-degree block, all conditions for A-V conduction are present but conduction does not take place. ATRIOVENTRICULAR B. delay or interruption in conduction of impulses through the A-V node and bundle of His; heart block; BUNDLE BRANCH B. complete or incomplete blockage of conduction in either right or left branch of the bundle of His (q.v.), or of both branches; COMPLETE HEART B. a blockage of conduction of all atrial impulses in the heart, often refers specifically to atrioventricular block; CONGENITAL HEART B. present at birth; due to defective development of the conduction tissues of the heart; HEMIBLOCK, of either the anterior or posterior branch of one of the fascicles of the left branch of the bundle of His; INTRA-ATRIAL B. interference with conduction through the atria; INTRAVENTRICULAR

B. delayed conduction through the ventricles or the myocardium; MOBITZ TYPE I B. impulses from the atria to the ventricles are delayed for increasingly longer periods of time until finally one impulse is not conducted at all and then the cycle starts over again. May be caused by certain drugs or be associated with myocardial infarction; sometimes hereditary. Usually transient and may not require treatment; MOBITZ TYPE II B. the block between the atria and ventricles is in one of the bundle branches; may be congenital but usually associated with the use of certain drugs or due to the effects of myocardial infarction, or of sclerosing, on the conduction system; MONOFASCICULAR B. a slowing of conduction velocity or a block in a fascicle of the right or left bundle branch; SINUS B. a block in the conduction system between the sinoatrial node and the atria; results in a complete cardiac cycle being stopped. See also WENCKE-BACH PHENOMENON.

heartburn: A vague scalding or burning sensation felt behind the sternum, usually associated with acid regurgitation after eating; caused by incompetence of the sphincter muscle at the lower end of the oesophagus; usually follows ingestion of fatty foods, caffeine, or nicotine; may be relieved by ingestion of certain medicinal substances, antacids in particular. Also called *pyrosis* and *waterbrash*.

heart–lung machine: A mechanical pump used in heart surgery; it shunts the blood from the venous circulation through the machine where it is oxygenated, and returns it to the arterial circulation.

heat: 1. The form of energy that produces a sensation of warmth opposed to cold. 2. To expose a substance, or the body, to a source of heat that characteristically causes an increase in the temperature of the substance or the body. 3. The sensation of an increase in temperature. H. CRAMPS spasms of voluntary muscles; usually occur in otherwise healthy persons following exercise during hot weather; due to loss of sodium chloride and water through excessive sweating; H. EXHAUSTION collapse, with or without loss of consciousness, suffered in conditions of heat and high humidity, resulting largely from loss of fluid and salt by sweating; if the surrounding air becomes saturated, heat stroke will ensue, characterized by pallor, cold clammy skin, rapid pulse, normal or subnormal temperature; H. FLASH a sudden transitory sensation of warmth; may involve the entire body; occurs as a symptom during menopause; H. OF VAPORIZATION the amount of heat needed to convert water into steam over and above that needed to bring it to the boiling point; this amount is released when steam is reconverted into water; H. PRODUCTION in the body, is accomplished chiefly by metabolism; H. RASH see MILIARIA. H. STROKE a serious condition produced by prolonged exposure to excessive temperatures; symptoms include hot, dry skin, headache dizziness, rapid pulse, high fever; in severe cases coma and death may ensue; see H. exhaustion; H. SYNCOPE dizziness, fatigue and sudden faintness after exercising in the heat; accompanied by weak pulse, sweaty pale skin, decrease in blood pressure; recovery follows removal from direct heat. LATENT H. excess body heat that is used up in the evaporation of sweat; PRICKLY H. see MILIARIA; RADIANT H., H. applied to the surface of the body from a source of infrared radiation; SENSIBLE H. heat that results in a rise in temperature of a body when absorbed; SPECIFIC H. The heat required to raise the temperature of 1 gram of a substance 1 degree as compared to that required to raise the temperature of water through 1 degree.

heat labile: Thermolabile (*q.v.*).

hedonism (hē´-don-izm): Excessive devotion to pleasure, so that a person's conduct is determined by an unconscious drive to seek pleasure and avoid unpleasant things.

heelcord: Achilles tendon, see under ACHILLES.

heel spur: A bony projection on the heel, caused by deposit of calcium during healing of chronic injury to the plantar fascia of the calcaneus (*q.v.*).

Hegar's sign: Marked softening of the cervix in early pregnancy. [Alfred Hegar, German gynaecologist, 1830–1914.] See GOODELL'S SIGN.

HEI: Abbreviation for higher education institutions.

Heimlich manoeuvre (hīm´-lik): An emergency procedure for dislodging an object in the trachea that is choking the person. The rescuer stands behind the person, who may be standing or sitting, wraps his arms about the victim, makes a fist with one hand, places it on the person's abdomen above the navel and below the rib cage, grasps the fist with the other hand and makes a quick upwards thrust against the victim's abdomen, causing the diaphragm to contract and force a column of air up against the obstruction. The manoeuvre may have to be repeated several times. If the person is lying down, the rescuer kneels beside the person and executes the same manoeuvre except that the heel of the hand is used instead of the fist. Also called *abdominal thrust man-*

oeuvre and *the hug of life*. [Henry J. Heimlich, American thoracic surgeon, 1920–.]

Heinz bodies: Small, round, oval, or irregularly shaped particles of denatured haemoglobin sometimes found in red blood cells; they indicate potential instability of the cells.

helcosis (hel-kō´-sis): Ulceration; ulcer formation.

heli-, helio-: Combining forms denoting (1) sun, sunlight; (2) solar energy.

helicotrema (hel´-i-kō-trē´-ma): The passage that connects the scala tympani and the scala vestibuli at the apex of the cochlea.

heliosensitivity (hē´-li-ō-sen-si-tiv´-i-ti): Sensitivity to the sun's rays.

helium (hē´-li-um): A colourless, odourless, tasteless, inert gas. Sometimes used in medicine as a diluent for other gases.

helix (hē´-liks): 1. The curved fold forming most of the rim of the external ear. 2. A coiled structure. WATSON–CRICK H., a double H. in which each chain contains information specifying the other chain; it represents the manner in which the genetic factors in DNA (deoxyribonucleic acid) reproduce themselves.

heloma (hē-lō-ma): A corn or callosity on the hand or foot.

hem-, hema-, hemat-, hemo-: For words beginning thus see HAEM-, HAEMA-, HAEMAT-, HAEMATO-.

hemeralopia (hem´-er-a-lō´-pi-a): Defective vision in a bright light with ability to see more distinctly in a dim light; day blindness.

hemi-: Prefix denoting (1) half of, or one-half; (2) affecting half of an organ or part.

hemiachromatopsia (hem´-i-a-krō-ma-top´-si-a): Colour blindness in one half of the visual field of each eye.

hemianaesthesia (hem´-i-an-es-thē´-zi-a): Loss of sensation on one side of the body; unilateral anaesthesia.

hemianalgesia (hem-i-an-al-jē´-zi-a): Loss of sensitivity to pain in one side of the body.

hemianopia (hem´-i-a-nō´-pi-a): Blindness or defective vision in one half of the field of vision, occurring in persons suffering from hemiparesis. BITEMPORAL H. blindness on the temporal side of the field of vision in one or both eyes; HOMONYMOUS H., H. that affects half of the visual fields of both eyes. Also called *heminopsia*.

hemiatrophy (hem-i-at´-ro-fi): Atrophy of one half or one side of the body or of an organ or part. H. FACIALIS a congenital condition, or a manifestation of scleroderma (*q.v.*), in which the structures on one side of the face are shrunken.

hemiblock (hem'-i-block): A block in either the anterior or posterior division of the left branch of the bundle of His.

hemibrachia (hem-i-brā'-ki-a): The congenital absence of one arm.

hemicardia (hem-i-kar'-di-a): A congenital anomaly in which (1) one lateral half of the heart is lacking, or (2) two of the four normal chambers of the heart are lacking.

hemicolectomy (hem'-i-kō-lek'-to-mi): Removal of approximately half the colon.

hemicrania (hem-i-krā'-ni-a): 1. Unilateral headache, as in migraine. 2. Congenital anomaly in which the cerebrum has not developed properly.

hemidiaphragm (hem'-i-dī'-a-fram): 1. One lateral half of the diaphragm. 2. Deficient muscular development of one lateral half of the diaphragm. 3. Paralysis of only half of the diaphragm.

hemidysaesthesia (hem'-i-dis-es-thē'-zi-a): A disorder of sensation affecting only one side of the body.

hemidystrophy (hem-i-dis'-trō-fi): A condition of underdevelopment of one side of the body.

hemihypertrophy (hem'-i-hī-per'-trō-fi): A congenital anomaly in which one half of the body is overdeveloped.

hemilateral (hem-i-lat'-er-al): Relating to or affecting one lateral half of the body or of an organ.

heminephrectomy (hem'-i-nef-rek'-to-mi): Surgical excision of part of a kidney.

hemiparaplegia (hem'-i-par-a-plē'-ji-a): Paralysis of one side of the lower half of the body, or of one lower extremity.

hemiparesis (hem-i-pa-rē'-sis): A slight paralysis or muscular weakness of one half of the body or face. — hemiparetic, adj.

hemiplegia (hem-i-plē'-ji-a): Paralysis of one side of the body, usually resulting from a cerebrovascular accident on the opposite side. FACIAL H., H. affecting one side of the face but not the rest of the body; FLACCID H., H. in which the muscles of the affected side lose their tone and tendon reflexes are lost; SPASTIC H., H. in which the muscles of the affected side are spastic and the tendon reflexes are increased.

hemisphere (hem'-i-sfēr): Half of a sphere or half of any spherical structure or organ; term commonly applied to either half of the cerebrum or the cerebellum.

Henry's law: States that when the temperature is constant, the solubility of any gas in a liquid is almost directly proportional to the pressure of the liquid; is applied in cases of nitrogen narcosis in deep-sea divers.

heparin (hep'-a-rin): A naturally occurring acid substance in several body tissues, especially the liver; it tends to prevent blood from clotting. In pharmacy, a preparation made from the livers and lungs of cattle, usually given by intravenous injection to inhibit coagulation of the blood; widely used in prevention and treatment of thrombosis.

heparin block: A device used for the intermittent administration of medications that are to be given intravenously; it consists of a scalp vein needle attached to a length of tubing that has a self-sealing diaphragm at the end; after the venepuncture, the needle is secured to the skin by its skin flaps; following an administration of medication a weak heparin solution is put into the needle and tubing to keep the line open.

heparinize (hep'-ar-i--nīz): To treat with administration of heparin for the purpose of increasing the clotting time of the blood. heparinization, n.

hepat-, hepatico-, hepato-: Combining forms denoting liver.

hepatectomy (hep-a-tek'-to-mi): Excision of part of the liver.

hepatic (hē-pat'-ik): Relating to the liver. H. COMA coma that accompanies H. encephalopathy. H. DUCTS right and left, unite to form the common hepatic duct which joins the cystic duct from the gallbladder to form the common bile duct; H. ENCEPHALOPATHY see under ENCEPHALOPATHY; H. FAILURE occurs when the liver is unable to carry out its normal functions due to damage from acute viral hepatitis, poisonings, or states of low cardiac output; clinical signs include jaundice, ascites; oedema; abnormal blood chemistry; tendency to spontaneous haemorrhage, often into the gastrointestinal tract and skin; and coma; H. FLEXURE see FLEXURE; H. VIRUS type A and type B, see under HEPATITIS.

hepatitis (hep-a-tī'-tis): Inflammation of the liver. Two main types are described: hepatitis A and hepatitis B. HEPATITIS A (infectious H.) caused by the hepatitis type A virus; is spread by the oral–faecal route; gives rise to epidemics in schools and among the armed forces, and is of worldwide distribution; is marked by jaundice occurring after an influenza-like illness, malaise, nausea, vomiting, clay-coloured stools, and the presence of bilirubin in the urine; confers indefinite immunity. HEPATITIS B (serum H.), caused by hepatitis B virus; may be transmitted by contaminated needles, blood, mucous membranes (sexual intercourse), or ingestion of contaminated food; has long incubation period and long duration; characterized by increase in aspartate transaminase and alanine transaminase levels and increased bilirubin in the blood; may be acute, chronic, or recurrent; produces carriers in 10% of patients. ALCOHOLIC H. occurs as a sequela of alcoholism; CHOLANGIOLITIC H. inflammation of the bile ducts and obstructive jaundice; CHRONIC H. persistent H., H. involving inflammation of the liver, sometimes cirrhosis, and may follow viral H.; ENZOIC H. Rift Valley fever (*q.v.*); EPIDEMIC H. infectious H.; FULMINANT H acute H., may cause death from acute yellow atrophy of the liver; HOMOLYGOUS H. symptoms as for infectious H. but is caused by a B virus and spread by contact, blood transfusion, or serum therapy, or by improperly sterilized needles or instruments; incubation period is 6 weeks to 6 months; can be severe, even fatal; an estimated 2% to 3% of the adult world population are carriers; INFECTIOUS H. hepatitis A; NEONATAL H. occurs soon after birth; cause often unknown; tends to be chronic and fatal; SERUM H. hepatitis B; TRANSFUSION H. usually caused by viral H., type B; VIRAL H. may be caused by H. A, or H. B virus.

hepatitis B surface antigen: Carried in patients with liver disease, including those who develop hepatitis after many transfusions; also carried in dirty syrings. Has been found in city areas frequented by alcoholics and drug addicts. Blood banks now screen for this antigen.

hepatization (hep'a-tī-zā'shun): Pathological changes in the tissues, which cause them to resemble liver. Occurs in the lungs in the exudative stages of lobar pneumonia.

hepatobiliary (hep'-a-tō-bil'-i-ar-i): Relating to the liver and the bile or bile ducts. H. SYSTEM composed of the liver, the hepatic duct system, the gall bladder, the cystic duct, and the common bile duct.

hepatocele (hep'-a-tō-sēl): A hernia or protrusion of a part of the liver through the diaphragm or the abdominal wall.

hepatocyte (hep'-a-tō-sīt): One of the cells of the epithelial type that make up most of the liver substance.

hepatogenous (hep-a-toj'-e-nus): Originating in the liver.

hepatolenticular (hep'-a-tō-len-tik'-ū-lar): Relating to the liver and the lenticular nucleus; see under LENTICULAR. H. DEGENERATION a rare inherited disorder due to a defect in metabolism of copper; characterized by a pigmented ring (Kayser–Fleischer ring) at the outer border of the cornea, cirrhosis of the liver, enlarged spleen, rigidity and contractures of muscles, dysphagia, progressive weakness, degeneration of the lenticular nucleus, and psychic disturbances; also called *Wilson's disease*.

hepatolith (hep'-a-tō-lith): A concretion within the liver.

hepatomegaly (hep'-a-tō-meg'a-li): Enlargement of the liver.

hepatorenal syndrome: Term originally used to describe death from hepatic and renal failure after cholecystectomy for prolonged obstructive jaundice. Now used to describe liver and kidney failure from any cause occurring simultaneously, and resulting from infection, dehydration, haemorrhage, or shock.

hepatotoxin (hep'-a-tō-tok'-sin): 1. Any substance that is destructive of or injurious to the liver cells. 2. A toxic substance elaborated in the liver.

hept-, hepta-: Combining forms denoting (1) seven; (2) division into seven units.

herbal medicine: 1. A system of healing based on the medicinal properties of plants. 2. A medication made from a herb or herbs.

herbicide (herb'-i-sīd): Any substance used to inhibit the growth of undesirable plants or weeds.

hereditary (he-red'-i-ter-i): Inherited; capable of being inherited. H. DISEASE a disorder passed from parent to child through genes; may be recessive or dominant; may not be observable at birth. Predisposition to certain diseases is also a hereditary trait; may or may not be detectable at birth.

heredity (hē-red'-i-ti): 1. The genetic factor responsible for the persistence of particular characteristics in successive generations. 2. The physical and mental components that are transmitted from parent to offspring at conception. 3. The transmission of particular traits and characters from parents to offspring.

heredofamilial (her'-e-dō-fa-mil'-i-al): Refers to a disease that occurs in more than one member of a family and is probably inherited.

Hering–Breuer reflex: See under REFLEX.

heritable (her'-it-a-b'l): Capable of being inherited.

Her Majesty's Stationery Office: A governmental office under the ministerial control of the Minister for the Cabinet Office. It delivers a wide range of services to the public, information industry, and government, relating to access to and re-use of government information.

hermaphrodite (her-maf′-rō-dīt): An individual possessing both ovarian and testicular tissue. Such a person may approximate either the male or female type, but is usually sterile from imperfect development of the gonads.

hermaphroditism (her-maf′-rō-dit-izm): The condition in which both ovarian and testicular tissue exist in the same individual. Also hermaphrodism.

hermeneutic (her-men-ū′-tik): Relating to an interpretive approach to the study of texts. A hermeneutic approach might look beyond the clear text written on the page to examine why the author was driven to write the text.

hermetic (her-met′-ik): Airtight. — hermetically, adv.

hernia (her′-ni-a): Rupture. The protrusion of an organ or part of an organ, through an abnormal aperture in the structure containing it; commonly the protrusion of an abdominal organ through a gap in the abdominal wall. Weakness of the wall may be caused by injury, general debilitation, old age, lifting, tumour, increased pressure from coughing. CEREBRAL H. protrusion of brain substance through the skull, usually occurs after surgery for brain tumour; DIAPHRAGMATIC H. protrusion through the diaphragm, most commonly involving the stomach at the oesophageal opening; FEMORAL H. protrusion of intestine through the femoral canal, alongside the femoral vessels as they pass into the thigh; HIATAL H. diaphragmatic H.; INCISIONAL H. may occur after abdominal surgery when there is a breakdown of sutures in the deep layers of tissue; may be caused by wound infection; INGUINAL H. protrusion of a sac of peritoneum through the inguinal canal, alongside the spermatic cord in the male; IRREDUCIBLE H. one that cannot be reduced by manual manipulation; OBTURATOR H. one through the obturator foramen; occurs rarely, usually in women; POPLITEAL H., H. of the synovial membrane at the back of the knee; occurs when the capsule is weakened by arthritis or infection; baker's cyst; REDUCIBLE H. one that can be corrected by manual manipulation; RICHTER′S H. one in which only a part of the intestinal wall is within the hernial sac; STRANGULATED H. one in which the blood supply to the herniated part is impaired; usually due to constriction by surrounding tissues or structures; UMBILICAL H. protrusion of part of the intestine through the umbilical scar area; VAGINAL H. a hernia into the vagina; VENTRAL H. a hernia through the abdominal wall.

herniated (her′-ni-ā-ted): 1. Having a hernia. 2. Descriptive of a structure that protrudes like a hernia. H. DISC an intervertebral disc in which the nucleus pulposus has ruptured through the surrounding fibrocartilage; most often occurs in the lumbar area; may cause pressure on spinal nerves, causing severe pain; also called *slipped disc* and *ruptured intervertebral disc*.

herniation (her-ni-ā′-shun): 1. Formation of a hernia. 2. A hernia.

heroin (her′-ō-in): A highly addicitive white crystalline powder derived from opium; favoured by drug users, may be sniffed, smoked or injected. Used medically as a narcotic and analgesic.

herpes (her′-pez): Name given to conditions that are caused by any one of five closely related herpesviruses and that are characterized by vesicular eruptions on the skin and mucous membranes of the facial and genital areas and by the ability to remain quiescent in the body until triggered by some event such as exposure to sunlight (herpes simplex, HSV-1) or a stressful event (genital herpes, HSV-2). H. GENITALIS (HSV-2), infectious recurring herpes of the genitalia; very contagious; transmitted by sexual intercourse; occurs in epidemics. Accompanied by fever, regional adenopathy, dysuria, possibly inflammation of the meninges of the brain and spinal cord. In women, the vesicles may develop into painful ulcers on the vulva, vaginal mucosa, perianal skin, and groin; other symptoms include vaginal discharge and sometimes neurological symptoms. In men, the lesions usually occur on the glans penis and scrotum. No known cure; treatment is symptomatic. Also called *H. progenitalis*; H. SIMPLEX (HSV-1), is characterized by the formation of blisters chiefly along the borders of the lips and external nares. Also called *fever blister*; VARICELLA-ZOSTER VIRUS appears as (1) chickenpox (*q.v.*), or (2) herpes zoster; H. ZOSTER is characterized by the eruption of vesicles that follow the course of a nerve, and severe pain; usually unilateral; also called *shingles*; fairly common in the elderly; H. ZOSTER OPHTHALMICUS a herpetic virus infection of the ophthalmic division of the trigeminal nerve ganglion; often accompanied by vesicular eruption along the ophthalmic branch of the nerve; may result in uveitis, glaucoma, keratitis; ZONA FACILIS herpes of the face. See also EPSTEIN–BARR VIRUS; CYTOMEGALOVIRUS; HERPETIC KERATITIS under KERATITIS.

herpesvirus (her'-pez-vī'-rus): See HERPETOVIR-IDAE.

herpetiform (her-pet'-i-form): Resembling herpes.

Herpetoviridae (her'-pe-tō-vir'-i-de): A group of similar viruses formerly referred to as herpesvirus; includes herpes simplex virus, varicella-zoster virus, cytomegalovirus, and Epstein–Barr virus.

Hers disease: Glycogen storage disease, Type VI. A rare herediatry condition characterized by the storage of large amounts of glycogen in the liver and hepatomegaly.

hertz (herts): In physics, a unit of frequency in a periodic process, equal to one cycle per second. Used in audiometry. Also known as *cycle per second.*

hesperidin (hes-per'-i-din): Functions as vitamin P; see CITRIN.

heter-, hetero-: Combining forms denoting (1) different; (2) other than usual; (3) containing several kinds.

heterocellular (het'-er-ō-sel'-ū-lar): Made up of different kinds of cells.

heterochromia (het'-er-ō-krō'-mi-a): A difference in the colour of two anatomical parts that are normally of the same colour, *e.g.*, the iris of the eye.

heterogeneous (het'-er-ō-jē'-nē-us): Made up of ingredients or constituents that are dissimilar.

heterogenous (het-er-oj'-e-nus): 1. Of unlike origin. 2. Not originating within the body. Opp. to autogenous (*q.v.*).

heterograft (het'-er-ō-graft): A graft of tissue from an individual of a species other than that of the recipient.

heterohypnosis (het'-er-ō-hip-nō'-sis): Hypnosis that is induced by the hypnotist as opposed to self-hypnosis.

heterokaryon (het'-er-ō-kar'-ē-on): A cell with two or more nuclei, each with a different genetic make-up.

heterokaryosis (het'-er-ō-kar-ī-ō'-sis): The formation of, or the state of containing, heterokaryons.

heterokinesia (het'-er-ō-kī-nē'-si-a): Movements that are the opposite of what the patient is told to make.

heterologous (het-er-ol'-o-gus): 1. Of different origin; from a different species. 2. Relating to or consisting of tissue that is not normal to that part of the body.

heterometropia (het'-er-ō-me-trō'-pi-a): A condition in which the degree of refraction is not the same in the two eyes.

heteromorphosis (het'-er-ō-mor-fo'-sis): The development of tissue or an organ that is different from the normal type, especially that which occurs in regeneration of tissue or of a structure that was destroyed or removed.

heteronymous (het-er-on'-i-mus): Having different names that are indicative of correlation, *e.g.*, male, female. H. HEMANIOPIA loss of vision in the inner or outer halves of the field of vision.

heterophasia (het-er-ō-fā'-zi-a): A speech disorder in which the person says one thing but means another.

heterophil (het'-er-ō-fil): A granular leukocyte of varying size and staining characteristics.

heterophilic (het'-er-ō-fil'-ik): Refers to a microorganism, cell, or tissue that stains with a stain other than the one usually used.

heterophthalmia (het'-er-of-thal'-mi-a): A difference in the colour of the two eyes.

heteroplasia (het'-er-ō-plā'-zi-a): The development of tissue in a place where it is not normally found or in a place where another type of tissue is normally found.

heteroplasty (het'-er-ō-plas-ti): Plastic surgery using a graft from an individual of another species, or a synthetic material that is not organic. — heteroplastic, adj.

heterosexual (het'-er-ō-seks'-ū-al): Relating to or characterized by heterosexuality (*q.v.*).

heterosexuality (het'-er-ō-seks-ū-al'-i-ti): Sexual attraction towards those of the opposite sex.

heterosome (het'-er-ō-sōm): A sex chromosome.

heterotransplant (het'-e-rō-trans'-plant): Xenograft (*q.v.*).

heterotropia (het'-er-ō'-trō'-pi-a): Strabismus (*q.v.*).

heterozygote (het-e-rō-zī'-gōt): In biology, refers to an organism or an individual in which one or more pairs of genes are unlike in regard to a given characteristic; the gene that produces its effect in the presence of the other is called dominant and the other is called recessive. See GENE. — heterozygous, adj.

hexachlorophene (heks-a-klō'-rō-fēn): An antiseptic used on the skin, as a bacteriostatic; and in some bactericidal soaps.

hexosamine (hek-sos'-am-in): A nitrogenous sugar in which a hydroxyl group has replaced an amine group; glucosamine is an important hexosamine.

hexose (hek'-sōs): A class of monosaccharides ($C_6H_{12}O_6$). The two chief hexoses are glucose and fructose; others are mannose and galactose.

Hg: Symbol for mercury.

HGC: Abbreviation for Human Genetics Commission (*q.v.*).

hiatus (hī-a′-tus): A space or opening. See HERNIA. — hiatal, adj.

Hib vaccine: Abbreviation for *Haemophilus influenzae* (*q.v.*) type B vaccine.

hibernation (hī′-ber-nā′-shun): The winter sleep of some animals. ARTIFICIAL H. lowering of the body temperature of human beings by the external application of cold packs (ice, etc.) in combination with drugs to control shivering. It reduces the oxygen requirements of vital tissues, and is used mainly in the treatment of head injuries and in cardiac surgery. Also called *hypothermia* (*q.v.*). See REFRIGERATION.

hiccough, hiccup (hik′-up): An involuntary inspiratory spasm with sudden closure of the glottis and contraction of the diaphragm resulting in a short inspiratory cough.

hidrosis (hī-drō-′-sis): 1. Sweat secretion. 2. Excessive sweating.

high blood pressure: Blood pressure that is above the normal range. See BLOOD PRESSURE, HYPERTENSION.

higher level practice: The standard of care provided by expert health-care professionals, who use their knowledge and skills as a basis from which to further develop practice. Practitioners working at a higher level of practice use complex reasoning, critical thinking, reflection and analysis to inform their health assesments, clinical judgements, and decisions. See CLINICAL NURSE SPECIALIST; CONSULTANT NURSE; NURSE CONSULTATNT.

Highmore: ANTRUM OF H.; the maxillary sinus, see under ANTRUM.

high-security hospitals: Hospitals where prisoners who had serious psychological disorders were detained (under the conditions of their prison sentence) and received treatment for their mental health problems. These hospitals have now been incorporated into NHS Trusts.

hilum (hī′-lum): Hilus (*q.v.*.).

hilus (hī′-lus): A depression on the surface of an organ where vessels, ducts, etc. enter and leave. — hilar, adj.; hili, pl.

HImP: Abbreviation for Health Improvement Programme (*q.v.*).

hindbrain (hīnd′-brain): See RHOMBENCEPHALON.

hindgut (hīnd′-gut): The embryonic structure from which the colon is formed.

hinge joint: A synovial articulation that allows for movement in only one plane. Syn., *ginglymus.*

hip: The lateral part of the body on either side between the waist and the thigh. H. BONE the os coxae, a large, stable, irregular bone, one on either side of the body, which together form the pelvic girdle and to which the lower extremities are attached; consists of three parts, the ilium, ischium, and pubis; also called the *innominate bone*; TOTAL H. REPLACEMENT a surgical procedure in which the natural hip socket (the acetabulum) is replaced with a polyethylene cup and the head of the femur with stainless-steel ball-and-socket appliance; also called a *hip implant.*

hippocampus (hip-pō-kam′-pus): One of two curved bands, about 5 cm in length, consisting of a special type of cortex, on the floor of the inferior horn of the lateral ventricle on each side of the brain. It is an important functional part of the limbic system (*q v*). Also called *Ammon's horn.*

Hippocrates (hi-pok′-ra-tēz): Famous Greek physician and philosopher (460 to 370 BC) who established a school of medicine at Kos, his birthplace. He is often termed the Father of Medicine.

Hippocratic oath: An oath based on one attributed to Hippocrates and required of his students, which has been the ethical guide of the medical profession ever since.

hippuric acid (hip-ū′rik as′id): An acid formed in the body by synthesis in the liver, and in the kidney; is excreted in the urine; its salts have some therapeutic uses.

hippus (hip′-us): Abnormal spasmodic rhythmic contraction and dilation of the pupil independently of illumination or any other external stimulus.

hircus (hur′-kus): 1. A hair of the axilla. 2. The odour of the axilla.

Hirschsprung's disease: Megacolon. Congenital hypertrophy and massive enlargement of the colon. The affected part is sometimes removed surgically. [Harold Hirschsprung, Danish physician, 1830–1916.]

hirsute (her′-sūt): Being hairy or shaggy.

hirsutism (her′-sū-tizm): Excessive hairiness, especially in women, or the growth of hair in unusual places.

His (hiss): See BUNDLE OF HIS.

hist-, hista-, histio-, histo-: Combining forms denoting relationship to tissue.

histaminase (his-tam′-i-nās): An enzyme that is widely distributed in body tissues and that inactivates histamine (*q.v.*).

histamine (his′-ta-mēn): A naturally occurring chemical substance in body tissues which, in small doses, has profound and diverse actions on muscle, blood capillaries, and gastric secretion. Its sudden excessive release from the tissues, into the blood is believed to be the cause of the main symptoms and signs in anaphylaxis (*q.v.*). — histaminic, adj.

histidase (his′-ti-dās): An enzyme found in the liver.

histidine (his′-ti-dēn): An essential amino acid which is widely distributed and is present in haemoglobin. It is a precursor of histamine.

histiocyte (his′-tē-ō-sīt): A tissue cell; a macrophage found in connective tissue.

histiocytoma (his′-tē-ō-si-tō′-ma): A tumour that contains histiocytes.

histiocytosis (his′-tē-ō-sī-tō′-sis): A condition marked by an excessive number of histiocytes in the blood. H. X is a group of diseases characterized by proliferation of histiocytes; includes Letterer–Siwe disease and eosinophilic granuloma of bone.

histocompatibility (his′-tō-kom-pat-a-bil′-i-ti): 1. The ability of the cells or tissue of a graft that enables the graft to be accepted and become functional following transplantation to another organism. 2. The quality of transfused blood cells to survive and remain functional in the recipient without immunological interference.

histology (his-tol′-o-ji): Microscopic study of the structure of cells and tissues. — histological, adj.; histologically, adv.

histopathology (his′-tō-pa-thol′-o-ji): The study of microscopically visible changes in diseased cells or tissue.

histrionic (his-tri-on′-ik): Refers to theatrical or hysterical behaviour such as uncontrolled weeping or laughing and other kinds of attention-getting actions.

HIV: Abbreviation for human immunodeficiency virus (*q.v.*).

hives (hīvs): Nettle-rash; urticaria (*q.v.*).

HMSO: Abbreviation for Her Majesty's Stationery Office, now the Stationery Office (*q.v.*).

H₂O: Chemical formula for water.

H₂O₂: Chemical formula for hydrogen peroxide.

hoarse (hors): Harsh and grating; said of the voice. — hoarseness, n.

hobnail liver: Describing the appearance of the liver in one form of cirrhosis; the surface of the liver is covered with small nodules while the body of the organ is shrunken and hard.

Hodgkin's disease: Lymphadenoma. Progressive, painless, frequently fatal disease in the reticulo-endothelial system, shown in generalized enlargement of the lymphatic glands and splenomegaly; of unknown cause. Other features are recurring fever, anaemia, and occasionally cutaneous manifestations. Also called *lymphosarcoma, lymphadenoma, anaemia lymphatica, malignant lymphoma.* [Thomas Hodgkin, English physician, 1798–1866.]

Hoffman's sign: May be elicited in patients with upper motor neuron lesions. The patient's hand is held with fingers extended and pressure is applied to the nail of the middle finger; the thumb adducts and the other fingers flex.

hoist: A mechanical device or apparatus, such as a winch or elevator, designed for lifting people or heavy objects.

hol-, holo-: Combining forms meaning (1) all or entire; or (2) denoting relationship to the whole.

holarthritis (hol-ar-thrī′-tis): Arthritis in all or many of the joints; polyarthritis.

holism (hō′-lizm): The idea that the properties of a system cannot be determined or explained by its components alone. It is often regarded as opposite to reductionism (*q.v.*).

holistic (hō-lis′-tik): Including or involving all of something. In health-care, acknowledging all of an individual's physical, mental, and social conditions, not just physical symptoms, in the treatment of illness.

Hollenhorst bodies or plaques: Small pieces of atheromatous plaques that have broken off and become lodged as emboli in retinal vessels; an indication of a serious cardiovascular problem.

hollow-back: See under BACK.

hologram (hōl′-ō-gram): The negative produced on a photographic plate in a type of lensless photography that utilizes the laser beam; a three-dimensional image.

Holter monitor: A cardiac monitor worn around the waist or on the shoulder of patients undergoing cardiac rehabilitation; usually worn for 24 hours only to identify any arrhythmias or to assess the effectiveness of antiarrhythmic drugs.

Holter pump: A motor-driven device designed to deliver an accurate volume of parenteral fluid or medication.

Holtzman inkblot technique: A technique similar to the Rorschach technique utilizing inkblots to test disorders of thought and emotion.

hom-, homo-: Combining forms denoting (1) alike, similar, one and the same, corresponding in structure or type; (2) from or of the same species.

Homan's sign: Pain in the calf muscles when the foot is passively dorsiflexed, with the patient lying flat on the bed; indicative of incipient or established venous thrombosis of the leg. [John Homans, American surgeon, 1877–1954.]

home help: Person paid by a local authority to provide general household help (cleaning, shopping, etc.) for the disabled or elderly for a few hours per week.

homeo-: Combining form denoting the same, alike, similar, unchanging.

homeodynamics (hō'-mē-ō-dī-nam'-iks): The process by which an individual maintains emotional balance in the presence of stress factors that have the potential to disturb emotional and/or physical stability.

homeopathy (hōm-ē-op'-a-thi): A complementary disease treatment system which holds that a medicinal substance that can evoke certain symptoms in healthy individuals may be effective in the treatment of illnesses having similar symptoms, if given in very small doses. The patient is given minute doses of naturally occurring medicines that in larger doses would produce symptoms of the disease itself. The system was created by Dr Samuel Hahnemann, German physician (1755–1843).

homeoplasia (hō-mē-ō-plā'-zi-a): The growth of new tissue that is similar to the adjacent tissue.

homeostasis (hō-'-mē-ō-stā'-sis,-os'-ta-sis): The state of relative stability or equilibrium of the internal environment of the body, including the various functions, such measurable conditions as blood pressure, temperature, heart rate, etc., and the chemical composition and reactions of tissues and fluids; or the physiological process by which this stasis is maintained.

homeotherm: A warm-blooded animal (such as *Homo sapiens*). Also called *endotherm*.

homicide (hom'-i-sīd): Killing of a human being; manslaughter; murder. A murder.

homocystine (hō-mō-sis'-tin): An amino acid containing sulphur; produced synthetically.

homoeroticism (hō'-mō-ē-rot'-i-sizm): Homosexuality. Eroticism directed towards another of the same sex.

homogenate (hō-moj'-e-nāt): A substance produced by homogenization (*q.v.*).

homogeneous (hom-ō-jē'-nē-us): Of the same kind; of the same quality or consistency throughout.

homogenization (hō-moj'-pen-ī-zā'-shun): The process of breaking down and blending the particles of a substance with those of another substance with which it is not normally miscible to form a uniform suspension or emulsion. — homogenize, v.

homogenize (hō-moj'-e-nīz): To reduce the particles of a substance so that they are uniformly

small and evenly distributed throughout the substance.

homogenous (hō-moj'-e-nus): 1. Having a structural resemblance because of having a common progenitor. 2. Having a like nature, *e.g.*, a bone graft from another human being.

homogentisic acid (hō'-mō-jen-tis'-ik as'-id): An intermediate product in the oxidation of tyrosine and phenylalanine. Found in urine of persons with alkaptonuria. Formerly called *glycosuric acid*.

homograft (hō'-mo-graft): A tissue or organ that is transplanted from one individual to another of the same species.

homolateral (hō-mō-lat'-er-al): On the same side. — homolaterally, adv.

homologous (hō-mol'-ō-gus): Corresponding in origin and structure, but not necessarily in function.

homologue (hom'-ō-log): 1. A part or organ of the body that is similar in structure to another part of organ. 2. Any part of an organ or structure of an animal that is similar in structure to that of another animal but which may differ in function.

homophilic (hō-mō-fil'-ik): Descriptive of an antibody that reacts with, or has affinity for, a specific antigen.

homophobia (hōm-ō-fō'-bi-a): Fear of homosexuals, of one's own homosexual tendencies, or of being considered a homosexual.

homophonia (hō-mō-fō'-ni-a): A speech defect characterized by lack of ability to produce vocal sounds, resulting in whispering speech.

homoplasty (hō'-mō-plas-ti): Surgical replacement of lost parts or tissue by similar parts or tissue from another of the same species.

homosexual (hō-mō-seks'-u-al): 1. Relating to the same sex. 2. An individual who exhibits homosexuality (*q.v.*).

homosexuality (hō'-mō-seks-ū-al'-i-ti): A sexual orientation characterized by sexual attraction towards members of the same sex. The term usually implies an exclusive or predominant orientation, and is distinguished from bisexuality as well as heterosexuality. See BISEXUAL; LESBIAN.

homotransplantation (hō'-mō-trans-plan-tā'-shun): Transfer of tissue or organ to a member of the same species. Syn., *homograft*.

homozygosis (hō-mō-zī-gō'-sis): The formation of a zygote by the union of like gametes.

homozygote (hō-mō-zī'-gōt): An individual produced by the union of two gametes having identical alleles (*q.v.*). at a given locus. — homozygous, adj.

homunculus (hō-mung'-kū-lus): **1.** A midget. **2.** A small-scale model of the human body or a part of it. **3.** A miniature human body, once thought to pre-exist as such in sperm or ovum.

honeycomb lung: Descriptive of the change that occurs in fibrosing alveolitis when the advancement of the disease causes solidification of the alveoli and the air spaces consist mainly of dilated bronchioles.

HoNOS: Abbreviation for Health of the Nation Outcome Scale (*q.v.*).

hookworm: Any one of a number of parasitic nematode worms (including ANCYLOSTOMA and UNCINARIA) that infest the intestinal tract of human; transmitted by faeces. H. DISEASE a chronic debilitating disease, characterized by severe anaemia; caused by the blood-sucking hookworm, which enters the body through the skin, usually that of the feet. The disease is found mostly in warm areas where disposal of faeces is inadequate and people do not wear shoes.

hordeolum (hor-dē'-ō-lum): A stye. A purulent inflammation of one or more of the sebaceous glands of the eyelid; may be external, occurring on the skin at the edge of the lid; or internal, occurring on the conjunctival surface of the lid.

horizontal violence (ho-ri-zon'-tal): Hostile and aggressive behaviour by a member or members of a group towards another member or members of the larger group. This aggression may include verbal abuse, character assassination, gossip, intimidation, and humiliation. This has been described as inter-group conflict.

hormone (hor'-mōn): A complex chemical substance produced in one part or organ of the body that initiates or regulates the activity of an organ or a group of cells in another part of the body. Hormones secreted by the endocrine glands are carried through the bloodstream to the target organ. See also ENDOCRINE. — hormonic, hormonal, adj.

hormone replacement therapy: The administration of hormones prepared in drug form as a substitute for those hormones that the body no longer produces or which have been lost through surgery; replacement must be continued through out life. Most commonly a combination of oestrogenic hormones given to women for the relief of menopausal symptoms and the prevention of osteoporosis; administered by implant, transdermally or orally. Popularly known as HRT.

hormonopoiesis (hor'-mō-nō-poy-ē'-sis): The production of hormones. — hormonopoietic, adj. Also *hormopoiesis*.

Horton's syndrome: Severe headache with pain in the eye, temple, neck, and face; nasal discharge, tearing. Due to release of histamine in the body. To be differentiated from migraine. [Bayard Taylor Horton, American physician, 1895–1980.]

hospice (hos'-pis): An institution for terminally ill people, where treatment focuses on the patient's well-being rather than providing a cure, and includes drugs for pain management and often spiritual counselling. It provides a centralized programme of palliative (*q.v.*) and supportive services to dying people and their families, usually in a small residential setting. These services are provided by an interdisciplinary team of professionals and volunteers.

hospital: An institution that is devoted to the diagnosis, treatment, and rehabilitation of persons who are mentally or physically ill or injured. BASE H. a military hospital at a large military base that receives the wounded from smaller hospital units nearer the fighting front; COMMUNITY H. any small general hospital providing services to a specific community; DAY H. one that patients attend daily, returning to their homes at night; recreational and occupational therapy are often provided; used mostly for psychiatric and geriatric patients; FIELD H. a first aid station near the fighting front; GENERAL H. a large hospital that cares for medical/ surgical, obstetrical, and emergency patients; MATERNITY H. a H. for women in childbirth; PRIVATE H. a H. owned and operated by an individual or corporation for profit.

hospital-acquired infection: See NOSOCOMIAL.

hospital at home: The provision of services usually given in a hospital in an individual's home environment; for example intermittent positive pressure ventilation.

hospitalization (hos'-pi-tal-ī-zā'-shun): Placement of an individual in a hospital for observation, diagnostic tests, or treatment for some disease or disorder.

host: 1. An organism that receives a transplant of tissue from another organism. **2.** In biology, the organic structure upon which a parasite lives or grows. INTERMEDIATE or INTERMEDIARY H. one in which a parasite passes its larval or cystic stage.

hot: 1. Have a relatively high temperature. **2.** Term is used colloquially to describe something that is charged with electricity or that contains dangerous radioactive material. H. DESKING The practice of allocating limited workspace according to the needs of the workers who do not have their own desks, and store their personal belongings in lockers or filing cabinets when not in the office; the system is heavily dependent on computers to route telephone calls, allocate resources, and maintain individual working files. H. FLUSH a phenomenon usually associated with the menopause, and due to vasodilation of the vessels of the head and neck particularly; accompanied by a visible flush and sweating, and sometimes, a feeling of suffocation. H. LINE a telephone assistance service for those in need of advice or support, usually provided by voluntary organizations.

house: H. PHYSICIAN a registered medical practitioner who cares for hospital patients under the supervision of the consultant medical staff. H. SURGEON a registered medical practitioner who cares for patients under the supervision of the consultant surgeon.

housemaid's knee: Propatellar bursitis. A traumatic condition in which there is marked swelling of the bursa in front of the patella, the result of kneeling.

House of Commons: One of the three Estates of UK Parliament (*q.v.*). It plays a major part in the process that makes new laws, by debating and looking in detail at proposals for new legislation. The Commons is responsible for scrutinizing the work of the government and questioning Ministers and Civil Servants about the work that they do. Unlike the House of Lords (*q.v.*), the House of Commons examines the financial work of the government and must approve spending and taxation. Also referred to as the *Lower House*.

House of Lords: Two of the three Estates of UK Parliament (*q.v.*). The Lords considers legislation, debates issues of importance, and provides a forum for government ministers to be questioned. It spends about two-thirds of its time revising Bills (*q.v.*) sent from the House of Commons (*q.v.*). The House of Lords also acts as a check on the government and is the ultimate Court of Appeal. Also referred to as the *Upper House*.

HPC: Abbreviation for Health Professions Council (*q.v.*).

HPV: Abbreviation for human papilloma virus, see under PAPILLOMAVIRUS.

HRT: Abbreviation for hormone replacement therapy (*q.v.*).

HSV-2: Herpes simplex virus, type 2. See under HERPES.

HTLV: Human T-cell leukaemia–lymphoma virus: a retrovirus group which includes the human immunodeficiency virus (HIV) shown to cause AIDS (*q.v.*). May be transmitted through sexual contact, transfusion, and by pregnant women to fetuses.

HTML: Abbreviation for hypertext markup language (*q.v.*).

Hubbard tank: A large tank used in physiotherapy, especially for underwater exercises. Also used for underwater treatment of patients with extensive burns.

huffing: Forced expiration; a technique used in chest physical therapy.

Huhner's test: A test involving post-coital examination of mucus from the cervical canal to determine the number and motility of the sperm.

human chorionic gonadotrophin: See under GONADOTROPHIN. Abbreviated hCG.

Human Fertilisation and Embryology Authority (em-brē-ol'-o-ji): A statutory body that regulates, licenses, and collects data on fertility treatments such as *in vitro* fertilization (*q.v.*) and donor insemination (*q.v.*) in the NHS and private fertility clinics, as well as human embryo research in the UK.

Human Genetics Commission: The UK government's advisory body on social, ethical, and legal implications of developments in genetics and their likely impact on people and healthcare. It also engages the public in considering these issues.

Human Genome Project: An international research project to map each human gene and to completely sequence human DNA.

human growth hormone: A secretion of the anterior part of the hypophysis; promotes growth and directly influences the metabolism of fats, proteins, and carbohydrates in the body. Can be produced artifically for treatment in disorders that interfere with normal growth.

human immunodeficiency virus: Virus shown to cause acquired immunodeficiency syndrome (*q.v.*).

human placental lactogen: A protein hormone elaborated by the placenta; its actions resemble somewhat those of the pituitary growth hormone and prolactin.

human rights: The equalities and freedoms that should be inherent to all people alike. They refer to a wide continuum of values or capabilities thought to enhance human agency and declared to be universal in character. See HUMAN RIGHTS ACT 1998; RIGHTS.

Human Rights Act 1998: A legal document incorporating into domestic law the European Convention on Human Rights to which the UK has been committed since 1951. Convention principles are therefore already reflected in government legislation and policies and have been informing best practice in health and social care. The Act modernizes relationships between people, and between people and the state, and will embed in a new way, values of fairness, respect for human dignity, and inclusiveness in the heart of public services. The following are examples of public bodies covered by the Act: general practitioners, dentists, opticians and pharmacists when undertaking NHS work; Primary Care Trusts; a body that has functions of a public nature (e.g. a professional regulatory body).

humectant (hū-mek′-tant): 1. A substance that promotes the retention of moisture. 2. Moist.

humerus (hū-mer-us): The bone of the upper arm between the elbow and shoulder joint; it articulates with the glenoid cavity of the scapula at the proximal end and with the radius and ulna at the distal end. — humeral, adj.; humeri, pl.

humidification (hū-mid′-i-fi-kā′-shun): The process of moistening air; in respiration, by moisture from the mucous membrane lining the respiratory tract.

humidifier (hū-mid′i-fi-er): An apparatus for adding humidity to the air in a specific area.

humidity (hū-mid′-it-i): The amount of moisture in the atmosphere as measured by a hygrometer. POSITIVE H. the actual amount of vapour present in the air; expressed in grams per cubic metre; RELATIVE H. the ratio of the amount of moisture present in the air to the amount which would saturate it (at the same temperature); H. TENT an enclosure placed over the patient, or just over the head, when administering humidity in the form of a mist. — humidification, n.

humour (hū′-mor): Any normal fluid or semifluid of the body. AQUEOUS H. the fluid filling the anterior and posterior chambers in front of the optical lens; VITREOUS H. the gelatinous mass filling the interior of the eyeball from the lens to the retina. — humoral, adj.

hunger (hun′-ger): A longing, desire, or urgent need, especially for food. AIR H. see AIR; H. PAIN epigastric pain which is relieved by taking food; associated with duodenal ulcer.

Hunner's ulcer: A lesion in the bladder wall characterized by dysuria that is relieved by voiding; occurs in chronic interstitial nephritis; is difficult to detect.

Hunter–Hurler syndrome: An inherited form of mucopolysaccharidosis, but the symptoms are less severe; closely resembles Hurler's syndrome (q.v.).

Hunterian chancre: The hard sore of primary syphilis. [John Hunter, Scottish anatomist, 1728–1793.]

Huntington's chorea or disease: See under CHOREA.

Hunt's syndrome: 1. A condition characterized by intention tremor, which begins in an extremity and gradually increases in intensity as more parts of the body become involved. 2. A condition resulting from a viral infection of the seventh cranial nerve; signs and symptoms include herpes zoster, facial paralysis, otalgia.

Hurler's syndrome: An inherited disorder of metabolism marked by skeletal deformities, causing a grotesque appearance, gargoylism, mental handicap, enlarged liver and spleen. Mucopolysaccharidosis (q.v.).

Hutchinson–Gilford syndrome: Premature ageing in children; marked by accelerated growth, severe atherosclerosis, hyperlipidaemia, collagen disorders. See also PROGERIA.

HV: Abbreviation for health visitor (q.v.).

HVCert: Abbreviation for Health Visitor's Certificate.

hyaline (hī′a-līn-lēn): Like glass; transparent. H. MEMBRANE see under MEMBRANE; H. MEMBRANE DISEASE or H. MEMBRANE SYNDROME see RESPIRATORY DISTRESS SYNDROME.

hyaloid (hī′-a-loyd): Resembling hyaline; glassy. H. MEMBRANE the transparent capsule enclosing the optical vitreous humour.

hyaluronic acid (hī′-al-ū-ron′-ik): A polysaccharide that occurs as a gelatinous substance in the intercellular spaces, especially of the skin; it holds the cells together.

hyaluronidase (hī′-al-ū-ron′-i-dās): An enzyme found in some pathogenic bacteria, sperm and some venoms; it breaks down hyaluronic acid (q.v.) and thus increases the permeability of tissues. When injected subcutaneously, it promotes the absorption of fluid; given with or immediately before a subcutaneous infusion.

hybrid (hī′-brid): An offspring of parents belonging to different strains, varieties or species.

hydatid (hī′-da-tid): 1. Any cyst-like structure. 2. The cyst formed by a tapeworm and found in various parts of the body, especially the liver. It may rupture and give rise to daughter cysts.

hydatid disease (hī′-da-tid): An infection caused by the larval forms of tapeworms of the genus Echinococcus characterized by the formation of multiple expanding cysts.

hydatidiform (hī-da-tid′-i-form): Resembling a hydatid cyst. H. MOLE see MOLE.

hydr-, hydra-, hydro-: Combining forms denoting (1) water, or water-loving organism, (2) hydrogen.

hydraemia (hī-dre′-mi-a): A relative excess of plasma volume compared with the red cell volume of the blood; it is normally present in late pregnancy. — hydraemic, adj.

hydragogue (hī′-dra-gog): 1. A purgative which produces a watery evacuation of the bowel. 2. Producing a watery discharge, particularly from the intestines.

hydramnios (hī-dram′-ni-os): An excess of amniotic fluid.

hydranencephaly (hī′-dran-en-kef′-a-li,-sef′-): Congenital absence, or partial absence, of some or all of the cerebral hemispheres, with the space they would normally occupy being filled with cerebrospinal fluid.

hydrarthrosis (hī-drar-thrō′-sis): A collection of watery fluid in a joint cavity. INTERMITTENT H. appears periodically, develops spontaneously, lasts a few days, and disappears. The joint may be normal between attacks. Affects young women mostly; may be due to an allergy.

hydrate (hī′-drāt): 1. A compound made up of water in chemical union with another substance. 2. To combine with or take up water. — hydration, n.

hydration (hī-drā′-shun): The union or combining of water with another substance.

hydraulic lift: A mechanical device for lifting a completely helpless person from the bed to a stretcher, wheel chair, toilet, etc.

hydroa (hī-drō′-a): A skin condition marked by the eruption of vesicles or bullae; dermatitis herpetiformis (*q.v.*). H. AESTIVALE a vesicular or bullous skin disease of children; the vesicles appear upon reddened patches of the skin. It may recur every summer; affects exposed parts and probably results from photosensitivity; often associated with porphyrinuria (*q.v.*). H. VACCINIFORME is a more severe form of H. AESTIVALE in which scarring occurs.

hydrocarbon (hī′-drō-kar′-bon): Any compound that contains only hydrogen and carbon.

hydrocele (hī′-drō-sēl): A swelling due to accumulation of serous fluid, especially in the tunica vaginalis of the testis, or along the spermatic cord. COMMUNICATING H. a H. in which the tunica vaginalis testis is filled with fluid and connects directly with the peritoneal cavity.

hydrocephalus (hī′-drō-kef′-a-lus, sef′-): Literally, water on the brain. An excess of cerebrospinal fluid within the ventricles of the brain or within the subdural spaces; usually a con-genital condition but may also result from injury, infection, tumour, or developmental anomalies. COMMUNICATING H. a H. in which there is no obstruction in the ventricles and the cerebrospinal fluid passes into the spinal canal but is not absorbed; EXTERNAL H., H. in which the fluid is mainly in the subarachnoid space; INTERNAL H., H. in which the fluid excess is mainly in the ventricles of the brain; NON-COMMUNICATING H., H. in which there is a block in the passage from the ventricles of the brain where the cerebrospinal fluid is produced and the subarachnoid space from which it is absorbed. — hydrocephalic, adj.

hydrochloric acid (hī-drō-klor′-ik): A colourless compound of hydrogen and chlorine; it is caustic when undiluted. Also secreted by the stomach lining and normally present in gastric juice in 0.2% solution.

17-hydrocorticosteroids (hī′-drō-kor′-ti-kŏ-stē′-royds): The metabolites or breakdown products of hydrocortisone, cortisone, and small amounts of aldosterone; their presence is increased in the urine of patients with Cushing's syndrome, adrenal cancer, polycystic ovaries, some adrenal tumours, and in late pregnancy; and decreased in Addison's disease and hypopituitarism.

hydrocortisone (hī′-drō-kor′-ti-sōn): The pharmaceutical name for the adrenocortical steroid commonly called cortisol; used for its anti-inflammatory action.

hydrogel (hī′-dro-jel): A semi-occlusive gel dressing or filler, used as wound dressing. It is absorptive, can be adhesive or non-adhesive, and is moisture-retentive. It is used in light to moderately exudative wounds and for autolytic débridement (*q.v.*).

hydrogen (hī′-drō-jen): A colourless, odourless, flammable gas, explosive when mixed with air; found in all organic compounds and water. The lightest element known. H. ION CONCENTRATION a measure of the acidity or alkalinity of a solution, expressed as pH and ranging from pH 1 to 14, 7 being approximately neutral; the lower numbers denote acidity, the higher ones alkalinity. H. PEROXIDE (H_2O_2), an oxidizing agent used diluted for cleansing wounds.

hydrogenation (hī′-drō-jen-ā′-shun): The addition of hydrogen to a compound, especially to an unsaturated fat or fatty acid, causing soft fats and oils to be solidified.

hydrolabyrinth (hī′-drō-lab′i-rinth): An excess of fluid (endolymph) in the inner ear.

hydrolysis (hī-drol′-is-sis): The splitting of a substance into more simple substances by the addition of water. — hydrolytic, adj.; hydrolyse, v.

hydromassage (hī'-drō-ma-sazh'): Massage by a whirlpool device or some other form of moving water.

hydrometer (hī-drom'-it-er): An instrument for determining the specific gravity of a liquid as compared to that of an equal volume of water.

hydronephrosis (hī'-drō-ne-frō'-sis): Distension of the kidney pelvis with urine, from obstructed outflow. If unrelieved, pressure eventually causes atrophy of kidney tissue and impaired renal function. — hydronephrotic, adj.

hydropericarditis (hī'-drō-pe-ri-kar-dī'-tis): Pericarditis with serous effusion.

hydroperitoneum (hī'-drō-pe-ri-tō-nē'-um): Ascites (q.v.).

hydrophilia (hī-drō-fil'-i-a): The property of readily absorbing and holding water. — hydrophilic, adj.

hydrophilic (hī-drō-fil'-ik): 1. Having the property of readily absorbing water; water soluble. 2. A substance that is attracted to water and readily absorbs it.

hydropneumothorax (hī'-drō-nū-mō-thō'-raks): Pneumothorax further complicated by effusion of fluid in the pleural cavity. Often tubercular.

hydrorrhoea (hī-drō-rē'-a): Copious watery discharge from any organ or part. H. GRAVIDARUM the intermittent discharge of a clear fluid from the uterus during the last months of pregnancy.

hydrostatic (hī-drō-stat'-ik): Relating to the study of hydrostatics. H. PRESSURE in physiology, the pressure exerted by blood and other body fluids.

hydrotherapy (hī'-drō-ther'-a-pi): Treatment of disease by the scientific application of water externally; hydrotherapeutics. — hydrotherapeutic, adj.

hydrothorax (hī'-drō-thō'-raks): The presence of serous fluid in the pleural cavity. May be caused by famine, oedema, heart failure, renal disorders.

hydroureteronephrosis (hī'-drō-ū-rē'-ter-ō-nef-rō'-sis): Distention and dilatation of one or both kidneys and ureters with urine or other watery fluid; due to an obstruction in outflow.

hydrous (hī'-drus): Describes a substance containing chemically bound water.

hydroxybutyric acid (hī-drok'-si-bū-tir'ik): An intermediate product formed during fat metabolism; one of a group of compounds called collectively *ketone* or *acetone bodies*, which are found in the urine of patients with ketosis.

hydroxyl (hī-drok'-sil): The univalent group OH, consisting of a hydrogen atom linked with an oxygen atom; when combined with certain other radicals, hydroxides are formed.

hydroxyl group (hī-drok'-sil): The OH group in an organic compound.

hydroxyproline (hī-drok'-si-prō'-lin): An amino acid produced in the digestion of certain proteins, including collagens.

hydruria (hī-drū'-ri-a): Polyuria (q.v.). See DIABETES INSIPIDUS.

hygiene (hī'-jēn): 1. The science dealing with health and its maintenance. 2. A condition or practice, such as cleanliness, that is conducive to the preservation of health. COMMUNITY H. maintenance of the health of the community by the provision of a pure water supply, good sanitation, housing, etc.; INDUSTRIAL H. (occupational H.), includes all measures taken to preserve the individual's health while at work; MENTAL H. deals with the establishment of healthy mental attitudes and emotional reactions; OCCUPATIONAL H. industrial H.; ORAL H. deals with the proper care of the mouth and teeth for the maintenance of health; PERSONAL H. deals with those measures taken by the individual to preserve his own health; PUBLIC H. community H.; SOCIAL H. deals with sex education, marriage, family relations, and the promotion of sexual health. — hygienic, adj.

hygienist (hī'-ji-en-ist): One who specializes in the science of health. DENTAL H. one trained to give dental prophylactic treatment.

hygr-, hygro-: Combining forms denoting moisture, humidity, or relationship to water.

hygroscopic (hī'-grō-skop'-ik): Readily absorbing water, *e.g.*, glycerin.

hymen (hī'-men): A membranous, perforated structure partially covering the vaginal entrance. IMPERFORATE H. a congenital condition leading to haematocolpos. See CRYPTOMENORRHOEA. — hymenal, adj.

hyoid (hī'-oyd): A U-shaped bone at the root of, and supporting, the tongue.

hypaemia (hī-pēm'-i-a): Lack of blood supply to a part.

hypalgesia (hī-pal-jē'-zi-a): Decreased sensitiveness to pain. Also called *hypalgia*; *hypoalgesia*. — hypalgesic, adj.

hyper-: 1. Excessive; above normal. 2. Located above. Opp. to hypo-.

hyperacidaminuria (hī'-per-as'-id-am-i-nū'-ri-a): An excess of amino acids in the urine.

hyperacidity (hī'-per-a-sid'-i-ti): Excessive acidity. See HYPERCHLORHYDRIA.

hyperactivity (hī´-per-ak-tiv´-i-ti): Excessive activity or restlessness as may sometimes be seen in children with minimal brain dysfunction.

hyperacusis (hī´-per-a-kū´-sis): 1. Abnormal acuteness of hearing. 2. Painful sensitivity to sounds. Also called *hyperacusia*.

hyperadrenalism (hī´-per-a-drē´-nal-izm): A condition in which the adrenal cortex secretes abnormally large amounts of glucocorticoid, mineralocorticoid, oestrogen, or androgen; may occur without apparent cause or may be due to excessive administration of the adrenal cortical hormones. See CUSHING'S DISEASE.

hyperadrenocorticism (hī-per-a-drē´-nō-kor´-ti-sizm): Cushing's syndrome (*q.v.*).

hyperaemia (hī-per-ē´-mi-a): Excess of blood in an area. ACTIVE H. caused by an increased flow of blood to a part. PASSIVE H. occurs when there is restricted flow of blood from a part. — hyperaemic, adj.

hyperaesthesia (hī´-per-es-thē´-zi-a): Excessive sensitiveness of the skin or another special sense organ. — hyperaesthetic, adj. Cf. ANAESTHESIA.

hyperalbuminaemia (hī´-per-al-bū-mi-nē´-mi-a): Abnormally high percentage of albumin in the blood.

hyperaldosteronism (hī´-per-al-dos´-ter-o-nizm): Excessive secretion of aldosterone, causing disturbance of electrolyte metabolism; may be primary in Conn's syndrome or secondary to another disease condition such as hypertension, heart failure, cirrhosis, low serum potassium levels, hypoproteinaemia.

hyperalgesia (hī´-per-al-jē´-zi-a): Excessive sensivity to pain. Also called *hyperalgia*. — hyperalgesic, adj.

hyperalimentation (hī´-per-al-i-men-tā´-shun): Administration or ingestion of more than the optimal amount of nutrients; may be temporary therapy or permanent for patients whose absorptive capabilities are inadequate. Usually refers to administration through an indwelling catheter in the subclavian vein; the solution given contains the substances for complete nutrition when the patient cannot take these via the usual route; has been used for patients with such conditions as oesophageal obstruction, ulcerous conditions, cancer of different parts of the digestive tract and accessory organs, enteritis, ulcerative colitis, burns, pancreatitis, and acute renal, hepatic, or respiratory failure. ENTERAL H. the special nutrient formula is introduced into the intestine through a tube that is inserted through the nose and passed to the small intestine.

hyperandrogenism (hī´-per-an-droj´-en-izm): The state characterized by or resulting from over-secretion of androgens.

hyperaphia (hī-per-ā´-fi-a): Abnormal acuteness of the sense of touch.

hyperasthenia (hī´-per-as-thē´-ni-a): Extreme weakness. — hyperasthenic, adj.

hyperbaric (hī-per-bar´-ik): At greater pressure, specific gravity, or weight than normal. H. OXYGEN CHAMBER sealed cylinder containing oxygen under pressure. Accommodates patient, attendant, and equipment. In some units surgery can be performed, as anaerobic organisms and their ability to produce toxins are adversely affected by oxygen; oxygen-saturated tissues also respond better to radiotherapy; H. OXYGEN TREATMENT has been suggested for treatment of burns, refractory osteomyelitis, cerebral oedema, soft tissue infections, peripheral vascular disease, gas gangrene, carbon monoxide poisoning, and any other condition in which the oxygen content of the blood is deficient.

hypercalcaemia (hī-per-kal-sē´-mi-a): An excessive amount of calcium in the circulating blood; occurs in osteoporosis, hyperparathyroidism, and other conditions marked by resorption of bone.

hypercalciuria (hī´-per-kal-si-ū´-ri-a): Greatly increased calcium excretion in urine, as seen in hyperparathyroidism. Of importance in pathogenesis of nephrolithiasis. IDIOPATHIC H., H. for which there is no known metabolic cause.

hypercapnia (hī-per-kap´-ni-a): Excessive amounts of carbon dioxide in the circulating blood. — hypercapnic, adj.

hypercellular (hī-per-sel´-ū-lar): Characterized by an abnormally large number of cells or an increase in the number of cells present. — hypercellularity, n.

hyperchloraemia (hī´-per-klō-rē´-mi-a): Excessive amounts of chloride in the circulating blood. — hyperchloraemic, adj.

hyperchlorhydria (hī´-per-klor-hid´-ri-a): Excessive hydrochloric acid in the gastric juice. — hyperchlorhydric, adj.

hypercholesterolaemia (hī´-per-ko-les´-ter-ōl-ē´-mi-a): Excessive cholesterol in the blood. Predisposes to atheroma and gallstones. Also found in myxoedema. — hypercholesterolaemic, adj.

hyperchromatism (hī´-per-krō´-ma-tizm): 1. Excessive pigmentation of the skin. 2. A condition in which parts of a cell accept more than a normal amount of stain. 3. An increased amount of chromatin in the nuclei of cells.

hyperchromia (hī'-per-krō'-mi-a): 1. Hyperchromatism (*q.v.*). 2. An increase in the normal amount of haemoglobin in the red blood cells.

hyperchylia (hī'-per-kī'-li-a): Excessive secretion of gastric juice.

hypercoagulability (hī'-per-kō-ag'-ū-la-bil'-i-ti): The state of being more than normally coagulable; usually refers to the blood.

hypercorticism (hī'-per-kor'-ti-sizm): Hyperadrenocorticism. See CUSHING'S SYNDROME.

hypercortisolism (hī'-per-kor'-ti-sol-izm): A condition characterized by excessive secretion of hydrocortisone (cortisol) by the adrenal cortex, as occurs in Cushing's syndrome.

hypercryalgesia (hī'-per-krī-al-jē'-zi-a): Abnormal sensitiveness to cold. Also called *hyperaesthesia*.

hypercythaemia (hī'-per-sī-thē'-mi-a): An abnormal number of red blood cells in the circulating blood.

hypercytosis (hī'-per-sī-tō'-sis): An abnormal increase in the number of cells in the circulating blood; term is sometimes used synonymously with leukocytosis (*q.v.*).

hyperemesis (hī'-per-em'-e-sis): Excessive vomiting. H. GRAVIDARUM the pernicious vomiting in pregnancy.

hyperendemic (hī'-per-en-dem'-ik): Refers to a disease that is present in a community at all times and with a high incidence rate.

hyperextension (hī'-per-ek-sten'-shun): Overextension of a limb or part, *i.e.*, extreme or excessive straightening of a limb beyond its normal limit.

hyperflexion (hī'-per-flek'-shun): Excessive flexion of a limb or part beyond its normal limit.

hypergalactia (hī'-per-ga-lak'-shi-a): Excessive secretion of milk.

hyperglycaemia (hī'-per-glī-sē'-mi-a): An excessive amount of glucose in the circulating blood; hyperglycosaemia. — hyperglycaemic, adj.

hyperinvolution (hī'-per-in-vo-lū'-shun): Reduction to below normal size, as of the uterus after parturition.

hyperkalaemia (hī'-per-ka-lē'-mi-a): Excessive potassium in the circulating blood; may be caused by renal pathology, adrenal insufficiency, oral or intravenous intake in excessive amounts; symptoms include flaccidity of muscles, shallow respirations, depression of myocardium, arrhythmias.

hyperkinesia (hī'-per-kī-nē'-si-a): Excessive movement; abnormal restlessness, or excessive muscular activity. Also called *hyperkinesis*. — hyperkinetic, adj.

hyperkinetic (hī'-per-kī-net'-ik): Characterized or relating to hyperkinesia (*q.v.*). H. SYNDROME a form of minimal brain dysfunction (*q.v.*) characterized by excessive energy and motor activity, emotional instability, distractibility, lack of fear; seen mostly in children with brain injuries or learning disability.

hyperleukocytosis (hī'-per-lū'-kō-sī-tō'-sis): An increase in the number of leukocytes in the blood greater than that usually seen in leukocytosis.

hyperlipaemia (hī'per-līp-ē'mi-a): An excess of one or more of the lipaemic substances in the blood, particularly cholesterol and triglycerides; may be a primary condition in disorders of metabolism or secondary as occurs in diabetes mellitus.

hyperlipidaemia (hī'-per-lip-i-dē'-mi-a): Hyperlipaemia.

hyperlipoproteinaemia (hī'-per-lip-o-prō'-tē-in-ē'-mi-a): A disorder of fat metabolism characterized by the presence of more than the normal amount of lipoproteins in the circulating blood; associated with a large group of inherited and acquired disorders in which large amounts of lipoproteins and cholesterol appear in the blood.

hypermagnesaemia (hī'-per-mag-ne-sē'-mi-a): An abnormally high level of magnesium in the blood serum, occurs most often in people who habitually take large amounts of antacid drugs containing magnesium.

hypermetabolism (hī'-per-me-tab'-ō-lizm): An abnormal increase in the utilization of food materials by the body, resulting in the production of excessive heat. Characteristic of thyrotoxicosis. — hypermetabolic, adj.

hypernatraemia (hī'-per-nā-trē'-mi-a): An unusual high level of sodium in the blood. May occur either when an excessive water loss follows an excessive water intake, or in diabetes insipidus. — hypernatraemic, adj.

hyperopia (hī'-per-ō'-pi-a): A condition is which the rays or light entering the eye are focused behind the retina; usually due to flattening of the eyeball from front to back. Farsightedness. — hyperopic, adj. Syn. hypernetropia.

hyperosmolar (hī'-per-oz-mō'-lar): Relating to a solution with osmotic pressure greater than that of normal blood plasma. — hyperosmolarity, adj.

hyperostosis (hī′-per-os-tō′-sis): Thickening or overgrowth of bone. *Exostosis.*

hyperoxaemia (hī′-per-ok-sē′-mi-a): A condition in which the blood is excessively acid.

hyperoxia (hī′-per-ok′-si-a): An excess of oxygen in the tissues or the system. — hyperoxic, adj.

hyperparathyroidism (hī′-per-par-a-thī′-roydizm): A condition due to overaction of the parathyroid glands resulting in loss of calcium from the bones and an increase in serum calcium levels; may result in osteitis fibrosa cystica with decalcification and spontaneous fracture of bones.

hyperphenylalaninaemia (hī′-per-fen′-il-al-a-ni-nē′-mi-a): A condition in which the blood levels of phenylalanine are abnormally high; seen in premature and full-term infants; may be associated with phenylketonuria (q.v.); symptoms may include aminoaciduria, jaundice, splenomegaly, cataracts, cerebral and liver damage.

hyperphrenia (hī-per-frē′-ni-a): 1. Excessive mental activity. 2. An unusually high intellect.

hyperpiesis (hī-per-pī-ē′-sis): High blood pressure of unknown origin, especially essential hypertension; see under HYPERTENSION.

hyperpigmentation (hī′-per-pig-ment-tā′-shun): Increased or excessive pigmentation of a tissue or part. H. of the skin, may be due to exposure to sunlight, use of certain drugs, or adrenal insufficiency.

hyperpituitarism (hī′-per-pi-tū′-i-ta-rizm): Overactivity of the anterior lobe of the pituitary, producing gigantism or acromegaly.

hyperplasia (hī′-per-plā′-zi-a): Excessive formation of cells resulting in overgrowth of tissue. CONGENITAL ADRENAL H. a group of disorders caused by enzymatic defects that result in excessive secretion of the adrenal androgens; the congenital form of adrenogenital syndrome (q.v.); GINGIVAL H. enlargement of the gums until they cover portions of the teeth. — hyperplastic, adj.

hyperpnoea (hī′-perp-nē′-a): Rapid, deep, laboured breathing; panting; gasping. — hyperpnoeic, adj.

hyperpotassaemia (hī′-per-pot-a-sē′-mi-a): Increased potassium in the blood, a condition that, theoretically, can cause heart block, cardiac arrest, and muscle paralysis. Syn., *hyperkalaemia.* — hyperpotassaemic, adj.

hyperprolactinaemia (hī′-per-prō-lak′-tin-ē′-mi-a): An excess of prolactin in the blood, a normal condition in lactating women, but otherwise abnormal; may be associated with pituitary tumours; often accompanies amenorrhoea.

hyperproteinaemia (hī′-per-prō′-tē-in-ē′-mi-a): More than the normal amount of protein in the circulating blood.

hyperpsychosis (hī′-per-sī-kō′-sis): Excessive mental activity.

hyperpyrexia (hī′-per-pī-rek′-si-a): Extremely high fever. MALIGNANT H. a rare, often fatal, possibly hereditary condition usually affecting young people; marked by high fever and muscular rigidity; most often seen in postoperative patients who have been given certain drugs.

hyperreflexic (hī′-per-rē-flek′-sik): Spastic or hypertonic, or pertaining to hyperreflexia. H. BLADDER see NEUROGENIC BLADDER under NEUROGENIC.

hypersensitivity (hī′-per-sen-si-tiv′-i-ti): A state of being unduly sensitive to a stimulus or an allergen (q.v.). — hypersensitive, adj.

hypersomnia (hī′-per-som′-ni-a): A condition in which one sleeps for long periods of time but is normal in the intervals between sleeping. — hypersomniac, n.; adj.

hypertension (hī′-per-ten′-shun): 1. Transient or persistently high blood pressure, by custom referring to blood pressure readings in which either or both systolic and diastolic pressure readings are significantly higher than the mean for the population. 2. Persistent elevation of blood pressure that is over 140 systolic and 90 diastolic (WHO definition). H. is a symptom rather than a disease and the cause is often unknown, but it may indicate change in the condition of the blood vessels or the heart muscle, or a kidney disorder, it is likely to increase during periods of emotional stress and decrease during periods of rest and sleep. H. is not usually considered curable, but can be controlled by appropriate medication; it can sometimes be controlled by weight loss and a low salt, low fat diet. ESSENTIAL H. that which occurs without pre-existing disease or demonstrable change in kidneys, heart, or blood vessels; also sometimes called *primary* or *benign H.*; symptoms include headache, dizziness, tinnitus, nosebleed, fainting; MALIGNANT H. usually develops at a comparatively early age, runs a rapid course, and has a poor prognosis; PORTAL H. abnormally high blood pressure in the portal venous system; often seen in cirrhosis of the liver; PULMONARY H. increased blood pressure within the pulmonary circulation; RENAL H. that due to damaged or defective kidney function; RENOPARENCHYMAL H.

that due to disease of the renal parenchyma; cause obscure; usually chronic and bilateral; RENOVASCULAR H. that resulting from interference with blood supply to the kidney.

hypertensive (hī´-per-ten´-siv): 1. Relating to, affected with, or characterized by hypertension. 2. A person affected with hypertension. H. CRISIS a sudden rise in blood pressure to measurements over 200/120 mmHg; occurs most often in patients who have not been treated or who have stopped taking prescribed medications; H. ENCEPHALOPATHY a condition occurring in persons with advanced arterial hypertension; symptoms include headache, vomiting, somnolence, and sometimes convulsions; H. HEART DISEASE a condition characterized by enlarged ventricles, altered pulse rate, nocturnal dyspnoea; H. RETINOPATHY see under RETINOPATHY.

hypertext markup language (hī´-per-tekst): A set of computer protocols used to write web sites.

hyperthelia (hī´-per-thē´-li-a): The presence of one or more supernumerary nipples.

hyperthermia (hī´-per-ther´-mi-a): 1. Extremely high temperature; hyperpyrexia. 2. A method of treating disease by raising the temperature of the body, either by external applications, the introduction of disease organisms into the body, or the injection of foreign proteins. See THERMODIALYSIS. MALIGNANT H. a rare complication of anaesthesia; the temperature rises very rapidly, with muscular rigidity, cardiac arrhythmia, circulatory collapse, and often coma and death.

hyperthymia (hī´-per-thī´-mi-a): 1. An overactive mental state with a tendency to perform impulsive acts. 2. Oversensitiveness. 3. Cruel or foolhardy behaviour as sometimes seen in patients with mental disorders.

hyperthyroidism (hī´-per-thī´-roy-dizm): Thyrotoxicosis (q.v.).

hypertonic (hī´-per-ton´-ik): 1. Having hypertonia 2. Having an osmotic pressure greater than a solution used for comparison, e.g., normal saline has a greater osmotic pressure than normal physiological (body) fluids. — hypertonicity, n.

hypertoxic (hī´-per-tok´-sik): Very poisonous.

hypertrophy (hī-per´-trō-fi): Increase in the bulk of a tissue or structure; due to increase in size of the cells, not to tumour formation; usually the result of functional activity, e.g., the H. of a muscle. — hypertrophia, n; hypertrophic, adj.

hyperuricaemia (hī´-per-ū-ri-sē´-mi-a): Excessive uric acid in the blood. Characteristic of gout. — hyperuricaemic, adj.

hypervascular (hī-per-vas´-kū-lar): Containing an abnormally large number of blood vessels. — hypervascularity, n.

hyperventilation (hī´-per-ven-ti-lā´-shun): 1. Over-breathing; more than 20 inspirations per minute. 2. A state in which there is a decrease of carbon dioxide in the blood as a result of rapid and deep breathing; symptoms may include dizziness, confusion, and muscle cramps. H. SYNDROME rapid and laboured breathing, as occurs in persons affected with depression or anxiety, leading to alkalosis.

hyperviscosity (hī´-per-vis-kos´-i-ti): The state of being excessively glutinous, sticky, or viscous.

hyperviscous (hī´-per-vis´kus): The condition of being abnormally viscous. See VISCOUS.

hypervolaemia (hī´-per-vō-lē´-mi-a): An abnormal increase in the volume of blood circulating in the body. Plethora (q.v.). — hypervolaemic, adj.

hypha (hī´-fa): One of the filaments that make up the mycelium (q.v.) of a fungus. — hyphae, pl.

hyphaemia (hī-fē´-mi-a): A deficiency of blood; oligaemia.

hyphidrosis (hīp-hīd-rō´-sis): A decrease in the secretion of sweat.

hypn-, hypno-: Combining forms denoting: 1. Sleep. 2. Hypnosis or hypnotism.

hypnagogic (hip-na-goj´-ik): Producing sleep or induced by sleep. In psychiatry, refers to hallucinations that occur during the period just before falling asleep.

hypnoanalysis (hip´-nō-a-nal´-a-sis): Psychoanalysis with the patient under hypnosis (q.v.).

hypnolepsy (hip´-nō-lep-si): Uncontrollable, abnormal drowsiness. Narcolepsy.

hypnosis (hip-nō´-sis): A state resembling sleep, brought about by the hypnotist utilizing the mental mechanism of suggestion H. can be used to produce painless labour and dental extractions; is occasionally utilized in minor surgery and in psychiatric practice. — hypnotic, adj.; hypnotize, v.t.

hypnotherapy (hip´-nō-ther´-a-pi): Treatment by prolonged sleep or hypnosis.

hypnotic (hip-not´-ik): 1. Relating to hypnotism. 2. A drug that produces sleep.

hypnotism (hip´-nō-tizm): 1. The process of inducing a condition in which a person appears to be asleep but is susceptible to suggestion and carries out commands. 2. The study or practice of hypnosis.

hypo-: Prefix denoting: 1. Deficient; less than normal. 2. Located beneath or below. Opp. to hyper-.

hypoactivity (hī′-pō-ak-tiv′-i-ti): Abnormally diminished activity; said of glands, nerves, muscles, or of the entire organism.

hypoadrenalism (hī′-pō-a-drē′-na-lizm): The condition of reduced adrenocortical function; adrenal insufficiency.

hypoadrenocorticism (hī′-pō-a-drē′-nō-kor′-ti-cizm): A condition characterized by a decrease in the activity of the adrenal gland; Addison's disease.

hypoaesthesia (hī′-pō-es-thē′-zi-a): Abnormally diminished sensitiveness of a part.

hypoalbuminaemia (hī′-pō-al-bu-min-ē′-mi-a): An abnormally low amount of albumin in the circulating blood. — hypoalbuminaemic, adj.

hypobaric (hī′ pō-bar′ik): 1. Referring to atmospheric pressure that is significantly lower than usual. 2. Referring to an anaesthetic in solution that has a lower specific gravity than that of cerebrospinal fluid.

hypobaropathy (hī′pō-bar-op′a-thi): A condition caused by diminished air pressure or decrease in oxygen in the air. Examples are altitude sickness, mountain sickness, aviator's sickness, caisson disease (q.v.).

hypocalcaemia (hī′-pō-kal-sē′-mi-a): Abnormally low levels of calcium in the circulating blood; occurs in such conditions as hypoparathy roidism, inadequate intake of calcium, vitamin D deficiency, kidney and pancreatic pathology; chief symptoms are tetany of the hands, feet, tongue and lips, and cardiac arrhythmias. See TETANY.

hypocalciuria (hī′-pō-kal-si-ū′-ri-a): An abnormal diminution in the amount of calcium excreted in the urine.

hypocapnia (hī-pō-kap′-ni-a): Less than the normal amount of carbon dioxide in the circulating blood. — hypocapnic, adj.

hypocellular (hī-pō-sel′-ū-lar): Characterized by an abnormally low number of cells or a decrease in the number of cells present. — hypocellularity, n.

hypochloraemia (hī′-pō-klō-rē′-mi-a): Less than the normal amount of chlorides in the circulating blood. A form of alkalosis. — hypochloraemic, adj.

hypochlorhydria (hī′-pō-klor-hid′-ri-a): Less than the normal amount of hydrochloric acid in the gastric juice. — hypochlorhydric, adj.

hypochlorite (hī-pō-klō′-rīt): Any salt of hypochlorous acid. Such salts are easily decomposed to yield active chlorine, have antiseptic and disinfectant properties, and have been widely used on that account in treating wounds and for the disinfection of equipment and infant feeding utensils (e.g., Milton and Dakin's solution).

hypocholesterolaemia (hī′-pō-kō-les′-ter-ē′-mi-a): Less than the normal amount of cholesterol in the blood.

hypochondria (hī-pō-kon′-dri-a): A fixed mental attitude involving the erroneous conviction that the body or organ is diseased. Excessive anxiety about one's health; common in depressive and anxiety states. — hypochondriac, adj.

hypochondriac (hī-pō-kon′-dri-ak): One suffering from hypochondria (q.v.).

hypodermic (hī-pō-der′-mik): 1. Below the skin; subcutaneous. 2. An injection into or under the skin. 3. A small syringe with a hollow needle used for injecting drugs or other agents into or under the skin. — hypodermically, adv.

hypodermis (hī-pō-der′-mis): The layer of tissue lying immediately beneath the corium of the skin (q.v.).

hypofunction (hī′-pō-funk′-shun): Diminished or inadequate function.

hypogammaglobulinaemia (hī′-pō-gam-ma-glob′-ū-li-nē′-mi-a): Decreased gamma globulin in the blood; may be acquired or congenital; several types are identified, all of which are characterized by immunodeficiency (q.v.). See IMMUNE RESPONSE under IMMUNE.

hypogastric (hī-pō-gas′-trik): Refers to the area immediately below the stomach. See ABDOMINAL REGIONS under REGION.

hypogastrium (hī′-pō-gas′-tri-um): That area of the anterior abdomen which lies immediately below the umbilical region. It is flanked on either side by the iliac regions. — hypogastric, adj.

hypogenitalism (hī-pō-jen′-i-tal-izm): Underdevelopment of the genitalia.

hypoglossal (hī-pō-glos′-al): Situated under the tongue. H. NERVE one of the twelfth pair of cranial nerves; the fibres arise in the medulla and go to the muscles of the tongue.

hypoglycaemia (hī′-pō-glī-sē′-mi-a): Abnormally low blood glucose levels; usually due to insulin overdose, dietary mismanagement, or an abnormal secretion of insulin, but may also result from anxiety, excitement, overactivity; symptoms include excessive perspiration, delirium, possible coma. H. is sometimes produced intentionally in treatment of schizophrenia. POSTPRANDIAL H. occurs in normal persons following the ingestion of a meal high in carbohydrates; a sharp insulin release is followed by a fall in the blood glucose level; also called *reactive glycaemia*.

hypoglycaemic (hī´-pō-glī-sē´-mik): Relating to hypoglycaemia. H. AGENT a drug or substance that lowers the glucose content of the blood; of two main types: (1) a drug that lowers the blood glucose and controls the various metabolic effects of the diabetes, *e.g.*, the sulphonylureas; and (2) a drug that assists patients who have some capacity to produce their own insulin to control their blood glucose, *e.g.*, the biguanides. H. CRISIS or SHOCK see INSULIN SHOCK.

hypokalaemia (hī´-pō-ka-lē´-mi-a): Abnormally low level of potassium in the blood. Symptoms are variable but may include muscle weakness and fatigue, nausea and/or vomiting, paralytic ileus, constipation or diarrhoea, apnoea, shallow breathing, respiratory arrest, arrhythmias. May be due to administration of potent diuretics or steroids, loss of body fluids by vomiting or diarrhoea, or decreased intake of dietary potassium.

hypokinesia (hī´-pō-kī-nē´-si-a): Abnormally decreased motor activity or function.

hypokinetic (hī´-pō-kī-net´-ik): Characterized by or pertaining to hypokinesia (*q.v.*). H. SYNDROME a form of minimal brain dysfunction (*q.v.*) in which motor activity is decreased.

hypoleukocytosis (hī´-pō-lū´-kō-sī-tō´-sis): Less than the normal number of leukocytes in the circulating blood. Syn., *leukocytopenia*.

hypomagnesaemia (hī´-pō-mag-ne-sē´-mi-a): Decreased magnesium content in the blood; may occur concurrently with hypercalcaemia.

hypomania (hī-pō-mā´-ni-a): A psychopathological state characterized by optimism, excitability, a marked hyperactivity and talkativeness, quick anger and irritability, and a decreased need for sleep.

hypomanic disorder (hī-pō-man´-ik): An atypical bipolar disorder (*q.v.*) in which a patient who previously had a depressive episode has a minor manic episode that is not serious enough to be classed as bipolar II.

hypometabolism (hī´-pō-me-tab´-ō-lizm): An abnormal decrease in the body's utilization of food materials, with resulting diminution in the production of heat; low metabolic rate. Characteristic of myxoedema (*q.v.*). — hypometabolic, adj.

hypomnesis (hī-pom-nē´-sis): Impaired memory.

hyponatraemia (hī´-pō-na-trē´-mi-a): Abnormally low concentration of sodium in the blood plasma; symptoms include muscle weakness, fatigue, possibly convulsions. May be (1) DILUTIONAL when it results from the intake of large amounts of water as is some-

times seen in schizophrenic and alcoholic patients or in those receiving excessive water enemas or electrolyte-free intravenous solutions, or (2) DEPLETIONAL when it is due to inappropriate use of diuretics, loss of body fluids, adrenal insufficiency, or renal disease. — hyponatraemic.

hypoperfusion (hī´-pō-per-fūzh´-un): Lack of adequate perfusion of the tissues with blood, due to decreased blood volume or inability of the heart to pump effectively.

hypophrenia (hī-pō-fre´-ni-a): Below the diaphragm.

hypophyseal (hī-pō-fiz´-ē-al): Relating to a hypophysis, particularly the pituitary gland.

hypophysectomy (hī´-pof-i-sek´-to-mi): Surgical removal of the pituitary gland. TRANSSPHENOID H. a H. performed through the sphenoid bone, a procedure that makes it possible for the posterior lobe of the pituitary gland to retain its function.

hypopiesis (hī´-pō-pī-ē´-sis): Abnormally low pressure, especially blood pressure.

hypopituitarism (hī´-pō-pi-tū´-i-tar-izm): Pituitary gland insufficiency, especially of the anterior lobe. Absence of gonadotrophins leads to failure of ovulation, uterine atrophy, amenorrhoea. Loss of trophic hormones often produces mental inertia, weakness, lack of sweating, sensitivity to cold, oliguria, loss of pubic and axillary hair, hypoglycaemia, pale skin, depigmentation of mammary areolae and perineum.

hypoplasia (hī-pō-plā´-zi-a): Defective or incomplete development of any tissue or organ due to a decrease in cell formation. CONGENITAL ADRENOCORTICOID H. caused by a defect in adrenal function, with absence or decrease in secretion of hydrocortisone; results in anomalies and abnormal development of reproductive organs, abnormal growth patterns, excessive hairiness, and skin pigmentation.

hypopnoea (hī-pop´-nē-a): An abnormal decrease in the rate and depth of respirations. Opp. to hyperpnoea.

hyposensitive (hī-pō-sen´-si-tiv): Having a deficient response to stimuli.

hyposensitiveness (hī-pō-sen´-si-tiv-nes): Subnormal sensitiveness in which (1) reponses to stimuli are lessened or delayed; or (2) there is greater than normal power of resistance to a pathogenic agent.

hyposensitization (hī´-pō-sen-si-tī-za´-shun): Reduction of the sensitiveness of an individual, especially to allergens; usually achieved by repeated injections of small amounts of the particular allergen.

hyposomnia (hī-pō-som′-ni-a): Insomnia (*q.v.*).

hypospadias (hī-pō-spā′-di-as): A congenital malformation in which the male urethra opens on the undersurface of the penis, that of the female opens into the vagina instead of externally from the bladder. Also called *hypospadia*. — hypospadiac, adj.

hypostasis (hi-pos′-ta-sis): 1. Congestion of blood in a part; due to impaired circulation. 2. The formation or deposit of a sediment resulting from impairment of flow of blood or other body fluid.

hypostatic (hī-pō-stat′-ik): 1. Caused by or pertinent to hypostasis (*q.v.*). 2. Abnormally static; said of certain inherited characteristics that are hidden or suppressed by other characteristics. H. CONGESTION see CONGESTION; H. PNEUMONIA see PNEUMONIA.

hyposthenuria (hī-pos-the-nū′ri-a): The secretion of urine that is of lower than normal specific gravity; often associated with chronic nephritis.

hypotension (hī-pō-ten′-shun): Lowered blood pressure, primary or secondary. May result from a decrease in cardiac output, total blood volume, or peripheral resistance, or from an endocrine disturbance, haemorrhage, fever, shock, Addison's disease, or drug toxicity. A person is said to be hypotensive when the systolic pressure is below 110 mmHg and the diastolic pressure is below 70 mmHg. ESSENTIAL H. may exist without apparent cause; seen most often in women and the undernourished; ORTHOSTATIC or POSTURAL H. a fall in blood pressure that occurs when a person stands up after being in a supine position, or stands erect for a long time.

hypotensive (hī-pō-ten′-siv): 1. A drug or agent that lowers blood pressure. 2. A person suffering from hypotension. 3. Characterized by low blood pressure.

hypothalamus (hī′-pō-thal′-a-mus): Below the thalamus. The part of the midbrain nearest to the pituitary gland; important because the nuclei of this region control the body temperature, visceral activities, sleep, water balance, and the metabolism of fats and carbohydrates; also important in emotional and motivational behaviour. — hypothalamic, adj.

hypothermia (hī-pō-ther′-mi-a): 1. A temperature below normal body temperature (below 98.6°F, or 37°C). 2. Artificially induced H. (86°F or 30°C) can be used in the treatment of head injuries and in cardiac surgery. It reduces the oxygen consumption of the tissues and thereby allows greater and more prolonged interference of normal blood circulation. ACCI-

DENTAL H. unexpected drop in body temperature; develops over a period of time, usually in old people in a cool but not cold environment; the temperature will continue to fall and death will result unless there is a change in the environment; H. BLANKET (1) a covering used to conserve the body heat of a person suffering from hypothermia, or (2) a blanket that has built-in hollow coils carrying cold water and alcohol or other cooling solution kept in circulation by a pump; used to reduce prolonged high fever or for its anaesthetic action on patients undergoing brain or heart surgery; NEONATAL H. precipitous fall in body temperature in the neonate; the common causes are prematurity, infection and hypoxic brain damage.

hypothesis (hī-poth′-ē-sis): A proposed explanation for a phenomenon. In the scientific method, a hypothesis should be falsifiable, meaning that it can be disproven by further observation.

hypothetico-deductive method (hī-pō-thet′-i-kō-di-duk′-tiv): A technique in which the investigator proposes hypotheses and tests their acceptability by determining whether their logical consequences are consistent with observed data. This method is used to construct a scientific theory that will account for results obtained through direct observation and experimentation and that will, through inference, predict further effects that can then be verified or disproved by empirical evidence derived from other experiments.

hypothrombinaemia (hī′-pō-throm-bin-ē′-mi-a): A deficiency of thrombin in the blood; resulting in a tendency towards bleeding.

hypothyroidism (hī′-pō-thī′-royd-izm): A group of symptoms caused by deficiency of thyroid secretion; characterized by low metabolic rate, slowing of all bodily functions, fatigue, lethargy, hoarseness, intolerance of cold, constipation, weight gain, rough skin; occurs most often in women. INFANTILE H. may result from agenesis of the thyroid gland or inadequate intake of iodine by the mother during pregnancy. See CRETINISM; MYXOEDEMA.

hypotonia (hī-pō-tō′-ni-a): 1. Flaccid muscle tone or muscle weakness. When present at birth the infant is referred to as 'floppy'. 2. Lack of tone in the muscle walls of arteries. 3. Reduced tension, as in the eyeball.

hypotonic (hī-pō-ton′-ik): 1. Having a low osmotic pressure; less than isotonic. 2. Lacking in tone, tension, strength. H. SOLUTION a solution having an osmotic pressure lower than that of physiological saline.

hypotrophy (hī-pot' -ro-fi): Progressive degeneration of cells and tissues with loss of function.

hypoventilation (hī' -pō-ven-ti-lā' -shun): 1. Diminished breathing or underventilation. 2. Less than the normal amount of air entering the lungs; results in less oxygen reaching the alveoli than the body needs for normal metabolism, and an elevation of the carbon dioxide content of the blood, thus causing hypoxaemia and hypercapnia.

hypovolaemia (hī' -pō-vō-lē' -mi-a): An abnormal decrease in the amount of blood circulating in the body. Opp. to hypervolaemia. — hypovolaemic, adj.

hypovolaemic (hī' -pō-vō-lē' -mik): Relating to or characterized by hypovolaemia. H. SHOCK shock caused by a reduced amount of blood in circulation, as may occur in perforating wounds, burns, or other types of trauma.

hypoxaemia (hī-pok-sē' -mi-a): Less then the normal amount of oxygen in the arterial blood. — hypoxaemic, adj.

hypoxia (hī-pok' -si-a): Diminished amount of oxygen in the tissues. ANAEMIC H. due to a decrease or alteration in the haemoglobin content of the blood; HISTOLYTIC H. the condition existing when the cells' ability to utilize required amounts of oxygen is impaired; HYPOXIC H. due to a reduced amount of arterial oxygen, caused by interference with the passage of oxygen over the alveolar membrane; ISCHAEMIC H. is due to inadequate perfusion of the tissues with blood; STAGNANT H. a condition in which the oxygen tension in peripheral vessels is less than normal while that in the arterial blood is normal; occurs in congestive heart failure, shock, and when venous return is interfered with.

hypoxin (hī-poks' -in): A deficiency of oxygen at the cellular or tissue level.

hyster-: Combining forms denoting: 1. Hysteria. 2. Uterus.

hysterectomy (his-te-rek' -to-mi): Surgical removal of the uterus. ABDOMINAL H. effected via a lower abdominal incision; RADICAL H.

Wertheim's H. (*q.v.*); SUBTOTAL H. removal of the uterine body, leaving the cervix in the vaginal vault; TOTAL H. complete removal of the uterine body and the cervix; VAGINAL H. effected through the vagina; WERTHEIM'S H. total removal of the uterus, the adjacent lymphatic vessels and glands, and a cuff of the vagina. See PANHYSTERECTOMY.

hysteria (his-tēr' -i-a): A psychoneurosis or neurosis characterized by a physical disorder such as blindness or paralysis, brought on by psychological rather than organic disorder. Marked by conversion of anxiety into such symptoms as nervousness, uncontrollable laughing, crying, convulsions, intense muscular activity, psychic disorders. CONVERSION H. a condition in which hysteria is used to symbolize intrapsychic conflict.

hysterical (his-ter' -i-kal): Related to or affected with hysteria (*q.v.*). H. NEUROSIS see HYSTERIA; H. PSYCHOSIS in psychiatry, refers to acute episodes marked by sudden violent behaviour or reaction in a person of H. personality; see PERSONALITY.

hysterics (his-ter' -iks): An uncontrollable fit of laughing or crying, or both. See HYSTERIA.

hysteropexy (his' -ter-ō-pek-si): Fixation of a displaced or abnormally placed uterus; may be fastened to the vaginal or abdominal wall.

hysteroptosis (his' -ter-op-tō-sis): Prolapse of the uterus.

hysterosalpingectomy (his' -ter-ō-sal-pin-jek' -to-mi): Excision of the uterus and usually both uterine tubes (oviducts).

hysterosalpingo-oophorectomy (his-ter-ō-sal' -ping-gō-ō' -of-o-rek' -to-mi): Removal of the uterus, uterine tubes, and ovaries.

hysteroscope (his' -ter-o-skōp): An instrument used in visual examination of the uterine cervix and cavity.

hysterotomy (his-ter-ot' -o-mi): Incision into the uterus, usually in order to remove a fetus in midpregnancy when it is too late to perform a therapeutic abortion.

Hz: Hertz (*q.v.*).

I

I: The chemical symbol for iodine.

^{131}I, ^{132}I: Radioactive isotopes of iodine.

-iasis: A combining form denoting (1) a morbid condition; disease produced by something specific, *e.g.*, amoebiasis (2) a disease having the characteristics of a specific thing, *e.g.*, elephantiasis.

-iatrics: Combining form denoting a special field of medical practice.

-iatrist: A combining form denoting a doctor, *e.g.*, psychiatrist.

iatro-: Combining form denoting relationship to a doctor or to medicine, *e.g.*, iatrogenic.

iatrogenesis (ī-at-rō-jen'-e-sis): The inadvertent development of a secondary illness or condition through medical or surgical treatment for a primary disorder. iatrogenic, adj.

IBD: Abbreviation for inflammatory bowel disease (*q.v.*).

IBS: Abbreviation for irritable bowel syndrome (*q.v.*).

ICAS: Abbreviation for Independent Complaints Advocacy Service (*q.v.*).

ICD: Abbreviation for: International Classification of Diseases of the World Health Organization (*q.v.*).

ichor (ī'-kor): A thin, watery discharge, as from a raw wound or ulcer. — ichorous, adj.

ichthyosis (ik-thi-ō'-sis): A congenital chronic condition of keratin formation in which the skin becomes rough, dry, and scaly over the entire body, the hair is lustreless, and cold weather causes intense itching; also called *fish skin or alligator skin*. I. CONGENITA NEONATORUM a severe form of I. in the newborn; the skin and mucous membranes of the body are thickened, dry, and cracked; the skin may peel off; the eyelids may be everted; the fetus may be stillborn or die soon after birth; also called *Harlequin fetus* because of the effect produced by the cracking of the skin; I. VULGARIS a form of I. that is inherited as an autosomal dominant trait; onset is in childhood; characterized by fine scales on most of the body; tends to improve with age; SEX-LINKED I., I. that appears at birth or soon thereafter; seen only in males; marked by the presence of large brown scales on most of the body except the face, palms, and soles; does not improve much with age.

ICN: Abbreviation for International Council of Nurses (*q.v.*).

ICPs: Abbreviation for integrated care pathways (*q.v.*).

ictal (ik'-tal): Relating to a stroke or seizure, *e.g.*, an acute epileptical seizure.

icteric (ik-ter'-ik): Relating to or affected with jaundice.

icterus (ik'ter-us): Jaundice (*q.v.*).

icterus index (ik'-ter-us in'-deks): An index, expressed in units, representing the bilirubin concentration in the blood plasma; used in diagnosis of jaundice. The normal range is 4–6 units.

ictus (ik'-tus): A stroke or blow; a sudden attack or fit; an epileptic seizure.

ICU: Abbreviation for intensive care unit (*q.v.*). ICU PSYCHOSIS, see under PSYCHOSIS.

id: In psychoanalysis, that part of the unconscious mind that consists of a system of primitive urges (instinctual drives), including sexuality and aggression, and that persists unrecognized into adult life as the source of basic desires operating for self-gratification; man's inner drives.

IDDM: Abbreviation for insulin-dependent diabetes mellitus, see under DIABETES.

ideation (ī-dē-ā'shun): The process concerned with the highest function of awareness, the formation of ideas. It includes thought, intellect, and memory.

idée fixe (ē-dā-fēks): A fixed idea, an obsession; a delusion.

identical twins: Monozygotic twins; two offspring developed from a single fertilized egg. They are always of the same sex and commonly much alike in appearance. See BINOVULAR, UNIOVULAR.

identification (i-den'ti-fi-kā'shun): In psychology, the way in which personality is formed by modelling it on a chosen person, *e.g.*, identification with the parent of the same sex in helping to form one's sex role, or identification with a person of one's own sex, as in the hero worship of adolescence.

identification band or **bracelet:** A band that is placed on the wrist or ankle when a patient enters a hospital and worn throughout the hospital stay; the patient's name and other identification information is on it.

identity (ī-den′ -ti-ti): The group of characteristics that distinguish an individual from others. I. CRISIS loss of the sense of one's self and inability to adopt the role one perceives as being expected; is most likely to occur when one moves from one age group to another, as during adolscence or as one grows older and one's status in the community changes.

ideology (ī′ dē-ol′o-ji): An idea that forms the basis of political thought, often defining political parties and their policy. The thoughts and beliefs of a social group.

ideomotor (ī′dē-o-mō′tor): Descriptive of auto-mative muscular activity that is aroused by thoughts or ideas, such as moving the lips while reading silently. Agitated movements of parts of the body resulting from mental agitation.

idio-: Combining form denoting: (1) self-pro-duced, self-producing, arising within the self; (2) separate, distinct, peculiar.

idioglossia (id-i-ō-glos′ -si-a): Any form of invented speech that is unique to the individual but is incomprehensible to others except in close siblings or twins in whom it often develops.

idiographic (id′ -i-ō-graf′ -ik): In research, refers to a study of events or subjects in which a great deal of data is acquired from a few people, perhaps only one. Opp. of nomothetic (q.v.).

idiopathic (id′ -i-ō-path′ik): **1.** Self-originated; of unknown cause. **2.** Relating to a peculiar individual characteristic.

idiopathy (id-i-op′ -a-thi): A pathological state of unknown or spontaneous origin. — idiopathic, adj.

idiophrenic (id′ -i-ō-fren′ -ik): Related to or originating solely in the mind.

idiosyncrasy (id′ -i-ō-sin′kra-si): A peculiar variation of constitution or temperament. Unusual individual response to certain drugs, proteins, etc., whether administered by injection, ingestion, inhalation, or contact.

idiosyncratic reaction (id-i-ō-sin-krat′ -ik): A reaction that is completely different from the one expected; usually refers to drugs which may produce a reaction that is completely opposite to the one which the drug was expected to produce.

idioventricular (id′ -i-ō-ven-trik′ū-lar): Relating to the cardiac ventricles and not affecting the atria.

IgG: The symbol for immunoglobulin G, which comprises about 80% of the serum antibodies in the adult.

ileal (il′ -ē-al): Relating to or involving the ileum. I. BYPASS the formation of an anastomosis between a part of the ileum and a part farther on; decreases the area for absorption; sometimes done in treatment of obesity; I. CONDUIT a surgically constructed passageway for urine in which a section of the ileum is separated from the rest of the bowel and one end is closed; the two ureters are attached to this segment which serves as a bladder; the unclosed end is brought to the surface of the abdominal wall in a stoma where the urine is collected in a special bag. Also called *ileal bladder, ileal loop*, and *ileal loop diversion*.

ileectomy (il-e-ek′ -to-mi): Surgical excision of the ileum.

ileitis (il-ē-ī′ -tis): Inflammation of the ileus, characterized by ulceration, possible formation of adhesions, pain in the umbilical area and right lower quadrant, vomiting, alternating constipation and diarrhoea. REGIONAL I. acute or chronic I., marked by diarrhoea, anaemia, abdominal pain, greyish or brownish coloured stools; may give rise to intestinal obstruction. Also called *Crohn's disease* (q.v.).

ileo-: A combining form denoting the ileum.

ileocaecal (il′ē-ō-sē′kal): Relating to the ileum and the caecum. I. VALVE the sphincter muscle that guards the opening between the ileum and the large intestine, allowing material to pass from the small to large intestine, but not in the reverse direction.

ileocolic (il′ -ē-ō-kol′ -ik): Relating to the ileum and the colon.

ileocolostomy (il′ -ē-ō-kō-los′to-mi): The creation of an anastomosis between the ileum and the colon; usually the transverse colon. Most often done to bypass an obstruction or inflammation of the caecum or ascending colon.

ileoileostomy (il-ē-ō-il-ē-os′ -to-mi): The surgical creation of an anastomosis between two parts of the ileum.

ileostomy (il-ē-os′ -to-mi): A surgically made fistula between the ileum and the surface of the anterior abdominal wall; usually a permanent form of artificial anus when the whole of the large bowel has to be removed, *e.g.*, in severe ulcerative colitis. I. BAGS rubber or plastic bags worn on the body to collect the liquid discharge from the ileum.

ileoureterostomy (il′ -ē-ō-ū-rēt-er-os′to-mi): Transplantation of the lower ends of the ureters from the urinary bladder to an isolated loop of small bowel which, in turn, is made to open on the abdominal wall. See BLADDER.

ileum (il′-ē-um): The lower three-fifths of the small intestine, lying between the jejunum and the caecum; about 3.7 metres long. — ileal, adj.

ileus (il′-ē-us): Intestinal obstruction. Usually restricted to paralytic as opposed to mechanical obstruction and characterized by abdominal distension, vomiting, fever, and dehydration. MECONIUM I. occurs in the newborn; due to blockage of the bowel by thick meconium; usually an indication of fibrocystic (*q.v.*); disease, PARALYTIC I. an intestinal obstruction that may result from hypokalaemia, toxaemia, or trauma, especially that caused by handling during abdominal surgery; characterized by intense pain and abdominal distension; SPASTIC I. obstruction resulting from persistent contraction of the intestinal muscles.

ili-, iliu-: Combining forms denoting relation ship to the ilium or flank.

iliac (il′-i-ak): Relating to the ilium. I. ARTERY the large artery that transports blood to the pelvis and the legs.

iliococcygeal (ll′l-ō-kok-sij′i-al): Relating to the ilium and the coccyx.

iliofemoral (il′-i-ō-fem′-or al): Relating to the ilium and the femur.

ilium (il-i-um): The large, flaring, lateral, and uppermost of the three bones that compose the innominate (hip) bone; it is a separate bone in fetal life. The flank. — iliac, adj.

Illich, Ivan (il′-lich): A Viennese-born libertarian philosopher, social critic, and former Roman Catholic priest. His critique of economic development suggests that people have become increasingly dependent on professionals, and experts for many of their fundamental needs, for example health care and compulsory schooling. Subsequently, valuable vernacular skills have been lost. He talks about iatrogenic disease; that is, an illness caused by doctors or medicine. [1926–2003.]

illness: Disease, sickness, or the condition of being in poor health, either physically or mentally. I. NARRATIVES The stories people tell about their experience of sickess; these are used increasingly as a research method. There are three types: restitution narrative, where the illness is seen as transitory; chaos narrative is the opposite to restitution, the narrator imagines life never getting better; and the quest narrative presents illness as a learning experience.

illusion (i-lū′-zhun): **1.** A sensory experience that is different from reality, causing the individual to misidentify a sensation, *e.g.*, of sight, whereby a white sheet is mistaken for a ghost;

an apparition. **2.** The state of being deceived. **3.** A false impression, or misconception of a sensory stimulus, often with difficulty in focusing and with increased colour vision and hearing acuity, and disturbance of depth perception. **4.** A perception that does not give the true character of an object; may be normal as in certain optical illusions, or abnormal as occurs in insanity.

image (im′-ij): **1.** A reasonably accurate representation or imitation of a person or thing, *e.g.*, a statue. **2.** An optical picture transferred to the brain by the optic nerve. **3.** A mental representation of a precept, or a thing, not actually present but that is recalled by memory or created by imagination, as a taste or smell.

imagery (im′-ij-ri): Imagination. The recall of mental images of various types depending on the special sense organs involved when the images were formed. In behaviour therapy, imagery is used as a technique by which the person is conditioned to recall or imagine pleasant situations or experiences that counter feelings or memories that are unpleasant or painful.

imaging (im′-ij-ing): The production of diagnostic images, *e.g.*, radiography (*q.v.*), magnetic resonance imaging (*q.v.*), ultrasonography (*q.v.*).

imagocide (i-mā′-gō-sīd): An agent that kills adult insects, especially mosquitoes.

IM&T: Abbreviation for information management and technology.

immature (im-a-tūr′): Not fully developed or grown. I. INFANT one of less than 37 weeks' gestation. — immaturity, n.

immersion (i-mer′-zhun): The plunging of a body or part into a fluid. I. FOOT a condition resulting from long exposure to cold and dampness, or of actual immersion of the feet in water causing damage to the skin, blood vessels, and nerves; also called *trench foot*.

immobility (im-mō-bil′-i-ti): Inability to move separate parts of the body (especially the limbs or the whole body) easily and without pain.

immobilization (im-mō-′bi-lī-zā′shun): The act of making immovable. In medicine or surgery, the act of making a normally movable limb or part immovable by splints, bandages, surgical procedures, etc. — immobilize, v.t.

immune (im-ūn′): **1.** Not susceptible to a particular infection. **2.** A sensitivity reaction that indicates immunity following exposure to an antigen. I. BODY antibody (*q.v.*); I. REACTION that which causes a body to reject a transplanted organ; I. RESPONSE specifically altered reactivity of the body following exposure to an antigen, and which is manifested as antibody production, cell-mediated immunity, or immunological tolerance; term is often used synonymously with I. reaction; I. SYSTEM a complex system that is involved with maintaining homeostasis in which potentially harmful invading organisms are inactivated or eliminated, mutated cells that may become malignant are destroyed, and toxins are neutralized; also called *immuno defence system*.

immunity (im-ū'-ni-ti): A state of relative resistance to a disease. Immunity can be NATURAL (acquired from inherited qualities) or it can be acquired, actively or passively, naturally or artificially. ACTIVE I. is acquired naturally during a disease (infectious), or artificially by vaccination with dead or living organisms of the disease. Such immunity is long-lasting. PASSIVE I. is acquired naturally when maternal antibodies pass to the child via the placenta or breast milk, or artificially by administering immune sera containing antibodies obtained from animals or human beings. ARTIFICIAL PASSIVE I. is more temporary than active I. A simple classification based on the way immunity is produced, lists four types. 1. Artificial active I. produced by the introduction of *antigens* into the body. 2. Artificial passive I. produced by the introduction into the body of *antibodies*. 3. Natural active I. produced by having the disease. 4. Natural passive I. acquired by heredity.

immunization (im'ū-nī-za'shun): The process of making an individual immune, or of becoming immune.

immunocompetence (im'ū-nō-kom'pe-tens): The competence or ability to develop an immune reaction or response, *e.g.*, the production of antibodies.

immunocyte (im'ū-nō-sīt): A lymphoid cell that can react with an antigen to produce antibody.

immunodeficiency (im'-ū-nō-dē-fish'-en-si): A deficiency in the immune response of the body.

immunodepression: See IMMUNOSUPPRESSION.

immunoelectrophoresis (im'-ū-nō-i-lek'-trō-fō-rē'-sis): A technique for distinguishing proteins from one another on the basis of their electrophoretic mobility and their specific immune reactions. See ELECTROPHORESIS.

immunogenesis (im'-ū-nō-jen'e-sis): The process of producing immunity. — immunogenetic, adj.

immunogenetics (im'ū-nō-jen-et'iks): A branch of genetics that is concerned with the study of immunology, including the inheritance of genetic factors that control an individual's immune response and the transmission of these factors to offspring.

immunoglobulins (im'ū-nō-glob'ū-lins): Any of five structurally and antigenically distinct antibodies present in the serum and external secretions of the body. Kinds of immunoglobulins are IgA, IgD, IgE, IgG and IgM. See also GAMMA GLOBULIN.

immunohaematology (im'-ū-nō-hē-ma-tol'-o-ji): A branch of the science of haematology that deals with antigen–antibody reactions and other phenomena related to the pathogenesis of blood dyscrasias.

immunology (im'-ū-nol'-o-ji): The special branch of medicine that deals with the body's natural defence systems and with immunity to disease.

immunopathology (im'-ū-nō-path-ol'-o-ji): 1. The study of the phenomena associated with immunity. 2. Abnormal immune reaction, as when a person becomes sensitized.

Initial immunization schedule.

Immunization	Schedule
Diphtheria	
Tetanus	
Pertussis	Primary course given at 2, 3 and 4 months
Haemophilus influenzae	
Oral polio	
Measles/mumps/rubella	Given at 12–18 months
BCG	May be given to infants under certain circumstances

immunoprophylaxis (im'-ū-nō-pro-fi-lak'-sis): The prevention of disease by the use of vaccine to produce immunity.

immunosensitivity (im'ū-nō-sen-si-tiv'i-ti): The state produced by immunopathology (*q.v.*).

immunosuppression (im'-ū-nō-su-presh'un): Modification of the body's immune response so that its reaction to a foreign substance is diminished; may be produced by any one of several immunosuppressive agents; including drugs, radiation, and antilymphocytic serum. Used to enhance the survival of allografts.

immunosuppressive (im'ū-nō-su-pres'-iv): 1. Relating to immunosuppression. 2. An agent that prevents the occurrence of an immune reaction; used therapeutically following organ transplant and in treatment of autoimmune disease.

immunotherapy (im'ū-nō-ther'a-pi): 1. Passive immunity conferred to one individual by administration of serum containing antibodies formed by another individual. 2. Therapy utilizing chemicals, drugs, or x-rays for suppressing immunological reactions in the body.

immunotransfusion (im'-ū-nō-trans-fū'-zhun): Transfusion of blood from a donor previously rendered immune by repeated inoculations with a given agent from the recipient.

impacted (im-pak'-ted): Firmly wedged or pressed together so as to be immovable; said of a fracture when the jagged ends of bone are wedged together; of faeces in the rectum; of a fetus in the uterus; of a tooth in its socket; or of a calculus in a duct. — impaction, n.

impaction (im-pak'-shun): Compressed material in a confined space, as hardened faeces in the colon.

impairment (im-par'-ment): A physical or anatomical loss, deterioration, or weakening; due to disease or trauma.

impalpable (im-pal'-pa-b'l): Not palpable. Incapable of being felt by touch (palpation).

impatent (im-pā'-tent): Closed or obstructed; not patent.

imperforate (im-per'-fō-rāt): Lacking a normal opening. I. ANUS absence of an opening from the rectum; I. HYMEN a fold of mucous membrane at the vaginal entrance, which has no natural outlet for the menstrual fluid.

impermeable (im-per'-mē-a-b'l): Not penetrable; not permitting passage, as of a fluid through a membrane.

impetigo (im-pe'-tī'-gō): A common, acute, inflammatory skin disease, characterized by pustules that rupture and become crusted, usually appearing around the mouth and nostrils, most often caused by staphylococci or streptococci, or a combination of both. I. CONTAGIOSA a highly contagious form of I., commonest on the face and scalp; starts with a small red spot, quickly develops into rapidly spreading, superficial vesicles that rupture; the escaped serum dries into honey-coloured gummy crusts; I. HERPETIFORMIS a rare form of I. occurring in pregnant women; characterized by pustules on the trunk and thighs, vomiting, fever, delirium, prostration; potentially fatal.

impinge (im-pinj'): To encroach or press upon.

implant (im'-plant): 1. To insert or to graft. 2. Any material that is implanted into a host's intact tissues; for example, a metal pin, electronic device, mucous or bony tissue, or certain drugs. Drugs administered in this way provide for slow, steady release over a definite period of time; examples include (1) the use of testosterone in treatment of carcinoma of the breast; (2) deoxycortocosterone acetate (DOCA) in Addison's disease; (3) insulin in diabetes, (4) certain drugs for treatment of bronchial asthma; (5) certain contraceptives. INTRAOCULAR I. a plastic lens placed in the anterior and posterior chamber of the eye as a substitute for a lens extraction for cataract; PENILE I. a procedure to counteract impotence; several devices are available, including a sponge-filled silicone rod, and inflatable prostheses.

implantation (im-plan-tā'-shun): 1. The insertion of living cells or solid materials into the tissues, as in (a) surgical implantation of radium, solid drugs, or a pacemaker; or (b) accidental implantation of tumour cells in a wound. 2. The attachment of the fertilized ovum to the epithelial lining of the uterus.

implementation (im-ple-men-tā'-shun): 1. In research, the process where recommendations and planned interventions are put into practice in order to achieve a given outcome. 2. The third stage of the nursing process (*q.v.*).

implosion (im-plō'-zhun): In psychiatry, treatment by exposing the patient to his or her severest phobias, first in imagination, then in actual life situations. Also called *imaginative flooding*. See FLOODING.

impotence (im'-pō-tens): Lack of sexual power, by custom referring to the inability of the male to have an erection or to ejaculate following an erection, may be due to a physiological or psychological condition.

impotent (im'-pō-tent): 1. Barren or sterile. 2. Unable to copulate. — impotence, n.

impregnate (im-preg'-nāt): Fill. Saturate. Make pregnant.

impulse (im´-puls): 1. A sudden uncontrollable urge to act without deliberation. 2. A sudden push or communicated force. — impulsive, adj.

in-: A prefix denoting; 1. Into, in, inside, on, towards. 2. Non-: not. Appears as il before l; ir before r; and im before m, p, and b.

inaccessibility (in´-ak-ses-i-bil´-i-ti): In psychiatry, denotes absence of patient response.

inactivate (in-ak´-ti-vāt): To destroy the active principle or the biological activity of an agent or a substance. — inactivation, n.

inanimate (in-an´-i-māt): 1. Not alive. 2. Bereft of life or consciousness. 3. Dull, inert, stolid.

inanition (in-a-nish´-un): Exhaustion and wasting from lack of food or from lack of proper assimilation of food. 1. FEVER occurs during the first few days of life; high fever with rapid weight loss and restlessness; also called *dehydration fever*.

inappropriate antidiuretic hormone syndrome: A syndrome characterized by hyponatraemia and water intoxication, caused by elevated blood levels of antidiuretic hormone; may be associated with hypoalbuminaemia, major trauma, the use of certain drugs, or decreased blood volume which may result from haemorrhage, decreased cardiac output, or dehydration; treated by administration of sodium chloride, diuretics, and fluid restriction.

inarticulate (in-ar-tik´-ū-lāt): 1. Not jointed. 2. Said of speech that is not intelligible. 3. Not able to speak distinctly or clearly. 4. Inability to express oneself in speech.

inborn (in´-born): Descriptive of physical and mental characteristics that are present at birth and that have developed or been implanted while the fetus was *in utero*. Innate.

inborn error of metabolism: A disorder resulting from a defect in the genetic material; most commonly involves the chemical processes involved in metabolism, as occurs in phenylketonuria in infants, and in diabetes mellitus, cystic fibrosis, sickle cell anaemia, Down's sydrome, goitre. Also called *genetrophic disease* and *enzymopathy*.

incapacity (in-ka-pas´-i-ti): 1. A lack of full legal competence (*q.v.*) in any respect; for example, the incapacity of mentally disordered persons to conclude valid contracts 2. The inability to perform the activities of daily living (*q.v.*). A person suffering from incapacity is frequently referred to as a person under disability (*q.v.*).

incarcerated (in-kar´-ser-āt-ed): In medicine, the abnormal imprisonment of a part, as in a hernia that is irreducible, or a pregnant uterus that is held beneath the sacral promontory.

incest (in´-sest): Sexual intercourse between near kin, whose marriage is prohibited by law.

incidence (in´-si-dens): The rate of occurrence of an event or of a condition, *e.g.*, the number of new cases of a specific disease occurring in a population over specified time, usually one year.

incident: An event that may be either unpleasant or unusual. See CRITIAL INCIDENT; CRITICAL INCIDENT TECHNIQUE; RISK ASSESSMENT. I. REPORT a required report to the administrative staff of a health-care institution regarding the occurrence of any injury to a patient or visitor; cardiac arrest; error of omission or commission; of medications or treatments; theft or loss of a patient's belongings; or any other untowards event involving a patient.

incipient (in-sip´-i-ent): Initial, beginning, or in early stages; often said of symptoms.

incise (in-sīz´): To cut or cut into.

incision (in-sizh´-un): A cut or wound produced by cutting into body tissue, using a sharp instrument. — incise, v.; incisional, adj.

incisors (in-sī´-zers): The eight front cutting teeth, four in each jaw.

incisure (in-sī´-zhur): In anatomy, a notch, groove, or fissure.

inclusion bodies: Minute particles found in the cells of tissues that are affected by a virus, *e.g.*, the virus of measles. They are stainable and vary (in size, appearance, and quantity) with different diseases.

incoherent (in-kō-hēr´-ent): 1. The state or fact of being confused, disjointed, inconsistent, rambling, incongruous, or without proper sequence. 2. Being unable to express oneself in an intelligible and understandable manner. — incoherence, n.; incoherently, adj.

incompatibility (in´-kom-pat-i-bil´-i-ti): In medicine and pharmacology, a situation in which two substances cannot be used together without producing undesirable reaction. Usually refers to the bloods of donor and recipient in transfusion, when antigenic differences in the red cells result in reactions such as haemolysis and agglutination. See BLOOD GROUPS. May also refer to tissue transplants that are rejected by the recipient because certain antibody factors involved are not compatible.

incompetence (in-kom´-pe-tens): Inadequacy to perform a natural or required function, often said of cardiac valves. — incompetency, n.; incompetent, adj.

incontinence (in-kon´-ti-nens): Inability to control the evacuation of any excretory product, particularly urine and faeces; may be due to loss of sphincter control or to a cerebral or spinal lesion. DRIBBLING I. continuous outflow of urine; may be associated with neurological pathology; FAECAL I. inability to postpone defecation; due to loss of control of the anal sphincter; may be caused by ulcerative colitis, disorders of the central nervous system, impaction, cancer, muscular deficiency; NOCTURNAL I. enuresis (*q.v.*); OVERFLOW I. dribbling of urine from a fully distended bladder; due to an obstruction or damage to pelvic nerves; PARADOXICAL I. dribbling of urine due to chronic retention or a flaccid bladder; STRESS I. of urine, occurs when intra-abdominal pressure is raised, as in coughing or sneezing; due to relaxation or incompetence of the sphincter muscle of the urethra, or injury to the pelvic floor; TRUE I. of urine, occurs when there is a fistulous connection between the urinary and genital tracts, usually between the bladder and the vagina; URGE I. of urine, occurs when a hypertonic bladder contracts strongly even when there is only a small amount of urine in it; the urge to void is followed immediately by voiding.

incontinent (in-kon'-ti-nent). Inability to resist yielding to normal impulses, such as the sexual impulse, or normal urges such as the urge to defaecate or urinate.

incoordination (in' kō-or-di-nā'-shun): 1. Inability to produce smooth, harmonious muscular movements. 2. Failure of organs to work together harmoniously.

incrustation (in'-krus-tā'-shun): The formation of a scab on a wound.

incubate (in'-kū-bāt): To promote the growth of microorganisms by placing them in an incubator (*q.v.*).

incubation (in'kū-bā'shun): In medicine, the maintenance of organisms in conditions that are optimal for their growth and reproduction. I. PERIOD the time that elapses between entry of infection and the appearance of the first symptom of disease.

incubator (in'-kū-bā-ter): A temperature-regulated apparatus in which: (1) pre-term or sick babies may be placed; (2) microorganisms can be cultivated.

incus (ing'-kus): The central one of the chain of three small bones of the middle ear, taking its name from the Latin for anvil, which it resembles in shape.

Independent Complaints Advocacy Service: Nationwide service provided by patients' forums to help patients pursue formal complaints through the NHS complaints procedure.

Independent Reconfiguration Panel: An advisory group with the remit of examining proposals for NHS reconfigurations and service changes in England. It ensures that decisions about future services are sustainable and they support the process of modernization; and result in improved services for patients.

independent sector: Providers of health care that do not fall under the jurisdiction of the NHS, including commercial and charitable organizations. Although it does not usually cover all the services provided by the NHS, this sector includes facilities for acute and long-term care, *e.g.*, nursing and residential care homes; screening units; pathology laboratories; and mental health units; making a significant contribution to health and social care. Also known as the *private sector*.

independent variable: In a study of the cause and effect of one factor on another, the independent variable is the causal or 'predictor variable', producing the effect seen in the outcome or 'dependent variable' (*q.v.*).

index: 1. The second finger; the pointer. 2. The ratio of measurement (size, capacity, or function) of one substance, thing, or part of a thing compared with a standard that is fixed after a series of observations and usually represented as 1 or 100.

Index Medicus: A compilation of medical journal articles published throughout the world, listed by author and subject; published monthly by the US National Library of Medicine, and as a cumulative index at the end of each year.

indicator (in'-di-kā-ter): In chemistry, a substance used to make visible the completion of a chemical reaction.

indigenous (in-dij'-i-nus): Native to a certain locality or country.

indigestion (in-di-jes'-chun): Dyspepsia. Lack or failure of digestion (*q.v.*).

indirect contact: Refers to the transfer of infection by such conveyers as milk, water, air, contaminated hands, and inanimate objects.

indisposition (in-dis-po-zi'shun): In medicine, a slight or temporary illness, malaise.

individuation (in'di-vid-ū-ā'shun): The process of developing individual parts or characteristics of a whole that become increasingly distinct and independent.

indolent (in'-dō-lent): Lazy, sluggish, inert. In medicine, a sluggish ulcer that is generally painless and slow to heal.

induction (in-duk'-shun): 1. The act of bringing about something, especially at an early time; for example, labour or anaesthesia. 2. A formal entry into a position or office, such as preparation for commencing a new post.

inductive reasoning: The process of reasoning from a part to a whole, or from particular to general. Opp. of deductive reasoning (*q.v.*).

induration (in-dū-rā′-shun): 1. A hard swollen area beneath the surface of the skin. 2. The hardening of tissue as in hyperaemia, infiltration by neoplasm, etc. — indurated, adj. BRAWNY I. inflammatory thickening and hardening of tissue; BROWN I. OF THE LUNG a condition of firmness and brown colour of the lung which is associated with haemosidrin-pigmented macrophages in the alveoli; due to long-standing congestion occurring with heart disease.

indwelling (in′-dwel-ling): Relating to a drainage or feeding tube, or a catheter, that is fastened in position and allowed to remain fixed for a period of time. See FOLEY CATHETER under CATHETER.

inebriation (in-ē′brē-ā′shun): Drunkenness.

inebriety (in-ē brī′-e-ti): Habitual drunkenness.

inequality: Social or economic disparity between people or groups. See SOCIAL EXCLUSION; SOCIAL INCLUSION.

inert (in-ert′): 1. Slow, sluggish, inactive; having no physical or mental activity. 2. Term used to denote drugs that have no pharmaceutical or therapeutic action.

inertia (in-er′-shi-a): Lack of activity or force, physical or mental. I. UTERI sluggishness of uterine muscles during labour; may be primary due to constitutional weakness, or secondary due to exhaustion from frequent and forcible contractions.

in extremis (ineks-trē′-mis): At the point of death.

infant (in′-fant): A child less than one year of age. I. RESPIRATORY DISTRESS SYNDROME acute difficulty in breathing; seen most often in preterm infants, those delivered by Caesarean section, or those born of diabetic mothers; see under RESPIRATORY DISTRESS SYNDROME; PREMATURE I. one born before term but capable of life; PRETERM I. see PRETERM.

infant Hercules syndrome: Adrenogenital syndrome. A condition in a male child in whom an excessive amount of androgens is produced, causing great acceleration of physical and sexual growth.

infanticide (in-fan′-ti-sīd): The killing of a child by its mother during the first year of its life.

infantile (in′-fan-tīl): Relating to an infant. Childish. I. UTERUS term used to describe a uterus that is undeveloped or underdeveloped.

infantile paralysis: See POLIOMYELITIS.

infantilism (in-fan′-ti-lizm): 1. A condition in which childish physical, intellectual, and emotional characteristics persist into adolescence and adult life; may be idiopathic or the result of underdevelopment of certain organs or systems of the body. 2. A condition of psychological origin occurring in adults that is characterized by the use of childish patterns of speech and voice.

infant mortality rate: The number of children per 1000 live births in a specific area who die during the first year of life.

infarct (in′-farkt): The area of tissue, organ, or part that dies when the end artery supplying it, or the vein that carries blood from it, is occluded, *e.g.*, in the kidney or heart; a common complication of subacute endocarditis. MYOCARDIAL I. see MYOCARDIAL INFARCTION under INFARCTION.

infarction (in-fark′-shun): 1. Formation of an infarct. 2. Death of a section of tissue because the blood supply has been shut off. CEREBRAL I. ischaemia of a part of the brain due to lack of blood supply in an area of distribution of one of the cerebral arteries; MYOCARDIAL I. necrosis of part of the myocardium as a result of lack of blood supply to that part, as occurs in coronary thrombosis; PULMONARY I. necrosis of a localized area of the lung due to obstruction of the blood spply, as occurs in pulmonary embolism.

infect (in-fekt′): To cause infection; to contaminate with disease-producing organisms.

infection (in-fek′-shun): 1. The successful invasion, establishment, and growth of microorganisms in a degree sufficient to cause symptoms of disease in the host. 2. The condition produced by the introduction and growth of microorganisms in the tissues of the body. AIRBORNE I. one transmitted by the air, *e.g.*, organisms transmitted from one person to another by droplets discharged in coughing or sneezing; COMMUNITY-ACQUIRED I. one due to a pathologic organism common in the community; CONCURRENT I. one occurring at the same time as another; CONTAGIOUS I. one that is communicable by contact with a person suffering from it, or with articles the ill person has handled; CROSS INFECTIONS. those transmitted to each other by persons with differing infections; DIRECT CONTACT I. one caused by direct transmission from one person to another, as by kissing; DROPLET I. airborne I.; ENDOGENOUS I. one transferred from a body site where the organism is commensal to another site where it acts as a pathogen; EXOGENOUS I. one transmitted from sources outside the body, such as infected materials or people; enters by ingestion, inhalation, or inoculation; FOCAL I. one confined to one part of the body; INDIRECT CONTACT I. one transmitted by inanimate objects that have been contaminated by a person suffering from it; MASS I. one produced by invasion of a large number of disease-producing organisms MIXED I. one occurring concurrently with one or more others caused by different organisms; seen in abscesses; NOSOCOMIAL I. one acquired by a person while a patient in a health-care institution, also known as *hospital-acquired* I.; PYOGENIC I. one due to a pus-producing organism; SECONDARY I. one I. imposed upon another; SLOW VIRUS I. an I. caused by any of several viruses that remain in the body for a long time before symptoms appear; now thought to be causative in certain rare degenerative diseases, subacute sclerosing panencephalitis, multiple sclerosis; SUBCLINICAL I. one not severe enough to have clinical symptoms; URINARY TRACT I. bacterial infection of the kidney, collecting system of the kidney, or the bladder, or of all of these; usually caused by *Escherichia coli*; VIRAL I. may be caused by any one of a score of viruses that are pathogenic to humans and that may enter the body through the skin, respiratory or digestive tract, or by transfusion, and that may or may not confer immunity to the particular virus.

infection control committee: A multi-disciplinary group in a health-care institution organized for the purpose of developing, maintaining, and monitoring a programme of infection control; members usually include representatives from the administrative and medical staff, housekeeping staff, dieticians, nursing service, medical laboratory, and operating theatre. It is responsible for setting policies, developing protocols, conducting surveillance programmes, and educating personnel.

infection control nurse: A professional nurse with a good understanding of microbiology, and knowledge of epidemiology and specialist training. Is involved in the education of staff and investigating, implementing, and enforcing infection control measures in the facility.

infectious (in-fek'-shus): 1. Communicable; capable of being transmitted by direct or indirect contact. 2. Denoting a disease caused by a specific, pathogenic organism and capable of being transmitted to another individual. I. HEPATITIS an endemic type of hepatitis caused by hepatitis A virus; I. MONONUCLEOSIS see MONONUCLEOSIS.

infective (in-fek'-tiv): 1. Relating to an infection. 2. Infectious. — infectivity, n.

inferior (in-fe'ri-or): In anatomy, denotes lower, beneath, or below a point of reference. I. VENA CAVA main vein returning blood to the right atrium of the heart from the trunk and lower extremities.

inferiority complex: See under COMPLEX.

infertile (in-fer'-til): Unable to conceive or to maintain a pregnancy; term is not usually applied until a person has engaged in sexual intercourse for a year or longer.

infertility (in'-fer-til'-i-ti): Lack of ability to reproduce; not necessarily irreversible.

infest (in-fest'): To occupy a site and dwell on the surface of the body, usually by macroscopic parasites, as opposed to dwelling within the body, *i.e.*, to infect.

infestation (in-fes-tā'-shun): The presence of such animal parasites as insects, ticks, fleas, mites, lice, or worms in or on the body. — infest, v.

infibulation (in-fib-ū-lā'-shun): The act of buckling or fastening; may refer to the procedure of fastening the edges of a wound together by a clasp. May also refer to the most extensive form of female circumcision, which it is illegal to perform in the UK.

infiltrate (in-fil'-trāt): 1. To permeate a substance by penetrating the spaces between the particles of a tissue or of a substance. 2. Cells or material that passes into body tissues by infiltration.

infiltration (in'fil-trā'shun): Penetration of the surrounding tissues by a fluid, as from an intravenous line, or by some other foreign substance; the leaking or oozing of a fluid into the tissues. I. ANAESTHESIA analgesia produced by infiltrating the tissues with a local anaesthetic.

infirm (in-firm'): Weak or feeble, either physically or mentally, because of old age or illness.

infirmity (in-fir'-mi-ti): An unhealthy or debilitated condition of body or mind.

inflamed (in-flāmd'): Hot and swollen; affected with inflammation (*q.v.*).

inflammation (in-fla-mā'-shun): The protective, characteristic chemical or physical reaction of living tissues to injury, infection or irritation; characterized by pain, swelling, redness and heat. — inflammatory, adj.

inflammatory bowel disease: A group of chronic intestinal diseases characterized by inflammation of the bowel — the large or small intestine. The most common types of I.B.D. are Crohn's disease (*q.v.*) and ulcerative colitis, see under COLITIS. Abbreviated IBD.

inflation (in-flā'shun): In medicine, the distension of a part with liquid or gas.

influenza (in-floo-en'-za): An acute, highly contagious infection, marked by inflammation of the nasopharynx and respiratory tract, fever, prostration, muscular and neurologic pains, gastrointestinal disturbances, headache, and depression; primarily caused by a filterable virus and occurring in epidemic and pandemic form. Syn., *la grippe, the grip, flu.* — influenzal, adj.

Information for Health Strategy: A policy introduced as part of the modernization of the NHS (1998–2005). Its purpose is to ensure that information is used to help patients receive the best possible care.

information management and technology: A process by which any sort of information is managed using technology, in order to ensure the effective running of any organization.

information technology: Term referring to the use of computer technology to collect, store, process, and manage information. See also APPENDIX 7.

informed consent: See under CONSENT.

infra-: Prefix denoting a position or status under or below the part named.

infrared rays: Long, invisible rays beyond the red end of the visible spectrum. Used therapeutically for the production of heat in tissues.

infrasternal (in-fra-ster'-nal): Below the sternum. I. NOTCH the slight depression in the anterior abdominal wall that overlies the xiphoid process of the sternum.

infraversion (in'-fra-ver'-zhun): The downwards rotation of one or both eyes.

infusion (in-fū'-zhun): 1. An aqueous solution containing the active principle of a drug, made by steeping the crude drug in water. 2. Fluid other than blood, flowing by gravity into the body. AMNIOTIC FLUID I. see AMNIOTIC; I. PUMP a device for injecting a specific amount of fluid within a specific time span; INTRAVENOUS I. usually refers to the intravenous administration of more than 100 ml of a fluid substance.

ingrowing, ingrown toenail: A nail whose edges have grown into the tissue on either side of it, causing inflammation and pain.

inguinal (ing'-gwi-nal): Relating to the groin. I. CANAL a tubular opening through the lower part of the anterior abdominal wall, parallel to and a little above the I. (Poupart's) ligament. It measures 4 cm. In the male it contains the spermatic cord; in the female, the uterine round ligaments; I. HERNIA one occurring

through the internal abdominal ring of the I. canal; I. LIGAMENT a strong cord of fibrous tissue that extends from the anterior superior iliac spine to the pubic spine; forms a firm edge of the abdominal wall across the groin; Poupart's ligament.

inhalant (in-hā'-lant): 1. That which is inhaled; may be something in the atmosphere or a medication. 2. A substance that occurs as an inhalant or one that is used medicinally as an inhalant.

inhalation (in-ha-lā'-shun): 1. The act of breathing in of air, or of a vapour. 2. A medicinal treatment substance that is inhaled, such as a gas anaesthetic, water vapour, etc.

inhale (in-hāl): To draw in breath; to inspire.

inhaler (in-hā'-ler): 1. An apparatus that provides for the breathing in of medicinal substances. 2. An apparatus that can be worn to prevent breathing in dust, smoke, dirt, etc. 3. An atomizer. METERED DOSE I. a device used in administering medications to the bronchial tree that ensures the medication gets to the desired part of the airway.

inherent (in-hēr'-ent, in-her'-ent): Innate; inborn.

inheritance (in-her'-i-tans): The process of acquiring characters or qualities by transmission from parent to offspring, or the characters and qualities so acquired.

inherited (in-her'-i-ted): Descriptive of mental and physical characteristics that one has received from one's parents; inborn.

inhibition (in'-hi-bish'-un): Loss or partial loss of function or activity, due to restraint, arrest, or being held back. In psychiatry, the restraint of a function or activity as a result of mental (psychic) influences, *e.g.*, failing to 'speak up' for fear of making unimportant or incorrect statements.

inhibitor (in-hib'-i-tor): A substance or agent that interferes with a physiological function or a chemical reaction.

inject (in-jekt'): To force into. In medicine, to force fluid, gas, air, or other substance into tissue, a cavity, or an organ of the body.

injectable (in-jek'-ta-b'l): 1. Capable of being injected. 2. A substance that can be injected.

injected (in-jek'-ted): 1. Congested; with full vessels. 2. Forced in by injection (*q.v.*).

injection (in-jek'-shun): 1. The act of introducing a fluid (under pressure) into the tissues, a vessel, cavity or hollow organ. (Air can be injected into a cavity. See PNEUMOTHORAX.) 2. The substance injected. See HYPODERMIC, INTRA-ARTERIAL, INTRADERMAL, INTRAMUSCULAR, INTRATHECAL, INTRAVENOUS, SUBCUTANEOUS.

3. Congestion; referring especially to dilatation of vessels in the vascular bed.

injury (in'-jer-i): A wound or damage to a person or thing, specifically any disruption to the continuity of body tissue that may or may not involve the skin. BIRTH I. The impairment of a body function as a result of some damage to the child during the birth process.

inkblot test: See RORSCHACH TEST.

inlet (in'-let): A means of entrance, particularly to a body structure. PELVIC I. the upper limit of the pelvic cavity.

in loco parentis (in lō'-ko pa-ren'-tis): A Latin term meaning 'in absence of the parents' which is invoked by school authorities and other responsible persons when a person who is under legal age requires medical care or surgery and the parents are not available to sign or make decisions about treatment.

inmate medical record: A prisoner's medical notes.

innate (in-āt'): Inborn; dependent on genetic constitution; congenital; hereditary; inherent.

inner ear: See EAR.

innervation (in'-er-vā'-shun): The nerve supply to or in a part.

innidiation (i-nid-i-ā'-shun): The development of cells within a tissue to which they have been carried by lymph or the bloodstream.

innocent (in'-ō-sent): Benign; not malignant; apparently not harmful.

innocuous (i-nok'-ū-us): Harmless.

innominate (i-nom'-i-nāt): Unnamed. I. ARTERY the largest branch of the aortic arch; it divides into the right common carotid and the right subclavian arteries; I. BONE one of the bones forming the pelvis; it is composed of the ilium, ischium and pubis; the os innominatum; I. VEINS formed by the union of the subclavian and internal jugular veins on either side.

inoculate (in-ok'-ū-lāt): To introduce a disease-producing agent or an antigenic material into the body for the purpose of creating immunity, treating a disease, or making a diagnosis.

inoculation (in-ok'-ū-lā'-shun): **1.** Introduction of material (usually vaccine) into the tissues, often done to create immunity by giving the person a mild form of the disease. **2.** Introduction of microorganisms into culture medium for propagation.

inoperable (in-op'-er-a-b'l): Describing a condition that under other circumstances could be relieved or cured by surgery, but for which, because of the location or advanced stage of the pathology, surgery would be either ineffective or unsafe.

inorganic (in'-or-gan'-ik): Neither animal nor vegetable in origin. In chemistry, the term refers to compounds that do not contain carbon.

inotropic (in-ō-trōp'-ik): Having an effect on the contractility of muscle tissue, usually referring to drugs, some of which have a weakening negative effect while others have a positive strengthening effect.

inpatient (in'-pā-shent): A person who receives food and lodging in a hospital while receiving care, treatment, or undergoing tests.

inquest (in'-qwest): A legal inquiry, held by a coroner, into the cause of sudden or unexpected death.

insane (in-sān'): **1.** Of unsound or deranged mind. Usually implies inability to manage one's own affairs or conduct oneself in a socially acceptable manner. **2.** Relating to insanity.

insanitary (in-san'-i-ter-i); Unclean to such a degree as to be injurious to health.

insanity (in-san'-i-ti): Old term for severe mental illness. In law, the term is used to designate the degree of mental illness that renders a person incapable of conduct or judgement that is legally regarded as normal.

insecticide (in-sek'-ti-sīd): An agent that kills insects. — insecticidal, adj.

insemination (in-sem-in-ā'-shun): Introduction of semen into the vagina, normally by sexual intercourse. ARTIFICIAL I. instrumental injection of semen into the female genital tract, sperm being donated by a partner or a donor.

insensible (in-sen'-si-b'l): **1.** Without sensation or consciousness. **2.** Imperceptible. Too small or gradual to be perceived, as I. perspiration (*q.v.*). I. LOSS usually refers to loss of fluids from the body in ways that cannot be measured by ordinary means, *e.g.*, in sweat.

insertion (in-ser'-shun): **1.** The act of setting or placing in. **2.** The attachment of a muscle to the bone it moves.

insidious (in-sid'-i-us): Having an imperceptible commencement, as of a disease with a late manifestation of definite symptoms.

insight (in'-sīt): Clear and immediate understanding; keen discernment. In psychiatry, means: (1) knowing that one is emotionally ill; (2) a developing knowledge of one's present attitudes and past experiences and the connection between them.

in situ (in si'-tū): In the normal or natural place; in the correct position; undisturbed by neighbouring tissues.

insolation (in-sō-lā'-shun): **1.** Sunstroke. **2.** Treatment of disease by exposure to the sun's rays.

insoluble (in-sol' -ū-b'l): Incapable of being dissolved.

insomnia (in-som'ni-a): Sleeplessness, especially when chronic, or difficulty in falling asleep or remaining asleep during the period when sleep normally occurs.

inspection (in-spek' -shun): Examination of persons or things by the eye.

inspersion (in-sper' -shun): The act of sprinkling, as with a powder or a fluid.

inspiration (in-spi-rā'shun): The drawing of air into the lungs; inhalation. — inspire, v.; inspiratory, adj.

inspiratory (in-spī' -ra-to-ri): Relating to inspiration, or breathing in. I. CAPACITY the sum of respiratory reserve volume and tidal volume; I. RESERVE VOLUME the maximum amount of air that can be exhaled after exhalation of the tidal volume.

inspire (in-spīr'): To breathe in; inhale.

instability: 1. Lack of stability or support; insecure support. **2.** Lack of purpose; changeable in beliefs or opinions.

instep (in' -step): The arch of the foot on the dorsal surface.

instillation (in' -sti-lā' -shun): The pouring, drop by drop, of a fluid into a body cavity or opening, e.g., the conjunctival sac or external auditory meatus. — instil, v.

instinct (in'stinkt): An inborn tendency, present in all normal members of a species, to act in a certain way that is usually helpful and beneficial, e.g., PATERNAL I. the I. to protect children. HERD I. the urge to copy standards of thinking and behaviour of a group. — instinctive, adj.; instinctively, adv.

institution (in-sti-tū' -shun): **1.** An established order or custom. **2.** A society or association for the promotion of a particular subject. **3.** A building for the recipients of public help or relief. See INSTITUTIONALIZATION.

Institutionaization (in-sti-tū' -shun-al-ī-zā'-shun): The process by which individuals who have lived or worked in institutions become acclimatized to a rigid routine and have difficulty adjusting to new situations and making decisions.

insufficiency (in-su-fish' -en-sē): The condition of being unable to perform an allotted duty or function. Term is used to describe failure to function properly of such organs and parts as the heart, cardiac valves, liver, stomach, kidney, adrenal or thyroid glands, muscles.

insufflation (in' -sū-flā' -shun): The act of blowing into; often refers to blowing air into the lungs of the newborn; blowing a powder, gas, or vapour into a body cavity; or blowing air along a tube (auditory or uterine) to establish patency. — insufflate, v.

insula (in'sū-la): An island, particularly the islets of Langerhans in the pancreas or the island of Reil, a triangular area of the cerebral cortex. See ISLAND.

insulation (in-sū-lā' -shun): The surrounding of a body or a space with non-conducting material to prevent the escape or entrance of radiant energy, electricity, sound or heat; also, the material so used.

insulin (in'sū-lin): A pancreatic hormone produced in the islet (beta) cells of the islets of Langerhans, secreted into the bloodstream in response to glucose in the blood; promotes utilization of glucose, synthesis of protein, and the formation and storage of neutral lipids. The hormone is obtained from animals and prepared commercially in several forms and strengths which vary in their speed, length, and potency of action, and which are used in treatment of diabetes mellitus; most forms are given subcutaneously. Insulin is now also produced by bacteria via genetic engineering. Excess dosage results in hypoglycaemia and insulin shock; inadequate dosage results in hyperglycaemia and diabetic ketoacidosis.

insulinase (in' -sū-lin-ās): An enzyme in the liver that is capable of inactivating insulin.

insulin pump: A device that is powered by batteries and worn by patients with diabetes; it is programmed to deliver a set amount of insulin at regular intervals; is connected to the infusion site, which is usually on the abdomen. The patient can control the amount of insulin delivered when blood sugar tests indicate the need for change in dosage.

insulin shock: A condition resulting from severe hypoglycaemia caused by overdose of insulin, insufficient intake of food, or excessive physical exertion; symptoms include sweating, chills, pallor, hunger, thirst, extreme nervousness and fear, fainting, possibly convulsions; treatment consists of immediate intake of sugar or intravenous injection of glucose. Also called *hypoglycaemic crisis or shock*.

insult (in' -sult): **1.** An injury or trauma. **2.** To injure or traumatize.

insusceptibility (in'su-sep-ti-bil'i-ti): Immunity. The incapability of becoming infected with a specific pathogen.

intake (in'tāk): In medicine, usually refers to substances taken into the body, by mouth or otherwise, and expressed in amounts such as ml of fluid intake, or calorie content of food intake. The nursing record of measured liquid intake and output is the Fluid Balance Chart.

integrated care pathways (in'-te-grā-ted): Multi-disciplinary plans of care; they may involve both clinical and non-clinical interventions. Care pathways are one of the tools used for continuous quality improvement in healthcare. They are developed by a multi-disciplinary team; based on evidence; designed to meet local needs and constraints; and consistent.

integrated medicine: Therapy incorporating orthodox, allopathic, and complementary medicines. It emphasizes collaborative, multidisciplinary team working.

intellect (in'-te-lekt): The power or facility of reasoning, thinking, and understanding; intelligence.

intellectualize (in-tel-lck'-tū-a-līz): To examine or analyse rationally; to reason.

intelligence (in-tel'-i-jens): The ability to comprehend or understand relationships, to think, to solve problems, and to adjust to new situations. Inborn mental ability. I. QUOTIENT, or IQ the ratio of mental age to chronological age; obtained by dividing the mental age by the chronological age and multiplying the result by 100; I. TESTS tests designed to determine one's level of intelligence or mental age.

intensive care unit: A special area in a hospital where critically ill patients who need close observation and frequent ministrations can be cared for by highly qualified, specially trained staff. Also called *intensive therapy unit*.

intention: A natural process of healing involving the union of the edges of a wound. FIRST I. healing of a wound by immediate union and scar formation without granulation or suppuration. SECOND I. healing of a wound after suppuration, by union of the two granulated surfaces and formation of a larger scar than forms in healing by first I. THIRD I. healing of a wound with extensive granulation and the formation of a still larger scar. I. TREMOR see TREMOR.

inter-: Prefix denoting among, between, together, within, in the midst.

interaction (in-ter-ak'-shun): A mutual or reciprocal action or influence. In pharmacotherapeutics, the modification of the action of one drug by one or more other drugs; may be detrimental or beneficial to the patient. I. may also occur between a drug and certain foods.

inter-agency: A term denoting a relationship between two or more agencies, especially government agencies. It concerns agencies and professionals working collaboratively together in order to achieve the best outcome for the patient/client, *e.g.*, in child protection.

interarticular (in-ter-ar-tik'ū-lar): 1. Between two articulating surfaces. 2. Between two joints.

intercellular (in-ter-sel'-ū-lar): Between the cells of a structure.

intercerebral (in'-ter-ser'-e-bral): Located between or connecting the two cerebral hemispheres.

intercostal (in-ter-kos'-tal): Between the ribs. I. MUSCLES those located between the ribs. EXTERNAL I. MUSCLES those that act to increase the size of the thoracic cavity; INTERNAL I. MUSCLES those that act to decrease the size of the thoracic cavity during breathing; I. SPACE the space between two adjacent ribs.

intercourse (in-ter-kōrs): Communication, interchange or exchange. SEXUAL I. coitus.

interdisciplinary: 1. Denoting the overlapping interests of different fields of health and social care. 2. Collaboration between two or more academic subjects or fields of study. See INTER-AGENCY; INTER-PROFESSIONAL; MULTI-DISCIPLINARY.

interest group: 1. An organization that supports a cause, and attempts to influence decisions made at local and national level through lobbying. 2. A group of people who share an interest in something, such as a subject of study.

interferon (in-ter-fēr'on): A class of small soluble glycoproteins produced naturally in most body cells in response to viral infections; discovered in 1957 and still under investigation. Called the body's first line of defence against infections, especially viral infections. Interferon is not itself antiviral but is thought to initiate RNA and protein synthesis, yielding a new protein that has an antiviral effect and prevents further spread of the infection; also appears to be effective against certain bacteria, protozoa, and rickettsias, and in certain types of cancer.

interictal (in'-ter-ik'-tal): Between attacks or paroxysms, *e.g.*, epileptic seizures.

interlobar (in-ter-lō'-bar): Between the lobes of an organ, *e.g.*, interlobar pleurisy.

intermediate care (in-ter-mē'-di-at): The care of people who do not need acute tertiary care in hospitals but are not sufficiently independent to be self-caring in their own home. Has specific outcomes for rehabilitation, reablement or recuperation, and is provided for a time limited period of up to six weeks. See CONTINUING CARE.

intermenstrual (in-ter-men′ -stroo-al): Between menstrual periods.

intermittent (in-ter-mit′ent): Occurring at intervals; characterized by periods of complete cessation of activity. I. CLAUDICATION see CLAUDICATION; I. fever one in which the symptoms of the disease disappear between attacks of fever, as occurs in malaria and undulant fever; I. INFUSION SET an apparatus that delivers intravenous solution into a vein at preset intervals; heparin lock; I. POSITIVE PRESSURE BREATHING a useful technique when weaning a patient from a respirator; the patient breathes spontaneously while still on the respirator which delivers a breath of air or oxygen at set intervals which are gradually lengthened until the patient is breathing entirely on his own; I. POSITIVE PRESSURE VENTILATION a temporary measure to ensure adequate ventilation, e.g., in treating patients with asthma, until other therapies can bring an acute attack under control; usually administered by endotracheal intubation along with sedatives and muscle relaxants; I. PULSE one in which there is an absence of beat at intervals; I. VENTILATION may be (1) mandatory, whereby the patient breathes at his normal rate but is helped by a respirator that is set to deliver a certain volume of air at a pre-set rate, or (2) demand, the same as mandatory except that the ventilator is set to deliver a certain amount of air at the patient's respiratory rate.

intermuscular (in-ter-mus′ -kū-lar): Situated between muscles.

internal (in-ter′ -nal): Located or occurring on the inside. I. EAR that part of the ear that comprises the vestibule, semicircular canals, and the ossicles; I. ENVIRONMENT the extracellular fluid that immediately surrounds the cells of the body; I. HAEMORRHAGE bleeding into a cavity or organ of the body; I. MARKET a system based on the economic theories of supply and demand, where knowledgeable consumers use their disposable income to purchase goods and services at a price that gives best value for money; I. SECRETIONS those produced by the ductless (endocrine) glands and passed directly into the bloodstream; hormones; I. VERIFIER an individual, approved by an awarding body (*q.v.*) for National Vocational Qualifications (*q.v.*) but working for an approved centre (an organization or group of organizations (consortium) which has been approved by an Awarding Body to offer NVQs/SVQs), who monitors and supervises the operation of the NVQs and ensures that all appropriate proced-

ures and quality control mechanisms required by the awarding bodies are adhered to; in effect, the I. verifier will act as the assessors' supervisor. — internally, adj.; internality, n.

internalization (in-ter′ -nal-ī-zā′ -shun): The unconscious adoption, as one's own, of another's values, characteristics; and attitudes.

International Classification of Diseases: The official list of disease categories, issued by the World Health Organization.

International Council of Nurses: A federation founded in 1899, the oldest healthcare association in the world. Ninety-four nations are now members; meets every four years. Purpose is to develop the highest level of health for all peoples of the world; to improve the status and competency of nurses; to improve the standards of nursing care; to promote the development of strong national nursing organizations; and to serve as the authoritative voice for nurses internationally. Publishes the International Nursing Review. Abbreviated ICN.

International Red Cross: A worldwide voluntary relief organization founded in Switzerland in 1864, largely through the efforts of Henri Dunant, who had visited the battlefields of the Crimean War and had seen the great need for care for wounded soldiers. The original purpose of the IRC was to aid the wounded and other victims of war but its activities now include disaster relief and the sponsorship of many health-related and social programmes. The national Red Cross Societies and the Red Crescent Societies of Moslem countries make up the international organization. See also RED CROSS.

International System of Units, International Unit: see SI UNITS.

Internet (in′ -ter-net): A network connecting computer networks that enables access to information from, and communication between, computers all over the world. Also known as the *information superhighway*. See E-MAIL; WORLD WIDE WEB.

interoceptor (in′ -ter-ō-sep′ -tor): A sensory nerve terminal or end organ situated in the walls of organs or in viscera and which responds to stimuli that arise within the body. — interoceptive, adj.

interosseous (in-ter-os′ -ē-us): Lying between bones, as some muscles and ligaments.

interpersonal: Usually refers to forces or relationships between people.

interpretative enquiry (in-ter′ -pre-tā-tiv): A method of investigation based on the idea that understanding an individual's behaviour involves knowing the meaning that the individual attributes to his or her actions and those of others.

inter-professional: Collaboration between health and social care practitioners working with patients, clients, and carers. See INTER-AGENCY; INTER-DISCIPLINARY; MULTI-DISCIPLINARY.

inter-professional education: A learning process in which different professionals learn from and about each other, in order to develop collaborative practice. See also MULTI-PROFESSIONAL EDUCATION.

interrupted: Lacking continuity; broken at intervals; I. STERILIZATION that which is done at intervals in order to allow any spores to develop in the periods between applications of the procedure; I. SUTURES a technique of closing a wound with stitches that are each made with a separate piece of suture material.

intersex (in'ter ueks): A congenital condition in which the sex of the individual is not clear. Two types are recognized: (1) true hermaphrodism, in which the individual possesses a mixture of both male and female gonads; and (2) pseudohermaphrodism, which occurs in individuals whose gonads are either basically male or female, but whose external genitalia did not develop accordingly in embryonic life. See HERMAPHRODITE.

intersexuality (in'ter-seks-ū-al'-i-ti): The possession of both male and female characteristics. See TURNER'S and KLINEFELTER'S SYNDROME.

interstitial (in-ter-stish'-al): 1. Related to or situated in the interstices of a tissue or part. 2. Distributed throughout the connective tissue. I. FLUID see under FLUID. — Syn., *intercellular*.

interstitium (in-ter-stish'-i-um): The supporting framework between organs that binds them together; may consist of various kinds of intercellular connective tissue, fibres, and so on.

intervention: Planned action to alter or correct an undesirable condition or situation.

interventricular (in-ter-ven-trik'-ū-lar): Between ventricles, as those of the brain or heart.

intervertebral (in-ter-ver'te-bral): Between two adjacent vertebrae, as discs or foramina. I. DISC a flattened cartilaginous disc lying between vertebrae, preventing friction and absorbing shock; it is spoken of as ruptured when accident or strain causes the soft central part of the disc to protrude through the surrounding ligament. — see NUCLEUS, PROLAPSE.

interviewing: A method of data collection, where communication skills are used to elicit the required information.

intestinal (in-tes'-tin-al): Of or relating to the intestine. I. JUICE *succus entericus*, secreted by the intestine; its function is to complete the hydrolysis of carbohydrates and proteins; consists of water, salts, and the enzymes enterokinase, peptidase, maltase, sucrase, lactase, and lipase; I. OBSTRUCTION stoppage of the passage of food or faeces through the intestine; may be due to physical blockage, lack of peristalsis, adhesions, tumours, stricture, volvulus, strangulation; symptoms include intense localized pain, vomiting, constipation, abdominal distension.

intestine (in-tes'-tin): The bowel; that part of the alimentary canal that extends from the pyloric end of the stomach to the anus. The SMALL I. is separated from the stomach by the pyloric valve, is about 6 metres in length, and consists of the duodenum, jejunum and ileum, in that order. Between the small I. and the large I. is the ileocaecal valve. The LARGE I. about 1.8 metres in length, is composed of the caecum, colon (ascending, transverse, and descending), and rectum, in that order. The function of the intestine is to complete digestion of foods, and to allow for absorption of digested food material, by blood and lymph vessels, through its walls, and to eliminate waste products of digestion. — intestinal, adj.

intima (in'-tim-a): The internal layer of a blood vessel. — intimal, adj.

intolerance (in-tol'-er-ans): In medicine, an idiosyncrasy (*q.v.*) to certain drugs, etc.

intortion (in-tor'-shun): 1. Inward rotation of the eye so that it moves towards the nose. 2. Inward rotation of a body part.

intoxicant (in-tok'-si-kant): An agent that decreases the individual's control over mental and physical functioning and causes intoxication.

intoxication (in-tok-si-kā'-shun): 1. The pathological state of being poisoned by alcohol, a drug, or any toxic substance that gains entrance to the body. 2. The state of being intoxicated, usually referring to the condition produced by overindulgence in alcohol; drunkenness. WATER I., see under WATER.

intra-: Prefix denoting within, on the inside, internal, between the layers of.

intra-aortic (in'-tra-ā-or'-tik): Within the aorta. I. BALLOON PUMP a device consisting of a balloon attached to the end of a catheter that is inserted into the aorta via a skin incision, and connected to an external pump mechanism that alternately inflates the balloon during diastole and deflates it during systole. This improves blood flow to the coronary arteries and reduces afterload. Used to treat acute left ventricular failure and artery angina before cardiac surgery.

intra-arterial (in′-tra-ar-tē′-ri-al): Within an artery. — intra-arterially, adj.

intra-articular (in′-tra-ar-tik′-u-lar): Within a joint.

intracapsular (in-tra-kap′sū-lar): Within a capsule, *e.g.*, that of the lens or of a joint. Opp. to extracapsular.

intracardiac (in-tra-kar′-di-ak): Within the heart.

intracellular (in′-tra-sel′-ū-lar): Within a cell. Opp. to extracellular. I. FLUID fluid within the cell membranes.

intracerebral (in-tra-ser′e-bral): Within the cerebrum. I. STEAL refers to a situation in which blood drains from one area of the cerebrum because of lowered cerebrovascular resistance in another area.

intracostal (in-tra-kos′-tal): Refers to the inner surface of the ribs.

intracranial (in-tra-krā′-ni-al): Within the skull.

intractable (in-trak′-ta-b′l): Resistant to treatment; not easily cured.

intradermal (in-tra-der′-mal): Within the skin. Often refers to an injection into or between the skin layers. — intradermally, adj.

intradural (in-tra-dū′-ral): Within the dura mater, *e.g.*, haemorrhage.

intramedullary (in′tra-med′ū-lar-i): **1.** Within the medulla oblongata or the spinal cord. **2.** Within the marrow cavity of a bone or the bone marrow. I. NAIL a nail or metal rod inserted into the intramedullary canal of a long bone to provide internal fixation. It extends on both sides of the fracture, thus holding the two parts of the fractured bone in proper position for healing.

intramembranous (in-tra-mem′bran-ous): Between membranes. Descriptive of a type of bone formation that differs from endochondral bone formation.

intramuscular (in-tra-mus′kū-lar): Within or into the substance of a muscle, as an intramuscular injection. — intramuscularly, adj.

intraocular (in′-tra-ok′-ū-lar): Within the globe of the eye. I. LENS TRANSPLANT the substitution of an artificial lens for one that has to be removed, usually for cataract. I. PRESSURE the pressure of the fluid within the eye, as measured by a tonometer.

intraorbital (in-tra-or′-bi-tal): Within an orbit, as of the eye.

intrapartum (in-tra-par′-tum): During labour or delivery, as asphyxia, haemorrhage, or infection. — intrapartal, adj.

intrapleural (in-tra-ploo′-ral): Within the pleural cavity. — intrapleurally, adv.

intrastitial (in-tra-stish′-al): Within the cells of a tissue.

intrasynovial (in-tra-si-nō′vi-al): Within a synovial membrane or sac.

intrathecal (in-tra-thē′-kal): Within a sheath. Within or going under or between the meninges of the brain or spinal cord, as an injection. I. THERAPY the introduction of a therapeutic agent into the spinal subarachnoid space. — intrathecally, adj.

intrathoracic (in′-tra-thō′-ras′-ik): Within, or occurring within, the cavity of the thorax.

intrauterine (in-tra-ū′-ter-in): Being or occurring within the uterus. I. CONTRACEPTIVE DEVICE a device placed within the uterus to prevent conception. Devices may be made in a variety of shapes, either of plastic or metal material. The precise mode of contraceptive action is not known but the device is thought to interfere with the implantation of the fertilized ovum.

intravasation (in-trav-a-zā′-shun): The introduction of foreign or abnormal matter into a blood vessel.

intravenous (in-tra-vē′-nus): Within, or going directly into, a vein or veins. I. INFUSION see under INFUSION; I. PYELOGRAM see under PYELOGRAM.

intrinsic (in-trin′-sik): Inherent or inside; from within; real; innate; innate; natural. Often used in reference to certain muscles, *e.g.*, certain eye muscles. I. FACTOR a glycoprotein secreted by the gastric mucosa; essential for the satisfactory absorption of vitamin B_{12}.

intro-: Prefix denoting into, within, inward, inwardly, to or on the inside.

introjection (in-trō-jek′-shun): In psychiatry, an unconscious defence mechanism whereby a person identifies with another loved or hated person or object.

introspection (in-trō-spek′-shun): The act of looking inwards to one's thoughts and feelings; self-examination. — introspective, adj.

introversion (in-trō-ver′-shun): **1.** Reclusiveness. **2.** The tendency to be overly concerned with one's thoughts, to be reflective rather than overtly expressive. **3.** The turning 'outside in' of a part, more or less completely, as invagination. — introvert, n.; introverted, adj.

introvert (in′-trō-vert): **1.** To turn one's thoughts inward towards one's own mental processes. **2.** A person who is self-centred and introspective, and who tends to be thoughtful, self-sufficient, and interested more in his own thoughts and feelings than in those of others. Tends to withdraw in social situations and to be a poor mixer. Opp. to extrovert (*q.v.*).

intubation (in-tū-bā′ -shun): The insertion of a tube into an organ or passage, usually through the nose or mouth, into a part of the body, especially a canal and particularly the trachea or intestine. DUODENAL I. a procedure for instilling barium into the duodenum prior to fluoroscopy; ENDOTRACHEAL I., I. done to maintain an airway by keeping the trachea open to administer anaesthesia, or to restore patency in cases of obstruction.

intuition (in-tū-ish′ -un): The quality or state of having quick insight or immediate comprehension or of having untaught knowledge.

intussusception (in′ tus-sus-scp′ -shun): A condition in which one part of the bowel slips or telescopes into the part immediately adjacent (invaginates). It occurs in infants and most frequently at the junction of the ileum and the caecum; causes obstruction. Usual therapy is surgery. ILEOCAECAL I., I. in which the ileocaecal valve prolapses into the caecum; ILEO-COLIC I., I. in which the ileum prolapses into the colon.

in utero (in ū′te-rō): Within the uterus; unborn.

invagination (in-vaj′ -i-nā′ -shun): The act or condition of being ensheathed; a pushing inward; telescoping; forming a pouch. — invaginate, v.t.

invasion (in-vā′ -zhun): 1. The entry of bacteria into the body. 2. The beginning or onset of a disease. 3. The spreading of a malignancy into surrounding tissue.

invasive (in-vā′ -siv): 1. Tending to invade healthy surrounding tissues; said of neoplasms or microorganisms. 2. Referring to a procedure that involves penetration of an organ or deeper tissues of the body. I. MONITORING monitoring of conditions existing within the body, utilizing devices that are placed within the body; I. PRESSURE MONITORING direct measurement of blood pressure, pulmonary artery pressure, venous pressure, or intracranial pressure; a cannula is inserted into the pressure source and connected to a transducer, which converts the pressure into an electric signal that can be seen on a monitor.

inversion (in-ver′ -zhun): 1. A turning inside out, upside down, outside in, or in any direction that is the reverse of normal. 2. Position in which a part is turned towards the midline of the body. 3. Outward turning of the ankle. 4. In obstetrics, I. of the uterus, an obstetric emergency that may follow delivery; may also be caused by the uterus attempting to expel a tumour. 5. A deviant or abnormal psychosocial preference leading to anti-social behaviour, *e.g.*, paedophilia, bestiality.

invert (in′ -vert): I. SUGAR the mixture of glucose and fructose obtained by hydrolysing sucrose.

invertebrate (in-ver′ -te-brāt): An organism without a backbone.

inverted (in-ver′ -ted): Turned upside down, inwards, or any direction contrary to normal.

in vitro (in vē′ -trō): In glass, as in a test tube. Outside of the living body.

in vitro **fertilization:** A method of assisted reproduction in which the man's sperm and the woman's egg (oocyte) are combined in a laboratory dish, where fertilization occurs. The resulting embryo is then transferred to the uterus to develop naturally. See INSEMIN-ATION. Abbreviated IVF.

in vivo (in vē′ -vō): In living tissue or in a living body.

involuntary (in-vol′ -un-ta-ri): Independent of the will, as the smooth muscle of the abdominal organs.

involution (in-vō-lū′ -shun): 1. A normal process characterized by a decrease in the size of an organ and a decrease in the size of its cells, such as post-partum involution of the uterus. 2. The period of progressive alteration in the body occurring with advancing age when glandular activity lessens and degenerative changes set in. 3. A rolling or turning inward.

involve: To include a person in an experience. — involvement, n.

iodine (ī′ -ō-dēn): A non-metallic element with several industrial and medicinal uses; obtained chiefly from seaweed. I. is also found in the body, chiefly in the form of thyroglobulin in the thyroid gland; protein-bound iodine is estimated in thyroid investigations. I. TEST a test for starch; when I. is added to a compound containing starch a deep blue colour is produced; the colour disappears when the substance is heated and reappears when it is cooled; LUGOL'S SOLUTION a 5% aqueous solution of iodine given orally in thyrotoxicosis, usually for preoperative stabilization; RADIOACTIVE I. (^{131}I) used in investigation and treatment of thyrotoxicosis; TINCTURE OF I. a 2% to 5% solution of iodine in alcohol, used as an antiseptic and disinfectant for small wounds.

iodize (ī′ -ō-dīz): 1. To treat with iodine or an iodide. 2. To impregnate with iodine, as table salt. — iodized, adj.

ion (ī′ -on): An atom, or group of atoms, that has either a positive or negative charge of electricity and which, in electrolysis, passes to one pole or the other.

ionization (ī-on-ī-za′ -shun): **1.** The breaking up of a substance into its component ions when in solution. **2.** Treatment whereby ions of various substances, *e.g.*, zinc, chlorine, iodine, histamine, are introduced into the skin by means of a constant electrical current.

iontophoresis (ī-on′ -tō-fo-rē′ -sis): The introduction, through the skin, of ions of various salts for therapeutic purposes; accomplished by electrical means.

ipecac (ip′ -e-kak): The dried roots and rhizome of a Central and South American tree; used in medicine as an emetic and in expectorants. Ipecacuanha.

IPPB: Abbreviation for intermittent positive pressure breathing. See under INTERMITTENT.

IPPV: Abbreviation for intermittent positive pressure ventilation. See under INTERMITTENT.

ipsilateral (ip-si-lat′ -er-al): Situated or appearing on the same side, or affecting the same side. — ipsilaterally, adv.

IPV: Abbreviation for inactivated poliovirus vaccine, See SALK VACCINE.

IQ: Abbreviation for intelligence quotient.

irid-, iridio-: Combining forms denoting the iris of the eye.

iridectomy (ir-i-dek′to-mi): Excision of part of the iris, thus enlarging the pupil or creating an artificial one.

iridocele (ir′i-dō-sēl): Protrusion of part of the iris through a defect or wound in the cornea.

iridodonesis (ir′ -i-dō-dō-nē′ -sis): Quivering movements of the iris; seen in patients with aphakia

iridology (ī-ri-dol′ -ō-ji): A study of the markings and changes in colour that are said to occur in the iris in the course of systemic disease, the assumption being that every organ of the body has a representative area in the iris.

iridotomy (ir′ -i-dot′ -om-i): A small incision into the iris, as in the operation to create an artificial pupil. LASER I. utilized in treatment of glaucoma.

iris (ī′ -ris): The coloured circular membrane forming the anterior one-sixth of the middle coat of the eyeball. It consists of two layers of muscle and is perforated in the centre by an opening called the pupil. Contraction of its muscle fibres regulates the amount of light entering the eye. I. BOMBÉ bulging forward of the iris due to pressure of aqueous humour behind it when posterior adhesions are present. — irides, pl.; iridal, iridian, iridic, adj.

iritis (ī-rī′ -tis): Inflammation of the iris, often with pain, tearing, photophobia, decreased vision, irregular pupils; due to local or systemic infection.

iron: A common metallic element found in some soils and waters and in certain minerals. Present in the body in small amounts, most of it in the red blood cells; important in the physiological process of transporting oxygen to the tissues. Some of it is stored in liver, spleen, or bone marrow, but since a certain amount is excreted in faeces, it must be supplied daily in the diet. Some of its salts are used in treating various forms of anaemia.

iron-deficiency anaemia: See under ANAEMIA.

IRP: Abbreviation for Independent Reconfiguration Panel (*q.v.*).

irradiation (ir-rā′dē-ā′ -shun): **1.** Subjection of a patient to the action of such rays as those of heat, light, radium, etc. for diagnostic or therapeutic purposes. **2.** Subjection of a substance, especially a food, to certain rays, *e.g.*, ultraviolet, to increase its vitamin potency. **3.** A spreading out, as of nerve impulses. — irradiate, v.

irreducible (irrē-dūs′i-b′l): **1.** Term applied to a hernia, fracture, or dislocation that is not capable of being brought into the desired position; opp. of reducible. **2.** Incapable of being made smaller or less in amount. **3.** In chemistry, incapable of being made simpler or reduced. I. HERNIA one in which the contents of the sac cannot be returned to the appropriate cavity without surgical intervention.

irreversible (ir-rē-ver′ si-b′l): Not capable of being reversed; said of a disease or process from which recovery is not possible.

irrigate (ir′ -i-gāt): In medicine, to wash out a body cavity or part with a continuous stream of water, or other fluid, for therapeutic purposes.

irritable (ir′ -i-ta-b′l): In medicine, capable of responding to stimuli; responding easily to stimuli. — irritability, n.

irritable bowel syndrome: A collection of symptoms, including tenderness over the small intestine and the ascending and transverse colon; also, alternating constipation, diarrhoea, and normal bowel movements; anxiety; fatigue; dysuria; excessive secretion of mucus; bloating. Also called *mucous colitis, spastic colon,* and *irritable colon syndrome.*

irritant (ir-i-tant): Any agent that causes irritation (*q.v.*). — irritative, adj.

irritation (ir-i-tā′ -shun): **1.** The normal response of a muscle or nerve to a stimulus. **2.** An exaggerated response of a nerve or tissue to stimulus. **3.** Greater than normal response of tissues to injury or trauma.

ischaemia (is-kē′mi-a): Local temporary reduction of blood supply of an area due to obstruction in the blood vessels supplying the area or due to vasoconstriction. MYOCARDIAL I. inadequate blood supply to the myocardium due to coronary artery disease. — ischaemic, adj.

ischaemic (is-kē′-mik): Relating to or affected by ischaemia (*q.v.*). I. CONTRACTURE see VOLKMANN'S CONTRACTURE under CONTRACTURE; I. HEART DISEASE caused by reduced blood supply to the myocardium; usually due to obstruction of flow in the coronary arteries; I. STROKE see TRANSIENT ISCHAEMIC ATTACK.

ischi-, ischio-: Combining forms denoting the ischium (*q.v.*).

ischial (is′ki-al): Relating to the ischium. I. SPINE one that lies above the ischial tuberosity and divides the greater and lesser sciatic notches; I. TUBEROSITY the body of the ischium; the part of the pelvis that the trunk rests on when one is sitting.

ischium (is′-ki-um): The lower, heavy, posterior part of the innominate bone of the pelvis; the bone on which the body rests when sitting. — ischia pl.; ischial, adj.

ischo-: Combining form denoting suppression or relationship to suppression.

ischocholia (is-kō-kō′-li-a): Suppression of bile formation or failure of the bile to reach the intestine. Also called *ischolia*.

Ishihara's test: A test for colour vision; consists of a series of plates with dots of differing sizes and colours.

island: In anatomy, a group of cells or a mass of tissue, separated in some way, or marked off, from surrounding tissue. I. OF REIL see INSULA.

islet (ī′-let): An island, as one of the I.S OF LANGERHANS, clusters of special cells scattered through the pancreas; they secrete insulin (*q.v.*), which pours directly into the bloodstream.

iso-: Prefix or combining form denoting equal, like, uniform, homogeneous.

ISO 9000: A standard specifying the requirements for a quality management system (*q.v.*) overseeing the production of a product or service. It does not directly specify what activities are required for the product/service to be of quality, rather it puts requirements on the way the production process will be managed and reviewed.

isoenzyme (ī′sō-en′zīm): One of a group of enzymes occurring in a given species that have similar catalytic characteristics but differing other physical properties. Also called *isozyme*.

Isogel (ī′sō-jel): Proprietary, bulk-forming laxative prepared from the husks of mucilaginous seeds. Used in chronic constipation.

isograft (ī′-sō-graft): A graft of tissue that has been obtained from another individual of the same species. Also called *isotransplant*.

isohaemagglutinin (ī′-sō-hē-ma-gloo′tin-in): A haemagglutinin in one person's blood serum that will agglutinate another person's red blood cells.

isoimmunization (ī′sō-im-ū-nī-zā′shun): The development in an individual of antibodies in response to antigens from another individual of the same species, *e.g.*, the development of anti-Rh agglutinins in the blood of an Rh-negative person who has been given an Rh-positive transfusion, or who is carrying an Rh-positive fetus.

isolation (ī-sō-lā′-shun): The act of setting a person with an infectious disease apart from those who do not have the disease. I. TECHNIQUE measures and precautions taken to prevent the spread of infection from a patient in isolation to others; REVERSE I. the use of strict isolation technique to protect the patient from infection caused by organisms in the environment, or that may be carried into the unit by caregivers or through articles used in the patient's care; the precautions are taken when entering the unit instead of when leaving it after giving care. May involve the use of laminar airflow. Also called *protective isolation*.

isologous (ī-sol′o-gus): **1.** Relating to any one or both of two compounds that are similar in structure but have differing compositions. **2.** Characterized by an identical genotype (see **2.** under GENOTYPE). I. TRANSPLANT a tissue transplant between identical twins.

isomers (ī′sō-merz): Compounds made up of the same elements but in different arrangements of their atoms, which gives them different physical or chemical properties, although the elements are present in the same proportions.

isometric (ī-sō-met′rik): Of equal length or dimensions. In physiology, a muscle contraction that occurs without shortening of the muscle, as it is fixed at both ends, but with increase in tone of the muscle fibres. Opp. of isotonic. I. EXERCISE active muscular exercise in which the muscle contraction does not reduce its length, due to the force exerted by an opposing muscle at the same time.

isomorphous (ī-sō-mor'-fus): Having the same form or shape.

isopropyl alcohol (ī'-sō-prō-pil): An alcohol similar to, but more toxic than ethyl alcohol; used in manufacture of cosmetics and medicinal preparations for external use. Rubbing alcohol contains about 70% isopropyl alcohol in water.

isosensitization (ī'sō-sen-sit-ī-zā'shun): See AUTOSENSITIZATION.

isotherapy (ī'-sō-ther'-a-pi): Treatment of a disease by administering its active causal agent, as is done in the treatment for prevention of rabies.

isotonic (ī'-sō-ton'-ik): 1. Having equal tension; applied to any solution that has the same osmotic pressure as blood. I. SALINE (syn., normal saline), 0.9% solution of salt in water. 2. Descriptive of muscular contraction that takes place without significant increase in tone but with shortening of the fibres. Opp. of isometric.

isotope (ī'-sō-tōp): One of two or more forms of the same element that have identical chemical properties but differing physical properties. Isotopes with radioactive properties emit their excess energy in three forms — alpha rays, beta rays, or gamma rays; they are used in medicine for research, diagnosis, and treatment of disease. I. SCAN see RADIOSOTOPE SCAN under RADIOISOTOPE.

isthmus (is'-mus): In anatomy, a connecting part between two larger parts. I. UTERI the constricted part of the uerus where the cervix and body of the uterus join.

IT: Abbreviation for information technology (*q.v.*).

itch: A name given to a wide variety of skin conditions that arouse a sensation of pricking or stinging and an intense desire to scratch or rub the affected part.

ITU: Abbreviation for intensive therapy unit, see INTENSIVE CARE UNIT.

-itis: Suffix denoting disease, usually inflammatory. — itises, itides, pl.

IU: Abbreviation for International Unit, see SI UNITS.

IUCD: Abbreviation for intrauterine contraceptive device, see under INTRAUTERINE.

IUD: Abbreviation for intrauterine device, see INTRAUTERINE CONTRACEPTIVE DEVICE under INTRAUTERINE.

IV: Abbreviation for intravenous (*q.v.*).

IVF: Abbreviation for *in vitro* fertilization.

IVI: Abbreviation for intravenous infusion, see under INTRAVENOUS.

IVP: Abbreviation for intravenous pyelogram, see under PYELOGRAM.

IVT: Abbreviation for intravenous therapy, see under THERAPY.

J

J: Symbol for joule (*q.v.*).

J point: Refers to the point where the QRS complex of the electrocardiogram meets the T segment.

J receptors: Sympathetic vagal nerve endings located deep in the parenchyma of the lung; thought to respond to the presence of pulmonary embolism or pulmonary oedema.

jacket: In medicine, a fixed bandage or covering for a part of the body, especially the thorax or trunk; sometimes made of plaster of Paris. STRAIT J. see under STRAITJACKET.

Jacksonian epilepsy: See EPILEPSY. [John Hughlings Jackson, English neurologist, 1835–1911.]

Jacquemier's sign (zhak'-mē-ās): Blueness of the vaginal mucosa just below the urethral orifice, sometimes seen in early pregnancy. [Jean Marie Jacquemier, French obstetrician, 1806–1879.]

jactitation (jak'-ti-tā'-shun): Excessive restlessness; constant turning or tossing about as seen in patients with high fever or serious illness.

Jaeger chart: A chart for testing near vision; uses a series of different sizes of printers' type. Also called *Jaeger's test types*. [Edward Jaeger von Jastthal, Austrian oculist, 1818–1911.]

Jakob–Creutzfeldt disease (yak'-ob-kroyts'-feld): See CREUTZFELDT–JAKOB DISEASE.

jamais vu (zha'-mā-voo): Literally, never having seen. A psychic phenomena in which the patient feels an absolute stranger in surroundings with which he is normally familiar; usually due to a lesion in the temporal lobe or to epilepsy.

Janeway's lesions: Circumscribed, slightly raised, erythematous, haemorrhagic, nodular or macular lesions; usually painless and occurring on the palms and soles; may be symptomatic of subacute bacterial endocarditis or mycotic aneurysm.

jargon (jar'-gon): **1.** unintelligible or confused speech. **2.** The technical terms used by specialists working in a particular field of knowledge.

jaundice (jawn'dis): A condition characterized by a raised level of bilirubin in the blood (hyperbilirubinaemia): due to deposition of bile pigments resulting from obstruction in bile passageways, excess destruction of red blood cells, or disturbance in liver function. Minor degrees are detectable only chemically and are most often referred to as LATENT J. Major degrees are recognized by yellow skin, sclerae and mucosae and are referred to as OVERT or CLINICAL J., J. may be due to (1) obstruction anywhere in the biliary tract (OBSTRUCTIVE J.); (2) excessive haemolysis of red blood cells (haemolytic J.); or (3) toxic or infective damage of liver cells. (HEPATOCELLULAR J.) ACHOLURIC J., J. without bile in the urine; usually reserved for congenital haemolytic anaemia, a familial disease characterized by abnormally fragile, small, spheroid cells haemolyse readily. Congenital spherocytosis. HAEMOLYTIC J. occurs in erythroblastosis fetalis or from excessive transfusion reactions; HEPATIC J. occurs in cirrhosis, and in infectious, viral, and toxic hepatitis; HEPATOCELLULAR J., J. due to impaired function or destruction of liver cells; INFECTIOUS OR INFECTIVE J. most commonly due to a virus; J. OF THE NEWBORN icterus neonatorum. MALIGNANT J. acute yellow atrophy of the liver; see under ACUTE. OBSTRUCTIVE J. occurs when a gallstone becomes lodged in the bile duct leading from the gallbladder, thus preventing the flow of bile into the duodenum. PHYSIOLOGIC J. OF THE NEWBORN yellowness of the skin and sclera, and hyperbilirubinaemia; seen in some neonates; usually mild and disappears in 7 to 14 days. Medical name: ICTERUS.

jaundiced (jawn'-disd): Of a yellowish colour; marked by jaundice.

jaw: Either the maxillary or mandibular bone, which together form the bony framework of the mouth into which the teeth are set.

jawbone: Either the maxilla (upper jaw) or mandible (lower jaw).

jejun-, jejuno-: Combining forms denoting jejunum.

jejunal (jē-joo'-nal): Of or relating to the jejunum. J. ULCER an ulcer in the mucous membrane lining the jejunum.

jejunectomy (jē-joo-nek'-to-mi): Surgical excision of the jejunum, or part of it.

313

jejunitis (jē-joo-nī′tis): Inflammation of the jejunum.

jejunogastric (jē-joo′-nō-gas-trik): Relating to the jejunum and the stomach.

jejunoileal shunt (jē-joo′-nō-il′-ē-al): A bypass procedure in which the upper jejunum is anastomosed to the terminal part of the ileum, and a blind loop is created; done for patients who are morbidly obese, to decrease available area for absorption of food in the intestine.

jejunoileum (jē-joo′nō-il′ē-um): The part of the small intestine between the duodenum and the caecum. — jejunoileal, adj.

jejunostomy (jē-joo-nos′-to-mi): A surgically made fistula between the jejunum and the anterior abdominal wall; used temporarily for feeding in cases where passage of food through the stomach is impossible or undesirable.

jejunotomy (jē-joo-not′o-mi): An incision into the jejunum.

jejunum (jē-joo′num): The part of the small intestine between the duodenum and the ileum. It is about 2.5 metres in length. — jejunal, adj.

Jellineck's sign: The brownish pigmentation, particularly of the upper eyelids, seen in hypoparathyroidism.

Jenner, Edward: English physician [1749–1823], in 1796 developed the method of preventing smallpox by inoculation with cowpox vaccine.

jerk: A sudden involuntary muscular movement; a reflex. Describes certain reflex actions that follow tapping or striking a muscle or tendon, e.g., knee-jerk.

Jervell and Lange-Nielsen syndrome: A condition occurring in certain congenitally deaf children; characterized by sudden attacks of syncope, ventricular fibrillation, and electrocardiographic anomalies.

Jesuits' balsam: Compound of tincture of benzoin. See BENZOIN.

Jesuits' powder or **bark:** See PERUVIAN BARK.

jet injection: The administration of medication by injection, intrasubcutaneously or subcutaneously, using a device that injects the fluid with great velocity and penetrates the skin painlessly.

jigger (jig′-ger): (*Tunga penetrans*) A flea, prevalent in the tropics. It burrows under the skin to lay its eggs, causing intense irritation. Secondary infection is common.

job description: Statement of requirements, qualifications, salary range, and any special conditions expected of an employee. See also PERSON SPECIFICATION.

jogger's heel: A painful traumatic condition of the heel, caused by repeatedly striking the heel forcefully on the ground or a hard surface when jogging.

jogging: Running at a slow, even pace.

joint: The articulation or connection of two or more bones for mobility and stability: consists of two cartilage-covered articular surfaces, a synovial membranous sac, and a capsule that thickens and becomes a ligament; provides for flexion, extension, abduction and adduction. Three main designated classes are: (1) SYNARTHROSES (fibrous) consisting usually of two bones bound together by fibrous material when little movement is desirable; further classified as (a) SUTURA, e.g., the sutures of the skull; (b) SYNDESMOSES, e.g., the union of the distal ends of the tibia and fibula; and (c) GOMPHOSES, e.g., the articulation of the teeth in the gums; and (2) CARTILAGINOUS in which two bones connected by cartilage allow for limited motion, e.g., the joints between the ribs and the sternum; further classified as (a) SYNCHONDROSES, as between the epiphyses and diaphyses of the long bones, in which the opposing surfaces are eventually converted into bone; and (b) SYMPHYSES, which are connected by a disc of fibrocartilage (as in the pubis, where the disc remains unossified throughout life); and (3) DIARTHROSES OR SYNOVIAL which are freely moveable joints, e.g., the hip and elbow joints.

joint capsule: The fibrous sheath that encloses a synovial joint.

joint cavity: The closed space in a synovial joint formed by synovial membrane that contains synovial fluid.

joint mouse: A small, loose, often calcified concretion in a synovial joint cavity.

joule (jool): Term used in nutritional science for calorie. It denotes the quantity of heat released when food is utilized in the body. One large calorie (kilocalorie) equals 4.184 kilojoules. JOULE'S EQUIVALENT the mechanical equivalent of the amount of heat or energy expended in raising one pound of water 1 degree Fahrenheit; 772 foot pounds. [J. P. Joule, English physicist, 1818–1889.]

jowl: The fleshy hanging part under the lower jaw.

jugal (jū′-gal): Relating to the cheek, the zygomatic bone in particular.

jugular (jug′-ū-lar): Relating to the throat. J. VEINS two veins passing down either side of the neck.

jugulum (joo′-gū-lum): The neck or throat.

juice: Any fluid from a body tissue; succus. DI-GESTIVE J. secreted by the glands in the walls of the small intestine; *succus entericus*; GAS-TRIC J. secreted by glands in the stomach walls; *succus gastricus*; PANCREATIC J. secreted by the pancreas; discharged into the duodenum; *succus pancreaticus*.

junction: The point or line where two parts meet. — junctional, adj.

junctional (junk'shun-al): Relating to a junction. J. RHYTHM a cardiac rhythm for which the pacemaker is in the atrioventricular junctional tissues; J. TACHYCARDIA an arrhythmia with a heartbeat of 140 to 220 per minute, for which the impulse arises in the atrioventricular tissues.

Jung: Carl Gustav Jung, Swiss psychiatrist. [1875–1961.] Founder of the school of analytical psychology. See JUNGIAN PSYCHOLOGY under PSYCHOLOGY.

jungian (yoon'-gi-an, joon'-): Relating to or characteristic of C. G. Jung, his theories, methods, or doctrines. See under PSYCHOLOGY.

jungle fever: 1. Malaria (*q.v.*). 2. Yellow fever (*q.v.*).

jurisprudence (jur-is-prū'-dens): The science or philosophy of law. MEDICAL J. see under MEDICAL.

jury mast (joo'-ri mast): An upright bar inserted into a plaster of Paris jacket to support the head in spinal fracture, or in spinal disease, as Pott's disease.

justo minor pelvis: A pelvis that is like the normal female pelvis in every way except that it is in miniature. All pelvic measurements are in the correct proportion but diminished.

juvenile (joo'-ve-nīl): Relates to childhood, immaturity, or youth, J. KYPHOSIS Scheuermann's disease (*q.v.*); J. MUSCULAR ATROPHY a hereditary disease marked by slowly progressive muscle weakness and wasting beginning in the lower extremities and pelvic girdle, with onset usually between 2 and 17 years of age; evidence of lower motor neuron disease; J. MUSCULAR DYSTROPHY limb-girdle dystrophy, see under DYSTROPHY; J.-ONSET DIABETES see under DIABETES; J. OSTEOMALACIA rickets; J. RHEUMATOID ARTHRITIS see STILL'S DISEASE.

juxta-: Combining form denoting situated near.

juxta-articular (juks'ta-ar-tik'ū-lar): Near a joint.

juxtaglomerular (juks'-ta-glō-mer'-ū-lar): Adjacent to or near the glomerulus. J. APPARATUS a cuff of tissue surrounding the arteriole leading into the glomerulus; J. CELLS cells found within the cuff of the apparatus surrounding the arteriole that supplies the glomerulus; their function is unknown.

juxtamedullary (juks'ta-med'ū-lar i). Relating to the part of the kidney cortex that is adjacent to the medulla.

juxtapose (juks'-ta-pōz): To place side by side.

juxtaposition (juks'ta-pō-zish'-un): The position of objects in relation to one another, being side by side; adjacent; in apposition; close at hand.

K

K: Chemical symbol for potassium.

Kahler's disease: Multiple myeloma; see under MYELOMA.

kakidrosis (kak-i-drō'-sis): Extremely unpleasant smelling sweat.

kakotrophy (kak-ot'-rō-fi): Undernutrition. Also spelled *cacotrophy*.

kalaemia (ka-lē' mi-a): The presence of potassium in the blood.

kalimeter (ka-lim'-i-ter): A device for measuring the alkalinity of a substance. Also called *Alkalimeter*.

kaliopenia (kal-i-ō-pē'-ni-a): An insufficiency of potassium in the body. — kaliopenic, adj.

kaliuresis, kaluresis (kal-i-ū-re'-sis, kal-ū-rē'-sis): The presence of potassium in the urine.

kaliuretic, kaluretic (kal-i-ū-ret'-ik, kal-ū-ret'-ik): 1. Relating to kaliuresis. 2. An agent that promotes kaliuresis.

kallidin (kal'-i-din): A kinin liberated by the action of kallikrein on a globulin in the blood plasma; of two varieties, K.-I and K-II. They increase capillary permeability.

kallikrein (kal-li-krē'-in, krīn): One of several proteolytic enzymes present in blood plasma, salivary glands, lymph glands, pancreas, urine, and lymph. It acts on a globulin in blood plasma to release kinins, such as bradykinin, from kininogens.

kallikreinogen (kal-i-krē'-nō-jen, -krīn'-): The precursor of kallikrein, normally present in the blood plasma.

Kandahar sore: Cutaneous leishmaniasis, see LEISHMANIASIS.

kaolin (kā'-ō-lin): Powdered dehydrated aluminium silicate; used internally as an absorbent in the treatment of diarrhoea and externally as a protective application that absorbs moisture.

kaolinosis (kā'ō-lin-ō'-sis): A form of pneumoconiosis caused by inhalation of particles of kaolin.

Kaposi: (ka-pō'-si): K'S DISEASE a rare condition marked by dermatosis, discoloration of the skin that may give rise to keratosis, ulcers, neoplastic growth, and a fatal termination; usually starts in childhood; K'S SARCOMA a malignant neoplasm of the skin marked by the development of purplish nodules or papules on the skin, lymphadenectomy, excessive weight loss, and immune deficiency; see ACQUIRED IMMUNO DEFICIENCY SYNDROME; K'S VARICELLIFORM ERUPTION a viral skin infection occurring in the presence of another skin disease such as eczema or herpes simplex. [Moritz K. Kaposi, Hungarian dermatologist, 1837–1902.]

karaya (ka-rā'-a): A vegetable gum with nonirritating and protective qualities; used especially for sealing ostomy appliances to the skin; also sometimes used as a laxative.

Kartagener's syndrome (kah-taj'-en-erz): A hereditary condition in which dextrocardia is present along with bronchiectasis and sinusitis.

kary-, karyo-: Combining forms denoting the nucleus of a cell.

karyochrome (kar'-i-ō-krōm): A nerve cell with a nucleus that takes a stain easily but has few, if any, Nissl bodies (*q.v.*).

karyoclasis (kar-i-ok'-la-sis): The breaking down of a cell nucleus, an early stage in necrosis.

karyocyte (kar'-i-ō-sīt): Any nucleated cell; usually refers to a young red blood cell.

karyogenesis (kar-i-ō-jen'-e-sis): The formation of a cell nucleus.

karyokinesis (kar'i-ō-ki-nē'sis): Equal division of nuclear material, as occurs in cell division.

karyolymph (kar'-i-ō-limf): The clear fluid part of a cell nucleus in which the other elements are dispersed.

karyolysis (kar-i-ol'-i-sis): The dissolution or destruction of a cell nucleus. — karyolytic, adj.

karyomegaly (kar-i-ō-meg'a-li): Abnormal enlargement of the nucleus of a cell.

karyon (kar'-i-on): Nucleus of a cell.

karyoplasm (kar'-i-ō-plazm): The protoplasm of a cell that is contained within the nucleus, *i.e.*, the nucleoplasm.

karyopyknosis (kar'i-ō-pik-nō'sis): Shrinkage of a cell nucleus with condensation of the chromatin content.

karyorrhexis (kar-i-ō-rek'-sis): Fragmentation of the chromatin mass in the nucleus of a cell, a stage in necrosis that precedes karyolysis.

karyosome (kar'-i-ō-sōm): The spherical mass of chromatin in the cell nucleus.

karyotheca (kar-i-ō-thē'-ka): The membrane around the nucleus of a cell.

karyotype (kar'-i-ō-tīp): The total chromosomal make-up of the nucleus of a single cell as to number, size, shape, and location of the centromere, and which is characteristic of an individual, species, or other grouping.

Kashin–Beck disease: A slowly progressive form of osteoarthritis of the peripheral joints and spine, occurring chiefly in young children in Eastern Siberia and Northern China; caused by eating fungus-contaminated grain.

Katz–Wechtel sign (Kats-vek'-tel): A change in the QRS complexes as shown on the electrocardiogram; indicates a defect in the ventricular spectrum.

Kawasaki's disease (ka-wa-sah'-kiz): A rare, acute, arthritis-like disorder, first described in 1967; endemic in Japan; usually occurs in children under two years of age, more often in boys than girls. Cause and mode of transmission not known; may be a sequela to a viral infection. Symptoms include a rash of red flat spots followed by desquamation, especially of the fingertips; sore throat, conjunctivitis, cervical lymphadenopathy, and, in 30% of cases, cardiac complications. Also called *mucocutaneous lymph node syndrome.*

Kayser–Fleischer ring (kā'-zer-flī'-sher): A ring of grey-green to red-gold colour at the outer margin of the cornea; seen in hepatolenticular degeneration (*q.v.*).

kcal: Kilocalorie. Also abbreviated kcal and C. The quantity of energy required to raise the temperature of one kilogram of water 1°C. Has 1000 times the value of a small calorie. Also known as large calorie.

Kehr's sign: Radiating shoulder pain occurring when the diaphragm is irritated by blood in the peritoneal cavity; may be a sign of ruptured spleen.

Kell blood group system: First described in 1946. Red blood cells that are antibodies to the K antigen have been observed in infants with haemolytic disease of the newborn and in association with haemolytic transfusion reactions. Also referred to as *K* or *k blood group system.*

Keller's operation: Arthroplasty of the metatarsophalangeal joint of the great toe, for removal of the bursa and for treatment of exostosis; bunionectomy.

Kelly forceps: See under FORCEPS.

keloid (kē'-loyd): An overgrowth of scar tissue, consisting of a shiny, firm, usually elevated, benign, thickened mass of fibrous tissue forming at the site of a burn, skin wound, or surgical incision; has a predilection for the face and trunk; may produce a constriction deformity. Most common in pigmented skin.

keloidosis (kē'-loy-dō'-sis): A condition marked by the formation of keloids.

keloma (kē-lō'-ma): A keloid.

kelotomy (kē-lot'-o-mi): An operation for the relief of strangulated hernia.

Kennedy Report (ken'-ne-di): A report recommending a framework of standards and professional regulation to provide effective management and professional accountability, resulting from the inquiry into children's heart surgery at Bristol Royal Infirmary, UK (published July 2001).

Kennedy's syndrome: Retrobulbar optic neuritis, a condition usually seen in tumours of the frontal lobe or sphenoid crest; symptoms include optic nerve atrophy, unilateral blindness, sometimes anosmia. Also called *Foster Kennedy syndrome.* [Robert Foster Kennedy, American neurologist, 1884–1952.]

Kenny method, treatment: A method of treating patients with anterior poliomyelitis to prevent paralysis; involves the use of hot wet packs, positioning, and muscle re-education. [Sister Elizabeth Kenny, Australian nurse, 1886–1952.]

Kent's bundle: A muscular bundle which, in some people, forms an abnormal direct connection between the atrial and ventricular walls.

kerat-, kerato-: Combining forms denoting (1) the cornea; (2) horny tissue.

keratalgia (ker-a-tal'-ji-a): Pain in the cornea.

keratectasia (ker-a-tek-tā'-zi-a): Protrusion of the cornea.

keratectomy (ker-a-tek'-to-mi): Removal of a portion of the cornea.

keratiasis (ker-a-tī'-a-sis): The presence of horny warts on the skin.

keratin (ker'-a-tin): A relatively insoluble protein found in all horny tissue; a principal constituent of the epidermis, where it serves to waterproof and toughen the skin. In pharmacology, used to coat pills given for their intestinal effect, since keratin can withstand the action of gastric juice.

keratinization (ker'a-tin-ī-zā'shun): 1. The formation of keratin in body tissues. 2. The development of a horny quality in tissues by the excess formation of keratin; occurs as a pathological process in vitamin A deficiency.

keratinocyte (ke-rat'-in-ō-sīt): The epidermal cell which synthesizes keratin in the skin.

keratinous (ke-rat′ -in-us): Horny.

keratitis (ker-a-tī′ -tis): Inflammation of the cornea. ACNE ROSEACEA K. severe K. associated with acne roseacea of the eyelids and cornea; HERPETIC K., K. characterized by simultaneous appearance with herpes simplex; fairly common in the elderly; INTERSTITIAL K. marked by deposits in the corneal substance giving it a hazy ground glass appearance; associated with congenital syphilis; K. NUMMULARIS a benign, slowly developing type of K. in which deposits in the cornea form into circles with sharply defined areas, surrounded by less dense areas forming a halo.

keratoacanthoma (ker′a-tō-ak′an-thō′ma): A rapidly growing firm skin nodule, usually singular, appearing on hairy parts of the body, especially on exposed areas; has a dome-shaped centre of keratotic material; resembles squamous cell carcinoma. Usually occurs in sun-damaged skin, but may also be due to exposure to tars and mineral oil products.

keratocele (ker′ -a-tō-sēl): Hernial protrusion of Descemet's membrane, the innermost layer of the cornea.

keratochromatosis (ker′a-tō-krō-ma-tō′sis): Discoloration of the cornea.

keratoconus (ker′ -a-tō-kō′ -nus): An inherited, degenerative, non-inflammatory condition marked by conical protrusion of the central part of the cornea; usually bilateral; results in astigmatism. Seen more often in women. May be associated with Down's syndrome. In advanced cases the cornea becomes scarred and a corneal transplant is required.

keratocyte (ker′ -a-tō-sīt): One of the flattened cells between the lamellae of the cornea, with branching processes that communicate with those of other cells.

keratoderma (ker′a-tō-der′ma): Hypertrophy of the horny layer of the skin (stratum corneum), marked by the appearance of cone-shaped horny lesions, affecting primarily the palms and soles. K. BLENNORRHAGICUM characterized by pustular, crusted, cone-shaped lesions on the palms and soles; may be associated with gonorrhoeal arthritis; K. CLIMACTERICUM occurs in menopausal women; marked by lesions on the hands and feet; may be associated with obesity.

keratogenesis (ker′ -a-tō-jen′ -e-sis): The formation of horny growths.

keratogenous (ker-a-toj′ -e-nus): Causing formation of horny tissue.

keratoglobus (ker′a-tō-glō′bus): Prominent globular protrusion of the cornea; seen in congenital glaucoma.

keratohelcosis (ker′a-tō-hel-ko′sis): Ulceration of the cornea.

keratoid (ker′ -a-toyd): 1. Hornlike. 2. Resembling corneal tissue.

keratoiritis (ker′ -a-tō-ī-rī′ -tis): Inflammation of the cornea and the iris.

keratoleukoma (ker′ -a-tō-lū-kō′ -ma): Areas of white opacity in the cornea.

keratolysis (ker-a-tol′ -i-sis): 1. Shedding of the epidermis. 2. A congenital anomaly characterized by the periodic shedding of skin. — keratolytic, adj.

keratoma (ker-a-tō′ -ma): An overgrowth of horny tissue. Callosity. — keratomata, pl.

keratomalacia (ker′a-tō-ma-lā′shi-a): Softening of the cornea with possible ulceration; frequently caused by lack of vitamin A.

keratome (ker′ -a-tom): A knife used in surgery on the cornea. Also called *Keratotome*.

keratometer (ker-a-tom′ -i-ter): An instrument for measuring the curvature of the surface of the cornea; used in fitting contact lenses.

keratomycosis (ker′ -a-tō-mī-kō′ -sis): A fungal disease of the cornea.

keratonyxis (ker′ -a-tō-nik′ -sis): Surgical puncture of the cornea, as in the procedure of needling the lens in treatment of soft cataract.

keratopathy (ker-a-top′ -a-thi): Any disease of the cornea. — keratopathic, adj.

keratoplasty (ker′ -a-tō-plas-ti): Corneal grafting. Replacing of unhealthy corneal tissue with healthy tissue obtained from a donor. — keratoplastic, adj.

keratoprosthesis (ker′ -a-tō-pros-thē′ -sis): An acrylic plastic corneal implant that replaces an area of the cornea that has become opaque.

keratorrhexis (ker′ -a-tō-reks′ -is): Rupture of the cornea; may be caused by trauma or be due to ulceration.

keratoscleritis (ker′ -a-tō-sklē-rī′ -tis): Inflammation of the cornea and the sclera.

keratoscope (ker′ -a-tō-skōp): An instrument for examining the cornea.

keratose (ker′ -a-tōs): Horny.

keratosis (ker-a-tō′ -sis): Thickening or overgrowth of the horny layer of the skin, such as a callosity or wart. ACTINIC K. slowly developing warty lesion in areas that are long exposed to sunlight; affects chiefly the middle-aged and elderly; potentially malignant; also called *senile keratosis, solar keratosis, keratoderma*; ARSENICAL K. precancerous hard, wart-like lesions seen in persons who have received medications containing arsenic or been long exposed to pesticides, dyes, or other substances containing arsenic; may not appear until 10 years after exposure; K. FOLLICULARIS a rare congenital condition marked by areas of symmetrical crusting and papular growths on the trunk, axillae, face, and scalp; K. NIGRICANS *acanthus nigricans*; see under ACANTHUS; K. PALMARIS ET PLANTARIS (tylosis) a congenital thickening of the horny layer of the palms and soles; K. SENILIS dry, harsh condition of the skin seen in the aged; also descriptive of the pigmented elevated papules seen in the skin of patients long exposed to sunlight; SEBORRHOEIC K. a coarse waxy benign neoplasm of the skin characterized by the formation of multiple shiny tan to brown dome-shaped lesions of varying size; usually develops in middle life; SOLAR K. actinic k. — keratoses, pl.; keratotic, adj.

keratotomy (ker-a-tot′-o-mi): A surgical incision into the cornea.

kerion (kē′-ri-on): A boggy suppurative swelling, often associated with ringworm of the scalp.

Kerley lines: Horizontal stepladder like lines that appear on chest x-rays and are associated with certain disease conditions, such as congestive heart failure and pleural lymphatic engorgement.

kernicterus (ker-nik′-ter-us): A serious form of icterus neonatorum; caused by high levels of bilirubin in the blood, bile staining, and widespread destructive lesions in various parts of the brain; may result in severe neurological defects; often a sequela to erythroblastosis fetalis (*q.v.*).

Kernig's sign (ker′nigs): Inability to straighten the leg at the knee joint when the thigh is flexed at right angles to the trunk. Occurs in meningitis. [Vladimir Kernig, Russian physician, 1840–1917.]

keto acid: A chemical compound that is both an acid and a ketone. See KETONE.

ketoacidosis (kē′-tō-as-i-dō′-sis): Acidosis accompanied by an increase of acetone bodies in the blood; due to incomplete metabolism of fatty acids; commonly seen in diabetes mellitus, starvation, pregnancy, or after ether anaesthesia. DIABETIC K. due to insulin deficiency, characterized by dehydration, electrolyte depletion, hyperpnoea, acetone odour to the breath, dry mouth and hyperglycaemia, followed by glycosuria and polyuria and, possibly, death.

ketoaciduria (ke′-tō-as-i-dū′-ri-a): The presence of excessive keto acids in the urine.

ketogenesis (kē-tō-jen′-i-sis): The production of ketone bodies.

ketogenic (kē-tō-jen′-ik): Producing or capable of producing ketone bodies. K. DIET consists of foods that cause a ketogenic state as a result of changes in the acid–base balance, *i.e.*, large amount of fats and minimal amounts of protein; used in treatment of epilepsy in young children.

ketohexose (kē-tō-hek′-sos): A monosaccharide that contains a six-carbon chain and a ketone group.

ketolysis (kē-tol′-i-sis): The dissolution or splitting up of acetone or ketone bodies. — ketolytic, adj.

ketonaemia (kē-tō-nē′mi-a): An excess of ketone bodies in the blood as occurs in starvation or diabetes mellitus.

ketone (kē′-ton): Any organic compound that contains the carbonyl group CO. The product of incomplete oxidation of fat in the body; when present in the bloodstream K.s upset the acid–base balance of the body and produce ketosis. See ACETONE BODIES under ACETONE.

ketone bodies: Acetone, acetoacetic acid, and β-hydroxybutyric acid; normal products of metabolism of lipids and pyruvate in the liver, occurring in increased amounts in the blood and urine of persons with certain conditions, *e.g.*, pregnancy, starvation, and diabetic acidosis.

ketonuria (kē-tō-nū-ri-a): Excessive ketone bodies in the urine. — ketonuric, adj.

ketosis (ke-tō′-sis): A condition that arises when incomplete oxidation of fatty acids results in an accumulation of ketone bodies in the blood; symptoms include drowsiness, headache, and deep respirations. A complication of diabetes mellitus and of starvation when it is the result of decreased carbohydrate intake. — ketotic, adj.

ketosteroids (kē-tō-stē′roidz): Steroid hormones that contain a keto group, formed by the addition of an oxygen molecule to the basic ring structure. The 17-K. (which have this oxygen at carbon 17) are produced by the adrenal cortex and excreted in normal urine; they are present in excess in overactivity of the adrenal glands and the gonads, and in renal and ovarian tumours; hyper- or hyposecretion is indicative of an endocrine disorder.

key informant: A long-standing member of a culture or group who has expert knowledge of its rules, customs, and language.

key worker (kē′-wor-ker): The current carer for a particular mental health patient, in charge of the patient's immediate treatment as determined by the Care Programme Approach (*q.v.*).

kg: Abbreviation for kilogram.

Kidd blood group: Red blood cell antigens that react with antibodies designated anti-Jk^a, first found in the mother of an infant with erythroblastosis; occasionally cause transfusion reactions or erythroblastosis fetalis (*q.v.*).

kidney (kid' -ni): One of two bean-shaped organs, situated on the posterior abdominal wall, behind the peritoneum in the lumbar region, one on either side of the vertebral column. Function is to secrete urine. FLOATING K. one that is misplaced and more or less freely movable; HORSESHOE K. a congenital malformation in which the K. has the shape of a horseshoe; K. STONE a calculus (*q.v.*) that forms, usually in the pelvis of the kidney, composed mostly of calcium oxalate. When small, calculi may pass down through the ureters and bladder and cause agonizing pain as they pass through the urethra; POLYCYSTIC K. a hereditary condition characterized by the formation of multiple cysts on both kidneys.

Kienböch's disease or atrophy (kēn' -berks, kēn' -boks): Osteochondrosis (*q.v.*) of the lunate bone of the wrist; marked by pain, loss of grip, limitation of motion. [Robert Kienböch, Austrian roentgenologist, 1871–1953.]

Kiernan's spaces: Triangular spaces in the liver formed by the invagination of Glisson's capsule; they contain the larger branches of the portal vein, hepatic artery, and the hepatic duct.

Kiesselbach's area (kē' -s'l-bahks, kē' -s'l-baks): An area on the anterior inferior part of the nasal septum; often the site of epistaxis.

killer cells: Lymphocytes developed in the bone marrow that, in the presence of an antibody, attack certain cells directly.

Killian's operation: The removal of a part of the frontal bone to allow for drainage from a suppurating frontal sinus.

kilo-: Combining form denoting one thousand; used chiefly in names of units in the metric system.

kilocalorie (kil' -ō-kal-o-ri): Large calorie; see under CALORIE.

kilogram (kg) (kil' -ō-gram): One thousand grams.

kilometre (km) (ki-lom' -e-ter): One thousand metres.

kilovolt (kv) (kil' -ō-vōlt): One thousand volts.

Kimmelstiel–Wilson syndrome (kim' -m'l-stīn-wil' -son): A condition that occurs in diabetics of long standing when glomerulosclerosis has occurred; characteristic signs are hypertension, oedema, proteinuria, and renal failure.

kin-, kine-, kinesi-, kinesio-, kino-: Combining forms denoting motion, action.

kinaesthesia (kin-es-thē' -zi-a): Muscle sense; perception of movement, weight, and position. — kinaesthetic, adj. Also called *kinaesthesis.*

kinaesthesiometer (kin'es-thē'zi-om' -i-ter): An instrument for measuring proprioception (*q.v.*).

kinanaesthesia (kin-an-es-thē'zi-a): Loss of the sense of movement.

kinase (kī'nās): An enzyme involved in the transfer of a phosphate group, usually from ATP.

kinematics (kin-e-mat' -iks): The science of motion of the body and of the body parts.

kinemometer (kī-nē-mom' -i-ter): An electromagnetic device used to measure the reflex time of a tendon reflex.

kineplastic surgery: Operative measures utilized in amputations whereby certain muscle groups are isolated and utilized to work certain modified prostheses.

kinescope (kin' -e-skōp): An instrument used in testing ocular refraction.

kinesia (kī-nē' -si-a): Motion sickness.

kinesialgia (kī-nē' -si-al' -ji-a): Pain caused by muscular movements.

kinesiatrics (kī-nē' -si-at-riks): The therapeutic use of active or passive movements; movement therapy. Kinesitherapy.

kinesics (kī-nē' -siks): The study of non-verbal bodily activity in communication, including posture, facial expression, and body movements.

kinesiology (kī-nē-si-ol' -o-ji): The science or study of human motion.

kinesis (kī-nē' -sis): Physical movement.

kinesitherapy (kī-nē' -si-ther-a-pi): Treatment by massage and therapeutic exercises. Kinesiatrics.

kinetic (kī-net' -ik): Relating to, or producing, motion.

kinetism (kin' -e-tizm): The ability to consciously initiate and perform movement.

kinetogenic (ki-nē-tō-jen' -ik): Causing or resulting in movement.

kinetoplasm (ki-nē' -tō-plazm): The chromophilic substance present in the nerve cells only at the time the cells begin to perform their specific functions.

kinetosis (ki-nē-tō' -sis): Any illness due to motion.

King's Fund: An independent charitable foundation, the goal of which is to improve health, especially in London.

kinin (kī' -nin): Any of a group of several peptides that appear to have a direct action on the blood vessels, cause contraction of smooth muscle, act as hypotensives, increase capillary permeability, and have certain other properties in common. VENOM K. found in the venom of snakes; WASP K. found in the venom of wasps. See also BRADYKININ.

kink: Angulation. An unnatural bend, twist, or angle in, structure, particularly in a duct or tube.

kinked carotid syndrome: A strong arterial pulsation felt just above the right clavicle; occurs chiefly in older women with systolic hypertension; to be differentiated from carotid aneurysm.

kinomometer (kin-ō-mom-i-ter): An instrument for measuring the degree of motion in a joint.

kinotoxin (kin-ō-tok'-sin): Toxin produced by fatigue.

kiotomy (kī-ot'-o-mi): Excision of the uvula or part of it.

Kirschner's wire (kirsch'-ner). A wire drilled into a bone to apply skeletal traction. [Martin Kirschner, German surgeon, 1879–1942.]

kissing: K. DISEASE infectious mononucleosis, see under MONONUCLEOSIS; K. ULCER an ulcer caused by pressure of apposing parts.

Klebsiella (kleb-si-el'-ah): A genus of the family Enterobacteriaceae, anaerobic, non-spore-forming, Gram-negative rods which may or may not be pathogenic; found in the respiratory, intestinal, and urogenital tracts; may be the causative agent in bronchitis, sinusitis, and certain pneumonias. K. PNEUMONIAE Friedländer's bacillus; a large Gram-negative rod bacterium occasionally found in the upper respiratory tract; may be the cause of lobar pneumonia and other inflammations of the respiratory tract.

kleptolagnia (klep'-tō-lag'-ni-a): Sexual gratification derived from the act of stealing.

kleptomania (klep'-tō-mā'-ni-a): Compulsive stealing due to mental disturbance, usually of the obsessional neurosis type.

kleptomaniac (klep'-tō-mā'-ni-ak): 1. Pertaining to kleptomania. 2. A person who is a compulsive thief.

Klinefelter's syndrome: A condition associated with abnormality of the sex chromosomes; in most instances the cells have an extra X chromosome. The individual appears to be male but has large breasts, small genitalia, atrophied testes, and is sterile; genetic female, pragmatic male. Frequently recognized in sterility clinics. [Harry F. Klinefelter, American physician, 1912–.]

Klippel–Feil syndrome: A condition occurring in infants with congenital hemivertebra; the neck is short and its movement is limited due to either a reduction in the number of cervical vertebrae or to fusion.

knee (nē): The hinge joint formed by the lower end of the femur and the head of the tibia. HOUSEMAID'S K. inflammation of the prepatellar bursa; K. JERK a reflex contraction of the relaxed quadriceps muscle elicited by a tap on the patellar tendon; usually performed with the lower femur supported from behind, the knee bent and the leg limp. Persistent variation from normal usually signifies organic nervous disorder; KNOCK-K. abnormal closeness of the knees while the ankles are abnormally far apart; genu valgum. See VALGUS.

kneecap: The patella (q.v.).

knee replacement: A surgical procedure in which diseased surfaces within the knee joint are removed and replaced with a hinged prosthesis that is cemented to the femur and tibia; usually done to relieve pain and to restore loss of range of motion due to osteoarthritis or some other pathological condition.

knismogenic (nis-mo-jen'-ik): Causing a tickling sensation.

knit (nit): Term used to describe the growing together of the ends of bones after a fracture.

knuckle (nuk'l): The dorsal aspect of any of the joints between the phalanges and the metacarpal bones, or between the phalanges.

Koch: K'S BACILLUS *Mycobacterium tuberculosis*, the causative organism of tuberculosis; K'S POSTULATES a list of requirements that an organism must meet before it can be considered the cause of a disease; also called *Koch's law*. [Robert Koch, German physician and bacteriologist, 1843–1910.]

Koch–Weeks bacillus: A small, Gram-negative rod; the cause of infective conjunctivitis (pinkeye).

Köhler's disease (ker'-lerz): 1. Osteochondritis of the navicular bone. 2. Osteochondritis of the second or third metatarsal head. [Alban Köhler, German physician, 1874–1947.]

Kohlrausch's folds (kōl'-rowsh): Horizontal folds of the rectal mucosa; rectal valve. Syn., *Houston's valves*.

koilo-: Combining form denoting hollowed, depressed, concave.

koilonychia (koy-lō-nik'-i-a): Spoon-shaped nails, characteristic of iron-deficiency anaemia.

koilorrhachic (koy-lō-rak'-ik): Having a spinal column in which the lumbar vertebrae curve anteriorly.

kola (kō'la): The dried cotyledons of the *Cola* species of plants; contain caffeine, theobromine, and cotalin; used in medicine as a nerve and heart stimulant.

kolp-, kolpo-: See words beginning COLP-.

konio-: See words beginning CONIO-.

Koplik's spots: Small, bluish-white spots, each surrounded by a bright red ring, that appear bilaterally on the mucous membrane inside the mouth, opposite the juncture of the molars, during the first 10 days of measles; they appear before the rash and are diagnostic. [Henry Koplik, American paediatrician, 1858–1927.]

Kopp's asthma (kops az'-ma): Spasm of the glottis in children under two; thought to be due to enlarged thymus gland.

kopr-, kopra-: See words beginning COPR-, COPRA-.

Korean haemorrhagic fever: Caused by a togavirus, endemic in Korea; spreads directly from animals to humans. Symptoms include prostration, chills and fever, headache and backache, conjunctivitis, severe proteinuria, and, in severe cases, shock and renal failure.

Korotkoff's sounds: The five distinct phases of sound heard through a stethoscope placed over the brachial artery below the pressure cuff of the sphygmomanometer during the procedure for determining the blood pressure. [Nicolai Korotkoff (Korotkov), Russian physician, 1874–1920.]

Korsakoff's psychosis or syndrome: A chronic condition that follows delirium and toxic states. Often due to alcoholism or dietary deficiencies. The consciousness is clear and alert, but the patient is disoriented as to time and place, especially for recent events; hallucinates and often confabulates to fill in the gaps in memory. Afflicts more men than women in the 45–55 age group. Also called *alcoholic dementia, cerebropathica psychica toxaemia, chronic alcoholic delirium, polyneuritic psychosis.* [Sergei S. Korsakoff, Russian neurologist, 1853–1900.]

kosher (kō'-sher): Clean or fit to eat according to Judaic dietary laws. Term is used to describe food that is prepared according to Jewish law.

Krabbe's disease: Globoid cell leukodystrophy; a rapidly progressing hereditary disease with onset early in infancy; symptoms include stupor, apathy, vomiting, rigidity, fretfulness, blindness, dysphagia, and mental handicap; death usually occurs within a year of onset.

kraurosis (kraw-rō-sis): Progressive atrophy, shrinking, and sclerosing of the skin. K. OF THE PENIS see BALANITIS XEROTICA OBLITERANS under BALANITIS; K. VULVAE a degenerative

condition of dryness, itching, and atrophy of the vaginal introitus associated with postmenopausal lack of oestrogen; may be precancerous; often occurs in conjunction with leukoplakia.

Krebs cycle: A cyclic series of reactions in the metabolism of fats, carbohydrates, and proteins in which enzymes act as catalysts in the formation of oxaloacetate, which in turn is oxidized into carbon dioxide and water with the release of energy. Also called *citric acid cycle, tricarboxylic acid cycle, TCA cycle.*

Krönig's isthmus: (krer'-nigz): A narrow area of resonance heard both anteriorly and posteriorly when percussing the apices of the lungs just above the clavicles; also called *Krönig's fields,* and *Krönig's area.*

Krukenberg's tumour: A secondary malignant tumour of the ovary, usually bilateral. The primary growth is usually in the stomach. [Friedrich Ernst Krukenberg, German pathologist, 1871–1946.]

kry-, kryo-: See CRY-, CRYO-.

krymotherapy (krī'mō-ther'a-pi): See CRYOTHERAPY.

Kuf's disease: A hereditary disorder of lipid metabolism with symptoms developing in adolescence or early life; marked by dementia, seizures, ataxia, and sometimes retinal pigmentation. Syn., *late juvenile amaurotic familial idiocy.* See SPHINGOLIPIDOSIS.

Küntscher nail (koon'-tcher): See under NAIL.

Kupffer's cells: Large intensely phagocytic cells found in the lining of the sinusoids of the liver.

kuru (koo'-roo): A chronic, progressive degenerative disorder of the central nervous system, of viral origin: found among natives of certain areas of New Guinea; most cases occur in women and children; characterized by tremor, ataxia, strabismus, dementia, and usually death within a year of onset.

Kussmaul: K.'S APHASIA voluntarily refraining from speaking, as practised by certain individuals suffering from a psychosis or insanity; K.'S RESPIRATIONS paroxysms of deep inspirations with sighing expirations, often a forerunner of diabetic acidosis and coma; also called *air hunger* and *Kussmaul–Kien respirations*; K.'S SIGN seen when the neck veins distend rather than collapse with inspiration; may occur in patients with cardiac tamponade and constrictive pericarditis. [Adolph Kussmaul, German physician, 1822–1902.]

kwashiorkor (kwa-shi-or'-kor): A nutritional disorder of infants and young children when the diet is persistently deficient in essential protein. Most common in Africa. Characteristic features are anaemia, wasting, dependent oedema, fatty liver, changes in hair colour, delayed wound healing; often accompanied by parasitic or viral infections. Untreated, it progresses to death.

K. Y. jelly: A tradename for a lubricating jelly.

kymatism (kī'-ma-tizm): Quivering of the muscles or a twitching of an isolated segment of a muscle.

kymograph (kī'-mō-graf): An apparatus for recording movements, *e.g.*, of muscles, columns of blood. Used in physiological experiments. — kymographic, adj.; kymographically, adj.

kymoscope (kī'-mo-skōp): An apparatus for measuring variations in pulse wave and in blood flow and pressure.

kyphorachitis (kī-fō-ra-kī-tis): A rachitic deformity involving both the thorax and the spine and marked by an anteroposterior hump.

kyphos (ki'-fos): The 'hump' of an individual with kyphoscoliosis.

kyphoscoliosis (kī'-fō-skō-li-ō'-sis): A backward and lateral curvature of the spine; seen in Scheuermann's disease (*q.v.*), in which there is necrosis of the epiphyses of the vertebrae.

kyphosis (kī'-fō-'-sis): An excessive backward convex curvature of the spine, usually in the thoracic region. Also called *Pott's curvature*, *humpback*, and *hunchback*. See also POTT'S DISEASE.

kyrtorrhachia (kir-tō-rak'-ki-a): Old term for a curved lumbar spine characterized by a backward concavity.

L

labia (lā'-bi-a): Lips. L. MAJORA two large lip-like folds extending from the mons veneris to encircle the vaginal opening. L. MINORA two smaller folds lying within the L. MAJORA. — labium, sing; labial, adj.

labile (lā'-bīl): Unstable, readily changed, as happens to many drugs when in solution. In psychology, emotionally unstable.

lability (la-bil'-i-ti): Instability. EMOTIONAL L. rapid change in mood; frequently occurs in the elderly with mental disorders or following stroke, when the patient's emotional reactions may include anxiety, anger, frustration, denial of illness, depression, disorientation, childishness.

labio-: Combining form denoting relationship to a lip or lips.

labioglossolaryngeal (lā'bi-ō-glos'ō-la-rin'jē-al): Relating to the lips, tongue, and larynx. L. PARALYSIS a nervous system disease characterized by progressive paralysis of the lips, tongue, and larynx.

labioglossopharyngeal (lā'bi-ō-glos'ō-fa-rin'jē-al): Relating to the lips, tongue, and pharynx.

labiomancy (lā'-bi-ō-man-si): Lip reading.

labour (lā'-bor): The act of giving birth to a child; parturition, confinement. The first stage lasts from onset of regular painful contractions until there is full dilatation of the cervical os; the second follows full dilatation of the cervix until the baby is delivered; the third follows delivery of the baby until expulsion of the placenta and membranes. COMPLICATED L. that in which convulsions, haemorrhage or some other untowards event occurs; DRY L. that which occurs after most of the amniotic fluid has been expelled; FALSE L. uterine contractions that occur before the onset of true L.; INDUCED L. that which is brought on by mechanical or other extraneous means; PREMATURE L. that which occurs between the 28th and 37th weeks of pregnancy after the fetus is viable but before the gestation period is complete.

labour market: The supply of available labour considered with respect to the demand for it.

labrum (lā'-brum): In anatomy, a lip, brim, or edge. ACETABULAR L. the ring of fibrocartilage attached to the rim of the acetabulum, increas-ing its depth; GLENOID L. the ring of fibrocartilage attached to the glenoid cavity of the scapula, increasing its depth. — labra, pl.

labyrinth (lab'-i-rinth): An intricate communicating passageway, particularly the tortuous cavities of the internal ear. BONY L. that part which is directly hollowed out of the temporal bone; MEMBRANOUS L. the membrane which loosely lines the bony labyrinth. — labyrinthine, adj.

labyrinthectomy (lab-i-rin-thek'-to-mi): Surgical removal of part or the whole of the labyrinth of the internal ear.

labyrinthitis (lab-i-rin-thī'-tis): Inflammation of the labyrinth of the ear. Syn., otitis interna (q.v.).

labyrinthotomy (lab-i-rinth-ot'-o-mi): A surgical incision into the labyrinth of the ear.

lac (lak): Any liquid with a whitish, milky appearance.

lacerated (las'-er-āt-ed): Torn. — lacerate, v.

laceration (las-er-ā'-shun): A wound made by tearing with a blunt object; the edges are torn and ragged. — lacerate, v.

lacrimal (lak'-ri-mal): Relating to tears. L. APPARATUS consists of the structures that secrete tears and drain them from the surface of the eyeball; lacrimal glands, ducts, sac, and nasolacrimal ducts; L. BONE a tiny bone at the inner side of the orbital cavity; L. DUCT connects L. gland to upper conjunctival sac; L. GLAND situated above the upper outer canthus of the eye; secretes tears; L. SAC situated in a groove in the L. bone at the upper end of the nasolacrimal duct; NASOLACRIMAL DUCT extends from the L. sac to the inferior meatus of the nose.

lacrimation (lak-ri-mā'-shun): An outflow of tears; weeping.

lacrimator (lak'-ri-mā-tor): A substance that increases the flow of tears.

lacrimonasal (lak-ri-mō-nā'-zal): Relating to the lacrimal and nasal bones and ducts.

lacrimotomy (lak-rim-ot'-o-mi): Incision of a lacrimal gland, duct, or sac.

lact-, lacti-, lacto-: Combining forms denoting relationship to (1) milk; (2) lactose.

lactacidaemia (lak-tas-i-dē'-mi-a): The presence of lactic acid in the blood.

lactalbumin (lac'-tal-bū'-min): An albumin found in milk; resembles serum albumin. It is the more easily digested of the two milk proteins. See CASEINOGEN.

lactase (lak'-tās): A sugar-splitting enzyme of intestinal juice, it splits lactose into glucose (dextrose) and galactose.

lactated Ringer's solution: Ringer's solution to which sodium lactate has been added; it is administered intravenously to replenish fluids and electrolytes and to create a condition of alkalinity in the body. See RINGER'S SOLUTION.

lactation (lak-tā'-shun): Secretion of milk by the breasts. Suckling; the period during which the child is nourished from the breast; MIME-LACTIC L., L. in which the infant is allowed to be at breast only at specified times and for a limited time; weaning begins at about three months; PRIMOLACTIC L., L. in which the infant is allowed frequent and unlimited opportunity to nurse; weaning beginning at about six months.

lacteal (lak'-tē-al): 1. Resembling or relating to milk. 2. Any one of the lymphatic ducts in the intestinal villi that take up split fats and convey them to the cisterna chyli (q.v.).

lactescent (lak-tes'-ent): 1. Milky in appearance. 2. Secreting milk or a fluid resembling milk.

lactic (lak'-tik): Relating to milk. L. ACID an acid formed by the action of certain bacteria on lactose and responsible for the souring of milk; in the body, this acid is found in muscles during exercise; L. ACIDOSIS a condition in which lactic acid accumulates in the tissues; occurs in association with circulatory failure, hypotension, and hypoxia.

lactic acid dehydrogenase (lak'-tik as'-id dē-hī-droj'-e-nas): An enzyme widely distributed in the tissues of mammals; it catalyses the dehydrogenation of lactic acid to pyruvic acid; measuring the level present in the blood is useful in diagnosing myocardial infarction. Also called *lactate dehydrogenase*.

lactiferous (lak-tif'-er-us): Conveying or secreting milk. L. DUCTS ducts that carry the secretion of the mammary gland; they open on the nipple.

lactifuge (lak'-ti-fūj): Any agent that suppresses milk secretion. — lactifugal, adj.

Lactobacillus (lak-tō-ba-sil'-us): A genus of bacteria of the family Lactobacillaceae occurring as Gram-positive rods that are active in fermenting carbohydrates, with the production of acid; found in dairy products, beer, wine, grain and meat products, fruits and fruit juices; seldom pathogenic. L. ACIDOPHILUS fer-ments the sugars in milk, producing lactic acid; found in milk and in the faeces of bottle-fed infants; L. BULGARICUS the species that ferments milk to produce yoghurt.

lactoferrin (lak-to-fer'-in): An iron-binding protein found in human milk, tears, saliva, and the secretions of the respiratory and intestinal tracts; prevents bacteria from metabolizing iron and assists antibodies to resist certain infectious diseases.

lactoflavin (lak'-tō-flā-vin): Riboflavin (q.v.).

lactogen (lak'-tō-jen): Any substance that promotes lactation. HUMAN PLACENTAL L. a hormone secreted by the placenta until delivery of the fetus; promotes lactation and growth; also called placental growth hormone. — lactogenic, adj.

lactogenesis (lak-tō-jen'-e-sis): The establishment of the secretory state in the mammary glands.

lactogenic (lak-tō-jen'-ik): Stimulating milk production; milk producing.

lactogenic hormone (lak-tō-jen'-ik hor'mōn): Prolactin (q.v.).

lactose (lak'-tōs): Milk sugar; a dissaccharide that is less soluble and less sweet than ordinary sugar. Used in infant feeding to increase the carbohydrate content of diluted cow's milk.

lactosuria (lak'-tō-sū'-ri-a): The presence of lactose in the urine. — lactosuric, adj.

lactotherapy (lak'-tō-ther'-a-pi): Treatment by milk diet.

lactotrophin (lak-tō-trō'-pin): Prolactin (q.v.).

lacuna (la-kū'-na): A small depression or hollow, or a space between cells; sinus. — lacunae, pl.; lacunar, adj.

lacunar (la-kū'-nar): Pertaining to a lacuna. L. STROKES small strokes resulting from damage to vessels scattered throughout the brain.

Ladin's sign: An area of elasticity that develops just above the cervix on the anterior wall of the uterus; can be felt on palpatation through the vagina as early as the fifth week of pregnancy; increases in size as the pregnancy progresses.

Laennec's cirrhosis: See under CIRRHOSIS.

lagophthalmos (lag'-of-thal'-mos): A condition marked by inability to close the eye completely. Also called *lagophthalmia*.

laissez faire (les-sā-fair', lā-sā-fair'): 1. The principle that government should allow matters to run their course without interference, especially in industrial affairs and in trade. 2. A hands-off management style in which the leader can abdicate responsibility, delay decisions, and provide little feedback.

lalling (lal'-ing): 1. A form of stammering in which babbling makes speech almost unintelligible; infantile speech. 2. Pronouncing *r* like *l*.

Lamaze method: A method of education for natural childbirth through a series of classes in which the pregnant woman and her partner are trained in controlled breathing and neuromuscular exercise; partner remains throughout labour.

lambda (lam'-da): The point in the skull where the sagittal and lambdoidal sutures meet.

lambdoidal suture (lam-doyd'-al): The line of union between the occipital and parietal bones.

lambliasis (lam-blī'-a-sis): Infestation with the parasite *Giardia lamblia* (*q.v.*). Can be symptomless, or can produce persistent dysentery and occasionally steatorrhoea.

lamella (la-mel'-a): 1. A thin plate-like scale or partition. 2. A gelatin-coated disc containing a drug; it is inserted under the eyelid. 3. Any of the tiny circular plates of bone between the Haversian systems in compact bone. — lamellae, pl.; lamellar, adj.

lamina (lam'-in-a): A thin plate or layer, usually of bone. — laminae, pl.

lamina cribrosa sclerae (lam'-in-a krib-rō'sa sklē'rē): The perforated portion of the sclera through which the axons of the ganglion cells of the retina pass.

laminectomy (lam-i-nek'-to-mi): Removal of laminae of one or more vertebrae — to expose the spinal cord and meninges. Most often performed in lumbar region, for removal of degenerated intervertebral disc.

laminogram (lam'-i-nō-gram): An x-ray photograph of a selected layer of the body obtained by sectional radiography.

laminography (lam-i-nog'-ra-fi): Body section roentgenography. A special x-ray technique used to show in detail the structures at a certain plane of the body while dimming or obliterating the details of structures in other planes.

lance (lans): 1. A short, two-edged knife; also called *lancet*. 2. To incise with a knife, as a boil or abscess.

Lancefield's groups or classification: A serological classification of haemolytic streptococci into groups A to O, according to their antigenic actions. Most streptococci that are of major importance to human health are in Group A; strains from Group F and nonpathogenic strains from G and H may also be found in the human throat; those from the other groups are found in certain foods and lower animals or animal products. [Rebecca Craighill Lancefield, American bacteriologist, 1875–1981.]

lancet (lan'-set): A small, sharp two-edged surgical knife.

lancinating (lan'-si-nā'-ting): Sharp, cutting, tearing; term used to describe a certain type of pain.

Landau reaction or response: When a normal infant is held suspended in the air, with the examiner's hands supporting him around the chest, the infant raises his head and extends his legs; then, when the head is flexed, the leg muscles lose their tone; the 'floppy' infant will not give his response while the hypertonic infant will give an exaggerated response.

Landry's disease: A form of paralysis that starts in the legs, ascends gradually to the arms, chest, and trunk, and then progresses to the circulatory and respiratory centres. See GUILLAIN–BARRÉ SYNDROME.

Langerhans' islets: See ISLET. [Paul Langerhans, German pathologist, 1847–1888.]

languor (lan'-ger): Listlessness, lack of vigour.

lanolin (lan'-ō-lin): Wool fat containing 30% of water. ANHYDROUS L. the fat obtained from sheep's wool. It is used in ointment bases, as such bases can form water-in-oil emulsions with aqueous constituents, and are readily absorbed by the skin.

lanugo (lan-ū-gō): The fine down or hair on the fetus from about the fifth month until birth. Also sometimes used to describe fine, downy hair on a child or adult.

laparo-: Combining form denoting relationship to the (1) loin or flank; (2) the abdominal wall, particularly an incision into it.

laparohysterectomy (lap'-a-rō-his-ter-ek'-to-mi): Removal of the uterus through an incision in the abdominal wall.

laparoscope (lap'a-ro-skōp): A lighted instrument used for viewing the interior of the abdomen and for performing certain surgical procedures.

laparoscopy (lap-a-ros'-ko-pi): The insertion of a laparoscope through a small abdominal incision for diagnostic purposes, lysis of adhesions, or tubal division. In tubal division, the laparoscope is inserted through a small incision near the navel, and the uterine tubes are located, cauterized, and separated; the operation takes little time and the patient is not incapacited for long.

laparotomy (lap-a-rot'-o-mi): Surgical opening into the flank; term commonly used to describe any opening into the abdominal wall.

LaPlace's law: States that the pressure produced in the ventricles of the heart depends on the size and shape of the heart as well as the tension produced by the ventricular myocardium when it contracts.

large-for-dates: Refers to a baby whose birth weight is above the 90th percentile. Large-for-gestational-age.

larva (lar'-va): An embryo that is independent before it has assumed the characteristic features of its parents. — larvae, pl.; larval, adj.

larvicide (lar'-vi-sīd): Any agent that destroys larvae. — larvicidal, adj.

larvivorous (lar-viv'-ō-rus): Usually refers to fishes that are the natural enemy of mosquitoes; used in malarial control programmes.

laryngeal (la-rin'-jē-al): Relating to the larynx. L. STRIDOR a noisy crowing sound made on inspiration; in the infant may be congenital, due to immaturity of the larynx; see STRIDOR.

laryngectomy (lar-in-jek'-to-mi): Excision of the larynx.

laryngismus stridulus (lar-in-jiz'-mus strī'dū-lus): Momentary attack of laryngeal spasm, inspiration producing a crowing sound and followed by a period of apnoea caused by the spasmodic closure of the glottis. Associated with low blood calcium in infantile rickets.

laryngitis (lar-in-jī'tis): Inflammation of the mucous membrane lining of the larynx; may be acute or chronic; may be associated with a cold or be caused by heavy smoking, exposure to irritating fumes, overuse of the voice. Usual symptoms are dryness and soreness of the throat, difficulty in swallowing, pain. ACUTE SPASMODIC L. croup; a mild inflammation of the larynx with spasm of the laryngeal muscles, causing partial obstruction; seen most often in young children; attacks often occur at night; symptoms dramatic with dyspnoea, coughing, high-pitched rasp with inspiration, cyanosis of lips and nails, rapid pulse, elevation of temperature.

laryngo-: Combining form denoting relationship to the larynx.

laryngocele (la-ring'gō-sēl): A congenital condition in which an air sac communicates with the laryngeal cavity; may appear as a tumour on the outside of the neck.

laryngofissure (la-ring'gō-fish'ūr): The operation of opening the larynx at midline.

laryngologist (lar'-ing-gol'o-jist): A specialist in laryngeal diseases and disorders.

laryngology (lar'-ing-gol'o-ji): The branch of medical practice that deals with diseases of the larynx.

laryngoparalysis (la-ring'gō-pa-ral'i-sis): Paralysis of the muscles of the larynx.

laryngopharyngectomy (la-ring'gō-far-in-jek'to-mi): Excision of the larynx and the lower part of the pharynx.

laryngopharyngitis (la-ring' gō-far-in-jī'tis): Inflammation of the larynx and the pharynx.

laryngopharynx (la-ring'gō-far'inks): The lower portion of the pharynx. — laryngopharyngeal, adj.

laryngoscope (la-ring'gō-skōp): A lighted instrument for exposing and visualizing the larynx. — laryngoscopy, n.; laryngoscopic, adj.

laryngoscopy (lar-ing-gos'ko-pi): Examination of the interior of the larynx with a laryngoscope.

laryngospasm (la-ring'gō-spazm): Convulsive involuntary muscle contraction of the larynx, usually accompanied by spasmodic closure of the glottis.

laryngostenosis (la-ring'gō-ste-nō' sis). Narrowing of the glottic aperture, or of the lumen of the larynx.

laryngostomy (lar'ing-gos'to-mi): The surgical creation of an artificial opening from the neck into the larynx.

laryngotomy (lar'ing-got'-o-mi): The operation of opening the larynx.

laryngotracheal (la-ring'gō-tra'kē-al): Relating to the larynx and the trachea.

laryngotracheitis (la-ring'gō-tra-kē-ī'tis): Inflammation of the mucous membrane lining of the larynx and the trachea.

laryngotracheobronchitis (la-ring'gō-tra'kē-ō-bron-kī'tis): Inflammation of the larynx, trachea, and bronchi. Usually refers to an acute respiratory condition in young children; attended by fever, toxaemia, laryngeal obstruction, hoarseness, dyspnoea, inspiratory stridor, barking cough. Syn., viral croup. See CROUP.

larynx (lar'inks): The organ of voice situated below and in front of the pharynx and at the upper end of the trachea. It is composed of muscular and cartilaginous tissue and is lined with mucous membrane. The vocal cords pass from front to back across the lumen of the structure. It also serves as a passageway for air entering the trachea. — laryngeal, adj.

lascivia (la-siv'i-a): Abnormal degree of sexual desire.

Lasègue's sign: Pain in the hip when the knee is extended but no pain on flexion; it differentiates sciatica from hip disease.

laser (lā'zer): An electron device containing a gaseous, solid, or liquid substance in which atoms that are stimulated by focused light rays magnify and concentrate these waves which may then be emitted as a very narrow, concentrated, powerful beam of light. L. BEAM the precisely aimed, high-intensity beam of light emitted by a laser and which transmits energy as heat; it permits visual examination of body cavities and allows for greater precision in surgery; has been used in treatment of iridectomy, detached retina, and cataract surgery as well as in a variety of surgical procedures to destroy tissue, to fix tissue in place, or to divide or create adhesions.

laserbrasion (lā-zer-brā-zhun): The bloodless removal of layers of sun-damaged skin utilizing a carbon dioxide laser; done under local anaesthesia.

Lassa fever: Named for the Nigerian town in which several fatal cases of an unknown disease occurred among American missionary nurses in 1969. Caused by the exceptionally virulent arenavirus, of which the rat is a carrier; isolated and identified during the same year. A viral haemorrhagic fever, incubation period 3–16 days. Symptoms vary widely and include very high fever, skin rash and tiny haemorrhages, mouth ulcers, pharyngitis, dysphagia, oedema, pneumonia, pleural effusion, kidney damage, infection of the heart leading to heart failure. Not limited to the tropics or Africa.

Lassar's paste: A paste used in treating several skin conditions; composed of starch, salicylic acid, and zinc oxide in a white petroleum base.

lassitude (las'i-tūd): Exhaustion; lack of energy.

latency (lā'ten-si): The period between the application of a stimulus and the reaction or response to the stimulus.

latent (lā'tent): Concealed, hidden, not active. L. STAGE the period in development of the libido, from about the sixth to the thirteenth year, when the endocrine activity slows down and the child's need for sexual gratification is slight but the need for belonging and social acceptance by peers is increased.

lateral (lat'er-al): 1. Relating to a side. 2. Denoting a position away from the midline or the median plane, either to the right or left.

lateral geniculate body: A small flattened area of nerve cells in the thalamus that receive impulses from the optic tract and relay them to the occipital area of the cortex.

lateralization (lat'er-al-ī-zā'shun): Localization on one side of the body or one part of the body, as in one cerebral hemisphere.

lateroversion (lat'er-ō-ver'zhun): A turning to one side or the other; said especially of the uterus.

latex agglutination test: A widely used test to detect the presence of rheumatoid factor in verifying the diagnosis of rheumatoid arthritis; also used to test for presence of antibodies to Hashimoto's disease (q.v.) Also called *latex fixation test*.

latissimus dorsi (la-tis'si-mus dor'si): A large, broad, flat muscle of the back; it arises from the spinous processes of the six lower thoracic vertebrae, the lumbar vertebrae, sacrum, and the posterior iliac crest (all via the lumbosacral fascia), and is inserted into a groove on the under side of the humerus. Its action is to adduct and medially rotate the arm.

laughing gas: Nitrous oxide (q.v.).

Laurence–Moon–Beidl syndrome: A recessive hereditary disorder characterized by obesity, mental handicap, visual disturbances, genital atrophy, and polydactyly.

lavage (la-vazh'): The irrigation of or washing out of an organ such as the stomach or colon, or the instillation and withdrawal of a rinsing fluid from a body cavity such as the peritoneal or pelural cavity. In BRONCHIAL L. small amounts of warm water or saline solution are injected into the airway to clear tenacious bronchial material. ENDOMETRIAL L. see under ENDOMETRIAL; GASTRIC L., L. of the stomach; LUNG L. the instillation and draining out of isotonic saline solution via a catheter inserted into the bronchi, to assist in removing collected mucus; used primarily in cystic fibrosis patients; PERITONEAL L. the rinsing out of the peritoneal cavity by instilling and then with drawing a dialysing solution.

laxative (laks'a-tiv): A mild cathartic (q.v.); an aperient.

lay: Not professionally qualified, especially in law and medicine, and with respect to clergy. Most frequently used when referring to user/consumer involvement.

layer: A sheet of substance lying upon another sheet of substance, but not connected or continuous with it, and differentiated by cellular structure, function, or some other characteristic, e.g., one of the three primary layers of the early embryo — the ectoderm, endoderm, or mesoderm.

LDH: Abbreviation for lactic acid dehydrogenase (q.v.).

L-Dopa: Levodopa. A drug used to control the symptoms of Parkinson's disease.

LDP: Abbreviation for Local Delivery Plan (q.v.).

lead (lēd): **1.** A wire carrying electricity to or from a device. **2.** A pair of electrodes that are placed in or on the body and are connected to an instrument that measures and records the difference in electrical potential between them. **3.** One of the electrical connections for the records made in electrocardiography; the pattern of the lead varies with the body site to which the electrode is attached.

lead (led): A metal, the salts of which are astringent when applied externally. L. POISONING rarely occurs in the acute form, but, in children, may be the cause of acute encephalopathy; the chronic form, due to absorption of small amounts of lead over a period, is fairly common, causing damage to brain function, headache and abnormal behaviour: it can happen to children who suck on articles made of lead alloys or painted with lead paint. It may also be an occupational danger to painters, the usual symptoms being anaemia that is due to interference with production of haem and to short life of red blood cells, leading to loss of appetite; abdominal cramps; metallic taste; and the formation of a blue line around the gums. Sometimes called *painter's colic.*

leadership: 1. The dignity, office, or position of a leader. **2.** Ability to lead. **3.** The position of a group of people leading or influencing others within a given context. **4.** The action or influence necessary for the direction or organization of effort in a group undertaking.

leadpipe rigidity: An increase in the tone of the skeletal muscles, making the limb appear stiff; due to pathology in the extrapyramidal tract. Also called *plastic rigidity.*

league tables: A list ranking competitors according to their performance. In the UK this refers to hospitals and institutes of education.

learning difficulty: See LEARNING DISABILITY.

learning disability: A generic term referring to the inability to easily attain a rounded intellectual development, encompassing a wide range of learning and social difficulties. Depending on the specific problem, difficulties may be encountered in one or more of the following areas: understanding, remembering or producing language (e.g. speaking, writing, reading, listening, spelling); reasoning; motor coordination; mathematics; noticing and remembering social information; emotional maturation; processing information; organization of things, time, and/or space.

Learning Disability Taskforce: A group in charge of improving services for the learning impaired, established in the UK, March 2001.

Leber's disease: 1. A hereditary form of optic atrophy, transmitted through the female; occurs chiefly in young men; progresses rapidly to blindness of central vision, with preservation of peripheral vision. **2.** Leber's congenital amaurosis, a rare type of blindness occurring in early infancy characterized by diffuse pigmentation and optic atrophy.

Leboyer method: An approach to childbirth advocated by a French doctor, Leboyer, that emphasizes avoidance of trauma, pain, and fear in the transition from uterine to extrauterine life; includes dimming of lights, silence insofar as possible; patience, warmth, and loving tender handling of the infant. It is claimed that the baby will cry less and become a more contented child and adult because the shock of delivery is minimized.

LE cells: Characteristic cells found in the bone marrow of patients with lupus erythematosus, together with a special globulin in the plasma.

lecithin (les'-i-thin). A nitrogenous, fatty substance in cell protoplasm; widely distributed throughout the body, being found in nerve tissue, semen, bile, and blood. Also found in egg yolk, soy beans, and other seeds.

leech (lēch): *Hirudo medicinalis.* A bloodsucking aquatic worm formerly much used for sucking blood from local areas. Its saliva contains hirudin, an anticoagulant.

left handedness: The use of the left hand in preference to the right in performing various tasks. Also called *sinistrality.*

Left ventricular failure: A disorder where the left side of the heart fails to pump blood effectively, resulting in a backflow of pressure leading to congestion in the lungs. Symptoms include shortness of breath with activity and while lying flat, cough, palpitations and fatigue.

legal: 1. Relating to law. **2.** Falling within the province of law.

Legg–Calve–Perthes disease: Osteochondritis (*q.v.*) of the head of the femur occurring in children. Also called *Legg's disease, Perthe's disease, Waldenström's disease,* and *coxa plana.*

Legionella pneumophila (lē-je-nel'-la-nū-mof'-i-la): A bacterium thought to be one cause of atypical pneumonia; see LEGIONNAIRES' DISEASE.

legionnaires' disease: Term coined to describe a disease affecting many who attended an American Legion meeting in Philadelphia in 1976; many cases were fatal. Sporadic outbreaks have occurred elsewhere since that time with the causative organism being cited as a pneumonia-like bacteria called *Legionella pneumophila*; which can propagate in warm, moist places such as air conditioning towers and ducts. Symptoms include acute onset, chills, fever, tachypnoea, cough, pleuritic pain, bradycardia, abdominal pain, diarrhoea. Also called *legionellosis*.

legume (leg-ūm): A plant belonging to the family Leguminosae, and the food produced by these plants, e.g., peas, beans, lentils, peanuts.

legumin (le-gū′-min): A storage protein resembling casein, found in plant foods.

leiodermia (lī-ō-der′-mi-a): A skin disorder characterized by abnormal glossiness and atrophy.

leomyoma (lī′-ō-mī-ō′ma): A benign tumour originating in smooth muscle tissue. L. UTERI a benign tumour of the uterus; see FIBROID.

leiomyosarcoma (lī′ō-mī-ō-sar-kō′ma): A malignant tumour derived from smooth muscle tissue.

Leishmania (lēsh-mā′-ni-a): A flagellated protozoan that is responsible for several recognized types of leishmaniasis (*q.v.*).

leishmaniasis (lēsh′ma-nī′a-sis): Any of several communicable protozoan diseases caused by *Leishmania* (*q.v.*); spread by sand flies. Generalized (or visceral) manifestation is kala-azar. CUTANEOUS L., L. caused by *Leishmania tropica*; also called *Aleppo boil. Delhi boil*, or *oriental sore*, characterized by nodules and ulcerating lesions on the skin. The nasopharyngeal manifestation causes ulceration of the nose and throat; espundia. The disease occurs in the Mediterranean and Near East areas, China, and some parts of Africa, and is occasionally brought to the UK by persons who have visited these areas.

Lenegre's disease: Atrioventricular dissociation caused by degeneration of the conduction system of the heart; due to small lesions in both the right and left bundle branch.

lenitive (len′-i-tiv): 1. Relieving discomfort or pain; soothing. 2. An agent that relieves discomfort or pain; a demulcent (*q.v.*).

lens (lenz): 1. The small, transparent, biconvex crystalline body that is supported in the suspensory ligament immediately behind the iris of the eye. On account of its elasticity, the lens can alter in shape, enabling light rays to focus exactly on the retina. 2. A piece of transparent material, usually glass, with a regular curvature of one or both surfaces, used for conveying or diffusing light rays, as in a camera, microscope or eyeglasses. CONTACT

L. a thin, usually plastic, curved lens that fits over the cornea and is used instead of an eyeglass; L. IMPLANT a thin artificial lens to correct any visual abnormality such as myopia, following a cataract operation.

lentectomy (len-tek′-to-mi): Surgical removal of the lens of the eye.

lenticonus (len-ti-kō′-nus): A conical prominence on the anterior or posterior surface of the lens; may be congenital.

lenticular (len-tik′-ū-lar): 1. Relating to or shaped like a lens. 2. Shaped like a lentil. L. NUCLEUS a mass of grey matter on the outer surface of the caudate nucleus, with which it unites to form the corpus striatum.

lentiform (len′-ti-form): Shaped like a lens. L. NUCLEUS the globus pallidus and the putamen considered together.

lentigines (len-tij′-i-nēz): Plural of lentigo (*q.v.*). L. LEPROSAE the pigmented lesions that occur in leprosy.

lentigo (len-tī′-gō): A smooth, brownish pigmented spot on the skin, usually seen on normally exposed areas and in people of middle age or older; caused by changes in the skin rather than sunlight; a freckle. L. MALIGNA, appears as a tan spot that becomes dark and nodular and often malignant; usually occurs on the face after age 60; also called *Hutchinson's freckle*; L. SENILIS flat dark-coloured spots that appear on exposed areas after middle age; usually benign; syn., *liver spots*.

leontiasis (lē′on-tī′a-sis): Enlargement of face and head giving a lion-like appearance, in such diseases as elephantiasis and leprosy.

Leopold's manoeuvres: A series of four manoeuvres performed with the hands, for palpating the abdomen to determine the position and presentation of the fetus *in utero*.

leper (lep′-er): A person who has leprosy.

lepidosis (lep-i-dō′-sis): Any skin eruption accompanied by scaling or desquamation, *e.g.*, pityriasis (*q.v.*).

leproma (lep-rō′-ma): A granulomatous nodule in the skin; seen in some patients with leprosy. — lepromata, pl.; lepromatous, adj.

leprosy (lep′-rō-si): A chronic, progressive, communicable disease; endemic in warmer climates; infrequently seen in the UK. Caused by *Mycobacterium leprae* (Hansen's bacillus) and very resistant to treatment. One of the two types of disease affects the peripheral nerves, resulting in anaesthesia in areas of the skin; the other type affects the skin, causing the formation of nodules in skin and mucous membrane that become granulomatous. Transmission of the disease results only from prolonged and intimate contact with an infected person; the incubation period is estimated at two to four years. Also called *Hansen's disease*. — leprous, adj.

lept-, lepto-: Combining forms denoting small, thin, weak, fine.

leptocephaly (lep-tō-kef´-a-li,-sef-): Abnormal height and narrowness of the skull.

leptocyte (lep´-tō-sīt): A red blood cell that is abnormally thin and flattened, has a central area of pigmented material surrounded by an area of clear unpigmented material, and is enclosed by an outer pigmented rim; sometimes referred to as a '*target*' or '*Mexican hat*' cell.

leptocytosis (lep'tō-sī-tō'sis): The presence of thin, flattened red cells circulating in the blood (leptocytes). Characteristic of thalassaemia (*q.v.*). Also seen in jaundice, hepatic disease, and sometimes after splenectomy.

leptodermic (lep´-tō-der´-mik): Having a thin skin.

leptomeninges (lep-tō-me-nin´-jēz): The pia mater and the arachnoid membranes considered together. — leptomeningeal, adj.

leptomeningitis (lep'to-men-in-jī'tis): Inflammation of the two inner covering membranes of the brain and spinal cord. See LEPTOMENINGES.

Leptospira (lep-tō-spī´ra): A genus of bacteria. Very thin, coiled spirochetes. Common in water as saprophytes; many pathogenic species may infect both humans and animals, producing leptospirosis. *L. icterohaemorrhagiae* causes Weil's disease in humans. *L. canicola* causes 'yellows' in dogs and pigs; transmissible to humans. See CANICOLA FEVER.

leptospirosis (lep-tō-spī-rō'sis): Infection by *Leptospira* organisms; transmitted to humans by water in swamps or ponds, infected rats, dogs, and swine; usual symptoms include hepatitis, nephritis, lymphocytic meningitis; may occur in epidemics. See LEPTOSPIRA, WEIL'S DISEASE.

Leriche's syndrome: A syndrome occurring mostly in males; marked by fatigue and coldness of hips and lower extremities following exercise, by lack of femoral pulsation, and sometimes impotence; caused by an obstruction, usually atheromatous, at the bifurcation of the aorta.

Lermoyez's syndrome (ler-moy´-āz): Unexplained attacks of loss of hearing followed by dizziness after which hearing returns to normal or near normal.

lesbian (lez´-bi-an): **1.** A homosexual (*q.v.*) woman. **2.** Relating to homosexual relations between women.

lesbianism (lez´-bi-an-izm): Homosexuality between women.

Lesch–Nyhan syndrome: A rare inherited disorder of purine metabolism marked by severe mental and physical retardation, choreoathetosis, self-mutilation particularly of the fingers and lips by biting; also neurological problems similar to cerebral palsy, failure to thrive, and defective kidney function.

lesion (lē'zhun): Any pathological change in the continuity or structure of a bodily tissue; may be caused by trauma or disease. SPACE-OCCUPYING L. a L. within a confined space, as the skull, that compresses the contents, interferes with blood supply, and may lead to loss of function; most often refers to tumours of the brain substance.

lethal (lē'thal): Deadly, fatal. L. DOSAGE the amount of a drug or other agent that will cause death. — lethality, adj.

lethargy (leth´-ar-jē): Abnormal drowsiness; torpor; apathy. Characteristic of certain diseases, *e.g.*, encephalitis. — lethargic, adj.

lethe (lē´-the): Loss of memory; amnesia.

lethologica (lēth-ō-loj'i-ka): Temporary inability to recall a proper name or noun.

Letterer–Siwe disease: A fatal disease of infancy and early childhood involving the reticuloendothelial system; cause unknown. Characterized by erythematous skin eruptions; a tendency to haemorrhage and purpura; enlarged spleen, liver, and lymph nodes; progressive anaemia; osseous defects, especially of the skull; bone marrow involvement; anorexia and weight loss. Also called *systemic aleukaemic reticuloendotheliosis*.

leuc-, leuco-: See leuk-, leuko-.

leucine (lū´-sēn): One of the essential amino acids that is obtained from protein; it is required for optimal growth and development in infants and for maintaining the nitrogen balance in adults. L. SENSITIVITY seen more often in infants than adults; characterized by the occurrence of hypoglycaemia following high protein intake; also occurs on fasting.

leuk-, leuko-: Combining forms denoting (1) white; (2) a type of blood cell; (3) white matter of the brain.

leukaemia (lū-kē´-mi-a): A disease of the blood-forming cells; many forms are recognized, both chronic and acute. The chief symptom is an increase in the number of white blood cells, along with the presence of immature leukocytes. Symptoms include poor appetite, lesions in the mouth, enlarged spleen and lymphatics, and bone marrow changes. Classified according to the kind of leukocyte found and whether the condition is acute or chronic. ACUTE L. characterized by rapid onset, anaemia, susceptibility to infection and haemorrhage; blast forms of cells predominate in the bone marrow; ALEUKAEMIC L. refers to a leukaemic condition in which the white cell count in the blood remains normal or is below normal; CHRONIC LYMPHOCYTIC L. characterized by proliferation and enlargement of the lymphocytes in any lymphoid tissue such as the spleen, lymph nodes, bone marrow; MONOCYTIC L., L. in which the predominating cells are monocytes; in the Naegeli type, many of the cells closely resembling myelocytes; in the Schilling type they resemble monocytes; MYELOGENOUS L., L. involving the bone marrow, especially that of the ribs, sternum, and vertebrae.

leukaemoid (lū-kē′-moyd): Resembling leukaemia but due to some other cause; usually refers to a condition that is marked by the presence in the blood of immature cells but that is not leukaemia.

leukoagglutinin (lū′kō-a-gloo′ti-nin): An antibody that acts against leukocytes; see AGGLUTININS.

leukocidin (lū-kō-sī′-din): A substance produced by certain bacteria that is toxic to polymorphonuclear leukocytes.

leukocyte (lū′-kō-sīt): A white corpuscle of the blood; a spherical, colourless, nucleated mass that has amoeboid movement; produced in lymph nodes and in the lymphatic tissue of the spleen, liver, and other organs; chief function is to produce antibodies and act as scavengers in protecting the body from invading organisms. May be classified into two categories, (1) granulocytes, including neutrophils, basophils, eosinophils; and (2) agranulocytes, including monocytes and lymphocytes. See BASOPHIL, EOSINOPHIL, LYMPHOCYTE, MONONUCLEAR, POLYMORPHONUCLEAR. — leukocytic, adj.

leukocythaemia (lū′-ko-sī-thē′-mi-a): An increase in the number of white blood cells; leukaemia.

leukocytolysis (lū-ko-sī-tol′-i-sis): Destruction and disintegration of white blood cells. — leukocytolytic, adj.

leukocytometer (lū-ko-sī-tom′-i-ter): An instrument for counting white blood cells.

leukocytosis (lū-ko-sī-tō′-sis): Increased number of leukocytes in the blood. Often a physiological response to infection. — leukocytotic, adj.

leukocyturia (lū-ko-sī-tū′-ri-a): Presence of leukocytes in the urine.

leukoderma (lū-kō-der′ma): Defective skin pigmentation, especially when it occurs in patches or bands.

leukoedema (lū′kō-ē-dē′ma): A condition of the buccal mucosa, characterized by thickness and oedema; resembles early leukoplakia (q.v.).

leukoencephalitis (lū′-kō-en-kef-a-lī′tis,-sef-): Inflammation of the white matter of the brain. SUBACUTE SCLEROSING L. subacute sclerosing panencephalitis; see under PANENCEPHALITIS.

leukoencephalopathy (lū′-kō-en-kef′-a-lop′-a-thi,-sef-): Any inflammatory or degenerative pathological condition involving chiefly the white matter, occurs most often in patients with leukaemia, lymphoma, granulomatosis; usually fatal. PROGRESSIVE MULTIFOCAL L. usually occurs secondary to certain neoplastic diseases; probably caused by a virus; characterized by demyelination in the white matter but is also seen in the brain stem and cerebellum; usually fatal.

leukoerythroblastosis (lū′kō-ē-rith′rō-blastō′sis): A condition characterized by the presence of immature leukocytes and erythrocytes in the peripheral blood.

leukokoria (lū-kō-kor′-i-a): A condition in which a whitish mass appears in the area behind the lens. Also spelled *leucocoria*.

leukoma (lū-kō′-ma): White opaque spot on the cornea. — leukomata, pl.; leukomatous, adj.

leukonychia (lū-kō-nik′-i-a): White spots on the nails.

leukopenia (lū-kō-pē′ni-a): A white blood cell count that is below normal; less than 5000 per cu mm. — leukopenic, adj.

leukopheresis (lū-kō-fer-ē′-sis): A procedure by which leukocytes, particularly granulocytes, are collected from the blood of a healthy donor for transfusion to patients with severe granulocytopenia, which is sometimes due to leukaemia, cancer, chemotherapy, or toxic drugs.

leukoplakia (lū-kō-plā′ki-a): A disease characterized by the occurrence of white, thickened patches on mucous membrane, usually on the lips and inside of the mouth; may also occur on genitalia. Often seen in smokers, but also due to bad fitting dentures, vitamin A deficiency, or uncleanliness. Sometimes becomes malignant.

leukopoieses (lū-kō-poy-ē′sis): The formation of white blood cells. — leukopoietic, adj.

leukorrhoea (lū-kō-rē′-a): A sticky, whitish vaginal discharge containing mucus and pus cells. — leukorrhoeal, adj.

leukosarcoma (lū′kō-sar-kō′ma): A blood condition that may develop in patients originally diagnosed as having lymphocytic malignant lymphoma; characterized by the presence in the bloodstream of lymphocytes that are morphologically different from those found in chronic lymphocytic leukaemia.

leukotoxic (lū-kō-tok′-sik): Relating to any substance that is toxic to leukocytes.

levator (le-vā′-tor): **1.** A muscle that acts by raising a part. **2.** An instrument for lifting a depressed part. — levatores, pl.

levatores ani (lev-a-tō′-rēz-ā′-ni): A pair of broad muscles extending from the back of the pubis to the sacrum and coccyx and to the lateral pelvic walls; forms the strongest part of the pelvic floor.

Levine scale: A scale used to describe the intensity of a heart murmur, from Grades I through IV, from faint to extremely loud.

levodopa (lev-ō-dō-pa): An antiparkinson drug. L-Dopa.

levoversion (lē′-vō-ver′-zhun): Turning to the left. In ophthalmology, the simultaneous movement of the eyes to the left.

Lev's disease: A condition in which lesions develop in the fibrous tissues of the heart and its valves and interfere with the functioning of the conduction system; may lead to complete heart block.

levulose (lev′-ū-lōs): Fructose or fruit sugar. Sweeter and more easily digested than ordinary sugar; useful in treatment of diabetes.

Lewy bodies: Round bodies found in the cytoplasm of some of the neurons of the midbrain of patients with paralysis agitans.

-lexia: Combining form denoting (1) speech; (2) word; (3) a type of incapacity to read.

Leydig cell: One of the interstitial cells of the testis that produce the male sex hormone.

LFT: Abbreviation for liver function test (*q.v.*).

LH: Abbreviation for luteinizing hormone (*q.v.*).

Lhermitte's sign (ler′-mits): A condition seen in multiple sclerosis and certain diseases of the cervical cord; when the head is flexed a transient electric shock-like sensation spreads down the arms and legs; may persist for a few days or weeks and then disappears without treatment.

LHRH: Abbreviation for luteinizing hormone releasing hormone (*q.v.*).

liberalism (lib′-er-al-izm): The holding of liberal opinions in politics.

libidinous (li-bid′-i-nus): Relating to libido; erotic; lustful; lascivious.

libido (li-bē′-dō): The vital force or energy that results in purposeful actions. Freud's name for the urge to obtain sensual satisfaction which

he believed to be the mainspring of human behaviour. Sometimes more loosely associated with the meaning of sexual urge. Freud's meaning was satisfaction through all the senses. In Jungian psychology the term denotes psychic energy. — libidinal, adj.

lice (līs): See LOUSE.

lichen (lī′-ken): In medicine, aggregates of papular skin lesions. L. AMYLOIDOSIS a form of localized cutaneous amyloidosis; seen most often on the shins; L. NITIDUS characterized by minute, shiny, flat-topped, pink papules of pinhead size; most frequently seen on the abdomen, breasts, and on the genitalia of males; L. PLANUS aggregates of small, persistant, polygonal papules, flat-topped with a characteristic sheen, and of reddish-purple colour, occurring in well defined patches on the wrists, ankles, and abdomen; greyish patches on mucous membranes; and may involve hair follicles and nails; L. SCLEROSIS ET ATROPHICUS a chronic skin condition in which flat papules appear and later coalesce into large white areas, and the skin becomes thin, hyperpigmented, and telangiectasic; cause unknown; occurs most often in women as kraurosis vulvae; in men it is known as *balanitis xerotica obliterans*; L. SCROFULOSUS small flat-topped papules that may occur as an allergic phenomenon in tuberculosis; L. SIMPLEX or L. SIMPLEX CHRONICUS a psychosomatic condition characterized by the development of localized areas of irritating, leathery, shiny papules (lichenification); skin abrasions and dry scaling are kept going by itching, rubbing, scratching; Syn., *chronic neurodermatitis*; L. SPINULOSIS characterized by small spines protruding from the openings of the hair follicles; seen especially around the anogenital area, dorsa of the hands and feet, bend of the elbow or knee, and back of the neck; appears to be a result of vitamin A deficiency; L. TROPICUS characterized by redness and inflammation of the skin; also called *malaria rubra* and *prickly heat*; L. URTICATUS papular urticaria; see URTICARIA. — lichenoid, adj.

lichenification (lī′-ken-i-fi-kā′-shun): Thickening and hardening of the skin; is usually secondary to pruritus, and due to scratching and excoriation of the skin.

lid lag: A condition in which a rim of sclera may be seen between the upper lid and the sclera when the patient gazes downward; usually a sign of hyperthyroidism.

Lieberkühn's crypts, glands, or follicles (lē′-ber-künz): Simple tubular glands in the mucous membrane of the small intestine. [Johann Nathaniel Lieberkühn, German physician and anatomist, 1711–1756.]

lien (lī′-en): The spleen. — lienal, adj.

lien-, lieno-: Combining forms denoting the spleen. See also SPLEN-, SPLENO-.

lienculus (lī-en′-kū-lus): A small accessory spleen.

lienorenal (lī′-en-ō-rē′-nal): Relating to the spleen and kidney: splenorenal; splenonephric.

life event: A descriptive term used by sociologists for a major event in a person's life, such as going to school for the first time, starting work, leaving home, getting married, retirement, etc.

life expectancy: The number of years a person can expect to live, based on statistical averages.

lifelong learning: A process of personal, social and professional development throughout the life span of the individual.

lifting: 1. The action or act of raising to a higher position. 2. (nursing) Relating to techniques for moving a patient around.

ligament (lig′-a-ment): A strong band of fibrous connective tissue serving to bind bones or other parts together, to support a structure or organ, and to strengthen joints. — ligamentous, adj.

ligate (lī′-gāt): 1. To constrict a blood vessel or a duct or the pedicle of a tumour by tying a thread or like material very tightly around it. 2. To apply a ligature. — ligation, n.

ligation (lī-gā′-shun): The application of a ligature (q.v.). TUBAL L. sterilization of the female by applying a ligature to the uterine tubes to constrict them; the tubes may or may not be severed or crushed; when performed through the vagina, it is referred to as VAGINAL TUBAL L.

ligature (lig′-a-chūr): The material used for tying tightly around a blood vessel to constrict blood flow, or around part of a body structure or a tumour to constrict it, or for sewing tissues. Silk thread, horsehair, catgut, silver wire, synthetic fibres, cotton, linen, kangaroo tendon, sheep intestine, or strips of the patient's own fascia are used. See SUTURE.

light adaptation: The adaptation by the eye to vision in bright light with a reduction in the concentration of the photosensitive pigments.

lightening: Term used to denote the relief of pressure on the diaphragm by the abdominal viscera when the presenting part of the fetus descends into the pelvis in the last two or three weeks of pregnancy.

lightning (līt′-ning): Descriptive of paroxysmal, stabbing pains, as those that occur in the lower limbs in tabes dorsalis.

Likert scale (lik′-ert): A gauge of attitude that indicates an individual's degree of agreement or disagreement with a statement according to a three-or five-point scoring system, for example strongly agree, no opinion, or strongly disagree.

limb-girdle dystrophy: A form of muscular dystrophy most often seen in late childhood or early adulthood; first affects the shoulder girdle or the pelvic girdle, then spreads to other parts of the body.

limbic system: A term loosely applied to a group of structures in the rhinencephalon (q.v.) of the brain, including the hippocampus, amygdala, and hypothalamus, that have to do with various senses, emotions, and feelings, and certain automatic functions. Lesions in this system result in a wide range of abnormal behaviours.

limbus (lim′-bus): A border. In anatomy, a border or edge of certain structures, e.g. the edge where the cornea joins the sclera. — limbic, adj.

limen (lī′-men): In physiology, a threshold, as of a stimulus. — limina, pl.; liminal, adj.

liminal (lim′-i-nal): The lowest intensity of a stimulus that can be perceived by the human sense. See SUBLIMINAL.

linctus (link′-tus): A sweet, syrupy liquid, made of a powdered drug combined with honey or other syrup; has a soothing effect on the mucous membrane of the pharynx; should be taken undiluted and sipped slowly.

Lindau's disease: von Hippel–Lindau disease (q.v.).

linea (lin′-ē-a): A line. L. ALBA the white line between the two rectus muscles, visible after removal of skin from the centre of the abdomen, stretching from the ensiform cartilage to the pubis, its position being indicated by a slight depression on the surface. The transversalis and parts of the oblique muscles are inserted into it; L. ALBICANTES white lines that appear on the abdomen after reduction of tension caused by stretching such as occurs in tumours, pregnancy, oedema, etc.; L. ASPERA roughened line on posterior aspect of the femur; L. NIGRA a pigmented line from umbilicus to pubis that appears in pregnancy; L. TERMINALIS PELVIS a line on the inner surface of either iliac bone; runs from the sacroiliac joint to the eminence of the symphysis pubis; it marks the division between the false and true pelves. — lineae, pl.

lingua (ling´-gwa): The tongue. — lingual, adj.

lingual (ling´-gwal): Relating to the tongue. L. GOITRE, an enlargement at the back of the tongue.

lingula (ling´-gū-la): General term used to describe a small tongue-shaped structure extending from a body part or organ.

liniment (lin´-i-ment): A medicinal oily liquid to be applied to the skin by friction.

linked (linkt): In genetics, descriptive of characters that are as inherited together. In nucleated cells this usually indicates that genes for the characters are on the same chromosome.

linoleic acid (lin-ō-lē´-ik): An unsaturated, essential fatty acid. Found in the glycerides of linseed and vegetable oils.

liothyronine (lī´ō-thī´rō-nēn): One of two thyroid hormones, normally present in the thyroid gland and the blood; it is important in tissue metabolism. Also prepared synthetically and used in treatment of hypothyroidism.

lip-, lipo-: Combining forms denoting (1) fat; (2) fatty tissue.

lipaemia (li-pē´-mi-a): Increased lipid (especially cholesterol) in the circulating blood. — lipaemic, adj.

lipase (lī´-pās): Any fat-splitting enzyme. LIPOPROTEIN L. an enzyme that promotes the storage of fat in the fat cells of the body; this activity seems to be reduced in cigarette smokers but becomes more active when the individual stops smoking. PANCREATIC L. the enzyme of the pancreatic juice, which splits fats into fatty acids and glycerine following emulsification of bile salts.

lipectomy (lī´-pek-to-mi): Operative removal of fatty tissue neoplasms or of the subcutaneous fatty tissue.

lipid (lip´-id): Any one of a widely varying group of fats and fat-like organic substances that are insoluble or only slightly so in water but are soluble in alcohol, ether, chloroform and other such substances, and that can be metabolized and easily stored in the body; obtained from plants and animals. Along with carbohydrates and proteins, lipids are important constituents of living cells and an important source of fuel in the body.

lipidosis (lip-i-dō´-sis): Overall term for disorders of fat metabolism that result in the accumulation of abnormal amounts of lipids in the body tissues.

lipochondrodystrophy (lip´-ō-kon´-drō-dis´-tro-fi): A congenital abnormality of fat metabolism involving the bones, skin, cartilage, brain, and other organs; characterized by short stature, kyphosis, and possibly mental handicap. Syn., *Hurler's syndrome*.

lipocyte (lip´-ō-sīt): A fat or fat-storing cell.

lipodystrophy (lip-ō-dis´-trō-fi): Any disturbance of fat metabolism. INTESTINAL L. a condition characterized by diarrhoea, fatty stools, emaciation, arthritis, and deposits of fat in intestinal lymphatic tissue.

lipofibroma (lip´ō-fi-brō´ma): A fibrous fatty tumour.

lipofuscin (lip-ō-fūs´sin): A brown pigment that accumulates in neural cells and is found in many body tissues; may be a product of degenerated lyosomes; has been associated with senile confusion.

lipogenesis (lip´-ō-jen´-e-sis): 1. The production of fat. 2. The deposition of fat in the body. 3. The conversion of protein or carbohydrate into fat.

lipogenous (li-poj´-e-nus): Producing fat or fatness.

lipogranuloma (lip´ō-gran-ū-lō´-ma): A nodule made up of fatty tissue with a necrotic centre; occurs in granulomatous inflammation.

lipogranulomatosis (lip´-ō-gran´-ū-lō-ma-tō´sis): A condition characterized by the occurrence of several lipogranulomas.

lipoidosis (lip-oy-dō´-sis): Disease that is due to disorder of fat metabolism.

lipolysis (li-pol´-i-sis): The chemical breaking down of fat.

lipolytic (lip-ō-lit´-ik): Relating to or causing lipolysis.

lipoma (li-pō´-ma): A benign tumour containing fatty tissue, usually multiple but not metastatic. — lipomata, pl.; lipomatous, adj.

lipomatosis (lip´ō-ma-tō´sis): A condition marked by an abnormal accumulation of fat in a localized area.

lipophilic (lip-ō-fil´-ik): 1. Having an affinity for lipids. 2. Absorbing fat.

lipoprotein (lip´ō-prō´ tē-in): A conjugated protein formed by the combination of a lipid and a protein, and having the general properties of proteins. ALPHA L. tiny particles, rich in protein and apparently not related to atherosclerosis. BETA-L., L. rich in cholesterol, therefore of significance in atherosclerosis.

liposarcoma (lip´-ō-sar-kō´-ma): A rare malignant tumour seen most often in the elderly; usually occurs in the retroperitoneal or mediastinal fat deposits.

lipotrophic (lip´-ō-trō´-pik): Acting on fat metabolism by promoting the reduction of fat deposit in the liver, or an agent that has this effect.

lipuria (li-pū′-ri-a): The presence of lipids in the urine. — lipuric, adj.

liquefaction (lik-we-fak′-shun): The conversion of a solid or gas into a liquid.

liquid (lik′-wid): A substance that flows freely, is neither a solid nor a gas, has no definite shape, but takes the shape of its container.

liquor (lik′-er): A solution. In anatomy, refers to certain body fluids; in pharmacology, refers to an aqueous solution. L. AMNII the fluid surrounding the fetus; L. FOLLICULI the fluid surrounding a developing ovum in a Graafian follicle; L. SANGUINIS the fluid part of the blood (plasma).

Lissauer's paralysis (lis′-sow-erz): A rapidly progressive general paralysis; characterized by seizures and by symptoms of unilateral frontal or temporal lobe disease. Also called *Lissauer's cerebral sclerosis.*

Lister, Lord Joseph: English surgeon 1827–1912. In 1867 Lister published *On the Antiseptic Principle in the Practice of Surgery* which, along with his own practice of surgery, laid the foundation for the development of modern surgery.

Listeria (lis-tēr′-i-a): A genus of coccoid and bacillary microorganisms that occur in lower animals as the cause of septicaemia or encephalitis and in humans as the cause of septicaemia, conjunctivitis, lymphadenitis, and upper respiratory infections. L. MONOCYTOGENES a cause of sporadic cases of purulent meningitis, septicaemia, and sometimes mononucleosis.

listeriosis (lis-tēr′-i-ō′-sis): Infection caused by *Listeria* organisms. See LISTERIA.

lith-, litho-,-lith: Combining forms denoting calculi (stones).

lithagogue (lith′a-gog): An agent that promotes the expulsion of calculi, especially urinary calculi.

lithiasis (li-thī′-a-sis): Formation of calculi, or concretions. L. BILIARIS gallstones; L. RENALIS kidney stones.

lithicosis (lith-i-kō′-sis): Pneumonoconiosis (*q.v.*).

lithium carbonate (lith′-i-um): A soft, silver-white metallic element, the salts of which are solvents of uric acid. Used in drug therapy for individuals with manic depressive illness. Contraindicated in cardiac or renal disease. Serum levels of lithium should be monitored regularly during treatment.

litholysis (li-thol′-i-sis): The dissolving of calculi, especially urinary calculi in the bladder.

lithonephrotomy (lith′ō-ne-frot′ō-mi): Surgical incision of the kidney for the removal of a calculus.

lithopaedion (lith-ō-pē′-di-on): A fetus that has died and calcified *in situ*; often extrauterine.

lithosis (li-thō′-sis): Pneumonoconiosis (*q.v.*).

lithotomy (lith-ot′-o-mi): An operation on a duct or organ for the removal of a calculus, especially from the urinary tract or bladder. L. POSITION that in which the patient lies in the dorsal position with the thighs raised and the knees supported and widely separated.

lithotripsy (lith′-ō-trip-si): The operation of crushing a stone in the urinary bladder and removing the fragments by irrigation. Also called *litholapaxy* and *lithotrity.*

lithotrite (lith′-ō-trīt): An instrument for crushing a stone in the urinary bladder, or in the urethra.

lithous (lith′-us): Relating to or resembling a calculus.

lithuria (lith-ū′ri-a): The presence of small stones or uric acid crystals in the urine.

litmus (lit′-mus): A vegetable pigment, obtained from lichen, used as an indicator of acidity or alkalinity. Blue L. paper turns red when in contact with an acid. Red L. paper turns blue when in contact with an alkali.

litre: (lē′-ter): A unit of liquid measurement in the metric system, being 1000 ml.

litter: A portable stretcher or couch used for transporting the sick or wounded.

Little's disease: Diplegia of spastic type causing scissor-leg deformity. Congenital disease in which there is cerebral atrophy or agenesis. [William John Little, English surgeon, 1810–1894.]

livedo (li-vē′-dō): A bluish discoloration of the skin; may occur in localized patches or generally. L. RETICULARIS cutis marmorata; see under CUTIS. May indicate the presence of an acute disease or a serious failure of the circulation; characterized by reddish-blue mottling of the skin, occurring particularly in the extremities.

liver: The largest gland in the body, lobular in structure, weighing from 1.36 to 1.8 kg in the adult male, less in women. It is dark red in colour and is situated in the upper right section of the abdomen; dome-shaped from fitting closely under the diaphragm. It produces bile, converts most sugars into glycogen, which it also stores, and is essential to life. The liver of some animals is used as food and as the source of pharmaceutical preparations used in treatment of certain anaemias. L. SPOTS yellowish-brown patches or spots on the skin. See also CIRRHOSIS, HOBNAIL LIVER.

liver function test: A test that measures the blood serum level of several enzymes produced by the liver. An elevated liver function test is a sign of possible liver damage.

livid (liv'-id): Ashen, cyanotic. Blue discoloration due to bruising, congestion of blood, or insufficient oxygenation; black and blue. — lividity, n.

living will: A written statement by a mentally competent adult that, should that person ever be in such a condition as to be unable to make decisions regarding his or her care and is clearly dying, no extraordinary measures be used to prolong life.

LMP: Abbreviation for last menstrual period.

loading dose: In pharmacotherapeutics, the administration of a drug in larger doses than the body can eliminate in order to bring the concentration of the drug to an effective level; usually by giving several doses close together; when this has been achieved the daily dose is reduced to the amount that equals the amount of drug that is eliminated each day.

Loa loa (lō'-a lō'-a): A species of nematode found mostly in West Africa; it penetrates the subcutaneous tissues, particularly around the eye and under the conjunctiva; flies are the intermediate host. Also called the *African eye worm*. See LOIASIS.

lobar (lō'-bar): Relating to a lobe. L. PNEUMONIA see PNEUMONIA.

lobate (lō'-bāt): Divided into or made up of lobes.

lobe (lōb): 1. The lower part of the external ear. 2. A more or less well-defined section of an organ, separated from neighbouring sections by a fissure, sulcus, or connective tissue. 3. A subdivision of the lung. — lobar, adj.

lobectomy (lō-bek'-to-mi): Excision of a lobe, as of the lung, brain, thyroid, or liver.

lobotomy (lō-bot'-o-mi): Incision into a lobe. FRONTAL or PREFRONTAL L. cutting through the nerve fibres that pass from the frontal lobe of the cerebrum to the thalamus; done to relieve certain mental states or intractable pain.

lobster-claw hand: An inherited deformity in which the middle digits of the hand are missing and the structures are fused so as to form a hand that resembles a lobster's claw. When only the first and fifth fingers are present, the condition is referred to as *bidactyly*.

lobule (lob'-ūl): A small lobe or a subdivision of a lobe. — lobular, lobulated, adj.

local: Not general; restricted to one part or area of the body; L. ANAESTHETIC, see ANAESTHETIC; L. INFECTION one restricted to a relatively small area, *e.g.*, a boil.

Local Delivery Plan: A three-year action plan to improve the health status and healthcare of a local population, and to modernize the health service; formerly Health Improvement and Modernisation Plan (HIMP) (*q.v.*).

local government: The administration of a particular county or district, with representatives elected by residents.

Local Implementation Team: A group of individuals given the remit to ensure that various healthcare initiatives are carried out at a local level.

localize (lō'-kal-īz): 1. To limit the spread. 2. To determine the site of a lesion. — localization, n.; localized, adj.

localized: Restricted to one area or spot; not spread throughout the body. Opp. to systemic.

Local Research Ethics Committee: A group including both lay people and medical practitioners, set up to monitor local research that involves the use of human subjects (UK).

Local Strategic Partnership (stra-tē'-jik): A cooperative scheme for bringing together different parts of the public sector as well as private and voluntary organizations, to ensure that related services work together and support each other.

lochia (lō'-ki-a): The discharge from the uterus following childbirth or abortion consisting of blood from the placental site, shed vaginal epithelial cells, shreds of decidua and initially debris from the uterus. L. ALBA (whitish) contains white blood cells and mucus. L. RUBRA (red) is mostly fresh and then staler blood. L. SEROSA (pinkish) contains more white cells and fewer red. Lochia may continue for 2–3 weeks or longer. — lochial, adj.

lochiometra (lō-ki-ō-mē'-tra): Retention of lochia in the uterus.

lockjaw: Tonic muscle spasm making it impossible to open the jaws. See TRISMUS.

locomotion (lō-kō-mō'-shun): The act of or ability to move from place to place.

locomotor (lō-kō-mō'-tor): Can be applied to any tissue or system used in human movement. Most usually refers to nerves and muscles. Sometimes includes the bones and joints. L. ATAXIA the disordered gait and loss of sense of position in the lower limbs that occurs in tabes dorsalis (*q.v.*). Tabes dorsalis is sometimes referred to, still, as locomotor ataxia.

loculated (lok'-ū-lā-ted): Divided into numerous cavities or pockets.

loculation (lok-ū-lā'-shun): The formation of loculi in the tissues. See LOCULUS.

loculus (lok′-ū-lus): A small depression, cavity, or space. — loculi, pl.; locular, adj.

locus (lo′-kus): A specific site or place. — loci, pl.

Löffler's syndrome: (lerf′-lerz): Löffler's eosinophilia, a condition characterized by an increase in the eosinophilic leukocytes in the blood, accompanied by transient infiltration of the lungs.

log-, logo-, -log, -logue: Combining form denoting (1) speech; (2) discourse.

logoclonia (lō-gō-klon′-i-a): The spasmodic repetition of the final syllables of words. Also called *logoclony*.

logopaedics (log′ō-pē′ diks): The study and treatment of speech defects.

logopathy (log-op′-ath-i): Any speech disorder of central nervous system origin.

logorrhoea (log′ō-rē′a): Excessive talkativeness; garrulousness.

-logy: Combining form denoting (1) science, theory, doctrine; (2) speaking, saying.

loiasis (lō-ī′-a-sis): A chronic disease caused by a nematode; transmitted by a fly of the genus *Chrysops*; found in central Africa. After as long as two or three years, the larvae of the organism *Loa loa* mature and move into the connective tissue, producing a creeping sensation, intense itching, and pain. Also spelled *loaiasis*.

loin: The lower part of the back, between the lower ribs and the iliac crest; the area immediately above the buttocks.

longevity (lon-jev′-i-ti): 1. Length of life. 2. Long individual life.

longsightedness: Hyperopia (*q.v.*).

long-term care: Medical and personal care that extends over a long period of time, often years, for patients who require some nursing care, who may or may not be bedridden, and whose chronic illnesses may improve somewhat or become controllable.

lophotrichous (lō-fot′-ri-kus): Having two or more flagella at one or both ends; said of bacteria.

Lorain's infantilism: Pituitary dwarfism; see under DWARFISM.

lordosis (lor-dō′-sis): An exaggerated forward, convex curve of the lumbar spine; sometimes called hollow back or saddle back.

lotion (lō′-shun): A liquid preparation, usually medicated, used externally on the skin.

Lou Gehrig's disease: Popular name for amyotrophic lateral sclerosis (*q.v.*).

Louis-Bar syndrome: Ataxia-telangiectasia (*q.v.*).

loupe (loop): A magnifying lens worn on the eyeglasses or a headband by the surgeon when operating on very small structures or by the ophthalmologist when examining the eye.

louse: A small parasitic insect; three species of which infest humans. — lice, pl. See PEDICULUS.

low birth weight: A weight at birth that is below 2.5 kg (5 1/2 pounds) regardless of gestation; the baby may be either preterm or small-for-dates.

lower motor neuron: An efferent neuron with a nucleus either in the anterior horn of the spinal cord or in the corresponding grey matter of the brain stem, and an axon that terminates in a skeletal muscle. See UPPER MOTOR NEURON.

lower respiratory tract: Composed of the right and left bronchi and their subdivisions, and the right and left lungs; abbreviated LRT. LRT INFECTION infection involving the bronchi and lungs; often an extension of an upper respiratory tract infection.

Lowe's syndrome: A hereditary condition characterized by mental handicap, decreased ammonia production by the kidneys, cataract, glaucoma, osteomalacia, rickets, retardation of growth, myotonia. Has been observed only in male infants.

Lown–Ganong–Levine syndrome: An electrocardiographic syndrome in which the P–R interval is short, but the QRS interval is normal; often associated with paroxysmal tachycardia.

low salt diet: See under DIET.

low salt syndrome: A syndrome caused by a drop in the salt concentration of the serum; occurs in heat exhaustion as well as in chronic heart and renal disorders; symptoms include nausea, vomiting, muscle cramps, hypotension, and tachycardia, possibly convulsions.

lozenge (loz′-inj): A medicated, sweetened tablet that is held in the mouth until it is dissolved; a troche.

LREC: Abbreviation for Local Research Ethics Committee (*q.v.*).

LRT: Abbreviation for lower respiratory tract (*q.v.*).

LSD: Lysergic acid diethylamide. Derivative of an alkaloid found in ergot. Has potent hallucinogenic action and produces mind-changing experiences. Although not addictive, abuse of the drug does occur by those who wish to achieve a state of euphoria and escape reality. Also called *acid tabs*.

LSP: Abbreviation for Local Strategic Partnership (*q.v.*).

lubb-dupp (lubb-dupp′): The sounds heard through the stethoscope when listening to the normal heartbeat. *Lubb* is heard when the atrioventricular valves close and *dupp* when the semilunar valves close. The first sound is longer and of lower pitch than the second. Also called *lupp-dupp*.

lubricant (loo′-bri-kant): Any substance such as oil, that lessens or prevents friction when applied between two solid surfaces.

lucent (lū′-sent): Clear; transparent.

Lucey–Driscoll syndrome: A type of congenital jaundice occurring in infants as a result of defective conjugation of bilirubin.

lucid (lū′-sid): Clear, particularly in reference to the mind. — lucidity, n.; lucidly, adv.

Ludwig's angina: See ANGINA.

Luer syringe: A glass syringe for injecting substances hypodermically or intravenously.

lues (lū′-ēz). Syphilis. — luetic, adj.

Luft's disease: A disorder of striated muscle, characterized by muscle weakness, profuse sweating, and increased rate of metabolism.

Lugol's solution: A deep brown, transparent solution consisting of iodine and potassium iodide, in purified water; used as a source of iodine in treating hyperthyroidism because it inhibits the release of thyroid hormone.

lum-, lumbo-: Combining forms denoting (1) the loin; (2) the lumbar area.

lumbago (lum-bā′-gō): Incapacitating low back pain, usually of muscular origin.

lumbar: Relating to the loins. L. NERVE one of the five pairs of spinal nerves; L. PUNCTURE puncture into the subarachnoid space of the spinal cord, usually between the fourth and fifth lumbar vertebrae, to remove an excess of fluid, to obtain fluid for examination, or to inject a medicament; L. SYMPATHECTOMY surgical removal of the sympathetic chain in the lumbar region; used to improve the blood supply to the lower limbs by allowing the blood vessels to dilate.

lumbocostal (lum′-bō-kos′-tal): Relating to the loins and ribs.

lumbosacral (lum′-bō-sā′-kral): Relating to the loin or lumbar vertebrae and the sacrum.

lumen (loo′-men): The channel of a tubular structure. — lumina, pl.; luminal, adj.

lumpectomy (lum-pek′-to-mi): Removal of a tumour, usually refers to breast surgery for removal of a lump only, leaving the surrounding tissues and lymph glands largely intact.

lunacy (lū′-na-si): An old fashioned term for insanity; so called because it was thought to be due to the moon's influence.

lunate (lū′-nāt): One of the bones of the wrist.

lunatic (lū′-na-tik): A term formerly much used to describe a mentally ill person.

Lund and Browder's chart: A chart for estimating the surface area involved in burns of children; it indicates percentages for four growth periods from age one to sixteen. An adaptation of Wallace's rule of nines (*q.v.*).

lung: One of the two main organs of respiration which occupy the greater part of the thoracic cavity. They are made up of an arrangement of air tubes terminating in air vesicles; connect with the outside by the bronchi and the trachea; and are divided into lobes, the right lung being composed of the superior, middle, and inferior lobes and the left lung of the superior and inferior lobes. The lungs are separated from each other by the heart and other organs in the mediastinum. Together they weigh about 1.2 kg and they are concerned with oxygenation of the blood.

lunula (lū′-nū-la): A small semicircular area, especially the semilunar pale area seen at the root of the nail.

lupoid (lū′-poyd): Relating to or resembling lupus. L. HEPATITIS a chronic form of hepatitis in which the serological reactions are similar to those occurring in lupus erythematosus.

lupus (lū′-pus): A destructive, chronic nodular skin condition with many manifestations. L. ERYTHEMATOSUS; see COLLAGEN, LE CELLS. The discoid variety is characterized by a superficial inflammation of the skin with disc-like patches that have reddish edges and depressed centres; commonest on the nose where the eruption appears in a butterfly pattern extending over the adjoining cheeks. The disseminated type is characterized by large areas of erythema on the skin, pyrexia, toxaemia, enlargement of lymph nodes, involvement of serous membranes (pleurisy, pericarditis) and renal damage; may be an autoimmune process; often fatal. L. PERNIO a form of sarcoidosis (*q.v.*); lesions of the hands and ears resembling those of frostbite; usually accompanied by a pulmonary disorder; granulomatous nodules may appear on the skin, especially in old scars; L. VULGARIS the commonest form of skin tuberculosis; ulceration occurs over cartilage (nose or ear) with necrosis and facial disfigurement; SYSTEMIC L. ERYTHEMATOSUS the disseminated variety of lupus. — lupiform, lupous, adj.

lutein (lū′-tē-in): Yellow pigment in the corpus luteum (*q.v.*): also in egg yolk and fat cells.

luteinizing hormone (lū′-tē-in-īz-ing hor′-mōn): A gonadotrophic (*q.v.*) hormone of the anterior pituitary, which acts with the follicle-stimulating hormone to cause ovulation and the secretion of sex hormones; is also involved in the formation of corpus luteum (*q.v.*). In males, it stimulates the interstitial cells of Leydig in the testes to produce testosterone.

Luteinizing hormone releasing hormone: A hormone that controls sex hormones in both men and women.

Lutembacher's syndrome (loo'-tem-bak-erz, loo'-tem-bahk-erz): A combination of atrial septal defect and mitral stenosis.

luteotrophin (lū'-tē-ō-trō'-fin): Hormone secreted by the anterior pituitary gland; it assists the fermentation of the corpus luteum in the ovary. Stimulates milk production after parturition.

luxation (luk-sā'-shun): Dislocation. — luxated, adj.

LVF: Abbreviation for left ventricular failure (*q.v.*).

lying-in: L. PERIOD the puerperium (*q.v.*). The term postnatal is now preferred; L. HOSPITAL an old term for a maternity hospital.

Lyme disease or arthritis An acute, transient disease thought to be caused by a virus transmitted by the bite of a tick; characterized by skin lesions, erythema, fever, headache, stiff neck, malaise; sequelae include cardiac and neurological disorders and actue arthritis affecting the knees and other large joints. So called because it was first identified in Lyme, Connecticut, USA.

lymph (limf): The pale, colourless or slightly yellow fluid that exudes from the blood through the capillaries, bathes the cells, and passes into lymphatic ducts which return the fluid to the blood-stream. Its function is to serve as the medium of exchange of nutrients and wastes between the blood and the cells. It resembles plasma, but contains only one type of blood cell, the lymphocyte. L. GLAND OR NODE see under NODE.

lymph-, lympho-: Combining forms denoting (1) lymph; (2) lymphatic tissue; (3) lymphocytes.

lymphadenectasis (lim'-fad-e-nek'-ta-sis): Enlargement of one or more lymph nodes.

lymphadenectomy (lim-fad'-e-nek'-to-mi): Excision of one or more lymph nodes.

lymphadenitis (lim'-fad-e-nī'-tis): Inflammation of one or more lymph nodes; usually produced by bacteria or their products; may be acute or chronic. The gland swells and there may be suppuration; the surrounding area may be red, hot, and tender to the touch. MESEN-

TERIC L., L. of the mesenteric lymph nodes; TUBERCULOUS L. tuberculosis of the lymph glands, particularly those of the neck and mediastinum, by metastasis from the lungs; suppuration may occur and form draining sinuses; formerly called *scrofula*.

lymphadenogram (lim-fad'-e-nō-gram): Radiography of lymph glands; a radiopaque dye is inserted into the gland before x-ray films are made; the dye is retained for several months, making it possible to take follow-up films.

lymphadenoid (lim-fad'-e-noid): Relating to or having the characteristics of a lymph gland.

lymphadenoma (lim-fad'-e-nō'-ma): An old term for an enlarged lymph node. MULTIPLE L. Hodgkin's disease.

lymphadenopathy (lim-fad' e-nop' a-thi): Any disease of the lymph glands. IMMUNOBLASTIC L. a serious progressive L. marked by fever, sweats, splenomegaly, thrombocytopenia, pruritus, haemolytic anaemia; proliferation of the smaller blood vessels; and generalized lymphadenopathy. — lymphadenopathic, adj.

lymphangiectasis (lim-fan'-ji-ek'-ta-sis): Dilation of the lymph vessels, resulting from some obstruction in the flow of lymph. May cause formation of lymphangioma. — lymphangiectatic, adj.

lymphangiectomy (lim-fan'-ji-ek' to-mi): The surgical removal of a lymph vessel.

lymphangiogram (lim-fan' ji-ō-gram): Radiograph demonstrating the lymphatic system after injection of an opaque medium. — lymphangiography, n.; lymphangiographical, adj.; lymphangiographically, adv.

lymphangioma (lim-fan' ji-ō'-ma): A fairly well circumscribed swelling or simple tumour consisting of lymph vessels; frequently associated with similar formation of blood vessels. May be present at birth or soon afterwards; occurs most commonly on the head, neck, axilla, L. CAVERNOSUM usually appears before two years of age and disappears in late childhood; characterized by dilatation of lymph vessels, forming cavities that are filled with fluid; seen mostly in the neck, axilla and mediastinum; L. CIRCUMSCRIPTUM L. present at birth or occurring in childhood; marked by appearance of one or more yellow to red patches; L. SIMPLEX small L. due to dilation of a lymph vessel in a circumscribed area.

lymphangioplasty (lim-fan'-ji-ō-plas-ti): Replacement of lymphatics by artificial channels (buried silk or nylon threads) to drain the tissues. Relieves the 'brawny arm' after radical mastectomy. — lymphangioplastic, adj.

lymphangiosarcoma (lim-fan'-ji-ō-sar-kō'-ma): A malignant tumour of lymphatic vessels, usually occurring in a limb that has been the site of chronic lymphoedema following radical mastectomy.

lymphangitis (lim-fan-ji'-tis): Inflammation of lymph vessel or vessels. May be due to infection through the skin, usually by streptococci; in fingertip infections a red line may be seen running up the arm. The condition usually terminates at the lymph node into which the vessel empties, but may result in septicaemia. Symptoms include headache, chills, fever, malaise, increased white blood cell count.

lymphatic (lim-fat'-ik): 1. Relating to, or conveying or containing lymph. 2. A vessel that conveys lymph. L. SYSTEM the vessels and glands (nodes) through which the lymph passes as it returns to the bloodstream.

lymphoblast (lim' fō-blast): An immature lymphocyte (*q.v.*).

lymphoblastoma (lim-fō-blas-tō' ma): Any one of several types of malignant lymphoma in which single or multiple tumours arise from lymphoblasts in lymph nodes. Sometimes associated with acute lymphatic leukaemia. Term is sometimes used synonymously with lymphosarcoma (*q.v.*). L. MALIGNUM Hodgkin's disease (*q.v.*).

lymphocyte (lim' fō-sīt): A variety of white blood cell formed in the lymphoid tissues of the body; round, colourless, somewhat motile, with a single nucleus and no cytoplasmic granules. Classified as large and small. They make up 20% to 30% of the total white blood cells and serve as a defence mechanism for the body. Their function is to produce antibodies. B-LYMPHOCYTES are those that migrate directly into the tissues without passing through the thymus, while T-LYMPHOCYTES are preprocessed in the thymus, especially in early life; thus children in whom the thymus is congenitally absent are highly susceptible to infections. — lymphocytic, adj.

lymphocythaemia (lim'-fō-sī-thē'-mi-a): Excess of lymphocytes in the blood. Seen in such infectious diseases as infectious mononucleosis, undulant fever, measles, mumps, whooping cough.

lymphocytic choriomeningitis (lim-fō-sit' ikkōr-i-ō-men-in-jī' tis): Acute meningitis due to a specific virus; benign; runs a short course with symptoms resembling those of aseptic meningitis; occurs chiefly in young adults.

lymphocytoma (lim'-fō-sī-tō'-ma): A malignant lymphoma characterized by the presence of cells that closely resemble mature lymphocytes. L. CUTIS a benign collection of lymphocytes in the dermis.

lymphocytopenia (lim' fō-sī-tō-pē' ni-a): A reduction in the normal number of lymphocytes in the blood.

lymphocytopoiesis (lim' fō-sī-tō-poy-ē'sis): The formation of lymphocytes.

lymphocytosis (lim'fō-sī tō'sis): An excess of normal lymphocytes in the blood. ACUTE INFECTIOUS L. an acute communicable disease of children in which there is an excess of normal small lymphocytes in the blood without disorder of the lymph glands or spleen.

lymphoedema (lim-fē-dē'-ma): Swelling of the subcutaneous tissues with excess lymph fluid due to faulty lymph drainage. May be congenital or hereditary, or may result from trauma or excision of lymph nodes L. PRAECOX gradual enlargement of the lower extremities of girls, starting in the feet; begins between the age of 10 and 25. See ELEPHANTIASIS; L. SLEEVE a tight-fitting elastic sleeve that extends from the wrist to the shoulder, or a sleeve that alternately inflates and deflates, thus providing intermittent compression; enhances venous return, and improves circulation; used in treatment of lymphoedema following mastectomy.

lymphoepithelioma (lim' fō-ep-i-thēl-i-ō' ma): A rapidly growing malignant tumour arising in the modified epithelial tissue in the area of the tonsil and nasopharynx; often metastasizes to the cervical lymph nodes. — lymphoepitheliomata, pl.

lymphogram (lim'-fō-gram): X-ray demonstration of the lymphatic system or part of it after the injection of a radiopaque medium into the lymph system of an arm or leg.

lymphogranuloma (lim'-fō-gran-ū-lō'-ma): Term descriptive of several diseases in which the chief pathological change is the development of lesions resembling granulomas (*q.v.*). L. VENEREUM an important contagious venereal disease, transmitted by sexual contact; primary lesion on genitalia may go unnoticed; later, regional lymph nodes enlarge and typical buboes form followed by formation of draining sinuses that leave thick scars when they heal. General symptoms are fever, malaise, joint pains. May cause elephantiasis of genitalia, ischiorectal abscesses and rectal stricture, the latter particularly in women. Also called *lymphogranuloma inguinale; Nicolas-Favre disease, sixth venereal disease, climatic* or *tropical bubo*.

lymphography (lim-fog′-ra-fi): A diagnostic x-ray procedure used in diagnosis of Hodgkin's disease and lymphoma; consists of injecting a dye, usually between the toes, which makes the lymph vessels and nodes visible on x-ray. — lymphographical, adj.

lymphoid (lim′-foyd): Relating to or resembling lymph or the tissues of the lymphatic system.

lymphokines (lim′-fō-kīns): Soluble chemical factors released by T-lymphocytes in response to an antigen; they are hormone-like substances produced by the thymus, the best known one being interferon (q.v.).

lymphokinesis (lim′-fō-kī-nē′-sis): 1. The circulation of lymph through the lymph channels and nodes. 2. The movement of endolymph in the semicircular canals of the internal ear.

lymphoma (lim-fō′-ma): Term includes several tumours of lymphatic tissue, the three main types being Hodgkin's disease, lymphosarcoma, and reticulum sarcoma. Of unknown cause, the tumour starts as an enlargement of lymph nodes, usually cervical or inguinal; later extends to adjacent lymphatic chains, liver, and spleen. May be transformed into one of the malignant types including Hodgkin's disease. The benign form remains localized and does not recur after surgical removal. BURKITT'S L. a type of malignant L. that occurs in children in certain parts of Africa; NODULAR L. a malignant L. that occurs chiefly in people over 40; asymptomatic at first followed by slowly progressive painless growth of nodules primarily in the axillary, inguinal, or femoral regions. — lymphomatous, lymphomatoid, adj.

lymphopenia (lim-fō-pē′-ni-a): A reduction in the proportion of lymphocytes in the circulating blood.

lymphoplasmia (lim-fō-plaz′-mi-a): A cell condition in which the red blood cells lack haemoglobin.

lymphoproliferative (lim′-fō-pro-lif′-e-ra-tiv): Referring to or characterized by proliferation of lymphoid tissue.

lymphoreticular (lim′-fō-re-tik′-ū-lar): Relating to the reticuloendothelial cells of the lymph nodes. L. SYSTEM the reticuloendothelial system; see RETICULOENDOTHELIUM.

lymphorrhagia (lim-fō-rā′ji-a): An outpouring of lymph from a severed or ruptured lymphatic vessel.

lymphosarcoma (lim-fō-sar-kō′ ma): A malignant tumour of unknown cause, arising in the lymphatic tissue and tending to metastasize freely. — lymphosarcomata, pl.; lymphosarcomatous, adj.

lymph-vascular (limf-vas′-kū-lar): Relating to lymphatic vessels.

lyophilization (lī-of′ i-lī-zā′ shun): The process of creating a stable preparation of a biological substance such as blood or plasma by first freezing it rapidly and then dehydrating it. — liophilize, v.

lys-, lysi-, lyso-,-lysis: Combining forms denoting (1) disintegration, decomposition, dissolution, lysis; (2) a loosening.

lyse: To produce, cause, or undergo lysis (q.v.).

lysergic acid: See LSD.

lysergide (lī-ser′-jīd): A hallucinogenic compound derived from lysergic acid; see LSD.

lysin (lī′ sin): An antibody that has the capability of causing the dissolution of cells. See BACTERIOLYSIN, HAEMOLYSIN.

lysine (lī′-sēn): An essential amino acid necessary for growth in infants and to maintain nitrogen balance in adults. Deficiency may cause nausea, dizziness, and anaemia. It is destroyed by dry heating, e.g., as in toasted bread and cereals such as puffed wheat.

lysinogen (lī-sin′-ō-jen): A substance that is capable of inducing the formation of lysins. Also spelled lysogen.

lysis (lī-′-sis): 1. A gradual return to normal, used especially in relation to pyrexia. Opp. to crisis. 2. Dissolution and disintegration of bacteria and cells by the action of a lysin. 3. Loosening of an organ from adhesions. — lytic, adj.

lysogen (lī′-sō-jen): See LYSINOGEN.

lysogenicity (lī′ sō-je-nis′ i-ti): 1. The ability to produce lysins. 2. The ability of a bacterium to perpetuate a bacteriophage (q.v.) in the prophage state.

lysosome (lī′-sō-sōm): One of a group of minute, cytoplasmic, intracellular, digestive bodies having a single membrane and containing a large number of powerful enzymes; found in saliva, tears, egg white, and many animal tissues. Shock, sepsis, or trauma may cause lysosomes to break down and release the enzymes which may damage the cells and, consequently, are an important factor in such wasting diseases as muscular dystrophy.

lysozyme (lī′ sō-zīm): A bacteriolytic enzyme present in tears, saliva, nasal mucus and many animal fluids; also found in egg white.

lyssic (lis′-ik): Relating to rabies.

lytic (lit′-ik): 1. Relating to lysis. 2. Producing lysis.

-lytic: A suffix denoting lysis. In pharmacology, it refers to the ability of a drug to block or inhibit the actions of the autonomic nervous system.

M

MA: Abbreviation for Master of Arts.

Maastricht Treaty (mah'-strikt, mah-strikt'): The treaty that established the European Union (*q.v.*).

Mackenrodt's ligament: The lateral cervical ligament of the uterus. [Alwin Karl Mackenrodt, German gynaecologist, 1859–1925.]

macr-, macro-: Combining forms denoting (1) large size (opp. to micro-); (2) abnormally large, *e.g.*, macrocolon; (3) visible to the naked eye.

macrencephaly (mak'-ren-kef'-a-li,-sef-): A condition in which the head and brain are abnormally large in relation to the rest of the body; a congenital anomaly. Also called *macrencephalia*.

macroaesthesia (mak'rō-es-thē'zi-a): A sensation that things seen or felt are larger than they really are.

macroaggregate (mak'-rō-ag'rē-gāt): An unusually large accumulation of a substance.

macroamylase (mak'-rō-am'-i-lās): A blood serum amylase in which the molecules have a high molecular weight and a tendency to combine with molecules of other proteins in the blood serum, forming a complex too large for the kidney to excrete.

macroangiopathy (mak'rō-an-ji-op'a-thi): Disease of the larger blood vessels.

macrobiosis (mak'-rō-bī-ō' sis): Longevity.

macrobiotic (mak'-rō-bī-ot'ik): 1. Having a long life. 2. Tending to prolong life. M. DIET a diet that began to be popular in the 1960s that emphasizes whole grains and foods native to one's environment, with gradual elimination of highly refined foods, sugar, and dairy products; was thought to reduce blood pressure and cholesterol levels. Some nutritionists held that the diet was injurious to health. Also called *Zen macrobiotic diet*.

macroblast (mak'-rō-blast): An abnormally large nucleated red blood cell.

macrocephalia (mak'rō-ke-fā'li-a,-se-): The condition of having an excessively long or large head. — macrocephalic, macrocephalous, adj.

macrocnemia (mak-rō-nē'-mi-a): Excessive development of the legs below the knees.

macrocyte (mak'-rō-sīt): A large red blood cell, found in the blood in some forms of anaemia, especially pernicious anaemia. — macrocytic, adj.

macrocythaemia (mak'-rō-sī-thē'-mi-a): A condition characterized by the presence of unusually large numbers of macrocytes in the circulating blood. Macrocytosis.

macrodactyly (mak-rō-dak'-ti-li): Excessive development of the fingers or toes. Also called *macrodactilia* and *megadactyly*.

macrodrip (mak'rō-drip): An IV apparatus that delivers intravenous solutions, with the drops being larger than those in the microdrip, the drop size being regulated by the calibre of the delivery tubing.

macroencephaly (mak'rō-en-kef'-a-li,-sef-): See MACRENCEPHALY.

macrogenesy (mak-rō-jen'-e-si): Gigantism.

macrogenitosomia (mak'-rō-jen-i-tō-sō'-mi-a): Excessive development of the body in general, and especially of the sex organs. When this occurs at an early age it is called M. *praecox*.

macroglobulin (mak'ro-glob'ū-lin): A globulin (*q.v.*) of high molecular weight; found in blood in certain diseases, particularly those affecting the lymphoid plasma cells and the reticuloendothelial system. See RETICULOEN-DOTHELIUM.

macroglobulinaemia (mak'rō-glob'ū-li-nē'mi-a): A condition characterized by an increase in macroglobulins in the blood. WALDEN-STRÖM'S M. a rare progressive syndrome involving the reticuloepithelial system; usually seen in elderly males; marked by an increase in macroglobulins and Bence-Jones proteins, adenopathy, splenomegaly, hepatomegaly, anaemia, anorexia, plasmacytosis (*q.v.*) of the bone marrow, and neurological manifestations; in some patients it resembles cancer and may be fatal; cause unknown.

macrogyria (mak-rō-jī'-ri-a): A congenital anomaly in which the convolutions of the brain are greatly enlarged; often associated with mental handicap.

macrolides (mak'-rō-līdz): A class of antibiotics of the genus *Streptomyces*; erythromycin is one of them.

macromolecule (mak'-rō-mol'-e-kūl): A molecule of very large size, as found in such substances as proteins, nucleic acids, and polysaccharides.

macrophage (mak'-rō-fāj): A large 'wandering' phagocytic cell that ingests foreign matter; plays an important part in resisting infection and in the organization and repair of tissue.

macroplasia (mak-rō-plā'zi-a): Overgrowth of a tissue or part. Gigantism.

macropsia (ma-krop'-si-a): A disorder of vision in which things appear larger than they really are.

macroscopic (mak'rō-skop'-ik): Visible to the naked eye; gross. Opp. to microscopic.

macroscopy (ma-kros'-ko-pi): Examination with the naked eye.

macrosurgery (mak'-rō-ser'-jer-i): Surgery that can be performed without the use of a microscope or miniature instruments. Opp. of microsurgery (q.v.).

macula (mak'-ū-la): A spot or stain on a body tissue, not elevated but differentiated from surrounding tissue. M. DENSA a dense collection of cells in the distal convoluted tubule of the nephron; its function is to regulate the reabsorption of sodium ions; M. LUTEA the yellow spot on the retina, the area of clearest vision; M. SOLARIS a sunspot; a freckle. — maculae, pl.; macular, adj.; maculation, n.

macular (mak'-ū-lar): **1**. Of, or relating to the macula lutea of the retina. **2**. Of, or relating to the presence of macules. M. DEGENERATION irreversible loss of central vision due to pathological changes in the macula lutea causing a gradual loss of clear central vision; may occur early in life but usually starts at about age 60; may be due to trauma, atherosclerosis, or senility, in which case it increases with age and may lead to total blindness. Individuals at high risk appear to be those with blue eyes, far-sightedness, cardiovascular disease, and lengthy exposure to sunlight. Early treatment is imperative; the laser beam has been used to seal off the affected area to prevent the spread of the disease.

macule (mak'-ūl): A small, circumscribed spot or stain on the skin, not raised above the skin surface; usually refers to an area up to 1 cm in diameter. — macular, adj.

maculopapular (mak'ū-lō-pap'ū-lar): The presence of macules and raised palpable spots (papules) on the skin.

maculopathy (mak-ū-lop'-a-thi): Any disease or disorder of the macula lutea (q.v.).

madarosis (mad'-a-rō'-sis): Loss of eyelashes and/or eyebrows.

mad cow disease: Colloquial term for bovine spongiform encephalopathy (q.v.), the human form of which is believed to be Creutzfeldt–Jakob disease (q.v.).

Madura foot: A fungus disease of the foot found in India and the tropics. Characterized by swelling and the development of nodules and sinuses from which there is a characteristic exudate containing granules that may be white, yellow, red, brown, orchid or black. See MYCETOMA.

magnesium (mag-nē'-zi-um): A silvery metallic substance, salts of which are found in bone, muscle, and blood; considered essential to nutrition and growth. Present in many animal and vegetable foods; deficiency in the diet causes disturbance in bone development and irritability of the nervous system that may result in convulsions and tetany. Chemical symbol is Mg. M. SULPHATE small, colourless, bitter tasting crystals, soluble in water, used as a cathartic and anti-inflammatory; Epsom salt.

magnetic resonance imaging (mag-net'-ik-rez'-o-nans-im'-a-jing): See NUCLEAR MAGNETIC RESONANCE IMAGING.

magnum (mag'-num): Large or great, as the foramen M. in the occipital bone.

Mahaim fibres: Fibrous connections between the atrioventricular node and the ventricular septum.

maidenhead (mā'-den-hed): The hymen.

maim (mām): To disable or wound by violence.

mainlining (mān'-līn-ing): Slang term used to describe the injection of a drug directly into a vein.

Makaton (mak'-a-ton): A unique language programme offering a structured, multimodal approach for the teaching of communication, language and literacy skills. Devised for children and adults with a variety of communication and learning disabilities, it is used extensively throughout the UK and has been adapted for use in over 40 other countries.

Making a Difference: A policy document published in 1999 by the Department of Health in England, which outlined a new curriculum for pre-registration nurse education. The aim of the policy was to develop and strengthen the nursing, midwifery and health visiting contribution to healthcare.

mal: Disease or disorder. M. DE MER seasickness. GRAND M. major epilepsy. PETIT M. minor epilepsy.

mal-: Combining form denoting (1) ill, bad, badly, poor, poorly, inadequate; (2) abnormal, irregular.

mala (mā′-la): The cheek or cheek bone. — malar, adj.

malabsorption (mal′-ab-sorp′-shun): Inadequate or disordered absorption of nutrients from the intestinal canal. M. SYNDROME refers to a group of disorders including giardiasis, Whipple's disease, cystic fibrosis of the pancreas, Hirschprung's disease, and adult onset sprue, which are characterized by malabsorption of essential nutrients, including electrolytes, vitamins, iron, and calcium; symptoms include pallor, lassitude, anorexia, failure to gain weight, weakness, large foul-smelling stools, and diarrhoea.

malac-, malaco-: Combining forms denoting a condition of abnormal softness or softening.

malacia (ma-lā′-shi-a): 1. Abnormal softening of a part. See KERATOMALACIA, OSTEOMALACIA. 2. Abnormal craving for certain foods, especially spicy foods.

maladaptation (mal′a-dap-tā′shun): The inability to make normal adjustments in personal relationships and in society, with resulting abnormal or anti-social behaviour.

maladie de Roger (mal′-a-di-de-roj′-ā): The murmur produced by ventricular septal defect; is most likely to be heard in children and disappears as the child matures and the defect corrects itself; also called *Roger's disease*.

maladjustment (mal′a-just′ment): Bad or poor adjustment to environment socially, mentally, emotionally, or physically; often results in conflict-producing behaviour.

malady (mal′-a-di): A disease, disorder or indisposition.

malaise (ma-lāz′): A feeling of discomfort and uneasiness; often a sign of developing disease or infection.

malalignment (mal′a-līn′-ment): Faulty alignment, as of the teeth, or of a fracture.

malar (mā′-lar): Relating to the cheek. M. or ZYGOTIC BONE forms the prominence of the cheek.

malaria (ma-lai′-ri-a): An infectious, febrile, tropical disease caused by one of the genus *Plasmodium*, and carried by mosquitoes of the genus *Anopheles*. Characterized by anaemia, toxaemia, splenomegaly, and intermittent paroxysms of fever, chills, and sweating that occur at intervals corresponding to the time it takes for a new generation of the parasites to develop in the blood. If the paroxysms occur every 24 h, the malaria is known as quotidian; if every 48 h, tertian; if every 72 h, quartan. Sometimes classified on the basis of ocurrence as (1) UNSTABLE M. in which the amount of transmission varies from year to year and epidemics are possible; and (2) STABLE M. in which the amount of transmission is generally high and epidemics are likely. ALGID M. a condition resembling surgical shock; the skin is pale, cold, clammy; the respirations are slow, pulse is weak, and blood pressure low; often fatal; CEREBRAL M. falciparum M. caused by localization of the causative organism in the brain; symptoms include delirium and coma; FALCIPARUM M. the most serious form of M., caused by *Plasmodium falciparum*; often fatal; TRANSFUSION M. caused by transfusion of blood from a symptomless infected donor.

malariologist (ma-lai-ri-ol′o-jist): A person knowledgeable about or engaged in the study of malaria.

malariology (ma-lai-ri-ol′-ō-ji): The study of malaria.

malassimilation (mal′a-sim-il-ā′shun): Poor or disordered assimilation.

malaxation (mal′-ak-sā′-shun): 1. A kneading manoeuvre in massage. 2. The act of kneading the materials to be made up into pills or plasters.

maldigestion (mal′-dī-jes′-chun): Imperfect or disordered digestion.

maleficence (mal-ef′-i-sens): Evil, harm, or mischief. Regarding an unlawful, wrongful act. See CONSENT.

maleness (māl′-nes): Anatomical and physiological characteristics that relate to a male person's procreative capacity.

malformation (mal′-for-mā′-shun): Abnormal or incorrect shape or structure; deformity.

malignancy (ma-lig′-nan-si): 1. Virulence. 2. A life-threatening disorder or neoplasm as opposed to a benign condition.

malignant (ma-lig′-nant): Virulent and dangerous; that which is likely to become progressively worse and to have a fatal termination. M. GROWTH or TUMOUR cancer or sarcoma; M. HYPERTENSION see under HYPERTENSION; M. PUSTULE anthrax. — malignancy, n.

malinger (ma-lin′-ger): To feign, induce, or deliberately prolong an illness or incapacitation to avoid work or a duty or to excite sympathy. — malingerer, n.; malingering, n.

malleolus (mal-lē′-ō-lus): A part of process of a bone shaped more or less like a hammer. EXTERNAL M. the process at the lower end of the fibula; INTERNAL M. the process at the lower end of the tibia. — malleoli, pl.; malleolar, adj.

Mallet finger: A tearing away of the extensor tendon of the distal phalanx of the finger; caused by a sudden blow on its tip as when catching a cricket ball or other type of hard ball.

malleus (mal'-ē-us): The hammer-shaped lateral bone of the middle ear.

Mallory's bodies: 1. Round or ovoid hyalin inclusion bodies found in the cytoplasm of some of the degenerated cells of the liver in certain nutritional disorders of the liver. **2.** Bodies found in the lymph spaces and epidermal cells in some cases of scarlet fever.

Mallory–Weiss syndrome: The vomiting of blood or melaena following prolonged vomiting, hiccups, or coughing; due to small lacerations in the gastric mucosa or submucosa, most often near the junction of the oesophagus and the stomach. Also called *Mallory–Weiss tear*.

malnutrition (mal-nū-trish'-un): The state of being poorly nourished. May be caused by inadequate food or of one of the essential nutrients, by malassimilation, or by a metabolic defect that prevents the body from utilizing nutrients properly.

malocclusion (mal'o-kloo' zhun): Failure of the upper and lower teeth to meet properly when the jaws are closed.

malodorous (mal-ō'-dor-us): Having an offensive or unpleasant odour.

Malpighian (mal-pig'-i-an): M. CORPUSCLES or CAPSULES the renal glomeruli with Bowman's capsule enclosing them (see GLOMERULUS). **2.** Name given to certain small lymphoid bodies or patches distributed throughout the spleen. [Marcello Malpighi, Italian anatomist, founder of microscopic anatomy 1628–1694.]

malposition (mal-pō-zish'-un): Any abnormal position of a part; in midwifery, a fetus whose occiput is directed towards either posterior quadrant of the pelvis.

malpractice (mal'-prak'-tis): In healthcare, the failure of a health-care professional to meet the accepted standards of care for professionals licensed to practise in a specific area, or the committment by a health-care professional of acts considered improper, negligent, or injurious to another; referred to as unethical M. when the misconduct involves actions or behaviour that is considered improper or immoral, and criminal M. when the action or behaviour involved is criminal in nature.

malpresentation (mal'-prē-zen-tā'-shun): **1.** Any unusual presentation of the fetus in the pelvis. **2.** Abnormal or faulty position of the body or any part of it.

malrotation (mal'-rō-tā'-shun): **1.** Abnormal position of the child at birth, making natural delivery difficult or impossible. **2.** A developmental anomaly in which the intestine becomes fixed to the mesentery in an abnormal way.

Malta fever: See BRUCELLOSIS.

maltase (mawl'-tās): A sugar-splitting (saccharolytic) enzyme found in the body, especially in intestinal juice. Also known as α-*glucosidase*.

Malthusian (mal-thū'-zi-an): Refers to the theory that populations tend to increase faster than their means of subsistence, unless intentionally checked and controlled. [Thomas Malthus, English economist, 1766–1834.] — Malthusianism, n.

maltose (mawl'-tōs): Malt sugar, a disaccharide; produced by the hydrolysis of starch during digestion.

malunion (mal-ūn'-yon): Union of a fracture in faulty position.

mamma (mam'-a): The breast; milk-secreting gland. — mammae, pl.; mammary, adj.

mammal (mam'-al): An individual belonging to the highest class of vertebrates; including man; a warm-blooded animal, usually hairy, that suckles its young. — mammalian, adj.

mammary (mam'-e-ri): Relating to the breasts. M. GLAND the specialized tuboalveolar glands of the female breast that secrete milk.

mammectomy (mam-mek'-to-mi): Surgical removal of one or both breasts; mastectomy (*q.v.*).

mammilla (ma-mil'-a): **1.** The nipple. **2.** A small papilla or nipple-like structure. — mammillae, pl.; mammillated, mammillary, adj.

mammilliplasty (mam-mil'i-plas-ti): Plastic reconstruction of a nipple and areola. — Syn., *theleplasty*.

mammillitis (mam'il-ī' tis): Inflammation of the nipple.

mammitis (mam-ī'-tis): Mastitis (*q.v.*).

mammogenesis (mam-mō-jen'-e-sis): The development of the mammary glands of the breast to their functional state.

mammogram (mam'-ō-gram): A roentgenogram of the breast.

mammography (mam-og'-ra-fi): X-ray examination of the breast after injection of an opaque agent. ULTRASOUND M. a technique used in breast examination that does not require the use of x-ray; said to be 80% to 90% accurate in determining whether a lesion is present. Syn., *mastography*. — mammographic, adj., mammographically, adv.

mammoplasty (mam'-ō-plas-ti): An operation to correct pendulous or sagging breasts; skin and glandular tissue is removed and the glands are fixed in their ordinary position. AUGMENTATION M. plastic surgery to increase the size and shape of the breast.

mammose (ma'mōs): Having large breasts.

mammotrophic (mam-ō-trōf'-ik): 1. Having an effect on the breast. 2. Having a stimulating effect on the mammary gland.

managed care: Systems and techniques used to control the use of health-care services; includes a review of medical necessity and case management; designed to ensure the provision of appropriate health-care services in a cost-efficient manner.

management: 1. A division of a company or group that organizes the rest, to make it run more effectively and efficiently. 2. The process of organization and leadership of others.

mandible (man'-dib'l): The lower jawbone. — mandibular, adj.

mandibulectomy (man-dib'-ū-lek-to-mi): Surgical removal of the mandible.

mandibulofacial (man-dib'-ū lō-fā'-shul): Relating to the mandible and some other parts of the face. M. DYSOSTOSIS a hereditary disorder characterized by underdevelopment of the mandible and zygoma, defects of the ear, abnormally large mouth, and downwards slant of the angles of the eyelids, giving a person a peculiar, fish-like appearance. Also called *Treacher Collins syndrome.*

manganese (mang'-ga-nēs): A metallic element that resembles iron and is often associated with it in ores; some of its salts are used in medicine.

mania (mā'-ni-a): A mood disorder that occurs as one phase in major affective disorders, bipolar disorders in particular, and in certain organic mental disorders such as dementia and delirium; characterized by undue elation and excitement, pronounced psychomotor activity, flight of ideas, talkativeness, anger, and destructiveness. M. Á POTU delirium tremens; a pathological intoxication in which the patient has hallucinations following alcoholic intake.

-mania: Formerly denoted any kind of madness. Currently used to denote a morbid preoccupation with some idea or activity, or a compulsive need to carry out a certain kind of behaviour.

maniac (mā'-ni-ak): A person affected with mania (*q.v.*). A person who is insane or violently disturbed. — maniacal, adj.

manic (man'-ik): Relating to or affected with mania (*q.v.*).

manic-depressive: Refers to a serious mental illness characterized by a cyclic, recurring

pattern of short periods of mania alternating with longer periods of depression.

manikin (man'-i-kin): A model of the human body, used in teaching anatomy and also for demonstrating and teaching nursing procedures.

manipulation (ma-nip'ū-lā'shun): 1. In medicine, using the hands skilfully, as in reducing a fracture or dislocation, or changing the fetal position. 2. In physical therapy, the movement of a joint beyond the limit to which the individual can move it voluntarily. 3. A means of influencing others' behaviour; methods may be overt or covert.

manipulative (ma-nip'-ū-lā-tiv): Usually refers to an individual who tries to control the behaviour of others in order to meet his or her own needs and desires regardless of the others' needs and desires; sometimes seen in psychiatric patients.

mannerism (man'-er-izm): A way of speaking, acting, or behaving that is unusual or peculiar, and characterizes a particular person.

mannitol (man'-i-tol): An alcohol derived from the manna ash (*Fraxinus ornus*) and other plant sources; has various uses in medicine, especially in kidney disorders, when it may be used in kidney-function testing and as an osmotic diuretic.

manoeuvre (man-nū'-ver): 1. A skilful procedure or act. 2. Special movement or procedure, using the hand or an instrument for a specific purpose. See HEIMLICH MANOEUVRE, LEOPOLD'S MANOEUVRES, and VALSALVA MANOEUVRE.

manometer (ma-nom'-i-ter): An instrument for measuring the pressure exerted by liquids or gases or the tension of blood vessels. See SPHYGMOMANOMETER.

Mantoux test (man-too'): A test for tuberculosis; a minute amount of diluted tuberculin (Purified Protein Derivative) (*q.v.*) is injected intradermally. If the person has, or has had tuberculosis, hyperaemia and a wheal will develop at the site of the injection. See TUBERCULIN.

manual (man'-ū-al): Related to or involving use of the hands. M. EXPRESSION OF URINE pressure on the abdominal wall at regular intervals to assist the patient to void when the bladder is paralysed because of an interruption in the spinal cord; M. THERAPY treatment performed by the hands *e.g.*, massage, manipulation; M. TRACTION, see under TRACTION.

manubrium (ma-nū'-bri-um): A handle-shaped structure; the upper part of the breast bone or sternum.

manus (mā'-nus): The hand, including the fingers.

MAO inhibitors: See under MONOAMINE OXIDASE.

maple bark disease: A type of pneumonitis caused by the spores of a mould found under the bark of maple logs.

maple syrup urine disease: A familial metabolic disorder, of unknown origin, with urine smelling of maple syrup, and with involvement of the central nervous system, sometimes resulting in mental handicap. Usually fatal within the first few months of life.

marantic (ma-ran'-tik): Relating to or resembling marasmus (q.v.).

marasmus (mar-az'-mus): Wasting away of the body, especially that of a baby, without apparent cause. — marasmic, adj.

marble bones: Osteopetrosis (q.v.).

Marburg disease: A severe haemorrhagic fever due to the Marburg/Ebola virus causing a wide range of symptoms including encephalitis, a morbilliform rash and renal failure. The incubation period is three to seven days. First reported from Marburg, Germany amongst laboratory workers handling monkey tissue from Uganda, later cases reported from Zaire. There is no specific treatment other than supportive therapy. Mortality is high, from 75% to 90%.

marche à petits pas (marsh'ah-ptē'pa): A slow, uncertain gait with small steps, usually with a slightly flexed posture, seen mostly in the aged who are senile.

March fracture: A hairline break in a long bone of the foot due to repeated trauma caused by heavy stamping in long marches or in jogging. The bone will usually heal without immobilization if the stress is removed.

Marchiafava–Bignami disease (mah-ki-a-fah'-va-bēn-yah'-mi): A degenerative disorder involving the corpus callosum; occurs chiefly in alcoholics who drink excessive amounts of red wine.

Marfan's syndrome: Hereditary congenital disorder caused by defect in the fibrillin gene. There is dislocation of the optic lens, congenital heart disease, and arachnodactyly, with hypotonic musculature and lax ligaments, occasionally excessive height, and abnormalities of the iris. [B. J. A. Marfan, French physician, 1858–1942.]

margin: An edge or border, as of an organ or structure. — marginal, adj.

marihuana, marijuana (mar-i-wah'-na): The dried leaves and buds of *Cannabis sativa* (q.v.).

market economy: A system characterized by free trade, where supply and demand control resources without interference.

marmorization (mar'mo-rī-zā'shun): A marble-like mottling of the skin. See CUTIS MARMORATA under CUTIS.

marrow: See BONE MARROW.

Marshall–Marchetti operation: A procedure that fixes the urethra to the back of the pubic bone; one treatment for stress incontinence.

marsupialization (mar-sū'-pia-lī-zā'shun): The surgical creation of a pouch by evacuating a cyst and exterioralizing it by suturing the cyst walls to the cut edges of the skin, which heals by granulation, thus creating a pouch.

Marxism (marks'-izm): School of socialism named after Karl Marx. Marx argued that society is stratified into classes according to the distribution of capital or the means of production.

masculine (mas'-kū-lin): Referring to the qualities and role behaviour that are considered characteristic of a male person, *e.g.*, strength, manliness, vigour, virility.

masculinize (mas'-kū-lin-īz): To confer or produce so-called male characteristics in a female. — masculinization, n.

mask: 1. A covering for the nose and mouth, sometimes the entire face, used to protect either the wearer or a patient, to prevent the inhalation of toxic substances or pathogenic organisms, or to administer oxygen or other medications in gas form. 2. An expression characteristic of a certain disorder or condition. AEROSOL M. a M. similar to a face M. but which has a nebulizing attachment that humidifies the inspired air; PARKINSON'S M. a fixed expression with staring and infrequent winking; characteristic of patients with Parkinson's disease; M. OF PREGNANCY a brownish patchy discoloration on the face and neck; occurs during pregnancy and disappears after delivery. SURGICAL M. a mouth and nose mask worn by operating room personnel to deflect the air from the nose and mouth and filter out any droplets that may contain pathogenic organisms; also worn for self-protection by those caring for patients with communicable disease; VENTURI M. a M. that delivers precise fixed concentrations of oxygen.

masochism (mas'-ō-kizm): A form of sexual perversion in which one has a pathological desire to inflict pain upon oneself or to suffer pain, abuse, or humiliation at the hands of another. Opp. of sadism. [Leopold von Sacher-Masoch, Austrian novelist, 1836–1895.]

masochist (mas'-ō-kist): One who derives sexual pleasure from humiliation, pain, or abuse inflicted by another.

mass: 1. A lump. 2. A mixture so prepared that it can be made up into pills.

massage (mas-sahzh'): Physical therapy that consists of manipulating the tissues of the body by the use of friction, stroking, kneading, etc. CARDIAC M. see under CARDIAC; CAROTID ARTERY M. a procedure sometimes used for patients with paroxysmal atrial tachycardia; gentle pressure in small circular motion is applied to one carotid artery for a short period of time.

masseter (mas-sē'-ter): The chief muscle of mastication; situated at the side of the face. It raises the lower jaw.

masseur (ma-ser'): A man who gives massage.

masseuse (mas-sūz'): A woman who gives massage.

mast-, masto-: Combining forms denoting: 1. The breast. 2. The mastoid process.

mastadenoma (mast-ad-e-nō'ma). A benign tumour of the breast.

mastalgia (mas-tal'-ji-a): Pain in the breast.

mastatrophia (mas-ta-trō'-fi-a): Atrophy or shrinking of the breasts.

mast cell: A large, round or ovoid, plump, granulated cell normally found in connective tissues; specific function undetermined; thought to contain heparin, histamine, bradykinin, and serotonin.

mastectomy (mas-tek'-to-mi): Surgical removal of the breast. ADENOMASTECTOMY subcutaneous M.; MODIFIED RADICAL M. one in which part of the pectoralis major or minor is preserved; RADICAL M. removal of the breast with the overlying skin and underlying pectoral muscles, together with the axillary lymph nodes; SIMPLE M. removal of the breast only with the overlying skin; SUBCUTANEOUS M. involves removing all of the breast tissue and usually some of the axilla but leaves the breast skin and sometimes the areola; a silicone prosthesis may be inserted during surgery or later; SUPER RADICAL M. in addition to the procedure of a radical M. the sternum is split and the lymph nodes in the mediastinum are also removed; TOTAL M. removal of the breast and axillary lymph nodes, leaving the pectoral muscles intact.

mastication (mas-ti-kā'-shun): The act of chewing food.

masticatory (mas'-ti-kā-to-ri): Relating to mastication. 1. A medication to be chewed. 2. An agent affecting the muscles of mastication. M. SPASM OF THE FACE trismus (q.v.).

mastitis (mas-tī'-tis): Inflammation of the mammary gland, common in women who are breastfeeding; characterized by fever, chills, lethargy, pain on palpation; usually caused by a staphylococcus. CHRONIC CYSTIC M. the name formerly applied to nodular and cystic changes in the breast, now usually called *fibrocystic disease of the breast*; M. NEONATORUM any of several abnormal conditions of the breast in the newborn, including hypertrophy, inflammation, engorgement with secretion, abscess formation.

mastocarcinoma (mas'-tō-kar-si-nō'-ma): Carcinoma of the breast.

mastocytoma (mas'-tō-sī-tō'-ma): A nodular, circumscribed accumulation of mast cells that resembles a neoplasm.

mastocytosis (mas'-tō-sī-tō'sis): Excessive local or systemic proliferation and accumulation of mast cells in the tissues. The systemic form is marked by urticaria pigmentosa (q.v.) and may involve the spleen, liver, lymph nodes, bones, digestive system.

mastodynia (mas-tō-din'-i-a): Pain in the breast.

mastography (mas-tog'-ra-fi): See MAMMOGRAPHY. — mastographic, adj.

mastoid (mas'-toyd): 1. Nipple-shaped. 2. Relating to the M. process, antrum, cells, etc. M. ANTRUM the air space within the mastoid process, lined by mucous membrane continuous with that of the tympanum and mastoid cells; M. CELLS small intercommunicating cavities in the mastoid process that empty into the mastoid antrum; M. PROCESS the rounded prominence on the mastoid portion of the temporal bone just behind the ear.

mastoidectomy (mas-toy-dek'-to-mi): Drainage of the mastoid air cells and excision of diseased mastoid tissue.

mastoiditis (mas-toy-dī'-tis): Inflammation of any part of the mastoid process; usually the result of an extension of a middle ear infection.

mastoidotomy (mas-toy-dot'-o-mi): Incision into the mastoid process of the temporal bone.

mastoptosis (mas-to-tō'-sis): Sagging or ptosis of the breasts.

masturbation (mas-tur-bā'-shun): Stimulation of the genital organs, manually or by other contact, but not sexual intercourse, usually resulting in orgasm.

maté (ma-tā'): A medication prepared from the dried leaves of a South American tree; contains caffeine and tannins; used as a laxative, tonic, diuretic, and stimulant.

mater (mah'-ter): The Latin word for mother. DURA M. the fibrous outer covering of the brain and spinal cord; PIA M. the vascular delicate membrane that immediately invests the brain and spinal cord. Between it and the dura M. lies the arachnoid (*q.v.*).

materia medica (ma-tē′i-a med′i-ka): The science dealing with the origin, preparation, action, and dosage of drugs.

maternal (ma-ter′-nal): Relating to the female parent.

maternity (ma-ter′-ni-ti): Motherhood.

matriarchy (mā′-tri-ark-i): A social system in which inheritance is traced through the female line; often the family life is dominated by the wife, mother, or other significant female who also has priority in certain other areas such as inheritance of property.

matrix (mā′-triks): The foundation substance in which the tissue cells are embedded. The basic material from which a thing develops.

matter: 1. Any material substance that occupies space and has weight. **2.** Pus; material discharged from a suppurative process. GREY M. found in the cortex of the brain; composed mainly of nerve cell bodies and unmyelinated nerve fibres; INORGANIC M. substances that are not living and never have been; ORGANIC M. substances that are or have been alive; WHITE M., M. composed mainly of myelinated nerve fibres; the conducting tissues of the brain and spinal cord.

maturation (mat ū-rā′shun): The process of attaining full development and maturity. — maturate, v.

mature (ma-tūr′): To be fully developed, or to reach full development; to ripen.

maturity (ma-tūr′-i-ti): The state of completed growth or ripeness.

Maurer's dots: Characteristic coarse reddish dots seen in erythrocytes infected with *Plasmodium falciparum*.

maxilla (mak-sil′-a): The jawbone; in particular the upper jaw. — maxillary, adj.; maxillae, pl.

maxillary (mak′-si-ler-i): Relating to the maxilla. M. SINUS either of a pair of large air cells that form a pyramidal cavity in the maxilla; lined with mucous membrane that is continuous with that of the nasal cavity.

maxillectomy (mak-sil-ek′-tō-mi): Partial or complete removal of the upper jaw.

maxillofacial (mak-sil-ō-fā′shal): Relating to the maxilla and the face. A subdivision in plastic surgery.

maximum (mak′-si-mum): The largest; utmost; the greatest possible size, quantity, value or degree. — maximal, adj.

maze (māz): A labyrinth consisting of blind alleys and one correct path, used in the study of animal and human learning processes.

mazoplasia (mā-zō-plā′-zi-a): Degenerative hyperplasia of the acini of the breast. See ACINI.

MBA: Abbreviation for Master of Business Administration.

McArdle's disease: Glycogen storage disease, Type V; most commonly seen in adults; characterized by pain, fatigability, and stiffness of muscles following exertion.

McBurney's point: A point about one-third of the way between the anterior superior iliac spine and the umbilicus, the site of maximum tenderness in cases of acute appendicitis. [Charles McBurney, American surgeon, 1845–1913.]

McDowell's operation: The operation for removal of an ovarian cyst through an abdominal incision. Named after the surgeon who first performed it in 1809. [Ephraim McDowell, American surgeon, 1771–1830.]

MCH: Abbreviation for mean cell haemoglobin (*q.v.*).

McMurray's test: A test involving rotation of the tibia on the femur; diagnostic for tears in the meniscus of the knee joint.

McNaughten, McNaghten rules: A set of rules established in 1843 for determining the circumstances in which insanity may exempt an individual from legal responsibility for a criminal act.

MCV: Abbreviation for mean cell volume (*q.v.*).

M.D.: Abbreviation for Doctor of Medicine.

MDMA: Abbreviation for methylenedioxymethamphetamine

ME: Abbreviation for myalgic encephalomyelitis, see CHRONIC FATIGUE SYNDROME.

Meals-on-Wheels: A voluntary community service provided for those who cannot do their own cooking in their home.

mean cell haemoglobin: The haemoglobin content of the average cell; the average haemoglobin concentration in a given volume of packed red cells. Also known as *mean corpuscular haemoglobin*; *mean corpuscular haemoglobin concentration*.

mean cell volume: An estimate of the volume of red blood cells; useful for determining the degree of anaemia (*q.v.*).

measles (mē′-zlz): Rubeola. Morbilli. An acute, highly contagious, febrile, exanthematous viral disease; spread by droplets; characterized by fever, a blotchy rash, and catarrhal inflammation of the mucous membranes; associated with a high rate of complications. Endemic and worldwide in distribution. See KOPLIK'S SPOTS and RUBELLA.

meatotomy (mē-a-tot'-o-mi): An operation for enlarging the external urethral opening; sometimes done on infants with hypospadias (q.v.).

meatus (mē-ā'-tus): An opening or channel, usually referring to the external opening of a passageway into or out of the body. AUDITORY M. the external opening into the auditory canal; also called *external acoustic M.*; URINARY M. the external orifice of the urethra; situated at the end of the penis in the male and between the clitoris and the vagina in the female. — meati, pl.

mechanoreceptors (mek'-an-ō-rē-sep'tors): Receptors that are sensitive to differences in pressure, such as those experienced through the sense of touch or hearing.

mechanotherapy (mek'-an-ō-ther'-a-pi): The treatment of disease by the use of various kinds of mechanical apparatus, especially as in physiotherapeutics.

Meckel's diverticulum (mek'-els dī-ver-tik'ū-lum): A blind, pouch-like sac somtimes arising from the free border of the ileum. It may be 5 to 7.5 cm in length and is a remnant of the duct which, in the embryo, connects the yolk sac with the primitive alimentary canal. [Johann Friedrich Meckel, German anatomist and gynaecologist, 1781–1833.]

meconium (mē-kō'-ni-um): The discharge from the bowel of a newly born baby. It is greenish-black, viscid, and contains epithelial cells, mucus, and bile. M. ASPIRATION SYNDROME characterized by severe asphyxia resulting from failure of the lungs to expand at birth because of the presence of aspirated meconium in the trachea or lungs; aspiration of meconium *in utero* is thought to be due to hypoxia. M. ILEUS obstruction in the ileum of the newborn caused by impaction of unusually thick tenacious meconium; may be the earliest sign of cystic fibrosis; also called *meconium plug syndrome.*

MEd: Abbreviation for Master of Education.

media (mē'-di-a): **1.** In anatomy, the middle coat of an artery. **2.** Nutritive jellies used for culturing bacteria. **3.** Plural of medium (q.v.).

mediad (mē'-di-ad): Toward the middle; towards a median line or plane of the body.

medial (mē'-di-al): Relating to or near the middle. — medially, adv.

median (mē'-di-an): The middle. In statistics, the value midway in a distribution of frequencies, that is, half of the observations fall above and half below the median value; M. (or medial) LINE an imaginary line passing through the centre of the body from a point between the eyes to between the closed feet; M. NERVE runs down the inner side and middle of the arm; innervates the flexor muscles of the wrist and hand.

mediastinal (mē'-di-as-tī'-nal): Relating to the mediastinum. M. SHIFT a complication of certain respiratory conditions and of sucking wounds of the chest; because inspired air cannot escape, the intrapleural pressure builds up, the lung collapses, and the heart and great vessels shift to the side of decreased pressure; may lead to shock.

mediastinitis (mē'-di-as-ti-nī'-tis): Inflammation of the mediastinum.

mediastinopericarditis (mē'-di-as-tī'-nō-per'-i-kar-dī'-tis): Inflammation of the pericardium and its surrounding mediastinal tissues.

mediastinoscope (mē'di-as-tī'-no-skōp): An instrument used in direct visual examination of the tissues in the mediastinal area.

mediastinoscopy (mē'di-as-tī-nos'ko-pi): Examination of the mediastinum by means of a tubular instrument which makes it possible to directly view the tissues of the area and to take tissue for biopsy.

mediastinum (mē-di-as-tī-num): The space between the lungs; bounded by the lungs on either side, the sternum in front, the vertebrae at the back, and the diaphragm at the bottom; contains all the organs of the chest except the lungs, *i.e.*, the heart, great vessels, and the oesophagus. — mediastinal, adj.

medical (med'-i-kal): Relating to medicine or the treatment of disease. M. JURISPRUDENCE the application of medical science and facts to legal problems. Forensic medicine.

Medic-Alert: An identification bracelet or necklet worn by persons with medical problems; inscription includes telephone number of a central office that has relevant health information about the person, regarding allergies etc. Medical history is available in emergencies anywhere in the world at any hour. Further information from 12 Bridge Wharf, 156 Caledonian Road, London N1 9UU. Tel: 0207 833 3034. Fax: 0207 278 0647.

medicalization (med'-i-kal-ī-zā'shun): Refers to a health-care system that emphasizes inpatient services and the sick role.

medical laboratory technician: A person who works in a pathological laboratory testing and analysing specimens of body tissue, fluids, or excretions. A medical technologist.

medical model: The framework of assumptions underpinning the relationship between doctor and patient.

medical officer: A doctor in charge of the health services of a civilian or military authority or other organization.

Medical Research Council: A national organization in the UK, funded by the government to promote research into all areas of medical and related sciences.

medical social worker: A health-care professional who is concerned with social aspects of illness; assists patients with many practical problems that may influence their emotional states and affect the course of their illnesses, treatments, and recovery.

medicate (med'i-kāt): 1. To impregnate with a drug or medicine. 2. To treat disease by administering a drug or drugs. — medicated, adj.

medication (med-i-kā'-shun): 1. Administration of a medicine or remedy. 2. A medicinal substance or agent. HYPODERMIC M. one given by hypodermic under the skin; ORAL M. a M. given by mouth; SUBLINGUAL M. one placed under the tongue and allowed to dissolve before it is swallowed.

medicinal (me-dis'-i-nal): 1. Relating to a medicine. 2. Having healing or curing effects or properties.

medicine (med'-i-sin): 1. The science or art of treating or preventing disease. 2. That branch of the healing art that deals with the treatment of disease by the administration of internal remedies as distinguished from such specialties as surgery. 3. A drug. 4. A therapeutic agent.

medicolegal (med'-i-kō-lē'-gal): Term referring to legal problems arising in the practice of medicine; e.g., problems that may be associated with such procedures as therapeutic abortion, or those that may arise in the treatment of minors or mentally incompetent persons.

medionecrosis (mē'-di-ō-ne-krō'-sis): Necrosis of the tunica media of an artery.

meditation: TRANSCENDENTAL M. an exercise in contemplative relaxation that induces changes in physiological functions including lowered metabolic rate, reduced oxygen consumption, decreased cardiac output, and altered brain wave activity, and resulting in a feeling of exaltation and well-being.

Mediterranean fever: See BRUCELLOSIS.

medium (mē'-di-um): A substance used in bacteriology for the growth of organisms. — media, pl.

MEDLARS: Medical Literature Analysis and Retrieval System A computerized system of the National Library of Medicine and part of the National Institutes of Health, Bethesda, USA from which the *Index Medicus* is produced. This is available in the UK in the larger libraries.

MEDLINE: An on-line service that is linked with a computer retrieval system (MEDLARS) that can furnish, in a short period of time, a printout of literature related to health.

medulla (me-dul'a): 1. The marrow in the centre of a long bone. 2. The soft, internal portion of glands, as distinguished from the outer part, as seen in the kidneys, adrenals, lymph nodes, etc. M. OBLONGATA the upper part of the spinal cord between the foramen magnum of the occipital bone and the pons varolii; contains the automatic control centres for breathing, arterial blood pressure, and vomiting. — medullary, adj.

medullary (me-du'-lar-i): Relating to (1) a medulla; (2) bone marrow; or (3) the medulla oblongata. M. CANAL the central cavity of a long bone; contains yellow bone marrow.

medullated (me'-du-lā-ted): Containing or surrounded by a covering or sheath, particularly referring to nerve fibres.

medulloblastoma (med'-u-lō-blas-tō'-ma): A malignant, rapidly growing tumour, seen mostly in children; usually appears in the midline of the cerebellum obstructing the flow of cerebrospinal fluid through the fourth ventricle and producing hydrocephalus.

meg-, mega-, megal-, megalo-: Combining forms denoting great size, powerful, enlarged. MEGA denotes one million units (metric system).

megacolon (meg'-a-kō'-lon): A condition of dilated and elongated colon; most common in males. In an adult the cause is unknown. In a child, the parasympathetic ganglion cells are absent in the distal part of the colon; Hirschsprung's disease (*q.v.*). Also called *congenital m.* and *aganglionic m.*

megakaryocyte (meg'-a-kar'-i-ō-sīt): Giant multinucleated cells in the bone marrow from which the mature blood platelets originate.

megalencephaly (meg'-a-len-kef'-a-li,-sef'-): Having an abnormally enlarged head.

megaloblast (meg'-a-lō-blast): A large, nucleated, primitive red blood cell. — megaloblastic, adj.

megalocardia (meg'-a-lō-kar'-di-a): Cardiomegally (*q.v.*).

megalokaryocyte (meg'a-lō-kar'i-ō-sīt): Megakaryocyte (*q.v.*).

megalomania (meg'-a-lō-mā'ni-a): Delusions of grandeur or self-importance.

megalopsia (meg-a-lop′-si-a): Macropsia (*q.v.*).

megaoesophagus (meg′-a-ē-sof′-a-gus): A markedly dilated or enlarged oesophagus; see ACHALASIA.

megaphonia (meg-a-fō′-ni-a): Abnormal loudness of the voice.

megavitamin (meg-a-vī′-ta-min): Usually refers to a type of therapy characterized by the administration of massive doses of vitamins.

meibomian (mī-bō′-mi-an): M. GLANDS sebaceous glands lying in grooves on the inner surface of the eyelids, their ducts opening on the free margins of the lids; M. CYST chalazion (*q.v.*). [Heinrich Meibom, German anatomist, 1638–1700.]

meiosis (mī-ō′-sis): 1. The division occurring in the last two stages of cell division in the maturation of sex cells when the cell bodies divide twice but the chromosomes are replicated only once, thus halving the number in the mature cells. 2. Constriction of the pupil as a result of contraction of the ciliary muscle. Also spelled *miosis*.

Meissner's corpuscles: Important receptors for the sense of touch; consist of elongated bodies enclosing the terminal ends of several afferent nerve fibres; lie just beneath the epidermis. Most numerous on the finger tips, palms of the hands and soles of the feet, tip of the tongue, and in the skin around the mouth and nipples. Sensitive to light touch and pressure. Also called *Wagner–Meissner corpuscles*.

mel-, melo-: Combining forms denoting: 1. An extremity or limb. 2. Cheek.

melaena (mel′-e-na,me-lē′-na): Dark, tarry stools resulting from the action of intestinal juices on free blood. M. NEONATORUM melaena of the newborn, resulting from the extravasation of blood into the alimentary canal during the first few hours after birth.

melan-, melano-: Combining forms denoting (1) melanin; (2) black, dark.

melancholia (mel-an-kō′-li-a): Extremely unhappy state, usually accompanied by inhibition of mental and physical activity. In psychiatry the term is reserved to mean severe forms of depression. — melancholic, adj. INVOLUTIONAL M. a major affective disorder, chiefly of the middle-aged and elderly; marked by anxiety, agitation, insomnia, feelings of guilt and hypochondria.

melanemesis (mel-a-nem′-e-sis): Black vomit that has been coloured as a result of the action of gastric juices on blood.

melanin (mel′-a-nin): A dark brown or black pigment found normally in hair, skin, choroid and retina of the eye, pia mater, cardiac muscle, and in some tumours. Accounts for racial differences in skin colour.

melanism (mel′-a-nizm): Excessive deposit of pigment in tissues or the skin.

melanization (mel-a-nī-zā′-shun): The formation and deposition of melanin in the body tissues or organs.

melanocarcinoma (mel′-a-nō-kar-si-nō′-ma): A malignant tumour believed to be of epithelial origin. A malignant melanoma (*q.v.*).

melanocyte (mel′a-nō-sīt, me-lan′-): A pigment-containing cell located between the epidermis and dermis; is responsible for the synthesis of melanin and provides for different colours of the skin, as yellow, brown, black.

melanoderma (mel′-a-nō-der′-ma): 1. The appearance of pigmented spots on the skin resulting from deposition of an abnormal amount of melanin. 2. Discoloration of the skin due to the administration of metallic substances such as silver or iron. 3. SENILE M. cutaneous pigmentation as occurs in the aged.

melanoglossia (mel′-a-nō-glos′-i-a): Black tongue. See under TONGUE.

melanoma (mel-a-nō′-ma): A deep-seated tumour occurring usually in individuals over 30; derived from cells that are capable of forming melanin. MALIGNANT M. often starts from a pigmented mole on the skin; also arises in mucous membranes of the mouth, anus, genitalia; has a strong tendency to metastasize; can be fatal if not recognized and treated early. In people with deeply pigmented skin, the toes and soles of the feet are often affected. In older people, should be differentiated from senile lentigo; see under LENTIGO.

melanosarcoma (mel′-a-nō-sar-kō′-ma): One form of malignant melanoma. — melanosarcomata, pl.; melanosarcomatous, adj.

melanosis (mel-a-nō′-sis): A condition characterized by the appearance of dark brown or brownish-black pigmentation in tissues of the body, as in the skin in sunburn or Addison's disease, or around the nipples and elsewhere during pregnancy. — melanotic, adj.

melanuria (mel′-a-nū′-ri-a): The presence of melanin in the urine which causes it to be dark or to turn dark upon standing.

melasma (me-laz′-ma): Any dark, discoloration of the skin, as in Addison's disease.

melatonin (mel′-a-tō′-nin): A hormonal secretion of the pineal gland; is thought to depress gonadal function, to affect the functioning of several other endocrine glands, and to decrease pigmentation of the skin.

meli-: Combining form denoting (1) sweetness; (2) honey.

-melia: Combining form denoting a condition of the limbs.

melioidosis (mē'-li-oy-dō'-sis): An often fatal disease; affects rats and transmissible to humans by the rat flea; occurs in certain parts of Asia and the Far East. The causative organism is *Pseudomonas pseudomallei*.

melitis (me-lī'-tis): Inflammation of the cheek.

meloplasty (mel'-ō-plas-ti): 1. Plastic surgery of the cheek. 2. Plastic surgery of an extremity.

member: An organ or a part of the body, particularly a limb.

membrane (mem'-brā-n): A thin, soft, pliable sheet of tissue that lines a tube or cavity, covers an organ or structure, or divides a space or organ. There are four major types in the body; cutaneous, mucous, serous, synovial. All are protective in function and secrete a fluid. — membranous, adj. BASEMENT M. a thin layer beneath the epithelium of mucous surfaces; CELL M. the thin, semipermeable M. that surrounds the cytoplasm of cells; CROUPOUS M. a yellow-white false M. that forms on the tracheal surfaces in laryngotracheobronchitis; CUTANEOUS M. the skin; DIPHTHERITIC M. a thick, tough fibrinous false M. that forms on mucous surfaces, characteristic of diphtheria; HYALINE M. a thin sheet of material lining the alveoli, alveolar ducts and bronchioles, sometimes found in postmortem examination of infants whose death was due to idiopathic respiratory distress; HYALOID M. that surrounding the vitreous humour of the eye; MUCOUS M. contains glands that secrete mucus. Lines cavities and passages that communicate with the exterior of the body; SEMIPERMEABLE M. one that allows the passage through it of a solvent such as water, but not any of the substances held in solution; SEROUS M. a lubricating M. lining closed cavities, and reflected over their enclosed organs; SYNOVIAL M. that lining the intra-articular parts of bones and ligaments; secretes synovial fluid for lubrication; TYMPANIC M. that which separates the middle ear from the external auditory canal; the ear drum.

memory: The mental faculty of being able to retain and consciously or unconsciously recall or relive that which has been learned or experienced in the past. ANTEROGRADE M., M. for things that occurred in the distant past but not for recent events; PRIMARY M. short-term M. acquired by shallow processing of information; does not last unless rehearsed; RETRO-GRADE M., M. for things that occurred recently but not for those that occurred in the distant past; SECONDARY M. permanent M. acquired by deep processing of information; limitless amounts can be acquired and used, both in the present and the future; SENILE M., M. for events that occurred in the distant past, characteristic of the aged; SHORT-TERM M. primary M.; VISUAL M. the ability to recall visual impressions that are unusually vivid and exact.

men-, meno-: Combining forms denoting menstruation; the menses.

menacme (me-nak'-mi): The period of a woman's life during which menstruation persists.

menadiol (men-a-dī'-ol): A yellow crystalline chemical substance, soluble in vegetable oils; promotes synthesis of prothrombin in conditions characterized by hypoprothrombinaemia; used as a supplement for vitamin K.

menarche (me-nar'-kē): 1. The first menstrual period. 2. When the menstrual periods commence and other bodily changes occur. — menarcheal, adj.

Mendelian (men-dē'-li-an): Relating to Mendel's theory. See MENDEL'S LAW.

Mendel's law: A theory of heredity which deals with the interaction of dominant and recessive characters in crossbreeding. Foundation of the present theory of heredity. [Gregor Johann Mendel, Austrian monk, 1822–1884.]

Mendelson's syndrome: Postoperative chemical pneumonitis due to inhalation of vomited or regurgitated gastric contents; marked by bronchospasm, dyspnoea, cyanosis, pulmonary oedema.

Ménière's disease, syndrome (mān-ē-airz'): A disorder of the membranous labyrinth of the inner ear; occurs in adult life. May accompany such disorders as drug poisoning, blood dyscrasias, circulatory disorders, neuritis or tumour, although the exact cause of the symptoms may be unknown. The most characteristic and disturbing symptoms are sudden dizziness; and tinnitus; nausea, vomiting, and progressive deafness may also occur. [Prosper Ménière, French otologist, 1799–1862.]

mening-, meningi-, meningo-: Combining forms denoting membrane, particularly one of the membranes (meninges) that cover the brain and spinal cord.

meningeal (me-nin'-jē-al): Relating to or affecting the meninges. M. CARCINOMATOSIS infiltration of the leptomeninges by a malignant tumour, *e.g.*, melanoma, medulloblastoma, or leukaemia; M. GLIOMATOSUS proliferation of a glioma into the subarachnoid space; M. SARCOMA a sarcomatous tumour of the meninges, arising in the dura; M. SPACES the space between the dura mater and the arachnoid and that between the arachnoid and the pia mater.

meninges (men-in'-jē-s): Membranes, specifically the three protective and nutritive membranes surrounding the brain and spinal cord: the dura mater (outer); the arachnoid (middle); the pia mater (inner). — meninx, sing.; meningeal, adj.

meningioma (me-nin'-ji-ō'-ma): A slowly growing benign extracerebral encapsulated tumour; arises from the dura but may also occur on the spinal cord, accounts for 15% of all brain tumours, usually occurring after age 30. Tends to remain localized; may cause damage by pressing on the brain and adjacent tissues. Symptoms include headache, seizures, and signs of optic nerve compression. Recurrence after surgical removal is rare.

meningism, meningismus (me-nin'jizm, men-in jiz'mus): Condition presenting with signs and symptoms of meningitis (e.g., neck stiffness) but meningitis does not develop. It may be hysterical in origin; may also result from irritation of the meninges at the onset of acute febrile diseases, particularly in children.

meningitis (men-in-jī'-tis): Inflammation of the meninges. Inflammation of the dura mater is called PACHYMENINGITIS. The arachnoid and pia mater are most commonly affected and the condition is known as LEPTOMENGINITIS. May be caused by any one of several microorganisms, the most common being meningococcus, pneumococcus, streptococcus, and the tubercle bacillus. Presence of the organism in the spinal fluid is diagnostic. Fever, malaise, stiff neck, vomiting, severe headache, stupor, confusion, delirium, convulsions, and unconsciousness are among the symptoms. Sometimes only the cerebral meninges are involved, sometimes only those of the spinal cord, and sometimes both. See LEPTOMENINGITIS. An epidemic form of M. is often called *cerebrospinal fever*; the infecting organism is *Neisseria meningitidis* (meningococcus). ASEPTIC M. most often caused by an enterococcus but also by the various herpes viruses, and by non-viral infections such as syphilis, leptospirosis, and lupus erythematosus; symptoms include headache, nausea, fever, malaise, stiff neck; course is short and usually uncomplicated; BENIGN LYMPHOCYTIC M. viral

M.; MENINGEAL M. the only type of bacterial M. that occurs in epidemic form; PURULENT M., M. that is suppurative; RECURRENT BACTERIAL M. recurring infections in the subarachnoid space; may be associated with a persistent suppurative focus in the skull, ears, or paranasal sinuses, or to lack of immunity to bacterial infections; TUBERCULOUS M. a severe form caused by *Mycobacterium tuberculosis*; VIRAL M. caused by various viruses, including the coxsackieviruses; characterized by fever, malaise, headache, stiff neck, increased number of lymphocytes. Also called *aseptic m.* and *benign lymphocytic m.* — meningitides, pl.; meningitic, adj.

meningocele (me-ning'-gō-sēl): Protrusion of the meninges through a bony defect in the skull or spinal column. It forms a cyst filled with cerebrospinal fluid. See SPINA BIFIDA.

meningococcaemia (me-ning'-gō-kok-sē'-mi-a): The presence of meningococci in the bloodstream. ACUTE FULMINATING M. Waterhouse–Friderichsen syndrome (*q.v.*).

meningococcus (me-ning'-gō-kok'-us): An individual organism of the species *Neisseria meningitidis*. — meningococcal, adj.

meningoencephalitis (me-ning'-gō-en-kef'-a-lī'-tis,-sef'-): Inflammation of the brain and the meninges. May follow such infections as measles, mumps, tularaemia, influenza, and some types of pneumonia.

meningomyelitis (me-ning'-gō-mī'-e-lī'-tis): Inflammation of the spinal cord and its coverings.

meningomyelocele (me-ning-gō-mī'-e-lō-sēl): A malformation that results from failure of the bone and tissues over the dorsal aspect of the spine to develop, allowing a portion of the spinal cord and its enclosing membranes to protrude through the defect; usually occurs in the lumbar area. — Syn., *myelomeningocele*.

meningopathy (men'-ing-gop'-a-thi): Any disease of the meninges of the brain or spinal cord.

meninx (mē'-ninks): 1. The singular of meninges. 2. Any membrane but particularly one of the coverings of the brain and spinal cord.

meniscectomy (men'-i-sek'-to-mi): The removal of a semilunar cartilage, especially from the knee joint, following injury and displacement. The medial cartilage is damaged most commonly.

meniscocytosis (me-nis-kō-sī-tō'-sis): Sickle cell anaemia; see under ANAEMIA.

meniscus (me-nis'-kus): 1. A fibrocartilaginous structure found between the articulating surfaces of some joints. 2. The curved upper surface of a column of liquid; may be concave or convex. DISCOID M. swelling of the lateral M. of the knee joint observed when the knee is slightly fixed; more painful on pressure and during the night; LATERAL M. a crescent-shaped fibrocartilage attached to the lateral superior end of the tibia; MEDIAL M. a crescent-shaped fibrocartilage attached to the medial surface of the superior end of tibia.

menometrorrhagia (men'-ō-met-rō-rā'-ji-a): Heavy bleeding from the uterus at irregular intervals as well as during regular menstrual periods.

menopause (men'-ō-pawz): The permanent cessation of menstruation, occurring normally between the ages of 45 and 50; involves hormonal changes, vascular phenomena, psychological and physical disturbances; characterized by such symptoms as flushing, sweating, headache, dizziness, fatigue, irritability, palpitations, insomnia, vaginal pruritus. ARTIFICIAL M. an earlier menopause induced by surgery or radiotherapy for a pathological condition; NATURAL M. that which occurs spontaneously without any medical or surgical treatment; PREMATURE M. that which occurs before the age of 35–40. — menopausal, adj.

menorrhagia (men-ō-rā'-ji-a): An excessive regular menstrual flow. Syn., *menorrhoea.*

menostasis (me-nos'-ta-sis): Amenorrhoea (*q.v.*).

menses (men'-sēz): The sanguineous fluid discharged from the uterus during menstruation; menstrual flow.

menstrual (men'-stroo-al): Relating to the menses. M. CYCLE the cyclical chain of uterine and ovarian changes that result from hormonal influence and that occur in the time from the beginning of one menstrual period to that of the next; M. EXTRACTION extraction of the products of menstruation, utilizing a soft double-walled cannula that is inserted through the vagina; usually done to avoid the inconvenience of blood flow.

menstruation (men-stroo-ā'-shun): The periodic physiological shedding of blood, secretions, and the functional layer of endometrium from the non-pregnant uterus; occurs at approximately four-week intervals; lasts four–five days; commences at about age 13 and ceases at about age 45. — menstrual, menstrous, adj.

menstruum (men'-stroo-um): 1. Menstrual fluid. 2. A solvent; a solution that contains another solution.

mental: 1. Relating to the chin. 2. Relating to intellect or the mind. M. AGE see under AGE; M. CONFUSION a state characterized by mingling of ideas leading to disturbed comprehension; to be differentiated from senility; M. DISEASE one that affects the mind or intellect; M. HANDICAP failure of or incompetent mental development first recognized in childhood, affects social adjustment and learning skills. Not curable and increasingly considered as a learning disability or disorder; M. HYGIENE the science of maintaining mental health and preventing development of mental disorders such as neuroses and psychoses; M. INCOMPETENCE inability to manage one's own life or affairs; M. TELEPATHY ESP; mind reading; M. TEST one given to determine an individual's mental capacity.

mental disorder: Descriptive of an emotional or behavioural disturbance that is characterized by symptoms that may have their origin in genetic, organic, psychological or psychosocial factors.

mental health: A state of well-being characterized by the absence of mental or behavioural disorder; the condition existing when the individual has made an adjustment satisfactory to himself and the community in regard to his emotional, behavioural, and social reactions. MENTAL HEALTH NURSING, see PSYCHIATRIC NURSING under NURSING.

Mental Health Act (1983): The principal Act governing the treatment of people with mental health problems in England and Wales. It covers all aspects of compulsory admission and subsequent treatment. Other sections of the Act cover situations beside emergencies under which a person can be detained in hospital without his or her consent. The Act is currently under revision. See COMPULSORY POWERS; COMPULSORY TREATMENT.

mentality (men-tal'-i-ti): Mental power or learning ability.

mentation (men-tā'-shun): Mental activity; the process of thinking.

mentor (men'-taw): One who provides an enabling relationship that facilitates another's personal growth and development. The relationship is dynamic, reciprocal and intense. Within such a relationship the mentor assists with career development and guides the mentoree through the organizational, social and political networks of a given profession or occupation.

mentorship (men'-taw-ship): 1. A system of support provided to pre- and post-registration students by more experienced colleagues to facilitate their professional and personal development. **2.** The office or function of a mentor.

mentovertical diameter (men-tō-ver'tik-al): The measurement from the point of the chin to above the posterior fontanelle; it is the presenting diameter in a brow presentation of the fetus.

mentum (men' -tum): The chin.

mephitic (mē-fit' -ik): Noxious; poisonous; foul.

meralgia (mer-al' -ji-a): Pain in the thigh. M. PARAESTHETICA a disorder marked by paraesthesia, tingling, and burning pain over the outer lower aspect of the thigh; due to entrapment of the femoral cutaneous nerve by the inguinal ligament; common in obese women and those who wear tight belts or corsets.

mercurial (mer-kū' -ri-al): Relating to mercury. M. DIURETICS potent diuretic drugs that contain mercury in organic combination.

mercurialism (mer-kū' -ri-al-izm): Chronic poisoning from misuse of mercury as a drug or from industrial exposure to the metal or its fumes. Symptoms include stomatitis with ulceration and sloughing of the mucous membrane of the mouth, salivation, loosening of the teeth, gastroenteritis with griping and diarrhoea, sometimes bloody stools, skin eruptions. In severe cases prognosis is grave.

mercury (mer' -kū-ri): Quicksilver. A heavy metallic element, liquid at ordinary temperatures. M. and its salts formerly much used as purgatives, antisyphilitics, intestinal antiseptics, and astringents. An important medical use is in the manufacture of various types of manometers and thermometers. Symbol is Hg. — mercurial, adj.

merotomy (me-rot' -o-mi): **1.** The sectioning of a cell for the purpose of studying its different segments. **2.** Experimental division of unicellular organisms such as amoebas.

merozoite (mer' -ō-zō' -ite): Any one of the segments resulting from the splitting up of the schizont (q.v.) during the life cycle of the malarial parasite; it is released into the blood where it invades the erythrocytes.

mes-, meso-: Prefix denoting (1) in or towards the middle; (2) an intermediate connecting part; (3) the mesentery or a membrane that supports a specific part.

mesangium (mes-an' -ji-um): The thin suspensory membrane containing sponge fibres that helps to support the capillary loops in the glomerulus.

mesaortitis (mes-a-ōr-tī' -tis): Inflammation of the middle coat of the aorta.

mesarteritis (mes-ar-ter-ī'tis): Inflammation of the middle coat of an artery.

mescaline (mes' -ka-lēn): Peyote. A hallucinogenic agent derived from small tubercles on the mescal cactus, native to Mexico and southwestern USA. Produces hallucinations similar to those produced by LSD.

mesencephalon (mes'en-kef'a-lon, sef-): The midbrain (q.v.).

mesenchyme (mes' -en-kīm): Embryonic connective tissue from which the connective tissue of the body and the vessels of the circulatory and lymphatic systems develop.

mesenteritis (mes'en-te-rī'tis): Inflammation of the mesentery (q.v.).

mesentery (mes'en-ter-i): A large fold of peritoneum that invests the intestines and attaches them to the posterior abdominal wall; it holds the organs in place and carries blood vessels, nerves and lymphatics to them. Usually refers specifically to the fan-shaped fold of peritoneum that encircles the small intestine (particularly the jejunum and the ileum) and attaches it to the posterior abdominal wall.

mesial (mē' -zi-al): Situated at the middle. Toward the midline of the body.

mesioclusion (mē-si-ō-klew' -zhun): A malrelation of the teeth in which the mandible is farther forward than normal, thus causing the lower teeth to be farther forward than in normal occlusion.

mesmerism (mes' -mer-izm): **1.** The induction of hypnosis by the method practised by Mesmer and believed to involve animal magnetism; broadly hypnotism. **2.** Intense fascination. — mesmerize, v. [Franz A. Mesmer, Austrian physician, 1733–1815.]

mesoblast (mes' -ō-blast): The mesoderm, particularly during its early stage of development.

mesocephalic (mes' -ō-ke-fal' -ik,-se-): Having a head of medium length, or an individual with such a head. See MICROCEPHALIC and MACROCEPHALIA.

mesocolon (mes'ō-kō'lon): The fold of peritoneum that attaches the colon to the posterior abdominal wall — mesocolic, adj.

mesoderm (mes'-ō-derm): The middle one of the three primary germ layers of the embryo; from it are developed all connective tissues, bone, muscle, cartilage, circulatory and lymphatic tissues, the lining of serous cavities and of the organs of the genitourinary tract. It lies between the ectoderm and the endoderm (q.v.). — mesodermal, adj.

mesometrium (mes'-ō-mē'-tri-um): The part of the broad ligament that lies below the mesovarium (*q.v.*); it is made up of layers of peritoneum that separate to enclose the uterus, and extends to the lateral wall of the pelvis.

mesomorph (mes'-ō-mōrf): A person whose tissues are derived mostly from mesoderm, *i.e.*, muscle, bone, and connective tissues predominate. A well-proportioned individual.

mesonephros (mes'-ō-nef'-rōs): The excretory organ of the fetus; consists of a long tube in the lower part of the body cavity, parallel to the spinal axis.

mesosalpinx (mes'-ō-sal'-pinks): The upper free part of the broad ligament that is above its attachment to the uterus; it encloses the uterine tube.

mesothelioma (mes'-ō-thē-li-ō'-ma): A rare, painful, progressive tumour originating in the mesothelium (*q.v.*). One type is a rapidly fatal tumour that spreads over the pleural covering of the lung; it has frequently occurred in workers and others who had been exposed to asbestos particles.

mesothelium (mes'-ō-thē'-li-um): The squamous epithelium that develops from the mesoderm (*q.v.*) of the embryo and forms the epithelial layer of membranes that line serous cavities. — peritoneal, pleural, pericardial, and scrotal. — mesothelial, adj.

mesovarium (mes'-ō-vai'-ri-um): The part of the broad ligament that encloses the ovary and holds it in place; it lies between the mesosalpinx (*q.v.*) and the mesometrium (*q.v.*).

mestranol (mes'-tra-nōl): A synthetic oestrogen used in various combinations as an oral contraceptive.

meta-: Prefix denoting: (1) change, transformation in; (2) between, among, after, over, along with.

meta analysis: A quantitative method of combining the results of independent studies (usually drawn from published literature) and synthesizing summaries and conclusions which may be used to evaluate therapeutic effectiveness or to plan new studies.

metabolic (met-a-bol'-ik): Relating to metabolism. BASAL M. RATE (BMR) the figure that expresses the amount of energy (heat) released in the body, based on the amount of oxygen utilized and carbon dioxide produced in a given period of time when the body is at complete rest in a warm atmosphere at least 12 hours after the ingestion of food. See METABOLISM; M. ACIDOSIS see ACIDOSIS; M. alkalosis see ALKALOSIS; M. DISEASE any condition that interferes with metabolism.

metabolism (me-tab'-o-lizm): The sum of physical and chemical changes in the body by which nutrition is effected, energy is provided for life processes, and life is maintained. The tissues are broken down by wear and tear (catabolism) and rebuilt (anabolism) continuously. BASAL M. the energy used by the body at complete rest, being the minimum necessary to maintain life; ERROR OF M. see INBORN ERROR OF METABOLISM. — metabolic, adj.

metabolite (me-tab'-o-līt): Any product of metabolism. ESSENTIAL M. a substance necessary for proper metabolism, *e.g.*, vitamins.

metacarpal (met'-a-kar'-pal): 1. Relating to that part of the hand called the metacarpus (*q.v.*). 2. Any one of the five bones of the metacarpus.

metacarpophalangeal (met'a-kar'pō-fa-lan'jē-al): Relating to the metacarpus and the phalanges.

metacarpus (met-a-kar'-pus): The part of the hand between the wrist and the fingers.

metachromasia (met-a-krō-mā'-zi-a): 1. The taking on of different colours by different elements of a substance when treated with a given stain. 2. A change in colour produced by application of a stain.

metamorphopsia (met'a-mor-fop'si-a): A disturbance of vision in which the shapes of objects seen are distorted; caused by retinal oedema or damage.

metamorphosis (met'-a-mor'-fō-sis): 1. A change in the shape, size, function or structure of a substance. 2. A transition from one stage of development to another.

metamyelocyte (met'-a-mī'-e-lō-sīt): An immature granular leukocyte.

metaphase (met'-a-fāz): The middle stage in mitotic cell division; it is the stage at which the chromosomes are aligned an the equator of the spindle. See MITOSIS.

metaphyseal (met-a-fiz'-ē-al): Relating to a metaphysis. M. CHONDRODYSPLASIA a rare condition in which x-ray photographs show the metaphyses to consist largely of cartilaginous material and to be unevenly calcified. M. DYSOSTOSIS an abnormal condition characterized by defective mineralization of the metaphyseal area of bones, resulting in dwarfism; several types are recognized.

metaphysis (me-taf'-i-sis): That part of a long bone that lies between the shaft (diaphysis) and the extremity (epiphysis). During the growth period it consists of spongy bone; after growth is completed, it is continuous with the epiphysis. — metaphyses, pl.; metaphyseal, adj.

metaplasia (met-a-plā'-zi-a): Conversion of one type of tissue into another, *e.g.*, cartilage into bone. MYELOID M. a condition characterized by splenomegaly, anaemia, the formation of red blood cells outside of the bone marrow, and the presence of immature red and white blood cells in the peripheral blood. — metaplastic, adj.

metapsychology (met'a-sī-kol'ō-ji): That branch of speculative or theoretical psychology that deals with the purpose and structure of the mind, mental processes, the nature of the body–mind relationship, and other hypotheses that cannot be verified by experiment or observation.

metarterioles (met'-ar-tē'-ri-ōls): Small peripheral blood vessels between the arterioles and capillaries.

metastasis (me-tas'-ta-sis): 1. The transference of bacteria or body cells, especially cancer cells, from the original site to another part of the body, usually by blood or lymph, and resulting in development of a similar lesion at the new site. 2. A secondary growth that results from the transference of disease to a site distant from the original lesion. Term is used particularly with reference to malignant growths. — metastases, pl.; metastatic, adj.; metastasize, v.

metatarsal (met'-a-tar'-sal): 1. Relating to that part of the foot called the metatarsus (*q.v.*). 2. Any one of the five bones of the metatarsus.

metatarsalgia (met'-a-tar-sal'-ji-a): Pain in the forefoot due to osteochondrosis of the heads of the metatarsal bones or to a structural abnormality of the foot; causes include arthritis, weakness of foot muscles, ill-fitting shoes; seen most often in older women. Also called *Morton's metatarsalgia, Morton's toe, Morton's neuralgia.*

metatarsophalangeal (met'a-tar'so-fa-lan'jē-al): Relating to the metatarsus and the phalanges.

metatarsus (met'-a-tar'-sus): The five bones that form the skeleton of the foot between the ankle and the toes. M. ABDUCTUS or M. VALGUS a congenital deformity in which the forepart of the foot deviates away from the midline of the body; M. ADDUCTUS a congenital deformity in which the front part of the foot deviates towards the midline of the body; M. ATAVICUS a congenital abnormality in which the first metatarsal is shorter than normal so that it must bear more than the normal amount of weight; M. LATUS a broad spread-out foot; widened forefoot; M. VARUS a congenital de-

formity in which the sole of the foot turns inward and the person walks on the outer border of the foot.

meteorism (mē'-tē-o-rizm): Excessive accumulation of gas in the intestines. Tympanites.

-meter: Combining form denoting relationship to (1) a measurement; (2) an instrument for making a measurement.

meter (mc'-tcr): An apparatus for measuring the quantity of anything passing through it.

methadone treatment: The treatment of a person addicted to a drug, usually heroin, with methadone, a narcotic that is also addicting but less socially disabling than heroin.

methaemoglobin (met-hē-mō-glō'-bin): A form of haemoglobin consisting of a combination of globin with an oxidized haem, containing Fe(III) iron. This pigment is unable to transport oxygen M. may be formed following the administration of a wide variety of drugs, including the sulphonamides. M. may be present in blood as a result of a congenital abnormality.

methaemoglobinaemia (met-he'-mo-glo-bi-ne'-mi-a): Methaemoglobin in the blood. If large quantities are present, individuals may show cyanosis, but otherwise no abnormality except, in severe cases, breathlessness on exertion, because the methaemoglobin cannot transport oxygen. — methaemoglobinaemic, adj.

methaemoglobinuria (met-hē'-mō-glō-bi-nū-ri-a): Methaemoglobin in the urine. — methaemoglobinuric, adj.

methane (meth'-ān): Marsh gas; the colourless, odourless, flammable gas that is given off by decomposing organic matter.

methanol (meth'-a-nōl): Methyl alcohol; see under ALCOHOL.

methicillin-resistant *Staphylococcus aureus*: A bacterium that is resistant to antibiotics.

methionine (me-thī'-o-nēn): One of the sulphur-containing amino acids; essential for growth in infants and for maintenance of nitrogen equilibrium in adults. Occasionally used therapeutically in hepatitis and other conditions associated with liver damage.

method: The manner of performing any act; a procedure. RHYTHM M. a method of contraception that involves abstinence from sexual intercourse during the period of the menstrual cycle when ovulation is most likely to occur.

methodology (meth-o-dol'-ō-ji): 1. A set of principles and methods that govern or regulate a discipline. 2. The principles and procedures involved in a study in a particular area.

methyl alcohol: Wood alcohol. See ALCOHOL.

methylene blue (meth'-i-lēn): A basic dye used in histological and microbiological studies. Used in medicine as a urinary antiseptic and as an antidote for cyanide poisoning. Also used as an antidote for methaemoglobinaemia. M. B. TEST may be (1) a test for renal function; (2) a test for the presence of vitamin C; or (3) a test for the presence of bilirubin in the urine.

methylenedioxymethamphetamine: A centrally active phenethylamine derivative related to amphetamine and methamphetamine.

methylprednisolone (meth'-il-pred-nis'-ō-lōn): An adrenocortical steroid that has the actions and uses of prednisolone (*q.v.*).

metopic (mē-top'ik): Relating to or relating to the forehead.

metra-, metro-: Combining forms denoting the uterus.

metralgia (mē-tral'-ji-a): Pain in the uterus; metrodynia.

metratrophia (mē-tra-trō'fi-a): Atrophy of the uterus.

metre (mē'-ter): The basic unit of length in the metric system.

-metria: A combining form denoting condition of the uterus.

metric system: A system of weights and measures, invented and first used in France in the late 18th century. Now used in most countries. Employs a decimal scale. The unit of weight is the gram, of length is the metre and of capacity is the litre.

metritis (mē-trī'-tis): Inflammation of the uterus.

metrocele (mē'-trō-sēl): Hernia of the uterus.

metrocolpocele (mē'trō-kol'-pō-sēl): A hernia of the uterus into the vagina; prolapse of the uterus.

metrodynia (mē-trō-din'-i-a): Pain in the uterus.

metrofibroma (mē'-trō-fī-brō'-ma): A fibroma of the uterus.

metropathia haemorrhagica (mē-trō-path'-i-ahem-or-aj'-ik-a): Irregular episodes of uterine bleeding due to excessive and unopposed oestrogen (*q.v.*) in the bloodstream. Usually associated with a follicular cyst in the ovary.

metropathy (mē-trop'-a-thi): Any disorder of the uterus.

metroptosis (mē'trō-tō'sis): Prolapse of the uterus.

metrorrhagia (mē-trō-ra'ji-a): Uterine bleeding between the menstrual periods.

metrorrhexis (mē-tro-rek'-sis): Rupture of the uterus.

mg: Abbreviation for milligram.

MI: Abbreviation for myocardial infarction, see under MYOCARDIAL.

micelles (mi-sel'-lez): Small, spherical, water soluble structures formed by the aggregation of bile salt molecules during digestion of lipids; they diffuse into the epithelial cells of the small intestine where they are concerned with the synthesis of phospholipids and protein and the absorption of fat and cholesterol.

Michel's clips (mi'-shels): Small metal clips used instead of sutures for the closure of a wound.

micr-, micro-: Combining forms denoting (1) small or minute size or amount; (2) abnormal smallness, *e.g.*, microcephalia; (3) instruments or objects used in dealing with minute objects, *e.g.*, microscope, microtome; (4) one millionth part (metric system).

micrencephaly (mī'kren-kef'-a-li-sef-): Abnormal smallness of the brain. — micrencephalic, adj. Also *micrencephalia, microencephaly.*

microaerophil(e) (mī'-krō-ai-er-ō-fil): An aerobic organism that grows best in an atmosphere with an oxygen content lower than that of the air. — microaerophilic, adj.

microanalysis (mī'krō-nal'i-sis): The analysis of minute quantities of material.

microanatomy (mī'krō-a-nat'o-mi): Histology (*q.v.*).

microaneurysm (mī'krō-an'ū-rizm): An aneurysm occurring in a capillary; often seen in diabetic retinopathy and in thrombotic purpura. See RETINOPATHY and PURPURA.

microbe (mī'-krōb): A microscopic unicellular organism, especially one capable of causing disease. Syn., *microorganism.* — microbial, microbic, adj.

microbicide (mī-krō'-bi-sīd): An agent that destroys microbes. — microbicidal, adj.

microbiologist (mī'-krō-bī-ol'-o-jist): A person who specializes in the study of microbes.

microbiology (mī'krō-bī-ol'o-ji): The branch of biology that is concerned with the study and science of microbes. DIAGNOSTIC M. is concerned with tests done to aid in diagnosis and in prescribing medications, and to check for freedom from pathogenic microorganisms.

microbiosis (mī'-krō-bī-ō'-sis): 1. Shortness of life. 2. The condition of being infected with microbes.

microbrachia (mī-krō-brā'ki-a): A congenital anomaly consisting of abnormal shortness of the arms.

microcephalic (mī-krō-kef-al'-ik,-sef-): 1. Relating to an abnormally small head. 2. An individual with an abnormally small head.

microcephalus (mī-krō-kef'-a-lus, -sef-): An individual with an abnormally small or imperfectly formed head.

microcephaly (mī-krō-kef′-a-li,- sef-): Abnormal smallness of the head. — microcephalic, adj.

microcirculation (mī′-krō-sir-kū-lā′-shun): Circulation in the smallest of the blood vessels, that is, the arterioles, capillaries, and venules.

Micrococcus (mī′krō-kok′-us): A genus of saprophytic Gram-positive spherical bacteria occurring in irregular masses. They comprise saprophytes, parasites, and pathogens.

microcolorimeter (mī′-krō-kol-o-rim′-i-ter): A colorimeter used for examining small blood samples.

microcornea (mī′krō-kor′-ni-a): An unusually thin flat cornea; usually bilateral and often associated with other inherited or developmental anomalies or disorders of the eye.

microcyte (mī′-krō-sīt): An undersized red blood cell found in anaemic blood. — microcytic, adj.

microcythaemia (mī′krō-sī-thē′mi-a): The presence of abnormally small erythrocytes in the blood.

microcytosis (mī-krō-sī-tō′-sis): A blood condition characterized by the presence of large numbers of microcytes (*q.v.*).

microdactylia (mī′-krō-dak-til′-i-a): Abnormal smallness of the fingers and toes.

microdissection (mī′-krō-di-sek′-shun): Dissection of cells or tissues under the microscope.

microdrip (mī′-krō-drip): An apparatus for delivering intravenous solutions by small drops; refers particularly to the administration of small amounts of solution slowly. See MACRO-DRIP.

microembolus (mī-krō-em′bō-lus): A embolus of microscopic size. — microembolism, n.

microgenitalia (mī′krō-jen-i-tā′li-a): The condition of having unusually small genitalia, particularly external genitalia.

microgram: One thousandth of a milligram; one millionth of a gram. Represented by the symbol μg.

microgyrus (mī-krō-jī′ rus): An unusually small convolution of the brain.

microlens (mī-krō-lens): A small thin corneal contact lens.

microlipoinjection (mī′-krō-lī′-pō-in-jek′-shun): A procedure whereby fat tissue is suctioned by needle from one part of the body and injected into the tissues of the face or other part of the body. M. corrects the deep skin furrows caused by ageing; also used to raise depressed areas of scars caused by surgery or injury.

microlithiasis (mī′-krō-li-thī′-a-sis): The formation of multiple small concretions or stones in an organ.

micrometer (mī-krom′-i-ter): An instrument for measuring objects being viewed under the microscope.

micron (mī′-kron): **1.** A metric unit of length equal to one millionth of a metre. **2.** (In physical chemistry), a colloidal particle with a diameter of between 0.2 and 10 microns.

micronodular (mī-krō-nod′ū-lar): Marked by the presence of small nodules; often said of the liver.

micronystagmus (mī′krō-nī-stag′mus): Very fine movements of the eye, normally present at all times.

microorganism (mī′krō-or′gan-izm): A microscopic cell. Often synonymous with bacterium but includes virus, protozoon, rickettsia, fungus, algae, and lichen.

microphage (mī′-krō-fāj): A very small phagocyte (*q.v.*).

microphallus (mī-krō-fal′-us): An abnormally small penis; also called *micropenis*.

microphobia (mī-krō-fō′-bi-a): **1.** Morbid dread of microbes. **2.** Morbid dread of small things.

microphotograph (mī-krō-fō′tō-graf): A small photograph of a microscopic object; usually magnified for viewing and interpreting.

microphysics (mī-krō-fiz′-iks): That branch of physics that deals with molecules, atoms, and elementary particles of matter.

microplasia (mī-krō-plā′-zi-a): Dwarfism.

micropsia (mī-krop′-si-a): A pathological condition in which objects appear to be smaller than they actually are. Micropia. — microptic, adj.

microsaccades (mī′-krō-sa-ka′-dez): Imperceptible jerks of the eye that occur during fixation.

microscope (mī′-krō-skōp): An instrument consisting of a lens or an arrangement of lenses for making enlarged images of minute cells or objects. BINOCULAR M. one that has two eyepieces; COMPOUND M. one that has two lens systems; DARK FIELD M. a M. modified to permit lateral lighting; ELECTRON M. one in which an electric beam causes an image to be projected on a fluorescent screen, where it may be viewed or photographed; SIMPLE M. one that has only one lens; a magnifying glass. Many special types of microscopes are available including those that utilize infrared and ultraviolet radiation, x-rays, ultrasound, laser beam, television, and scanning techniques. See also MICROSURGERY.

microscopic (mī-krō-skop′ik). Extremely small; visible only with the aid of a microscope.

microscopy (mī-kros'-ko-pi): Examination by means of a microscope.

microspherocytosis (mī'-krō-sfē-rō-sī-tō'-sis): A condition in which most of the red blood cells are more round and smaller than usual; seen in haemolytic icterus.

Microsporum (mī-kros'-pō-rum): A genus of fungi that causes various superficial cutaneous infections; it is parasitic, living in the keratin-containing tissues of humans and animals. M. AUDOUINII the commonest cause of scalp ringworm (tinea tonsurans) in children; M. CANIS the species of M. that causes dermatophytosis (q.v.) in children and adults; usually contracted from infected cats or dogs.

microsurgery (mī-kro-ser'-jer-i): Dissection, or the performance of surgery, under a high-powered microscope capable of magnifying nerves and blood vessels up to 40 times, using specially developed miniature instruments; the microscope is often hooked up to television screens so that other members of the operating team can see what the surgeon is doing. — microsurgical, adj.

microthrombus (mī-krō-throm'bus): A small thrombus located in a capillary or other small vessel.

microtia (mī-krō'-shi-a): The condition of having ears with exceptionally small pinnae but which are of normal shape.

microtome (mī'-krō-tōm): An instrument for making thin sections of tissue for microscopic study.

microvilli (mī-krō-vil'lī): Microscopic processes on the surface of a cell, which increase the area available for absorption of nutrients or for excretion; found particularly in the cells of the proximal renal tubule and the intestinal epithelium.

microwave (mī-krō-wāv): An electromagnetic wave of very short length and high frequency.

micturate (mik'-tū-rāt): To void or pass urine (v.).

micturating urethrogram: An x-ray photograph of the bladder after injection of a radio-opaque substance; taken when the patient is at rest and while actually voiding.

micturition (mik-tū-rish'-un): The act of passing urine. M. SYNCOPE syncope following rapid emptying of a distended bladder; results from sudden drop in blood pressure; may be associated with postural hypotension, but may also occur in otherwise healthy persons.

midaxillary line (mid-ak'-si-lar-i): An anatomical landmark consisting of an imaginary line drawn vertically on the surface of the body from the apex of the axilla, dividing the body into an anterior and a posterior portion.

midbrain: The mesencephalon, that short portion of the brain stem that lies just above the pons and just below the cerebrum; it connects the cerebrum with the pons and the cerebellum and is involved in motor coordination.

midclavicular line (mid-kla-vik'-ū-lar): An anatomical landmark consisting of an imaginary line drawn vertically on the surface of the body from the outer end of the clavicle through the centre of the nipple.

middle age: Commonly considered to be the years between 40 or 45 and 60, but usually defined by psychosocial rather than physiological events and changes.

middle ear: The space on the medial side of the tympanic membrane; connects with the mastoid cells and the auditory tube; contains the auditory ossicles. See OSSICLE.

middle ear disease: A condition common in the elderly; starts with a feeling of fullness in the ear and general discomfort; may be a sign of developing nasopharyngeal cancer, lymphoma, or leukaemia.

midget (mij'-et): An individual who is smaller than normal, but whose organs and parts are perfectly formed.

midgut (mid'-gut): The region between the foregut and the hindgut in the developing embryo.

midline (mid'-līn): An imaginary line that divides the body into right and left halves.

midriff (mid'-rif): 1. The diaphragm (q.v.). 2. The middle region of the human torso, particularly the front external aspect.

midsternal line: An anatomical landmark consisting of a vertical line drawn from the cricoid cartilage through the sternum to the xiphoid process.

midstream specimen: See CLEAN-CATCH SPECIMEN.

midwife (mid'-wīf): A specialist health professional who is qualified to give total care to a woman and her baby during pregnancy, labour and after the birth.

midwifery (mid'-wif-ri): The practice of delivering babies or of assisting women in childbirth.

migraine (mī'-grān): Hemicrania. A syndrome characterized by recurring throbbing headache, usually bilateral. Symptoms include photophobia, phonophobia, nausea, vomiting. More common in women than men; often there is a family history of M. dietary factors and emotional stress may contribute but the cause is not fully understood; when severe may result in incapacitation. CLASSIC M. of three types: (1) MUSCLE CONTRACTION M. formerly called *tension headache*; differs from vascular M. in that the pain is occipital, dull, aching, and bilateral; (2) TRACTION AND INFLAMMATORY M. caused by some disease or disorder of the skull contents; and (3) VASCULAR M. the most common type of M. due to depression and conversion reactions; two classes are identified: (a) HEMIPLEGIC M. in which there is slight paralysis of one side of the body; may occur two or three times a day and last for about 45 minutes; and (b) OPHTHALMOPLEGIC M. recurrent vascular headache that occurs periodically on one side only; characterized by transient oculomotor palsy (see under PALSY).

migrainous (mī'-gran-us): Relating to or resembling migraine. M. NEURALGIA characterized by attacks of severe pain over the eye and forehead, with fever, rhinorrhoea, and lacrimation, tending to occur in clusters and lasting from 15 to 30 minutes; also called *cluster headache*, histamine cephalalgia, and Horton's headache. See HEADACHE.

migration (mī-grā'-shun). In physiology, the passage of leukocytes through the walls of vessels into tissue spaces in order to combat organisms that have invaded tissues.

Mikulicz's disease or syndrome (mik'-ū-lichs): Chronic hypertrophic enlargement of the lacrimal and salivary glands; of unknown aetiology, but sometimes occurs as a syndrome in association with certain other diseases such as leukaemia or lymphosarcoma. [Mikulicz-Radecki, Romanian surgeon, 1850–1905.]

milia (mil'i-a): Whiteheads. Tiny white epidermal cysts appearing usually over the face, nose, upper eyelids and neck, and sometimes over the chest; due to blocked pilosebaceous glands. M. NEONATORUM M. occurring in the newborn, thought to be due to blocked hair follicles and sweat glands; the whiteheads are filled with keratinous material and disappear without specific treatment.

miliaria (mil-i-ār'i-a): An inflammatory skin condition characterized by vesicular and erythematous eruption caused by blocking of sweat ducts and their subsequent rupture, or their infection by bacteria or fungi. Often accompanied by burning, itching, prickling sensation. Common in the tropics. Also called *heat rash, prickly heat, summer rash, wildfire rash, strophulus*.

miliary (mil'-i-er-i): Resembling a millet seed. M. TUBERCULOSIS a form in which minute tu-

berculous nodules are widely disseminated throughout the organs and tissues of the body.

milieu (mil-yu'): Environment; surroundings. M. THERAPY treatment, usually psychiatric, in a carefully structured environment in which all elements such as furnishings, equipment, staff, etc., enhance the medical therapy, encourage acceptable and responsible behaviour, and help the patient towards rehabilitation.

milium (mil'-i-um): A small pearly epidermal cyst, thought to be due to a blocked pilosebaceous gland. Usually referred to in the plural, milia. Whitehead.

milk: The liquid nourishment secreted by female mammals from the mammary glands. Milk is a basic food, containing most of the nutrients necessary for the early stages of growth and development. The constituents of breast milk, particularly fat levels, vary according to the time of day and even during a feed.

milk line: In anatomy, an imaginary line extending from the axilla to the groin; so called because extra nipples sometimes develop at points along the line.

milk sugar: Lactose (*q.v.*).

milk teeth: The first set of teeth.

Miller–Abbott tube: A double-lumen rubber tube with an inflatable balloon at the distal end; used in diagnosis and treatment of obstructive lesions of the small intestine.

Miller–Kurzrok test: A test to determine the ability of the sperm to penetrate the mucous plug normally present in the cervix of the uterus.

milli-: Prefix denoting one thousandth part of the root to which it is affixed (metric system).

milliampere (mA) (mil'li-am'pair): One thousandth of an ampere.

millicurie (mCi, mc) (mil'li-kū'rē): The unit of radioactivity used to determine dosage; one thousandth of a curie.

milliequivalent (mEq) (mil'li-i-qwiv'-a-lent): Term used to express the concentration of a substance in a litre of solution; the number of grams of a solvent in one millilitre of normal solution.

milligram (mg) (mil'li-gram): One thousandth of a gram.

milligrams-percent (mg%): In biochemistry, milligrams of a substance in 100 millilitres of solution.

millilitre (ml) (mil'li-lē-ter): One thousandth of a litre; in liquid measure, equivalent to a cubic centimetre.

millimetre (mm) (mil-li-mē'ter): One thousandth of a metre.

millimicron (mμ) (mil-li-mī'kron): One thousandth of a micron (*q.v.*).

millimole (mM) (mil'i-mōl): One thousandth of a mol.

millirad (mil' -li-rad): One thousandth of a rad. A measurement of a unit of absorbed radiation dose.

millisecond (ms, msec) (mil'li-sek-ond): One thousandth of a second.

millivolt (mV) (mil'li-volt): One thousandth of a volt.

Milroy's disease: Congenital lymphoedema. Hereditary lymphoedema of the legs caused by chronic obstruction of lymphatic vessels; may also affect other parts of the body.

Milwaukee brace: A splint used for children; it extends from the back of the head to the hips and maintains extension of the spine from fixed points on the pelvis, chin, and occiput; longitudinal struts are utilized in such a way that they can be lengthened as the child grows; used in treatment of scoliosis, lordosis, kyphosis, and requires careful fitting.

mimesis (mi-mē'sis): 1. Mimicry. 2. The appearance of symptoms of one disease in a person with another, different, disease.

-mimetic Combining form denoting the ability of a drug to mimic the action of the autonomic nervous system.

MIND: National Association for Mental Health; www.mind.org.uk

mineralocorticoid (min'er-al-ō-kor'ti-koyd): A secretion of the adrenal cortex that affects the fluid and electrolyte balance of the body, chiefly through its influence on sodium retention and potassium loss from the body. See ALDOSTERONE.

miner's anaemia: See HOOKWORM DISEASE.

miner's elbow: Inflammation of the olecranon bursa over the point of the elbow; caused by leaning on the elbow; also called *student's elbow*.

Minerva jacket or brace: A cast that covers the head, with cutouts for the face and ears, and reaching to the hips; used in cases of cervical and/or thoracic vertebral fracture.

minilaparotomy (min'i-lap-a-rot'o-mi): A sterilization procedure for women that can be done under local anaesthesia; consists of ligation of the uterine tubes through a small suprapubic incision.

minimal brain dysfunction syndrome: Usually occurs in children with some functional disorder of the central nervous system; the child is of near average intelligence but may have difficulty with language and memory and con-

trolling his emotions and impulses. Occurs more often in boys than girls; may be caused by peri-natal or post-natal disease or injury, genetic factors, or pathological biochemical conditions. Also called *hyperkinesis, hyperkinetic syndrome*, attention deficit hyperactivity disorder (*q.v.*).

minimum lethal dose: The smallest dose of a medication or drug that will cause death.

minor: 1. In surgery, an operation that can be done under local anaesthesia and in which the risk of death and the death rate are negligible. 2. A person under full legal age.

minute respiratory volume: The total amount of air breathed in during one minute.

miosis (mī-ō'sis): Contraction of the pupil of the eye.

miotic (mī-ot'ik): 1. Relating to or producing miosis. 2. A medication that causes constriction of the pupil.

mirror writing: Backward writing that resembles ordinary writing as reflected in a mirror.

misalignment (mis-a-līn'ment): The condition of being out of line or improperly adjusted.

misanthropy (mis-an'thro-pi): Hatred, distrust of, or contempt for mankind. — misanthrope, n.; misanthropic, adj.

miscarriage (mis-kar'ij): Expulsion of the fetus before it is viable, *i.e.*, before the 24th week.

misce: A term used in prescription writing; means to mix.

miscegenation (mis'e-je-nā'shun): Intermarriage or cohabitation between persons of different races.

misdiagnosis (mis'diag-nō'sis): An incorrect diagnosis.

miso-: Combining form denoting hatred of.

misogyny (mi-soj'e-ni): Hatred of women.

misopaedia (mis-ō-pē'di-a): Hatred of children.

mission statement: A formal summary of the aims, general principles and values of an organization.

Misuse of Drugs Act (1971): Legislation for the control of manufacture, distribution and possession of potentially addictive drugs. Controlled drugs include natural opiates and their synthetic substitutes, many stimulants and hallucinogens. These drugs are available on medical prescription only. Severe penalties may be incurred following conviction for the illegal sale or supply of any of these controlled drugs. Amended on 17 January 2001 to include rescheduling of certain drugs.

mit-, mito-: Combining forms denoting: 1. Thread or thread-like. 2. Mitosis.

mite (mīt): A minute arthropod, related to the spiders, that is parasitic on humans and that produces various skin irritations. Some mites are intermediary hosts for certain pathogenic organisms, *e.g.*, that causing scrub typhus.

mitochondria (mī'tō-kon'dri-a): Organelles in the cytoplasm of cells, disclosed by differential staining; in the presence of oxygen they convert nutrients into carbon dioxide and water and during this process adenosine triphosphate is formed. — mitochondrion, sing.

mitosis (mī-tō'sis): A complicated method of division occurring in cells; usually consists of a series of stages. — prophase, metaphase, anaphase and telophase. — mitotic, adj.

mitral (mī'tral): 1. Mitre-shaped. 2. The biscuspid valve between the left atrium and left ventricle of the heart. M. INCOMPETENCE a defect in the closure of the mitral valve, whereby blood tends to flow backward into the left atrium when the valve is closed; M. MURMUR a murmur produced at the mitral valve orifice; M. STENOSIS narrowing of the mitral orifice, usually done to the formation of fibrous tissue as a result of rheumatic fever; M. VALVE a valve with two flaps, located in the septum between the left atrium and left ventricle; it allows blood to flow from the atrium into the ventricle and prevents backflow into the atrium. Also called *bicuspid v.* and *atrioventricular valve*; M. VALVULOTOMY the operation of splitting the cusps of a stenosed mitral valve.

mittelschmerz (mit'-el-shmertz): Pain or discomfort in the lower abdomen experienced by some women midway in the intermenstrual interval; thought to be the result of irritation of the pelvic peritoneum caused by the escaping fluid or blood from the ovarian follicle.

mixture (miks'tūr): A combination of two or more substances, usually in liquid form, with each substance retaining its particular physical characteristics.

mmHg: Symbol for millimetres of mercury.

mmol: Symbol for millimole.

MMR: Abbreviation for measles, mumps, and rubella vaccine.

Mobile Coronary Care Unit: A specially equipped vehicle, available on an emergency basis, manned by personnel trained to detect heart failure, carry out cardiopulmonary resuscitation at the site of the attack, and to transfer the patient safely to a hospital.

mobility (mō-bil'-i-ti): The ability to move or be moved.

mobilization (mō'-bi-li-za'shun): The process by which a fixed part is made movable, or

motion is restored to an ankylosed joint. STAPES M. surgery to correct immobility of the stapes; has been used in treating certain types of deafness.

Mobitz heart block, types **I** and **II**. See under HEART BLOCK.

modality (mō-dal'-i-ti): A method of applying or using a therapeutic agent or procedure.

model: A simplified representation of a phenomenon, with fundamental properties that are explicitly defined and from which other properties can be observed or deduced.

modernism: Twentieth-century movement in art, architecture, design and literature that, in general, concentrates on space and form, rather than content or ornamentation.

Modernization Agency: A government department that supports health and social care agencies in their efforts to deliver improvements in their services. It helps to identify some of the best-performing organizations, rewarding them with more power to make decisions at a local level and assists where services are poor or failing.

modiolus (mō-dī'-ō-lus): The central, bony pillar of the cochlea, around which the spiral canal winds.

modus (mō'-dus): Manner. M. OPERANDI a way of performing an operation or of working.

moiety (moy'-i-ti): 1. A portion or part of a molecule that has a characteristic pharmacological or chemical effect. 2. One of two equal parts into which something is divided.

mol (mōl): Abbreviation for mole (*q.v.*).

molality (mo-lal'-i-ti): The concentration of a solution expressed as mols per 1000 grams of solvent.

molar (mo'-lar): 1. The double teeth or grinders; three on either side of the jaw. 2. A solution containing one mole of solute per litre of solution.

molarity (mō-lar'-i-ti): The concentration of a solution expressed in gram molecular weight of solute per litre of solution.

mole (mōl): The molecular weight in grams of a compound or the atomic weight in grams of an element. See GRAM MOLECULE.

mole (mōl): Lay term for a naevus; a circumscribed, pigmented, elevated area on the skin. CARNEOUS M. the dead and organized remains of a fetus that has died *in utero*; HYDATIDIFORM M. a condition in which the chorionic villi of the placenta undergo cystic degeneration and the fetus is absorbed; may be a harmless condition safely corrected, but a proportion of these moles are active and if remnants are left in the uterus after abortion of the mole, malignant changes may ensue, giving rise to a chorionepithelioma (*q.v.*).

molecular (mo-lek′-ū-lar): Relating to a molecule. M. BIOLOGY the branch of biology that deals with the function and structure of the molecular constituents of biological systems and their physical and chemical roles in living tissues; M. CLOCK HYPOTHESIS the assumption that senescence and death are the final steps in a programme that begins with the development of the embryo.

molecule (mol′-e′-kūl): The smallest particle into which matter can be divided and still retain its identity. — molecular, adj.

mollities (mol-ish′-i-ēz): Softness. Malacia.

molluscum (mō-lus′-kum): A soft tumour. M. CONTAGIOSUM a mildly contagious type of wart that appears especially on the face, buttocks, and perineum as a waxy papule, often umbilicated; spread is by autoinoculation; M. FIBROSUM the superficial tumours of Recklinghausen's disease.

mon-, mono-: Combining forms denoting (1) involving, having, or affecting a single element or part; (2) restricted to one. In chemistry, denotes combination with one atom.

monarticular (mon′-ar-tik′-ū-lar): Relating to or affecting only one joint.

monaural (mon-aw′-ral): 1. Relating to one ear. 2. One ear functioning alone. 3. Hearing with one ear.

monilial vaginitis (mō-nil′-i-al vaj-in-ī′-tis): Candidiasis (*q.v.*).

moniliasis (mō-ni-lī′-a-sis): Candidiasis (*q.v.*.). ORAL M. *Candida* infection of the mouth; seen in the very young and the very old; also called *thrush* (*q.v.*).

moniliform (mo-nil′-i-form): Like a string of beads; beaded. Used to describe the arrangement of microorganisms, or such manifestations as skin rash.

monitor (mon′-i-tor): 1. To watch, observe, or check constantly on a state or condition. 2. An electronic apparatus that is attached to the patient and automatically records on a screen such physical signs as respiration, pulse, and blood pressure; may be employed in caring for an anaesthetized person who is undergoing or recuperating from surgery or other procedure.

monitoring (mon′-i-tor-ing): The continuous or periodic observing, reporting and/or controlling of certain physiological, biochemical, or bacterial processes, activities, or conditions. INVASIVE M. involves instrumental penetration of the body, *e.g.*, central venous monitoring;

NONINVASIVE M. is based on observations, *e.g.*, blood pressure, pulse rate, respiratory rate.

monoamine (mon-ō-am′-ēn): An amine compound that contains only one amine group. See AMINES.

monoamine oxidase (mon-ō-am′-ēn oks′-i-dās): An enzyme present in most tissue cells; its function is to act as a catalyst in the deamination of certain monoamines such as adrenaline and serotonin. MAO INHIBITOR any drug or chemical that inhibits the action of monoamine oxidase with the result that the amines normally acted on by the enzyme accumulate in the body. Drugs in this class are sometimes used as psychic energizers in the treatment of fairly severe depression, but under close medical supervision because of their side effects and incompatibilities with certain other drugs and foods.

monoblast (mon′-ō-blast): A large immature monocyte.

monoblepsia (mon-ō-blep′-si-a): 1. A condition of vision in which one is able to see better with only one eye than with two. 2. Colour blindness in which all colours appear to be the same.

monochromatic (mon′ō-krō-mat′ik): 1. Existing in one colour only. 2. Staining with only one dye at a time. 3. A person who exhibits monochromatism (*q.v.*).

monochromatism (mon′ō-krō′ma-tizm): Complete colour blindness; all colours appear as shades of grey. A rare disorder.

monoclonal (mon-ō-klō′-nal): Relating to a single group of cells, or a clone, involving an identical cell product.

monococcus (mon-ō-kok′-us): A coccus that occurs singly, not in pairs, chains, or groups.

monocular (mon-ok′-ū-lar): Relating to or affecting one eye only.

monocyte (mon′-ō-sīt): A large mononuclear leukocyte. The monocytes are phagocytic; they make up about 5% of the total white blood cell count.

monocytopenia (mon′ō-sī-tō-pē′ni-a): Less than the normal number of monocytes in the circulating blood.

monocytosis (mon′-ō-sī-tō′-sis): An abnormal increase in the proportion of leukocytes in the circulating blood.

monogenesis (mon-ō-jen′-e-sis): Non-sexual reproduction.

monoideism (mon-ō-ī-dē′-izm): Inability to stop talking or thinking about a certain idea or group of ideas; a degree of monomania.

monomania (mon′ō-mā′ni-a): Obsessed with a single idea or group of ideas.

monomer (mon'ō-mer): A simple molecule that is capable of combining with other similar or unlike molecules to form a polymer.

mononeuritis (mon'-ō-nū-rī'-tis): Neuritis affecting only one nerve. See NEURITIS.

mononeuropathy (mon'-ō-nū-rop'a-thi): A condition in which pain and weakness develop suddenly in the areas of distribution of one or two nerves; usually occurs in the leg with the femoral or sciatic nerve being involved; may be seen in diabetics and in cases of herniated vertebral disc. CRANIAL M. a disease involving one of the cranial nerves.

mononuclear (mon'-ō-nū'-klē-ar): With a single nucleus. Usually refers to the largest type of blood cell, characterized by a round or oval shape and idented nucleus. Monocyte.

mononucleosis (mon'-ō-nū-klē-ō'-sis): An increase in the number of circulating monocytes (mononuclear cells) in the blood. INFECTIOUS M. is an acute infectious type of M. caused by a virus; characterized by sudden onset, fever, malaise, sore throat, enlargement of lymph nodes and spleen. Occurs most frequently between the ages of 20 and 30 and is usually self-limited and benign.

monoparesis (mon'-ō-par-ē'-sis): Weakness of the muscles of one arm or one leg.

monophasia (mon'ō-fā'zi-a): Aphasia in which the individual is able to utter only one word or phrase and repeats it constantly.

monoplegia (mon-ō-plē'-ji-a): Paralysis of only one limb, or of one muscle or group of muscles. — monoplegic, adj.

monorchidism (mon-or'-ki-dizm): Having only one testis, or the condition of only one testis having descended into the scrotum. Monorchism.

monosaccharide (mon-ō-sak'-a-rīd): A simple sugar ($C_6H_{12}O_6$). Examples are glucose, fructose, and galactose.

monosexual (mon-ō-seks'-ū-al): Having the characteristics of only one sex.

monosodium glutamate (mon-ō-sō'-di-um glū'-ta-māt): A salt of glutamic acid; used as a food additive for flavouring and also in the treatment of encephalopathy associated with liver disease.

monotrichous (mo-not'-ri-kus): Having a single flagellum at one end; said of a bacterial cell.

monovular (mon-ov'-ū-lar): Relating to a single ovum; or derived from a single ovum, as identical twins.

monoxide (mon-ok'-sīd): An oxide in which the molecules have only one atom of oxygen.

Commonly used by the general public to mean carbon monoxide.

monozygotic (mon'ō-zī-got'ik): Referring to twins that develop from the same fertilized ovum, *i.e.*, identical twins.

mons veneris (mons ven'-er-is): The eminence formed by the pad of fat that lies over the symphysis pubis in the female. Also called *mons pubis*.

Montgomery's tubercles: Name given to the sebaceous glands on the areola of the breast when they become enlarged during pregnancy.

mood: A prevailing attitude or state of mind. In psychiatry, a sustained emotional state such as melancholia or mania.

moon face: The rounded full face that is characteristic of hyperadrenocorticism, see CUSHING'S SYNDROME.

Moore pin: A metal pin used in hip surgery.

morbid (mor'-bid): 1. Diseased. Relating to, affected by, or productive of disease. 2. Grisly or gruesome. M. ANATOMY that branch of anatomy that is concerned with the study of diseased tissues and organs.

morbidity (mor-bid'-i-ti): 1. The state of being sick or diseased. 2. The incidence of disease. 3. The sick rate; the ratio of sick persons or of cases of disease to the number of well persons in a specified geographic area during a specific period of time.

morbific (mor-bif'-ik): Causing disease; pathogenic.

morbilli (mor-bil'ī): Measles (*q.v.*).

morbilliform (mor-bil'-i-form): Descriptive of a rash resembling that of measles.

morbus (mor'-bus): Disease.

mordant (mor'-dant): In microbiology, a substance used to fix a dye or stain.

mores (maw'-rēz): The fixed values and customs of a particular group. Habits; manners; moral code.

morgue (morg): A place where bodies of the deceased are placed temporarily until they are identified or claimed for burial.

moribund (mor'-i-bund): Dying; having no vital force left.

morning-after pill: A contraceptive pill that is taken after sexual intercourse, usually the next morning. It blocks the formation of corpus luteum following ovulation and presumably prevents implantation of the fertilized ovum. Has been used after rape, or incest, or when there is undue anxiety about the possibility of pregnancy.

morning sickness: Nausea and vomiting when arising in the morning, especially that which occurs during the first 4 to 16 weeks of pregnancy. Occurs in about 50% of pregnant women.

Moro reflex: See under REFLEX.

morph-, morpho-: Combining forms denoting form, shape, type, structure.

-morph,-morphous: Combining forms denoting shape, form.

morphea (mor' -fē-a): Localized scleroderma; see under SCLERODERMA.

morphine (mor' -fēn): The active principle of opium and a valuable opioid hypnotic, and analgesic. Habit-forming.

morphinism (mor' -fin-izm): Addiction to morphine.

morphogenesis (mor' -fō-jen' -e-sis): The morphological changes, including growth and cell differentiation, during human development.

morphology (mor-fol' -o-ji): The science that deals with the form and structure of living things, regarded as a whole, and apart from their function. — morphological, adj.; morphologically, adv.

morphometry (mor-fom' -e-tri): Measurement of the forms of organisms.—morphometric, adj.

mortal: 1. Fatal; causing or resulting in death. **2.** Human.

mortality (mor-tal' -i-ti): **1.** The quality of being mortal (*q.v.*). **2.** The death rate; the number of deaths in a unit of population occurring within a prescribed time. Mortality rates for deaths from all causes are usually expressed as number of deaths per 1000 population. INFANT M. RATE the number of deaths during the first year of life per 1000 live births for the year; MATERNAL M. RATE the number of deaths due to pregnancy or childbearing per 1000 registered births per year; PERINATAL M. RATE the number of stillbirths and babies that die during the first week of life per 1000 registered births in a year.

Mortenson's syndrome: Haemorrhagic thrombocythaemia; a blood disorder characterized by increased thrombocytic count, prolonged bleeding time, haemoptysis, easy bruising, and enlarged spleen; may occur in association with leukaemia or polycythaemia, or following splenectomy.

mortification (mor' -ti-fi-kā' -shun): Local death of tissue. See GANGRENE.

Morton's syndrome or neuralgia: A painful condition in which congenital shortness of the first metatarsal causes hypertrophy and pain in the second metatarsal; the pain is caused by irritation of the nerve between the heads of the

metatarsals. If the nerve becomes thickened and hypertrophied, the condition is referred to as MORTON'S NEUROMA. See METATARSALGIA.

morula (mor' -ū-la): In embryonic development, the solid mass that results from cleavage of a fertilized ovum; consists of blastomeres (*q.v.*).

mosaicism (mō-zā' -i-sizm): The presence of cells with differing genetic make-up in the same individual.

Mosenthal test: (mō' -zen-tahl): A kidney function test involving measuring the variability of the specific gravity of the urine over 24 hours.

mosquito (mo-skē' -tō): A large family of blood-sucking arthropods, several varieties of which are carriers or vectors of infectious disease.

mother complex: Oedipus complex (*q.v.*).

motile (mō' -til): Capable of spontaneous movement. — motility, n.

motion sickness: Nausea and usually vomiting due to stimulation of the semicircular canals caused by the irregular or rhythmic motion of an aeroplane, car or boat, or by swinging.

motivation (mō-ti-vā' -shun): Drive; incentive; need; attitude and expectation that results in action.

motor: Relating to (1) action or motion; or (2) a muscle, nerve, or centre that is concerned with motion. See NEURON. M. APHASIA see under APHASIA; M. APRAXIA ideomotor apraxia (*q.v.*); M. AREA the area in the cerebral cortex that controls the contraction of voluntary muscles.

motor end plate: A specialized structure at the terminus of a motor nerve fibre where it makes functional contact with a muscle fibre.

motor fibres: Nerve fibres that are responsible for voluntary movement; consist of (1) pyramidal fibres that originate in the cortex of the brain, cross in the medulla oblongata, descend in the pyramidal tract of the spinal cord and end in roots that enervate skeletal muscles; and (2) extrapyramidal fibres that originate in the brain stem and descend in close association with the pyramidal fibres.

motor neuron, upper and lower: See under NEURON.

motor point: A point on the skin over a muscle where the application of an electric current will cause the muscle to contract.

motor unit: An anatomical unit consisting of an anterior horn cell, its axon with all of its branches, the motor end plates, and the muscle fibres that are innervated.

mottling (mot' -ling): Spotty discoloration of the skin without a distinct pattern; patches have varying sizes, shapes, and depth of colour.

mould (mōld): 1. Multicellular fungus; a member of the plant kingdom with no division into root, stem, or leaf, and without chlorophyll. Structurally consists of hyphae which aggregate into a mass of cobwebby filaments called a mycelium. Propagation is by means of spores. Occurs in infinite variety, commonly as saprophytes contaminating foodstuffs, and more rarely as pathogens. 2. The process of changing the shape of something, referring particularly to the change in shape of the fetal head to accommodate to the birth canal. 3. A shaped receptacle into which a malleable substance is poured or placed, in making a cast.

moulding (mōl′-ding): The shaping of the fetal head in adjustment to the shape and size of the birth canal during the passage of the fetus through the canal in labour.

mountain: M. FEVER see ROCKY MOUNTAIN SPOTTED FEVER; M. SICKNESS symptoms of sickness, dyspnoea, and tachycardia; due to low oxygen content of rarefied air at high altitudes.

mourning: See BEREAVEMENT.

mouth: An aperture or opening into a cavity; specifically the opening through which food passes into the body.

mouth sticks: Sticks of varying lengths that are held in the mouth and can be manipulated by handicapped persons, e.g., quadriplegics, to assist in such activities as typing, drawing, using keypads, etc.

movement: 1. Motion; the act of moving. 2. The act of emptying the colon; defecation. 3. The material evacuated from the rectum during one bowel movement; the stool.

MPhil: Abbreviation for Master of Philosophy.

MRC: Abbreviation for Medical Research Council (q.v.).

MREC: Abbreviation for Multi Research Ethics Committee (q.v.).

MRI: Abbreviation for magnetic resonance imaging (q.v.).

MRSA: Abbreviation for methicillin-resistant *Staphylococcus aureus* (q.v.).

MRV: Abbreviation for minute respiratory volume (q.v.).

MS: Abbreviation for multiple sclerosis, see under SCLEROSIS.

MSc: Abbreviation for Master of Science.

MSU: Abbreviation for midstream specimen of urine, see CLEAN-CATCH SPECIMEN.

mucin (mū′-sin): A mixture of mucopolysaccharides found in or secreted by many cells and glands. The chief constituent of mucus. — mucinous, adj.

mucobuccal (mū-kō-buk′-al): Relating to the mucous lining of the mouth and cheek.

mucocele (mū′-kō-sēl): 1. Distention of a cavity with mucus. 2. A cyst or cyst-like structure that contains mucus.

mucocutaneous (mū-kō-kū-tā′nē-us): Relating to mucous membrane and skin.

mucoid (mū′-koyd): Resembling mucus.

mucolysis (mū-kol′-i-sis): Dissolution or liquefaction of mucus. — mucolytic, adj.

mucolytic (mū-kō-lit′-ik): 1. Capable of destroying or dissolving mucus. 2. An agent that liquefies or dissolves mucus.

mucopolysaccharide (mū′-kō-pol-i-sak′-a-rīd): A polysaccharide widely distributed in nature; a complex material that makes up the amorphous substance in the intercellular material in the body.

mucopolysaccharidosis (mū′kō-pol-i-sak′a-ri-dō′sis): An inherited disorder of mucopolysaccharide metabolism; characterized by mental handicap, skeletal deformities, clouding of the cornea, and the secretion of mucopolysaccharides in the urine. Several types are identified on the basis of findings, including *Hurler's syndrome, Hunter's syndrome, Morquio's syndrome, Sanfilippo's syndrome,* and *Scheie's syndrome.*

mucoproteins (mū′kō-prō′tē-ins): Glycoproteins (q.v.) that often have a lubricating function.

mucopurulent (mū′kō-pū′roo-lent): Containing mucus and pus.

mucopus (mū-kō-pus): Mucus containing pus.

Mucor (mū′-kor): A genus of moulds that are frequently found on dead or decaying vegetable matter; some of them are pathogenic to man.

Mucorales (mū-kor-ā′-lez): An order of fungi, including the bread moulds; the majority are saprophytic; the cause of mucormycosis, which is often a complication of debilitating disease, diabetes in particular. See MUCORMYCOSIS.

mucormycosis (mū′-kor-mī-kō′-sis): An acute, usually fulminating, infection by a fungus of the Mucorales order; usually accompanies a systemic disorder such as diabetes, lymphoma, or leukaemia; often starts in the respiratory tract and metastasizes to other parts of the body, including the skin, brain, and gastrointestinal tract.

mucorrhoea (mū-kō-rē′-a): An increase in the discharge of mucus from the cervix at the time of ovulation; usually continues for three to four days and has the general appearance of egg white. See SPINNBARKEIT.

mucosa (mū-kō′-sa): A mucous membrane; see under MEMBRANE. — mucosal, adj.; mucosae, pl.

mucosanguineous (mū′-kō-sang-gwin′-ē-us): Composed of both mucus and blood.

mucositis (mū-kō-sī′-tis): Inflammation of a mucous membrane.

mucous (mū′-kus): Relating to, secreting, or containing mucus. See MEMBRANE. M. COLITIS mucomembranous colitis; possibly a functional disorder, manifested by passage of mucus in the stool, obstinate constipation and occasional colic; M. POLYPUS condition in which the mucous membrane becomes pedunculated and projects from the surface in polypoid masses.

mucoviscidosis (mū′kō-vis′-i-dō′sis): A congenital hereditary disease with failure of development of normal mucus-secreting glands, sweat glands and pancreas. May be present in a newborn as meconium ileus; in infancy with septic bronchitis and steatorrhoea. Stools contain excess fat; trypsin is absent from stool and duodenal juice. See CYSTIC FIBROSIS.

mucus (mū′-kus): The viscid fluid secreted by the mucous glands. Contains mucin and such other substances as inorganic salts, epithelial cells, leukocytes, and water. Serves as a protective lubricant coating.

Müllerian ducts (mool-ē′-ri-an): Embryonic structures from which the urinary system develops; in the female, the origin also of the uterine tubes, uterus, and most of the vaginal canal.

multi-: Combining form denoting (1) multiple, many, much; (2) affecting many parts.

multi-agency working: A collaborative approach to the provision of services for specific patient groups which involves workers from a range of agencies. See INTER-DISCIPLINARY; INTER-PROFESSIONAL.

multiarticular (mul′-ti-ar-tik′ū-lar): Relating to or affecting several joints.

multicellular (mul-ti-sel′-ū-lar): Constructed of many cells.

multi-disciplinary: Combining or involving several separate academic disciplines. M. TEAM professionals and providers from different specialties who work together to provide services to an individual or group.

multifocal (mul-ti-fō′-kal): Arising from, relating to, or having several foci.

multiform (mul′-ti-form): Having many forms or shapes.

multiglandular (mul-ti-glan′-dū-lar): Relating to or affecting several glands.

multigravida (mul-ti-grav′-i-da): A woman who has been pregnant more than once. — multigravidae, pl.

multilobar (mul-ti-lō′-bar): Possessing several lobes.

multilobular (mul-ti-lob′-ū-lar): Possessing many lobules.

multilocular (mul-ti-lok′-ū-lar): Possessing many small cysts, loculi or pockets.

multinuclear (mul-ti-nū′-klē-ar): Possessing many nuclei. — multinucleate, adj.

multipara (mul-tip′-a-ra): A woman who is having or has had two or more pregnancies resulting in viable children. Written Para II, III, etc. GRANDE M. name given to a woman who has had seven or more children. — multiparae, pl.; multiparous, adj.

multiparity (mul-ti-par′-i-ti): 1. The production of more than one child in the same gestation. 2. The condition of being a multipara (*q.v.*).

multiple sclerosis: See SCLEROSIS.

multi-professional education: A process in which people from different professional backgrounds learn together.

Multi Research Ethics Committee: A group including both lay people and medical practitioners, set up to monitor research that involves the use of human subjects. It is responsible for ensuring that subjects are adequately informed of the procedures involved in a research project.

multi-variant analysis: A statistical method involving the comparison of several variables.

multivitamin (mul-ti-vi-ta-min): Relating to a preparation that contains several vitamins, especially those considered to be essential to life and health.

mummification (mum-i-fi-kā′-shun): 1. Dry gangrene. 2. The drying up of a dead fetus in the uterus.

mumps: Infectious parotitis; an acute, infectious disease, communicable and statutorily notifiable, characterized by inflammation of one or both parotid (*q.v.*) glands; caused by a filterable virus. The chief symptom is a sensitive swelling below and in front of the ear and oedema of the surrounding tissues, distorting the features. The most common complication in the adult male is orchitis; in the female, ovaritis and mastitis. Syn., *epidemic parotitis*.

Münchausen's syndrome (muntsh′-how-zenz): A condition characterized by repeated presentations with fictitious symptoms and an untrue history; these individuals often produce symptoms by various means and willingly undergo any suggested treatment or tests to get attention or, sometimes, drugs. M.'s BY PROXY a paediatric situation in which a parent (usually the mother) or other adult responsible for a young child provides details of an imaginary illness leading to unnecessary medical interventions and treatment in which fatal outcomes have been reported. Overlaps with other forms of child and self-abuse.

mural (mū'-ral): Relating to or occurring in the wall of a cavity, organ or vessel.

muriatic acid (mū-ri-at'ik as'id): Hydrochloric acid (*q.v.*).

murmur (mur'-mur): An abnormal, usually soft, blowing sound, but may be rasping, harsh, or musical, caused by vibration produced by the turbulent flow of blood between two pressure areas and/or within the heart or the adjacent great vessels; not necessarily significant. AORTIC M. one heard at the aortic orifice of the heart; may be regurgitant or obstructive; DIASTOLIC M. one that occurs during ventricular diastole and may be classified as (1) regurgitant, a high-pitched long M. or (2) filling, a low-pitched rumbling M.; FUNCTIONAL OR INNOCENT M. one commonly heard in young children; not associated with a heart lesion; MILLWHEEL M. a churning M. produced by air embolism to the heart; MITRAL M. one heard at the mitral valve, due to obstruction or regurgitation; ORGANIC M. a M. caused by an organic lesion; PRESYSTOLIC M. one that occurs just before the systole and is usually due to stenosis of one of the atrioventricular orifices; PULMONARY M. a M. heard at the pulmonary orifice of the heart; may be due to obstruction or regurgitation; SYSTOLIC M. an abnormal quality of the first heart sound, usually related to the area of one of the heart valves, *e.g.*, systolic mitral murmur; may be classified as (1) SYSTOLIC EJECTION M. produced by the blood moving over the pneumonic and aortic valves, heard early in systole at the base of the heart, and in older people without signs of heart disease; or (2) REGURGITANT M. heard when there is backflow from ventricles to atria through a septal defect. Systolic M. may also be pansystolic or holosystolic, lasting throughout the entire phase of systole.

Murphy's sign: A sign of gall bladder disease when the patient cannot take a deep breath while the physicians fingers are pressed deeply beneath the right costal margin.

muscae volitantes (mus'-kē vol-i-tan'-tēz): The sensation of moving spots before the eyes. Caused by the presence of cells or cell fragments in the vitreous humour. See FLOATERS.

muscarine (mus'ka-rēn): A deadly alkaloid found in certain mushrooms and certain rotten fish.

muscle (mus'-el): Strong, contractile tissue that produces movement of the body. Depending on structure, muscle tissue is classified as striated (striped), non-striated (smooth), and indistinctly striated. Also classified according to whether it is voluntary (under conscious control) or involuntary (under control of the autonomic nervous system). Characteristics of muscle tissue are contractility, excitability, extensibility, and elasticity. CARDIAC M. forms the walls of the heart, is indistinctly striated and involuntary; SKELETAL M. surrounds the skeleton, is striated and voluntary; VISCERAL M. (internal) is non-striated (except for the heart) and involuntary. — muscular, adj.

muscle-bound: Having some of one's muscles enlarged, tense, and lacking in elasticity; usually due to over exercise.

muscle cramp: A sudden, involuntary, painful contraction of a skeletal muscle.

muscul-, musculo-; Combining forms denoting muscle, muscular.

muscular (mus'-kū-lar) 1. Relating to muscle or muscles. 2. Descriptive of an individual with well-developed muscles.

muscular dystrophy: See under DYSTROPHY.

musculature (mus'-kū-la-tūr): The muscular system of the body or part of it.

musculocutaneous (mus'-kū-lō-kū-tā-nē-us): Relating to both muscle and skin.

musculomembranous (mus'-kū-lō-mem'-bra-nus): Relating to both muscle and membrane. Descriptive of such muscles as the occipitofrontalis, which is largely membranous.

musculoskeletal (mus'-kū-lō-skel'-e-tal): Relating to the muscular and skeletal systems.

musculotendinous (mus'-kū-lō-ten'-di-nus): Relating to or composed of muscle and tendon.

musculotrophia (mus'-kū-lō-trō'-fi-a): Having an affinity for or affecting chiefly muscular tissue.

musicomania (mū'-zi-kō-mā'-ni-a): An insane preoccupation with music.

musicotherapy (mū'-zi-kō-ther'-a-pi): Music therapy. The use of music in treatment of disease, especially mental disorders.

Musset's sign (moo'-sāz): Subtle, rhythmic up and down movements of the head in synchronization with the heartbeat; seen in cases of aortic aneurysm and aortic insufficiency. Also called *de Musset's sign*.

mussitation (mus-i-tā'-shun): Movement of the lips without producing any sound; sometimes seen in delirious patients.

mustard: The powdered seed of a plant of the genus *Brassica*; has been used in medicine as an emetic and rubefacient. M. GAS a poisonous gas used in warfare; it causes vesication and corrosion of the skin and mucous membranes; is particularly damaging to the membranes of the respiratory system; NITROGEN M.S mustard compounds that have been used therapeutically in treatment of certain cancers.

mutagen (mū'-ta-jen): A physical or chemical agent that is capable of causing a heritable alteration in the deoxyribonucleic acid (*q.v.*), which induces a genetic mutation, *e.g.*, drugs, ultraviolet light, ionizing radiation.

mutagenesis (mū'-ta-jen'e-sis): The production of genetic change.

mutagenic (mū-ta-jen'-ik): Capable of causing genetic mutations. — mutagenicity, n.

mutant (mū'-tant): A cell that is the result of a genetic change. It has characteristics that are different from those of the parent cells and that can be passed on to the offspring.

mutation (mū-tā'-shun): 1. A transformation or change in form, quality, or some other characteristic. 2. A genetic change in the germ plasm of a cell which results in a change of the characters of the cell. This change is heritable, remaining until further mutation occurs. INDUCED M. a gene mutation produced by a known agent outside the cell, *e.g.*, ultraviolet radiation; NATURAL M. a gene mutation taking place without apparent influence from outside the cell.

mute (mūt): 1. Unable to speak. 2. A person who is unable to speak. DEAF M. a term used formerly for a person who is unable to speak or to hear, now called '*deaf without speech*'.

mutilate (mū'ti-lāt): To maim or disfigure the body by removing, destroying, or deforming some essential and conspicuous part. — mutilation, n.

mutilation (mū-ti-lā'shun): 1. The destruction or removal of a body part. 2. The loss of an important part of the body with consequent disfigurement.

mutism (mū'tizm): Dumbness; speechlessness. In psychiatry, refusal or inability to speak. May be conscious or unconscious, organic or functional. AKINETIC M. a type of M. in which the person makes no bodily or other response to sound.

mutualism (mū'tū-a-lizm): Symbiosis. Equally beneficial interactions between organisms, *e.g.*, between humans and certain bacteria.

my-, myo-: Combining forms denoting relationship to muscle.

myalgia (mī-al'ji-a): Pain in the muscles. — myalgic, adj.

myalgic encephalomyelitis (mī-al'jik en-kef-a-lo'-mī-e-lī'tis): See CHRONIC FATIGUE SYNDROME.

myasthenia (mī'as-thē'ni-a): Muscular weakness. M. GRAVIS a progressive disorder, seen mostly in adults, chiefly women, 20 to 50 years of age; characterized by marked fatigability of voluntary muscles, especially those of the face, lip, tongue, throat and neck, and eye. The patient has a characteristic sleepy expression due to ptosis of the eyelids and weakness of the facial muscles. Results from lack of acetylcholine or excess of cholinesterase at the myoneural junction.

myasthenic syndrome (mī-as-then'ik): Weakness of the limb girdle muscles; often associated with cancer, particularly of the lung; to be distinguished from myasthenia gravis, which it resembles.

myatonia (mī-a-tō'ni-a): Absence of tone in muscle. M. CONGENITA a form of congential muscular dystrophy in infancy. Child is unable to bear the weight of the head on the shoulders. — myatonic, adj.

myatrophy (mī-at'-rō-fi): Atrophy of muscle.

myc-, myceto-, myco-: Combining forms denoting fungus.

mycelium (mī-sē'li-um): The tangled mass of branching filaments (hyphae) that represents the body of a mould or fungus. — mycelial, mycelian, mycelioid, adj.

mycetoma (mī-si-tō'ma): A fungal infection, usually of the feet, occurring in tropical and subtropical regions. Similar to actinomycosis and aspergillosis. Syn., *Madura foot, maduromycosis*.

Mycobacterium (mī-kō-bak-tēr'i-um): Small slender rod bacteria, Gram-positive and acid-fast, both to a varying degree. Saprophytic, commensal, and pathogenic species. *M. BALNEI,* the cause of 'swimming pool' granuloma; see GRANULOMA; *M. BOVIS* the bovine variety of the tubercle bacillus; causes bovine tuberculosis, which may be acquired by humans, usually through infected milk. *M. LEPRAE* the cause of leprosy; *M. TUBERCULOSIS* the cause of tuberculosis.

mycology (mī-kol'o-ji): The study of fungi. — mycologist, n.; mycological, adj.; mycologically, adv.

Mycoplasma (mī'kō-plaz-ma): A genus of microorganisms intermediate in size between viruses and bacteria; includes the pleuropneumonia-like organisms; important in respiratory diseases. One type is associated with acute leukaemia. *M. HOMINIS* found in genital and rectal mucosa; associated with non-gonococcal urethritis; *M. ORALE* found in human saliva; *M. PNEUMONLAE* the cause of primary atypical pneumonia; also called *Eaton agent*; *M. SALIVARIUM* found in human saliva and the upper respiratory tract. — mycoplasmal, mycoplasmic, adj.

mycoplasmosis (mī'kō-plaz-mō'sis): Infection with *Mycoplasma* (*q.v.*).

mycoprotein (mī-kō-prō'te-in): The protein in fungi or bacteria.

mycopus (mī-kō'pus): Mucus that contains pus.

mycosis (mī-kō'sis): Any disease caused by a fungus; may be superficial, affecting only the skin, or systemic. M. FUNGOIDES a rare, chronic, usually fatal skin malignancy; characterized by pruritus and psoriasis-like dermatitis, followed by skin abscesses; in the late stages it spreads to the lymph nodes and the viscera resulting in the development of large painful tumours that ulcerate; seen most often in adult males and the elderly.

mydriasis (mi-drī'a-sis): Abnormal dilatation of the pupil.

mydriatics (mid-ri-at'iks): Drugs that cause mydriasis (*q.v.*).

myectomy (mī-ek'to-mi): Surgical removal of part of a muscle.

myel-, myelo-: Combining forms denoting: 1. Bone marrow. 2. Spinal cord.

myelencephalitis (mī'el-en-kef-a-lī'tis, -sef-): Inflammation of the brain and spinal cord.

myelencephalon (mī'el-en-kef'a-lōn,-sef-): The lower part of the embryonic hindbrain; it develops into the medulla oblongata.

myelic (mī-el'ik): Relating to: 1. Bone marrow. 2. The spinal cord.

myelin (mī'e-lin): The white, fatty substance constituting the medullary sheath of certain nerve fibres.

myelinization (mī'e-li-nī-zā'shun): The accumulation or supplying of myelin during the process of nerve development or repair.

myelinolysis (mī'e-lin-ol'i-sis): Disintegration of myelin. — myelinotic, adj.

myelinosis (mī'e-li-nō'sis): Necrosis or decomposition of fat, with the formation of myelin.

myelitis (mī-e-lī'tis): Inflammation of (1) the spinal cord; (2) bone marrow. TRANSVERSE M., M. that extends across the spinal cord.

myeloblast (mī'e-lō-blast): An immature cell in the bone marrow which develops into a granular leukocyte.

myeloblastoma (mī'e-lō-blas-tō'ma): A fairly well circumscribed malignant tumour consisting of a mass of myeloblasts (*q.v.*).

myeloblastosis (mī'e-lō-blast-tō'sis): Abnormally large number of myeloblasts in the blood or in the tissues, sometimes seen in acute leukaemia.

myelocele (mī'e-lō-sēl): A form of spina bifida (*q.v.*); the development of the spinal cord itself has been arrested, and the central canal of the cord opens on the skin surface, discharging cerebrospinal fluid. Incompatible with life.

myelocystomeningocele (mī'e-lō-sis'tō-mening'gō-sēl): A congenital anomaly in which a cystic tumour composed of spinal cord and meningeal tissues protrudes through a defect in the bony spinal column. Also called *meningomyelocele*.

myelocyte (mī'e-lō-sīt): 1. An immature bone marrow cell of the type from which leukocytes develop. Present in blood in some pathological conditions, *e.g.*, leukaemia. 2. Any cell in the grey matter (*q.v.*).

myelodysplasia (mī'e-lō-dis-plā'zi-a): Defective development of the spinal cord, occurs most often in the lumbosacral region — myelodysplastic, adj.

myeloencephalitis (mī'e-lō-en-kef a-lī'tis, -sef-): Acute inflammation of the brain and spinal cord. EPIDEMIC M. acute anterior poliomyelitis (*q.v.*).

myelofibrosis (mī'e-lō-fī-brō'sis): Excessive growth of bone marrow.

myelogenesis (mī'e-lō-jen'e-sis): Myelinization (*q.v.*).

myelogenous (mī-e-loj'e-nus): 1. Produced in or by the bone marrow. 2. Myelogenic.

myelogram (mī'e-lō-gram): An x-ray of the spine after injection of a radiopaque substance into the subarachnoid space. AIR M. a M. in which air or oxygen is injected into the subarachnoid space instead of a radiopaque substance.

myelography (mī-e-log'ra-fi): Visualization of the spinal cord after the injection of a contrast medium into the subarachnoid space. GAS M. radiographic examination of the spinal cord following the injection of gas into the subarachnoid space. — myelographic, adj.; myelographically, adv.

myeloid (mī'e-loyd): 1. Relating to or derived from bone marrow. 2. Relating to the spinal cord.

myeloma (mī-e-lō'ma): 1. A tumour of the medullary canal. 2. A tumour containing cells of the type normally found in the bone marrow.

MULTIPLE M. a primary tumour of bone marrow; usually malignant; associated with hyperplasia of the bone marrow, Bence Jones protein in the urine, neuralgic pain, sometimes spontaneous fracture; bone pain in the back or hip is the usual complaint; occurs most often in the elderly.

myelomalacia (mī'e-lō-ma-lā'shi-a): Softening of the spinal cord.

myelomatosis (mī'e-lō-ma-tō'sis): Multiple myeloma (q.v.).

myelomeningocele (mī'e-lō-me-ning'gō-sēl): Meningomyelocele (q.v.).

myelopathy (mī-e-lop'a-thi): Any disease or pathological change in the spinal cord.

myelophthisis (mī-e-lof'thi-sis): 1. Atrophy or wasting of the spinal cord. 2. A pathological condition in which the blood-cell forming tissues of the bone marrow are displaced by fibrous or bony tissue, resulting in anaemia that is characterized by the presence of immature granulocytes in the blood (myelopathic anaemia).

myelopoiesis (mī-e-lō-poy-ē'sis): The formation of bone marrow, or of the cells that arise in the bone marrow.

myeloproliferation (mī'e-lō-prō-lif-er-ā'shun): Proliferation of one or more elements of the bone marrow without other signs of neoplasia. — myeloproliferative, adj.

myelosclerosis (mī'e-lō-skle-rō'sis): Multiple sclerosis of the spinal cord. See SCLEROSIS.

myelosis (mī-e-lō'sis): 1. The development and presence of a tumour on the spinal cord. 2. A bone marrow condition characterized by proliferation of the tissue, or cellular elements resulting in changes in the blood, as seen in myelocytic leukaemia. ERYTHREMIC M. a malignant blood condition associated with anaemia, enlarged liver and spleen, haemorrhagic tendencies and the presence in the blood of erythrocytes in all stages of development, including megaloblasts.

myelotomy (mī'e-lot'o-mi): A surgical procedure in which nerve tracts in the spinal cord are severed.

myelotoxic (mī'e-lō-tok-sik): Depressing or destructive to the bone marrow or relating to diseased bone marrow.

myiasis (mī-i-a-sis): Any infection that develops as a result of invasion of a body tissue or cavity by the larvae of dipterous insects (houseflies, mosquitoes, gnats, etc.); may involve the eye, ear, nasal passages, intestinal tract, or skin.

mylohyoid (mī'lō-hī'oyd): Relating to molar teeth or the lower part of the jaw and the hyoid bone; denotes various structures as nerves, muscles.

myoasthenia (mī-ō-as-thē'ni-a): Lack or loss of muscle strength.

myoblastoma (mī'ō-blas-tō'ma): A neoplasm occurring in striated muscle, often in the tongue; made up of immature muscle cells.

myobradia (mī-ō-brā'di-a): Sluggish reaction of muscle to electrical stimulation.

myocardia (mī-ō-kar'di-a): A non-inflammatory disease of the myocardium. The term is often used to describe heart failure when the cause is unknown.

myocardial (mī-ō-kar'di-al): Relating to the myocardium. M. INFARCTION the formation of an infarct (q.v.) in the myocardium.

myocarditis (mī-ō-kar-dī'tis): Inflammation of the myocardium.

myocardium (mī'ō-kar'di-um): The middle and thickest of the layers of the heart wall; composed of indistinctly striated, involuntary muscle tissue. — myocardial, adj.

myocele (mī'ō-sēl): Protrusion of a muscle through its ruptured sheath.

myocelialgia (mī'ō-sē-li-al'ji-a): Pain in the abdominal muscles.

myocelitis (mī-ō-sē-lī'tis): Inflammation of the abdominal muscles.

myoclonus (mi-ok'lo-nus): Clonic contractions of individual muscles or groups of muscles. Twitching. M. MULTIPLEX a disorder characterized by rapid contractions of unrelated muscles, either simultaneously or consecutively; also called *paraclonus*.

myocytoma (mī'-ō-sī-tō'ma): A benign muscle tumour involving non-striated muscle.

myodegeneration (mī'ō-dē-jen-er-ā'shun): Degeneration of muscle tissue.

myodynia (mī'ō-din'i-a): Pain in a muscle; myalgia.

myodystonia (mī'-ō-dis-tō'-ni-a): Any disorder of muscle tone.

myoelectric (mī'-ō-ē-lek'-trik): Relating to the electrical properties of muscle. M. ARM an artificial arm that is activated by amplifying the electric currents produced by the patient's own muscles.

myoendocarditis (mī'-ō-en-dō-kar-dī'-tis): Inflammation of the heart muscle and of the endocardium.

myofacial pain dysfunction syndrome: Temporomandibular joint syndrome: see under TEMPOROMANDIBULAR.

myofascitis (mī'-ō-fa-sī'-tis): Musculoskeletal pain, probably due to inflammation of a muscle and its fascia.

myofibril (mī-ō-fī′ -bril): One of the long fibrils that make up a muscle fibre.

myofibroma (mī-ō-fī-brō′ -ma): A tumour of muscular and fibrous tissue.

myofibrosis (mī-ō-fī-brō′sis): Replacement of muscle with fibrous tissue; leads to inadequate functioning of the involved part. — myofibroses, pl.

myogenic (mī-ō-jen′ -ik): Originating in, or starting from, muscle.

myoglobin (mī-ō-glō′ -bin): Oxygen-transporting muscle protein. Syn., *myohaemoglobin*.

myoglobinuria (mī′ō-glō-bin-ū′ri-a): Excretion of myoglobin in the urine as occurs in crush syndrome. Syn., *myohaemoglobinuria*.

myogram (mī′ -ō-gram): A radiological or graphic study of muscle activity.

myohaemoglobin (mī′ō-hē-mō-glō′bin): A haemoglobin present in muscle, of much lower molecular weight than blood haemoglobin. It is liberated from muscle and appears in the urine in crush syndrome (*q.v.*).

myohaemoglobinuria (mī′ō-hē-mō-glō-bin-ū′ri-a): The presence of myohaemoglobin in the urine.

myohypertrophy (mī′ō-hī-per′trō-fi): Abnormal increase in muscle size.

myoid (mī′ -oyd): Resembling muscle.

myoischaemia (mī′ -ō-is-kē′ -mi-a): A deficiency of blood supply to a muscle.

myokymia (mī-ō-kim′ -i-a): Twitching of a few isolated muscle bundles within a single muscle; may be transitory or persistent; may occur after exercise or chilling, or may be a sign of infection or tumour of the brain stem.

myolipoma (mī-ō-li-pō′ma): A benign fatty tumour of smooth muscle tissue.

myolysis (mī-ol′ -i-sis): Degeneration or disintegration of muscle tissue.

myoma (mī-ō′ -ma): A benign tumour of muscle tissue; most often refers to tumour of uterine muscle. Also called *fibroid* or *fibroids*. — myomas, myomata, pl.

myomalacia (mī′ō-ma-lā′shi-a): Softening of muscle, as occurs in the myocardium after coronary occlusion.

myomatosis (mī-ō-ma-tō′ -sis): The presence of multiple myomas, as often occurs in the uterus. See LEIOMYOMA.

myomectomy (mī-ō-mek′to-mi): Surgical removal of a myoma, specifically a uterine myoma.

myomeningocele (mī′ -ō-me-ning′ -gō-sēl): A congenital anomaly in which there is a sac-like protrusion of meningeal and spinal cord substance; usually occurs in the lumbosacral region; may be associated with other abnormalities including mental handicap. See MENINGOCELE.

myometer (mī-om′ -i-ter): An instrument for measuring the strength of muscle contraction.

myometritis (mī-ō-me-trī′tis): Inflammation of the muscular wall of the uterus.

myometrium (mī′ō-mē′tri-um): The thick muscular wall of the uterus.

myonarcosis (mī′ -ō-nar-kō′ -sis): Numbness of muscles.

myonecrosis (mī′ō-ne-krō′sis): Death of individual muscle fibres. CLOSTRIDIAL M. gas gangrene; caused by the anaerobic *Clostridium perfringens*; seen in deep wound infections; early signs and symptoms include pain, tenderness, fever, accumulation of gas in the muscle tissue, shock with tachycardia, and hypotension.

myoneural (mī-ō-nū′ -ral): Relating to muscle and nerve. M. JUNCTION the place where a nerve ending terminates in muscle tissue.

myoneuralgia (mī′ō-nū-ral′ji-a): Muscular pain.

myoneurasthenia (mī′ō-nū-ras-thē′ni-a): A relaxed state of muscles, seen in neurasthenia (*q.v.*).

myoneuroma (mī′ō-nū-rō′ma): A neuroma (*q.v.*) that contains muscle tissue.

myopachynsis (mī-ō-pa-kin′sis): Abnormal enlargement or thickening of muscle.

myopalmus (mī-ō-pal′mus): Twitching of a muscle or muscles.

myopathy (mī-op′a-thi): Any disease or abnormal condition of muscle tissue. ALCOHOLIC M. M. occurring in alcoholics, marked by acute myoglobulinuria (*q.v.*) and weakness of the limbs; OCULAR M. slowly progressive muscular dystrophy characterized by ptosis and immobility of the eye.

myope (mī′ōp): A nearsighted person. — myopic, adj.

myopia (mī-ō′pi-a): Nearsightedness. The light rays come to a focus in front of, instead of on, the retina. — myopic, adj.

myoplasty (mī′ō-plas-ti): Plastic surgery of muscles, or the use of muscle tissue in plastic surgery. — myoplastic, adj.

myorrhaphy (mī-or′a-fi): Suturing of a wound in muscle, or of a divided muscle.

myorrhexis (mī-ō-rek′sis): Rupture or tearing of a muscle.

myosarcoma (mī′ō-sar-kō′ma): A malignant tumour derived from muscle. — myosarcomata, pl.; myosarcomatous, adj.

myosclerosis (mī′ō-skle-rō′sis): Fibrous myositis; see under MYOSITIS. — myosclerotic, adj.

myosin (mī'ō-sin): A globin that makes up about 68% of the muscle substance. Along with actin, it is responsible for contraction and relaxation of muscles.

myosis (mī-ō'sis): See MIOSIS.

myositis (mī-ō-sī'tis): Inflammation of a voluntary muscle. FIBROUS M., characterized by formation of fibrous tissue in muscle; INTERSTITIAL M. usually of viral origin; characterized by fever, headache, aching limbs, sore throat; also called *Bornholm disease*. M. OSSIFICANS deposition of active bone cells in muscle, resulting in hard swellings.

myospasm (mī'ō-spazm): Spasmodic contraction of a muscle.

myotenositis (mī'ō-ten-ō-sī'tis): Inflammation of a muscle and its tendon.

myotomy (mī-ot'om-i): Cutting, or dissection of, muscle tissue.

myotonia (mī-ō-tō'ni-a): A disorder characterized by increased muscular contractions and decreased relaxation; tonic muscle spasm. M. CONGENITA an inherited disorder characterized by early onset and by stiffness of muscles, which is accented by cold weather; the skeletal muscles become hypertrophied; M. DYSTROPHICA myotonic dystrophy; see under DYSTROPHY.

myotonic (mī-ō-ton'ik): Relating to myotonia. M. REACTION the delay in relaxation of a muscle after contraction.

myringa (mi-ring'ga): The eardrum or tympanic membrane.

myringitis (mir-in-jī'tis): Inflammation of the eardrum (tympanic membrane). M. BULLOSA viral otitis media characterized by the formation of serous or haemorrhage blisters on the tympanic membrane.

myringoplasty (mī-ring'-gō-plas-ti): A plastic operation on the eardrum (tympanic membrane). — myringoplastic, adj.

myringotome (mī-ring'gō-tōm): A delicate instrument for incising the eardrum (tympanic membrane).

myringotomy (mīr-in-got'o-mi): Incision of the eardrum (tympanic membrane).

mysophobia (mī-sō-fō'bi-a): A morbid fear of dirt or germs, or of touching even familiar objects, *e.g.*, doorknobs.

myx-, myxo-: Combining forms denoting mucus, mucous.

myxadenitis (miks-ad-e-nī'tis): Inflammation of a mucous gland or glands.

myxadenoma (miks-ad-e-nō'ma): A benign tumour with the structure of a mucous gland, or one that contains mucous elements.

myxoedema (mik-se-dē'ma): A syndrome resulting from hypofunction of the anterior pituitary, or deficiency of iodine in the diet, or to excessive use of antithyroid drugs; may also be secondary to removal of the thyroid gland. Symptoms include lethargy, mental dullness, bradycardia, subnormal temperature, dry skin, alopecia, oedema of the face and extremities. The basal metabolic rate is low, and blood cholesterol is elevated, but there is no enlargement of the thyroid gland. CONGENITAL M. see CRETINISM. — myxoedematous, adj.

myxoma (mik-sō'ma): A connective tissue tumour composed largely of mucoid material. — myxomata, pl.; myxomatous, adj.

myxosarcoma (mik-sō-sar-kō'ma): A malignant tumour of connective tissue with a soft, mucoid consistency. — myxosarcomata, pl.; myxosarcomatous, adj.

myxovirus (mik-sō-vī'rus): A group of RNA viruses including the parainfluenza virus, measles viruses, respiratory syncytial virus and mumps.

N

N: Chemical symbol for nitrogen.

NA: Abbreviation for Nomina Anatomica (*q.v.*).

Na: Chemical symbol for sodium (L. natrium).

nabothian: N. CYSTS tiny cysts that form in the cervical glands of the uterus when these become inflamed and their secretions are retained because of obstruction in the ducts. Also called *Naboth's follicles*. N. GLAND any of several small mucous glands in the uterine cervix. [Martin Naboth, German anatomist, 1675–1721.]

NaCl: Chemical formula for sodium chloride.

naevoid (nē'-voyd): Relating to or resembling a naevus.

naevolipoma (nē'vō-lī-pō'ma): A naevus that contains fibrofatty tissue; rare.

naevosarcoma (nē'vōsar-kō'-ma): A malignant melanoma presumed to have developed from a naevus.

naevus (nē'vus): 1. A general term used to describe any congenital circumscribed pigmented lesion on the skin; may be epidermal, connective tissue, or vascular in origin. 2. A mole. 3. A birthmark. N. FLAMMEUS a diffuse, poorly defined area of skin varying in colour from pink to deep purple; a portwine n.; N. MATERNUS a birthmark; N. PILOSUS a hairy naevus; SPIDER N. a congenital or acquired lesion composed of lines radiating from a centre, due to capillary dilatation; STRAW-BERRY N. a raised, bright red skin lesion; cavernous haemangioma; see HAEMANGIOMA. — naevi, pl.; naevoid, adj.

Naga sore (nah'-gah): One of several names for the chronic sloughing ulcer seen chiefly on the lower extremities of people living in tropical areas; thought to be due to a nutritional deficiency.

Nägele's rule (nā'-ge-liz): A method used to calculate the estimated date of confinement; calculated by subtracting 90 days from the first day of the last menstrual period and adding seven days. [Franz K. Nägele, German obstetrician, 1777–1851.]

NaHCO₃: Chemical formula for sodium bicarbonate.

nail: 1. A rod of material (usually bone or metal) used to hold pieces of fractured bones together.

2. The horny cutaneous plate that covers the dorsal surface of the distal ends of fingers and toes; the root is that part embedded in a deep fold of skin at the base, and the body is the exposed part lying on a bed of matrix of the skin from which the new substance develops. The white crescent at the base of the nail is called the lunula. Discoloration of the nails may occur due to haemorrhage, trauma, certain pathological conditions such as diabetes, anaemia, or certain poisonings, or in persons receiving certain substances such as silver. EGG SHELL N. a condition of thinning, softening and splitting of the nails; associated with several general pathological conditions; HANG N. a bit of skin hanging loose at one side or root of a N.; INGROWN N. a painful aberrant growth, usually of a toenail, with the edges pressing into the soft tissues at the side; KÜNTSCHER N. a stainless steel flanged nail used for intermedullary fixation of fractures; NEUFELD N. a N. used for fixation of an intertrochanteric fracture of the femur; REEDY N. a N. with lengthwise furrows; SMITH-PETERSEN N. a trifid, cannulated metal N., formerly much used to provide internal fixation of the head of the femur in fracture of the neck of the femur; SPOON N. a N. that is depressed in its central portion; TURTLEBACK N. a distorted nail that is more convex than normal.

nailing: The operation of fastening the ends of a fractured bone together with a nail.

nail–patella syndrome: A congenital condition characterized by absence of the nails, various skeletal abnormalities, including absence of the patella, and abnormalities of the eyes and ears.

nalidixic acid: An antibacterial agent frequently used in treatment of urinary tract infections caused by Gram-negative organisms.

nandrolone (nan'-drō-lōn): An anabolic steroid that promotes skeletal growth and protein metabolism.

nanism (nā'-nizm): Dwarfism; the condition of being much smaller than normal.

nano-: 1. A combining form denoting small or dwarfish. 2. A prefix denoting one-billionth (10^{-9}) of a measure.

nanocephaly (nā-nō-kef'-a-li, nā-nō-sef'-a-li): Abnormal smallness of the head. Also called

nanocephalia, nanocephalism, nanocephalus.
— nanocephalous, adj.

nanocurie (nā-nō-kū'-ri): A unit of radiation equal to one-billionth (10^{-9}) of a curie.

nanogram (nā'nō-gram): In the metric system, a unit of mass weight; one-billionth (10^{-9}) of a gram. Abbreviated ng.

nanomelus (nā-nom'-e-lus): An individual with unusually short extremities; often refers to a fetus. Also called nanomelia. — nanomelous, adj.

nanometre (nā-nom-e-ter): The official International Standard Unit of Wavelength, 10 ångströms; equal to one-billionth (10^{-9}) of a metre; a millimicron.

nanophthalmus (nan-of-thal'-mus): The condition of having abnormally small eyeballs. Microphthalmus.

nanus (nā'-nus): Of small stature; a dwarf. — nanoid, nanous, adj.; nanism, n.

NaOH: Chemical formula for sodium hydroxide.

nape (nāp): The back of the neck; the nucha.

napex (nā'-peks): The part of the scalp that is immediately below the occipital protuberance.

naphthol (naf'-thol): A substance obtained from coal tar; has antiseptic qualities.

nappy rash: A red, erythematous rash in the napkin area of an infant; if severe can lead to excoriation. Causes may include thrush, infantile psoriasis, diarrhoea and allergy to detergents/soaps.

naprapathy (na-prap'-a-thi): A school of folk medicine that utilizes diet, massage, and manipulation of muscles, ligaments, and joints of the spine, pelvis, and thorax.

narcissism (nar-sis'-izm): Self-love; absorption with one's own perfections. In psychiatry, the narcissistic personality is one in which the sexual love-object is the self; named for a character in Greek mythology who fell in love with his own image reflected in a pool. — narcissistic, adj.

narco-: Combining form denoting (1) stupor; (2) deep sleep; (3) numbness.

narcoanaesthesia (nar'-kō-an-es-thē'-zi-a): Anaesthesia resulting from a subcutaneous injection of a narcotic such as morphine and scopolamine.

narcoanalysis (nar-kō-a-nal'-a-sis): Psychotherapy conducted while the individual is under light anaesthesia produced by certain drugs, *e.g.*, sodium pentothal or sodium amytal. The purpose is to assist the person to recover repressed memories along with the emotion that accompanied the experience, with the idea of helping him or her to accept the memories and integrate them into his or her self-image.

narcohypnia (nar-kō-hip'-ni-a): A sensation of general numbness felt upon awakening.

narcohypnosis (nar-kō-hip-nō'-sis): A hypnotic state produced by some drugs and used sometimes in psychotherapy.

narcolepsy (nar'-kō-lep-si): An irresistible tendency to fall into deep sleep during the daytime, but from which an individual can be easily aroused; may occur several times a day and last for only a few minutes or for hours; seen in diverse clinical conditions. — narcoleptic, adj.

narcomania (nar-kō-mā'-ni-a): 1. Uncontrollable craving for narcotics. 2. Insanity resulting from alcoholism or from a narcotic drug habit.

narcose (nar'-kōs): Stuporous.

narcosis (nar-kō'-sis): Unconsciousness, stupor, or insensibility produced by a drug and from which recovery is possible. BASAL N. a state of unconsciousness produced by drugs prior to giving an anaesthetic; NITROGEN N., N. produced by (1) nitrogenous substances in the blood, as occurs in hepatic coma and uraemia, or (2) increased nitrogen pressure in the blood, as occurs in deep-sea divers; often called '*rapture of the deep*'.

narcosynthesis (nar-kō-sin'-the-sis): The building up of a clearer mental picture of an incident involving the patient by reviving memories of it under semi-narcosis, so that both patient and therapist can examine the incident in clearer perspective.

narcotherapy (nar-kō-ther'-a-pi): Narcoanalysis (*q.v.*).

narcotic (nar-kot'-ik): 1. Relating to or producing narcosis. 2. Any substance that in moderate doses relieves pain and produces profound sleep, particularly substances derived from opium; most are habit-forming.

narcotic addict: A person who has become physiologically or psychologically dependent on a narcotic drug.

narcotism (nar'-kō-tizm): 1. Addiction to narcotics. 2. A state of stupor produced by a narcotic drug.

narcotize (nar'-kō-tīz): To place under the influence of a narcotic drug.

nares (nā'-rēz): The nostrils. ANTERIOR N. the pair of openings from the exterior into the nasal cavities; POSTERIOR N. the pair of openings from the nasal cavities into the nasopharynx. Syn., *choanae*. — naris, sing.

narrative (nar'-ra-tiv): 1. A spoken or written account of connected events. 2. The descriptive part of a literary work, as distinct from dialogue. **3.** The practice or art of narration. **4.** In research, the description of experiences by participants.

narrative notes: A written record of a patient's progress or response to therapy; part of the patient's chart.

nasal (nā'-zal): Relating to the nose. N. BONE either of the two small oblong bones which together form the arch of the nose; N. CANNULA a cannula inserted through the nasal cavity for administering oxygen; N. CATHETER one inserted through the nose, to deliver oxygen; N. CAVITY that in the nose, separated into right and left halves by the N. SEPTUM; N. CONCHAE three long thin projections from the lateral walls of the N. CAVITY; identified according to position as superior, medial, and inferior; N. DECONGESTANT a drug that reduces local inflammation in nasal passages in ordinary rhinitis and sinusitis; many are antihistamines; N. DRIP see POSTNASAL DRIP; N. FOSSA one of the two parts of the N. cavity extending from the exterior to the nasopharynx; N. INTUBATION an endotracheal tube is inserted through the nostril and advanced through the vocal cords during inspiration, to establish an airway; N. MUCOSA the mucous membrane lining the nose; N. POLYP focal hyperplasia of the submucous connective tissue of the nose with accumulation of oedematous fluid; N. SEPTUM the thin bony cartilaginous structure that separates the nostrils; N. SINUSES any of several cavities in the bones of the skull that communicate with the N. cavity; in particular, the frontal, ethmoid, sphenoid, and maxillary (also called *antrum of Highmore*) sinuses; they are lined with mucous membrane that is continuous with that of the nasal cavity and are often irritated; N. SOUNDS so called because to produce them air is resonated in the nasal cavity; they are the sounds of *m, n,* and *ng.*

nasalis (nā-zal'is): Relating to the nose.

nascent (nā'-sent): **1.** At the moment of birth. **2.** Coming into existence or in the process of emerging.

nas-, nasi-, naso-: Combining forms denoting (1) the nose; (2) nasal.

nasoantral (nā'-zō-an'-tral): Relating to the nose and the maxillary antrum.

nasoantritis (nā'-zō-an-trī'-tis): Inflammation of the nose and the antrum of Highmore (maxillary sinus).

nasobronchial (nā-zō-bron'-ki-al): Relating to the nose and bronchi.

nasoduodenal (nā'-zō-dū-ō-dē'-nal): Relating to the nose and the duodenum; usually refers to a tube used for enteral nutrition.

nasofrontal (nā'-zō-frun'-tal): Relating to the nasal and frontal bones or forehead.

nasogastric (nā'-zō-gas'-trik): Relating to the nose and stomach. N. FEEDING see under FEEDING; N. TUBE a soft tube that is inserted through the nostril into the stomach; used for instilling liquids and foods and for withdrawing stomach contents.

nasojejunal feeding: See TRANSPYLORIC FEEDING under FEEDING.

nasolabial (nā'-zō-lā'-bi-al): Relating to the nose and the upper lip. N. SEBORRHOEA enlarged follicles at the sides of the nose; they contain plugs of sebaceous material.

nasolacrimal (nā'-zō-lak'-ri-mal): Relating to the nose and the lacrimal apparatus. N. DUCT carries the tears from the N. sac to the inferior meatus of the nose; see under LACRIMAL.

naso-oral (nā'-zō-or'-al): Relating to the nose and the mouth.

nasopalatine (nā'-zō-pal'-a-tīn): Relating to the nose and the palate.

nasopharyngeal (nā'-zō-fa-rin'-jē-al): Relating to the nasopharynx. N. ANGIOFIBROMA a relatively benign tumour of the nasopharynx, seen most often in teenage boys; characterized by nasal and auditory tube obstruction resulting in adenoidal speech.

nasopharyngitis (nā'-zō-far-in-jī'tis): Inflammation of the nasal passages and the pharynx; caused by a virus or group of viruses. The common cold.

nasopharyngoscope (nā'-zō-far-ing'-go-skōp): An endoscopic device for viewing the nasal passages and the postnasal space. — nasopharyngoscopic, adj.

nasopharynx (nā'-zō-far'-inks): The portion of the pharynx above the soft palate, which opens anteriorly into the nasal cavity. — nasopharyngeal, adj.

nasoscope (nā'zō-skōp): An instrument for examining the nasal cavity. Also called *Rhinoscope.*

nasoseptal (nā'-zō-sep'-tal): Relating to the nasal septum.

nasosinusitis (nā'-zō-sī-nu-sī'-tis): Inflammation of the nasal cavities and adjacent sinuses.

nasotracheal (nā'-zō-tra'-ki-al): Relating to the nasal cavity and the trachea. N. TUBE a tube that is inserted into the trachea via the nasal cavity and the pharynx.

nasus (nā'-sus): The nose.

natal (nā'-tal): Relating to: **1.** Birth. **2.** The buttocks.

natality (nā-tal' -i-ti): 1. The birth rate; the ratio of births to the population in a given area. 2. Birth.

nates (nā' -tēz): The buttocks.

natimortality (nā' -ti-mor-tal' -i-ti): The proportion of fetal deaths and stillbirths to the general birth rate.

National Beds Inquiry: A UK government investigation set up in response to the apparent inability of hospitals to deal with the high levels of demand experienced in winter months. It developed into a wider review of the future size and role of the acute hospital, particularly in respect of care for the elderly.

National Care Standards Commission: A regulatory body responsible for the registration and inspection of health and social care services; monitors the provision and quality of care in children's homes, independent hospitals, and care homes. Established by the Care Standards Act (2000).

National Council for Vocational Qualifications: A regulatory body established by government to provide for a national framework for vocational qualifications in England, Wales and Northern Ireland. The qualifications are generally known as NCVQs.

National Electronic Library for Health: An online database that provides access to a range of quality information resources to support better patient care and choice. It developed to provide health professionals and the public with the knowledge to support health-care decisions. www.nelh.nhs.uk

National Forum for People with Learning Disabilities: An organization that provides a voice for those with learning difficulties at a governmental level. Regional user forums have also been established.

National Framework for Assessing Performance: Guidelines established to review the NHS as a genuinely national service; to make delivery against national standards a local responsibility; to encourage the NHS to work in partnership with the private sector; to drive efficiency; to ensure that the quality of care guarantees excellence to all patients; and to rebuild public confidence in the NHS.

National Health Service: A comprehensive health service in the UK that aims to bring about the highest level of physical and mental health for all citizens, within the available resources. It promotes health; diagnoses and treats injuries and disease; and cares for those with a long-term illness or disability.

National Health Service Beacon services: A programme that identifies, shares, and cele-brates examples of good practice, providing an improved service for patients in the NHS. See BEACON SITES.

National Health Service Centre for Reviews and Dissemination: An organization that provides the NHS with important information on the effectiveness of treatments and the delivery and organization of healthcare. Established in January 1994.

National Institute for Clinical Excellence: A special health authority, providing formal advice for NHS clinicians and managers on the clinical and cost effectiveness of new and existing technologies such as medicines. It provides and disseminates guidance based on the relevant evidence, clinical audit methodologies, and information on good practice.

National Institute for Mental Health Excellence: A new organization based within the Modernisation Agency (*q.v.*) at the Department of Health. Aiming to improve the quality of life for people of all ages who experience mental distress.

National Patient Safety Agency: A special health authority created in July 2001 to coordinate the efforts of health-care providers across the UK to report, and to learn from, adverse events occurring in the NHS.

National Primary and Care Trust Development: Programme established to provide organizational development support to primary care teams.

National Research Register: A database of ongoing and recently completed research projects funded by, or of interest to, the NHS.

National Service Frameworks: A series of guidelines for the future of public healthcare. The key aims are: to set national standards and define service models for a specific service or care group, and to put in place strategies to support their implementation; establish performance milestones against which progress will be measured within an agreed time scale; and to raise quality and decrease variations in service. Frameworks are in place or are being developed for cancer, paediatric intensive care, mental health, older people, diabetes, renal services, and children's services.

National Survey of Patient and User Experience: A survey that catalogues the views of NHS patients about the service they receive.

National Training Organization: A government-recognized, industry-focused body established to support the development of skills and training within an industry. It is the recognized voice of employers on the skills and people development needs of UK industry and employment sectors.

National Treatment Agency (for Substance Misuse): A group that provides services to drug misusers through pooled budgets from health and other agencies. It also encourages good practice, sets standards, and monitors performance.

National Vocational Qualification/Scottish Vocational Qualification: Work-related, nationally recognized qualifications. The qualifications are comprised of occupational standards (*q.v.*) and are assessed through portfolios of evidence. The Scottish qualification takes into account differences in Scotland.

NatPaCT: Abbreviation for National Primary and Care Trust Development (*q.v.*).

natraemia (nā-trē′-mi-a): The presence of more than the normal amount of sodium in the blood.

natriuresis (nā′-tri-ū-rē′-sis): A condition in which there is an unusually large amount of sodium in the urine; occurs in certain diseases and following the administration of diuretic drugs.

natriuretic (nā′-tri-ū-ret′-ik): **1.** Relating to natriuresis. **2.** An agent that promotes natriuresis by inhibiting the reabsorption of sodium ions by the glomerulus.

natural: 1. Neither artificial nor pathological. **2.** Inborn. **3.** Normal. N. CHILDBIRTH a system of management for childbirth in which anaesthesia, sedation, and medical intervention are replaced by antenatal education. The educational process prepares the parents for active participation in the birth. N. DEFENCES OF THE BODY include the skin, lymphatic tissue, white blood cells, and antibodies in the blood; N. HEALING PROCESSES processes such as blood clot formation, scar tissue formation, bone repair after fracture, and cell division; N. IMMUNITY immunity resulting from the genetic composition of the host; may be manifested in individuals, families, or races.

naturopathy (nā′-tūr-op′-a-thi): A system of treatment that makes use of such physical agents as light, heat, water, massage, exercise, and diet; no surgical procedures are used and only such medications as are derived from herbs, vitamins, etc.

Nauheim bath (now′-hīm, naw′-hīm): A bath of all or part of the body in naturally hot carbonated water, followed by exercise; originated at the spas in Bad-Nauheim, Germany, for use in treating cardiac conditions.

naupathia (naw-path′-i-a): Seasickness.

nausea (naw′-zē-a): **1.** A sensation of discomfort or sickness in the area of the stomach often leading to the urge to vomit. Nausea may be a symptom of a variety of disorders, some minor and some more serious. **2.** Extreme disgust, loathing. — nauseating, adj.; nauseate, v.

nauseant (naw′-zē-ent): A drug that produces nausea.

nauseous (naw′-zē-us): Producing nausea, disgust, or loathing.

navel (nā′-vel): The umbilicus. The depression in the centre of the abdomen marking the place where the umbilical cord is attached to the fetus.

navicular (nav-ik-ū-lar): **1.** Shaped like a boat or canoe. **2.** Relating to a bone in the wrist or one in the ankle.

NBM: Abbreviation for nil (nothing) by mouth.

NCSC: Abbreviation for National Care Standards Commission (*q.v.*).

NCVQ: Abbreviation for National Council for Vocational Qualifications (*q.v.*).

NDU: Abbreviation for Nursing Development Unit, see under NURSING.

nearsightedness: Lay term for myopia (*q.v.*).

nebula (neb′-u-la): **1.** A greyish, corneal opacity. **2.** An oily mixture for use in a nebulizer (*q.v.*). **3.** A cloudiness in the urine.

nebulization (neb′-ū-lī-zā′-shun): **1.** Conversion into a spray. **2.** Treatment of an area by spraying.

nebulize (neb′-ū-līz): To convert into a fine spray or vapour.

nebulizer (neb′-ū-līz-er): An apparatus for converting a liquid into a fine spray. Syn., *atomizer.*

NEC: Abbreviation for necrotizing enterocolitis (*q.v.*).

Necator (nē-kā′-tor): A genus of nematodes (see Nematoda); *N. AMERICANUS* the hookworm found in the USA and Central and South America. See HOOKWORM.

neck: 1. The part between the head and the shoulders. **2.** The constricted portion of bone or an organ, *e.g.*, the neck of the femur, the neck of the uterus.

necr-, necro-: Combining forms denoting (1) death; (2) a dead body; (3) dead tissue.

necrectomy (nek-rek′-to-mi): Surgical removal of necrosed tissue.

necrobiosis (nek′-rō-bī-ō′-sis): The degeneration or death of cells followed by replacement; may be normal as in red blood cells and epithelial cells, or abnormal as in a pathological process. N. LIPOIDICA a skin disease characterized by the formation of the reddish yellow plaques, mostly on the legs; occurs most often in older women, especially those with diabetes; also called *necrobiosis lipoidica diabeticorum.*

necrocytosis (nek'-rō-sī-tō'-sis): The death of cells.

necrogenic (nek'-rō-jen'-ik): Caused by or productive of necrosis.

necrology (nek-rol'-o-ji): 1. The study of death statistics. 2. The science of collecting, classifying, and interpreting death statistics. — necrological, adj.

necrolysis (nek-rol'-i-sis): The dissolution or breaking down of dead tissue.

necromania (nek'rō-mā'ni-a): 1. Morbid interest in death or in corpses. 2. A form of mania in which one wishes to die.

necrophile (nek'-rō-fīl): A person who derives pleasure from dead bodies, who is sexually aroused by thoughts of death, or who derives pleasure from sexual activity with a dead body.

necrophilia (nek'-rō-fil'-i-a): 1. A morbid preoccupation with death and a liking for being in the presence of dead bodies. 2. A morbid desire to have sexual intercourse with a corpse. — necrophiliac, adj.

necrophobia (nek'-rō-fō'-bi-a): A morbid dread of dead bodies.

necropsy (nek'-rop-si): The examination of the internal organs of a dead body; autopsy.

necrose (ne-krōz'): 1. To become necrotic. 2. To be necrotic.

necrosis (ne-krō'-sis): Localized death of tissue or bone. When N. occurs in bone the dead part is referred to as a sequestrum; when it occurs in soft tissue it is referred to as slough; when large areas are affected the condition is referred to as gangrene. May be caused by lack of normal circulation to a part, trauma, radiant energy such as x-rays or radium, or bacterial invasion; and may be described according to cause, location, extent, and consistency of the dead tissue. AVASCULAR N., N. due to lack of normal circulation to a part; also called *anaemic* N.; CASEOUS N., N. in which the dead tissue has a cheesy consistency; DRY N., N. in which the dead material is dry, as compared with that which is termed MOIST; EPIPHYSIAL ASEPTIC N. usually occurs in the head of the femur, medial condyle, head of the humerus, or the tibial tubercle; associated with sickle cell anaemia and alcoholism; PUTREFACTIVE N., N. caused by bacterial invasion of tissue; TOTAL N., N. that destroys all or most of an organ or part; TUBULAR N., N. of the epithelial tissue along the kidney tubules. — necroses, pl.; necrotic, adj.

necrotic (ne-krot'-ik): Relating to or characterized by necrosis.

necrotize (nek'-rō-tīz): 1. To undergo necrosis. 2. To produce or cause necrosis. — necrotizing, adj.

necrotizing enterocolitis (nek'-rō-tī-zing-enter-ō-ko-lī'-tis'): A gastrointestinal disease that affects mostly premature infants. It involves infection and inflammation that causes destruction of the bowel.

necrotomy (nek-rot'-o-mi): An operation for the removal of a sequestrum (*q.v.*) or other necrotic tissue.

need: 1. A lack of something that is required for survival. 2. To require.

needle: 1. A slender, sharp, pointed instrument used for suturing wounds or for puncturing. Needles may be straight or curved, and have a cutting or rounded edge. 2. A hollow pointed instrument used to deliver medication into the body or to withdraw fluid from a tissue, blood vessel, or hollow organ. ASPIRATING N. a long, hollow N. used for removing fluid from a cavity; HYPODERMIC N. a short, hollow N. used for administering medications through the skin; SCALP VEIN N. a N. originally designed for use in administering intravenous fluids to infants, now often used for prolonged intravenous therapy for patients of all ages; is made in various lengths and gauges and fitted with plastic wings that fold flat on the skin to help anchor the N. in place; SWAGED N. has no eye; the suture material is fused to the needle. See NEEDLE BIOPSY under BIOPSY.

needling (nēd'-ling): Puncturing with a needle as in discission of the lens capsule in surgical treatment of cataract. Also called *Discission.*

negation (ne-gā'-shun): Denial.

negative (ne'-ga-tiv): 1. Not affirmative; the opposite of positive. 2. Denoting that a substance or microorganism tested for is not present in the material examined.

negativism (neg'-a-tiv-izm): 1. Habitual scepticism. 2. Tendency to do the opposite of what one is asked or expected to do. Occurs commonly in children at about the age of two, but not usual in adults. Often associated with schizophrenia.

negatron (neg'-a-tron): A negatively charged electron.

neglect: Fail to give proper care or attention to; fail to do something.

negligence (neg'-li-jens): In the health sciences, the basis for many lawsuits for malpractice. Includes actions of both commission and omission, *e.g.*, failure to provide care that a reasonably prudent healthcare professional would provide in the given circumstances, failure to provide care that meets the accepted standards of care, or giving care that results in harm or injury to the patient.

Negri bodies: Microscopic bodies found in the cytoplasm of certain nerve cells of animals or persons with rabies; of diagnostic importance.

Nélaton's line (nā'-la-tonz): A line that demonstrates the normal level of the greater trochanter of the femur, that is, the tip of the trochanter should lie just below or on a line from the anterior spine of the ilium to the tuberosity of the ischium; in dislocation of the hip the tip of the trochanter lies above this line.

NeLH: Abbreviation for National Electronic Library for Health (*q.v.*).

Nemathelminthes (nem-a-thel-min'-thēz): The roundworms.

nemathelminthiasis (nem'-a-thel min-thī'-a-sis): Infestation with roundworms of the phylum Nemathelminthes.

nematocide (nem'a-tō sid): An agent that destroys nematode worms.

nematoda (nem-a-tō'-da): A class of Nemathelminthes (*q.v.*) that includes the true roundworms, many are parasitic in humans. — nematode, sing.

nematode (nem'-a-tōd): Any member of the class Nematoda.

nematodiasis (nem'-a-tō-dī'-a-sis): Infestation with a nematode parasite.

nematoid (nem'-a-toid): Thread-like; refers to a nematode parasite.

nematosis (nem-a-tō'-sis): The condition of being infested with nematode parasites (roundworms).

neo-: Combining form denoting new, newness, strange.

neoarthrosis (nē'-ō-ar-thrō'-sis): Abnormal articulation; a false joint as at the site of a fracture. Also refers to a joint created in an operation for total joint replacement.

neocerebellum (nē'-ō-ser-e-bel'-um): The more recently evolved part of the cerebellum; is concerned with voluntary movement.

neocortex (nē-ō-kor'-teks): The more recently evolved part of the cerebral cortex, which is most highly developed in humans; contains a larger number of nerve cells than the allocortex. Also called *isocortex* and *neopallium*.

neocyte (nē'-ō-sīt): An immature leukocyte.

neocytosis (nē'-ō-sī-tō'-sis): The presence of neocytes in the blood.

Neo-Darwinism: A theory that extends the scope of the Darwinian idea of natural selection, specifically to include subsequent scientific discoveries and concepts unknown to Darwin, such as DNA and genetics, that allow rigorous, in many cases mathematical, analyses of phenomena.

neoformation (nē'-ō-for-mā'-shun): 1. A neoplasm (*q.v.*). 2. Regeneration, as of tissue or bone.

neogenesis (nē-ō-jen'-e-sis): The regeneration of tissue. — neogenicity, adj.

neoglottis (nē-ō-glot'-is): Name given to an artificial larynx, a prosthetic device for persons who have had the larynx removed.

neoglycogenesis (nē'-ō-glī-kō-jen'-e-sis): See GLYCONEOGENESIS.

neohymen (nē-ō-hī'-men): A new or false membrane.

neokinetic (nē'-ō-ki-net'-ik): Referring to movement, particularly to the nervous mechanism that regulates voluntary muscle activity.

neolalia (nē ō lal'-i-a): Speech in which neologisms are used freely, a common habit among schizophrenics.

neologism (nē-ol'-o-jizm): A specially coined word, phrase, or usage, often meaningless to everyone except the person who invented it.

neon (nē'-on): A colourless, odourless, tasteless, inert gas; found in minute quantities in the air; used in electric lamps.

neonatal (nē-ō-nā'-tal): Relating to the period immediately following birth and continuing through the first month of life. N. MORTALITY RATE the death rate of babies in the first month of life per 1000 live births in any one year; N. PERIOD the first 28 days of life.

neonate (nē'-ō-nāt): A newborn baby up to one month old.

neonatologist (nē'-ō-nā-tol'-o-jist): A physician who specializes in the care and treatment of the newborn.

neonatology (nē'-ō-nā-tol'-o-ji): That branch of medicine that is concerned with the care and treatment of the newborn.

neonatorum (nē'-ō-nā-tor'-um): Relating to the newborn.

neopathy (nē-op'-a-thi): 1. A new disease or condition arising in a patient who already has another disease. 2. A newly recognized disease.

neopenthic (nē-ō-pen'-thik): Having the effect of inducing peace and forgetfulness.

neophobia (nē-ō-fō'-bi-a): A morbid dread of newness or new things.

neoplasia (nē-ō-plā'-zi-a): Literally, the formation of new tissue. By custom refers to the pathological process in tumour formation. — neoplastic, adj.

neoplasm (nē'-ō-plazm): Any abnormal, progressive, uncontrolled growth of cells or tissues that serves no useful purpose; a tumour. May be benign, malignant, or potentially malignant. — neoplastic, adj.

neostomy (nē-os'-to-mi): The creation of an artificial opening into an organ or between two organs.

neovascularization (nē'ō-vas'kū-lar-ī-zā'shun): Formation of new blood vessels, as occurs in tumours or in abnormal places, as in the retinae of patients with diabetic retinopathy.

nephalism (nef'-a-lizm): Total abstinence from alcohol or alcoholic liquors.

nephelopia (nef-e-lō'-pi-a): Visual defect due to cloudiness of the cornea.

nephr-, nephro-: Combining forms denoting relationship to the kidney.

nephradenoma (nef'-rad-e-nō'-ma): Adenoma (*q.v.*) of the kidney.

nephralgia (ne-fral'-ji-a): Pain in the kidney. — nephralgic, adj.

nephrectasia (nef-rek-tā'-zi-a): Distension of the pelvis of the kidney. Also called *nephrectasis.*

nephrectomy (ne-frek'-to-mi): Removal of a kidney.

nephric (nef'-rik): Relating to the kidney.

nephridium (ne-frid'-i-um): The embryonic tube that is the excretory organ of the fetus and from which the kidney develops.

nephrism (nef'-rizm): Cachexia due to kidney disease or disorder.

nephritic (ne-frit'-ik): 1. Relating to (a) nephritis; (b) the kidney. 2. A person with nephritis.

nephritides (ne-frit'-i-dēz): Plural of nephritis; the term is used collectively to refer to all types of nephritis.

nephritis (ne-frī'-tis): A term embracing a group of conditions in which there is either an inflammatory or an inflammatory-like condition, focal or diffused, in the kidneys. ACUTE N. Bright's disease. A diffuse inflammatory reaction of both kidneys, usually following a streptococcal infection, and classically manifest by puffiness of the face and scanty blood-stained urine; CHRONIC N. a chronic condition in which there is widespread fibrous replacement of functioning kidney tissue, resulting in progressive renal failure and arterial hypertension, and terminating ultimately in death; INTERSTITIAL N., N. affecting the interstitial tissue of the kidney; LUPUS N. diffuse glomerulonephritis occurring in patients with lupus erythematosus or systemic lupus; character-ized by haematuria and progressing to renal failure; NEPHROTIC N. a chronic condition of unknown cause, characterized by massive oedema and heavy proteinuria.

nephritogenic (ne-frit'-ō-jen'-ik): Giving rise to nephritis.

nephroangiosclerosis (nef'-rō-an'-ji-ō-skle-rō'-sis): Necrosis of the renal arterioles; usually associated with high blood pressure; symptoms include headache, blurred vision, enlarged heart, retinal haemorrhage, and papilloedema; when untreated, progresses to heart and kidney failure.

nephroblastoma (nef'-rō-blas-tō'-ma): A malignant tumour of the kidney; occurs almost exclusively in children. Thought to develop from embryonic structures. Also called *embryoma* and *Wilms' tumour.*

nephrocalcinosis (nef'-rō-kal-sin-ō'-sis): A form of renal lithiasis (*q.v.*); characterized by calcium deposits in many areas of the kidney, resulting in renal insufficiency.

nephrocapsectomy (nef'-rō-kap-sek'-to-mi): Surgical removal of the kidney capsule. Usually done for chronic nephritis. Also called *nephrocapsulectomy.*

nephrocele (nef'-rō-sēl): A hernia of the kidney.

nephrocystanastomosis (nef'-rō-sist-an-as-to-mō'-sis): The surgical creation of a communicating passageway between the kidney and the urinary bladder to correct an irremovable obstruction in the ureter.

nephrocystitis (nef'-rō-sis-tī'tis): Inflammation of the kidney and the urinary bladder.

nephrocystosis (nef'-rō-sis-tō'-sis): The development of cysts in the kidney substance.

nephroedema (nef'-re-dē'-ma): Oedema caused by disease of the kidney. Rarely, oedema of the kidney.

nephrogenic (nef'-rō-jen'-ik): 1. Arising in a kidney. 2. Produced by the kidneys. 3. Capable of generating kidney tissue.

nephrogenous (nef-roj'-e-nus): Arising in a kidney.

nephrogram (nef'-rō-gram): X-ray of renal shadow following injection of opaque medium. — nephrography, n.; nephrographical, adj.; nephrographically, adv.

nephrography (ne-frog'-ra-fi): Roentgenography of the kidney.

nephrohaemia (nef-rō-hē'-mi-a): Congestion of the kidney.

nephrohydrosis (nef'-rō-hī-drō'-sis): Hydronephrosis (*q.v.*).

nephrohypertrophy (nef'-rō-hī-per'-tro-fi): Hypertrophy of the kidney.

nephrolith (nef'-rō-lith): A kidney stone.

nephrolithiasis (nef'-rō-lith-ī'-a-sis): The presence of stones in the kidney.

nephrolithotomy (nef'-rō-lith-ot'-o-mi): Removal of a stone from the kidney by an incision through the kidney substance.

nephrologist (ne-frol'-o-jist): A physician who specializes in diseases and disorders of the kidney.

nephrology (ne-frol'-o-ji): Scientific study of the kidneys and the diseases that affect them. — nephrological, adj.

nephrolysis (ne-frol'-i-sis): 1. Destruction of kidney substance. 2. The operation of freeing a kidney from adhesions. — nephrolytic, adj.

nephroma (ne-frō'-ma): A tumour that arises in the kidney.

nephromalacia (nef'-rō-ma-lā'shi-a): Softening of the kidney substance.

nephromegaly (nef'-rō-meg'-a-li): Enlargement of one or both kidneys.

nephron (nef'-ron): The basic structural and functional unit of the kidney, comprising a glomerulus (*q.v.*) within Bowman's capsule, proximal and distal convoluted tubules with the nephronic loop (loop of Henle) connecting them, and a straight collecting tubule via which urine is conveyed to the renal pelvis. There are more than a million nephrons in each kidney.

nephropathy (ne-frop'-a-thi): Any disease of the kidney(s). — nephropathic, adj.

nephropexy (nef'-ro-pek-si): Surgical fixation of a floating kidney.

nephrophthisis (ne-frof'-thi-sis): Tuberculosis of the kidney.

nephroptosis (nef-ro-tō'-sis): Downward displacement of the kidney; also called *floating kidney*.

nephropyelitis (nef'-rō-pī-e-lī'-tis): Inflammation of the pelvis and the parenchyma of the kidney.

nephropyelography (nef'rō-pī'e-log'-ra-fi): Roentgenography of the kidney including its pelvis.

nephropyelolithotomy (nef'-rō-pī'-e-lō-lith-ot'-o-mi): The surgical removal of a stone from the pelvic area of the kidney.

nephropyeloplasty (nef'-rō-pī'-e-lō-plas-ti): A plastic operation on the pelvis of the kidney.

nephropyosis (nef'-rō-pī'-ō'-sis): Pus formation in the kidney.

nephrorrhagia (nef'-rō-rā'-ji-a): Haemorrhage from a kidney or into the pelvis of the kidney.

nephrorrhaphy (nef-ror'-a-fi): Suturing a kidney or fixing a kidney in place by suturing. Nephropexy.

nephrosclerosis (nef'-rō-skle-ro'-sis): Hardening or sclerosis of the kidney. Seen in cardiovascular–renal disease. May be benign or malignant. ARTERIOLAR N. sclerosis of the small arteries of the kidney. — nephrosclerotic, adj.

nephrosis (ne-frō'-sis): A term descriptive of any degenerative change in the kidney, the tubules in particular, that is not associated with inflammation as occurs in nephritis, or with vascular involvement which may occur. ACUTE N., N. caused by certain chemical poisons, toxaemia of pregnancy, or obstructive jaundice; characterized by low urine output, and little or no oedema or proteinuria; HYPOXIC N. acute renal failure caused by hypovolaemia resulting from such conditions as burns, haemorrhage, or shock; LIPOID N., N. characterized by oedema and albuminuria, and increased blood cholesterol; occurs most often in children; TOXIC N. acute renal failure caused by ingestion of such poisons as mercuric chloride or by septicaemia. — Syn., *nephropathy; nephrodystrophy*.

nephrostomy (ne-fros'to-mi): A surgically established fistula from the pelvis of the kidney to the body surface. N. TUBE a tube inserted through the abdominal wall into the pelvis of the kidney to provide for drainage of urine.

nephrotic (ne-frot'ik): Relating to, resembling, or caused by nephrosis. N. SYNDROME a protein-wasting kidney condition; may be primary or secondary to some systemic disease; caused by damage to the glomerular membrane; characterized by fatigue, severe generalized oedema, ascites, proteinuria, hypoproteinaemia, hyperlipidaemia, lipiduria, hypoalbuminaemia, pleural effusion, lowered resistance to intercurrent infections. May be associated with diabetes mellitus, hypovolaemia, sickle cell disease, allergic reactions. Also called *nephrosis*.

nephrotomography (nef'rō-tō-mog'-ra-fi): An x-ray procedure for obtaining sectional views of the kidney.

nephrotomy (ne-frot'-o-mi): An incision into the kidney.

nephrotoxic (nef-rō-tok'-sik): Toxic or destructive to cells of the kidney. — nephrotoxicity, n.

nephrotoxin (nef-rō-tok'-sin): A cytotoxin that is destructive to kidney cells. — nephrotoxic, adj.

nephroureterectomy (nef'rō-ū-rē'-ter-ek'to-mi): Removal of a kidney along with a part or the whole of the ureter.

nephroureterocystectomy (nef'-rō-ū-rē'-ter-ō-sis-tek'-to-mi): Surgical excision of a kidney, ureter, and part or all of the urinary bladder.

nerve: An elongated bundle of fibres that may or may not be myelinated, along with blood vessels and connective tissue. The individual fibres are covered with a sheath called endoneurium; the individual bundles are covered with a sheath called perineurium; and the nerve is covered with a sheath called epineurium. AFFERENT N. a N. conveying impulses from the tissues to a nerve centre; also known as *receptor* and *sensory n.*; EFFERENT N. one that conveys impulses outward from a nerve centre; MIXED N. one that consists of both motor and sensory fibres. Nerves are also known as effector, motor, secretory, trophic, vasoconstrictor, vasodilator, etc., according to function and location. — nervi, pl.

nerve block: Regional anaesthesia produced by interruption of the passage of impulses over a nerve, usually by injection of an anaesthetic close to the nerve supplying the area to be anaesthetized.

nerve gas: A chemical compound in gaseous form which, following inhalation, ingestion, or application to the skin, is absorbed by the body, with serious effects on the nervous system and various body functions.

nervous (ner'vus): 1. Relating to nerves or nerve tissue. 2. Referring to a state of restlessness or timidity. 3. Easily excited or agitated. 4. Exhibiting undue irritation or excitability of the nervous system. N. BREAKDOWN a common non-medical term for an emotional illness or psychosis.

nervousness (nerv'us-nes): A state of unrest, jitteriness, and irritability.

nervous system: The structures that control the actions and functions of the body, which allow the individual to react and adjust to varying internal and external conditions. It comprises the central nervous system and the peripheral nervous system with its subsystems, the somatic and the autonomic systems. AUTONOMIC N.S. is concerned with regulating the activities of cardiac muscle, smooth muscle, and the glands of internal secretion. The autonomic system has two subsystems, (1) the PARASYMPATHETIC N.S. which consists of some of the cranial and sacral nerves that are concerned with the innervation of smooth and cardiac muscle and glands; and (2) the SYMPATHETIC N.S. which comprises a chain of ganglia on either side of the vertebral column in the thoracolumbar region; it sends fibres to all involuntary muscle tissue and glands. CENTRAL N.S. includes the brain and spinal cord; it is the integrative and control centre of the entire nervous system. PERIPHERAL N.S. consists of all parts of the nervous system outside of the pia arachnoid membrane of the brain and spinal cord; it includes the 12 pairs of cranial nerves and 31 pairs of spinal nerves and their many ganglia, branches, and fibres that reach out to the periphery of the body. SOMATIC N.S. consists of motor and sensory nerves that supply skeletal muscles and somatic tissues; it initiates voluntary actions.

nesidiectomy (nē-sid'i-ek'to-mi): Surgical removal of the pancreatic islets of Langerhans.

nesidioblastoma (nē-sid'i-ō-blas-tō'ma): A tumour of islet tissue of the pancreas.

nesidioblastosis (nē-sid'-i-ō-blas-tō'sis): Excessive proliferation of the islet cells and tissue of the pancreas.

nestia (nes'ti-a): Abstinence from food; starvation.

nestiostomy (nes-tē-os'tō-mi): The surgical creation of a permanent opening into the jejunum through the abdominal wall; jejunostomy.

nestis (nes'tis): The jejunum.

nettle rash (net'tl): 1. Popular term for urticaria; weals of the skin; see URTICARIA. 2. A fine, intensely itchy rash caused by contact with nettles; self-limited and of short duration.

network: In anatomy, a structure resembling a net; formed by intertwining fibres.

networking: Establishing professional contacts through social meetings. Networking is an active and dynamic and means of sharing innovations, disseminating practice developments, and sharing information.

Neufeld nail (nū'-feld, noy'-feld): A nail used in orthopaedic surgery for fixation of an intertrochantic fracture of the femur.

neur-, neuro-: Combining forms denoting (1) nerve; (2) neural tissue; (3) nervous system.

neural (nū'ral): Relating to a nerve or nerves. N. TUBE the embryonic epithelial tube from which the brain and spinal cord develop.

neuralgia (nū-ral'ji-a): Severe, paroxysmal pain occurring along the course of one or more nerves. Many varieties are distinguished and named according to the part affected or the nerve that supplies the part affected. GENICULATE N. severe pain in the middle ear and auditory canal, facial paralysis, lack of tearing and salivation, and loss of taste; due to a lesion of the facial nerve at the geniculate ganglion; often associated with herpes zoster; MIGRAINOUS N. characterized by severe burning pain over the eye and part of the face, with fever, rhinorrhoea, lacrimation; usually occurs in the morning and characteristically in clusters; POSTHERPETIC N. often follows herpes zoster in which the trigeminal nerve is involved; marked by burning, unrelenting pain; TRIGEMINAL N. may affect all or only one branch of the nerve; marked by excruciating episodic pain along the distribution of the nerve; also called *tic douloureux, cluster headache,* and *Horton's headache, facial neuralgia* and *Fothergill's neuralgia.*

neuralgic (nu-ral'jik): Relating to or resembling neuralgia.

neuranagenesis (nūr'an-a-jen'e-sis): The regeneration of a nerve following injury or destruction of part of the nerve.

neurapraxia (nū'ra-prak'si-a): Temporary loss of function in peripheral nerve fibres without interruption of the nerve. Most commonly due to crushing or prolonged pressure; recovery is usually rapid and complete.

neurasthenia (nū'ras-the'ni-a): A condition of nervous exhaustion characterized by lassitude, inertia, fatigue, loss of initiative, oversensitivity, and undue irritability; may be a sequela of psychiatric illness.

neurasthenic (nū-ras-then'ik): 1. One suffering from neurasthenia (*q.v.*). 2. Relating to neurasthenia.

neuraxis (nū-rak'sis): 1. An axon. Also called *neuraxon.* 2. The central nervous system.

neurectasis (nū-rek'ta-sis): The stretching of, or an operation for, the stretching of a nerve.

neurectomy (nū-rek'to-mi): The surgical division of a nerve or excision of part of a nerve to relieve pain.

neurectopia (nū'rek-tō'pi-a): A condition in which a nerve follows an abnormal course.

neurergic (nūr-er'jik): Relating to the action or activity of a nerve.

neuriatry (nū-rī'a-tri): The medical practice concerned with the treatment of the diseases and disorders of the nervous system.

neuricity (nū-ris'i-ti): The energy inherent in nervous tissue.

neurilemma, neurilema (nū-ri-lem'ma): The thin membranous layer of cells that cover the myelinated sheaths of the fibres of peripheral nerves or the axon of a non-myelinated nerve. See also ENDONEURIUM and SHEATH OF SCHWANN.

neurilemmitis, neurilemitis (nū'ri-lem-ī'tis): Inflammation of the neurilemma of one or more nerves.

neurilemmoma, neurilemoma (nū'-ri-lem-mō'ma): A benign, slow-growing tumour that arises from the neurilemma of certain cranial or spinal nerves. Also called *neurolemmoma* and *Schwannoma.*

neurinoma (nū-ri-nō'ma): A benign encapsulated fibroma (*q.v.*) which arises in the endoneurium of the sheath of Schwann of peripheral, autonomic, or cranial nerves. ACOUSTIC N. acoustic neuroma, see under NEUROMA.

neurinomatosis (nū'ri-nō-ma-tō'sis): A condition marked by the appearance of numerous neuromas.

neurite (nū'rīt): An old term for axon.

neuritis (nū-rī'tis): Inflammation of a nerve, accompanied by pain and tenderness over the nerve, sometimes by paraesthesias and loss of reflexes. DISSEMINATED N. polyneuritis; also called *multiple* N.; NUTRITIONAL N. beriberi (*q.v.*); OPTIC N. inflammation of the optic nerve; PERIPHERAL N., N. of nerve endings or of terminal nerves; RETROBULBAR N. acute impairment of vision, especially of central visual acuity, in one or both eyes; due to demyelination or other pathology of the orbital part of the optic nerve; SCIATIC N. inflammation of the sciatic nerve; sciatica, VESTIBULAR N. irritation of the vestibular part of the 8th cranial nerve; characterized by vertigo, vomiting, imbalance; to be differentiated from Ménière's disease (*q.v.*).

neuroanastomosis (nū'rō-an-as-to-mō'sis): The operation of joining or making a junction between nerves.

neuroanatomy (nū'rō-a-nat'o-mi): The anatomy of the nervous system. — neuroanatomical, adj.

neuroarthropathy (nū'rō-ar-throp'a-thi): A pathological joint condition occurring simultaneously with a disease of the nervous system.

neuroastrocytoma (nū'rō-as-trō-sī-tō'ma): A glioma (*q.v.*) made up chiefly of astrocytes; may arise in almost any part of the nervous system but most often occurs in the third ventricle of the brain.

neurobiology (nū'rō-bī-ol'o-ji): The biology of the nervous system.

neuroblast (nū'rō-blast): A primitive nerve cell.

neuroblastoma (nū-rō-blas-tō'ma): A malignant tumour seen mostly in infants and young children; composed of immature cells resembling neuroblasts; usually occurs in the retroperitoneal area, the adrenal medulla especially, and metastasizes to other organs and bones.

neurocanal (nū'-rō-kan-al): The vertebral column, which contains the spinal cord.

neuroceptor (nū'rō-sep-tor): A terminal branch of a dendrite that receives a stimulus from an adjoining neuron.

neurochemistry (nū'rō-kem'is-tri): The branch of neurology that deals with the chemistry of nerve substance.

neurochorioretinitis (nū-rō-ko'ri-ō-ret-i-nī'tis): Inflammation of the optic nerve, choroid and retina.

neurocirculatory (nū-rō-sir'kū-lā-tō'-ri): Relating to both the nervous and circulatory systems. N. ASTHENIA see under ASTHENIA.

neurocladism (nū-rok'la-dizm): The formation of new branches by a process of a neuron; said especially of the formation of a bridge between the two ends of a divided nerve.

neuroclonic (nū-rō-klon'ik): Relating to or characterized by nervous spasm.

neurocranium (nū'rō-krā'ni-um): The part of the cranium that contains the brain.

neurocutaneous (nū'rō-kū-tā'nē-us): Relating to (1) the nervous system and the skin; or (2) the nerves of the skin.

neurocyte (nū'rō-sīt): A nerve cell. Neuron.

neurocytoma (nū-rō-sī-tō'ma): A tumour made up of nervous system cells, usually ganglionic. See GANGLION.

neurodeatrophia (nū'rō-dē-a-trō'fi-a): Atrophy of the retina.

neurodendrite (nū'rō-den'drīt): A dendrite (q.v.).

neurodermatitis (nū'rō-der-ma-tī'tis): Lichen simplex (q.v.). Leathery, thickened patches of skin secondary to pruritus or anything that causes habitual scratching, e.g., insect bites, psoriasis, contact with chemicals. As the skin thickens, irritation increases, scratching causes further thickening and thus a vicious circle is set up.

neurodiagnosis (nū'rō-dī-ag-nō'sis): The diagnosis of nervous disorders. — neurodiagnostic, adj.

neurodynia (nū'rō-din'i-a): Pain in one or more nerves. Neuralgia.

neuroelectricity (nū'rō-e-lek-tris'i-ti): The electrical currents generated by the nervous system.

neuroencephalomyelopathy (nū'rō-en-kef'a-lō-mī-e-lop'a-thi, -sef'-): Pathology involving the nerves, brain, and spinal cord.

neuroendocrine (nū'rō-en'dō-krēn): 1. Relating to the relationship between the nervous and endocrine systems. 2. Relating to cells that release a hormone into the bloodstream following a neural stimulus, e.g., the beta cells of the islets of Langerhans in the pancreas.

neuroendocrinology (nū'rō-en'dō-krin-ol'o-ji): The study of relationships between the nervous and endocrine systems and their interactions.

neuroepithelium (nū'rō-ep-i-thē'li-um): Simple columnar epithelium made up of cells that act as receptors for external stimuli, as in the nose, tongue, and cochlea. — neuroepithelial, adj.

neurofibril (nū-rō-fī'bril): One of the many fine fibrils that run through the cytoplasm and the axons and dendrites of a nerve cell. It is thought that they may form the conducting element of the neuron. — neurofibrillary, adj.

neurofibrillary (nū-rō-fib'ri-lar-i): Relating to neurofibrils. N. TANGLE bundles of fibrillary material within the cytoplasm of neurons and projecting into the axon and dendrites, particularly those of the hippocampus; commonly seen in cerebral cortex of persons over 65 years of age.

neurofibroma (nū'rō-fī-brō'ma): A somewhat firm, benign tumour occurring on a peripheral nerve sheath and including portions of nerve fibres; often multiple; due to disorderly proliferation of Schwann cells. Also called *Schwann's tumour.*

neurofibromatosis (nū'rō-fī-brō-ma-tō'sis): A condition characterized by the formation of multiple neurofibromata and possible neuromas.

neurogangliitis (nū'rō-gang-gli-ī'tis): Old term for inflammation of a neuroganglion.

neuroganglion (nū-rō-gang'gli-on): A mass of nerve cell bodies in either the central or peripheral nervous system.

neurogastric (nū-rō-gas'trik): Relating to the nerves of the stomach.

neurogenesis (nū-rō-jen'e-sis): The development of nerve tissue.

neurogenic (nū-rō-jen'ik): 1. Originating within or forming nervous tissue. 2. Stimulating nervous energy. N. BLADDER a condition resulting from any defect in the functioning of the urinary bladder that is the result of damage to the nerve supply to that organ; N. SHOCK see under SHOCK.

neurogenous (nū-roj'e-nus): Arising from nervous tissue.

neuroglia (nū-rog'li-a): The tissue that supports elements of the central nervous system, especially the brain, spinal cord, and ganglia; of ectodermal origin; consists of a network of fine fibrils, stellate cells, and many radiating fibrillar processes. — neuroglial, adj.

neurogliacyte (nū-rog'li-a-sīt): A neuroglial cell.

neurogliocytoma (nū-rog'li-ō-sī-tō'ma): A tumour composed of neuroglial cells.

neuroglioma (nū-rōg'lī-ō'ma): A tumour composed of neuroglial tissue. Glioma.

neurogliosis (nū-rog'li-ō-sis): A condition characterized by formation of multiple foci of glioma in the brain and spinal cord.

neurogram (nū'rō-gram): The imprint that a mental experience makes on the brain; important in the development of memory and of personality.

neurohistology (nū'rō-his-tol'o-ji): The histology (*q.v.*) of the nervous system.

neurohormone (nū'rō-hor-mōn): A hormone that stimulates neuronal activity, *e.g.*, adrenaline.

neurohypophyseal (nū'rō-hīpō-fiz'i-al): Relating to the neurohypophysis (*q.v.*).

neurohypophysis (nū'rō-hī-pōf'i-sis): The posterior lobe of the pituitary gland. See also PITUITARY.

neuroid (nū'royd): Resembling a nerve.

neurolepsis (nū-rō-lep'sis): A state of consciousness in which anxiety and psychomotor activity are reduced and the individual is unresponsive to elements in the environment; sleep may occur but the individual responds to commands; may be induced by administration of analeptic (antipsychotic) drugs.

neuroleptanalgesia (nū'rō-lept-an-al-jē'zi-a): A state produced by the administration of a major tranquillizer and a narcotic analgesic together, most often after minor surgery, to produce somnolence and lessen the stress on the central nervous system that results from anaesthesia.

neuroleptic (nū-rō-lep'tik): 1. An agent that acts to produce symptoms resembling those of certain disorders of the nervous system. 2. An agent that acts on the nervous system to reduce anxiety and psychomotor activity; includes the tranquillizers and antipsychotics; used in psychotherapy for treating acute and chronic psychoses and the psychoses associated with old age.

neurologic (nū-rō-loj'ik): Relating to neurology or to the nervous system.

neurological observations leaflets (nū-rō-loj'-i-k'l): Leaflets offering information on neurological observations, particularly aimed at nurses working in accident and emergency, but they may also be relevant to others where neurological observation is an important assessment tool, particularly those treating patients following head injury. Sections include information on the Glasgow Coma Score (*q.v.*), eye opening, motor response, verbal response, pupil reaction, vital signs, and the importance of accurate scoring.

neurologist (nū-rol'o-jist): A physician who specializes in diseases of the brain, spinal cord, and nerves.

neurology (nū-rol'o-ji): The branch of medical science that deals with the nerves, their structure, function, and pathology, and with the diseases and disorders of the nervous system.

neurolymph (nū'rō-limf): Cerebrospinal fluid.

neurolysis (nū-rol'i-sis): 1. The breaking down of nerve substance. 2. The operation of freeing a nerve from adhesions. 3. Exhaustion of nerve from overstimulation. — neurolytic, adj.

neuroma (nū'rō'ma): A tumour made up of nerve cells and nerve tissue. An old general term for many neoplasms of the nervous system. ACOUSTIC N. a N. arising in the vestibular portion of the 8th cranial nerve; lies in the auditory canal and enlarges progressively, causing headache, dizziness, staggering gait, diplopia, and eventual hearing loss; may be unilateral or bilateral; is usually benign; JOPLIN'S N. perineural fibrosis of the plantar proper digital nerve; may result from bunionectomy or trauma to the first metatarsal joint; characterized by pain and paraesthesia on the plantar aspect of the joint; N. CUTIS a N. arising in the skin, nerve tissue may be involved, making the neoplasm extremely sensitive to painful stimuli.

neuromalacia (nū'rō-ma-lā'shi-a): Pathological softening of the nerves.

neuromatosis (nū'rō-ma-tō'sis): A condition characterized by the presence of numerous neuromas.

neuromuscular (nū'-rō-mus'kū-lar): Relating to nerves and muscles.

neuromyasthenia (nū'rō-mī-as-thē'ni-a): Muscular weakness associated with emotional lability. Cause unknown; symptoms usually include sore throat, headache, slight fever, malaise.

neuromyelitis (nū'rō-mī-e-lī'tis): Myelitis (*q.v.*) occurring in conjunction with neuritis. N. OPTICA demyelination of the optic nerve and spinal cord, marked by dimming of vision and possible blindness, flaccid paralysis of extremities, disturbances of sensation; more common in children than adults. Also called *Devic's disease*.

neuromyopathic (nū'rō-mī-op'a'-thik): Relating to a pathological condition of muscle and of the nerves supplying the muscles.

neuromyositis (nū'rō-mī-ō-sī'tis): Inflammation of both the nerves and muscles of a part.

neuron, neurone (nū'ron, nū'-rōn): The structural and functional unit of the nervous system comprising the fibres (dendrites) that convey impulses to the nerve cell, the nerve cell itself, and the fibres (axons) that convey impulses from the cell. May be classified according to function as (1) afferent, which carry impulses from receptors in all parts of the body to the central nervous system; (2) efferent, which carry impulses from the central nervous system to muscles and glands of the body; and (3) interneurons, which connect neurons within the nervous system. BIPOLAR N. one with two processes arising from opposite poles of the cell body; CONNECTOR N. one that serves as a link between a receptor and an effector neuron; INTERNUNCIAL N. a N. between two other N.S. connecting them; LOWER MOTOR N. a N. with the cell in the grey matter of the anterior horn of the spinal cord and the axon passing to skeletal muscle; UPPER MOTOR N. a N. with the cell in the cerebral cortex and the axon passing down the spinal cord to arborize with a lower motor N. — neural, adj.

neuronitis (nū-ro-nī′tis): Term applied to a disorder of the more proximal part of the peripheral nervous system; it involves breakdown of the fibres due to inflammation. VESTIBULAR N. may follow a viral infection; the patient feels dizzy when lying down and tends to fall or deviate to one side when walking; may persist for a few days or weeks; to be differentiated from Ménière's disease (*q.v.*).

neuronophage (nū-ron′ō-fāj): A phagocyte that destroys nerve cells.

neuro-ophthalmology (nū′rō-of-thal-mol′o-ji): The study of, or branch of medicine that deals with the diseases of the eye as related to the nervous system.

neuroparalysis (nū′rō-pa-ral′i-sis): Paralysis caused by disease of the nerve(s) supplying the affected part. — neuroparalytic, adj.

neuropathic (nū-rō-path′ik): 1. Relating to disease of the nervous system. 2. Having a nervous disease.

neuropathology (nū′-rō-path-ol′o-ji): A branch of medicine dealing with diseases of the nervous system. — neuropathological, adj.

neuropathy (nū-rop′-a-thi): A general term for any disease of the nerves, of known or unknown cause, in which there is functional disturbance in the peripheral nervous system. ASCENDING N., N. that progresses from the feet upward; DESCENDING N., N. that starts at the shoulders and progresses downward; DIABETIC N., N. that arises as a complication in diabetic patients; characterized by leg pain, abnormal burning sensation, tingling, and numbness; ENTRAPMENT N., N. due to compression of a nerve in a confined space such as the carpal tunnel in the wrist; characterized by pain, weakness; seen more often in women.

neuropharmacology (nū′rō-far-ma-kol′o-ji): The branch of pharmacology dealing with the drugs that affect the nervous system.

neurophonia (nū-rō-fō′ni-a): The involuntary uttering of peculiar cries or sounds often resembling the sounds produced by animals; characteristic of certain nervous disorders.

neurophysiology (nū′rō-fiz-ē-ol′-o-ji): The physiology of the nervous system. — neurophysiological, adj.

neuroplasm (nū′rō-plazm): The cytoplasm of a nerve cell.

neuroplasty (nū′rō-plas-ti): Surgical repair of nerves. — neuroplastic, adj.

neuropraxia (nū-rō-prak′si-a): Contusion or trauma to a nerve that results in temporary disruption of its function by blocking conduction of the nerve impulse.

neuropsychiatry (nū′ rō-sī-kī′a-tri): The combination of neurology and psychiatry; a specialty dealing with organic and functional diseases of the nervous system and utilizing the results of psychological tests in the diagnosis of neuropathology.

neuropsychology (nū′rō-sī-kol′-o-ji): A system in psychology that is based on neurology; it is the study of the relationships between the brain and behaviour.

neuropsychopathy (nū′rō-sī-kop′a-thi): Emotional illness that involves disease or disorder of the nervous system.

neuropsychosis (nū′rō-sī-kō′sis): Psychosis of neurological origin.

neuroradiology (nū′rō-rādi-ol′o-ji): Radiology of the central nervous system. Neuroroentgenology.

neuroretinitis (nū′rō-rō-ret-in-ī′tis): Inflammation of the optic nerve and the retina.

neuroroentgenography (nū′rō-rent-ge-nog′ra-fi): Neuroradiology (*q.v.*).

neurorrhaphy (nū-ror′a-fi): Suturing the ends of a divided nerve.

neurosarcoma (nū′-rō-sar-kō′ma): A sarcoma made up of nerve, connective, and vascular tissue.

neurosciences (nū′rō-sī′en-sis): The disciplines that are concerned with the anatomy, structure, function, development, and pathology of the various elements that make up the nervous system.

neurosclerosis (nū′rō-skle-rō′sis): The hardening of a nerve or of nerve tissue.

neurosecretory (nū′rō-sī′krē-to-ri): Relating to the secretory activity of nerves.

neurosensory (nū-rō-sen′so-ri): Relating to sensory nerves.

neurosis (nū-rō′sis): A functional emotional disorder, the commonest types being anxiety state, reactive depression, hysteria, and obsessional N. To be differentiated from psychosis by the fact that it arises from stresses and anxieties in the environment and that the individual usually retains his or her relation to reality. ANXIETY STATE N. an apprehensive state and feeling of uncertainty and helplessness without sufficient cause; occurs as a result of a threat to the person's self-esteem or identity; marked by recurrent anxiety attacks (panics) with symptoms that include all the signs of fear, leading up to fear of impending collapse and sometimes of death; CHARACTER N. a personality disorder in which the individual's character and lifestyle are abnormal and whose interpersonal relationships may or may not be normal; COMPULSIVE N., N. characterized by compulsion to perform certain acts against one's will to the extent that this interferes with living and functioning; DE-PERSONALIZATION N., N. in which the individual has strong feelings of unreality and estrangement, both physically and from the environment; DEPRESSIVE N., N. characterized by severe depression due to internal conflict; often follows the loss of a loved one or object; HYPO-CHONDRIACAL N. a condition characterized by the certainty that one has a physical illness although none can be detected; HYSTERICAL N., CONVERSION TYPE a form of psychoneurosis characterized by signs and manifestations that have no organic basis but arise from anxiety caused by some emotional conflict and which involve the special senses and the voluntary nervous system, *e.g.*, blindness, deafness, anaesthesia, pain, paralysis; INSTITUTIONAL N. apathy, non-participation, and withdrawal occurring in long-term patients in reaction to institutionalization; OBSESSIONAL N. of two types: (1) The patient has obsessive–compulsive thoughts, *i.e.*, is preoccupied with constantly recurring thoughts that cannot be eliminated; the thoughts are always painful and out of keeping with the patient's normal personality; (2) The patient has obsessive–compulsive thoughts and also engages in actions that are both obsessional and compulsive, such as handwashing, not touching doorknobs, etc. The ideas are often concerned with feelings of guilt; PHOBIC N., N. characterized by intense anxiety and unwanted fears that interfere with the adjustment to one's environment; SOMATIC N., N. in which the patient's anxiety is fixed on the body; SYMBOLIC N., N. in which the patient's anxiety is transformed into

bizarre behaviour; TRAUMATIC N. N. that results from injury; WAR N. shell shock; see under SHOCK.

neuroskeletal (nū′rō-skel′e-tal): Relating to the nervous system and the skeletal muscles.

neurospasm (nū′rō-spazm): Twitching of a muscle due to a disorder of the nerve supplying the muscle.

neurospongioma (nū′-rō-spon-ji-ō′ma): Medulloblastoma (*q.v.*).

neurostatus (nū-rō-stā′tus): The state of the patient's nervous system as shown in the case history.

neurosurgeon (nū-rō-sur′jun): A surgeon who specializes in surgery on nerves and other parts of the nervous system.

neurosurgery (nū-rō-ser′jer-i): Surgery involving any part of the nervous system. — neurosurgical, adj,

neurosyphilis (nū-rō-sif′i-lis): Infection of the brain or spinal cord, or both, by *Treponema pallidum*. The variety of clinical pictures produced is large, but the two common syndromes encountered are tabes dorsalis and dementia paralytica. The basic pathology is disease of the blood vessels, with later development of pathological changes in the meninges and the underlying nervous tissue. Very often symptoms of the disease do not arise until 20 years or more after the date of primary infection. See ARGYLL ROBERTSON PUPIL. — neurosyphilitic, adj.

neurotendinous (nū′rō-ten′din-us): Relating to both a nerve and a tendon.

neurotension (nū′rō-ten′shun): See NEURECTASIS.

neurothecitis (nū′rō-thē-sī′tis): Inflammation of the sheath of a nerve.

neurotherapy (nū-rō-ther′a-pi): The treatment of nervous diseases and disorders.

neurothlipsis (nū-rō-thlip′sis): Irritation or pressure on one or more nerves.

neurotic (nū-rot′ik): 1. Relating to neurosis. 2. Nervous. 3. A person suffering from a neurosis or from instability of the nervous system; usually characterized by over-reaction to stresses, but without loss of contact with reality.

neurotic disorders: Mental disorders in which there is no demonstrable organic disorder, and that are relatively enduring and/or recurring unless treated; the symptoms are not acceptable to the patient; anxiety states and panic states characterized by fear and apprehension may interfere with the person's social functioning.

neuroticism (nū-rot′i-sizm): The condition of being neurotic or suffering from abnormal nervousness.

neurotization (nū-rot′ī-zā′shun): 1. The regeneration of a nerve. 2. The implantation of a nerve into a paralysed muscle.

neurotmesis (nū-rot-mē′sis): Complete destruction of the connective tissue of a nerve causing interruption of the nerve; may be caused by scarring or cutting.

neurotomy (nū-rot′o-mi): Surgical cutting or division of a nerve.

neurotony (nū-rot′o-ni): The stretching of a nerve; sometimes done to relieve intractable pain. Neurectasis.

neurotoxic (nū-rō-toks′ik): Harmful or destructive to nerve tissue. — neurotoxicity, n.

neurotoxin (nū-rō-toks′in): Any toxic substance that acts directly on the nervous system and is destructive to nerve tissue, *e.g.*, the venom of certain snakes.

neurotransmission (nū′rō-trans-mish′un): The process by which a presynaptic cell releases a specific chemical agent to cross the synpase and stimulate or inhibit a postsynaptic cell.

neurotransmitter (nū′rō-trans-mi′ter): Any of several chemical substances that make possible the transmission of nerve impulses within the brain and from one nerve cell to another.

neurotrauma (nū-rō-traw′ma): Injury to a nerve or nerves.

neurotripsy (nū-rō-trip′si): The surgical crushing of a nerve.

neurotrophia (nū-rō-trō′fi-a): Impaired nutrition of the nervous system.

neurotrophic (nū-rō-tro′fik): 1. Relating to the influence of nervous impulses on the nutrition and normal condition of nerves. 2. Having a predilection for the nervous system, said especially of *Treponema pallidum*, some forms of which seem always to produce neurosyphilitic complications. N. VIRUSES (rabies, poliomyelitis, etc.) make their major attack on the cells of the nervous system.

neurovascular (nū-rō-vas′kū-lar): Relating to (1) both nerve and vascular tissues, or (2) the nerves that supply the walls of the blood vessels.

neurula (nū′roo-la): The period in the development of an embryo when the nervous system tissues begin to differentiate; occurs about 20 to 26 days after fertilization.

neutral (nū′tral): Having no positive properties or characteristics. In chemistry, neither acid nor basic in reaction.

neutralization (nū′tral-ī-zā′shun): 1. The conversion of an acid or basic substance into a neutral one. 2. The process of rendering any action or process ineffective. 3. In bacteriology, the action of an antibody in coating the membrane of a host cell, thus preventing a virus from attaching to it and invading the body.

neutralize (nū′tra-līz): 1. To render something neutral. 2. To render ineffective.

neutron (nū′tron): An elementary particle that is a constituent of the nuclei of all elements except hydrogen. It has no electric charge and is approximately the same size as a proton.

neutropenia (nū-trō-pē′ni-a): The condition in which there is a much lower percentage of neutrophils in the blood than normal.

neutrophil (nū′trō-phil): One form of polymorphonuclear leukocyte (*q.v.*); its nucleus has two or more lobes that are connected by strands of chromatin; stains readily with neutral dyes with the nucleus staining a dark blue and the cytoplasm pink. N.S constitute from 50% to 65% of the leukocytes in the blood and are essential for phagocytosis of bacteria and cellular debris. The number of N.S in the blood increases in certain pathological conditions and haemorrhage.

neutrophilia (nū-trō-fil′i-a): An increase in the percentage of neutrophils in a differential white blood cell count.

neutrophilic (nū-trō-fil′ik): Refers to cells that take up both acidic and basic stains.

newborn (nū′born): 1. A recently born infant. 2. Recently born.

Newcastle disease: A highly contagious viral disease of fowl, transmissible to humans; symptoms include those of severe follicular conjunctivitis and lymphangiitis.

NG: Abbreviation for nasogastric (*q.v.*).

NHS: Abbreviation for National Health Service (*q.v.*).

NHS central register: A central database for all NHS patients. Used to monitor changes when patients move from one GP to another, and flag populations for authorized health research purposes.

NHSCRD: Abbreviation for National Health Service Centre for Reviews and Dissemination (*q.v.*).

NHS Direct: A free health service supported by a 24-hour nurse advice and information helpline (Tel. 0845 4647), providing confidential information on: what to do if you are feeling ill; particular health conditions; local healthcare services, such as doctors, dentists, or late night opening pharmacies; and self-help and support organizations. Advice is also available online at http://www.nhsdirect.nhs.uk

NHS Information Authority: The body responsible for ensuring delivery of the Information for Health Strategy (*q.v.*).

NHS Plan: A framework, published in July 2000, outlining radical changes to the way the NHS is organized and managed.

NHS professionals: A national service to match health-care staff seeking temporary work with NHS employers who need them.

NHS University: An aid to learning available to all people working in the NHS. Learning materials are available online, and staff are able to access them through a variety of systems, including digital television. See E-LEARNING.

NHS walk-in centres: Clinics that provide treatment for minor injuries and illnesses seven days a week. An appointment is not required and patients are seen by an experienced NHS nurse.

niacin (nī'a-sin): Nicotinic acid; a member of the vitamin B complex; essential for glycolysis, fat synthesis, and prevention of pellagra. Found in high-protein diets that include meats, fish, poultry, organ meats, eggs, certain legumes, yeast, wheat germ, enriched or whole grain flour and cereals, nuts, peanuts, milk. Deficiency results in rough skin, loss of strength, gastrointestinal disturbances, pellagra, and depression. Niacin is not stored in the body and must be supplied daily.

NICE: Abbreviation for National Institute for Clinical Excellence (*q.v.*).

niche (nēsh): A depression or defect in an otherwise smooth surface, as in the wall of a hollow organ; is detected by x-ray.

nicking (nik'ing): Localized constriction of blood vessels in the retina; sometimes occurs in patients with arterial hypertension.

Nicolas–Favre disease (nē'kō-la-fav'ri): A venereal disease involving the inguinal lymph glands; see LYMPHOGRANULOMA VENEREUM under LYMPHOGRANULOMA.

nicotinamide (nik-ō-tin'a-mīd): Nicotinic acid amide; it has the same vitamin action as nicotinic acid, but is not a vasodilator. Deficiency occurs in alcoholics and is associated with the severe vomiting seen in cancer of the stomach, pancreas, and colon, and in intestinal obstruction. Also called *niacinamide*.

nicotine (nik'ō-tēn): A poisonous alkaloid (*q.v.*) derived from tobacco.

nicotinic acid (nik-ō-tin'ik): Niacin (*q.v.*); vitamin B₃. Occurs as a white crystalline powder; essential for metabolism of carbohydrate; used as a vasodilator and in the prevention and

treatment of pellagra. Occurs naturally in milk, cheese, liver, yeast, and cereals.

nicotinism (nik'ō-tin-izm): Poisoning caused by excessive use of tobacco or nicotine; characterized by stimulation of the central and autonomic nervous systems, followed by depression. Symptoms include nausea, vomiting, diarrhoea, salivation, weakness, mental confusion, sometimes shock and respiratory depression.

nictitation (nik-ti-tā'shun): Rapid and involuntary blinking of the eyelids. — nictitate, v.

NICU: Abbreviation for neonatal intensive care unit.

nidal (nī'dal): Relating to a nidus (*q.v.*).

nidation (nī-dā'shun): Implantation of the early embryo in the uterine mucosa.

NIDDM: Abbreviation for non-insulin-dependent diabetes mellitus, see under DIABETES.

nidus (nī'dus): 1. The focus of an infection. Septic focus. 2. A group of cells within the central nervous system.

Niemann–Pick disease (nē'-man-pik'): A hereditary disease of lipid metabolism, occurring chiefly in female Jewish infants. There is enlargement of the liver, spleen, and lymph nodes and mental subnormality. There is no effective treatment and the affected children die early. [Albert Niemann, German paediatrician, 1880–1921. Ludwig Pick, German paediatrician, 1868–1935.]

night: N. BLINDNESS nyctalopia (*q.v.*); reduced visual adaptation to darkness; may be associated with vitamin A deficiency; N. CRY a shrill cry uttered by children during sleep; may signify the beginning of hip joint disease when pain occurs in the relaxed joint; N. SWEAT sweating during sleep; often a symptom of tuberculosis; in debilitated children, a sign of rickets; N. TERRORS a disorder similar to nightmare; occurs most often in children who wake from sound sleep screaming in fright; the episode may last for some time, with the child remaining unconscious; N. VISION the ability to see at night or in a dim light.

night guard: A dental device worn at night to prevent and correct the effects of bruxism (*q.v.*).

Nightingale, Florence: Considered the founder of modern nursing; in 1860, established the Nightingale School at St. Thomas's Hospital, London, which set the pattern for nursing education throughout the world. [1820–1910.] See also under NOTES ON NURSING.

nightmare: A terrifying dream occurring during rapid eye movement sleep (*q.v.*) that arouses feelings of intense, inescapable fear, terror, distress or extreme anxiety and usually awakens the sleeper.

nightshade: A plant of the genus *Solanum*. DEADLY N. belladonna, the active principle in atropine, a drug used in medicine as a mydriatic, sedative, antispasmodic, antisudorific, and narcotic.

nightwalking: Walking during sleep. Somnambulism.

nigral (nī'gral): Relating to the substantia nigra; see under SUBSTANTIA.

nigrities (nī-grish'i-ēz): Blackness. N. LINGUAE black tongue; see under TONGUE.

nihilism (nī'il-izm): 1. In psychiatry, a form of delusion in which the patient denies the reality of everything, including that of the self, in whole or in part. 2. In medicine, THERAPEUTIC N. disbelief in the therapeutic value of drugs. 3. The performance of acts that are destructive to the world at large as well as to oneself.

Nikolsky's sign: A condition in which the external layer of skin 'slips' or rubs off with slight friction or injury; see in pemphigus vulgaris. [Pyotr V. Nikolsky, Russian dermatologist, 1858–1940.]

niphablepsia (nif-a-blep'si-a): Snow blindness. Also niphotyphlosis.

nipple (nip'l): 1. The conical eminence in the centre of the areola of the breast. The tip of the nipple has approximately 20 tiny openings to the lactiferous ducts. The skin of the nipple is surrounded by the lighter pigmented skin of the areola. 2. An artificial substitute for the human nipple used on an infant's nursing bottle. ACCESSORY N. a structure resembling a nipple occurring in an abnormal location; see MILK LINE.

NIPPV: Abbreviation for non-invasive positive pressure ventilation, see under VENTILATION.

nirvana (nir-vah'na): A state of bliss, with freedom from worry and the cares of the world; a Buddhist concept.

Nissl('s) bodies: Granular, stainable protein bodies within the cytoplasm of nerve cells and dendrites; they contain ribonucleoprotein, and are concerned with protein synthesis and metabolism.

nit: The egg of a louse. The nits of head lice are found firmly attached to the hair shaft.

nitrate (nī'trāt): Any salt of nitric acid.

nitric acid (nī'trik as'id): A colourless, corrosive inorganic acid that gives off choking fumes. It is exceedingly caustic; sometimes used for removing warts.

nitrite (nīt' -rīt): Any salt of a nitrous acid. Organic nitrites are used in treatment of certain

heart diseases; they cause the blood vessels to dilate and thus lower blood pressure.

nitrituria (nī-tri-tū'ri-a): The presence of nitrites in the urine.

nitrogen (nī'trō-jen): A colourless, tasteless, odourless, gaseous element; constitutes about 80% of the atmosphere and is an essential constituent of protein foods. N. is excreted mainly in the urine as urea; ammonia, creatine, and uric acid account for a further small amount; less than 10% total nitrogen is excreted in faeces; N. BALANCE the difference between the intake and output of N. by the body; a person is in positive N. balance when the intake exceeds the output, in negative balance when the intake of N. is less than the output; N. EQUILIBRIUM the condition that exists when the amount of N. excreted equals the amount taken into the body as foods; NON-PROTEIN N. (NPN) nitrogenous constituents in the blood that are not protein, *i.e.*, urea, uric acid, creatine, creatinine, amino acids, ammonia.

nitrogen mustard: A warfare agent (mechlorethamine hydrochloride) from which a series of therapeutic compounds are derived; has been used in medicine as antineoplastic agents in treatment of Hodgkin's disease, certain leukaemias, lymphosarcoma, and lymphoblastoma.

nitrogenous (nī-troj'en-us): Relating to or containing nitrogen.

nitroglycerin (nī'trō-glis'er-in): A vasodilating drug used in the prophylaxis and treatment of pain, particularly that of angina pectoris.

nitrosamines (nī-trōs-am'ēns): A group of derivatives of secondary amines, some of which appear to have carcinogenic properties.

nitrous (nī'trus): Relating to or containing nitrogen in its lowest valency. N. OXIDE a colourless, sweet-tasting gas with a not unpleasant odour; widely used in obstetrics, dental surgery, and for induction of anaesthesia. Laughing gas.

NMC: Abbreviation for Nursing and Midwifery Council (*q.v.*).

NMR: Abbreviation for nuclear magnetic resonance, see NUCLEAR MAGNETIC RESONANCE IMAGING.

N₂O: Chemical symbol for nitrous oxide, see under NITROUS.

Nocardia (nō-kar'di-a): A genus of branching aerobic microorganisms of the same family as *Actinomyces* (*q.v*); a few are pathogenic to humans. N. ASTEROIDES cause of a pulmonary infection resembling tuberculosis; N. BRASILIENSIS cause of mycetoma and nocardiosis;

N. MADUREA widely distributed in soil; causes maduromycosis.

nocardiosis (nō′kar-di-ō′sis): Infection caused by certain species of *Nocardia*; characterized by chills, sweating, anorexia, weight loss, dyspnoea.

nociassociation (nō′si-a-sō-si-ā′shun): The unconscious discharge of nervous energy following overstimulation of nociceptors (*q.v.*), as occurs in surgical shock, trauma, and some diseases.

nociceptive (nō-si-sep′tiv): 1. Relating to a neuron that is receptive to painful sensations. 2. Painful; injurious.

nociceptor (nō-si-sep′tor): A receptor that is stimulated by injuries that cause pain. Cf. BEN- ECEPTOR

noci-influence: A traumatic or harmful influence.

noct-, nocti-, nocto : Combining forms denoting night or during the night.

noctalbuminuria (nok′-tal-bū-min-ū′ri-a): The presence of large amounts of albumin in urine secreted during the night.

noctambulation (nok tam′bū-lā′shun): Sleep walking, somnambulism

noctiphobia (nok-ti-fō′bi-a): Morbid fear or dread of the night or darkness.

nocturia (nok-tū′ri-a): Excessive urination during the night. May or may not be a sign of kidney disease. Also called *nycturia*.

nocturnal ((nok-tur′nal): 1. Relating to the hours of darkness. 2. Nightly; during the night. 3. Descriptive of an individual or animal that is awake and active during the night and sleeps during the day. N. EMISSION 'wet dreams', expulsion of semen resulting from erotic dreams that culminate in orgasm; a common occurrence in males.

nodal (nō′dal): Relating to a node, often the atrioventricular node. N. RHYTHM see under RHYTHM.

node (nōd): 1. A small, rounded protuberance, mass, or swelling. 2. A constriction. ATROVEN- TRICULAR N. a small mass of neuromuscular fibres in the septa between the atria and the ventricles; conducts impulses from the atria to the bundle of His; LYMPH N. a mass of lymphoid tissue resembling a gland, found along the course of lymph vessels; N. OF RANVIER a constriction in the neurilemma of a nerve fibre. [Louis Antoine Ranvier, French pathologist 1835–1922.] SINOATRIAL N. situated at the opening of the superior vena cava into the right atrium; the wave of contraction begins here, then spreads over the heart; called the pacemaker of the heart; SINGER'S N. a small node that develops on the vocal cord(s) of singers as a result of overuse or improper use of the voice; SINUS N. sinoatrial N..

nodose (nō′dōs): Characterized by the presence of nodes; protuberances, or knotty swellings.

nodosity (nō-dos′i-ti): A node or protuberance.

nodular (nod′ū-lar): 1. Resembling or like a node or nodule. 2. Having nodules.

nodule (nod′ūl): A small, solid, palpable, elevated area, extending deeper into the dermis than a papule, and which moves when the skin is palpated.

noesis (nō-e′sis): Cognition; intellectual apprehension. — noetic, adj.

Nofnagel's syndrome (nof′-nā-g′lz): Unilateral third cranial nerve paralysis combined with ipsilateral cerebellar ataxia

Nolan principles (nō′-lan): Ideals governing public life drawn up by Lord Nolan's committee in 1995: selflessness, integrity, objectivity, accountability, openness, honesty and leadership.

noli me tangere (nō′li-mē-tan′jer-ē): Literally, 'touch me not'. An old term applied to destructive skin lesions; now used chiefly in referring to basal cell carcinoma (rodent ulcer).

noma (nō′ma): Gangrenous stomatitis; usually observed in malnourished children and debilitated adults. Starts with ulcers of the mucous membrane at the corners of the mouth and spreads to lips and cheeks, sometimes to the genitalia, and progresses with necrosis, sloughing of tissues and destruction of bone; marked by a foul odour. Also called *water canker, stomatonecrosis*, and *cancrum oris*.

nomenclature (nō′men-klā′chur): A system of words and terms used in a particular science or discipline.

Nomina Anatomica (nom′-i-na-an-a-tom′-i-ka): An international system of nomenclature for anatomy; approved by the Sixth International Congress of Anatomists in 1950 and amended several times since.

nomogram (nō′mō-gram): 1. A graphic representation, by any of various systems, of a numeric relationship. 2. A graph on which a number of variables are plotted in order that the value of a dependent variable can be read on the appropriate line when the values of other variables are given.

nomothetic (nō-mō-thet′ik): 1. In research, refers to a study in which a relatively small amount of data is collected from many people. Opp. of idiographic (*q.v.*). 2. Refers to general or universal laws concerned with the behaviour of people in groups rather than as individuals.

non-: Prefix denoting not, without, absence of.

nona-, noni-: Combining forms denoting nine or ninth.

non-accidental injury: Injury found on infants and young children occurring as a result of trauma inflicted upon them by caregivers, usually the parents.

nonan (nō'nan): Occurring every ninth day, as a symptom.

nonapeptide (non-a-pep'tīd): A peptide that contains nine amino acids.

non-compliance (non-kom-plī'ans): In healthcare, refers to the actions of a person who deviates from a prescribed therapeutic regimen or fails to keep appointments because of personal belief and who claims the right to some control over treatment.

non compos mentis (non kom'pos men'tis): Of unsound mind.

non-conductor (non-kon-duk'tor): A substance that does not readily conduct heat, light, sound, or electricity.

non-electrolyte (non-i-lek'trō-līt): A substance that in solution will not conduct electricity because the molecules do not dissociate into ions.

non-governmental organization: A group or company that does not belonging to, or associate with, any government.

non-granulocyte (non-gran'ū-lō-sīt): A nongranular leukocyte.

nonigravida (nō-ni-grav'i-da): A woman pregnant for the ninth time.

non-infectious (non-in-fek'shus): Not communicable; not spread by contact.

non-invasive (non-in-vā'siv): 1. Referring to a test or type of therapy that does not involve penetrating the skin or going into a body cavity. 2. Referring to a tumour that has not spread.

nonipara (nō-nip'a-ra): A woman who has given birth to nine viable offspring.

non-maleficence (non-mal-ef' -i-sens): 1. Do no harm. 2. Stringent duty not to injure others. See MALEFICENCE.

non-myelinated (non-mī' -e-lin-ā-ted): Referring to (1) a substance that contains no myelin, or (2) a nerve process that has no myelin sheath.

non-nucleated (non-nū'klē-ā-ted): Not having a nucleus.

non-parametric tests (non-pa-ra-met' -rik): Statistical analyses often used in place of their parametric (*q.v.*) counterparts when certain assumptions about the underlying population are questionable; for example, when it does not follow a normal distribution (*q.v.*).

non-pathogenic (non-path-ō-jen'ik): Not productive of or causing disease.

non-prescription (non-pre-skrip'shun): Referring to drugs that may be purchased over the counter, *i.e.*, without a doctor's prescription.

non-proprietary (non-prō-prī'e-tar-i): Refers to the name of a drug other than the trade name; may or may not be the same as the generic name.

non-purulent (non-pū'roo-lent): Non-pyogenic (*q.v.*).

non-pyogenic (non-pī-ō-jen'ik): 1. Not containing or associated with pus. 2. Not promoting the formation of pus.

non-rapid eye movements: Eye movements that occur during the early stages of sleep and which are not as rapid as those that occur during the later stage of deep sleep. NREM SLEEP that which begins as the person passes from wakefulness to deep sleep and no rapid eye movements occur; represents about 75% to 80% of one's total sleeping time.

non repetat: Do not repeat. Term used in ordering medications.

non-specific (non-spē-sif' -ik): 1. Not caused by a specific agent. 2. Referring to a disease for which the specific causative agent or organism has not been identified.

non-steroidal anti-inflammatory drugs: Medications that act as painkillers and reduce inflammation. They are the most commonly used drugs for arthritis and are particularly useful in the treatment of rheumatoid arthritis.

non-toxic (non-toks'ik): 1. Not poisonous. 2. Not capable of producing disease or injury. N. GOITRE simple or colloid G.; see under GOITRE.

non-tropical sprue: See COELIAC DISEASE.

non-union (non-ūn'yun): Failure of the ends of a fractured bone to unite or knit together.

non-urgent (non-ur'jent): In emergency department management or in triage, refers to a patient who presents for care but who does not require emergency service, and who is usually referred for appropriate routine medical attention.

non-viable (non-vī' a-b'l): Not capable of life, or of living independently. Often said of a fetus that is born before it is capable of living outside the uterus.

Noonan's syndrome: A condition of unknown cause occurring only in males; the individual is of short stature, webbed neck, low-set ears and often has valvular pulmonic stenosis. Testicular function may be normal, but fertility is often decreased. See also TURNER'S SYNDROME.

noradrenaline (nor-ad-ren'a-lin): A hormone secreted by the adrenal medulla; it acts to increase blood pressure by constricting the blood vessels; also available as an agent used in treatment of acute hypotension.

norepinephrine (nor'ep-i-nef'rin): Noradrenaline (q.v.).

norethindrone (nor-eth'in-drōn): A steroid hormone with action similar to that of progesterone; used in treatment of certain uterine conditions and, in combination with oestrogen or mestranol, as an oral contraceptive.

norm: A fixed standard or model.

norm-, normo-: Combining forms denoting normal.

normal: Natural, average, or healthy. N. SALINE or SALT SOLUTION see under SOLUTION.

normalcy (nor'mal-sĭ): The state of being normal.

normal distribution: A plot of a variable versus its frequency within a population that gives a symmetrical, bell-shaped curve. The assumption that the population from which a sample is taken follows this distribution is the foundation of many statistical tests.

normetanephrine (nor-met-a-nef'rin): A catabolite of adrenaline, found in some tissues and in urine, along with metanephrine.

normoblast (nor'mō-blast): A normal-sized nucleated red blood cell, the precursor of the erythrocyte. Normally present in the bone marrow, but appears in the blood in certain types of anaemia.

normocalcaemia (nor-mō-kal-sē'mi-a): The presence of a normal amount of calcium in the blood.

normocapnia (nor-mō-kap'ni-a): The condition in which the carbon dioxide tension in the blood is normal. — normocapnic, adj.

normocephalic (norm'ō-kef-al'ik,-sef-): Mesocephalic (q.v.).

normochromia (norm-ō-krō'mi-a): Normal colour and haemoglobin content of the red blood cells. — normochromic, adj.

normocyte (nor'mō-sīt): A nucleated red blood cell of normal size and haemoglobin content. — normocytic, adj.

normoglycaemia (nor-mō-glī-sē'mi-a): The condition of having the normal amount of glucose in the blood. — normoglycaemic, adj.

normokalaemia (nor-mō-kal-ē'mi-a): The presence of the normal amount of potassium in the blood. — normokalaemic, adj.

normoproteinaemia (nor-mō-prō'te-in-ē'mi-a): The presence of the normal protein content in the blood.

normoskeocytosis (nor-mō-skē'ō-sī-tō'sis): The presence of the normal number of leukocytes in the blood, many of which, however, are immature.

normotension (nor-mō-ten'shun): Normal tension, by current custom alluding to blood pressure. — normotensive, adj.

normotensive (nor-mō-ten'siv): 1. Relating to normal tone, tension, or pressure, by custom referring to blood pressure. 2. An individual with normal blood pressure.

normothermia (nor-mō-ther'mi-a): Normal body temperature, as opposed to hyperthermia and hypothermia. — normothermic, adj.

normotonia (nor-mō-tō'ni-a): Normal strength, tension, or tone, by current custom referring to muscle tissue. — normotonic, adj.; normotonicity, n.

normotopia (nor-mō-tō'pi-a): In anatomy, normal location.

normotrophic (nor-mō-trō'fik): Of normal size and development.

normouricuria (nor'mō-ū-ri-kū'ri-a): The presence of the normal amount of uric acid in the urine.

normovolaemia (nor-mō-vō-lē'mi-a): Having the normal volume of blood. — normovolaemic, adj.

North American Nursing Diagnosis Association: (NANDA) Formerly called the National Conference Group on Classification of Nursing Diagnoses. Has met at regular intervals since 1973 to develop a classification system for nursing diagnoses that are concerned with the alterations or potential alterations in individuals' health status and the human responses to these alterations to the extent that they involve the nursing process. At each meeting of the Association the list of previously approved nursing diagnoses is reviewed and corrected as necessary and the newly approved diagnoses are added.

Norton scale: A scoring chart devised by Norton, McLaren and Exton-Smith that lists five characteristics of elderly patients who are at risk of developing decubitus ulcers and rates them on a scale of 1 to 4, from good (4) to very bad (1); the characteristics are physical condition, mental condition, activity, mobility, and incontinence.

nos-, noso-: Combining forms denoting disease, pathology.

nosaetiology (nōs'ē-ti-ol' -o-ji): The study of the causes of disease.

nose: The prominent structure in the middle of the face; the organ of smell and the beginning of the respiratory tract; it warms and filters the inspired air.

nosebleed: Haemorrhage from the nose. Syn., *epistaxis.*

Nosema (nō-sēm' -a): A group of several spore-forming protozoan species that cause infections in invertebrates and, rarely, in humans.

nosematosis (nō-sēm-a-tō'sis): Infection with a *Nosema* organism which, in humans, causes necrotizing keratosis of the cornea and painful inflammation of the conjunctiva; may also be associated with meningoencephalitis and meningitis.

nosh: To eat or snack between meals, or the food taken as snacks between meals. (slang).

nosocomial (nōs'ō-kō'mi-al): Relating to a hospital. N. DISEASE a new disorder, not related to the original disease, that is caused or aggravated by hospital life; N. INFECTION an infection acquired during hospitalization; organisms commonly involved include *Staphylococcus, Pseudomonas, Escherichia coli, Candida albicans, Streptococcus,* and the viruses of herpes and hepatitis.

nosocomium (nōs' -ō-kō'mi-um): A hospital or infirmary. Also *nosocomion.*

nosogenesis (nōs'ō-jen'e-sis): Pathogenesis (*q.v.*).

nosology (nō-sol'o-je): The science of the systematic classification of diseases.

nosomania (nōs-ō-mā'ni-a): The unfounded and irrational belief that one is afflicted with a particular disease.

nosophilia (nōs'ō-fil'i-a): A morbid desire to be ill. — nosophiliac, adj.; n.

nosophobia (nōs'ō-fō'bi-a): A morbid dread or fear of disease, or of contracting a certain disease.

Nosopsyllus fasciatus (nōs'ō-sil'us fas-si-ā'tus): A species of the rat flea that transmits murine typhus and possibly plague.

nosotaxy (nōs-ō-tak'si): The classification of diseases.

nosotherapy (nōs-ō-ther'a-pi): Treatment that involves the introduction of another agent or organism into the body in addition to the one being treated.

nostrils (nos'trils): The anterior openings in the nose; the anterior nares.

nostrum (nos'trum): A quack or patent remedy; or a secret remedy that is recommended by its maker.

notalgia (nō-tal'ji-a): An old term for pain in the back.

notch: A rather deep impression or indentation; usually refers to such an indentation on the surface of a bone or organ. INFRASTERNAL N. a landmark depression in the anterior abdominal wall just above the xiphoid cartilage; SUPRASTERNAL N. or JUGULAR N. the depression in the centre of the upper part of the sternum; an anatomical landmark.

notencephalocele (nō-ten-kef'a-lō-sēl,-sef' -): A hernial protrusion of brain substance through a malformed occiput.

Notes on Nursing: What It Is and What It Is Not: A treatise on nursing by Florence Nightingale (*q.v.*), published in 1859. The first book on nursing written by a nurse; draws attention to the author's ideas concerning hospital construction, ventilation, cleanliness, diets for patients, the nurse's functions, and the need for careful observation of the patient in order to plan for prevention of disease and for care of the sick.

notifiable (nō-ti-fi'a-b'l): In healthcare, referring to those designated diseases that are required by law to be reported to health authorities.

notochord (nō'tō-kord): The long rod of cells that forms the longitudinal supportive structure in an embryo. Traces of it remain in the adult in the central portion of the intervertebral discs.

notomelus (nō-tom'e-lus): A congenital anomaly in which supernumerary limbs are attached to the back.

notomyelitis (nō' -tō-mī-e-lī'tis): Inflammation of the spinal cord.

nourish (nur'ish): To provide foods and other substances that are essential for maintaining and supporting growth and life.

nourishment (nur' -ish-ment): Food, vitamins, minerals, and other substances needed to maintain and support growth and life.

noxious (nok'shus): Harmful; not wholesome; injurious to health.

NPN: Abbreviation for non-protein nitrogen, see under NITROGEN.

NREM: Abbreviation for non-rapid eye movements (*q.v.*).

NRR: Abbreviation for National Research Register (*q.v.*).

NSAIDs: Abbreviation for non-steroidal anti-inflammatory drugs (*q.v.*).

NSFs: Abbreviations for National Service Frameworks (*q.v.*).

NTO: Abbreviation for National Training Organization (*q.v.*).

nubecula (nū-bek'ū-la): Cloudiness, especially that of the cornea or of urine. See NEBULA.

nubile (nu'-b'il): Marriageable; said of a girl or young woman, especially in regard to physical development or age.

nucha (nū'ka): The nape of the neck. — nuchal, adj.

nuchal (nū'kal): Relating to the nucha (q.v.). N. CORD an umbilical cord that is looped around the baby's neck as it is being born; occurs most often with long cords and can usually be slipped over the baby's head; N. RIGIDITY stiffness of the neck; may be associated with spasm and pain on movement; a common sign of meningeal irritation.

Nuck: Canal of Nuck, a diverticulum of the peritoneal membrane extending into the inguinal canal; in the female, the round ligament passes along it to the pubic region; in the male, it accompanies the testis into the scrotum; may be the seat of inguinal hernia or the development of cysts. [Anton Nuck, Dutch anatomist, 1650–1692.]

nuclear (nū'klē-ar): 1. Relating to or containing a nucleus. 2. Forming, or like, a nucleus. 3. Characterized by the use of atomic energy. 4. Relating to atomic nuclei. N. CHEMISTRY the branch of chemistry that deals with changes in the nucleus of the atom; N. ENERGY energy that is released in reactions involving the nuclei of atoms; N. FISSION the splitting of certain heavy atomic nuclei into large fractions, accompanied by conversion of part of the mass into energy; the principle of the atomic bomb; N. PHYSICS that branch of physics that deals with the structure and properties of the nuclei of atoms.

nuclear family: A family consisting only of a father, mother, and their children.

nuclear magnetic resonance imaging: A process that utilizes magnets to produce three-dimensional images of internal organs to locate tumours without using x-rays or radioactive elements.

nuclear medicine: That branch of medicine which deals with the use of radionuclides in diagnosis, therapy, and research.

nucleated (nū-klē-āt-ed): Possessing one or more nuclei.

nucleic acid (nū-klē'ik): Any of a large group of important chemical substances containing phosphoric acid, sugar, and purine and pyrimidine bases; found in the nuclei and cytoplasm of the cells of all living organisms; are concerned with the determination of genetic characteristics and their transmission. Two important types are ribonucleic acid and deoxyribonucleic acid.

nucleolus (nū-klē'ō-lus): A small, rounded, basophilic body within the cell nucleus; usually single but there may be several; rich in ribonucleic acid and protein; essential in the formation of ribosomes (q.v.). — nucleoli, pl.; nucleolar, adj.

nucleoplasm (nū'klē-ō-plazm): The protoplasm that makes up the nucleus of the cell. Also called karyoplasm.

nucleoproteins (nū'klē-ō-prō'tē-inz): The form in which nucleic acids are found in the nuclei of plant and animal cells; consist of conjugated proteins in which the protein molecules are closely associated with those of nucleic acid.

nucleoside (nū'klē-ō-sīd): A compound formed by the combination of a purine or pyrimidine base with a pentose sugar.

nucleotide (nū'klē-ō-tīd): The structural unit of a nucleic acid; consists of an ester of a nucleoside and phosphoric acid.

nucleotoxin (nū'klē-ō-tok'sin): Any agent that is toxic to cell nuclei, including drugs, toxins, and viruses. — nucleotoxic, adj.

nucleus (nū-klē-us): 1. The inner essential part of a tissue cell, being necessary for the growth, nourishment, and reproduction of the cell, and for the transmission of hereditary characteristics. 2. A circumscribed accumulation of nerve cells of the central nervous system having a particular function. 3. The central core of an atom. N. PULPOSIS the soft core of an intervertebral disc which can prolapse (q.v.) into the spinal cord and/or nerve roots. Most common in the lumbar region where it causes low back pain and/or sciatica. — nuclei, pl.; nuclear, adj.

nudomania (nū-dō-mā'ni-a): Obsessive desire to be naked.

nudophobia (nū-dō-fō'bi-a): Abnormal aversion to being nude or unclothed.

null hypothesis (nul-hī-poth'-ē-sis): In statistics, the hypothesis that the independent variable has no significant effect on the dependent variable.

nulligravida (nul-i-grav'i-da): A woman who has never been pregnant.

nullipara (nul-lip'a-ra): A woman who has not had a pregnancy that lasted to the stage of viability.

nulliparity (nul-li-par'i-ti): The condition of not having borne any children.

numb (num): 1. Lacking sensation, especially when caused by anaesthesia or cold. 2. Lacking emotion; indifferent.

numbers needed to treat: A way of stating the benefits of an intervention. The number of subjects who need to receive a treatment before one subject has a positive outcome.

numbness (num'nes): Lack or diminution of sensation in a part.

nummular (num'ū-lar): Coin-shaped; resembling rolls of coins, as seen in the sputum in pulmonary tuberculosis.

nummulation (num'ū-lā' shun): An aggregation of red blood cells in a row resembling a roll of coins; rouleau (*q.v.*).

nurse: 1. To care for the sick, wounded, or helpless. 2. To feed an infant at the breast. 3. A person who is specially prepared and registered to provide care for the sick, wounded, or helpless, as well as those with potential health problems. Only those whose names appear on the register maintained by the Nursing and Midwifery Council are entitled legally to be called nurse. CHARGE N. one who is in charge of a unit; CIRCULATING N. one who does not 'scrub' but who is responsible for many functions in preparing the operating room before surgery and following surgery, for providing various materials and services that may be required during surgery, and for seeing that sterility in the surgical field is maintained; DISTRICT N. a professional nurse who is prepared through special education and training to provide a nursing service to patients in their own homes; OCCUPATIONAL HEALTH N., one employed in industry who gives immediate care to ill or injured workers, follows up on the sick and injured, and helps develop accident prevention and health programmes for workers; PAEDIATRIC N. a registered nurse qualified in the nursing care of the sick child; PRIMARY CARE N. consistently represents the nursing staff to assigned patients and their families throughout their contact in the hospital; is responsible for providing comprehensive nursing care while on duty and for directing others who give such care when the primary care nurse is off duty; is accountable to both the patient and the institutional administration for all outcomes of nursing activities on behalf of the patient; PSYCHIATRIC N. a registered nurse qualified in the nursing care of the mentally ill; SCHOOL N. a registered nurse employed to work in educational institutions to participate in health programmes for school-aged children. Responsibilities also include monitoring growth and development, screening for health problems and supporting those pupils with special needs; 'SCRUB' N. a nurse who assists a surgeon by handing him things he needs during an operation, holding retractors, etc.; WET N.

any woman who suckles someone else's child. See also CLINICAL NURSE SPECIALIST; NURSE PRACTITIONER.

nurse consultant: A new role in the NHS referring to an expert clinician who has four core functions: (1) expert practice with a minimum clinical focus of 50%; (2) professional leadership and consultancy; (3) education, training, and development; (4) practice and service development, research, and evaluation. See CLINICAL NURSE SPECIALIST; CONSULTANT NURSE; EXTENDED ROLE; HIGHER LEVEL PRACTICE.

nurse educator: A registered professional nurse who has also had education in the discipline of teaching and who specializes in the teaching of nursing and in planning and implementing nursing education programmes.

nurse practitioner: 1. A nurse who is able to diagnose and manage diseases commonly seen in healthcare, directly or indirectly with general practitioners and other members of the primary health-care team. 2. A registered nurse who has undertaken advanced preparation to provide nurse-led services for specific patient groups.

nurse prescribing: See CROWN REPORT II.

nursery: A unit or department in a hospital where the newborn are cared for. DAY N. a place where children of preschool age are cared for during the daytime.

nurses' agency: A service where nurses can register their availability for employment, usually private commercial nursing, 'bank' nursing, or 'specialing' a patient.

nurses' aide: A person who assists nurses to care for the sick, wounded, or helpless; may have a course of instruction and training before starting work supported by on-the-job instruction in tasks that are less technical than those performed by nurses; works under the direct supervision of a professional nurse. Also called nursing assistant (*q.v.*) or *health-care assistant*.

nurse specialist: A registered nurse who has acquired additional specialist knowledge and experience. He or she will have the skills and competencies required for managing a clinical caseload within agreed boundaries and protocols in line with clinical governance.

nurses' station: A centrally located administrative office in a hospital ward, or unit where nurses meet to give and receive reports and assignments, where patients' records are kept, where the ward clerk or secretary handles the necessary paperwork and answers the telephones, and where, in some instances, the computer terminals for centralized monitoring of patients are located.

nurse theorists: A person who develops integrated concepts or frameworks of nursing roles, functions, objectives, and activities and their relationships to clients and the role of other health professionals. See NIGHTINGALE, FLORENCE; PEPLAU, HILDEGARD.

nursigenic (nurs-i-jen'ik): A recently coined word used to identify a state or condition thought to have been induced by nursing action.

nursing: 1. Strictly, the activities involved in giving physical care and emotional support to the sick, wounded, and helpless. 2. Broadly, all activities performed by nurses and concerned with restoration or maintenance of individual and community health, both physical and mental. BARRIER N. a nursing technique involving keeping the infectious person isolated in a private room or other personal space; everything used in this space is disinfected before removal; paper and other disposable products are used when available. Called REVERSE BARRIER N. when the techniques involved protect the patient from acquiring infections from others; CLINICAL N. direct interventions by a nurse on behalf of a client; involves observing, evaluating, diagnosing, treating, counselling, serving as a clinical advocate; COMMUNITY HEALTH N. nursing practice aimed at promoting and preserving the health of populations, and extending continuous comprehensive nursing care to individuals, families, and groups; includes the work of health visitors, school nurses and district nurses; N. DEVELOPMENT UNIT a unit or centre based in the community or hospital, managed directly by nurses who control the budget and staffing; NDUs are committed to providing patient-centred care based on nursing models of care; GERIATRIC N. is concerned with the assessment of nursing needs of elderly patients and with planning and implementing nursing care to meet these needs; INTERNATIONAL N. nursing in foreign countries, often under the auspices of some agency established for giving aid to countries with limited healthcare facilities, *e.g.*, Save the Children Fund, Oxfam; OCCUPATIONAL HEALTH N. the application of nursing principles to the conservation and maintenance of workers' health; usually carried out at the place of employment; PRIMARY N. continuous comprehensive nursing care by a professional nurse who is assigned complete responsibility for planning, implementing, coordinating, and de-livering care to the patient from the time of entering the hospital until discharge, for seeing that the patient's needs are met when the primary nurse is off duty, and for providing the teaching needed by the patient and the patient's family; PSYCHIATRIC N. the branch of nursing that is concerned with the care of patients with mental disorders and with the prevention of such disorders; often involves working with families and others associated with the patient. Those psychiatric nurses working in situations outside of institutions with their clients are known as COMMUNITY PSYCHIATRIC; TEAM N. a system of nursing care in which a group of nursing staff, led by a registered nurse who is appointed by the head nurse on a unit, is assigned specific patients for whom the various team members provide comprehensive nursing care services; TRANSCULTURAL N. cross-cultural nursing, *i.e.*, working with people from varying cultural backgrounds; some US universities offer masters and doctoral degrees in this field.

nursing action: An activity, stated in the nursing care plan (*q.v.*), that is to be carried out by the nurse during a nursing intervention to meet a specific physical, psychologic, or socioeconomic need of the patient and which is expected to have a salutary effect on the patient's behaviour and/or health status.

Nursing and Midwifery Council: The regulatory body for nursing, midwifery and health visiting in the UK. It was established in April 2002 and replaced the United Kingdom Central Council for Nurses, Midwives and Health Visitors.

nursing assessment: The systematic collection and analysis of data relating to a patient's current health or illness problem; the first step in the nursing process. In addition to a physical inspection and the nurse's close observations as to how the patient is responding to the health problem, data is collected from the patient, family and significant others, usually through structured interviews. Data collected concern not only the current or potential health problem but also the patient's social, economic, emotional, and spiritual status, and personal view of the illness. All of this data is entered on the patient's permanent record, and may be added to or amended as the patient responds to various nursing interventions. The nursing assessment furnishes part of the database on which nursing diagnoses and nursing care plans are formulated.

nursing assistant: A non-professional health-care worker who assists professional nurses and who has had training in performing such basic procedures as bathing and taking temperature, pulse, and respirations; works under the direct supervision of a registered nurse; the term may be applied to nurses' aides, health-care workers, and certain other attendants, *e.g.*, auxillaries.

nursing audit: A means of monitoring the results of the nursing process through a systematic, written appraisal of the formally constructed patient care plan and the nurses' notes on the patient's record; done for the purpose of implementing and maintaining a quality assurance programme. The findings are compared to a set of standards of nursing care, which may be set by the health authority or trust. The audit may be done concurrently, that is, while the patient is receiving nursing care, or retrospectively after the patient has been discharged; in the latter case the patient's chart is used to obtain the data for the audit. CONCURRENT N.A. one done during the time that care is being given; EXTERNAL N.A. one done by a group of peers who were not involved in the patient care; INTERNAL N.A. one done by the caregivers who were involved in the patient's care; OUTCOME N.A. one in which the focus in on the patient and the end results of care; PEER N.A. evaluation of one's performance by a group of one's peers; PROCESS N.A. an examination of the nature and sequence of the events that took place during the time the patient was receiving care; RETROSPECTIVE N.A. one done after the care has been given; STRUCTURAL NURSING A. an A. of the organizational and physical elements of a health-care system.

nursing-bottle-mouth syndrome: Extensive cavities and discoloration of the teeth in young children, particularly those who have prolonged bottle feedings and who take their bottles of milk or sweetened juice to bed, thus exposing the teeth to contact with the milk or juice for many hours. Also referred to as *nursing-bottle caries*.

nursing care plan: A written protocol for nursing care prepared by a professional nurse at the beginning of the nurse–patient relationship; it is kept updated and modified as the patient responds to treatment and it becomes part of the patient's permanent record. The plan identifies the patient's nursing care problems as they are revealed by the nursing assessment and nursing diagnosis, states the nursing actions and interventions to be undertaken to correct or ameliorate those problems, sets patient-centred goals and outcomes to be achieved by the nursing actions, and states the nurse's evaluation of the patient's responses to the nursing actions.

nursing diagnosis (dī-ag-nō′-sēz): A statement of a health problem or a potential problem in the client's health status that a nurse is licensed and competent to treat. See DIAGNOSE.

nursing education: Education for the practice of nursing. Several types of programmes are available through colleges of nursing and universities. These include Project 2000 courses at diploma level and degree courses. Postgraduate courses including modules and doctoral programmes are widely available and support the ongoing continuing professional development of practitioners.

nursing goal: A general goal that the nurse hopes to achieve through nursing interventions and activities in connection with the patient's treatment for a specific condition or disorder, *e.g.*, the development of the individual's ability to care for him or herself in regard to personal hygiene, nutrition, and compliance with a prescribed medical or health promotion regimen.

nursing history: Data obtained from the patient and the patient's family, regarding the present illness, previous illnesses and hospitalizations, any handicaps, marital status, religion, general life activities and interests, allergies, food preferences, sleeping habits, medicines taken regularly, use of habituating drugs including alcohol and tobacco, type of work engaged in and any hazardous conditions in the workplace, etc. Data are usually obtained at the time the nursing assessment is made and are useful in making nursing care plans and in understanding the patient's reactions to the current situation.

nursing home: A convalescent home or private facility for the care of individuals who do not require hospitalization but who cannot be cared for at home. Following the introduction of the Care Standards Act 2002, the term 'care home' is also used.

nursing informatics: See HEALTH INFORMATICS; APPENDIX 7.

nursing intervention: The nursing action selected and implemented by the nurse to meet or resolve a patient's current or potential health need or problem. The action is based on analysis of the need or problem as revealed in the first step of the nursing process, *i.e.*, the nursing assessment.

nursing orders: Written instructions for the nurse who makes nursing interventions and carries out nursing activities called for by the nursing care plan; they are written and signed by a professional nurse and are not to be confused with medical orders.

nursing process: The scientific system of assessing, planning, organizing, implementing, delivering, and evaluating nursing care that progresses in orderly steps taken by the nurse. These steps begin with the collection of data obtained through a physical examination and interviews with the patient and significant others, progresses to the assessment and analysis of the patient's nursing care needs, the establishment of a nursing diagnosis and the making of a nursing care plan, the determination of priorities in carrying out the nursing interventions for which professional nurses are qualified, the setting of goals for the outcome of the interventions and, finally, to the evaluation of the patient's responses to the nursing care and to the treatment. Thus, a structural framework for the nurse patient relationship is formulated. At each step the nurse works closely with the patient and, whenever possible, with the family and other involved persons in collecting significant data relative to the patient's health history, current health status, and response to treatment. See also NURSING ACTION, NURSING ASSESSMENT, NURSING AUDIT, NURSING CARE PLAN, NURSING DIAGNOSIS, NURSING INTERVENTION, NURSING ORDERS.

nursing research: A systematic enquiry to discover facts or to test theories for the purpose of obtaining valid answers to questions raised or hypotheses made regarding some aspect of nursing. Research in nursing may be categorized as nursing practice research or clinical research, or practitioner-based research, *e.g.*, research in the field of nursing education or nursing service administration. The eventual goal of nursing research is improved nursing practice and better patient care. See also PRACTITIONER-BASED RESEARCH and PRACTICE DEVELOPMENT.

nursing theory: Concepts, definitions, and propositions applied to the study of various phenomena relating to nursing and nursing research.

nursling (nurs'ling): An infant that is still being breast-fed; one that has not been weaned.

nurturance (nur'chur-ans): Affectionate care and attention. — nurturant, adj.

nutation (nū-tā'shun): Nodding; applied especially to uncontrollable head shaking.

nutmeg (nut'meg): The dried ripe seed of the *Myristica fragrans* tree; a carminative, stimulant, and condiment; source of N. oil which, if taken in large quantities, produces narcosis and delirium, headache, restlessness, visual hallucinations, palpitation, flushing, and numbness of extremities; overuse may be accidental or intentional.

nutrient (nū'tri-ent): 1. Food that supplies the elements necessary to nourish the body. 2. Nourishing. 3. Serving as or providing nourishment. N. ARTERY one that enters a long bone; N. FORAMEN hole in a long bone that admits the N. artery.

nutriment (nū'tri-ment): Nourishment.

nutrition (nū-tri'-shun): 1. The sum total of the processes by which the living organism receives and utilizes the materials necessary for survival, growth and repair of tissues, the creation and liberation of energy, and the elimination of waste products and of unusable portions of the materials. 2. The science that deals with the food requirements of the body. — nutritions, nutritive, adj.

nutritionist (nū-trish'un-ist): A health-care professional with special education in the field of human nutrition; may function as a dietitian.

nutritious (nū'trish'us): Containing elements needed for growth, development, and health.

nutritive (nū'tri-tiv): Relating to or supplying nutrition to the body.

NVQ/SVQ: Abbreviation for National Vocational Qualification/Scottish Vocational Qualification (*q.v.*).

nyct-, nycti-, nycto-: Combining forms denoting (1) night; (2) darkness.

nyctalgia (nik-tal'ji-a): Pain that occurs only during sleep.

nyctalopia (nik'ta-lō'pi-a): Imperfect or defective vision in a dim light or at night; may be caused by retinitis pigmentosum (see under RETINITIS), or other eye disorders, or by vitamin A deficiency. Night blindness.

nyctamblyopia (nik-tam-bli-ō'pi-a): Poor night vision that does not seem to be due to any change in the eyes.

nyctophilia (nik'tō-fil'i-a): An abnormal preference for night-time over daytime.

nyctophobia (nik'tō-fō'bi-a): Abnormal fear of the night and darkness.

nycturia (nik-tū'ri-a): Nocturia (*q.v.*).

nymphae (nim'fē): The labia minora. — Sing., nympha.

nymphectomy (nim-fek'tō-mi): Excision of the labia minora.

nymphitis (nim-fi'tis): Inflammation of the labia minora.

nymphohymeneal (nim-fō-hī′me-nē-al): Relating to the labia minora and the hymen.

nymphomania (nim-fō-mā′ni-a): Excessive sexual desire in a female. — nyphomaniac, adj., n.

nymphomaniac (nim-fō-mā′ni-ak): **1.** A woman who exhibits nymphomania. **2.** Relating to nymphomania.

nystagmogram (nis-tag′mō-gram): The tracing of movements of the eyeball, produced by a nystagmograph.

nystagmograph (nis-tag′mō-graf): An instrument similar to the cardiograph for measuring the involuntary movements of the eyeball and recording them graphically. — nystagmography, n.

nystagmus (nis-tag′mus): Constant, rhythmic, involuntary, rapid movements of the eyeball, a neurological sign useful in diagnosing certain nervous conditions and drug toxicity, particularly that resulting from anticonvulsants and barbiturates. JERKING N., N. marked by movements that are faster in one direction than the other; this is normal when watching a moving object but may indicate drug toxicity or neurological or vestibular disorder; MINERS' N. caused by working many years in the dark or in poor light; OPTOKINETIC N. jerking movements of the eyes normally caused by watching moving objects or in situations like watching things from a moving train; PENDULAR N. characterized by oscillations that are equal in length in both directions; occurs in miners' N., albinism, and retinal pathology; POSITIONAL N. occurs when the head is placed in an abnormal plane; ROTARY N., N. in which the eyes move about the visual axis.

O

O: In chemistry, the symbol for oxygen (O_2).

oat cell carcinoma: Carcinoma in which the cells are elongated and blunted at the ends and have long oval nuclei and very little protoplasm. The tumour is not formed into a mass, but the tightly packed cells spread along the the lymphatics; most often affects the lung; the prognosis is usually poor. Also called *small cell lung cancer.*

ob-: A prefix denoting toward, against, over; inward; completely; in reverse order; in the way of (something).

obdormition (ob-dor-mish'un): Numbness and tingling in an extremity due to pressure on a sensory nerve; the part is commonly referred to as being '*asleep*'.

obese (ō-bēs'): Excessively fat. Syn., *corpulent, fat.*

obesity (ō-bē'si-ti): The condition of excessive accumulation and storage of fat in the body; occurs when more calories are consumed than are expended in the form of energy, and is evidenced when one's weight is greater than 20% of the expected weight for males and 25% for females. ENDOGENOUS O. that due to certain endocrine or metabolic disorders with the fat being distributed in certain body areas, *e.g.*, the girdle area; EXOGENOUS O. that due to excessive calorie intake; HYPERPLASTIC O. that due to an increase in the number of fat cells in the body; HYPERTROPHIC O., that due to increase in the size of fat cells in the body; MORBID O., increase in body weight of at least 70% more than the ideal weight for that individual, or over 45 kg over that weight.

obfuscate (ob'fus-kāt): To make cloudy, dim, or confuse; to make obscure or unnecessarily complicated. — obfuscated, adj.; obfuscation, n.

obfuscation (ob-fus-kā'shun): 1. Clouding, as of the cornea. 2. Mental confusion.

obicularis oculi (ō-bik-ū-lar'is ok'-ū-li): The circular, sphincter-like muscle that surrounds the orbit of the eye; its function is to allow the eyelids to close tightly.

objective (ob-jek'tiv): 1. Aim, goal, or target. 2. Relating to the object or end as the cause of action. 3. Final cause. 4. A lens or series of lenses in a microscope. 5. Pertaining to things external to one's self. Opp. of subjective (*q.v.*). O. SIGNS signs of disease which the observer notes, as distinct from the symptoms of which the patient complains.

objectivity (ob-jek-tiv'-i-ti): 1. The absence of bias in making observations or interpreting data. 2. The quality or character of being objective. 3. Corresponding to a true representation of the world.

obligate (ob'-li-gāt): 1. Compulsory; required; bound; of necessity. 2. To make necessary or require. In bacteriology, refers to an organism that can survive and thrive in only one particular environment; said particularly of certain bacteria; opp. of facultative.

oblique (ō-blēk): Slanting. EXTERNAL O. MUSCLE, forms the outer side of the side wall of the abdomen; INTERNAL O. MUSCLE, forms the second layer of the side wall of the abdomen. — obliquity, n.

obliteration (ob-lit'er-ā'shun): 1. The complete closure of a lumen, as of a blood vessel. 2. The complete removal of a part by a pathological process or by surgery. 3. Complete loss of memory for certain events. — obliterative, adj.

oblongata (ob-long-ga'ta): The medulla oblongata (*q.v.*).

observation (ob-zer-vā'shun): The act or faculty of noticing or paying attention. In nursing, the active process of utilizing all of one's senses to note things about the patient for the purpose of collecting data needed for formulating a nursing diagnosis and making a nursing care plan.

obsession (ob-sesh'un): A persistent, recurring pathological concern with an overvalued idea or set of ideas that dominate the mind, often leading to irrational actions and/or compulsive performance of certain acts, *e.g.*, frequent handwashing; the person may wish to banish these ideas from the mind but cannot. A characteristic symptom of patients with a diagnosis of obsessive–compulsive disorder.

obsessive–compulsive: In psychiatry, a type of neurosis marked by insistent compulsion to repeatedly perform certain acts or rituals or to entertain unwanted ideas, which often interfere with performance of normal daily activities; the obsessional ideas usually have to do with dirt. Likely to occur in children whose parents stress cleanliness and neatness.

obstetrician (ob-ste-trish'un): A qualified medical practitioner who practises obstetrics.

obstetrics (ob-stet'riks): The branch of medicine dealing with the care of the pregnant woman during pregnancy, labour and the puerperium; midwifery. — obstetric, obstetrical, adj.

obstipation (ob-sti-pā'shun): Obstinate constipation, sometimes due to intestinal obstruction.

obstruction (ob-struk'shun): 1. The blockage, clogging, or closing of a natural passageway. 2. An obstacle that blocks a passageway. 3. The condition of being blocked or clogged; may occur in any tubular structure including the colon, common bile duct, larynx, intestine, pancreatic duct. — obstructive, adj.

obstructive (ob-struk'tive): Obstructing or tending to obstruct. O. ANOSMIA loss of the sense of smell, which may be due to an obstruction of the nasal cavity or to disorder of the olfactory nerve; O. ANURIA a urological condition in which an obstruction in the urinary tract results in scanty or almost complete lack of urination; O. GLAUCOMA glaucoma in which the outflow of aqueous humour from the anterior chamber of the eye is obstructed; see NARROW-ANGLE GLAUCOMA under GLAUCOMA; O. JAUNDICE a condition in which there is interference with the flow of bile in some part of the biliary system; may be due to the presence of gallstones or tumour, hepatitis, alcoholism, or use of certain drugs; O. PULMONARY DISEASE any condition or disorder in which an obstruction interferes with air flow through the respiratory tract; may be due to a structural change, spasm, or excess secretions as occur in such disorders as bronchiectasis, bronchiolitis, bronchitis, bronchial stenosis, asthma, emphysema, cystic fibrosis. The term is also sometimes used to describe cor pulmonale (*q.v.*), pulmonary emboli, and adult respiratory disease syndrome in which pulmonary ventilation is compromised; O. SHOCK a state of shock resulting from obstruction in some part of the mainstream of blood flow; may be due to cardiac tamponade, compression on the vena cava, or pulmonary embolism.

obstruent (ob'stroo-ent): 1. Obstructing or blocking a passageway. 2. An agent that blocks or obstructs the passage of a discharge; usually refers to a discharge from the bowels.

obtund (ob-tund'): To blunt or to dull, said especially of pain or of sensation. — obtundent, adj.; n.

obturation (ob-tū-rā'shun): Closure; occlusion. Usually said of an opening or a passageway. — obturate, v.

obturator (ob'tū-rā-tor): Any natural or artificial thing that closes an aperture or opening O. FORAMEN the opening in the innominate bone, largely filled in by the O. MEMBRANE which is made up of muscle and fascia; O. MUSCLES two muscles at each side of the pelvic area, the O. INTERNUS and the O. EXTERNUS; they rotate the thigh laterally; OESOPHAGEAL O. a single-lumen tube with a balloon attached; used as an airway in unconscious non-breathing patients; it occludes the oesophagus and prevents gastric regurgitation.

obtuse (ob-tūs'): Dense, stupid, dull, blunted; lacking awareness of perception or sensation. — obtuseness, adj.; obtusely, n.

occipital (ok-sip'it-al): Relating to the back part of the head. O. BONE the bone at the back of the head, characterized by the large hole (foramen magnum) through which the cranial cavity communicates with the spinal canal; O. LOBE the portion of the cerebral hemisphere that lies behind the parietal and temporal lobes.

occipitoanterior (ok-sip'it-ō-an-tē'ri-or): Denoting the position of the fetus when the occiput lies in the anterior half of the maternal pelvis.

occipitofrontal (ok-sip'i-tō-fron'tal): Relating to the occiput and forehead. O. DIAMETER the measurement from the root of the nose to the occipital protuberance.

occipitomental (ok-sip'i-tō-men'tal): Relating to the occiput and the chin.

occipitoposterior (ok-sip'it-ō-pos-tē'ri-or): Denoting the position of the fetus when the occiput is in the posterior half of the maternal pelvis.

occiput (ok'si-put): The posterior region of the head.

occlude (o-klood'): 1. To shut, close, or stop up so as to prevent the normal passage of something. 2. To bring together, as the upper and lower teeth.

occlusion (o-kloo'shun): 1. The closure of an opening, especially of ducts or blood vessels, due to obstruction. 2. In dentistry, the fit of the teeth as the two jaws meet.

occlusive (o-kloo'siv): Serving to cover or close; often refers to a dressing or bandage that closes a wound or prevents its exposure to air.

occult (o-kult'): 1. Hidden, concealed, obscure. 2. In medicine, not detectable except by microscopic or chemical means; used especially to describe conditions such as blood in the urine or faeces, but also to describe certain infections, lesions or neoplasms. O. BLOOD see BLOOD.

occupational: O. DELIRIUM psychiatric term for a condition occurring in dementia and consisting of purposeless over-activity relating to a patient's occupation; O. DERMATITIS see DERMATITIS; O. DISEASE one contracted by reason of occupational exposure to an agent known to be hazardous to health, *e.g.*, dust, fumes, chemicals, radiation, etc. Also called *industrial disease*; O. HEALTH NURSE see under NURSE; O. NEUROSIS a functional disorder of a part of the body caused by occupational activity, *e.g.*, writer's cramp; O. THERAPIST a person who practises occupational therapy; O. THERAPY see under THERAPY.

occupational standards: A statement of what someone is expected to achieve at work. The standards are developed by representatives from every field of work and form the basis of the National Vocational Qualification/Scottish Vocational Qualification (*q.v.*); described in terms of units and elements of competence and the evidence required to support the assessment.

ochlophobia (ok-lō-fō'bi-a): Abnormal dread of crowds.

ochrodermatosis (ō'krō-der-ma-tō'sis): Yellowness of the skin.

ochronosis (o-krōn-ō'sis): Bluish and/or brownish discoloration of the skin and of the cartilage and connective tissue, especially around joints; often associated with alkaptonuria and the long-time application of phenol compounds to the skin and mucous membrane.

octa-, octo-: Combining forms denoting eight.

octan (ok'tan): Occurring every eighth day, counting both the first and last day of the episode; said of certain fevers.

octipara (ok-tip'a-ra): A woman who has borne eight viable children.

octogenarian (ok'tō-je-nair'i-an): A person who is in his or her eighties.

ocul-, oculo-: Combining forms denoting (1) the eye; (2) ocular.

ocular (ok'ū-lar): **1.** Relating to the eye, or the sense of sight. **2.** The eyepiece of a microscope. O. BOBBING sudden downwards jerking of the eyes at irregular intervals followed by slow return to normal position; seen infrequently in otherwise normal newborns.

oculisics (ok-ū-lis'iks): Eye movements that convey non-verbal communication.

oculist (ok'ū-list): Ophthalmologist (*q.v.*).

oculocephalogyric (ok'ū-lō-kef-a-lō-jī'rik,-sef-): Pertaining to rotary movements of the head and eyes.

oculocutaneous (ok'ū-lō-kū-tā'nē-us): Relating to or affecting both eyes and the skin.

oculofacial (ok'ū-lō-fā'shi-al): Relating to the eye and the face.

oculography (ok'ū-log'ra-fi): A technique for recording eye movements and eye position.

oculogyration (ok'ū-lō-jī-rā'shun): Circular movement of the eyeball.

oculogyric (ok-ū-lō-jī'rik): Referring to rotary movements of the eyeball. O. CRISIS a spasm of eye muscles that occurs in some neurological disorders; the eyeballs become fixed in one position, usually upwards; seen sometimes in parkinsonism.

oculomotor (ok'ū-lō-mō'tor): Relating to or causing movements of the eyeball. O. NERVE one of the third pair of cranial nerves that control eye movement and also supply the eyelid; fibres of this nerve also go to the pupil to control pupillary dilatation and contraction.

oculonasal (ok'ū-lō-nā'zal): Relating to the eye and the nose.

oculus (ok'ū-lus): The organ of vision; the eye. O. DEXTER right eye; O. SINISTER left eye. — oculi, pl.; ocular, adj.

Oddi: Sphincter of O., see under SPHINCTER.

odditis (ō-dī'tis): Inflammation of the sphincter of Oddi at the junction of the duodenum and the common bile duct.

odds ratio (odz-rā'-shi-ō): A statistic used to summarize the possible association between an independent (*q.v.*) and a dependent (*q.v.*) variable, *e.g.*, a risk factor and the incidence of disease. Clinical trials typically look for treatments that have odds ratios of less than one.

odont-, odonto-: Combining forms denoting a tooth or teeth.

odontalgia (ō'-don-tal'ji-a): Toothache.

odontectomy (ō'don-tek'to-mi): Surgical removal of a tooth or teeth.

odonterism (ō-don'ter-izm): Chattering of the teeth.

odontitis (ō-don-tī'tis): Inflammation of the pulp of a tooth.

odontoclasis (ō-don-tō'kla-sis): The fracture or breaking of a tooth.

odontodynia (ō-don'tō-din'i-a): Toothache.

odontogenesis (ō-don'tō-jen'e-sis): The formation and development of teeth. — odontogenic, adj.

odontoid (ō-don'toid): Resembling a tooth. O. PEG or PROCESS the toothlike projection from the upper surface of the body of the second cervical vertebra or axis.

odontolith (ō-don'to-lith): Tartar; the concretions which are deposited around teeth.

odontology (ō-don-tol"o-ji): Dentistry.

odontoma (ō-don-tō'ma): A tumour developing from or containing tooth structures. — odontomata, pl.; odontomatous, adj.

odontonoid (ō-don'to-noyd): Relating to a tumour that contains tooth substance.

odontopathy (ō'don-top'a'-thi): Any disease of the teeth.

odontoprisis (ō'don-top'ri-sis): Grinding of the teeth. Bruxism (q.v.).

odontorrhagia (ō-don-tō-rā'ji-a): Haemorrhage following extraction of a tooth or other dental surgery.

odontotherapy (ō-don-tō-ther'a-pi): The treatment given for diseases of the teeth.

odour (ō'-der): A quality of a substance that affects the sense of smell. Odours are described as pure when only one sensation is produced, or mixed when more than one sensation is produced. One system of classifying odours lists six fundamental sensations — spicy, fruity, flowery, resinous, foul, and burnt.

-odynia,-dynia: Combining forms denoting pain in a specific location.

odynophagia (ō-din'ō-fā'ji-a): Painful swallowing; dysphagia.

oedema (i-dē'-ma): Localized or general swelling due to the accumulation of fluids in the cells, intercellular spaces, and serous cavities. ANGIONEUROTIC O. acute, localized, transitory swelling of the subcutaneous and submucosal tissues; may be a hereditary condition or due to a food or drug allergy, or may be of nervous origin; marked by sudden onset, sometimes fever and arthralgia; involves chiefly the face and lips, larynx, viscera, and extremities. CARDIAC O. often results fron congestive heart failure, reduced cardiac output, hypertension or hypotension; most marked in the extremities; DEPENDENT O., O. occurring in the extremities and lower part of the body; NUTRITIONAL O. occurs in starvation or prolonged malnutrition; results from protein deprivation along with excessive intake of water and salt; ORTHOSTATIC O., O. of the legs which may develop in psychiatric patients who exhibit catatonia and stand in one position for a long period of time; PERIORBITAL O. fluid which collects in the tissues around the eye; PITTING O., O. in which pressure on the tissues produces long-lasting depressions; PULMONARY O. a form of waterlogging of the lungs resulting from left ventricular failure or mitral stenosis; also sometimes due to overloading of intravenous solutions; RENAL O. results from disturbed kidney function in nephritis.

oedematogenic (e-dēm-a-tō-jen'-ik): Producing or resulting in oedema.

oedipal (ēd'i-p'l): Relating to the Oedipus complex. O. STAGE the stage in a child's development when there is a feeling of strong attachment for the parent of the opposite sex and envious and aggressive feelings towards the parent of the child's own sex. See O. COMPLEX.

oedipism (ēd'i-pizm): 1. Infliction of injury to one's own eyes. 2. Manifestation of the Oedipus complex (q.v.).

Oedipus complex (ēd'i-pus kom'pleks): [Oedipus, King of Thebes, unwittingly killed his father and married his own mother. When he discovered the true relationship he tore out his own eyes.] A strong attachment of a child for the parent of the opposite sex resulting in a feeling of jealousy towards the parent of the same sex, and guilt, producing emotional conflict; usually said of a male offspring. This process was described by Freud as part of his theory of infantile sexuality and considered to be normal in male infants.

oesogastritis (ēs-ō-gas-trī'-tis): Inflammation of the mucous membrane lining of the stomach.

oesophagalgia (ē-sof-a-gal'-ji-a): Pain in the oesophagus.

oesophageal (ē-sof-a-jē'-al): Belonging or pertaining to the oesophagus. O. ATRESIA congenital failure of the lumen of the oesophagus to develop fully; O. DIVERTICULUM a circumscribed pouch-like protrusion from the wall of the oesophagus; O. HIATUS the opening in the diaphragm through which the oesophagus passes before joining the stomach; O. REFLUX see GASTROESOPHAGEAL R. under REFLUX; O. PLEXUS a plexus surrounding the oesophagus; made up of branches of the right and left vagus nerves and visceral fibres from the oesophagus; O. SPASM strong contractions of the muscles of the oesophagus occurring after the individual swallows food; the contractions are not coordinated and do not propel the food towards the stomach; seen chiefly in the elderly; O. SPEECH produced by the vibration of the column of air in the oesophagus; used after removal of the larynx; O. TEAR see MALLORY–WEISS SYNDROME; O. TUBE a soft, flexible tube used for stomach lavage or forced feeding; O. VARICES varices in the oesophageal wall; see VARIX.

oesophagectasia (ē-sof-a-jek-tā'-si-a): Dilatation of the oesophagus.

oesophagectomy (ē-sof' -a-jek' -to-mi): Excision of a portion of the oesophagus.

oesophagism (ē-sof' -a-jizm): Spasmodic stricture of the oesophagus, due to contraction of the circular muscle fibres, causing dysphagia.

oesophagitis (ē-sof-a-jī' -tis): Inflammation of the oesophageal mucosa; may progress to ulceration, haemorrhage, and secondary infection. PEPTIC O. caused by reflux of acid and pepsin from the stomach; may be associated with hiatus hernia or duodenal ulcer; often occurs in the elderly; also called *oesophageal reflux.*

oesophagocardioplasty (ē-sof' -a-gō-kar' -di-ō-plas-ti): A plastic operation on the oesophagus and the cardiac end of the stomach.

oesophagocele (ē-sof' -a-gō-sēl): Hernia, diverticulum, or distension of the oesophagus.

oesophagoenterostomy (ē-sof' -a-gō-en-ter-os' -to-mi): The surgical formation of an anastomosis between the oesophagus and the intestine.

oesophagogastrectomy (ē-sof' -a-gō-gas-trek' -to-mi): Removal of the distal end of the oesophagus and the proximal part of the stomach.

oesophagogastric (ē-sof' -a gō-gas' -trik): Pertaining to the oesophagus and the stomach.

oesophagogastroduodenoscope (ē-sof' -a-gō-gas' -trō-dū-ō-dē' -nō-skōp): An instrument for examining the interior of the oesophagus, stomach, and duodenum.

oesophagogastroscopy (ē-sof' -a-gō-gas-tros' -ko-pi): Examination of the oesophagus and stomach with an endoscope.

oesophagogastrostomy (ē-sof' -a-gō-gas-tros' -to-mi): The creation of artificial communication between the oesophagus and stomach. Also called *oesophagogastronanastomosis.*

oesophagogram (ē-sof' -a-gō-gram): An x-ray view of the oesophagus after the administration of a radiopaque substance.

oesophagomalacia (ē-sof' -a-gō-ma-lā' -shi-a): Softening of the walls of the oesophagus.

oesophagomyotomy (e-sof' -a-gō-mī-ot' -o-mi): An incision through the muscular wall of the oesophagus.

oesophagoplasty (e-sof' -a-gō-plas-ti): Plastic surgery for the repair of damage to the oesophagus.

oesophagoptosis (e-sof' -a-gop-tō' -sis): Relaxation of the oesophageal walls and downwards displacement of the oesophagus.

oesophagoscope (e-sof' -a-gō-skōp): An endoscope (*q.v.*) fitted with a light and lenses; used for examining the oesophagus.

oesophagoscopy (e-sof-a-gos' -kō-pi): The examination of the internal surface of the oesophagus with an endoscopic type of instrument.

oesophagospasm (e-sof' -a-gō-spazm): Spasm of the muscles of the oesophagus.

oesophagostenosis (e-sof' -a-gō-stē-nō' -sis): Constriction or stricture of the lumen of the oesophagus.

oesophagostomy (e-sof-a-gos' -to-mi): A surgically created fistula between the oesophagus and the exterior; used temporarily for feeding after excision of some part of the throat, usually for cancer.

oesophagotomy (e-sof-a-got' -o-mi): An incision into the oesophagus.

oesophagus (ē-sof' -a-gus): A musculomembranous canal or tube, about 23 or 25 cm long, that extends from the pharynx through the diaphragm to join the cardiac end of the stomach. Serves as a passageway for food.

oestradiol (ēs-tra-dī' -ol, es-): A steroid hormone, produced by the Graafian follicles and placenta, stimulates follicle growth, proliferation of the endometrium, and uterine contractions. Also influences the pituitary gland, stimulating production of gonadotrophic hormones. Also prepared synthetically. Administered subcutaneously or intramuscularly.

oestrin (ēs' -trin, es' -): Oestrogen.

oestrinization (ēs-trin-ī-zā' -shun, es-): 1. Descriptive of the alterations that take place in the vaginal and uterine mucosa during oestrus. 2. Treatment with oestrogenic substances.

oestriol (ēs' -trē-ōl, es' -): A naturally occurring oestrogenic hormone secreted by the ovaries and found chiefly in the urine; makes up about 90% of the oestrogen eliminated during pregnancy; it is synthesized by enzymes of the placenta and the adrenal gland of the fetus, hence measurement of the amount eliminated indicates the status of the placenta, the fetus, and the mother.

oestrogen (ēs' -trō-jen, es' -): The collective name for the female sex hormones, whether natural or synthetic; in humans they are formed in the ovary, fetoplacental uterus, adrenal cortex, and testes. Oestrogens are responsible for the development of secondary sex characteristics in the female and for the changes that occur in the genitalia during menstruation. They are used therapeutically in treating hormonal deficiencies, to suppress ovulation, to prevent lactation, and to ameliorate the symptoms of breast cancer. See also OESTROGENIC.

oestrogenic (ēst-rō-jen' -ik, est-): Having the action of the female sex hormones. See OES-TROGEN. O. HORMONES any of the substances secreted within the ovary that stimulate activity of the female sex organs; those produced in animals (mare) may be used in medicine when the normal supply is lacking or deficient. The active ingredient of the contraceptive pill.

oestrus (ēs' -trus, es' -): The sexually receptive state in females. In humans, it occurs during that phase of the menstrual cycle when changes in the lining of the uterus prepare it for receiving the fertilized ovum, should conception occur.

Office for Information on Health-Care Performance: An agency set up to publish information on national patient and NHS staff surveys, clinical audits (*q.v.*) and performance assessment, including the revised star ratings system.

Office of National Statistics: The organization responsible for producing official UK statistics in relation to the economy, population, and society at national and local level. This government department is responsible for conducting national surveys and censuses. http://www.statistics.gov.uk

OH: The symbol that represents the hydroxyl ion in solution. When one or more OH groups unite with a metallic element, a base is formed.

ohm (ōm): A unit of measurement of electrical resistance; the resistance through which a potential difference of one volt can produce a current of one ampere.

Ohm's law: States that for a given resistance the current flowing through it will be proportional to the voltage across it.

-oid: A suffix denoting having the quality, form, and appearance of; resembling the item designated in the first part of the word, *e.g.*, epitheloid.

oil: A liquid of fatty consistency and greasy feel, insoluble in water but soluble in ether and some alcohols; classified as animal, vegetable, or mineral according to source, and as volatile or fixed according to its action on exposure to air or heat.

oil immersion objective: An objective for the microscope that is equipped for a special lens to be used when oil replaces the air between the objective and the object being studied.

ointment (oynt'ment): A semisolid fatty mixture that is applied externally as a protective covering or as a vehicle for a medicinal substance that is to be absorbed.

old: In statistics one who has lived for a long time; often refers to the years between about 65 and 75. O. AGE usually refers to the final years of one's life, most often any age over 75. The World Health Seminar on Aging (Kiev, 1965) developed the following definitions: *elderly*, persons 60–74 years old; *old*, those between 75–89; *very old*, those over 90. Another classification lists those 55–75 as *young old*, and those 75–89 as *old*, and still another classifies those 75 and older as *old-old*. The term old-old has also been used to identify elderly persons who have survived major debilitating illnesses or mental disorders and who require a range of health and social services.

older persons: Advanced in years; not young; elderly; in the final part of the individual life course. In the UK can be associated with the age a person is entitled to his or her state pension: for men at 65 years, for women 60 years. It is a social construct rather than a biological stage as its onset and significance vary historically and culturally.

ole-, olei-, oleo-: Combining forms denoting oil.

oleaginous (ō-lē-aj'i-nus): Greasy, oily.

oleate (ō'lē-āt): A combination of an alkaloid or a metallic base in oleic acid; used as an ointment.

olecranarthritis (ō-lek'ran-ar-thrī'tis): Inflammation of the elbow joint.

olecranon (ō-lek'ra-non): The large process at the upper end of the ulna; it forms the tip of the elbow when the arm is flexed and fits into the olecranon fossa when the forearm is extended.

oleic acid (o-lē'ik): An acid prepared for fats; occurs as a yellow liquid used in the preparation of lotions.

oleotherapy (ō-lē-ō-ther' -a-pi): The use of oil in therapeutics.

oleum (ōl'ē-um): Oil. O. RICINI castor oil, a purgative; O. MORRHUAE cod liver oil (*q.v.*).

olfaction (ol-fak'shun): 1. The act of smelling. 2. The sense of smell.

olfactology (ol'fak-tol'o-ji): The science or study of the sense of smell.

olfactometer (ol'fak-tom'i-ter): A device for determining the keenness of an individual's sense of smell.

olfactorium (ol-fak-tor' -i-um): An air-conditioned temperature-controlled room into which a known concentration of an odour is introduced; the subject reports when he or she first detects the odour and when he or she recognizes it. Used to test a person's sense of smell.

olfactory (ol-fak'to-ri): Relating to the sense of smell. O. NERVE one of the first pair of cranial nerves; some of the processes of the O. nerve are embedded in the mucosal lining of the nasal cavity, and others penetrate the cribriform plate of the ethmoid bone and join others in the O. BULB that lies just above the ethmoid bone, from which they leave as olfactory tracts that travel to the cerebral cortex on the medial sides of the temporal lobes; O. ORGAN the nose. — olfaction, n.

olig-, oligo-: Combining forms denoting (1) deficiency; (2) insufficiency; (3) little, few.

oligaemia (ol-i-gē′mi-a): Diminished total quantity of blood in the body. — oligaemic, adj. Also called *olighaemia* and *oligohaemia*.

olighydria (ol′-ig-hid′ri-a): Scanty perspiration. Also called *oligidria*.

oligocholia (ol′i-gō-kō′li-a): A deficiency in the secretion of bile.

oligochylia (ol′i-gō-kī′li-a): A deficiency of chyle or of gastric juice.

oligocythaemia (ol′i-gō-sī-the′mi-a): Deficiency in the cellular elements in the blood.

oligodactylla, oligodactyly (ol′i-gō-dak-til′i-a, ol-i-gō-dak′ti-li): Fewer than the normal number of fingers or toes. — oligodactylic, adj.

oligodendrocyte (ol′i-gō-den′drō-sīt): One of the non-neural cells that form part of the structure of the neuroglia of the central nervous system. See NEUROGLIA.

oligodendroglioma (ol′i-gō-den-drō-glī-ō′ma): An intracerebral malignant tumour; arises from the oligodendrocytes; usually occurs in the frontal lobe; characterized by calcification, which gives a honeycomb appearance on x-ray.

oligodipsia (ol′i-gō-dip′si-a): Abnormally diminished sensation of thirst.

oligodontia (ol′i-gō-don′shi-a): Congenital absence of one or more of the teeth.

oligoerythrocythaemia (ol′i-gō-rith′rō-sī-the′mi-a): A deficiency of red blood cells or of colouring matter in these cells.

oligogalactia (ol′i-gō-ga-lak′shi-a): Diminished or deficient secretion of milk.

oligohydramnios (ol′i-gō-hī-dram′ni-ōs): Deficient amount of amniotic fluid in the pregnant uterus. Also called *oligamnios*.

oligohydruria (ol′i-gō-hī-drū′ri-a): Excretion of small amount of highly concentrated urine.

oligohypermenorrhoea (ol′i-gō-hī-per-men-ō-rē′a): Infrequent menstruation but with excessive flow.

oligohypomenorrhoea (ol′i-gō-hī-pō-men-ō-rē′a): Infrequent menstruation with less than normal flow.

oligoleukocythaemia (ol′i-gō-lū′kō-sī-the′mi-a): A reduction in the number of leukocytes in the circulating blood. Leukopenia.

oligomenorrhoea (ol′i-gō-men-ō-rē′a): Scanty or infrequent menstruation.

oligophosphaturia (ol′i-gō-fos-fa-tū′ri-a): An abnormally small amount of phosphates in the urine.

oligophrenia (ol′i-gō-frē′ni-a): Mental handicap due to faulty development. PHENYLPYRUVIC O., O. characterized by excretion of phenylpyruvic acid in the urine; see PHENYLKETONURIA.

oligopnoea (ol-i-gop′nē-a): Abnormally slow or infrequent respirations.

oligoptyalism (ol′i-gō-tī′a-lizm): Diminished or deficient secretion of ptyalin.

oligospermia (ol′i-gō-sper′mi-a): Deficiency in the number of spermatozoa in the semen.

oligotrichia (ol′-i-go-trik′-i-a): Congenital thinness of the hair.

oliguria (ol-i-gū′-ri-a): Deficient urine secretion in relation to amount of fluid intake; a condition frequently seen in persons with low cardiac output or renal failure. — oliguric, adj. Also called *oliguresia* and *oliguresis*.

olivary (ol′-i-var-i): Olive shaped.

olive oil: The oil of the olive; used externally as an emollient and lubricant, internally as a lubricant, and as a food.

Ollier's disease: Dyschondroplasia (*q.v.*).

-oma: A suffix denoting a tumour or neoplasm of the part named in the stem.

omagra (ō-mag′-ra): Gout in the shoulder joint.

omalgia (ō-mal′-ji-a): Pain in the shoulder.

omarthritis (ō′-mar-thrī′-tis): Arthritic pain and inflammation of the shoulder joint.

ombudsman (om′-buds-man): In healthcare, an agent officially appointed to investigate complaints for which the client or complainant has not received a satisfactory response or explanation at local level.

omentectomy (ō-men-tek′-to-mi): Excision of all or part of the omentum.

omentitis (o-men-tī′-tis): Inflammation of the omentum.

omentorrhaphy (ō-men-tor′a-fi): Suturing of the omentum.

omentum (ō-men′tum): A double layer of peritoneum that covers the stomach and hangs down like an apron covering the anterior surface of the abdominal organs. The functions of the O. are protection, repair and fat storage. GREATER O. the fold which hangs from the lower border of the stomach and covers the front of the intestines; LESSER O. a smaller fold, passing between the transverse fissure of the liver and the lesser curvature of the stomach. — omental, adj.

omitis (ō-mī-tis): Inflammation of the shoulder.

omo-: Combining form denoting shoulder.

omodynia (ō-mō-din'i-a): Pain in the shoulder.

omohyoid (ō-mō-hī'oyd): 1. Relating to the shoulder and the hyoid bone. 2. Refers to a digastric muscle that is attached to the scapula and the hyoid bone.

omphal-, omphalo-: Combining forms denoting the umbilicus.

omphalectomy (om-fa-lek'-to-mi): Excision of the umbilicus.

omphalitis (om-fa-lī'tis): Inflammation of the umbilicus.

omphalocele (om-fal'-ō-sēl): Congenital umbilical hernia.

omphaloncus (om-fa-lon'-kus): A swelling or tumour of the umbilicus.

omphaloproptosis (om'-fal-ō-prop-tō'-sis): Abnormal protrusion of the umbilicus.

omphalorrhagia (om'fa-lō-rā'-ji-a): Haemorrhage from the umbilicus.

omphalotomy (om-fa-lot'-o-mi): The severing or cutting of the umbilical cord.

omphalus (om'-fa-lus): The umbilicus.

onanism (ō'-nan-nizm): 1. Incomplete sexual intercourse with withdrawal before the emission of semen. 2. Masturbation.

onc-, onco-: Combining forms denoting (1) tumour; (2) swelling or mass; (3) barb or hook.

onchocerciasis (on'-kō-ser-kī'-a-sis): Infestation of humans with worms of the genus *Onchocerca*; the adult worms are encapsulated in subcutaneous connective tissue; may migrate to the eye causing opthalmic problems including cataract and blindness.

oncogene hypothesis: The theory that cancer may be caused by certain DNA viruses that insert their DNA within the genetic material; ordinarily they are held in suppression.

oncogenesis (on'-kō-jen'-e-sis): The production of tumours.

oncogenic (on'kō-jen'-ik): 1. Capable of tumour production. 2. Pertaining to the origin and growth of a neoplasm: often used to describe the carcinogenic viruses.

oncogenous (on'-koj'-e-nus): Arising in, originating in, or inducing the development of a tumour.

oncologist (on-kol'-o-jist): A physician who specializes in oncology (*q.v.*).

oncology (on-kol'-o-ji): The scientific study of tumours. — oncological, adj.

oncolysis (on-kol'-i-sis): The destruction of a neoplasm. Sometimes used to describe reduction in size of a tumour. — oncolytic, adj.

oncometer (on-kom'-i-ter): An instrument for measuring the variations in size or delineating the form of certain viscera such as the kidney.

oncosis (on-kō'-sis): 1. Any condition characterized by the formation of a neoplasm. 2. Any swelling or tumour. 3. The formation of multiple tumours.

oncothlipsis (on'-kō-thlip'-sis): Pressure caused by a pathological growth or a tumour.

oncotomy (on-kot'o-mi): An incision into a tumour, an abscess, or a cyst.

Ondine's curse: Term sometimes used to describe a syndrome wherein the individual is apnoeic although the respiratory organs are able to function normally; due to a defect in the breathing control centres in the central nervous system which are sensitive to excess carbon dioxide. May occur following infections such as poliomyelitis or encephalitis, certain types of brain and spinal cord surgery, or overdose of certain drugs; may also be the condition causing infant apnoea syndrome. [Ondine, a water nymph in fable, caused the human male who loved her to sleep continuously.]

oneiric (ō-nī'rik): Relating to dreams or dreaming.

oneiroanalysis (ō-nī'rō-a-nal'a-sis): Psychoanalysis that involves the exploration of the personality through the interpretation of drug-induced dreams.

oneirophrenia (ō-nī'rō-frē'ni-a): A form of schizophrenia marked by hallucinations, amnesia, confusion and disorientation, stupour, prolonged sleeplessness.

onomatopoiesis (on'-ō-ma-tō-poy-ē'-sis): In psychiatry, the creation by the patient of meaningless words, phrases, or sounds.

ONS: Abbreviation for Office of National Statistics (*q.v.*).

ontic (on'tik): Relating to or having real being or existence.

ontogenic, ontogenetic (on-tō-jen'ik, on-tō-jenet'ik): Referring to the development of an individual or organism as distinguished from the evolutionary development of a species.

ontogeny (on-toj'e-ni): The life history of an individual from a one-celled ovum to birth.

ontology (on-tol'-o-ji): 1. The science or study of being. 2. That department of metaphysics which relates to the being or essence of things, or to being in the abstract.

onych-, onycho-: Combining forms denoting the nails.

onychatrophia (on'i-ka-trō'fi-a): Atrophy of the finger- and toenails.

onychauxis (on-i-kawk'sis): Hypertrophy of a nail or nails.

onychectomy (on-i-kek'to-mi): Surgical removal of a nail.

onychia (ō-nik'i-a): Acute inflammation of the nail bed; may become suppurative and result in loss of the nail.

onychocryptosis (on'ik-ō-krip-tō'sis): Ingrowing of a toenail.

onychogryphosis (on'-ik-ō-grī-fō'sis): A deformed overgrowth of the nails in which they become ridged, thickened, and elongated, sometimes with an inward curvature.

onycholysis (on-i-kol'i-sis): Loosening of toe- or fingernail. — onycholytic, adj.

onychomadesis (on'i-kō-ma-dē'sis): The separation or loosening of the nails, beginning at the base and continuing until the nails fall off.

onychomalacia (on'ik-ō-ma-lā'shi-a): Softening of the nails.

onychomycosis (on'ik-ō-mi-kō'sis): A fungal infection of the nails causing thickening and splitting. Also called *ringworm of the nails*.

onychophagia, onychophagy (on-i-ki-ō-fā'ji-a, on-i-kof'a-ji): Nailbiting.

onychorrhexis (on'i-kō-rek'sis): Spontaneous splitting of the nails at the free edge.

onychosis (on-i-kō'sis): Any disease or deformity of the nails.

onychotillomania (on-i-kot'-i-lō-mā'ni-a): A neurotic habit of picking or tearing at the nails.

onychotomy (on-i-kot'o-mi): Surgical incision of a fingernail or toenail, usually to remove a mass under the nail.

onyx (on'iks): 1. A finger- or toenail. 2. A collection of pus that resembles a nail, located between the layers of the cornea.

onyxis (o-nik'sis): Ingrowing of a nail or nails.

ooblast (ō'ō-blast): A cell from which an ovum develops.

oocyst (ō'ō-sist): The encysted zygote in the life of some sporozoa. See OOKINETE.

oocyte (ō'ō-sīt): An immature ovum.

oogenesis (ō'o-jen'e-sis): The production and formation of ova in the ovary. — oogenetic, adj.

ookinete (ō'ō-kī-nēt): The zygote in the life cycle of some protozoan parasites, as that of the malarial parasite; it bores into the female mosquito's intestinal wall where it develops into an oocyst (*q.v.*).

oophor-, oophoro-: Combining forms denoting (1) ovary; (2) ovarian.

oophoralgia (ō-of'or-al'ji-a): Pain in an ovary.

oophorectomy (ō-of'o-rek'to-mi): Excision of an ovary; ovariectomy.

oophoritis (ō-of-or-ī'tis): Inflammation of one or both ovaries.

oophorocystectomy (ō-of'or-ō-sis-tek'to-mi): Removal of an ovarian cyst.

oophorocystosis (ō-of'ō-rō-sis-tō'sis): The formation of an ovarian cyst.

oophorohysterectomy (o-of'ō-rō-his-ter-ek'to-mi): The surgical removal of the ovaries and the uterus.

oophoroma (ō-of-or-ō'ma): A malignant tumour of the ovary.

oophoron (ō-of'or-on): The ovary.

oophoropexy (ō-of'o-rō-pek-si): See OVARIO-PEXY.

oophorosalpingectomy (ō-of'-or-ō-sal-pin-jek'to-mi): Excision of an ovary and its associated uterine tube.

oosperm (ō'ō-sperm): A fertilized ovum.

opacification (ō-pas'i-fi-kā'shun): The process of becoming opaque.

opacity (ō-pas'i ti): Non-transparency; cloudiness; an opaque spot, as on the cornea or lens.

opaque (ō-pāk'): Not transparent.

open: 1. Exposed to the air. 2. Not covered by skin. 3. To puncture, as a boil or abscess. 4. To make an opening into a wound or cavity. O. CARE care given to a patient in a community where programmes aimed at supporting living in one's home are available. O. FRACTURE one in which an external wound leads to the fractured bone; O.-HEART SURGERY performed on the opened heart; involves incision into one or more of the chambers of the heart. The term is often loosely used to refer to all heart surgery, whether or not the heart itself is opened; O. HOSPITAL see under HOSPITAL; O. REDUCTION reduction of a fracture after incision into the site of the fracture; O. WOUND one that opens to the surface of the body.

open learning: A system of learning which is based on independent study or initiative rather than formal classroom instruction.

operable (op'er-a-b'l): Descriptive of a condition that it is thought can be cured or improved by surgery that will not endanger the patient's life or general health.

operant (op'er-ant): In behavioural experimentation, refers to the desired response or behaviour chosen by the experimenter; hopefully, pairing the behaviour with a reinforcer will either increase or decrease its occurrence, whichever is desired. O. BEHAVIOUR behaviour that operates on the environment; O. CONDITIONING see under CONDITIONING; O. LEARNING THEORY the theory that behaviour is solely the result of environmental cues and rewards.

operation (op-er-ā'shun): A procedure in which a surgeon uses his hands or instruments to correct or alter a pathological condition or state or for removing a tumour, limb, etc. ELECTIVE O. one for which haste is not required; can be performed at the patient's and surgeon's convenience; EMERGENCY O. one that must be done immediately in order to save the patient's life; EXPLORATORY O. one done for diagnostic purposes; MAJOR O. one involving risk to the patient's life; MINOR O. a relatively simple one that usually does not involve risk to the patient's life; RADICAL O. one done in an effort to effect a complete cure; SUBTOTAL O. one in which not all of the involved organ is removed.

operculum (ō-per'kū-lum): **1.** A lid or covering. **2.** Obstructive tissue or substance. In obstetrics, the plug of mucous and mucoid material that fills the cervical canal during pregnancy and helps to prevent infection of the genital tract.

ophiasis (ō-fī'a-sis): A type of baldness in which hair is lost in one or more winding streaks around the hair margin.

ophidiophilia (ō-fid-i-ō-fil'i-a): Abnormal fondness for snakes.

ophidiophobia (ō-fid-i-ō-fō'bi-a): A morbid dread of snakes.

ophidism (ō'fi-dizm): Poisoning caused by snake venom.

ophiotoxaemia (ō'fi-ō-tok-sē'mi-a): Poisoning by snake venom.

ophthal-, ophthalmo-: Combining forms denoting (1) the eyes; (2) the eyeball.

ophthalmacrosis (of-thal-ma-krō'sis): Abnormal enlargement of the eyeball.

ophthalmagra (of'thal-mag'ra): Sudden pain in the eye.

ophthalmalgia (of'thal-mal'ji-a): Pain in the eye.

ophthalmatrophia (of'-thal-ma-trō'fi-a): Atrophy of the eye.

ophthalmectomy (of-thal-mek'to-mi): Surgical removal of the eyeball by enucleation.

ophthalmia (of-thal'mi-a): Inflammation of the eye involving especially the conjunctiva. O. NEONA TORUM or PURULENT O. purulent infection of the eyes of an infant at birth as it passes through the genital tract; may be caused by gonococci; SYMPATHETIC O. inflammation of one eye secondary to injury or disease of the other.

ophthalmiatrics (of-thal-mi-at'riks): Treatment of diseases and disorders of the eye.

ophthalmic (of'thal'mik): Relating to the eye.

ophthalmitis (of-thal-mī'tis): **1.** Any inflammation of the eye. **2.** Ophthalmia (q.v.).

ophthalmoblenorrhoea (of-thal'mō-blen-ō-rē'a): Purulent ophthalmia (q.v.); often due to a gonococcal infection.

ophthalmocele (of-thal'mō-sēl): Exophthalmos (q.v.).

ophthalmocentesis (of-thal'mō-sen-tē'sis): Surgical puncture of the eye.

ophthalmocopia (of-thal-mō-kō'pi-a): Eyestrain or eye fatigue.

ophthalmodonesis (of-thal'mō-dō-nē'sis): Trembling movement of the eye or eyes.

ophthalmodynamometer (of-thal'mō-dī-na-mom'i-ter): An instrument for measuring (1) the arterial pressure in the retinal vessels, or (2) the power of convergence of the eye.

ophthalmodynamometry (of-thal'mō-dī-na-mom'i-tri): Use of the ophthalmodynamometer for making indirect measurements of (1) the blood pressure in the retinal arteries, or (2) the power of the extraocular muscles.

ophthalmodynia (of-thal'mō-di'ni-a): Pain in the eye.

ophthalmofundoscope (of-thal'mō-fun'do-skōp): An instrument for examining the fundus of the eye.

ophthalmograph (of-thal' -mō-graf): An instrument for photographing eye movements during reading.

ophthalmogyric (of-thal-mō-jī'rik): See OCULO-GYRIC.

ophthalmolith (of-thal'mō-lith): A calculus in the eye or lacrimal duct.

ophthalmologist (of-thal-mol'o-jist): A physician who specializes in the diseases and refractive errors of the eye; may also do eye surgery, examine eyes, and prescribe corrective lenses.

ophthalmology (of-thal-mol'o-ji): The science that deals with the structure, function and diseases of the eye, and with the diagnoses and treatment of the diseases and disorders of the eye.

ophthalmomalacia (of-thal'mō-ma-lā'shi-a): Abnormal softness of the eyeball.

ophthalmometer (of'thal-mom'i-ter): An instrument for measuring the eye, particularly its refractive powers. See KERATOMETER.

ophthalmometry (of'thal-mom'i-tri): Measurement of the acuity of vision and of the eye's refractive power.

ophthalmomyositis (of-thal´-mō-mī-ō-sī´tis): Inflammation of the muscles that move the eyeball.

ophthalmomyotomy (of-thal´mō-mī-ot´o-mi): The surgical division of one or more muscles of the eye.

ophthalmoneuritis (of-thal´mō-nū-rī´tis): Inflammation of the ophthalmic nerve.

ophthalmopathy (of-thal-mop´a-thi): Any disease or disorder of the eye.

ophthalmoplegia (of-thal´mō-plē´ji-a): Paralysis of either or both the extrinsic and intrinsic muscles of the eye. — ophthalmoplegic, adj.

ophthalmoptosis (of-thal´-mop-tō´sis): Protrusion of the eyeball; exophthalmos (*q.v.*).

ophthalmorrhagia (of-thal-mō-rā´ji-a): Haemorrhage from the eye.

ophthalmorrhexis (of-thal-mō-rek´sis): Rupture of the eyeball.

ophthalmoscope (of-thal´-mo-skōp): An instrument fitted with a lens and illumination for examining the posterior portion of the interior of the eye. — ophthalmoscopic, adj.

ophthalmoscopy (of-thal-mos´ko-pi): Examination of the interior fundus of the eyeball with an ophthalmoscope.

ophthalmosteresis (of-thal´mō-ste-rē´sis): Loss of an eye.

ophthalmotomy (of-thal-mot´o-mi): Incision into the eyeball.

ophthalmotonometer (of-thal´mō-tō-nom´it-er): Instrument for determining the intraocular tension.

-opia: Combining form denoting sightedness, or visual conditions, *e.g.*, myopia.

opiate (ō´pi-āt): 1. Any drug derived from opium. 2. In a broad sense, sometimes used to describe any drug that produces sleep.

OPCS: Abbreviation for Office of Population Censuses and Surveys (*q.v.*).

opioids (ō´pi-oyds): 1. Substances produced in the body which have actions similar to those of the opiate, morphine. 2. Synthetic substances that have actions similar to those of opium but are not derived from it.

opisthotonos (op-is-thot´on-ōs): Extreme extension of the body, occurring in tetanic spasm. The spine is bent forward to such a degree that the patient may be supported on his head and heels alone. The symptom may be present in meningitis and strychnine poisoning as well as tetanus. — opisthotonic, adj.

opium (ō´pi-um): The dried juice of the unripe o. poppy capsules; long used as an opioid analgesic, astringent, and diaphoretic. Contains valuable alkaloids such as morphine, codeine, and papaverine.

opiumism (ō´pi-um-izm): The habit of using opium or the physiological condition resulting from the habitual use of opium.

opodidymus (op-o-did-i-mus): Conjoined twins with a single body but two heads that are partly fused.

opotherapy (o-pō-ther´a-pi): The use of animals' organs, or the products of such organs, in treatment of disease.

oppilation (op´i-lā´shun): 1. Constipation. 2. An obstruction.

opponens (o-pō´nenz): 1. Opposing. 2. The name given to several small muscles of the hand or foot that act to draw the lateral digits across the palm or sole to oppose each other.

opportunistic (op´por-tū-nis´tik): 1. Said of infections that are capable of adapting to a host or environment other than the normal one for the particular organism. 2. Relating to a serious infection with a microorganism that normally has little or no pathogenic activity but which has been activated by a serious disease or a modern method of treatment, or lowered resistance of the host.

oppress (op-presh): 1. Tyrannize; keep subservient; inflict hardships or cruelties, or govern cruelly or unjustly. 2. Weigh down, overburden. — oppression, n.

opsin (op´sin): A protein in the rods and cones of the retina that is involved in the formation of the light-sensitive visual pigments.

opsinogen (op-sin´o-jen): A substance that induces the formation of opsonins (*q.v.*).

opsoclonia (op´sō-klō´ni-a): A condition characterized by irregular, jerking horizontal and vertical movements of the eyeball. Opsoclonus.

opsonic (op-son´ik): Relating to opsonins. O. ACTION the effect produced by opsonins on susceptible microorganisms and other cells; O. INDEX the numerical measure of opsonic activity of the blood serum; indicates the ability of phagocytes to ingest foreign bodies such as bacteria.

opsonin (op´son-in): Any of several substances including antibodies that unite with antigens and render bacteria and other cells more susceptible to phagocytosis. See ANTIBODIES. — opsonic, opsoniferous, adj.; opsonification, n.

opsonization (op-son-ī-zā´shun): In bacteriology, the rendering of bacteria and other cells susceptible to phagocytosis (*q.v.*).

-opsy: Combining form denoting examination of.

optic (op'tik): Relating to sight or to the eye. O. ATROPHY refers to atrophy of the optic nerve; LEBER'S O. ATROPHY a hereditary form of O. atrophy in which central vision is completely lost while peripheral vision is partially retained; is transmitted by the female and occurs in males; O. CHIASM or CHIASMA the X-shaped crossing on the ventral surface of the brain where some of the fibres of the two optic nerves cross to the opposite sides and continue in the optic tracts of those sides; see CHIASM; O. DISC the point at the back of the retina where the O. nerve fibres converge to form the O. nerve; O. GLIOMA a glioma of the optic nerve or the optic chiasm, characterized by slow growth, visual loss, protrusion of the eyeball, and strabismus; O. NERVE one of the second pair of cranial nerves; it conducts visual stimuli from the retina to the brain; O. NEURITIS involvement of any part of the optic nerve in a disease process that impairs nerve conduction; may be an inflammatory, vascular, or degenerative disease.

optical (op'ti-kal): Related to vision or the science of optics.

optician (op-tish'an): One who grinds lenses to prescription and dispenses spectacles to correct refractive errors in vision.

optics (op'tiks): The branch of physics that deals with light, its sources, transmission, refraction, absorption, etc., particularly as these phenomena relate to vision.

optimum (op'ti-mum): The quality of being the best or most favourable; conducive to the most favourable activity or result. In bacteriology, the temperature at which bacteria grow best. O. POSITION that which will be the least awkward and most useful should a limb remain permanently paralysed.

opto-: Combining form denoting: **1.** Vision. **2.** The eye. **3.** Optic.

optometer (op-tom'i-ter): An instrument used for measuring the power and range of vision.

optometry (op-tom'e-tri): **1.** Measurement of visual acuity with an optometer. **2.** An occupation consisting of examining the eye for refractive errors and prescribing lenses or any other means except drugs for the correction of these errors; non-medical visual care. — optometric, adj.

OR: Abbreviation for odds ratio (*q.v.*).

orad (ō'rad): Towards the mouth, or situated near the mouth.

oral (aw'-ral): Relating to the mouth. O. CONTRACEPTIVE pill taken orally to block the possibility of impregnation during sexual intercourse; O. HERPES herpes simplex (*q.v.*); O. HYGIENE care of the mouth tissues and structures including brushing of the teeth, use of dental floss, massaging the gums, and ensuring that dentures are properly fitted; O. HYPOGLYCAEMIC AGENTS chemicals taken by mouth and used in treating certain types of diabetes; O. PHASE the earliest phase of psychosocial (*q.v.*) development in which the child derives pleasure from sucking or biting; persists in adult life in sublimated form.

oral personality type: In psychiatry, refers to a person who seeks gratification by eating, drinking, smoking; usually is also very talkative, envious, nagging, insecure.

orb: A sphere. In medicine, the eyeball.

orbicular (or-bik'ū-lar): Resembling a globe; spherical or circular.

orbicularis (or-bik-ū-lar'is): Descriptive of a muscle that encircles an opening of the body. O. OCULI the muscle that surrounds the eye; O. ORIS the muscle that surrounds the mouth.

orbit (or'bit): In anatomy, the bony socket that encloses and protects the eyeball and its appendages. — orbital, adj. Also called *eye socket*.

orchi-, orchid-, orchio-: Combining forms denoting the testes.

orchialgia (or-ki-al'ji-a): Pain in a testis. Also called *orchidalgia*.

orchiatrophy (or-ki-at'rō-fi): Atrophy or shrinkage of the testes.

orchiauxe (or-ki-awk'sē): Enlargement of a testis.

orchidectomy (or-ki-dek'to-mi): Excision of one or both testes; castration. Also called *orchectomy, orchiectomy*.

orchidic (or-kid'ik): Relating to the testes.

orchidopexy (or'ki-dō-pek'si): The operation of bringing an undescended testis into the scrotum, and fixing it in this position. Also called *orchiopexy, orchiorrhaphy*.

orchidoptosis (or'-ki-dō-tō'sis): Ptosis of the testes.

orchidotherapy (or'-ki-dō-ther'a-pi): Treatment of disease with testicular extract. Orchiotherapy.

orchiepididymitis (or'ki-ep-i-did-i-mī'tis): Inflammation of the testis and an epididymis.

orchiocatabasis (or'-ki-ō-ka-tab'a-sis): The descent of the testes into the scrotum.

orchioncus (or-ki-on'kus): A tumour of the testis.

orchiopathy (or-ki-op'a-thi): Any disease of the testis.

orchiotomy (or-ki-ot'o-mi): Incision and drainage of a testis. Also called *orchotomy*.

orchis (or'kis): The testis. — orchitic, adj.
orchitis (or-ki'tis): Inflammation of a testis. GRANULOMATOUS O. a hard, painful testicular mass; develops suddenly or insidiously; seen mostly in older men.
orderly: An attendant in a hospital or other institution.
Order of Deaconesses: A church order that existed as early as the 4th century but which fell into abeyance by the Middle Ages; it was revived by Pastor Theodore Fliedner at Kaiserswerth, Germany, in 1833 with the aim of training women in the care of the sick; it was here that Florence Nightingale received her instruction in nursing.
ordure (or'dur): Excrement.
Orem's self-care model of nursing (aw'-rem): A client-based theory in which self-esteem is important in optimizing a patient's recovery. Using this model, nurses are able to design a plan of care for patients. [Dorothea Orem, American nursing theorist.]
orexia (ō-rek'sē a): Appetite.
orexigenic (ō-rek si-jen'ik): 1. Stimulating the appetite. 2. An agent that stimulates the appetite.
orf: A disease of sheep, transmissible to, but rare, in humans; caused by a filterable virus; characterized by dark red papules that become indurated, but most often confined to a single self-limited lesion of the finger.
organ: A differentiated part of the body that may or may not be grouped with other parts to perform a specific function. O. OF CORTI, see CORTI.
organelle (or'ga-nel): A specialized part of structure within the cytoplasm of a cell that is presumed to have a special function in the cell's overall activities in the life process.
organic (or-gan'ik): 1. Relating to an organ. 2. Associated with life. 3. Pertinent to or derived from animal or vegetable life. 4. In nutrition, refers to foods grown without use of manmade fertilizers, pesticides or herbicides. O. ACID an acid containing one or more COOH (carboxyl) groups, e.g., acetic acid, formic acid, and fatty acids; O. CHEMISTRY the study of substances that contain carbon; O. CONFUSIONAL STATE in psychiatry, refers to a state of disturbed orientation to time, place, or person which sometimes appears to be of organic origin; O. DISEASE one in which there is structural change in organs or tissues.
organic brain syndromes: A group of mental disorders caused by local or widespread cognitive impairment, these include (1) delirium and dementia in which the impairment is widespread; (2) amnestic syndrome and organic (or substance) hallucinosis in which selected areas of cognition are affected; (3) organic (or substance) delusional syndrome and organic (or substance) affective syndrome, which resemble schizophrenic or affective disorders; (4) organic (or substance) personality syndrome, in which the person's personality is affected; (5) intoxication and withdrawal, in which the disorder is associated with the ingestion or withdrawal of a substance, or which does not fit into any of the first four categories; (6) atypical or mixed organic brain syndrome, a category which includes any organic brain syndrome not included in the other five categories.
organic mental disorders: A large heterogeneous group of disorders that are characterized by behavioural and psychological abnormalities and which are associated with brain dysfunction.
organism (or'gan-izm): A living cell or group of cells differentiated into functionally distinct parts that are interdependent. Any living individual, either plant or animal.
organization (or-gan-ī-zā'shun): 1. The process of providing or assuming a structure. 2. The change in the structure of a blood clot in a vein whereby it becomes fibrous.
organogenesis (or'gan-ō-jen'e-sis): The formation and development of the organs and organ systems of the body.
organology (or-ga-nol'o-ji): The special study of the history and formation of organs of the body, including their anatomy, physiology, and functions.
organomegaly (or'gan-ō-meg'a-li): Abnormal enlargement of a viscus or of viscera. Also called *splanchnomegaly* and *visceromegaly*.
organopathy (or-ga-nop'a-thi): Organic disease. See ORGAN.
organopexy (or'ga-nō-pek'si): The surgical fixation of an organ; refers often to the uterus after removal of a tumour.
organotherapy (or'ga-no-ther'a-pi): Treatment of disease by administration of animal organs or the extracts of these organs.
organs of Zuckerlandl: Glandular cells of sympathetic origin found along the aorta in the abdominal cavity; they are chemoreceptors for oxygen, carbon dioxide, and hydrogen ion concentration; they help control and regulate respiration.
organ transplant: The replacement of a diseased or malfunctioning organ or part with one from another individual, either living or

recently deceased. Organs that have been transplanted include kidney, heart, liver, lung, pancreas, spleen, and an entire human eye. The principal problem in transplants is the rejection of the organ by the immunological defences of the recipient which treat the transplanted organ as foreign and try to destroy it. Corneal transplants are frequently successful.

orgasm (or'gazm): The climax of sexual excitement.

oriental sore (o-ri-en'tal sōr): Delhi boil. A form of cutaneous leishmaniasis producing papular, crusted, granulomatous eruptions of the skin. A disease of the tropics and subtropics. Also called *Aleppo boil*.

orientation (or-i-en-tā'shun): Clear awareness of one's position relative to time and the environment. In mental conditions o. in space and time means that the patient knows where he is and recognizes the passage of time, *i.e.*, can give the correct date. Disorientation means the reverse.

orifice (or'i-fis): 1. A mouth or opening. 2. The outlet or entrance of the body cavity or aperture, *e.g.*, the urethral meatus, vagina, anus, ducts of glands, and the mouth.

origin (or'i-jin): The commencement or source of anything. O. OF A MUSCLE the end that remains relatively fixed during contraction of the muscle.

ornithine (or'ni-thēn): An amino acid formed when arginine is hydrolysed; an important intermediate product in the urea cycle.

Ornithodoros (or-ni-thod'o-rōs): A genus of ticks which are the vectors of the organisms causing such diseases as spotted fever, Q fever, tick fever, tularaemia, relapsing fever, and certain types of encephalitis.

ornithosis (or-ni-thō'sis): A contagious virus disease of wild birds and some domestic fowl, sometimes transmitted to humans. Disease closely resembles psittacosis but is usually less severe.

orofacial (o-rō-fā'shi-al): Relating to the mouth and the face.

orolingual (or-ō-ling'gwal): Relating to the mouth and tongue.

oronasal (or-ō-nā'zal): Relating to the mouth and nose.

oropharyngeal (o'rō-far-in'jē-al): Relating to the mouth and the pharynx.

oropharynx (ō-rō-far'inks): 1. That portion of the pharynx that is below the level of the hyoid bone. 2. Relating to the mouth and pharynx. — oropharyngeal, adj.

orotic acid (ō-rot'ik): An acid found in milk.

orphan: O. DRUGS drugs that have been found useful in treating relatively rare diseases but which are not manufactured commercially; O. VIRUSES viruses that have been isolated from tissue culture in the laboratory but which do not appear to be associated with any particular disease.

orrhorrhoea (or-ō-rē'a): A copious serous or watery discharge.

orth-, ortho-: Combining forms denoting (1) straight or normal; (2) correct or corrective.

orthesis (or-thē'sis): An orthopaedic brace, splint, or other device used by patients with physical disability or impairment, but not a prosthesis. — orthetic, adj.

orthetics (or-thet'iks): Orthotics (*q.v.*).

orthobiosis (or-thō-bī-ō'sis): A lifestyle that is based on hygienic and moral principles and other factors that make for physical and mental well-being and longevity.

orthocephalic (or-thō-ke-fal'ik, -se-): Having a well-proportioned head.

orthodontics (or-tho-don'tiks): A branch of dentistry dealing with prevention and correction of irregularities and malocclusion of the teeth. Also called *orthodontia*.

orthodontist (or-tho-don'tist): A dentist who specializes in orthodontics (*q.v.*).

orthodromic (or-tho-drō'mik): Descriptive of fibres that conduct impulses over an axon in a normal direction.

orthograde (or'thō-grād): The upright position of the body in standing or walking.

orthokeratology (or'thō-ker-a-tol'o-ji): A method of improving vision by utilizing a contact lens to mould the cornea.

orthomolecular (or-thō-mo-lek'ū-lar): Referring to the chemical make-up of the body, both the substances formed endogenously and those taken into the body through diet and administration, including vitamins.

orthopaedics (or-thō-pē'diks): A branch of surgery dealing with deformities and diseases of the skeleton and its associated structures and their correction, whether by apparatus, manipulation, or surgery.

orthopantograph (or-thō-pan'-tō-graf): A radiographic device that makes possible the visualization of all of the teeth, the alveolar bone, and the surrounding tissues on a single film.

orthopnoea (or-thop-nē'a): Inability to breathe except in an upright, sitting position. Opp. to plabypnoea. — orthopnoeic, adj.

orthopsychiatry (or-thō-sī-kī'a-tri): That branch of psychiatry that deals with the amelioration of disorders of personality and behaviour in normal or near-normal persons, particularly in children and young adults.

orthoptic (or-thop'tik): Relating to orthoptics (*q.v.*). O. EXERCISES a system of eye exercises designed to strengthen the eye muscles and prescribed to help correct such conditions as strabismus (*q.v.*) or squint.

orthoptics (or-thop'tiks): The study and treatment of muscle imbalances of the eye, especially the treatment of strabismus by exercise of the ocular muscles.

orthosis (or-thō'sis): General term for an external device applied to a patient for supportive, preventive, or corrective purposes. — orthoses, pl.; orthotic, adj.

orthostatic (or-thō-stat'ik): Caused by or related to the upright stance. O. ALBUMINURIA occurs in some healthy subjects only when they take the upright position; when lying in bed the urine is normal; O. HYPOTENSION see under HYPOTENSION.

orthotics (or-thot'iks): The science of orthopaedic appliances and their use.

orthotist (or'tho-tist): One who makes and fits orthopaedic appliances.

Ortolani's sign: A positive click heard on abduction and external rotation of the hip; a sign of dislocated hip.

os: A mouth. EXTERNAL O. the opening of the cervix into the vagina; INTERNAL O. the opening of the cervix into the uterine cavity. — ora, pl.

os: A bone. O. CALCIS the heel bone; the calcaneus; O. COXAE or O. INNOMINATUM the hip bone. — ossa, pl.

osche-, oscheo-: Combining forms denoting the scrotum.

oscheal (os'kē-al): Relating to the scrotum.

oscheitis (os-kē-ī'tis): Inflammation of the scrotum.

oschelephantiasis (osk'el-e-fan-tī'a-sis): Enlargement of the scrotum.

oscheocele (os'kē-ō-sēl): Swelling, tumour, or hernia of the scrotum.

oscheoma (os-kē-ō'ma): A tumour of the scrotum.

oscheoncus (os-kē-on'kus): Tumour of the scrotum; oscheoma.

oscillating bed (os'il-āt-ing): A mechanical bed so designed that it may be tilted at regular intervals, thus changing the patient's posture and allowing for the alternate filling and drainage of the blood vessels of the lower extremities.

oscillation (os-il-ā'shun): A swinging or moving to and fro; a vibration.

oscillograph (o-sil'ō-graf): An instrument that records alternating current waves or other types of electrical oscillation (*q.v.*) that are used in recording heart action.

oscillometry (os-i-lom'-e-tri): Measurement of vibration, using a special apparatus (oscillometer, oscilloscope). Measures the magnitude of the pulse wave more precisely than palpation.

oscillopsia (os'i-lop'si-a): The sensation that stationary objects one is viewing are swaying back and forth.

oscilloscope (os-sil'-ō-skōp): An instrument that displays temporarily on a fluorescent screen the fluctuations in an electric quantity; used in monitoring various body functions, primarily heart function.

oscitation (os'i tā'shun): Yawning.

-oscopy: Combining form denoting a looking into.

osculum (os'kū-lum): A small opening or aperture; a pore.

-ose: Combining form denoting (1) full of, or having the quality of; (2) a carbohydrate substance.

Osgood–Schlatter disease: Osteochondrosis of the tuberosity of the tibia. See OSTEOCHONDROSIS. Also called *epiphyseal aseptic necrosis*.

osmatic (oz-mat'ik): Relating to the sense of smell.

osmesis (oz-mē'sis): The sense of smell; the act of smelling.

osmics (oz'miks): The science dealing with the sense and organs of smell.

osmolality (oz'mō-lal'i-ti): Osmotic pressure expressed in terms of osmoles or milliosmoles per kilogram of fluid; it reflects the concentration of a solute in a solution.

osmolarity (os'mō-lar'i-ti): The osmotic pressure exerted by a substance in aqueous solution, defined in terms of the number of active particles per unit of volume.

osmole (oz'mōl): The standard unit of osmotic pressure; based on the concentration of an ion in solution.

osmology (oz-mol'o-ji): 1. The science that deals with odours and the sense of smell. 2. The study of osmotics.

osmophilic (oz-mō-fil'ik): Readily stained with osmic acid.

osmoreceptor (oz'mō-re-sep'tor): 1. A sensory nerve ending that is responsive to stimulation by odours. 2. A sensory nerve ending that is responsive to changes in the osmotic pressure of the surrounding medium.

osmose (oz-mōs'): To pass through a membrane by osmosis.

osmosis (os-mō'sis): The movement of a pure solvent, such as water, through a semipermeable membrane from a solution that has a lower solute concentrations to one that has a higher solute concentration. Movement across the membrane continues until the concentrations of the solutions equalize.

osmotic fragility test: A laboratory test for determining the fragility of red blood cells.

osmotic pressure (os-mot'ik): The force with which the fluid part of a solution is drawn across a semi-permeable membrane that separates two solutions of different concentrations and that permits passage of the fluid but not of the solutes, the direction of flow being from the solution of lesser to the solution of greater concentration. When the pressure is due to the movement of protein molecules over a semipermeable membrane it is called colloidal osmotic pressure or oncotic pressure.

osphresiology (os-frē'zi-ol'o-ji): The science of odours and the sense of smell; osmology.

osphresis (os-frē'sis): Olfaction. — osphretic, adj.

osphyalgia (os-fi-al'ji-a): Pain in the lumbar region; see LUMBAGO.

osphyarthrosis (os'-fi-ar-thrō'sis): Inflammation of the hip or loins area.

ossein (os'ē-in): The organic matter in bone.

osseous (os'ē-us): Relating to, composed of, or resembling bone; bony.

ossi-: Combining form denoting relationship to bone.

ossicle (os'ik'l): A small bone, particularly one of those contained in the middle ear; the malleus, incus, and stapes. — ossicular, adj.

ossiculectomy (os-ik'-ū-lek'to-mi): Removal of one or all the ossicles of the middle ear.

ossiferous (o-sif'er-us): Producing or containing bone tissue.

ossification (os'i-fi-kā'shun): The formation of bone; the conversion of cartilage, etc. into bone. INTRACARTILAGINOUS O. the replacement of cartilaginous structures by bone; many bones are formed this way; INTRAMEMBRANOUS O. the replacement of dense connective tissue by deposits of calcium salts, forming bone; the skull bones are formed this way.

ossify (os'i-fi): To change or develop into bone.

ost-, oste-, osteo-, osti-: Combining forms denoting bone.

ostealgia (os-tē-al'ji-a): Pain in a bone or bones.

osteanabrosis (os'tē-an-a-brō'sis): See OSTEOANABROSIS.

ostearthritis (os'tē-ar-thrī'tis): Osteoarthritis (q.v.).

ostectomy (os-tek'to-mi): Surgical removal of a bone or part of a bone.

osteectopia (os'-tē-ek-tō'pi-a): Displacement of bone.

osteitis (os-tē-ī'tis): Inflammation of a bone. ALVEOLAR O. alveoalgia (q.v.); O. CONDENSANS ILII dense sclerosis on the iliac side of the sacroiliac joint, often leading to fibrositis syndrome or sciatica; O. DEFORMANS Paget's disease; rarefaction leading to bowing of long bones and deformity of flat bones; O. FIBROSA CYSTICA softening and resorption of bone and replacement of calcified bone with fibrous tissue; usually the result of excessive secretion of parathyroid hormone; Recklinghausen's disease; O. FRAGILITANS osteogenesis imperfecta; see under OSTEOGENESIS; O. OSSIFICANS condensing O. in which an entire bone eventually becomes more or less cancellated; O. PUBIS sclerosis of the pubic bones at the symphysis with pain radiating downwards in the thigh, tenderness, and eventual widening of the symphysis.

ostempyesis (os'-tem-pī-ē'sis): Suppuration of or within a bone.

osteoanabrosis (os'tē-ō-an-a-brō'sis): Atrophy of bone.

osteoarthritis (os'-te-ō-ar-thrī'tis): Degenerative arthritis. A chronic disease of weight-bearing joints and interphalangeal joints of the fingers particularly; occurring mostly in middle or old age, characterized by degenerative changes in the bone and cartilage of all of the joints, The articular cartilage becomes worn and osteophytes may form at the periphery of the joint and loose bodies result. Apparently no specific cause; may be primary, or follow disease or injury involving the articular surfaces of synovial joints; other factors may be heredity, occupation, obesity, faulty posture. — osteoarthritic, adj.

osteoarthropathy (os'tē-ō-ar-throp'a-thi): 1. Increased bone formation at joints. 2. Any disease involving bones, or joints, accompanied by pain. 3. Osteoarthritis. PULMONARY O. osteitis of the legs and arms, chiefly in the terminal epiphyses of long bones and in the phalanges; associated with dorsal kyphosis and joint abnormalities; often secondary to chronic pulmonary or cardiac disorders. Also called *hypertrophic pulmonary osteoarthropathy*.

osteoarthrosis (os'tē-ō-ar-thrō'sis): 1. Chronic arthritis. 2. Degenerative joint disease. 3. Osteoarthritis.

osteoarthrotomy (os'tē-ō-ar-throt'o-mi): Surgical removal of the articular end of a bone.

osteoarticular (os'tē-ō-ar-tik'ū-lar): Relating to or affecting bones and joints.

osteoblast (os'tē-ō-blast): A bone-forming cell.

osteoblastoma (os-tē-ō-blas-tō'ma): An uncommon tumour of osteoblasts; occurs chiefly in the spine in young people.

osteocachexia (os'tē-ō-ka-kek'si-a): Chronic disease of the bone that results in malnutrition. See CACHEXIA.

osteocarcinoma (os'-tē-ō-kar-sin-ō'ma): Carcinoma of a bone or bones.

osteocartilaginous (os'tē-ō-kar-til-aj'i-nus): Composed of both bone and cartilage.

osteocele (os'tē-ō-sēl): The presence in the scrotum of a mass that contains bony deposits.

osteochondral (os-tē-ō-kon'dral): Relating to or composed of both bone and cartilage.

osteochondritis (os'-tē-ō-kon-drī'tis): Inflammation of both bone and cartilage. Term most often applied to non-septic conditions, especially avascular necrosis involving a joint surface. O. DEFORMANS JUVENILIS a form of O. occurring most often in boys 5–10 years of age; disturbance of growth at the epiphyseal cartilage results in flattening of the head of the femur causing muscle spasm, limitation of movement, limping and sometimes shortening of the leg. Syn., *Legg's disease, Legg–Calvé–Perthes* disease; O. DISSECANS a form of O. in which small pieces of an articular joint may separate to form loose bodies in the joint; seen most often in the knee and shoulder.

osteochondrodystrophia (os'tē-ō-kon'drō-dis'trō-fi-a): Dysplasia of bone and cartilage with atrophy and abnormal development. See DYSPLASIA.

osteochondrofibroma (os'tē-ō-kon'-drō-fī-brō'ma): A tumour containing elements of osteoma, chondroma, and fibroma.

osteochondroma (os'-tē-ō-kon-drō'ma): A benign tumour made up of osseous and cartilaginous tissue.

osteochondromatosis (os'tē-ō-kon-drō-ma-tō'sis): Multiple cartilaginous tumours that form on the surface of bones.

osteochondropathy (os'-tē-ō-kon-drop'a-thi): A pathological condition of bone and cartilage.

osteochondrosarcoma (os'tē-ō-kon'drō-sar-kō'ma): A sarcomatous tumour of bone and cartilage.

osteochondrosis (os'-tē-ō-kon-drō'sis): A disease of the ossification centre in the bones of children. Usually begins with a degeneration that is followed by regeneration and calcification. May affect the femur, tibia, vertebrae,

bones of the wrist or hand and result in deformity. See SCHEUERMANN'S DISEASE.

osteoclasia (os-tē-ō-klā'zi-a): **1.** The destruction and absorption of bony tissue by osteoclasts. **2.** Osteoclasis.

osteoclasis (os-te-ok'la-sis): The intentional therapeutic fracture of a deformed or misshapen bone to correct the condition. Also called *osteoclasia, osteoclasty.* — osteoclastic, adj.

osteoclast (os'tē-ō-klast): A large multinucleated cell that is formed in the bone marrow; its function is to dissolve or remove unwanted or dead bone.

osteoclastoma (os'-tē-ō-klas-tō'ma): A tumour made up of cells resembling osteoclasts. May be benign, recurrent, or frankly malignant. The usual site is near the end of a long bone. See MYELOMA.

osteocope (os'tē-ō-kōp): Extreme pain in bone; usually related to syphilitic bone disease.

osteocystoma (os'tē-ō-sis-tō'ma): A cystic tumour of bone usually occurring in childhood or early adolescence. Site is most often the shaft of a long bone, particularly the upper part of the humerus.

osteocyte (os'tē-ō-sīt): A bone cell.

osteodermia (os-tē-ō-der'mi-a): A condition characterized by bony deposits in the skin.

osteodiastasis (os'tē-ō-dī-as'ta-sis): Separation of two adjacent bones.

osteodynia (os-tē-ō-din'i-a): Pain in a bone.

osteodystrophy (os-tē-ō-dis'tro-fi): Faulty formation or growth of bone. Osteodystrophia. RENAL O. renal rickets; see under RICKETS.

osteofibroma (os'tē-ō-fi-brō'ma): A tumour made up mostly of fibrous tissue but which has small foci of bony tissue.

osteogenesis (os'tē-ō-jen'e-sis): Formation of bone; development of bones. O. IMPERFECTA an inherited condition in which the bones are brittle and subject to repeated fractures, often resulting in such deformities as pigeon breast and curvature of the spine. The sclera has a blue colour and the person may be subject to bruising, hernias, constipation, deafness. Sometimes fractures occur in intrauterine life and sometimes not until the child is old enough to walk. Worldwide; affects both sexes. Also called *brittle bones; fagilitas ossium.*

osteogenic (os-tē-ō-jen'ik): Bone producing. O. SARCOMA a general term for a malignant tumour arising in cells whose normal function is the production of bone; usually occurring in children and young adults; characterized by pain, swelling, and early metastases especially to the lung.

osteohalisteresis (os′tē-ō-hal-is-ter-ē′sis): Softening of bone due to loss or deficiency of mineral elements.

osteoid (os′tē-oid): Resembling bone.

osteoma (os-tē-ō′ma): A bony tumour; usually developing on a bone, but may also be on some other organ, *e.g.*, lung or pleura; may be single or multiple. OSTEOID O. a circumscribed tumour, usually benign, seen mostly in the cortex of long bones, occasionally in the cancellous portion; occurs most often in younger persons.

osteomalacia (os′tē-ō-ma-lā′shi-a): A condition of adult life in which there is a softening of bone due to deficiency of vitamin D, calcium, and phosphate, or excessive absorption of calcium and phosphorus from the bones. May occur in malnutrition or pregnancy; often referred to as *adult rickets*.

osteomyelitis (os′-tē-ō-mī-e-lī′tis): Inflammation of bone caused by infection with a pyogenic organism such as staphylococcus, streptococcus, pneumococcus, gonococcus, or meningococcus. Usually begins in the bone marrow; may remain localized or spread to other parts of the bone. May be acute, chronic, or iatrogenic, or may follow injury to the bone, a skin infection, or an abscess in another part of the body. SCLEROSING NON-SUPPURATIVE O. chronic iatrogenic osteomyelitis involving especially the tibia and the femur, characterized by diffuse inflammation without suppuration, and pain, especially at night; affects mostly young adults; SUPPURATIVE O. may occur as a complication or sequela of typhoid fever or paratyphoid fever, other salmonella infections, or in association with sickle cell anaemia. Usually involves the long bones and occurs most often in children under 12 years of age.

osteomyelodysplasia (os-tē-ō-mī′e-lō-dis-plā′zia): A condition characterized by thinning of the osseous tissue of bones and accompanying increase in size of the marrow cavity, leukopenia, and fever.

osteoncus (os-tē-on′kus): A bone tumour. Osteoma.

osteonecrosis (os′tē-ō-ne-krō′sis): Death (necrosis) of bone when it occurs in areas considered large as compared with such small foci of necrosis as occur in dental caries.

osteonosus (os-tē-on′o-sus): Any disease of bone.

osteopath (os′tē-ō-path): One who practises osteopathy.

osteopathy (os-tē-op′a-thi): 1. Any disease of bone. 2. A theory that attributes a wide range of disorders to mechanical derangements of the skeletal system, which it claims can be rectified by suitable manipulations along with adequate nutrition and favourable environment. — osteopathic, adj.

osteopenia (os-tē-ō-pē′ni-a): Loss of bone mass which occurs when bone synthesis is not sufficient to compensate for bone lysis. The bones become less dense and there is a thinning of the cortex of the long bones. Seen in the elderly and in women more than men.

osteoperiostitis (os′tē-ō-per′i-os-tī′tis): Inflammation of periosteum and the bone under it.

osteopetrosis (os′-tē-ō-pe-trō′sis): A condition in which progressive sclerosis causes a generalized increase in the density of the bones and eventual obliteration of the marrow; may be fatal due to bone marrow failure. Characteristics are clubbing of the ends of long bones, retarded growth, anaemia, and a strong tendency to spontaneous fractures. Also called '*marble bones*' and *Albers-Schönberg disease*.

osteophage (os′tē-ō-fāj): Syn., *osteoclast* (*q.v.*).

osteophlebitis (os′tē-ō-flē-bī′tis): Inflammation of veins in a bone.

osteophone (os′tē-ō-fōn): A device for helping the deaf to hear. An audiophone.

osteophony (os′tē-of′on-i): The conduction of sound waves to the inner ear by bone.

osteophyma (os-tē-ō-fi′ma): A tumour or outgrowth on a bone.

osteophyte (os′tē-ō-fīt): A horny outgrowth or spur, usually at the margins of joint surfaces, *e.g.*, in osteoarthritis. — osteophytic, adj.

osteophytosis (os′tē-ō-fī-tō′sis): A condition characterized by the formation of osteophytes. See OSTEOPHYTE.

osteoplasty (os′tē-ō-plas-ti): Any plastic operation on bone. — osteoplastic, adj.

osteoporosis (os′tē-ō-po-rō′sis): Loss of density of bone and enlargement of the bone spaces due to disturbance of mineral metabolism, inadequate absorption of calcium into bone, and failure of the osteoclasts to lay down sufficient matrix; characterized by abnormal porousness, fragility, and reduction in quantity of bone. Cause is unknown; begins in the spine, causing compression of the vertebrae which results in low back pain, development of a 'dowager's hump', and loss of weight; progresses to the bones of the pelvis, ribs, arms, and legs. Spontaneous fractures may occur. Most often seen in women after menopause; may also accompany pathological conditions, *e.g.*, parathyroid tumour. ALVEOLAR O. involves the alveolar part of bone which serves as a reservoir for minerals needed to maintain vital functions; seen most often in the alveolar processes of older people following the extraction of teeth and resorption of the processes. — osteoporotic, adj.

osteoradionecrosis (os'tē-ō-rā'di-ō-ne-krō'sis): Necrosis of bone following irradiation.

osteorrhaphy (os-tē-or'a-fi): The suturing or wiring of bone.

osteosarcoma (os'tē-ō-sar-kō'ma): A malignant tumour originating in bone cells or containing bony tissue.

osteosclerosis (os'tē-ō-skler-ō'sis): Abnormal density or hardness of bone. — osteosclerotic, adj.

osteosis (os-tē-ō'sis): Metaplastic formation of bone. See METAPLASIA.

osteospongioma (os'tē-ō-spon'ji-ō'ma): A spongy tumour of bone.

osteosynovitis (os'tē-ō-sin-ō-vī'tis): Inflammation of the synovial membrane covering a joint, along with osteitis of adjacent bone.

osteosynthesis (os-tē-ō-sin'the-sis): Bringing the ends of a fractured bone into close apposition by means of a metal plate or other mechanical means.

osteotabes (os'-tē-ō-tā'bēz): Degeneraton of bone; begins with destruction of bone marrow cells, progresses to spongy bone, then to compact bone.

osteothrombosis (os'tē-ō-throm-bō'sis): Thrombosis of the veins of a bone.

osteotome (os'tē-o-tōm): An instrument for cutting bone; it is similar to a chisel, but bevelled on both sides of its cutting edge.

osteotomy (os-tē-ot'o-mi): The surgical division, cutting, or repositioning of bones in treatment of diseased or deformed joints or bones.

osteotropic (os'tē-ō-trō'pik): Relating to the nutrition of bone.

ostitis (os-tī'tis): Osteitis (*q.v.*).

ostium (os'ti-um): A mouth or opening; often refers to an opening between two cavities, *e.g.*, the entrance to the oviduct or uterine tube. — ostia, pl.; ostial, adj.

ostomate (os'tō-māt): One who has an artificial opening or stoma into the gastrointestinal canal.

ostomy (os'-to-mi): An informal term referring to a surgical procedure that involves making an artificial opening between two organs or between an organ and the surface of the body.

ot-, oto-: Combining forms denoting the ear.

otalgia (ō-tal'ji-a): Earache.

OTC: Abbreviation for over the counter (*q.v.*).

otiatrics (ō-ti-at'triks): The branch of medicine that deals with the science and treatment of ear diseases.

otic (ō'tik): Relating to the ear.

otitis (ō-tī'tis): Inflammation of the ear. O. EXTERNA inflammation of the external auditory canal; O. INTERNA O. of the inner ear, usually caused by extension of inflammation from the middle ear; main symptoms are dizziness, nausea, nystagmus, headache and possibly deafness; O. MEDIA O. of the middle ear; may be acute or chronic; may follow infectious disease such as measles or scarlet fever; chief symptoms are pain, fever, tinnitus, bulging of the tympanic membrane, possibly deafness; SEROUS O. MEDIA a common disorder of the middle ear; usually occurs in children; not pyogenic; may be due to a virus or allergy. Marked by a serous discharge; when chronic may lead to conductive deafness.

otoantritis (ō-tō-an-trī'tis): Inflammation of the mastoid antrum.

otoblennorrhoea (ō'tō-blen-ō-rē'a): A mucous discharge from the ear.

otocleisis (ō-tō-kli'sis): Closure of the auditory tube or of the external auditory canal; may be caused by a new growth or by the collection of cerumen in the external canal.

otodynia (ō-tō-din'i-a). Earache. Otalgia.

otoencephalitis (ō'tō-en-kef-a-lī'tis,-sef-): Inflammation of the brain resulting from an extension of inflammation of the middle ear.

otogenic (ō'tō-jen'ik): Originating within the ear, inflammation of the ear in particular.

otolaryngologist (ō'tō-lar-in-gol'o-jist): A medical practitioner who specializes in otolaryngology.

otolaryngology (ō'tō-lar-in-gol'o-ji): Strictly speaking, the branch of medical science that deals with the structure, function, and diseases of the ear, larynx, and laryngeal area; sometimes includes diseases of the upper respiratory tract and some diseases of the head and neck.

otoliths (ō'tō-liths): Tiny dustlike deposits of calcium carbonate within the membranous labyrinth of the inner ear.

otologist (ō-tol'ō-jist): One specializing in the functions and diseases of the ear.

otology (ō-tol'o-ji): The branch of medical science that deals with the structure, functions, and diseases of the ear. — otologic, adj.

-otomy: Refers to a surgical incision.

otomycosis (ō'-tō-mī-kō'sis): A fungal (*Aspergillus, Candida*) infection of the external auditory meatus and canal, accompanied by itching, pain, and scaling; usually bilateral. — otomycotic, adj.

otopathy (ō-top'a-thi): Any disease of the ear.

otopharyngeal (ō'tō-fa-rin'jē-al): Relating to the ear and pharynx.

otophone (ō'tō-fōn): An ear trumpet.

otoplasty (ō'tō-plas-ti): Plastic surgery for the correction of deformed, flattened, or protruding ears; done preferably during childhood.

otopyorrhoea (ō'-tō-pī-o-rē'a): Flow of purulent discharge from the ear; often results from chronic otitis media with perforation of the ear drum.

otopyosis (ō-tō-pī-ō'sis): Suppuration occurring in the external auditory canal; often associated with suppuration in the middle ear.

otorhinolaryngology (ō'tō-rī'nō-lar-in-gol'o-ji): The branch of medical science that deals with the structure, function, and diseases of the ear, nose and larynx.

otorhinology (ō'tō-rī-nol'o-ji): The branch of medicine that deals with the ear and nose.

otorrhagia (ō-tō-rā' -ji-a): A bloody or purulent discharge from the external auditory canal due to inflammation of the ear.

otorrhoea (ō-tō-rē'a): A discharge from the external auditory meatus, especially one that is mucopurulent.

otosalpinx (ō-tō-sal'pinks): The auditory tube.

otosclerosis (ō-tō-skle-rō'sis): A condition of progressive deafness marked by new bone formation affecting primarily the labyrinth of the inner ear and causing ankylosis of the stapes to the margin of the round window. Of unknown origin; heredity may be a factor. — otosclerotic, adj.

otoscope (ō'to-skōp): An instrument for examining the ear; auriscope (q.v.). — otoscopic, adj.

otoscopy (ō-tos'kō-pi): Visualization of the external auditory canal and the tympanic membrane by means of an otoscope.

otosis (ō-tō'sis): Mishearing spoken words.

otosteal (ō-tos'tē-al): Relating to the small bones of the middle ear.

ototomy (ō-tot'o-mi): 1. Incision of the drum membrane; myringotomy. 2. The anatomy of the ear.

ototoxic (ō-tō-tok'sik): Refers to a substance that has a toxic effect on the organs of balance and hearing, or on the eighth cranial nerve.

ototoxicity (ō-tō-tok-sis'i-ti): The quality of being toxic or damaging to the eighth cranial nerve or to the organs of equilibrium and hearing.

outcomes: Visible or practical result, effect, or product. See PATIENT OUTCOME.

outlet: An opening, usually in the nature of a passageway, by means of which something escapes.

outpatient: An ambulatory patient who does not require admission to a hospital bed, but who comes to the hospital outpatient department for consultation or treatment.

output: 1. The quantity of waste substance produced by a process such as metabolism and excreted from the body, e.g., the amount of urine voided in a given time. Opp. of intake. 2. The amount of a substance ejected from a given place, e.g., the cardiac output of blood.

outreach: The provision of an organization's services in the community in order to include the disadvantaged or those individuals who are socially excluded. ASSERTIVE O. WORKER a health-care professional who aims to establish a relationship with each client in a flexible, creative, and needs-focused way that enables the delivery of a health and social care package that fits each client's specific needs; MENTAL HEALTH CRITICAL CARE O. managing highly dependent patients in a ward setting.

ov-, ovi-, ovo-: Combining forms denoting ovum.

oval window: Fenestra ovalis: see under FENESTRA.

ovar-, ovari-, ovario-: Combining forms denoting (1) ovary; (2) ovarian.

ovarialgia (ō-var-i-al'ji-a): Pain in an ovary.

ovarian (ō-vair'i-an): Relating to the ovaries. O. CYST a tumour that forms on the surface of the ovary; may be benign or malignant; O. CYSTECTOMY the removal of cystic tissue from an ovary without disturbing the remaining tissue.

ovariectomy (ō-var-i-ek'to-mi): Excision of an ovary. Oophorectomy.

ovariocele (ō-vair' -i-ō-sēl): A hernia of an ovary.

ovariocentesis (ō-vair'i-ō-sen-tē'sis): Surgical puncture of an ovary usually for the drainage of an ovarian cyst.

ovariocyesis (ō-vair'i-ō-sī-ē'sis): Ovarian pregnancy.

ovarioncus (ō-var-i-on'kus): Tumour of the ovary.

ovariopexy (ō-vair'i-ō-pek' -si): The surgical procedure of elevating and fixing an ovary to the abdominal wall.

ovariorrhexis (ō-vair'i-ō-rek'sis): Rupture of an ovary.

ovariosalpingectomy (ō-vair'i-ō-sal-pin-jek'to-mi): The surgical removal of an ovary and uterine tube.

ovariotomy (ō-vair-i-ot'om-i): Literally means incision of an ovary, but it is the term usually applied to the removal of an ovary. Also called *oophorectomy*.

ovaritis (ō'var-ī'tis): Oophoritis (*q.v.*).

ovary (ō'va-ri): One of the paired sex glands of the female; an oval, flattened gland, about 4 cm long, suspended on the posterior surface of the broad ligament, one on either side of the uterus. The substance is vascular and fibrous and contains egg cells, one of which matures and is expelled periodically. Function of the gland is to develop the egg cells and also to produce the female sex hormones. CYSTIC O. retention cysts in the ovarian follicles; POLY-CYSTIC O. the ovary is enlarged and the cortex contains multiple small follicular cysts; associated with an endocrine disturbance.

overcompensation (ō'ver-kom-pen-sā'shun): Name given to any type of behaviour a person adopts in order to cover up a deficiency in his personality, of which he is aware. Thus a person who is afraid may react by becoming arrogant or boastful or quarrelsome.

overdosage (ō-ver-dōs'-aj): The administration or taking of an excessive dose of a drug; the amount considered overdose varies with the individual and the degree of tolerance he or she may have built up for the drug.

overextension (ō-ver-eks-ten'shun): Extension beyond the usual normal limit, said of a joint or muscle.

overflow: Continuous escape of fluid such as tears or urine.

overhydration (ō-ver-hī-drā'shun): The presence of excess fluids in the body tissues; often associated with congestive heart failure and renal pathology; signs and symptoms include oedema, puffy eyelids, tachypnoea, oversecretion of antidiuretic hormone.

overriding: 1. The slipping of one end of a fractured bone past the other end. 2. The moulding of the fetus's head during delivery.

overt (ō-vert'): Obvious, manifest; open to view.

over the counter: Refers to drugs sold without a doctor's prescription over the counter but within the law.

overtoe (ō-ver-tō): A condition in which the great toe lies over the adjacent toes. Hallux varus.

overventilation (ō'ver-ven-til-ā'shun): See HYPERVENTILATION.

oviduct (ō'vi-dukt): Uterine tube (*q.v.*).

ovotestis (ō-vō-tes'tis): A gonad that contains both ovarian and testicular tissue.

ovotherapy (ō-vō-ther'a-pi): Therapeutic use of ovarian secretion, particularly that from the corpus luteum.

ovulation (ov-ū-lā'shun): The process of maturation and rupture of a Graafian follicle, with the discharge of the ovum; should occur 14 days before the next menstrual flow is expected. O. METHOD see BILLING'S OVULATION METHOD.

ovule (ō'vūl): The ovum before it has been expelled from the ovary.

ovum (ō'vum): The female reproductive cell; a round cell about 0.1 mm in diameter that develops in the Graafian follicle and, when mature, is expelled by the follicle into the abdominal cavity whence it enters the uterine tube; unless fertilized it is cast off; this occurs approximately every 28 days during a female's life, from puberty to menopause. — ova, pl.; ovarian, adj.

oxalaemia (ok-sa-lē'mi-a): Presence of abnormally large amounts of oxalates in the blood.

oxalate (ok'sa-lāt): Any salt of oxalic acid.

oxalic acid (ok-sal'ik): An organic acid found in many plants that are used as foods.

oxidant (oks'i-dant): An oxidizing agent. See OXIDIZE.

oxidase (ok'si-dās): Any enzyme that promotes oxidation.

oxidation (ok'si-dā'shun): The process of converting a substance into an oxide by the addition of oxygen. The carbon in organic compounds undergoes O. with the formation of carbon dioxide when they are combusted in air, or when they are metabolized in living material in the presence of oxygen. Also used in biochemistry for the process of removing hydrogen from a molecule (*e.g.*, in the presence of air, ascorbic acid undergoes O. with the formation of dehydroascorbic acid). The loss of an electron with an increase in valency (*e.g.*, the conversion of ferrous to ferric iron) is also an O. The greater part of the energy present in foods is made available to the body by the process of O. in the tissues.

oxide (ok'sīd): Any compound of oxygen with another element or radical, usually a metal.

oxidize (ok'si-dīz): To combine oxygen with an element or a radical, or to cause such combination to take place.

oxidosis (ok-si-dō'sis): Acidosis (*q.v.*).

oximeter (ok-sim'i-ter): A photoelectric device for measuring the level of oxygen saturation of the circulating blood.

oximetry (ok-sim'i-tri): The use of an oximeter to determine the oxygen saturation level in the arterial blood.

oxy-: Combining form denoting: 1. The presence of oxygen in a substance. 2. Pointed. 3. Sharp. 4. Sour. 5. Quick.

oxyblepsia (ok-sē-blep'si-a): Unusual acuteness of vision.

oxycephaly (ok-sē-kef'a-li,-sef'-): A congenital deformity in which the head is more pointed than rounded.

oxygen (ok'si-jen): A colourless, odourless, gaseous element, necessary for life and combustion. The most abundant element on Earth; constitutes 20% by weight of air. Used medicinally as an inhalation, supplied in cylinders in which the gas is at a high pressure. See HYPERBARIC. O. MASK used mainly for administering oxygen when the patient requires it for only a short time, or intermittently; O. TENT transparent plastic tent which encloses the patient and part or all of the bed; used to provide a constantly oxygenated environment; O. THERAPY administration of oxygen in conditions resulting from oxygen deficiency, for example, pneumonia, congestive heart failure, coronary thrombosis; may be administered by mask, nasal catheter, tent, or special oxygen chamber.

oxygenation (ok'si-je-nā'shun): The saturation of a substance (particularly blood) with oxygen. — oxygenated, adj.

oxygenator (ok'si-je-nā'tor): A device for oxygenating the blood outside of the body. The artificial lung as used in heart surgery.

oxygen dissociation curve: The release of oxygen from the red blood cells in the capillaries into the interstitial fluid from which it can enter the cells, as demonstrated on a plotted curve.

oxygeusia (ok'si-gū'si-a): Abnormally keen sense of taste.

oxyhaemoglobin (ok'-si-hē-mo-glō'bin): Oxygenated haemoglobin, an unstable compound.

oxyhaemoglobinometer (ok'si-hē'mo-glō-binom'e-ter): An instrument for measuring the oxygen level in the blood.

oxylalia (ok-si-lā'li-a): Abnormally fast speech.

oxymyoglobin (ok'-si-mī-ō-glō'bin): Oxygen combined with myoglobin.

oxyntic (ok-sin'tik): Producing acid. O. CELLS the cells in the gastric mucosa which produce hydrochloric acid.

oxyopia (ok-si-ō'pi-a): Abnormally acute vision.

oxyosmia (ok-si-os'mi-a): Abnormally acute sense of smell.

oxytocic (ok-si-tō'sik): 1. Hastening parturition. 2. An agent promoting uterine contractions.

oxytocin (ok-si-tō'sin): One of two hormones formed in the posterior pituitary gland, the other being vasopressin (q.v.). Stimulates contraction of the uterine muscles.

oxyuriasis (ok-si-ū-rī'a-sis): Infestation with pinworms or threadworms.

ozena (ō-zē'na): An atrophic condition of the nasal mucous membrane with associated crusting and offensive-smelling discharge.

ozone (ō'zōn): 1. A modified and condensed form of oxygen; a slightly blue irritating gas, generated naturally by the action of ultraviolet light rays on oxygen; also made commercially; O_3. Has stronger oxidizing properties than oxygen; is used as an antiseptic and disinfectant, e.g., in the purification of water. 2. May be descriptive of air that contains a perceptible amount of O_3, e.g., seaside air.

ozostomia (ō'-zō-stō'mi-a): Foul breath; halitosis.

P

P: Chemical symbol for phosphorus. ^{32}P radioactive phosphorus.

pabulum (pab'ū-lum): Food or nourishment.

Pacchioni's bodies (pak-ē-ō'nēz): Projections of the arachnoid membrane through the dura mater into the superior sagittal sinus. Also called *arachnoid granulations.*

pacemaker: The sinoatrial node of specialized nervous tissue located at the junction of the superior vena cava and the right atrium. It originates the contractions of the atria, which transmit the impulse on to the atrioventricular node, thereby inhibiting the contraction of the ventricles. ARTIFICIAL P. an electrical device used to re-establish the muscular contractions of an arrested heart or to steady the heartbeat; consists of an electrode introduced into the right atrium or ventricle and attached to an electrical source that is either implanted within the body or located externally; it initiates an increase in the rate of contraction of the ventricle resulting in output adequate to allow the patient to participate in his or her usual activities; ASYNCHRONOUS P. a device that paces the heartbeat when the heartbeats too slowly or not at all without help; also called *fixed-rate P.*; ATRIAL P. used to stimulate atrial contraction when the conduction system between the atria and the ventricles is intact; DEMAND P. a P. that will provide or withhold stimulation depending on how the heart is functioning on its own; EXTERNAL P. a temporary P. placed outside the body until a permanent P. can be implanted; TEMPORARY P. used in certain emergency situations to correct severe cardiac arrhythmias; usually inserted into the subclavian, jugular, basilic, or femoral vein; WANDERING P. a condition in which the origin of the heartbeat is shifted from the head of the sinoatrial node to the lower or other part of the atrium.

pachy-: Combining form denoting thick.

pachydermoperiostosis (pak-i-der'mō-per'i-ostō'sis): A condition characterized by thickening of the skin over bones, especially those of the face and distal parts of the extremities, with clubbing of the fingers; may be hereditary or due to underlying pulmonary disease.

pachymeter (pa-kim'i-ter): An instrument for measuring thickness, especially of thin objects or tissues, *e.g.*, a membrane.

pachyonychia (pak'-i-ō-nik'i-a): Abnormal thickening of the fingernails or toenails, often congenital.

pachypleuritis (pak-i-ploo-rī'tis): Inflammation of the pleura accompanied by thickening of the membrane. Also called *productive pleurisy.*

pachysomia (pak-i-sō'mi-a): Abnormal thickening of parts of the body, especially of the soft parts, as seen in acromegaly.

pacifier (pas'i-fi-er): 1. A rubber nipple-shaped device for babies to suck, also known as a 'comforter' or 'dummy'. 2. A tranquillizer.

pacing (pas'ing): The application of an electric stimulus to the heart to initiate contractions.

Pacini's corpuscles (pa-chē'nēz): Oval bodies in the deep parts of the corium of the skin that act as end organs for the sense of pressure; found especially in the skin of the hands and feet, but also in tendon and some internal structures. [Filippo Pacini, Italian anatomist, 1812–1883.]

pack: 1. A collection of instruments or equipment needed for a certain medical or surgical procedure. 2. To fill a cavity or tubular structure. 3. A hot or cold, wet or dry dressing applied to the body or part of it.

packed cells: Refers to whole blood from which the plasma has been removed by centrifugation or sedimentation; the cells then have a haematocrit of about 80% and are used in certain blood transfusions; also called packed red cells. P. CELL VOLUME the volume of cells in 100 ml of a blood sample after it has been centrifuged.

paederasty: See PEDERASTY.

paediatrician (pē-di-a-trish'un): A medical practitioner who specializes in the health supervision and treatment of children.

paediatrics (pē-di-at'riks): The branch of medicine that deals with the development and care of the child and with the diseases of children and their treatment.

paedodontics (pē'-dō-don'tiks): The branch of dentistry that deals with the diagnosis and treatment of conditions of the teeth and surrounding tissues in children.

paedophilia (pē-dō-fil'i-a): Abnormal fondness for children. P. EROTICA sexual perversion in which children are the preferred objects.

paedophobia (pē-dō-fō'bi-a): An abnormal fear or dread of children.

PAF: Abbreviation for performance assessment framework (*q.v.*).

Paget's disease: 1. Osteitis deformans. A chronic disease of the bone that resembles arthritis; of unknown cause. Characterized by softening and thickening of the bones of the spine, skull, pelvis, thigh, and lower legs, and by degeneration of the joints, with consequent distortion and bowing deformity of the long bones. Occurs most often in people of Western European descent, particularly those from the British Isles, France and Germany and who are in the 60 or 70 year age group. **2.** A progressive, inflammatory, eczematous dermatosis of the nipple and surrounding area, seen most often in older women. There is itching, soreness, ulceration and retraction of the nipple. May be precancerous or associated with cancer of the breast. **3.** Paget's disease of the vulva, a rare condition seen mostly in postmenopausal women; usually malignant and occurring in association with carcinoma in some other part of the vulvorectal area; symptoms include pain, pruritus, and burning; treatment is usually vulvectomy. [Sir James Paget, English surgeon, 1811–1899.]

pagophagia (pā-gō-fā'ji-a): Ice eating; thought to be a sign of iron deficiency.

pagoplexia (pā'gō-plek'si-a): Frostbite.

pain: Physical or mental suffering. A state of localized or generalized discomfort that ranges from mild distress to acute agony; usually caused by injury to a part or disturbance of the normal condition or functioning of a part of the body. In the plural it usually refers to the pains experienced during childbirth. AFTERPAINS those due to contraction of the uterus following the birth of a child; FALSE P.S occur late in pregnancy and resemble labour pains but do not result in labour; GROWING P.S. those that sometimes occur in muscles and joints of adolescents and children; may be manifestation of rheumatic fever; HUNGER P.S. those that occur in the stomach when it is time for a meal; sometimes a sign of gastric disorder; INTERMENSTRUAL P. see MITTELSCHMERZ; LABOUR P.S. the progressively severe, involuntary, rhythmic pains that occur during childbirth; PHANTOM LIMB P. that which is felt as being in a limb although the limb has been amputated; PSYCHOGENIC P. imaginary P.; REFERRED P. that which is felt in a part other than where it is produced; VASCULAR P. results from dilatation of blood vessels, particularly those around the brain; most common in migraine headaches. See GATE CONTROL THEORY.

pain assessment: The biological, psychological, and social measurement of pain and its impact on an individual's daily living. A number of assessment tools are available for use with adults and children; they are primarily longitudinal scales which list 'no pain' at one end to 'intense pain' at the other.

painter's colic: See LEAD.

palaeogenetic (pā'lē-ō-je-net'ik): Having originated in the past; not newly acquired. Said of traits, structures, abnormalities, etc.

palaeopathology (pā'-lē-ō-pa-thol'o-ji): The study of diseases in bodies preserved from ancient times, *e.g.*, mummies.

palatable (pal'a-tab'l): Pleasant or agreeable to the taste; savoury.

palate (pal'at): The roof of the mouth, consisting of the structures that separate the mouth from the nasal cavity, with its upper surface forming the floor of the nasal cavity; formed by parts of the palatine bones and the maxillae. ARTIFICIAL P. prothesis for use in correcting cleft palate; CLEFT P. a congenital cleft between the palatal bones which leaves a gap in the roof of the mouth; usually associated with cleft lip; HARD P. the anterior part of the P., formed by parts of the palatine and maxillary bones; SOFT P. situated at the posterior end of the palate and consisting of muscle covered with mucous membrane; forms the pillars of the fauces and the uvula. — palatal, palatine, adj.

palatine (pal'a-tīn): Relating to the palate. P. ARCHES the bilateral double pillars or arch-like folds formed by the descent of the soft palate as it meets the pharynx; P. BONE one of two irregular bones that form the back part of the palate, the lateral walls of the nasal cavity, and the floor of the orbit; P. PROCESS OF THE MAXILLA a horizontal plate of bone extending from each side of the maxilla to form the hard palate; P. TONSIL see TONSIL.

palatitis (pal-a-tī'tis): Inflammation of the hard palate.

palatomaxillary (pal'-a-tō-mak'si-lar-i): Relating to the palate and the maxilla.

palatonasal (pal-a-tō-nā'zal): Relating to the palate and the nasal cavity.

palatopharyngoplasty (pal'a-tō-far-ing'-ō-plas-ti): The surgical removal of excess tissue in the upper throat which vibrates like a reed in a musical instrument, causing snoring.

palatoplasty (pal'a-tō-plas-ti): Plastic surgery of the palate, including operations to correct cleft palate. Also called *uraniscoplasty*.

palatoplegia (pal'at-ō-plē'ji-a): Paralysis of the muscles of the soft palate. — palatoplegic, adj.

palatorrhaphy (pal'a-tor'a-fi): An operation for the repair of a cleft palate. Syn., *staphylorrhaphy, uraniscoplasty*.

pali-, palin-: Combining forms denoting again.

palikinaesia (pal-i-kī-nē'si-a): Pathological, involuntary repetition of certain movements.

palilalia (pal-i-lā'li-a): The constant repetition of a word or phrase with increasing rapidity and with the speech becoming less and less audible. May occur in persons with parkinsonism following encephalitis, or those with Pick's disease (*q.v.*).

palindromia (pal-in-drō'mi-a): The worsening or recurrence of a disease. — palindromic, adj

palingenesis (pal'-in-jen'e-sis): 1. The restoration or regeneration of a body part that has been lost or removed. 2. The appearance of ancestral characteristics particularly abnormal ones, in successive generations.

palliate (pal'ē-āt): To reduce the severity of; allay; abate; mitigate; lessen. To ease pain or symptoms without curing the condition.

palliative (pal'ē-a-tive): 1. Anything which serves to alleviate but cannot cure a disease. 2. Providing relief but not cure.

pallid (pal'id): Lacking the normal amount of colour; wan.

pallidotomy (pal-i-dot'o-mi): Surgical severance of the fibres from the cerebral cortex to the corpus striatum. Done to relieve the tremor in Parkinson's disease.

pallor (pal'lor): Absence of normal colour in the skin, especially of the face; paleness.

palm: The anterior, somewhat concave, flexor surface of the human hand; extends from the wrist to the bases of the fingers. The flat of the hand.

palmar (pal'mar): Relating to the palm of the hand. P. ARCHES superficial and deep, formed by the anastomosis of the radial and ulnar arteries.

palmaris (pal-mā'ris): Referring or related to the palm of the hand. P. LONGUS and P. BREVIS, two of the muscles of the palm of the hand.

palpable (pal'pa-b'l): 1. Evident, plain. 2. Capable of being felt or touched.

palpate (pal'pāt): To examine by touching with the fingers or palms of the hands.

palpation (pal-pā'shun): The act of feeling or touching the external surface of the body in order to determine the condition of a part or organ lying underneath; a procedure used in making physical diagnoses, and involving the ability to interpret the significance of what is being sensed by touch.

palpebra (pal'pe-bra): The eyelid. INFERIOR P. the lower eyelid; SUPERIOR P. the upper eyelid. — palpebral, adj.; palpebrae, pl.

palpebral (pal'pe-bral): Relating to the eyelids. P. CARTILAGES the thin, cartilage-like plates of tissue that make up the framework of the eyelids; P. COMMISSURE the union of the upper and the lower eyelid, either medial or lateral; P. FISSURE the opening between the two eyelids.

palpebration (pal'pe-brā'shun): 1. Winking. 2. Abnormally frequent winking.

palpebritis (pal'pe-brī'tis): Old term for blepharitis.

palpitation (pal-pi-tā'shun): The sensation that accompanies a condition in which the heartbeats very rapidly or there is a change in rhythm of which the person is aware; flutter.

PALS: Abbreviation for Patient Advice and Liaison Service (*q.v.*).

palsy (pawl'zi): Paralysis, temporary or permanent. Term most often used in combination. BELL'S P. facial hemiparesis from a lesion in the seventh (facial) nerve, resulting in distortion of the facial features; cause unknown. [Charles Bell, Scottish physician, 1774–1842.]; BIRTH P., P. due to injury at birth; BRACHIAL P. cause may be unknown, but may be due to birth trauma or may follow administration of antitoxin, or an influenzal infection; marked by pain across the shoulder and upper arm, weakness and focal paralysis; often bilateral; BULBAR P. a chronic, usually fatal disease caused by degeneration of motor nuclei in the medulla oblongata; characterized by progressive paralysis of muscles of the mouth, pharynx, and larynx; CEREBRAL P. progressive persistent disorder of motor power and coordination, due to damage to the brain; CREEPING P. progressive muscular dystrophy, see under DYSTROPHY; CRUTCH P. paralysis of the extensor muscles of the wrist, thumb, and fingers, due to pressure of the crutch crosspiece on the radial nerve in the axilla; DUCHENNE'S P. bulbar P.; DYSKINETIC P. cerebral P., characterized by uncontrolled movements that disappear during sleep; ERB'S P. paralysis of a group of shoulder and arm muscles; caused by an injury to the brachial plexus or to the lower cervical nerve roots; the arm hangs loosely with the forearm pronated (waiter's tip position); also called *Erb–Duchenne paralysis*,

Duchenne–Erb paralysis. [William Erb, German neurologist, 1840–1921.]; FACIAL P. unilateral paralysis of muscles supplied by the seventh cranial nerve; OCULOMOTOR P. paralysis of the oculomotor nerve; accompanied usually by ptosis, dilatation of the pupil, and external deviation of the eye; PERONEAL P. due to compression of the peroneal nerve by tight garters or by sitting with legs crossed; weakness of the peroneal muscle results in dorsiflexion, eversion of the foot, and foot drop; PROGRESSIVE SUPRANUCLEAR P. characterized by staring facial expression, ocular dysfunction, dementia, and progressive spasticity; PSEUDOBULBAR P. resembles bulbar P., but not of bulbar origin; seen in arteriosclerotic parkinsonism when it is associated with emotional instability, dysphagia, dysarthria; marked by spastic weakness of facial muscles, tongue, and pharynx. SCRIVENER'S P. an occupational neurosis characterized by painful spasmodic cramps of the fingers, hands, and forearm whenever an attempt is made to write; often called writer's cramp; SHAKING P. paralysis agitans, (see PARKINSON'S DISEASE); ULNAR P. due to injury of the ulnar nerve; usually bilateral; may occur as a result of activities which involve leaning on the elbows for long periods of time; marked by weakness, wasting, and sensory loss in the ulnar area of the hand; WASTING P. progressive muscular dystrophy; see under DYSTROPHY.

pan-, pant-, panta-, pano-, panto-: Combining forms denoting (1) all, completely whole; (2) general.

panacea (pan-a-sē′a): A universal remedy; a cure-all. Term derived from Panacea, the daughter of Aesculapius, who, along with her sister Hygiea, assisted in caring for the sacred serpents and in carrying out rites in early Greek temples of healing.

panarteritis (pan′ar-ter-ī′tis): Periarteritis nodosa (*q.v.*).

panarthritis (pan-ar-thrī′tis): Inflammation of all the structures of a joint, or of all of the joints.

pancarditis (pan-kar-dī′tis): Inflammation of all the structures of the heart.

Pancoast's tumour: A malignant tumour of the apex of a lung; chracterized by neuritic pain in the arm and atrophy of the muscles of the arm and hand, due to involvement of the brachial plexus. Syn., *Pancoast's syndrome*.

pancreas (pan′krē-as): A large, long, narrow, tongue-shaped glandular organ lying below and behind the stomach. Its head or right end is encircled by the duodenum and its tail often touches the spleen. It secretes pancreatic juice which passes into the duodenum via the pancreatic duct and the common bile duct, and acts on all classes of foods. An internal secretion, insulin, produced in the islets of Langerhans, see under ISLET, is required for the regulation of carbohydrate metabolism. ANNULAR P. an anomaly in which the P. forms a ring that completely surrounds the duodenum.

pancreatalgia (pan′krē-a-tal′ji-a): Pain in the pancreas or in the area of the pancreas.

pancreatectomy (pan′krē-a-tek′to-mi): Excision of part or the whole of the pancreas.

pancreatic (pan-krē-at′ik): Of or relating to the pancreas. P. DUCT begins with the junction of small ducts from lobules in the tail of the pancreas and runs from right to left through the gland, receives other ducts along the way, and finally empties into the common bile duct; P. JUICE an external secretion of the pancreas; consists of clear alkaline fluid containing trypsinogen, which converts proteins to amino acids; amylase, which converts all starches to maltose and dextrin; and lipase, which converts fats to fatty acids and glycerol.

pancreatic function test: A test involving analysis of aspirated material from the stomach and second part of the duodenum to determine the response of the pancreas to various hormonal stimuli.

pancreatico-: Combining form denoting relationship to the pancreatic duct.

pancreaticojejunostomy (pan-krē-at′i-kō-jē-ju-nos′to-mi): The surgical anastomosis of the pancreatic duct, or of the divided end of the pancreas, with the jejunum.

pancreatin (pan′krē-a-tin): A mixture of pancreatic enzymes obtained from cattle or pigs; used as a digestive or in the preparation of predigested foods.

pancreatitis (pan′krē-a-tī′tis): Inflammation of the pancreas, acute or chronic; may be symptomless or characterized by pain and tenderness of the abdomen, nausea, vomiting, and tympanites. ACUTE HAEMORRHAGIC P. characterized by autolysis of pancreatic tissue by enzymatic action, which causes haemorrhage into surrounding tissues, often staining them; CHRONIC P. is of two types, (1) painless attacks progressing to loss of pancreatic function, and (2) recurring attacks of progressive severity with destruction of pancreatic tissues.

pancreato-: Combining form denoting relationship to the pancreas.

pancreatoduodenectomy (pan-krē-at′ō-dū-ō-dē-nek′to-mi): Excision of the head of the pancreas along with the encircling loop of the duodenum, done in cases of carcinoma of the head of the pancreas. Most of the pancreas, the pylorus, duodenum and the common bile duct are excised. Gastrojejunostomy is performed with anastomosis of the tail of the pancreas and gall bladder to the jejunum.

pancreatography (pan′krē-a-tog′ra-fi): X-ray examination of the pancreas during surgical exploration, after a contrast medium has been injected into the pancreatic duct.

pancreatolith (pan-krē-at′ō-lith): A pancreatic calculus.

pancreozymin (pan′krē-ō-zī′min): A hormone of the duodenal mucosa that stimulates the secretion of the pancreatic enzymes, amylase in particular.

pancytopenia (pan-sī-tō-pē′ni-a): A deficiency of all three types of blood cells — erthrocytes, lymphocytes, and platelets. Aplastic anaemia.

pandemic (pan-dem′ik): 1. An infection spreading over a whole country or the world. 2. Widely epidemic.

panencephalitis (pan′en-kef-a-lī′tis,-sef-): In flammation of all or most of the brain. SUBACUTE SCLEROSING P, a rare, progressive, often fatal form of P., characterized by lesions in the white matter, demyelination, and pathological changes in the nerve cells; probably caused by a virus, the measles virus in particular; symptoms include ataxia, seizures, blindness, progressive dementia; occurs most often in children and adolescents. Also called *Dawson's encephalitis*.

pang: A sudden piercing physical pain or feeling of mental anguish.

panhypopituitarism (pan′hī-pō-pi-tū′i-tar-izm): The condition of complete absence of pituitary secretion; results in pituitary dwarfism, absence of gonadal function, weight loss, hypotension, insufficient thyroid and adrenal function. See SIMMOND'S DISEASE.

panhysterectomy (pan′his-ter-ek′to-mi): Removal of the entire uterus, including the cervix.

panhysterosalpingo-oophorectomy (pan-his′ter-ō-sal-ping′ō-ō-of-ō-rek′tō-mi): Surgical removal of the uterus, cervix, uterine tubes, and ovaries.

panic (pan′ik): Sudden overwhelming and unreasoning fear resulting in hysteria and irrational behaviour. May be brought on by a trifling cause or a situation perceived to be of extreme danger; usually accompanied by frantic efforts to escape. In psychiatry, an attack of intense anxiety with distorted perceptions, loss of rational thought and often considerable disinte-

gration of the personality. P. ATTACK short-lived crescendo of anxiety.

panmyelopathy (pan-mī-e-lop′a-thi): A condition in which there is a proliferation of the bone marrow elements without visible evidence of neoplasm, along with extramedullary production of blood cells and the presence of immature cells in the circulating blood.

panniculectomy (pa-nik′ū-lek′tō-mi): Surgical removal of the abdominal panniculus adiposus; may be required after an obese person has had a significant weight loss. See PANNICULUS.

panniculitis (pa-nik′ū-lī′tis): Inflammation of the thin sheet of fatty subcutaneous connective tissue of the anterior abdominal wall. SYSTEMIC NODULAR P. recurrent crops of tender, movable subcutaneous nodules, most commonly seen on the legs, thighs, buttocks, abdomen, breasts, arms; accompanied by chills, fever, malaise, musculoskeletal aching, splenomegaly, sometimes leukopenia.

panniculus (pa-nik′ū-lus)· A layer or sheet of tissue. P. ADIPOSUS a sheet of superficial fascia that contains deposits of fat.

pannus (pan′us): Vascularization of the cornea, usually the upper half, resulting in thickening and opacity and causing dimness of vision; often caused by conjunctival irritation; frequently also a complication of trachoma.

panophthalmitis (pan′of-thal-mī′tis): Inflammation and infection, usually purulent, in all parts of the eye.

panoptosis (pan-o-tō′sis): General prolapse or ptosis of all of the abdominal organs.

panosteitis (pan′os-tē-ī′tis): Inflammation of all constituents of a bone, *i.e.*, medulla, bony tissue, and periosteum.

panotitis (pan-ō-tī′tis): Inflammation of all the parts of the ear.

panphobia (pan-fō′bi-a): Morbid fear of everything.

panproctocolectomy (pan-prok′tō-kō-lek′tō-mi): The surgical excision of all of the rectum and the colon, and the creation of an ileostomy for the elimination of faeces.

pant: 1. A short, quick, laboured breath. 2. To breathe quickly or with difficulty; to gasp for breath.

pantothenic acid (pan-tō-then′ik as′id): A constituent of the vitamin B complex. Widely distributed in plant and animal tissues; found in yeast, liver, heart, salmon, eggs, various grains; also produced synthetically. Is essential for nutrition of certain animal species but its importance to human nutrition is not fully understood. Also known as vitamin B_3.

pantropic (pan-trōp'ik): 1. Having affinity for many body tissues, often said of viruses. 2. Having affinity for many body organs or parts.

pap: Any soft, pulpy food for infants or invalids. PAP SMEAR Papanicolaou smear; P. TEST Papanicolaou test; see PAPANICOLAOU.

papain (pa-pā'in): An enzyme derived from the pawpaw; it acts as a catalyst in hydrolysis of proteins and polypeptides to amino acids; also has several uses in medicine.

Papanicolaou (pap-a-nik-ō-la'ow): P. SMEAR a vaginal smear prepared for microscopic examination of exfoliated cells. Can also be prepared from many other body secretions including sputum, gastric contents, mammary secretions, washings from a bronchoscope. P. TEST a cytological test for early detection of the presence of cancer cells utilizing cells scraped from the surface of a membrane, or from body secretions or fluids; most often done as a screen for cancer of the cervix. [George N. Papanicolaou, Greek physician and anatomist, 1883–1962.]

papilla (pa-pil'a): A small, nipple-shaped eminence. CIRCUMVALLATE P. the large papillae found at the base of the tongue; arranged in a V shape; contain taste buds; FILIFORM P. fine hair-like papillae at the tip of the tongue; FUNGIFORM P. fungus-shaped papillae found chiefly on the dorsocentral area of the tongue; MAMMARY P. the pigmented projection on the anterior aspect of the mammary gland into which the milk ducts open; OPTIC P. the terminus of the optic nerve at the point where it enters the eyeball; RENAL P. the summit of one of the renal pyramids; TACTILE P. one that projects into the true skin and contains an end organ for touch; VALLATE P. a circumvallate P. — papillae, pl.; papillary, adj.

papillary (pap'i-ler-i): Relating to or resembling a papilla or nipple. P. MUSCLES small cone-shaped muscles that project from the walls of the ventricles and attach to the chordae tendinae (q.v.); when the ventricles fill with blood and contract, these muscles also contract and tighten the chordae, pressing the valves shut but preventing them from being pushed back into the atria by the surging blood.

papilliferous (pap'i-lif'er-us): Containing or provided with papillae.

papillitis (pap'i-lī'tis): 1. Inflammation of a papilla. 2. Inflammation and oedema of the optic disc. CHRONIC LINGUAL P. painful glossitis that often extends to the palate and cheeks; characterized by redness, burning, and desquamation of the stratum corneum; most often

seen in middle-aged women; Also called *Moeller's glossitis*; NECROTIZING P. a necrosis of the renal papillae; seen in the most severe forms of pyelonephritis (q.v.).

papilloedema (pap-il-ē-dē'ma): Oedema of the optic disc; indicative of increased intracranial pressure.

papilloma (pap-i-lō'ma): A branching or lobulated, circumscribed epithelial neoplasm, usually benign, arising in the skin or mucous membrane; may appear as a wart, condyloma, or polyp. DUCTAL P. a benign tumour of the mammary duct system of the breast, characterized by atypical papillary structures; VILLOUS P., P. characterized by long slender processes, usually seen in the urinary bladder.

papillomatosis (pap'i-lō-ma-tō'sis): The simultaneous widespread development of several papillomata.

papillomavirus (pap'i-lō-ma-vī'rus): Any of a group of small viruses that cause papillomata in humans.

papovavirus (pa-po'-va-vī'rus): Any of a group of small viruses, many of which are thought to be the cause or potential cause of tumours, and some of which cause warts.

papule (pap'ūl): A small, solid, usually round or conical, circumscribed elevation on the skin. A pimple. — papular, adj.; papulation, n.

papulopustular (pap'-ū-lō-pus'-tū-lar): Relating to an eruption composed of both papules and pustules.

papulosis (pap-ū-lō'sis): A condition marked by the presence of multiple papules on the skin. LYMPHOMATOID P. a form of P. characterized by ulcerative lesions, with new lesions occurring as others recede.

papulosquamous (pap'ū-lō-skwā'mus): Both papular and scaly; pertains to certain dermatoses, including psoriasis, pityriasis rosea, and lichen planus.

papyraceous (pap-i-rā'shus): Like paper or parchment. P. FETUS a dead twin fetus that has been compressed by the other growing twin and which has a mummy-like, parchment appearance.

par-, para-: Prefixes denoting (1) beside, alongside, parallel; (2) closely resembling a true form, e.g., paratyphoid; (3) faulty, irregular, abnormal, perverted.

Para: A word used to designate the number of pregnancies a women has had that have resulted in viable births. It is usually capitalized and combined with the proper numeral, e.g., Para I, II, etc.

para-aminobenzoic acid (par-a-am'i-nō-benzō'ik as'id): Often occurs as a member of the vitamin B complex. Found in certain meats, cereal grains, milk products, and eggs; also occurs in small amounts in body fluids, particularly cerebrospinal fluid, blood, urine, and sweat; also known as *vitamin H₁*. Sometimes used as an antirickettsial drug, and in treatment of certain dermatoses.

para-aminosalicyclic acid (par-a-am'i-nō-sal-i-sil'ik as'id): A synthetic drug that acts as a tuberculostatic.

para-arthria (par-a-ar'-thri-a): The imperfect utterance of words.

Paracelsus: [Philippus Aureolus Theophrastus Bombastus Hohenheim Paracelsus, Swiss physician and alchemist, 1439–1541.] Introduced such substances as lead, iron, sulphur, and arsenic into medicine.

paracentesis (par'a-sen-tē'sis): Puncture, particularly the puncture of a fluid-filled body cavity by a needle or trocar for the purpose of drawing off fluid; designated according to the particular cavity that is punctured, *e.g.*, abdominal, thoracic, etc.

paracervical block: A form of regional anaesthesia used during labour; consists of the injection of an anaesthetic into the area on each side of the uterus.

paracholia (par-a-kō'li-a): A condition characterized by disordered secretion of bile.

parachroma (par-a-krō'ma): Abnormal or unusual coloration of the skin.

parachromatopsia (par'a-krō'ma-top'si-a): Partial colour blindness. Also called *dichromatopsia*.

paracolpitis (par-a-kōl-pī'tis): Inflammation of the tissues surrounding the vagina.

paracusia (par-a-kū'si-a): Impaired or disordered hearing. Paracusis.

paracyesis (par-a-sī-ē'sis): Extrauterine pregnancy.

paradigm: A pattern that may serve as a model or example. P. CASE a term used, specifically by Patricia Benner and recently other nursing theorists, to describe a powerful and memorable experience that can be employed to inform future practice. See also PATRICIA BENNER.

paradipsia (par-a-dip'si-a): A perverted and exaggerated appetite for fluids out of proportion to the needs of the body.

paradoxical (par-a-dok'si-kal): Occurring in a manner that is inconsistent with or contrary to the normal or usual. P. BREATHING occurs in patients whose chest is opened by severe injury; during inspiration the affected part is sucked in as the lung fills and during expir-

ation the affected part bulges out; P. BLOOD PRESSURE a diminution in systemic arterial pressure on inspiration and a strengthening on expiration; this is normal in deep breathing; otherwise it may indicate cardiac tamponade; P. PULSE see under PULSE.

paraesthesia (par-as-thē'zi-a): Abnormal tactile sensation such as burning, tingling, prickling, creeping; may be a symptom of psychosis or neurological disease.

paraffin (par'a-fin): A colourless, odourless, taste-less, white or somewhat translucent substance obtained from petroleum. P. BATH a physiotherapy treatment in which part or all of an extremity is dipped into or brushed with liquid paraffin repeatedly to form a thick coating.

parafollicular (par-a-fo-lik'ū-lar): Associated with or in the vicinity of a follicular structure. P. CELLS argyrophil cells, cells found between or among the follicles in the thyroid epithelium; they are thought to be the source of thyrocalcitonin and are rich in mitochondria.

paragammacism (par-a-gam'a-sizm): Faulty pronunciation of the letters *g* and *k* and of *ch*.

paraganglioma (par a-gang-gli-ō'ma): A benign neoplasm that occurs in the medullary portion of the adrenal gland.

paraganglion (par-a-gang'gli-on): Any of the small chromaffin (*q.v.*) cells or a group of them. They secrete adrenaline and noradrenaline. — paraganglia, pl.

paraglossia (par-a-glos'i-a): Swelling of the tongue.

paragnathus (par'ag-nath'us): A fetus with a supernumerary or malformed jaw.

paragraphia (par-a-graf'i-a): A psychological condition in which a person understands words and their meanings but is unable to write correctly from dictation, or uses the wrong word in writing, or makes mistakes in writing.

paraguesia (par-a-gū'si-a): 1. A disorder or perversion of the sense of taste. 2. An unpleasant taste in the mouth.

parahaemophilia (par'a-hē-mō-fil'i-a): An inherited tendency to haemorrhage due to absence of coagulation factor V.

parahormone (par-a-hor'mōn): A substance that acts to control the function of a distant part or organ but is not a true hormone. A common example is carbon dioxide which acts on the respiratory centre in the brain.

parainfluenza virus: Several serotypes are recognized. Infection in adults is associated with pharyngitis, hoarseness, and tracheitis; in children the virus is associated with croup.

parakeratosis (par'a-ker-a-tō'sis): Any disorder of the horny layer of the skin, particularly if it interferes with keratinization.

paralalia (par-a-lā'li-a): A disorder of speech in which sounds are distorted or one letter is substituted for another.

paralambdacism (par-a-lam'da-sizm): Inability to pronounce the letter *l* (ell), or the substitution of another letter for it.

paralanguage (par-a-lang'waj): Non-verbal aspects of speech, *i.e.*, voice quality, intonation, pitch, rhythm, loudness, silence, head nodding, position, body movements, facial expression, etc.; important in studies of personality. Also called *paralinguistics*.

paralepsy (par'a-lep-si): Psycholepsy (*q.v.*).

paralexia (par-a-lek'si-a): An impairment of reading ability, characterized by the transposition of words and syllables so that the resulting combinations are meaningless.

parallagma (par-a-lag' ma): The displacement of the ends or the fragments of a fractured bone.

parallergy (par-al'er-ji): A condition in which sensitization of the body with a specific allergen predisposes the individual to susceptibility to non-specific allergens.

paralogia (par'a'-lō'ji-a): Inability to reason, marked by illogical speech and self-deception.

Paralympics (par-a-lim'piks): An international sports contest, organized in 1952 for paraplegic patients; since 1976 non-wheelchair contestants have been admitted, including the blind and amputees. Events are held in conjunction with the regular Olympic Games.

paralyse (par' a-līz): To produce a state of paralysis (*q.v.*).

paralysis (pa-ral'i-sis): Complete or incomplete, temporary or permanent loss of motor function or of sensation in a part of the body; may be caused by damage to the central or peripheral nervous system by injury, disease, or certain chemical poisonings or drugs. Many types are described, usually according to aetiology, the part or parts affected or the extent to which they are affected, or muscle tone, *i.e.*, whether the muscles are flaccid or spastic. See also PALSY; PARESIS; ASCENDING P., P. that begins in the legs and ascends towards the head; BRACHIAL P., P. of the arm due to a lesion in the brachial plexus; see under PALSY; BULBAR P. involves the labioglossopharyngeal region; see under PALSY; DIPHTHERITIC P. affects the uvula and usually some other muscles; appears two or three weeks after an attack of diphtheria; due to toxic neuritis; DIVER'S P. see CAISSON DISEASE; EMOTIONAL P. occurs in hysterical

subjects; ERB'S P., ERB–DUCHENNE P. see under PALSY; FACIAL P. Bell's palsy, see under PALSY; FAMILIAL PERIODIC P. a condition characterized by episodes of weakness caused by a hereditary tendency to fluctuation in potassium balance; treated by correcting electrolyte balance; FLACCID P. results mainly from lower motor neuron lesions; tendon reflexes are diminished or absent; IMMUNOLOGICAL P. the absence of immune response to a specific antigen; INFANTILE P. anterior poliomyelitis; see POLIOMYELITIS; KLUMPKE'S P., P. and atrophy of forearm and hand muscles, along with sensory and pupillary disturbances; due to injury of the lower part of the brachial plexus, often a birth injury; see ERB'S PALSY under PALSY; LANDRY'S P. acute ascending P. beginning in the feet and rapidly progressing; characterized by fever; may terminate in respiratory stasis and death; P. AGITANS see PARKINSON'S DISEASE; PERIODIC P. a group of disorders characterized by attacks of muscular weakness beginning when the individual is exposed to cold or is at rest after exercise; there are no other symptoms and recovery between attacks is complete; PROGRESSIVE BULBAR P. bulbar P. that begins in later life; due to atrophic degeneration that is characteristic of ageing; PSEUDOBULBAR P., affects chiefly the facial muscles; there is gross disturbance in control of the tongue, bilateral hemiplegia, and mental changes following a succession of 'strokes'; resembles bulbar P.; SPASTIC P. results mainly from upper motor neuron lesions; there are exaggerated tendon reflexes, rigidity of muscles of the extremities with atrophy; TICK P. caused by the bite of a tick found in certain parts of the world; affects both animals and children; a flaccid ascending motor paralysis is the principal symptom, which usually disappears when the tick is removed.

paralytic (par-a-lit'ik): **1.** A person afflicted with paralysis. **2.** Pertaining to paralysis. P. ILEUS paralysis of the intestinal muscle, so that the bowel content cannot pass onward even though there is no mechanical obstruction; may be a complication of abdominal surgery. — See also APERISTALSIS.

paralytogenic (par'a-lit-ō-jen'ik): Causing paralysis.

paramania (par-a-mā'ni-a): A condition characterized by enjoyment of complaining.

paramedian (par-a-mē'di-an): Situated near the midline.

paramedic (par-a-med'ik): **1.** A person who is not a physician who works in a paramedical field; may be a pharmacist; technician; physiotherapist, occupational or speech therapist, or a medical social worker. **2.** A person who has had training in emergency intensive care; often utilized to staff ambulances and rescue squads; fire fighters and police officers often receive this training.

paramedical (par-a-med'i-kal): Having an indirect or secondary relationship to the practice of medicine. P. WORKERS include nurses, pharmacists, technicians, physiotherapists, occupational and speech therapists, social workers, dentists, chiropodists.

paramenia (par-a-mē' ni-a): Disordered menstruation.

parametrial (par-a-mē'tri-al): Relating to the parametrium (*q.v.*).

parametric (par-a-met'rik): Around the uterus.

parametric testing: Statistical testing that assumes that data (taken from a sample of the population) have a normal distribution curve.

parametritis (par-a-mē-trī'tis): Inflammation of the parametrium (*q.v.*).

parametrium (par-a-mē'tri-um): The connective tissues and smooth muscle of the pelvic floor and immediately surrounding the lower part of the uterus and extending laterally between the layers of the broad ligament. — parametrial, adj.

paramimia (par-a-mim'i-a): Faulty or incorrect use of muscles and gestures in the verbal expression of thoughts.

paramnesia (par-am-nē'zi-a): A disorder of the memory characterized by the belief that certain events that never took place actually occurred; it is involuntary falsification. Also sometimes denotes a person who remembers words but forgets their meanings so that use of them results in incomprehensible speech.

paramorphia (par-a-mor'fi-a): Any abnormality of structure or form.

paramyoclonus (par'a-mī-ok'lo-nus): A condition in which various unrelated muscles go into myoclonic contraction. See MYOCLONUS.

paramyotonia (par'a-mī-ō-tō'ni-a): A condition in which impaired muscle tone results in tonic muscle spasms. P. CONGENITA a congenital P. that is induced by exposure to cold, which causes intermittent flaccid paralysis but does not permanently affect the muscles.

paramyxovirus (par'a-mik-sō-vī'rus): A subgroup of the myxovirus group; includes the viruses that cause mumps, measles, parainfluenza, possibly syncytial virus disease. Infection with P. may have serious complications involving the breast, seminal vesicles, prostate gland, or pancreas.

paranasal (par-a-nā'zal): Near the nasal cavities, as the various sinuses; P. SINUSES air cavities in the skull bones which are lined with mucous membrane and communicate with the nasal cavity.

paranephric (par-a-nef'rik): **1.** Near the kidney. **2.** Referring to the adrenal gland.

paranoia (par-a-noy'a): A chronic, slowly progressive psychiatric disorder characterized by well-organized delusions of grandeur or of persecution, or attitudes of suspicion. Mental powers, including clear, orderly thinking are preserved. True paranoia occurs rarely but many other psychotic conditions resemble it. — paranoid, paranoiac, adj.

paranoiac (par-a-noy'ak): **1.** Resembling, pertaining to, or suffering from paranoia. **2.** A person suffering from paranoia. P. BEHAVIOUR, characterized by extreme suspicion of others delusions of persecution, megalomania.

paranoid (par'a-noyd): Resembling paranoia. Term often used to describe people who are overly suspicious or jealous. P. DISORDERS disorders characterized by the development of a delusional system in which one considers oneself endowed with superior and unique abilities, while one's thinking remains orderly and clear; P. SCHIZOPHRENIA see under SCHIZOPHRENIA.

paranomia (par-a-nō'mi-a): A type of aphasia characterized by inability to properly name objects seen or touched.

paraoesophageal (par' a-ē-sof-a-jē'al): Situated alongside the oesophagus. P. CYST a cyst that has its origin in a bronchus and ultimately connects with the oesophageal wall; P. HERNIA a hiatus hernia in which part of the stomach herniates into the thorax.

paraparesis (par-a-par'e-sis): Partial paralysis affecting particularly the legs and lower part of the back.

parapertussis (par-a-per-tus'sis): A disease that resembles pertussis but is much less severe in nature.

paraphasia (par-a-fā'zi-a): A speech disorder characterized by inability to use the right words, or to arrange words correctly in sentences; the result is unintelligible speech.

paraphemia (par-a-fē'mi-a): A type of aphasia in which the person consistently uses the wrong words.

paraphia (pa-rā'fi-a): A disorder of the sense of touch.

paraphilia (par-a-fil'i-a): An emotional disorder characterized by unusual sexual behaviour, including the practice of fetishism and sexual activities with unconsenting humans, or involving suffering or humiliation.

paraphiliac (par-a-fil′i-ak): 1. Relating to paraphilia. 2. A person who practises paraphilia (*q.v.*).

paraphimosis (par′a-fī-mō′sis): A painful condition in which the prepuce has been retracted behind the glans penis and cannot be replaced; the tight ring of skin interferes with the flow of blood in the glans. Surgical correction is possible.

paraphonia (par-a-fō′ni-a): Partial loss of the voice or any change in its quality. P. PUBERUM the harsh, deep, irregular quality that develops in boys' voices at puberty.

paraphrasia (par-a-frā′zi-a): A type of aphasia in which incorrect words or senseless combinations of words are used.

paraphrenia (par-a-frē′ni-a): A paranoid state characterized by delusions of grandeur but in which the person's thinking processes are not disturbed.

paraplasm (par′a-plazm): 1. The fluid part of the protoplasm. 2. Any malformed substance or growth.

paraplegia (par-a-plē′ji-a): Paralysis of the lower half of the body, including the lower trunk and both legs; usually due to disease or injury of the spinal cord; SENILE P., P. in the elderly which involves changes in gait; may be associated with cervical spondylitis or vascular disease. — paraplegic, paraplectic, adj.

paraplegic (par-a-plē′jik): Relating to paraplegia. Also sometimes used to denote a person suffering from paraplegia.

parapraxia (par-a-prak′si-a): A term used to describe such minor aberrations of behaviour as forgetfulness, a tendency to misplace things, or slips of the tongue or pen.

paraprotein (par-a-prō′tēn): 1. Any plasma protein that differs in one or more characteristics from normal plasma protein, usually refers to a globulin. 2. A protein that has been modified so that it is slightly different from the native protein.

paraproteinaemia (par′a-prō-tin-ē′mi-a): The presence of abnormal amounts of a paraprotein in the blood plasma.

parapsoriasis (par-a-sō-rī′a-sis): Name given to a group of rare skin diseases that are characterized by red scaly patches or papules that resemble those of psoriasis and are resistant to treatment.

parapsychology (par′a-sī-kol′o-ji): A term used to describe the branch of psychology dealing with motor and psychic phenomena that occur

without the apparent mediation of sensory or motor organs and that cannot be accounted for by currently known scientific methods, *e.g.*, clairvoyance and extrasensory perception.

pararectal (par-a-rek′tal): Near the rectum.

parasellar (par-a-sel′lar): Adjacent to or near the pituitary fossa.

parasigmatism (par-a-sig′ma-tizm): Imperfect pronunciation of the letter *s*, resulting in a lisp.

parasinusoidal (par′a-sī-nū-soy′dal): Near or around a sinus; usually refers to a cerebral sinus, the superior sagittal sinus in particular.

parasitaemia (par′a-sī-tē′mi-a): The presence of parasites in the blood; usually refers to malarial parasites. — parasitaemic, adj.

parasite (par′a-sīt): Any organism that lives in or on another organism and obtains all or part of its nourishment from its host without giving anything in return. — parasitic, adj. FACULTATIVE P. an organism that is parasitic on another but is also capable of existing independently; OBLIGATORY P. an organism that cannot live independently of its host.

parasiticide (par-a-sit′i-sīd): Any agent that destroys parasites.

parasitogenic (par′a-sī-tō-jen′ik): Caused by or due to parasites.

parasitology (par′a-sī-tol′o-ji): The science that studies parasites and their effects on other living organisms, especially the human body.

parasitophobia (par′a-sī-tō-fō′bi-a): Morbid dread of parasites.

parasitosis (par′a-sī-tō′sis): The condition of being infested or infected with parasites.

paraspadias (par-a-spā′-di-as): A condition in which the urethra opens on one side of the penis.

paraspasm (par′a-spazm): 1. Spasm of corresponding muscles on both sides of the body. 2. Spasm or paralysis of the muscles of the lower extremities.

parasuicide: A suicidal gesture such as self-mutilation. It maybe motivated by a desire to die. See ATTEMPTED SUICIDE.

parasympathetic (par-a-sim-pa-thet′ik): P. NERVOUS SYSTEM a division of the autonomic nervous system; see under NERVOUS SYSTEM.

parasympatholytic (par-a-sim′pa-tho-lit′ik): Opposing or blocking the action of parasympathetic nerve fibres, or an agent that has this physiological effect.

parasympathomimetic (par-a-sim′pa-thō-mi-met′ik): Producing effects similar to those produced by stimulation of parasympathetic nerve fibres, or an agent that has this physiological action.

parasystole (par-a-sis'to-li): An irregular cardiac rhythm in which the heartbeat is paced at different rates by two pacemakers that function independently of each other.

parataxia (par-a-taks'i-a): 1. An emotional state in which one views all events, persons, and objects as entirely separate without any relationship to other aspects of one's personal experience. 2. Behaviour that demonstrates lack of adjustment to emotions and desires.

paratendinitis (par'-a-ten-di-nī'tis): A common condition in young adults whose occupation involves repetitive movements of the hand and wrist which causes friction between the tendons; marked by swelling, local oedema, fine crepitation, and pain at the back of the wrist and in the forearm. Syn., *acute frictional tenosynovitis.*

paratherapeutic (par-a-ther-a-pū'tik): Refers to a condition caused by treatment for another condition or disease; iatrogenic.

parathormone (par-a-thor'mōn): A hormone secreted by the parathyroid glands; controls the metabolism of calcium and phosphorus. Excess hormone causes mobilization of calcium from the bones, which become rarefied.

parathyroid (par a thī'royd): Any one of several, usually four, small endocrine glands lying close to or embedded in the posterior surfaces of the lateral lobes of the thyroid gland. They secrete a hormone, parathormone (*q.v.*). P. OSTEODYSTROPHY a condition in which an excess of parathyroid secretion causes generalized osteoporosis and cystic changes in some bones, usually the clavicle, long bones, and skull; seen in adults.

parathyroidectomy (par'a-thī-roy-dek'to-mi): Excision of one or more parathyroid glands.

paratonia (par-a-tō'ni-a): A disorder of tension or tone, particularly of muscle, manifested in uneven resistance of limbs to passive movement; seen most often in stuporous patients or those with dementia. Syn., *gegenhalten.*

paratrigeminal syndrome (par'a-trīl jem'i-nal): A rare condition characterized by paroxysmal pain in the face, sensory loss on the affected side, ptosis of the upper eyelid, and weakness of the muscles of mastication. One cause is thought to be an aneurysm of the internal carotid artery.

paratrooper fracture: See under FRACTURE.

paratyphoid fever (par-a-tī-foydfē'ver): Descriptive of a variety of enteric fevers that closely resemble typhoid fever but which are less prolonged and severe. Usually contracted by eating food that has become contaminated with the bacteria of the genus *Salmonella.* See TAB.

paraurethral (par'a-ūrē'thral): Near the urethra. P. DUCTS the ducts from two small glands that open into the posterior wall of the female urethra at the orifice; Skene's ducts; P. GLANDS see SKENE'S GLANDS.

paravaginal (par-a-vaj'in-al): Near or alongside the vagina.

paravertebral (par-a-ver'te-bral): Alongside or near the vertebral column. P. BLOCK ANAESTHESIA induced by infiltration of local anaesthetic around the spinal nerve roots as they emerge from the intervertebral foramina; P. INJECTION of local anaesthetic into sympathetic chain; can be used as a test in ischaemic limbs to see if sympathectomy will be of value.

paregoric (par-e-gor'ik): Camphorated tincture of opium, frequently used in cough syrups and mixtures; also used in treatment of diarrhoea.

parencephalia (par'en-ke-fā'li-a,-se-): Imperfect development of the brain.

parencephalitis (par-en-kef-a-lī'tis,-sef-): Inflammation of the cerebellum.

parencephalocele (par-en-kef'al ō oēl,-sef'-): Protrusion of part of the cerebellum through a defect in the structure of the cranium.

parencephalon (par-en-kef'a-lon,-sef'-): The cerebellum.

parenchyma (pa-ren'kī-ma): The functional parts of any organ, as opposed to tissue that forms its stroma or framework. — parenchymal, parenchymatous, adj.

parenteral (pa-ren'ter-al): 1. Located or occurring outside of the intestine. 2. Refers to the administration of a substance by some manner other than via the alimentary tract, *e.g.*, delivering nutrition subcutaneously or intravenously. — parenterally, adj.

paresis (pa-rē'sis), (par'e-sis): 1. Slight or partial paralysis. 2. General paralysis, a condition due to neurosyphilis, with late and insidious onset, beginning with headache and fatigability with slowly progressive deterioration, involving personality changes, tremor, speech disturbances, Argyll Robertson pupil (*q.v.*), increasing muscular weakness. Also called *dementia paralytica.*

paretic (pa-ret'ik): 1. Relating to paresis. 2. A person afflicted with paresis.

pareunia (par-ū'ni-a): Sexual intercourse; coitus.

paries (pā'ri-ēz): A wall: by common usage refers to the wall of a hollow organ or cavity. — parietes, pl.; parietal, adj.

parietal (pa-rī'e-tal): Relating to or forming the outer wall of a body cavity. P. BONES the two bones that form the sides and vault of the skull; P. LOBE one of the five lobes of each hemisphere of the cerebrum; lies over the parietal bone; P. PLEURA see under PLEURA.

parietofrontal (pa-rī′e-tō-fron′tal): Relating to the parietal and frontal bones or the part of the cerebral cortex that lies under them.

parietooccipital (pa-rī′e-tō-ok-sip′i-tal): Relating to the parietal and occipital bones or regions.

parity (par′i-ti): Status of a woman with regard to the number of children she has borne. See PARA.

parkinsonian (par-kin-sōn′i-an): 1. Of, like, or referring to Parkinson's disease. 2. A person afflicted with Parkinson's disease. P. MASK a fixed, staring expression with eyebrows raised, infrequent winking, and immobility of facial muscles, the characteristic feature of parkinsonism; P. TREMOR a fine, slowly spreading, rhythmic tremor of three or four per second; most prominent in repose.

parkinsonism: See PARKINSON'S DISEASE and POSTENCEPHALITIC.

Parkinson's disease: Paralysis agitans (shaking palsy); a slowly progressive degenerative disease of the nervous system affecting especially the brain centres that control movement; seen more often in men than in women; cause unknown, but may follow encephalitis, various infections, head trauma, or use of psychotropic drugs. Disturbance in the production of dopamine in the brain results in the characteristic signs and symptoms, including onset in middle age, slowing of spontaneous movements, rigidity, peculiar shuffling gait with short steps, 'pill-rolling' tremor of the hands, mask-like facial expression, diminished blinking, narrowing of the palpebral fissures, slow and monotonous speech, difficulty in swallowing, salivation, weakness, and inability to initiate movements. [James Parkinson, English physician, 1755–1824.]

Parliament (pah′-la-ment): The supreme legislature of the UK, consisting of the three Estates, namely the Lords Spiritual and Temporal (forming together the House of Lords (q.v.)), and the representatives of the counties, cities, boroughs, and universities (forming the House of Commons (q.v.)).

parodynia (par-ō-din′i-a): Abnormal or difficult labour.

paronychia (par-ō-nīk′i-a): Suppurative inflammation around a fingernail. A whitlow (q.v.).

paroophoron (par-ō-off′o-ron): A group of vestigial tubular structures in the broad ligament of the uterus; usually disappear in the adult but may give origin to cysts.

parorexia (par′ō-rek′si-a): Morbid craving for certain foods or for substances that are not fit for food.

parosmia (par-oz′mi-a): Perverted or distorted sense of smell, usually of an hallucinatory nature.

parotic (pa-rot′ik): Situated or occurring near or about the ear.

parotid (pa-rot′id): Situated near the ear. P. GLAND one of the paired salivary glands located interior and anterior to the ears connected to the oral cavity via Stensen's duct that opens into the inside of the cheek opposite the upper second molar tooth.

parotidectomy (pa-rot′-i-dek′tol mi): Excision of the parotid salivary gland.

parotitis (par-ō-tī′tis): Inflammation one or both parotid glands. INFECTIOUS (SPECIFIC) P. mumps (q.v.); SEPTIC P. refers to ascending infection from the mouth via the parotid duct, when a parotid abscess may result. Also spelled *parotiditis*.

parous (par′us): Having borne a child or children.

paroxysm (par′ok-sizm): 1. A sudden, temporary attack or convulsive seizure. 2. A sudden exacerbation or intensification of the symptoms of a disease.

paroxysmal (par-ok-siz′mal): Coming on in attacks or paroxysms. P. DYSPNOEA occurs mostly at night in patients with cardiac disease; P. FIBRILLATION occurs in the atrium of the heart and is associated with a ventricular tachycardia and total irregularity of the pulse rhythm; P. TACHYCARDIA may result from ectopic impulses arising in the atrium or in the ventricle itself; of sudden onset and abrupt ending.

parrot disease or **fever:** Psittacosis (q.v.).

pars: A part or portion. In anatomy, a part of a structure that differs from the main part. P. FLACCIDA MEMBRANAE TYMPANI the small, thin, lax, triangular portion of the upper part of the tympanic membrane; P. TENSA MEMBRANAE TYMPANI the main portion of the tympanic membrane.

Parse, Rosemary (pahz): Founder of the Institute of Human Becoming which teaches the ontological, epistemological, and methodological aspects of the human becoming school of thought.

partial pressure: The pressure of any one gas in a mixture of gases or in a liquid; it relates to the concentration of that gas and to the total pressure of all gases in the liquid.

partial prothrombin time: A test for detecting coagulation defects and the presence of haemophilia.

participant observation (par-tis'-i-pant): A method of research in which an observer gathers information about a group while also belonging to the group under observation (utilized most often in the social sciences).

partograph (part'ō-graf): A graphic device for recording the salient features of labour.

parturient (par-tū'ri-ent): Relating to childbirth.

parturition (par-tū-rish'un): The act of bearing a child; labour.

Pascal's law: States that when pressure is exerted on one part of a fluid in an enclosed space, the increased pressure will be transmitted throughout the whole fluid. Also called *Pascal's principle*. [Blaise Pascal, French mathematician and scientist, 1623–1662.]

Paschen bodies (pash'en): Minute particles once thought to contain the virus of smallpox, found in great numbers in skin exanthemas. [E. Paschen, German bacteriologist, 1860–1936.]

passive (pas'iv): Neither active nor spontaneous. P. CARRIER one who harbours the causative organism of a disease without having the disease; P. IMMUNITY see under IMMUNITY; P. LEARNING incidental learning; learning without intention to learn; P. MOVEMENT or EXERCISE performed by the physiotherapist, the patient being relaxed; P. RANGE OF MOTION the limits of motion through which a joint can be put without use of the muscles that cross the joint; P. SMOKING inhaling cigarette or tobacco smoke produced by someone else.

passivism (pas'i-vizm): Sexual act in which the individual submits to the will of another.

passivity (pas-iv'i-ti): The absence of activity or initiative; submissiveness; inertia. In psychiatry, a state of dependency on others and failure to take the initiative or personal responsibility for making decisions.

Pasteur, Louis: Noted French chemist [1822–1895]; developed the germ theory of disease; discovered a treatment for rabies; and invented the process of pasteurization. With Robert Koch, considered to be a founder of modern bacteriology.

Pasteurella (pas-tur-el'a): A genus of bacteria. Short Gram-negative rods, staining more deeply at the poles (bipolar staining); pathogenic to humans and animals. P. PESTIS an obsolete name for YERSINIA PESTIS, the causative organism of classical plague; P. TULARENSIS an obsolete name for FRANCISELLA TULARENSIS see under FRANCISELLA.

pasteurization (pas'tūr-ī-zā'shun): A process whereby non-sporebearing pathogenic organisms in fluid (especially milk) are killed by heat without affecting the food properties or flavour of the fluid. Flash method of P. (HT, ST — High temperature, short time), the fluid is heated to 72°C, maintained at this temperature for 30 minutes, then rapidly cooled; a useful procedure when the materials to be treated might be altered or damaged by excessive heat.

Pasteur's method or treatment: The method devised by Pasteur for preventing the development of rabies by injecting repeated doses of attenuated virus of the disease, gradually increasing the strength of the virus.

Pastia's sign: Transverse lines of small petechiae on the skin surfaces of the antecubital area; seen in scarlet fever.

pastille (pas'-til): A medicated disc or lozenge intended to be held in the mouth until dissolved; used for local action on mucous membrane of mouth and throat.

Patau's syndrome: Trisomy 13. See TRISOMY.

patch: An area larger than a macule that differs in appearance from the surrounding surface. NICOTINE P. a nicotine-impregnated P. which delivers decreasing doses of nicotine to help overcome withdrawal symptoms on giving up smoking. P. TEST a test for hypersensitiveness to certain foods, pollens, or other substances; a small amount of the suspected substance is applied to an adhesive patch that is placed on the skin along with a plain patch which acts as a control; after about two days the patches are removed and if the skin under the one with the substance on it has reddened, it indicates that the individual is probably sensitive to that substance; PEYER'S PATCHES small oval masses of typhoid tissue found on the mucous membrane of the small intestine.

patella (pa-tel'a): The kneecap; a triangular sesamoid bone. — patellar, adj., patellae, pl.

patellectomy (pat'e-lek'to-mi): Excision of the patella.

patent (pā'tent): Open; apparent; evident; not closed or occluded. P. DUCTUS ARTERIOSUS failure of the ductus arteriosus to close soon after birth, so that the fetal shunt between the pulmonary artery and the aorta is preserved; P. FORAMEN OVALE a congenital heart defect; the oval hole between the left and right atria of the fetal heart fails to close at or soon after birth; P. INTERVENTRICULAR SEPTUM a congenital defect in the dividing wall between the right and left ventricles of the heart.

patent medicine (pat′ent): A medicine that has been patented and protected by a trademark. Can be sold without a prescription; must be labelled as to content and dosage.

paternity (pa-ter′ni-ti): The state of being a father. P. TEST a blood test in which the blood groups of the child, its mother and a certain man are compared to determine whether the man could be the father of the child; it does not always prove paternity.

Paterson–Kelly syndrome: Plummer–Vinson syndrome (*q.v.*).

-path: Combining form denoting: 1. One suffering from a specific ailment. 2. A physician who practises a specific kind of medicine, *e.g.*, a homeopath.

path-, patho-: Combining forms denoting: 1. Pathology; disease. 2. Emotion.

pathogen (path′ō-jen): A disease-producing agent, usually restricted to a living agent, as a microorganism or a virus. — pathogenic, adj. pathogenicity, n.

pathogenesis (path′ō-jen′e-sis): The origin and development of disease. — pathogenetic, adj.

pathogenicity (path′ō-jen-is′i-ti): The capacity to produce disease.

pathognomonic (pa-thog′no-mon′ik): Characteristic of or peculiar to a disease or pathological condition.

pathologist (path-ol′o-jist): A physician who is specially trained in the study of disease by laboratory examination of tissues and other body substances, for changes in structure or function caused by a disease process.

pathology (path-ol′o-ji): The branch of medical science that deals with the cause and nature of disease and the changes in structure and function that result from disease processes. — pathological, adj.; pathologically, adv.

pathomimesis (path′ō-mim-ē′sis): Intentional or unconscious mimicry of disease; malingering. See MÜNCHAUSEN'S SYNDROME.

pathophobia (path-ō-fō′bi-a): A morbid dread of disease.

pathophysiology (path′ō-fiz-i-ol′o-ji): The physiology of disordered function or of functions altered by disease, as distinguished from structural defects. — pathophysiological, adj.

pathopsychology (path-ō-sī-kol′o-ji): The study of causes and processes in the development of mental diseases and disorders.

pathway: In neurology and neurophysiology, usually refers to a structure that carries impulses to or from the central nervous system. MOTOR P. consists of afferent neurons that carry impulses from the brain to nerves that

supply muscles or glands; REFLEX P. bypasses the brain in transmitting impulses between efferent and afferent neurons; SENSORY P. consists of efferent neurons that transmit impulses from the body to the brain via the spinal cord.

-pathy: Suffix denoting: 1. Disease of a specific part. 2. A system of therapy. 3. A feeling, *e.g.*, empathy.

patient (pā′shent): A person who is physically or mentally ill or who is undergoing treatment for physical or mental illness.

Patient Advice and Liaison Service (lē-ā′-zon): A system established in every NHS Trust to provide information and contacts for patients.

patient advocate: A knowledgeable person who counsels a patient in regard to the law and their legal rights and obligations, or to act for the person who is incompetent to make his or her own decisions regarding healthcare.

Patients' Charter: A document issued by the Department of Health as an extension to the Citizens Charter initiative for the National Health Service. The Patient's Charter outlines the patient's rights to care within the National Health Service and also identifies national standards of patient care. Providers of care are required to set local standards. All standards are required to be regularly monitored and achievements or lack of progress reported to health authorities.

patient-controlled analgesia (an-al-jē′-zi-a): A system of pain control managed by the patient; usually refers to self-dosing with intravenous opioid (for example, morphine) administered by means of a programmable pump.

patient-focused care: An approach to care where the assessment, planning, implementation, and evaluation of clinical need is focused on the requirements of the patient rather than those of the health-care professional.

patient information: Authoritative guidelines, tips and resources designed to help users of healthcare to make sound decisions about their care. Increasingly, patients are responsible for making their own decisions about their care and treatment, and such sources of information can be useful.

patient outcome: The final effects of a course of treatment or intervention on a patient or patients.

patient satisfaction: The degree to which the individual regards the health-care service or product, or the manner in which it is delivered by the provider, as useful, effective, or beneficial.

patients' councils: Lobby groups capable of campaigning on behalf of patients across an NHS region and organizing lay (*q.v.*) complaints services.

patients' forums: Bodies set up in each NHS Trust and Primary Care Trust (*q.v.*) to represent the views of patients and users of the services. They have extensive powers to inspect all aspects of health service work.

patient's rights: These fall into three basic rights; the right to know; the right to privacy; the right to treatment. The first two rights are moral rights but not unconditional, and maybe modified by circumstances and/or professional judgement. The third right in the UK is both a legal and moral right.

patriarch (pā'tri-ark): The male head of a family, tribe, or other social organization.

patriarchy (pā'tri-ar-ki): A form of social organization in which the father is the supreme authority in the family or group and descent is traced through the male line with the children belonging to the father's group; or a society based on this type of social organization.

pavor (pā'vor): Dread; terror. P. NOCTURNUS night terrors during sleep.

Pb: Chemical symbol for lead.

PBL: Abbreviation for problem-based learning (*q.v.*).

p.c.: Abbreviation for *post cibum* [L.] meaning after meals.

PCA: Abbreviation for patient-controlled analgesia (*q.v.*).

PCG: Abbreviation for Primary Care Group (*q.v.*).

pCO₂: Chemical formula for partial pressure (*q.v.*) of carbon dioxide. The normal for arterial blood is about 40 mmHg; it is elevated in acidosis.

PCR: Abbreviation for practitioner-centred research (*q.v.*).

PCT: Abbreviation for Primary Care Trust (*q.v.*).

PD: Abbreviation for personality disorder (*q.v.*).

Peach Report: See FITNESS FOR PRACTICE.

peak flow meter: An instrument used to determine how rapidly a person who has had or is recovering from a respiratory disorder can expel air from the lungs.

peccant (pek'ant): Unhealthy; causing disease.

pecten (pek'ten): 1. Any body structure with comblike projections or processes. 2. The middle third of the anal canal.

pectin (pek'tin): A gelatinous substance found in fruits; used in preparing jams, jellies, and similar foods. In medicine, used as a plasma

expander and, in conjunction with other agents, to control diarrhoea.

pectinate line (pek'tin-āt): A sinuous or jagged line at the level of the anal valves that marks the junction of columnar epithelium and stratified epithelium that line the anal canal.

pectineus (pek-tin'ē-us): An anterior muscle of the femur; it acts to flex and adduct the thigh and to rotate it medially.

pectoral (pek'tor-al): Relating to the breast or chest.

pectoralgia (pek'to-ral'ji-a): Pain in the chest or breast.

pectoralis (pek-to-ra'lis): 1. Relating to the breast or chest. 2. Any one of the four muscles of the chest. P. MAJOR the large, fan-shaped muscle that covers the upper anterior chest; P. MINOR the thin, triangular muscle underlying the P. major.

pectoriloquy (pek-tō ril'ō kwi): The transmission of voice sound through the chest wall; can be heard on auscultation; indicates the presence of a large cavity in the chest or, when combined with bronchophony, consolidation of the lung. WHISPERED OR WHISPERING P. the transmission of whispered sounds through the chest wall.

pectus (pek'tus): The chest. P. CARINATUM pigeon chest; P. EXCAVATUM funnel breast.

ped-, pedi-, pedio-, pedo-: Combining forms denoting 1. The foot; or having foot-like projections. 2. Child; children.

pedal (ped'al): Relating to the foot.

pedatrophia (ped-a-trō'fi-a): Marasmus (*q.v.*); any wasting condition in children.

pederasty (ped'er-as-ti): Homosexual anal intercourse between men and boys.

pederosis (ped-er-ō'sis): A sexual interest in children; sexual abuse of children by adults.

pedicellate (ped'-is-e-lāt): Resembling a pedicle; pedunculated. See PEDUNCLE.

pedicle (ped'ik'l): 1. A stalk, *e.g.*, the narrow part by which a tumour is attached to the surrounding structures. 2. The two processes that extend backward from the body of a vertebra and connect the laminae with the body of the vertebra.

pedicterus (pē-dik'ter-us): Jaundice of the newborn; icterus neonatorum.

pediculicide (pē-dik'ū-li-sīd): An agent that destroys lice (pediculi).

pediculosis (pē-dik'ū-lō'sis): Infestation with lice (pediculi).

pediculous (pē-dik'ū-lus): Infested with pediculi; lousy.

Pediculus (pē-dik'ū-lus): A genus of wingless, blood-sucking insects (lice), important vectors of disease. P. CAPITIS the head louse; P.

CORPORIS the body louse; P. PUBIS (more correctly, PHTHIRUS) the pubic louse; also called the *crab louse*. — pediculi, pl.

pedogamy (ped-og'a-mi): Fertilization by the union of two cells with the same chromatin inheritance; inbreeding. Also called *endogamy*.

pedograph (ped'ō-graf): 1. An imprint of the weight-bearing surface of the foot. 2. A device for taking footprints.

pedojet (ped-ō-jet'): Apparatus for introducing vaccine under pressure into the skin. Avoids use of the needle with consequent danger of spreading serum hepatitis.

peduncle (pē-dun'kl): 1. A stalk-like narrow structure that serves as a support. 2. Any of several structures consisting of bands of nerve fibres that connect various parts of the central nervous system.

pedunculated (pē-dunk'ū-lāt-ed): Having a peduncle or stem. Opp. of sessile.

pedunculus (pē-dun'kū-lus): Peduncle (*q.v.*).

peeling: Desquamation (*q.v.*).

PEEP: Abbreviation for positive end expiratory pressure (*q.v.*).

peer review: In nursing, nurses of equal status review nursing care given by each other; accepted standards of care are used as the measuring tool.

pejorative (pe-jor'a-tiv): Changing for the worse; unfavourable.

Pel–Ebstein's fever: Recurring bouts of pyrexia in regular sequence found in lymphadenoma (Hodgkin's disease). [Pieter Klazes Pel, Dutch physician, 1852–1919. Wilhelm Ebstein, German physician. 1836–1912.]

pellagra (pel-ag'ra): A deficiency disease caused by lack of vitamin B complex (nicotinic acid) and protein. Syndrome includes glossitis, dermatitis, peripheral neuritis and spinal cord changes (even producing ataxia), anaemia and mental confusion.

Pellegrini–Stieda's disease (pel-leg-rē'-miste'-daz): A condition characterized by the formation of a semilunar bony deposit in the upper part of the medial lateral knee ligament; due to trauma; results in limitation of flexion.

pellet (pel'et): A small pill; may contain medication and be taken by mouth, or may contain pure steroid hormones and be implanted under the skin from which location it is slowly absorbed by the body.

pellicle (pel'i-kl): 1. A thin skin or membrane. 2. A film on the surface of a liquid.

pelmatogram (pel-mat'o-gram): A footprint; an imprint of the sole of the foot made by pressing the inked sole on a piece of paper.

pelotherapy (pē'lō-ther'a-pi): The use of mud in the treatment of disease.

pelvic (pel'vik): Relating to the pelvis. P. CAVITY the cavity within the bony pelvis; see PELVIS; P. ENDOSCOPY LAPAROSCOPY (*q.v.*); P. EXAMINATION see under EXAMINATION; P. EXENTERATION see under EXENTERATION; P. FLOOR muscular lower part of the pelvis; includes the levator ani and coccygeus muscles, and fascia; P. F. EXERCISE an exercise regimen for tightening certain perineal muscles to improve the ability to retain urine; it utilizes the squeezing action of stop-and-go voiding of urine, also called *Kegel's exercise*; P. GIRDLE the bony framework of the pelvis; consists of two innominate bones and the sacrum; P. INFLAMMATORY DISEASE inflammation of the internal female genital tract, caused by any of several microorganisms, including the *Neisseria gonorrhoeae*; marked by abdominal pain, fever, and tenderness in the uterine cervix; P. ROLL an exercise involving motion of the pelvis around its transverse axis; P. SLING a sling that encloses the hips and is suspended from an overhead bar; used in treatment of pelvic injuries; P. TILT an exercise in which the patient lies flat on the back with the knees flexed and feet on the bed, and then contracts the abdominal and gluteal muscles firmly, thus flattening the lumbar back.

pelvimeter (pel-vim'e-ter): An instrument specially designed to measure the pelvic diameters.

pelvimetry (pel-vim'e-tri): The measurement of the dimensions of the pelvis by means of a pelvimeter. Four measurements are taken; the distances between (1) the anterior superior spines of the ilia; (2) between the crests of the ilia; (3) between the greater trochanters of the femurs; (4) between the spinous process of the 5th lumbar vertebra and the anterior surface of the symphysis pubis.

pelvis (pel'vis): 1. A basin-shaped cavity, *e.g.*, pelvis of the kidney. 2. The large bony basin-shaped cavity formed by the innominate bones and sacrum, containing and protecting the bladder, rectum, and reproductive organs. ANDROID P. a male type P. with heavy bones and a heart-shaped brim; the cavity has a poor curve and the outlet has less space than the normal female pelvis, thus presenting difficulties in delivery; ANTHROPOID P. a female type pelvis characterized by an anterior–posterior diameter at the outlet that is as great or greater than the transverse diameter; most often seen in tall, long-legged women; CONTRACTED P. one in which one or more diameters are smaller than normal and this may result in difficulties in childbirth; FALSE P. the wide expanded part of the pelvis above the brim; GYNAECOID P. the normal female pelvis; rounded oval shape with rounded brim, and a well-rounded anterior and posterior segment; PLATYPELLOID P. has a short anterior–posterior diameter, lengthened transverse diameter, and a capacious outlet; seen as a sequela of rickets; TRUE P. that part of the pelvis that lies below the pelvic brim.

pen-, pent-, penta-: Combining forms denoting (1) five; (2) containing five atoms.

pendular (pen'dū-lar): 1. The movement of a pendulum. 2. Resembling a swinging pendulum.

pendulous (pen'dū-lus): Hanging down.

-penia: A combining form used in a suffix to denote deficiency.

penicillin (pen-i-sil'in): The first antibiotic; derived from cultures of certain moulds of the genus *Penicillium*; it is the parent substance of a large group widely used in treating diseases caused by most Gram-positive and some Gram-negative bacteria, some cocci and some spirochetes. Administered orally, topically, and intravenously.

penicillinase (pen-i-sil'in-āse): An enzyme produced in several strains of staphylococci that are resistant to penicillin; it inactivates penicillin and thus promotes resistance to it.

Penicillium (pen-i-sil'i-um): A genus of fungi comprising the blue moulds, the hyphae of which bear spores characteristically arranged like a brush. Common contaminant of food. Found chiefly on decaying non-living organic matter such as fruit. P. *CHRYSOGENUM* is now used for the commercial production of penicillin, along with P. *notatum*.

penile (pē'nīl): Relating to or affecting the penis. P. PROSTHESIS an inflatable device inserted into the penis; consists of a pump and a reservoir; used in cases of impotence.

penis (pē'nis): The male organ of copulation; in mammals a penis is also the organ of urination. P. ENVY in psychoanalytic theory, the desire of a female child to possess a penis. — penile, adj.

penitis (pē-nī'tis): Inflammation of the penis. Also called *phallitis, priapitis.*

pennate (pen'āt): Shaped like a feather or looking like a feather. Penniform.

Penrose drain: Also cigarette drain, consisting of a piece of rubber tubing containing a length of absorbent gauze. [Charles B. Penrose, American gynaecologist, 1862–1925.]

pentagastrin (pen-ta-gas'trin): A synthetic pentapeptide, see PEPTIDE, which has the same amino acids as the human gastrin; used thera-peutically to stimulate production of hydrochloric acid in the stomach.

pentose (pen'tōs): A class of monosaccharides with five carbon atoms in the molecule; abundant in some fruits.

pentosuria (pen-tō-sū'ri-a): The occurrence of one or more pentoses in the urine. The alimentary type is temporary and due to ingestation of large amounts of certain foods, *e.g.*, plums, cherries, or grapes. May be caused by a hereditary error of metabolism; Not significant except that it may be mistaken for diabetes.

peotomy (pe-ot'o-mi): Surgical amputation of the penis.

Peplau, Hildegard (pep' low, hil'-de-gard): A nurse who pioneered the development of the theory and practice of psychiatric and mental health nursing. Her ideas, including her notable work in patient–nurse relationships, have been incorporated into virtually every nursing speciality and into the practices of other health-care professionals.

pepsin (pep'sin): A proteolytic enzyme of the gastric juice; converts the native proteins of foods into proteoses and peptones. Along with dilute hydrochloric acid, it is the chief active ingredient of gastric juice.

pepsinogen (pep-sin'ō-jen): A pre-enzyme secreted by the peptic cells in the gastric mucosa and converted into pepsin by contact with hydrochloric acid.

peptase (pep'tās): An enzyme that splits peptides into amino acid.

peptic (pep'tik): Relating to the stomach, to pepsin or to digestion generally. P. ULCER a non-malignant ulcer in those parts of the digestive tract that are exposed to the gastric secretions; hence it usually occurs in the stomach or duodenum.

peptide (pep'tīd): A chemical combination of two or more amino acids; *e.g.*, dipeptide, tripeptide, polypeptide.

Peptococcus (pep'tō-kok'us): A genus of bacteria of the family Peptococcaceae; an anaerobic, spherical, Gram-positive organism; some species are found in the upper respiratory, gastrointestinal, and urinary tracts as non-pathogenic parasites.

peptone (pep'tōn): Substance produced when the enzyme pepsin acts upon the acid metaproteins produced in the first stage of digestion of proteins.

peptonuria (pep-tō-nū'ri-a): The excretion of peptones in the urine.

Peptostreptococcus (pep'tō-strep-tō-kok'us): One of a large group of anaerobic microorganisms of the tribe Streptococceae that occur in the intestinal tract of humans and as secondary invaders in necrotic and gangrenous wounds.

per-: Prefix denoting (1) by means of; through; (2) completely, throughout, extremely. In chemistry, it denotes the highest member of a series.

peracidity (per-a-sid′i-ti): Excessive acidity.

peracute (per-a-kūt′): Extremely acute.

per anum (per ā′num): By way of or through the anus.

percentile (per-sen′tīl): A point on a frequency scale above and below which a certain percentage of observations fall.

percept (per′sept): 1. An object perceived; the impression of an object obtained through the senses. 2. The mental product of a sensation; a sensation plus memories of similar sensations and their relationships.

perception (per-sep′shun): The reception of a conscious impression through the senses by which we distinguish objects one from another and recognize their qualities according to the different sensations they produce. Intelligent discernment; insight. — perceptual, adj.

perceptive hearing loss: Sensorineural (*q.v.*) type of hearing loss.

percolation (per′kō-lā″shun): The process by which fluid slowly passes through a hard but porous substance.

percussible (per-kus′i-b′l): Detectable on percussion.

percussion (per-kush′un): 1. A diagnostic procedure consisting of tapping or striking the surface of the body to produce sounds that reflect the size, position, and density of the underlying organs and tissues in order to determine the condition of these organs or tissues. Normally a finger of the left hand is laid on the patient's skin and the middle finger of the right hand is used to strike the left finger. Useful in detecting consolidation, fluid, or pus in a cavity, change in the size of an organ, etc; used especially over the chest and abdomen. 2. A movement in massage consisting of taps of varying force. 3. Striking the hand on the chest wall to produce vibration that loosens secretions retained in the lung. P. HAMMER see under HAMMER. — percuss, v.

percussor (per-kus′er): An instrument used in percussion, usually a hammer with a rubber or metal head.

percutaneous (per′kū-tā′nē-us): Through unbroken skin, as by absorption of substances applied by inunction. Also denotes procedures that are performed by needle puncture, *e.g.*,

intravenous injection or intraarterial catheterization.

perflation (per-flā′shun): The blowing of air into a cavity or canal to force its walls apart or to force out any secretions or other substances.

perforate (per′fō-rāt): To pierce through. May be applied to the fibres of a tendon, ligament, or muscle or to a nerve or blood vessel.

perforating ulcer: One that erodes through the wall of an organ such as the stomach or intestine; a serious development requiring immediate surgery.

perforation (per-fo-rā′shun): A hole in an intact sheet of tissue, or the act of making such a hole; may be pathogenic or intentional. Used especially in reference to the tympanic membrane or the wall of the stomach or intestine.

perforator (per′fō-rāt-er): 1. An instrument used to perforate a body tissue or structure. 2. A nerve, blood vessel, or tissue fibre that perforates a tissue or body structure.

performance assessment framework: Guidelines against which all NHS organizations are assessed, leading to a star rating. The main areas covered are health improvement; fair access to services; effective and appropriate delivery of healthcare; outcome from healthcare; efficient use of resources; high-quality experience for patients and carers.

performance criteria (krī-tē′-ri-a): Written descriptions of activities that an individual is expected to be able to perform. These will be used by an assessor to judge whether the individual has attained a certain level.

performance indicators: Statistical information based upon quantitative data related to patient-based activities and the use of resources available in the NHS, prepared by Health Authorities for the Department of Health. The information allows for the evaluation of performance from one Health Authority to another.

perfusate (per′fūz-āt): The fluid that is introduced during perfusion (*q.v.*).

perfuse (per-fūz′): To spread or pour over or through.

perfusion (per-fū′zhun): 1. The act of spreading or pouring over or through, specifically the artificial passage of fluid through an organ or tissue by way of the blood vessels. 2. The process whereby oxygen is carried from the lungs to body tissues and carbon dioxide is carried from tissues to the lungs.

peri-: Prefix denoting (1) all around, about; (2) near; (3) enclosing, surrounding.

periadenitis (per-i-ad-en-ī′tis): Inflammation in soft tissues surrounding a gland or glands.

perianal (per-i-ān'al): Around or surrounding the anus.

periapical (per-i-ap'i-kal): Relating to the tissues that enclose the apex of the tooth. P. ABSCESS one that forms at or near the apex of a tooth.

periarterial (per'i-ar-tē'ri-al): Around or surrounding an artery.

periarteriolar (per'i-ar-tē-ri-ō'lar): Around an arteriole.

periarteritis (per-i-ar-tē'rī'tis): Inflammation of the outer sheath of an artery and the periarterial tissue. P. NODOSA a widespread disease of the arteries; frequently produces renal damage and hypertension; see COLLAGEN, POLYARTERITIS.

periarthritis (per-i-ar-thrī'tis): Inflammation of the structures surrounding a joint. Sometimes applied to frozen shoulder (q.v.).

periarticular (per'i-ar-tik'ū-lar): Around or surrounding a joint. P. FIBROSITIS an inflammation of the fibrous tissues around a joint; P. OSSIFICATION deposits of calcium around a joint.

periauricular (per'i-aw-rik'ūlar): Around the external ear.

periblepsis (per-i-blep'sis): The characteristic staring expression of a mentally disturbed person.

peribronchial (per-i-bron'ki-al): Surrounding or occurring about a bronchus.

pericardectomy (per-i-kard-ek-to-mi): Surgical removal of a portion of the pericardium which has thickened from chronic inflammation and is embarrassing the heart's action. Also called *pericardiectomy*.

pericardial (per-i-kar'di-al): Relating to or affecting the pericardium. P. EFFUSION see under EFFUSION; P. FRICTION RUB see under RUB; P. TAMPONADE see under TAMPONADE.

pericardiocentesis (per-i-kar'-di-ō-sen-tē'sis): The withdrawal of fluid from the pericardial sac by insertion of a hollow needle or cannula.

pericarditis (per-i-kar-dī'tis): An acute or chronic inflammation of the outer, serous covering of the heart; caused by many agents; it may or may not be accompanied by an effusion and formation of adhesions between the two layers. ACUTE IDIOPATHIC P. causes interference with the filling of the ventricles which results in dyspnoea, ascites, fatigue, hepatomegaly, pain, peripheral oedema; ACUTE FIBRINOUS P. marked by a fibrinous exudate; ADHESIVE P., P. characterized by adhesions that form between the two layers of pericardium; CONSTRICTIVE P. thickening, fibrosis, and sometimes calcification of the pericardium and constriction of the heart chambers; may follow inflammation or tuberculosis; DRY P. inflam-

mation and roughening of the pericardium without formation of effusion, interferes with cardiac functioning; P. CALCULOSA, P. marked by deposits of calcium in the pericardium; P. OBLITERANS P. marked by adhesions between the two layers of pericardium and obliteration of the pericardial cavity; PYOGENIC P. inflammation of the pericardium by pyogenic bacteria such as staphylococcus, or by septicaemia or pneumonia; RHEUMATIC P. inflammation of the pericardium associated with rheumatic fever; TUBERCULAR P., P. caused by *Mycobacterium tuberculosis*; URAEMIC P. occurs in patients with renal failure and high blood urea levels. See also PERICARDECTOMY.

pericardium (per-i-kard'i-um): The double fibroserous membranous sac which envelops the heart. The layer in contact with the heart is called visceral; that reflected to form the sac is called parietal. Between the two is the pericardial cavity, which normally contains a small amount of serous fluid. — pericardial, adj.

pericholangitis (per-i-kō-lan-jī'tis): Inflammation of the tissues around the bile ducts.

pericholycystitis (per-i-kol-ē sis tī'tis). Cholecystitis extending to the tissues around the gall bladder.

perichondrial (per'i-kon'dri-al): Composed of or pertaining to the perichondrium.

perichondritis (per-i-kon-drī'tis): Inflammation of the perichondrium.

perichondrium (per-i-kond'ri-um): The membranous covering of cartilage. — perichondrial, adj.

pericolic (per'i-kō'lik): Around the colon.

pericolitis (per'i-ko-lī'tis): Inflammation of the tissues around the colon, especially of the peritoneal coat.

pericolpitis (per-i-kol-pī'tis): Inflammation of the tissues around the vagina.

pericoronitis (per-i-kor-o-nī'tis): Pain and inflammation around the crown of a tooth, especially around an erupting third molar (wisdom tooth).

pericranium (per'i-krān'i-um): The periosteal covering of the cranium. — pericranial, adj.

pericystitis (per-i-sis-tī'tis): Inflammation of the tissues around the urinary bladder.

pericyte (per'i-sīt): One of the peculiarly shaped elongated cells found outside the basement membrane of capillaries, usually having the power of contraction.

peridontoclasia (per'i-don-tō-klā'zi-a): 1. The loosening of one or more permanent teeth. 2. Any destructive disease of the periodontium.

peridural (per-i-dū'ral): Around or external to the dura mater.

perifollicular (per-i-fol-ik′ū-lar): Around a follicle.

perifolliculitis (per′i-fol-ik-ū-lī′tis): Inflammation around the root of a hair follicle.

perihepatic (per-i-he-pat′ik): Situated or occurring around or near the liver.

perihilar (per-i-hī′lar): Around a hilus (*q.v.*).

perikaryon (per-i-kar′i-on): The protoplasmic part of the cell body, exclusive of the nucleus and processes.

perilymph (per′i-limf): The fluid contained in the internal ear, between the bony and membranous labyrinth.

perimeter (pe-rim′i-ter): 1. An outer border or edge. 2. A device used to determine the characteristics and extent of one's visual field.

perimetritis (per′i-mē-trī′tis): Inflammation of the perimetrium (*q.v.*).

perimetrium (per′i-mē′tri-um): The peritoneal (serous) covering of the uterus. — perimetrial, adj.

perimetry (per-im′i-tri): The determination of the extent of an individual's peripheral visual field.

perimyocarditis (per-i-mī′-ō-kar-dī′tis): A condition in which the patient has symptoms of both pericarditis and myocarditis.

perimysium (per-i-mis′i-um): The delicate connective tissue sheath that envelops and separates the bundles of voluntary muscle fibres.

perinatal (per-i-nā′tal): Occurring at, or relating to, the time of birth. P. PERIOD considered to be the period between the 28th week of gestation, the birth, and between one to four weeks after delivery.

perinate (per′i-nāt): An infant in the perinatal (*q.v.*) period.

perineal (per-i-nē′al): Relating to or involving the perineum. P. BODY a wedge-shaped mass of tissue that lies between the anal canal and vagina in the female and between the anal canal and the corpus spongiosum of the penis in the male.

perineometer (per′i-nē-om′i-ter): An instrument for measuring the strength of the perivaginal muscles.

perineoplasty (per-i-nē′-ō-plas-ti): Reparative or plastic surgery of the perineum.

perineorrhaphy (per-i-nēor′a-fi): The operation for the repair of a torn perineum. Perineoplasty.

perineotomy (per-i-nē-ot′o-mi): A surgical incision into the perineum. See also EPISIOTOMY.

perinephric (per′i-nef′rik): Around or surrounding the kidney.

perinephritis (per′-i-nef-rī′tis): Inflammation of the peritoneal covering of the kidney and of the surrounding tissues. — perinephritic, adj.

perineum (per-i-nē′um): The area that lies between the vulva and the anus in the female and between the scrotum and the anus in the male. Often referred to as the *pelvic floor*, see under PELVIC. — perineal, adj.

perineurium (per-i-nū′ri-um): The connective tissue sheath that surrounds the separate bundles of fibres of peripheral nerves.

period: An interval or extent of time. GESTATION P. the period of pregnancy; in the human it is approximately 270 days; INCUBATION P. the time between the entrance of a pathogenic organism into the body and appearance of first symptoms of disease. MENSTRUAL P. menses (*q.v.*).

periodic table: A table in which the elements are arranged according to their atomic numbers.

periodontal (per′i-ō-don′tal): Refers to the area surrounding a tooth or teeth. P. DISEASE a chronic inflammatory condition that attacks the supporting structures of the teeth, including the ligaments, and destroys the bone.

periodontitis (per′i-ō-don-tī′tis): Inflammation of the tissues surrounding a tooth; may be due to gingivitis, faulty dental restoration, oral sepsis, malnutrition, diabetes, scurvy, or pellagra; when untreated usually leads to loss of the tooth.

periodontium (per′i-ō-don′shi-um): The tissues surrounding and supporting the teeth, including the cementum, bone, and gingivae; strictly speaking, the tissue between the teeth and their bony sockets.

periodontologist (per′i-ō-don-tol′o-jist): A dentist who practises in the field of periodontology.

periodontology (per′i-ō-don-tol′o-ji): The study of the tissues that surround and support the teeth, *i.e.*, the periodontium.

periomphalic (per′i-om-fal′ik): Around the umbilicus.

perionychia (per′i-ō-nik′i-a): Inflammation around a nail.

perioral (pe-ri-or′al): Around or surrounding the mouth.

periorbital (per-i-or′bit-al): 1. The periosteum within the orbit of the eye. 2. Situated around or near the eye socket.

periosteal (per-i-os′teal): Relating to the periosteum.

periosteitis (per-i-os-tē-ī′tis): Periostitis (*q.v.*).

periosteoma (per′i-os-tē-ō′ma): A neoplasm on the surface of a bone.

periosteomyelitis (per-i-os′-tē-ō-mī-e-lī′tis): Inflammation of the bone including the marrow and the periosteum.

periosteum (per'i-os'tē-um): The thick, fibrous membrane that covers bones except at their articulations; it is protective and essential for regeneration of bone. Consists of two layers, the inner one being concerned with formation of bone tissue and the outer one serving to convey nerves and blood vessels to the bone. — periosteal, adj.

periostitis (per'i-os-tī'tis): Inflammation of the periosteum. P. DIFFUSE that involving the periosteum of long bones; P. HAEMORRHAGIC that accompanied by bleeding between the periosteum and the bone.

periotic (per'i-ō'tik): Around the internal ear.

peripartum (per'i-par'tum): Relating to or occurring at or near the time of parturition.

peripatetic (per'i-pa-tet'ik): Walking around.

peripheral (per-if'er-al): Relating to the periphery (q.v.); situated away from the centre of a structure. P. LESION one in the periphery of the body, a peripheral nerve in particular; P. NERVE any of the nerves in the peripheral nervous system; P. NEUROPATHY pathology affecting any part of the peripheral nervous system; P. RESISTANCE opposition to the flow of blood through the small vessels and capillaries; P. VASCULAR DISEASE refers broadly to pathology of the blood vessels outside the heart, specifically to atherosclerosis affecting the legs, causing insufficient supply of blood to the feet; characterized by numbness, tingling, and cramplike pain in calf muscles; may lead to gangrene; see INTERMITTENT CLAUDICATION under CLAUDICATION; P. VISION vision in that area of the retina which is outside the macula lutea; less distinct than central vision but important to functioning in and adapting to the environment.

peripheral circulatory assist: A device for preventing decubiti; consists of an electrically monitored pad that creates pressure differentials in selected areas by introducing air into tubes in the pad.

periphery (per-if'er-i): The outward part or surface of the body; the parts away from the centre or midline.

periportal (per-i-por'tal): Surrounding the portal vein and its branches.

periproctitis (per'i-prok-tī'tis): Inflammation of the tissues around the rectum and anus.

perirectal (per'i-rek'tal): Around the rectum.

perirenal (per'i-rē'nal): Around the kidney.

perisalpingitis (per'-i-sal-pin-jī'tis): Inflammation of the peritoneum and tissues around the uterine tubes.

perisinusitis (per'i-sī-nū-sī'tis): Inflammation of the tissues around a sinus; often refers to a sinus of the dura mater.

perisplenitis (per-i-sple-nī'-tis): Inflammation of the peritoneal coat of the spleen and of the adjacent structures.

perispondylitis (per'-i-spon-di-lī'tis): Inflammation of tissues around a vertebra.

peristalsis (per'i-stal'sis): The characteristic movements of the intestine consisting of a wave of contraction preceded by a wave of relaxation; begins with swallowing and continues throughout the digestive tube until the contents are moved forward into the rectum. MASS P. strong peristaltic waves occurring several times a day in the large intestine and which move the contents from one division of the intestine to the next; REVERSED P., P. in which the wave is in a direction opposite to normal and the contents of the lumen are forced backward; may occur in malrotation of the bowel, duodenal ulcer or stenosis, gastrointestinal allergy, urinary tract infections, — peristaltic, adj.

peritectomy (per'i-tek'to-mi): Excision of a strip of conjunctiva at the edge of the cornea, a surgical treatment for pannus (q.v.).

peritendinitis (per'-i-ten-di-nī'tis): Inflammation of the sheath enclosing a tendon.

peritomy (per-it'o-mi): 1. Surgical incision of the conjunctiva around the entire circumference of the cornea; peritectomy. 2. Circumcision.

peritoneal (per'i-tō-nē'al): Referring or relating to the peritoneum. P. CAVITY the potential space between the parietal and visceral layer of the peritoneum; P. DIALYSIS the separating of particles from the blood by using the peritoneum as a semipermeable membrane through which a fluid is repeatedly introduced into and removed from the peritoneal cavity.

peritoneocentesis (per'i-tō-nē'ō-sen-tē'sis): Paracentesis of the abdominal cavity. Abdominocentesis.

peritoneoscopy (per'i-tō-nē-os'ko-pi): Inspection of the peritoneal cavity by means of an electrically lighted, tubular optical instrument (peritoneoscope) introduced through the abdominal wall. — peritoneoscopic, adj.; peritoneoscopically, adv.

peritoneum (per'i-tō-nē'um): The delicate, smooth, transparent, serous membrane that lines the abdominal and pelvic cavities and is reflected over the organs contained in them, thus forming a sac. PARIETAL P. the layer of P. that lines the abdominal walls; VISCERAL P. the layer of P. that invests the abdominal organs.

peritonitis (per'i-tōn-ī'tis): Inflammation of the peritoneum, usually secondary to disease of one of the abdominal organs.

peritonsillar (per'i-ton'si-lar): Around the tonsil or tonsils. P. ABSCESS caused by a streptococcal organism, characterized by pain, fever, malaise, and bulging of the tonsillar fauces; mediastinitis is a possible complication; see QUINSY.

perityphlitis (per'i-tif-lī'tis): Inflammation of the peritoneum around the caecum and the appendix; appendicitis.

periumbilical (per'i-um-bil'ik-al): Around or surrounding the umbilicus.

periungual (per'i-un'gwal): Around a finger or toenail.

periurethral (per'i-ū-rē'thral): Surrounding the urethra, as a P. abscess.

periuterine (per'i-ū'ter-in): Around the uterus.

perivascular (per'i-vas'kū-lar): Around a blood vessel.

perle (purl): A very small, thin glass ampoule containing one dose of a volatile drug; it is to be crushed in a handkerchief or sponge and the contents inhaled.

perlèche (per-lesh'): An inflammation at the angles of the mouth, sometimes with maceration, fissuring, or crust formation; causes lip licking and results in thickening and desquamation of the skin. Occurs mostly in malnourished children as a result of vitamin deficiency, thrush, bacterial infection, drooling or thumbsucking. In adults may result from poorly fitted dentures or from overclosure of the mouth in edentulous persons.

permeability (per'mē-a-bil'it-i): In physiology, the ability of cell membranes to allow salts, glucose, urea and other soluble substances to pass into and out of the cells from the body fluids.

permeable (per-mē-a-b'l): Capable of being traversed; pervious.

permissiveness (per-mis'siv-nes): The habitual or characteristic allowance or tolerance of behaviour that others might disapprove or forbid.

permit (per'mit, per-mit'): 1. Permission. 2. To allow.

pernicious (per-nish'us): Deadly, noxious, destructive. In medicine, usually denotes a disease of severe character and tending to a fatal outcome. P. ANAEMIA see ANAEMIA; P. VOMITING see VOMITING.

pernio (per'ni-ō): Chilblain. Congestion of the skin due to exposure to cold; may cause swelling, itching, burning, or even ulceration of the skin.

perniosis (per-ni-ō'sis): Chronic chilblains. The smaller arterioles go into spasm readily from exposure to cold.

pero-: Combining form denoting deformed.

peromelia (per-ō-mē'li-a): Severe congenital deformity of the limbs, including absence of hand or foot.

perone (per-ō'ne): Fibula. — peroneal, adj.

peroneal (per-ō-nē'al): Relating to the fibula or to the outer side of the leg, or to the muscles or tissues on the outer side of the leg. P. MUSCULAR ATROPHY a chronic familial condition characterized by wasting of the muscles of the foot and lower leg, with footdrop; also called *Charcot–Marie–Tooth disease*; P. NERVE a branch of the sciatic nerve; innervates the front of the leg and foot.

peroneotibial (per'o-nē'-ō-tib'i-al): Pertaining to both the fibula and the tibia.

peroral (per-ō'ral): By or through the mouth.

per os: (per ōs): By or through the mouth.

peroxide: See HYDROGEN PEROXIDE under HYDROGEN.

perseveration (per-sev-er-ā'shun): The continuation of an activity after the causative stimulus has been removed, or of a response that is no longer correct. In psychiatry, a mental symptom consisting of an apparent inability of the patient's mind to detach itself from one idea to another with normal speed. Thus, shown a picture of a cow, the patient repeats 'cow' when shown further pictures of different objects. Common in senile dementia and schizophrenia.

persona (per-sō'na): In psychiatry, the mask or assumed personality that a person presents to the outside world as opposed to the anima (*q.v.*) which is his or her inner personality or true character.

personality (per'son-al'i-ti): The total complex of individual mental attitudes, characteristics, and ways of behaving and reacting to the environment that distinguish a person. P. is sometimes classified as Type A, which includes competitive impatient persons with excessive drive; believed to be associated with high incidence of coronary disease; and Type B, which describes persons who are relaxed, easy-going and less competitive than those in Type A.

personality disorder: A set of traits that combine to negatively affect an individual's life. There are a number of such traits, including paranoid, schizoid, anti-social, borderline, histrionic, narcissistic, avoidant, dependent and obsessive–compulsive, which are further defined in DSM IV (*q.v.*).

personal professional profile: A system used by practitioners to keep a record of their own personal and professional development, in order to comply with Post-Registration Education and Practice requirements, see APPENDIX 8.

personhood (per'-son-hood): The quality or condition of being an individual person.

person specification (spes-i-fi-kā'-shun): Relating to a particular job, the list of characteristics ideally preferred to carry out that role or responsibility.

perspiration (per-spi-rā'shun): 1. The excretion of sweat through the skin pores. INSENSIBLE P. invisible P.; the P. evaporates immediately upon reaching the skin surface; SENSIBLE P. visible drops of sweat on the skin. 2. Sweat, the fluid secreted by the sweat glands.

perspire (per-spīr'): To sweat.

Perthes' disease: Syn., *Legg–Perthes–Calve's disease, pseudocoxalgia.* A vascular degeneration of the upper femoral epiphysis; revascularization occurs, but residual deformity of the femoral head may subsequently lead to arthritic changes. Occurs chiefly in male adolescents. [Georg Clemens Perthes, German surgeon, 1869–1927.]

Perthes' test: A test to determine whether the collateral circulation in the deep veins of the leg is adequate when the individual has varicose veins. A tourniquet or tight bandage is applied just below the knee and the person walks around with it on for a set period of time; when the bandage is removed the varicose veins will have been cleared if the collateral circulation is adequate.

pertussis (per-tus'is): Whooping cough. A highly communicable infectious disease of children with paroxsyms of coughing that reach a peak of violence ending in a long-drawn inspiration that produces a characteristic 'whoop'. The organism responsible is *Bordetella pertussis*. Prophylactic vaccination is responsible for the decrease in case incidence.

pertussoid (per-tus'soid): Resembling whooping cough or a cough resembling that of whooping cough.

Peruvian: P. BARK the dried bark of a South American tree of the *Cinchona* genus; discovered in the 17th century to be therapeutic for malaria and used widely throughout the world. Also called *Jesuits' bark, Jesuits' powder.*

perversion (per-ver'shun): A turning away from what is normal or right. In medicine, a pathological alteration of function. SEXUAL P. indulgence in what is traditionally regarded as unnatural sexual practices.

pervert: 1. (per-vert') To turn aside, or cause to be turned aside from what is considered right or normal; to lead astray. 2. (per'vert) A person who has turned aside from what is considered proper and normal behaviour; applied especially to one who exhibits sexual behaviour traditionally regarded as unnatural.

pes: A foot or foot-like structure. P. CAVUS 'hollow' foot, when the longitudinal arch of the foot is accented; clawfoot; P. PLANUS or P. PLANOVALGUS flatfoot, when the longitudinal arch of the foot is lowered.

pessary (pes'a-ri): 1. An article inserted into the vagina to support the uterus or to correct uterine displacements. 2. A medicated suppository used to treat vaginal infections or as a contraceptive.

pest: 1. An epidemic disease usually associated with high mortality, specifically the plague. 2. A destructive or annoying plant or animal.

pesticide (pes'ti-sīd): A poisonous agent used to destroy a pest, e.g., insect, rodent, fungus.

pestilence (pes'ti-lens): 1. A virulent, communicable, devastating disease, specifically the plague. 2. Something that is pernicious or extremely destructive. — pestilential, adj.

pestis (pes'tis): Plague.

petechia (pe-tē'ki-a): A pinpoint, reddish to brown spot of haemorrhage into the skin or a membrane. — petechiae, pl.; petechial, adj.

petit mal (pet'ē mal): Minor epilepsy (*q.v.*).

Petri dish: A round glass dish with a cover; used in the laboratory for growing bacterial cultures.

pétrissage (pā-tri-shazh'): A movement in massage that resembles kneading.

petrolatum (pet'rō-lah'-tum): A yellowish, semisolid substance obtained from petroleum; used as an emollient and as a base for many ointments. Petroleum jelly.

petroleum distillates: Gasoline, kerosene, charcoal igniting fluids, paint thinners, and other like substances, a frequent cause of poisoning.

petroleum jelly: Petrolatum (*q.v.*).

petrosa (pe-trō'sa): The hardened cone-shaped part of the temporal bone; it contains the structures of the inner ear.

petrositis (pe-trō-sī'tis): Inflammation of the petrous part of the temporal bone; usually associated with inflammation of the middle ear or with mastoiditis. Also spelled *petrousitis*.

petrous (pe'trus): 1. Resembling stone. 2. Relating to the petrosa.

Peutz–Jeghers syndrome (pertz-yā'-gerz): An inherited condition, thought to be transmitted by a dominant trait, characterized by the development of multiple cysts in the ileum, colon, or stomach, and excessive pigmentation, usually involving skin, lips, oral mucosa, fingers, palms, toes, and umbilical area; complications include colic, anaemia, intussusception.

-pexy: Suffix denoting fixation; a making fast.

Peyer's patches (pī'ers): Flat patches of lymphatic tissue situated in the small intestine but mainly in the ileum; they are the seat of infection in typhoid fever. [Johann Conrad Peyer, Swiss anatomist, 1653–1712.]

peyote (pā-yō '-tē): Mescaline (*q.v.*):

Peyronie's disease: A chronic condition, of unknown cause, in which the dense fibrous strands develop in the corpus cavernosum of the penis causing deformity of the penis and painful erections.

Pfannenstiel's incision: (pfan'-nen-shtēlz): A transverse incision above the pubes; used in operations on the pelvic organs. [Emil Pfannenstiel, German gynaecologist, 1862–1909.]

PFI: Abbreviation for Private Finance Initiative (*q.v.*).

pH: A symbol of the measure of the concentration of hydrogen ions in a solution. The pH scale extends from 0 to 14.0, with a value of 7.0 expressing neutrality, values lower than 7.0 expressing acidity, and values higher than 7.0 expressing alkalinity.

phac-, phaco-: Combining forms denoting: **1.** A lentil or thing shaped like a lentil. **2.** A lens. **3.** The crystalline lens of the eye.

phacoanaphylaxis (fak'ō-an-a-fi-laks'is): Hypersensitivity of the crystalline lens to protein.

phacoemulsification (fak'ō-ē-mul-si-fi-kā'shun): A surgical procedure for dissolution of a cataract utilizing ultrasound waves.

phacolysis (fak-ol'i-sis): **1.** The operation of breaking down the lens of the eye and then removing it. **2.** The dissolution of the crystalline lens by some means other than surgery.

phacomalacia (fak'-ō-ma-lā'shi-a): A soft cataract, or a softening of the crystalline lens.

phacomatosis (fak'ō-ma-tō'sis): Name given to several types of hereditary neurocutaneous syndrome which later develop into tuberous sclerosis, neurofibromatosis, and angiomatosis, involving particularly the brain, skin, and eye.

phacosclerosis (fak'o-skler-ō'sis): A hard cataract, or a hardening of the crystalline lens.

phaeochromocytoma (fē'-ō-krō-mō-sī-tō'ma): A tumour derived from the cells of the adrenal medulla; secretes adrenaline and noradrenaline, usually benign. Produces hypertension with palpitation, nausea, vomiting, pounding headache, sweating, tingling sensations in the extremities.

phag-, phago-: Combining form denoting something that eats, ingests, or devours.

phage (fāj): See BACTERIOPHAGE.

-phagia: Combining form denoting a desire to eat a certain substance or food.

phagocyte (fag'ō-sīt): A cell capable of engulfing, sometimes digesting, bacteria, foreign particles, cells, and other debris in the tissues. — phagocytic, adj.

phagocytose (fag-ō-sī'tōs): To engulf and possibly destroy bacteria or other foreign material.

phagocytosis (fag-ō-sī-tō'sis): The engulfment, and usually the isolation or destruction by phagocytes, of foreign or other particles or cells harmful to the body.

phagomania (fag-ō-mā'ni-a): Abnormal craving for or obsession with food. Morbid desire to eat continually.

phak-, phako-: See PHAC-, PHACO-.

phakitis (fa-kī'tis): Inflammation of the crystalline lens.

phakoma (fa-kō'ma): A microscopic greyish-white tumour occasionally seen on the retina in patients with tuberous sclerosis. Also spelled *phacoma*.

phalangeal (fa-lan'jē-al): Relating to a phalanx or phalanges.

phalangectomy (fal-an-jek'to-mi): Removal of one or more of the phalanges.

phalanges (fal-an'jēz): Plural of phalanx (*q.v.*).

phalanx (fā'lanks): Any one of the small bones of the fingers or toes; two in the thumb and great toe, and three in each of the other digits. — phalanges, pl.; phalangeal, adj.

phall-, phallo-: Combining forms denoting the penis.

phallectomy (fal-ek'to-mi): Amputation of the penis.

phallic (fal'ik): Relating to the penis. P. PHASE in psychoanalytic theory, the period in psychosocial development when a boy's interest is centred on the penis and a girl's, to a lesser extent, on the clitoris.

phallitis (fal-ī'tis): Inflammation of the penis.

phallodynia (fal-ō-din'i-a): Pain in the penis. Phallalgia.

phalloncus (fal-on'kus): An abnormal swelling or tumour of the penis.

phallorrhoea (fal-o-rē'a): **1.** A discharge from the penis. **2.** Gonorrhoea in the male.

phallus (fal'us): The penis. — phallic, adj.

phantasm (fan'tazm): A delusion or illusion. An impression not caused by an actual physical stimulus. Phantom.

phantasmatomoria (fan-taz'mat-ō-mō'ri-a): Silly fantasies, delusions, or childishness; seen in demented persons.

phantasy: See FANTASY.

phantom (fan'tom): **1.** A model of a part of the body, *e.g.*, a model of the pelvis, used in teaching obstetrics. **2.** An apparition; something that a person sees but which does not actually exist. P. LIMB term applied to a sensation that a patient has a limb although the limb has been amputated; P. PAIN pain felt as though it were in a limb that has been amputated.

pharmaceutical (far-ma-sū'tik-al): **1.** Relating to drugs. **2.** A medicinal drug.

pharmacist (far'ma-sist): One who is qualified and licensed to prepare and dispense drugs.

pharmaco-: Combining form denoting drug(s), medicine(s).

pharmacodynamics (far'ma-kō-dī-nam'iks): The study of the action of drugs on the human body.

pharmacogenetics (far'ma-kō-jen'et'iks): The study of genetically determined reactions of individuals to drugs.

pharmacogenic (far'ma-kō-jen'ik): Produced by drugs, usually referring to side effects.

pharmacognosy (far-ma-kog'nō-si): The branch of pharmacology dealing with the economic, biological, and chemical aspects of natural drugs and their constituents.

pharmacokinetics (farm'a-kō-kī-net'iks): The study of the action of drugs in the body and their movement through the body systems during absorption, distribution, biotransformation, and elimination, and including the time required for therapeutic or pharmacological responses to them.

pharmacologist (far-ma-kol'o-jist): One who studies drugs, their sources, uses, and actions.

pharmacology (far-ma-kol'o-ji): The science that deals with drugs in all their aspects and relations. CLINICAL P. the study of the action of drugs in humans.

pharmacomania (far'ma-kō-mā'ni-a): A morbid desire to give or take medicines.

pharmacopoeia (far'ma-kō-pē'a): A book in which accepted drugs and their preparations are listed and described, including dosages and other pertinent information. Prepared by an official authority of the government or of a medical group and accepted as a legal standard. See BRITISH NATIONAL FORMULARY and BRITISH PHARMACOPOEIA.

pharmacopsychosis (far'ma-kō-sī'-kō'sis): Psychosis due to addiction to alcohol, a drug, or a poison.

pharamcotherapeutics (farm'a-kō-ther-a-pū'tiks): The study of the uses of drugs in the treatment of disease.

pharmacotherapy (far'ma-kō-ther'a-pi): Treatment of disease with drugs.

pharmacothymia (farm'a-kō-thī'mi-a): Drug addiction.

pharmacy (far'ma-si): **1.** The practice of preparing and dispensing medications. **2.** A place where medications are prepared and dispensed; a chemist.

pharyng-, pharyngo-: Combining forms denoting the pharynx.

pharyngeal (fa-rin'jē-al): Relating to the pharynx.

pharyngectomy (far'in-jek'to-mi): Removal of part of the pharynx.

pharyngismus (far'in-jis'mus): Spasm of the muscles of the pharynx.

pharyngitis (far'in-jī'tis): Inflammation of the pharynx or tonsils, or both.

pharyngoconjunctival (fa-ring'gō-kon-junk-tī'val): Relating to the pharynx and the conjunctiva. P. FEVER a disease of children, characterized by pharyngitis, conjunctivitis, rhinitis, fever, and inflammation of cervical lymph nodes; caused by an adenovirus. Also called '*swimming-pool*' conjunctivitis: see under CONJUNCTIVITIS.

pharyngolaryngeal (far-ing'gō-la-rin'jē-al): Pertaining to the pharynx and larynx.

pharyngolaryngectomy (far-ing'gō-lar-in-jek'to-mi): Surgical removal of the pharynx and larynx.

pharyngolaryngitis (far-ing'gō-lar-in-jī'tis): Inflammation of both the pharynx and larynx.

pharyngoplasty (far-ing'gō-plas-ti): Any plastic operation on the pharynx.

pharyngoplegia (far-ing'gō-plē'ji-a): Paralysis of the muscles of the wall of the pharynx.

pharyngospasm (far-ing'gō-spazm): Pharyngismus (*q.v.*).

pharyngotomy (far'-ing-got'o-mi): The operation of making an opening into the pharynx, done from either the outside or the inside.

pharyngotonsillitis (fa-ring'gō-ton-sil-lī'tis): Inflammation of the pharynx and the tonsils.

pharyngotympanic (fa-ring'gō-tim-pan'ik): Relating to the pharynx and the tympanic cavity. P. TUBE see AUDITORY TUBE.

pharynx (far'inks): The upper expanded portion of the digestive tube that forms the cavity at the back of the mouth. It is cone-shaped, 7.5 to 10 cm long, and is lined with mucous membrane; at the lower end it opens into the oesophagus. The auditory tubes pierce its lateral walls and the posterior nares pierce its anterior wall. The larynx lies immediately below it and in front of the oesophagus. For descriptive purposes it is divided into the nasopharynx, that part above the level of the soft palate; the oropharynx, that part between the soft palate and the epiglottis; and the laryngopharynx, that part between the upper edge of the epiglottis and the larynx. It functions as a passageway for both food and air. — pharyngeal, adj.

Phase I trials: see DRUG TRIALS.

Phase II trials: see DRUG TRIALS.

Phase III Trials: see DRUG TRIALS.

-phasia, -phasy: Combining forms denoting a speech disorder, especially related to the symbolic use of language.

phen-, pheno-: Combining forms denoting: 1. Appearance; showing. 2. Derivation from benzene.

phencyclidine (fen-sī′kli-dēn): A white powder, colourless in solution; smoked, inhaled, or swallowed, it has a hallucinogenic effect.

phenocopy (fē′nō-kop-i): An effect produced experimentally that resembles an effect that is normally produced genetically.

phenol (fē′nol): Carbolic acid. Formerly widely used as a disinfecting agent. Strong solutions are caustic. — phenolic, adj. P. COEFFICIENT the disinfecting power of a chemical as compared with phenol.

phenolic (fē-nol′ik): 1. Relating to or derived from a phenol (q.v.). 2. Resembling phenol in action.

phenolsulphonphthalein (fē′nol-sull-fōn-thāl′ē-in): A bright red crystalline powder used in diagnostic tests. P. TEST a kidney function test; P. is administered intravenously and the rate and amount of excretion of the P. in the urine is a measure of the functional ability of the kidney; normally 50% to 70% is eliminated within 2 hours.

phenomenology (fē-nom′en-ol′o-ji): The science of phenomena as distinct from that of being (ontology, q.v.). A philosophy that explores the meaning of individuals' lived experiences through their description.

phenomenon (fe-nom′e-non): 1. Any unusual occurrence or fact. 2. In medicine, a symptom or any occurrence in relation to disease, whether or not it is unusual or extraordinary. — phenomena, pl.

phenothiazines (fē′-nō-thī′a-zēns): A group of drugs in the major tranquillizer category; administered orally or intramuscularly. They act as mood stabilizers and are used in both excited assaultative patients and those who are withdrawn and apathetic.

phenotype (fē′nō-tīp): 1. The outward observable expression of one's hereditary physical makeup. 2. Term applied to a group of persons who resemble each other but who have different genetic make-ups.

phenylalanine (fen-il-al′a-nēn): One of the essential amino acids; found in all natural protein foods.

phenylalanine 4-hydroxylase (fen-il-al′a-nēn hī-droks′-i-lās): An enzyme that converts phenylalanine to tyrosine (q.v.), a reaction requiring oxygen; a deficiency of this enzyme occurs in phenylketonuria, a hereditary metabolic disorder. See also PHENYLKETONURIA.

phenylketonuria (fen′il-kē′tō-nū′ri-a): An inherited disorder caused by a deficit of phenylalanine 4-hydroxylase, an enzyme that causes conversion of phenylalanine into tryosine; this results in an inborn error of metabolism of amino acids and an increase in the phenylalanine level in the blood which, if untreated, leads to severe mental handicap. Marked by the presence of phenylpyruvic acid in the urine. Other symptoms include tremor, convulsions, mental handicap, hyperactivity, eczema, offensive odour to faeces and urine. Appears most often in families of Irish or Mediterranean descent. Syn., *phenylpyruvic oligophrenia*. See also GUTHRIE TEST.

phenylpyruvic acid (fen′il-pī-rū′vik as′id): A product of the metabolism of phenylalanine (q.v.); its appearance in the urine is indicative of phenylketonuria.

pheresis (fe-rē′sis): 1. The separation of blood into its individual components and the removal of one or more selected components. 2. The removal of one or more selected components from a donor's blood, followed by return of the blood to the donor.

pheromone (fer′ō-mōn): Any substance that is elaborated in the body; secreted to the exterior, and has a characteristic odour that serves as a means of communication with other individuals of the same species and arouses certain behaviours.

phial (fī′al): A small glass bottle for medicine; a vial.

-phil, -phile, -philia, -philic: Combining forms used in the suffix position to denote (1) loving, having a fondness for; (2) one who loves or has an affinity for.

-philia: Suffix denoting (1) love or craving for; (2) tendency towards.

philtrum (fil′trum): Anatomical term for the vertical groove in the midline of the upper lip.

phimosis (fĭ-mō'sis): Tightness of the prepuce so that it cannot be retracted over the glans penis.

phi phenomenon: The sensation of motion when viewing a row of stationary lights that flash alternately.

phleb-, phlebo-: Combining forms denoting vein(s).

phlebangioma (flēb-an-ji-ō'ma): An aneurysm in a vein.

phlebarterectasia (fleb'ar-te-rek-tā'-zi a): A general dilatation of both veins and arteries.

phlebectasia (fleb-ek-tā'zi-a): The dilatation of a vein or veins; syn., *variscosity*. P. LARYNGITIS, P. affecting veins of the larynx, particularly the vocal cords; usually a permanent condition.

phlebectomy (fle-bek'to-mi): Excision of a portion of a vein, sometimes done to relieve varicose veins. MULTIPLE COSMETIC P. removal of varicose veins through little stab incisions that heal without scarring.

phlebitis (fle bī'tis). Inflammation of a vein, often one in the leg. P. MIGRANS recurrent attacks of thrombophlebitis, usually in the leg, characterized by pain, tenderness, and swelling of a segment of a superficial vein; occurs most often in men and may be an early sign of Buerger's disease.

phleboclysis (fle-bok'li-sis): The intravenous injection of a medicinal solution.

phlebogram (fleb'ō-gram): An x-ray picture of a vein, or the recording of the venous pulse, usually jugular, utilizing a contrast medium.

phlebolith (fleb'ō-lith): A concretion that forms in a vein.

phlebology (fle-bol'o-ji): The branch of medical science that deals with the anatomy and physiology of veins and their disorders and diseases.

phlebomanometer (fleb'ō-man-om'e-ter): An instrument for measuring blood pressure within the veins.

phlebophlebostomy (fleb'ō-flēb-os'to-mi): The surgical procedure of anastomosing vein to vein.

phleborrhagia (fleb-ō-rā'ji-a): Haemorrhage from a vein.

phleborrhaphy (fle-bor'a-fi): The procedure of suturing a vein; also called *venesuture*.

phleborrhexis (fleb-ō-rek'sis): Rupture of a vein.

phlebosclerosis (fleb'ō-skle-rō'sis): Loss of elasticity of the walls of a vein; due to fibrous hardening.

phlebostasis (fle-bos'ta-sis): 1. Retardation of blood flow in a vein. 2. The temporary shutting off of venous circulation in a part by compression on the veins; also called *bloodless phlebotomy*.

phlebostenosis (fleb'ō-ste-nō'sis): Narrowing or constriction of the calibre of a vein.

phlebothrombosis (fleb'ō-throm-bō'sis): Thrombosis in a vein due to sluggish flow, accompanied by relatively slight inflammation, occurring chiefly in bedridden patients and affecting the deep veins of the lower limbs or pelvis; may also occur as a complication of intravenous therapy. The loosely attached thrombus is likely to break off and lodge in the lungs as an embolus.

phlebotomize (fli-bot'o-mīz): To perform phlebotomy (incision into a vein) for the purpose of drawing blood.

Phlebotomus (fle-bot'o-mus): A genus of blood-sucking sandflies that transmit various forms of leishmaniasis, sandfly fever, Oroyo fever, kalazar, and bartonellosis; found chiefly in China, the Middle East, and India.

phlebotomy (fli-bot'o-mi): Venesection. A bleeding of 400 to 500 ml of blood; a therapeutic measure in pulmonary congestion to relieve the workload of the heart, to reduce the red cell volume in polycythaemia vera, or to reduce the total body iron in haemochromatosis. May also be done to obtain blood for a blood bank or for autotransfusion. BLOODLESS P. the temporary production of phlebostasis in the extremities by compression of the veins.

phlegm (flem): Thick, viscid mucus that is secreted in abnormal quantities in the respiratory tract and expectorated.

phlegmasia (fleg-mā'zi-a): Inflammation. P. ALBA DOLENS inflammation of the femoral vein; sometimes follows childbirth; marked by swelling of the leg, usually without redness; also called milk leg and white leg; P. CERULEA DOLENS acute fulminating thrombophlebitis involving both deep and superficial veins of the leg, characterized by severe pain, cyanosis, oedema, purpura; possibly circulatory collapse.

phlegmatic (fleg-mat'ik): 1. Emotionally stolid; not easily excited; apathetic. 2. Resembling phlegm.

phlegmon (fleg'mon): Inflammation of subcutaneous connective tissue, often terminating in ulceration or abscess formation. Cellulitis (*q.v.*).

phlogistic (flo-jis'tik): Relating to or inducing fever or inflammation.

phlyctena (flik'te-na): A small vesicle, such as occurs following a first-degree burn. — phlyctenae, pl.

phlyctenulae (flik-ten'ū-lē): Small vesicles, usually occurring on the conjunctiva or cornea, most often in debilitated or tubercular children. — phlyctenula, sing.; phlyctenular, adj.

phob-, phobo-: Prefix denoting (1) fear; (2) avoidance of.

-phobe: Suffix denoting a person with a phobia.

phobia (fō'bi-a): A persistent, unreasonable, exaggerated, irrational fear or dread that focuses on a definite subject. The term is often used as the termination of a word in which the main stem indicates the object of the person's fear. — phobic, adj.

-phobia: Combining form used as a suffix denoting fear, hatred, or aversion to a subject.

-phobic: Combining form denoting morbid fear of, or aversion to, something.

phon-, phono-: Combining forms denoting sound, voice, speech, tone.

phonal (fō'nal): Relating to speech or the voice.

phonasthenia (fō-nas-thē'ni-a): Weakness or hoarseness of the voice due to fatigue.

phonation (fō-nā'shun): The utterance of sounds produced by vibration of the vocal cord. — phonate, adj.

phonetic (fo-net'ik): Relating to the voice and pronunciation of speech. Phonic.

phonetics (fo-net'iks): The science of speech and of pronunciation. Syn., *phonology*.

phoniatrics (fō-ni-at'riks): The study and treatment of the voice and speech defects.

phonoangiography (fō'nō-an-ji-og'ra-fi): The process of recording and then analysing the sound produced by the blood passing through an artery; often used to measure the extent to which the vessel's lumen has been narrowed by atherosclerosis.

phonocardiogram (fō-nō-kar'di-ō-gram): A graphic record of heart sounds and murmurs.

phonocardiography (fō'nō-kar-di-og'ra-fi): The electronic recording of heart sounds, utilizing a highly sensitive stethoscope and microphone that detects sounds not otherwise available, displays the patterns on an oscilloscope screen, and makes a permanent record by photography.

phonopathy (fō-nop'a-thi): Any disease or disorder of the voice.

phonophobia (fōn-ō-fō'bi-a): 1. Abnormal fear of speaking or of one's own voice. 2. Abnormal fear of any sound.

phonophoresis (fō'nō-fo-rē'sis): The introduction of a medication through the skin by use of ultrasonic energy.

phonopsia (fō-nop'si-a): A sensation of seeing certain colours when one hears certain sounds.

-phoria: A combining form meaning (1) a turning; in ophthalmology, a turning of the visual axis; (2) an emotional state.

phosgene (fos'jēn): A suffocating, extremely poisonous gas, which was used extensively in World War I; now used in the production of several chemical and pharmaceutical products.

phosphataemia (fos-fa-tē'mi-a): The presence of a higher than normal concentration of phosphates in the blood.

phosphatase (fos'fa-tās): One of a group of enzymes that hastens the hydrolysis and synthesis of organic esters of phosphoric acid; essential in the absorption and metabolism of carbohydrates, phospholipids, and nucleotides, and in the calcification of bones.

phosphate (fos'fāt): A salt or ester of phosphoric acid; has a minor buffering action in the blood; important in maintaining the acid–base balance in the blood. Phosphates eliminated in the urine are decreased in nephritis and hypoparathyroidism, and increased in starvation, extreme prolonged muscular exercise, and in those on high protein diets.

phosphaturia (fos-fa-tū'ri-a): The presence of an excess of phosphates in the urine; may be the cause of renal calculi. Also called *phosphoruria* and *hyperphosphaturia*.

phosphene (fos'fēn): The subjective sensation of light due to stimulation of the retina by pressure on the eyeballs or any stimulus other than light.

phosphofructokinase (fos'fō-fruk-tō-kī'nas): An enzyme of importance in glycolysis (*q.v.*).

phospholipase (fos-fō-lī'pās): Any one of four enzymes that act as catalysts in the splitting of a phospholipid (*q.v.*). Formerly called *lecithinase*.

phospholipid (fos-fō-lip'id): A class of greasy or waxy compounds widely distributed in plants and animals, particularly in membranes; on hydrolysis they yield phosphoric acid and several carbon compounds, including lecithin, cephalin, and sphingomyelin.

phosphonecrosis (fos-fō-nē-krō'sis): 'Fossy-jaw', necrosis of the jaw with loosening of the teeth, occurring in workers engaged in the manufacture of products made with white phosphorus, *e.g.*, matches.

phosphorus (fos'fo-rus): A non-metallic constituent of bones, teeth, and nerve tissue, not found in the pure form in the body but in combination with alkalis. Important in conversion of glucogen to glucose, in the metabolism of proteins and calcium, and as a source of energy in muscle contraction. Vitamin D is required for its absorption and metabolism. Phosphorus compounds are found in the protein in many foods such as dairy products, eggs, legumes and many other vegetables, some nuts, liver, many cereals, figs, pineapple, and prunes. Deficiency in the diet results in perverted appetite, weight loss, retarded growth, rickets, anaemia, and imperfect development of teeth and bones. RADIOACTIVE P. (^{32}P) is used in treating certain pathological conditions, e.g., leukaemia and polycythaemia vera, and as a tracer substance in certain physiological studies.

phosphorylase (fos-for'i-lās): An enzyme that acts as a catalyst in the formation of glucose from glycogen.

phot-, photo-: Combining forms denoting: 1. Light. 2. Photograph or photographic.

photalgia (fō-tal'ji-a): Pain in the eyes from exposure to intense light.

photic (fō'tik): Of, related to, or caused by light.

photoallergy (fō'tō-al'er-ji): Hypersensitization to sunlight following ingestion of certain plant foods or certain drugs. See HYPERSENSITIVITY.

photobiotic (fō'tō-bī-ot'ik): Capable of living and growing only in the presence of light, said of certain microorganisms.

photocoagulation (fō'tō-kō-ag-ūlā'shun): The use of controlled light rays to treat such conditions as intraocular tumour or detached retina, or to destroy abnormal retinal blood vessels. See LASER.

photodermatitis (fō'tō-der-ma-tī'tis): Skin lesions due to exposure to sunlight or ultraviolet rays.

photodissociation (fō'tō-dis-sō-si-ā'shun): The chemical decomposition of a substance due to exposure to light.

photodynia (fō-tō-din'-i-a): Pain in the eyes caused by too great intensity of light; see PHOTOPHOBIA.

photoerythema (fō'tō-er-i-thē'ma): Erythema (q.v.). caused by exposure to light.

photokeratosis (fō'tō-ker-a-tō'sis): Mild corneal irritation due to overexposure to the ultraviolet rays of the sun.

photomania (fō'tō-mā'ni-a): 1. A morbid desire for light. 2. Insanity or maniacal symptoms induced by prolonged exposure to bright light.

photometer (fō-tom'i-ter): A device for determining (1) the intensity of light, or (2) the degree of sensitivity of the eye to light.

photophobia (fō-tō-fō'bi-a): 1. Profound intolerance for light; may be a significant symptom of central nervous system disorder, e.g., meningitis. 2. Dread or avoidance of light places. — photophobic, adj.

photopsia (fō-top'si-a): The subjective sensation of seeing sparks or flashes of light before the eyes; may be due to irritation of the retina, or certain diseases of the brain or optic nerve. Also called photopsy.

photoreceptor (fō'tō-rēsep'tor): A sensory end organ capable of receiving stimuli caused by light, i.e., the rods and cones of the retina.

photoscan (fō'tō-skan): A two-dimensional photograph showing the distribution and concentration of a radioactive isotope that has been administered internally.

photosensitive (fō-tō-sen'si-tiv): 1. Sensitive to light, as the retina of the eye. 2. Exhibiting an increased reactivity of the skin to sunlight. — photosensitivity, n.

photosensitization (fō'tō-sens-i-tī-zā'shun): Hypersensitivity of the skin to light, sunlight or ultraviolet rays in particular; due to the presence in the body of certain drugs, hormones, or heavy metals that have been used, either internally or externally; may occur immediately after ingestion (or use) of such substances for weeks, even months, afterwards.

photosynthesis (fō-tō-sin'the-sis): The process by which plants, utilizing light energy, synthesize carbohydrate (glucose) from carbon dioxide and water in the presence of chlorophyll.

phototherapy (fō-tō-ther'a-pi): Therapeutic treatment by exposure to sunlight or artificial light, ultraviolet in particular; often used in treatment of skin disorders such as acne, psoriasis, and decubitis ulcer.

phototoxic (fō-tō-tok'sik): Relating to the harmful reaction caused by exposure to light, particularly the reaction of the skin to exposure to the ultraviolet rays in sunlight.

phototoxis (fō-tō-tok'sis): A disorder caused by over-exposure to ultraviolet light or from exposure to light in combination with a phototoxic substance. See PHOTOSENSITIZATION.

phren (fren): 1. The diaphragm. 2. The mind. — phrenic, adj.

phren-, phreni-, phreno-: Combining forms denoting: 1. The mind. 2. The diaphragm. 3. The phrenic nerve.

phrenasthenia (fren-as-thē'ni-a): 1. Loss of muscle tone of the diaphragm. 2. Feeblemindedness; mental handicap.

phrenetic (fren-et'ik): 1. Frenzied. 2. A person who is maniacal or frenzied.

-phrenia: Combining form denoting a disordered condition of mental functioning.

phrenic (fren'ik): 1. Relating to the diaphragm. 2. Relating to the mind. P. NERVE a general motor and sensory nerve originating in the cervical plexus and distributed to the pleura, pericardium, diaphragm, and peritoneum.

phrenicectomy (fren-i-sek'to-mi): Resection of all or part of the phrenic nerve.

phrenicotomy (fren-i-kot'o-mi): Division of the phrenic nerve to paralyse one half of the diaphragm, done to produce compression of a diseased lung.

phrenitis (fren-ī'tis): 1. Inflammation of the diaphragm. 2. Inflammation of the brain. 3. Frenzy; delirium.

phrenology (fre-nol'o-ji): A pseudoscience based on the belief that the external configurations of the skull indicate areas of development in the brain of certain mental faculties, and that therefore one's mental characteristics can be determined by examination of the various prominences of the skull.

phrenoplegia (fren'ō-plē'ji-a): 1. Paralysis of the diaphragm. 2. Paralysis or sudden loss of mental faculties.

phrynoderma (frin'ō-der'ma): A dry eruption of the skin; possibly due to vitamin A deficiency. Also called *Follicular keratosis.*

phthiriasis (thi-rī'a-sis): Infestation with the crab or pubic louse.

Phthirus (thir'us): A louse. P. PUBIS the crab louse; infests pubic area primarily but also the axillae, eyebrows, and beard on occasion.

Phycomycetes (fī'kō-mī-sē'tēz): A class of fungi, including black bread mould and water mould; may be pathogenic to humans, particularly diabetics and debilitated individuals.

phycomycosis (fī'kō-mī-kō'sis): An acute or chronic systemic infection caused by one of the *Phycomycetes,* often *Mucor.* The central nervous system, blood vessels, or lungs may be affected; usually occurs in debilitated individuals.

phylaxis (fi-laks'is): The body's action in protecting or defending itself against infection.

physiatrics (fiz-i-at'riks): The branch of medicine that utilizes physical agents such as heat, cold, light, water, and electricity in the prevention, diagnosis, and treatment of disease. Physical medicine.

physic (fiz'ik): 1. Old term for the art and science of medicine. 2. A purgative or laxative drug.

physical (fiz'i-kal): Relating to: (1) the body; (2) natural science; (3) material things; (4) physical science. P. ASSESSMENT the process of evaluating a client's health status utilizing data obtained from the client and the findings of a physical examination; P. MEDICINE a medical specialty that utilizes physiotherapy and occupational therapy and physical reconditioning in the management of the sick and injured.

physician (fi-zish'un): A person fitted by knowledge and training to care for the sick and licensed by the proper authorities as a doctor and who practises medicine as distinct from surgery. COMMUNITY P. a doctor who practises community medicine; CONSULTANT P. an experienced, well-qualified hospital doctor who has overall charge of patients allocated to their care, and also has responsibility for the supervision and guidance of junior medical staff; HOUSE P. a newly qualified doctor who lives in the hospital and is responsible for patients' care under the supervision and guidance of the consultant physician.

physicochemical (fiz'-i-kō-kem'ik-al): Relating to physics and chemistry.

physics (fiz'iks): A fundamental science that deals with the phenomena and laws of nature, particularly with the properties of matter and energy.

physiognomy (fiz-i-o'-no-mi): The facial appearance, facial features, and expression that are thought by some to reveal inner character and quality.

physiological (fiz-i-ō-loj'ik-al): 1. Of or related to physiology. 2. Denoting the action of a drug in a healthy person as distinguished from its therapeutic action. 3. Normal as opposed to pathological; in accordance with natural processes of the body. Adjective often used to describe a normal process or structure, to distinguish it from an abnormal or pathological feature. P. SALINE a solution consisting of 0.9 gram sodium chloride per 100 ml distilled water; it has the same osmotic pressure as plasma; also called *physiological salt solution,* normal saline, and normal salt solution.

physiology (fiz-i-ol'ō-ji): The branch of biology that deals with the normal vital processes, activities, and functions of living organisms.

physiopathology (fiz'-i-ō-pa-thol'o-ji): The science of body functions in disease or as modified by disease.

physiopsychic (fiz-i-ō-sī'kik): Pertinent to or involving both the body and the mind.

physiotherapist (fiz'i-ō-ther'a-pist): One skilled or trained in physiotherapy (*q.v.*).

physiotherapy (fiz'i-ō-ther'a-pi): Treatment of disease, injury, or disability by physical means, *e.g.,* light, heat, electricity, water, massage, regulated exercises.

physique (fi-zēk'): The general bodily structure or type. Syn., *body build.*

pia (pē'a): Soft, tender. P. MATER the innermost of the three meninges (*q.v.*); the vascular membrane that lies in close contact with the substance of the brain and spinal cord. See MATER.

pia-arachnitis (pē'a-ar-ak-nī'tis): Leptomeningitis (*q.v.*).

pia-arachnoid (pē'-a-ar-ak'noid): Relating to the pia mater and the arachnoid membrane.

pica (pī'ka): 1. The habit of eating non-food substances such as plaster, chalk, ashes, etc., after the age when it might be considered natural behaviour. Often indicates a nutritional deficiency. 2. The desire for extraordinary articles of food. See GEOPHAGIA.

Pick's disease: A progressive type of presenile dementia in which atrophy of the cerebral cortex occurs, especially in the frontal and temporal lobes; a hereditary condition with onset in the 4th to 6th decade, characterized by apathy, mutism and altered speech pattern, personality changes; patients are often bedridden. [Arnold Pick, Czechoslovakian physician, 1851–1924.]

Pickwickian syndrome: A condition characterized by obesity, sleepiness, hypoventilation, cyanosis, erythrocytosis, hypoxia. Named after an obese character in Charles Dickens' writings.

picogram (pī'kō-gram): Micromicrogram. One trillionth (10^{-12}) of a gram.

piebaldism (pī'bawl-dizm): An inherited condition in which some areas of the skin, and sometimes of the hair, are white, due to hypomelanosis; partial albinism. — piebald, adj.

Pierre Robin syndrome: A congenital condition in which micrognathia, with a high arched palate and glossoptosis, occurs; congenital glaucoma and retinal detachment are often present.

piesaesthesia (pī-es-es-thē'zi-a): Sensitivity to pressure.

pigeon breast: A deformity in which a narrow chest causes the sternum to bulge anteriorally resulting in an increased anterior–posterior diameter; occurs especially in rickets. *Pectus carinatum.*

pigeon toe: A condition in which the toes permanently turn inward towards the median line. — pigeon-toed, adj.

piggy-back: Refers to the simultaneous administration of two or more intravenous solutions.

pigment (pig'ment): In anatomy, any colouring matter in the body.

pigmentation (pig'men-tā'shun): The deposit of pigment in any of the body tissues, especially when abnormal or excessive.

pigmentum nigrum (pig-men'tum nī'grum): The black pigment that lines the choroid coat of the eye.

piitis (pē-ī'tis): Inflammation of the pia mater.

pil-, pili-, pilo-: Combining forms denoting hair(s).

pilar (pī'lar): Related to hair. Covered with hair. P. CYST an epidermal cyst of the scalp; a wen (*q.v.*).

piles: See HAEMORRHOID.

pili (pī'lī): Plural of pilus (*q.v.*).

pill: 1. A small, usually rounded mass of some cohesive substance containing a medication; may or may not be coated; to be swallowed whole. BREAD P. one made of bread crumbs pressed into a ball; usually a placebo; ENTERIC COATED P. one coated with a substance that will not dissolve until the pill reaches the intestine; PEP P. one that contains a drug with a stimulating effect, especially benzedrine. 2. A contraceptive substance taken orally.

pillar: In anatomy, a supporting structure or part that resembles a column, usually in pairs, *e.g.*, the pillars of the fauces.

pilocarpine (pī-lō-kar'pōn): An alkaloid obtained from the leaves of *Pilocarpus* sp., a shrub native to Central America; it stimulates perspiration, the flow of saliva, and intestinal motility when given internally; used externally as a miotic and for treatment of glaucoma.

pilocystic (pī-lō-sis'tik): Denoting a cyst that contains hair.

piloerection (pī'lō-ē-rek'shun): Raising up of the hair accompanying chilling of the body; 'goose pimples'.

pilomotor (pī-lō-mō'tor): Causing the hair to move. P. MUSCLES the arrectores pili of the skin; P. NERVES tiny nerves attached to the hair follicle; innervation causes the hair to stand upright and give the appearance of 'goose flesh'.

pilonidal (pī-lō-nī'dal): Hair-containing. P. CYST see under CYST; P. SINUS see under SINUS.

pilose (pī'los): Covered with hair, especially that of a soft texture; hairy.

pilosebaceous (pī'lō-sē-bā'shus): Relating to the hair follicle and the sebaceous gland opening into it.

pilosis (pī-lō'sis): An abnormal growth of hair.

pilot study: An experimental undertaking prior to full-scale operation, activity, or use. A small-scale trial run of a research interview, questionnaire, or observation.

pilula (pi-loo'la): A pill.

pilus (pī'lus): A hair. — pili, pl.

pimple: A small, circumscribed, usually pointed, erythematous elevation on the skin; often suppurated. See pustule; papule.

pin: A slender metal rod used in the surgical fixation of the ends of fractured bones.

pinch gauge: An instrument for measuring the strength of a finger pinch. Pinch meter.

pineal (pin'ē-al): 1. Having a shape like a pine cone. 2. Pertaining to the pineal body (*q.v.*).

pineal body (pin'ē-al): The small reddish-grey conical structure extending from the posterior part of the third ventricle of the brain; it apparently secretes the hormone melatonin which is thought to influence the metabolic actions of several hormones. Also called *pineal gland* and *epiphysis cerebri*.

pinealoma (pin'ē-a-lō'ma): A tumour of the pineal gland; usually occurs in young people in association with obesity and early puberty.

pinguecula (ping-gwek'ū-la): A small slightly elevated fat pad on the conjunctiva near the junction of the cornea and the inner canthus, or sometimes the outer canthus; usually does no harm but may disturb the individual who fears loss of vision. — pingueculae, pl.

pinkeye: Popular name for acute contagious conjunctivitis.

pinna (pin'a): That part of the ear which is external to the head; the auricle. — pinnae, pl.

pinocytosis (pīn'ō-sī-tō'sis): The absorption of liquids by cells with phagocytic properties such as the macrophage.

pinta (pin'ta): A chronic, non-venereal disease caused by a spirochaete; characterized by the eruption of patches of varying colour that finally become white. Occurs mostly in children. Is endemic among dark-skinned peoples of the tropics and sub-tropics.

pinworm: Threadworm; *Enterobius vermicularis* (*q.v.*).

pipette (pi-pet'): A glass tube with a small lumen used in the laboratory for transferring and measuring small amounts of fluid.

piriform (pir'i-form): Having the shape of a pear.

Pirquet's reaction: (pēr'-kāz,per'-kāz): A local inflammatory reaction in response to the application of tuberculin to scarified skin to determine the presence of tuberculosis; used especially with children. [Baron Clemens von Pirquet, Austrian paediatrician, 1874–1929.]

pisiform (pis'-i-form): 1. Having the shape or size of a pea. 2. One of the bones of the carpus.

pit: 1. Any hollow or depression on the surface of the body or of an organ. 2. A dimple or pockmark. 3. A depression in the enamel of a tooth. 4. To make an indentation, as occurs when a finger is pressed against oedematous tissue.

pitchblende (pich'blend): A brown to black lustrous mineral that contains a large amount of uranite; it is the principal source of uranium and the elements produced from its breakdown, chiefly radium.

pith: 1. The spinal cord and medulla oblongata. 2. The centre of a hair shaft. 3. To destroy the spinal cord or the entire central nervous system.

pitting: 1. Depressed scars left on the skin, especially after chickenpox. 2. Indentations remaining temporarily in oedematous tissue after pressure with a finger.

pituitarism (pi-tū'-i-tar-izm): Any dysfunction of the pituitary gland.

pituitary (pit-ū'i-tar-i): Relating to the hypophysis cerebri or the pituitary gland. P. GLAND a small, two-lobed, oval endocrine gland located at the base of the brain in the sella turcica of the sphenoid bone; often called the *master gland* because it influences the secretory activity of all the endocrine glands except the adrenals. The larger anterior part (adenohypophysis) secretes several hormones that have an effect on other endocrine glands: the follicle-stimulating hormone, adrenocorticotrophic hormone, growth hormone, prolactin, thyroid-stimulating hormone, luteinizing hormone. The smaller posterior lobe (neurohypophysis) furnishes a secretion that stimulates lactation, and vasopressin (antidiuretic hormone) which has an effect on the fluid and electrolye balance in the body; it also acts to regulate and stimulate smooth muscle tissue, thus affecting blood pressure and the activity of the intestinal and uterine musculature. P. DWARFISM dwarfism due to hypofunctioning of the anterior lobe of the pituitary gland.

pituitectomy (pi-tū-i-tek'to-mi): Surgical removal of the pituitary gland.

pituitrin (pi-tū'i-trin): 1. A secretion of the posterior lobe of the pituitary gland; it acts specifically on the smooth muscle of the uterus increasing tone and contraction. 2. Trademark for a preparation of pituitary extract made from the pituitary gland of certain animals.

pityriasis (pit-i-rī'a-sis): Name given to a group of skin diseases characterized by scaly (branny) eruption of the skin; P. ALBA a very common skin disorder of children; characterized by the appearance of one or many round or oval finely scaling macules; may last for several years and apt to recur if untreated; also called *impetigo sicca*; P. CAPITIS dandruff; P. ROSEA a slightly scaly eruption of ovoid erythematous lesions widespread over the trunk and proximal parts of the limbs. There may be mild itching. It is a self-limiting condition; P. RUBRA a form of exfoliative dermatitis; P. RUBRA PILARIS a chronic skin disease characterized by tiny red papules of perifollicular distribution; P. VERSICOLOR, also called *tinea versicolor*, is a fungus infection which causes the appearance of buff-coloured patches on the chest.

Pityrosporum (pit-i-ros'pōr-um): A fungus associated with dandruff and seborrhoeic dermatitis.

placebo (pla-sē'bō): An inactive substance given for its psychological or suggestive effect. In experimental research; an inert substance, identical in appearance with the material being tested; neither the physician nor the patient knows which is which.

placenta (pla-sen'ta): Afterbirth. A plate-shaped spongy, vascular structure measuring 17.5–20 cm in diameter and 2.5 cm in thickness tapering to 1.2 cm at the periphery. It weighs approximately one-sixth of the baby's birthweight at full term. It is developed from the trophoblastic layers with a lining of mesoderm in which the blood vessels develop. It is formed by the 12th week of pregnancy, and is composed of large numbers of chorionic villi grouped together in cotyledons, and embedded in the decidua basalis of the uterus. The umbilical cord usually arises from a place near its centre, and is the means by which the fetus is supplied with oxygen, nutrients and other substances and excretes its waste products. It also produces several hormones including oestrogen and progesterone, which are responsible for many of the physical changes that occur in the mother during pregnancy. The time between the delivery of the infant and the expulsion of the placenta is the third and last stage of labour. P. ACCRETA a P. that is morbidly adherent to the uterine wall; BATTLEDORE P. a P. that develops in the shape of a battledore when the umbilical cord arises in the periphery instead of the centre; P. PRAEVIA a P. that is abnormally situated in the lower segment of the uterus, either completely or partially covering the internal os; RETAINED P. one that is not expelled within the normal time after childbirth; P. SUCCENTURIATA a P. in which one or more accessory lobules form at some distance from the placenta but still with the membranes and connected with it by vascular channels.

placental (pla-sen'tal): Relating to the placenta. P. ABRUPTION premature separation of a normally affixed placenta from the wall of the uterus; *abruptio placentae*; P. BARRIER the tissues between the maternal and fetal blood of the placenta which prevent certain substances from passing from the mother to the fetus; P. INSUFFICIENCY inefficiency of the placenta, may be due to maternal disease or postmaturity of the fetus producing a 'small for dates' baby;

P. TRANSFUSION SYNDROME occurs in twin pregnancies; one twin is anaemic at birth and the other is plethoric resulting from the forcing of placental blood into its circulation from that of the other twin.

placentography (plas-en-tog'ra-fi): X-ray examination of the placenta after delivery, using a contrast medium.

plague (plāg): Any disease of wide prevalence and high mortality, but particularly the very contagious epidemic disease caused by *Yersinia pestis*, and spread by infected rats that transfer the infection to humans through the agency of fleas. It is characterized by high fever, prostration, a petechial eruption, glandular swellings. The main clinical types are bubonic, pneumonic, septicaemic, and sylvatic. Also called *pest, black death, oriental plague*. See BUBO, BUBONIC PLAGUE.

plane (plān): A flat smooth surface. In anatomy, an assumed or imaginary surface extending from certain landmarks through an axis of the body, *e.g.*, the SAGITTAL P. extends from the sagittal suture downwards and divides the body into right and left portions, the FRONTAL P. (often referred to as the CORONAL P.) runs at right angles to the sagittal P. and divides the body into anterior and posterior portions; the TRANSVERSE P. divides the body into superior and inferior portions.

planned parenthood: The practice of measures (including contraception) that limit the number of offspring and determine the time interval between pregnancies.

planta (plan'ta): The sole of the foot.—plantae, pl.

plantar (plan'tar): Relating to the sole of the foot. P. ARCH the union of the P. and dorsalis pedis arteries in the sole of the foot; P. FLEXION downwards movement of the big toe; opp. of dorsiflexion; P. WART one that occurs on the sole of the foot; usually very painful and difficult to cure; thought to be caused by a specific virus that attacks irritated tissue. Also called *Verruca plantaris*.

planus (plan'us): Flat. Refers to a foot having a low arch; flatfoot.

plaque (plak): **1.** A small flattened localized abnormal area or patch on a body surface or part. **2.** A blood platelet. ARGYROPHILIC P. microscopic areas of degeneration in the cerebral cortex which stain readily with silver; a diagnostic sign of Alzheimer's disease; ATHEROMATOUS P. a deposit of fatty or fibrous material in the walls of a blood vessel, as occurs in atherosclerosis; DENTAL P. deposit of material which may or may not contain colonies of bacteria on the surface of a tooth; it causes fermentation of carbohydrates with the formation of acids which demineralize the tooth enamel, then the dentin, resulting in a cavity; SENILE P. areas of incomplete necrosis in the cerebral cortex of persons with senile dementia.

-plasia: Combining form denoting formation, development.

plasm (plazm): 1. Plasma. 2. That part of the germ cell that contains the substance by which individual characteristics are transmitted from generation to generation.

plasm-, plasmo-: Combining forms denoting: 1. The blood plasma. 2. The substance of a cell.

plasma (plaz'ma): 1. Cytoplasm or protoplasm. 2. The liquid fraction of lymph. 3. The liquid fraction of the circulating blood; to be differentiated from serum (*q.v.*). It is clear, straw-coloured and 90% water. Suspended or dissolved substances in it include the blood corpuscles, fibrinogen, electrolytes, proteins, hormones, vitamins, various waste products, and gases.—plasmic, adj.

plasma cell: See B LYMPHOCYTE.

plasmacyte (plaz'ma-sīt): Plasma cell.

plasmacytoma (plaz'ma-sī-tō'ma): A focal neoplasm consisting of plasma cells. See also MULTIPLE MYELOMA under MYELOMA.

plasmacytosis (plaz'ma-sī-tō'sis): An abnormal number of plasmacytes in (1) the peripheral blood, or (2) in the lymph nodes, spleen, liver, kidney, or bone marrow.

plasmin (plaz'min): The active substance in fibrinolysin that has the particular ability to dissolve fibrin clots.

plasminogen (plaz-min'ō-jen): The inactive precursor of plasmin; found in many body fluids and tissues; the release of inactivators from damaged tissues promotes its conversion into plasmin.

Plasmodium (plaz-mō'di-um): A genus of protozoa; parasitic in the red blood cells of warm-blooded animals; they complete their sexual cycle in blood-sucking arthropods. Four species cause malaria in humans. — P. FALCIPARUM, P. MALARIAE, P. OVALE, and P. VIVAX.

plasmolysis (plaz-mol'i-sis): Contraction or shrinking of a cell due to loss of water by osmosis; occurs when the cell is suspended in a hypertonic solution.

plasmoptysis (plaz-mop'ti-sis): The swelling of a cell and bursting of its wall with the escape of protoplasm; occurs when the cell is suspended in a hypotonic solution.

plaster: A fabric or similar material, spread with a mixture or substance that may or may not

contain a medication, to be applied externally. ADHESIVE P. fabric coated with a gummy substance, used to hold dressings in place, to protect wounds, sometimes for immobilization of a part; COURT P., P. made of isinglass spread on fine fabric; used for covering small lesions; MUSTARD P. made of mustard and flour mixed with water and spread on a cloth; a counterirritant. See also PLASTER OF PARIS.

plaster of Paris: Gypsum cement (calcium sulphate), which forms a quick-setting paste when mixed with water; used for casts and stiff bandages to immobilize a part.

plastic (plas'tik): 1. Tending to build up or regenerate tissue. 2. Capable of taking the form of a mould. 3. A substance that has been produced chemically. P. SURGERY a surgical procedure in which healthy tissue is transferred, or tissues are reconstructed or repaired in order to correct deformities or abnormalities present at birth or caused by injuries, burns, etc.

-plasty: Combining form denoting (1) moulding or shaping; (2) repair, reconstruction, plastic surgery.

plate: 1. In anatomy, a thin, flat structure, especially a bone. 2. A narrow, flat piece of metal that is screwed to the ends of fractured bones to keep them in alignment. 3. Common term for a denture.

plateau level: In drug administration, refers to the time when the amount of drug eliminated remains at the same level regardless of the amount of the drug that is in the body.

platelet (plāt'let): Small, oval, disc-like colourless cell found in the blood plasma; does not contain haemoglobin; is essential for clotting. A thrombocyte. P. PHERESIS the removal of platelets from the whole blood and immediate return of the red cells, white cells, and plasma to the donor.

plating (plāt'ing): The cultivation of bacteria on solid medium in a Petri dish.

platy-: Combining form denoting broad or flat.

platybasia (plat'i-bāz'i-a): A developmental anomaly in which the cervical spine appears to have pushed the floor of the occipital bone upward, producing a short neck, torticollis, and features of Arnold–Chiari malformation.

Platyhelminthes (plat'i-hel-min'thēz): Flatworm; fluke.

platymorphic (plat'i-mor'fik): Having a flattened shape; used especially in reference to the eyeball.

platyopic (plat'i-op'ik): Having a broad face.

platypnoea (pla-tip'nē-a): Dyspnoea occurring when the person is in the upright position and which is relieved when a recumbent or semi-recumbent position is assumed; the opposite of orthopnoea.

platypodia (plat-i-pō'di-a): Flatfootedness.

platysma (pla-tiz'ma): The broad, thin sheet of muscle on each side of the neck; it acts to depress the lower jaw and draw down the corners of the mouth.

play therapy: See under THERAPY.

pleasure principle: The tendency to direct one's behaviour towards immediate satisfaction of innate drives and immediate relief from any pain or discomforting situation.

-plegia: Combining form denoting paralysis.

pleio-, pleo-, plio-: Combining forms denoting more.

pleocytosis (plē'ō-sī-tō'sis): 1. An increase of cells in any place in the body. 2. An increase in the number of lymphocytes in the cerebrospinal fluid.

pleomastia (plē-ō-mas'ti-a): The condition of having supernumerary breasts or nipples.

pleonexia (plē-ō-nek'si-a): Greediness.

pleoptics (plē-op'tiks): A system of eye exercises to improve vision of a poorly functioning eye.

plethora (pleth'o-ra): Fullness; overloading. Used especially to describe a condition of overfullness of the blood vessels accompanied by congestion of tissues, a feeling of tension in the head, flushed complexion, bounding pulse. — plethoric, adj.

plethysmograph (pleth-iz'mō-graf): A device for measuring the volume variations in an organ, an extremity, or other body part. OCULAR P. a device for measuring the systolic pressure in the ophthalmic artery.

plethysmography (pleth'iz-mog'ra-fi): 1. The determination of variations in the size of an organ or part by measuring change in its volume. 2. Determination of the variation in size of a body part by measuring the volume of blood contained in it or passing through it.

pleura (ploo'ra): A thin serous membrane covering the surface of the lung and reflecting, at the root of the lung, on to the chest wall. PARIETAL P. that portion of the pleura that lines the inner surface of the chest wall and covers the top of the diaphragm. VISCERAL P. that portion of the pleura that is closely adherent to the lung surface. It is separated from the parietal P. by a very thin layer of fluid. — pleurae, pl.; pleural, adj.

pleuracentesis (ploor'a-sen-tē'sis): Surgical puncture of the chest wall for drainage of fluid. Pleurocentesis. Also called *thoracocentesis*.

pleural (ploor'al): Of or relating to the pleura. P. CAVITY the potential space between the parietal and visceral pleura; P. EFFUSION the presence of fluid in the pleural space; heard on auscultation as a crackling, grating sound during both inspiration and expiration; P. FRICTION RUB see under RUB; P. SPACE the potential space between the parietal and visceral layers of pleura; it contains a very small amount of serous fluid which prevents friction on breathing; P. TAP thoracentesis (*q.v.*).

pleuralgia (ploo-ral'ji-a): Pain in the pleura or in the side of the chest. — pleuralgic, adj.

pleurisy (ploor'-i-si): Inflammation of the pleura. Pleuritis. May be fibrinous (dry), associated with an effusion (wet), or complicated by empyema. DIAPHRAGMATIC P. inflammation of the pleura of the diaphragm; DRY P. a painful type of P. in which the two pleural surfaces are covered with a fibrinous exudate resulting in acute pain, especially when coughing, PURULENT P., P. marked by high fever, chills, and sweating; aspirated fluid is purulent. — pleuritic, adj.

pleuritic (ploo-rit'ik): Relating to the pleura or to one suffering from pleurisy.

pleuritis (ploo-rī'tis): Pleurisy (*q.v.*).

pleurocele (ploo'rō-sēl): A hernia of the lungs or of the pleura.

pleurodynia (ploo'rō-din'ē-a): Intercostal myalgia; muscular rheumatism, with pain and fever; symptoms are increased by movement and coughing; may appear in epidemic form. See BORNHOLM DISEASE.

pleurolysis (ploo-rol'i-sis): Loosening of the pleura from the thoracic wall to allow for collapse of the lung in treatment for pulmonary tuberculosis.

pleuropericardial (ploo'rō-per-i-kar'di-al): Relating to or affecting both the pleura and pericardium.

pleuropericarditis (ploo'rō-per-i-kar-dī'tis): Inflammation of the pleura and the pericardium.

pleuropneumonia-like organisms (ploo'rō-nū-mo'ni-a): A widely distributed group of minute organisms that cause atypical pneumonia. See MYCOPLASMA.

pleuropulmonary (ploo'rō-pul'mo-nar-i): Relating to the pleura and lungs.

pleurothotonos (ploo'rō-thot'o-nos): A bending of the body to one side, due to tetany of the muscles.

pleurotomy (ploo-rot'o-mi): An incision into the pleural cavity to allow escape of effused fluid. Also called *thoracotomy*.

pleximeter (plek-sim'i-ter): A finger or small, thin oblong plate of hard material that is held against the skin to receive the stroke of a finger or percussion hammer in indirect percussion; also called *plessimeter*. See PERCUSSION.

plexor (plek'sor): 1. A percussion hammer; see HAMMER. 2. The finger that applied the tap in the indirect method of percussion, usually the third right finger.

plexus (pleks'us): A network of vessels or nerves. AUERBACH'S P. a network of nerves and ganglia located between the circular and longitudinal muscle fibres of the oesophagus, stomach, and intestine; BRACHIAL P. one located at the side of the neck and extending into the axilla; made up of branches of three of the cervical nerves and the first two thoracic nerves; supplies the upper arm; CERVICAL P. one made up of branches of the upper four cervical nerves; supplies nerves to the muscles of the neck and shoulders; CHOROID P. projections of tufts of blood vessels from the pia mater into each of the ventricles of the brain; concerned with the secretion of cerebrospinal fluid; COELIAC P. one located in the peritoneal cavity at the level of the first lumbar vertebra; consists of a large mass of sympathetic nerves and ganglia which supply nerves to the abdominal viscera; OESOPHAGEAL P. one surrounding the oesophagus; formed by branches of the vagus nerve and sympathetic trunks; LUMBAR P. one located in the posterior part of the psoas major muscle; made up of branches of the 4th and 5th lumbar nerves; LUMBOSACRAL P. the lumbar and sacral plexuses considered together because of their contiguity; MEISSNER'S P., one in the submucosal coat of the intestine; consists of nerves and ganglia that supply the muscles and submucous membrane of the intestine; SACRAL P. one made up of sacral nerves and parts of the 4th and 5th lumbar nerves; supplies nerves to the pelvic structures, buttocks, and lower limbs; gives off the sciatic nerve; SOLAR P. the coeliac P.

-plexy: Combining form denoting seizure or stroke.

plica (plī'ka): A fold. — plicate, adj.; plication, n.

plica syndrome (plī'ka): Inflammation of the folds in the synovium of the knee joint; marked by pain and effusion; caused by a blunt or twisting injury.

plication (plī-kā'shun): The taking of tucks in a structure to shorten it or in the walls of a hollow organ to make it smaller.

-ploid: Suffix denoting: 1. Multiple in form. 2. Number of chromosomes.

plombage (plom-bazh'): The use of an inert material to fill the space between the lungs and the chest wall in order to compress the lung in treatment for pulmonary tuberculosis.

plosive (plō'siv): The speech sound heard when the air stream is blocked for a moment and then suddenly released, as in pronouncing the letters *p* and *t*.

plumbism (plum-bizm): Chronic lead poisoning; see under LEAD.

plumbum (plum'bum): Lead.

Plummer–Vinson syndrome: Combination of severe glossitis with dysphagia caused by degeneration of the muscle of the oesophagus, atrophy of the papillae of the tongue, and secondary (nutritional) anaemia. [Henry Stanley Plummer, American physician, 1874–1937. Porter Paisley Vinson, American surgeon, 1890–1959.]

Plummer's disease: Hyperthyroidism occurring in patients having a toxic adenoma of the thyroid gland.

pluralism (plū'-ral-izm): 1. A theory that opposes monolithic state power and advocates instead increased devolution and autonomy for the main organizations that represent human involvement in society. 2. The belief that power should be shared among a number of political parties.

pluri-: Prefix denoting (1) several; (2) more.

pluriglandular (plū'ri-gland'ū-lar): Relating to or affecting several glands, as mucoviscidosis (*q.v.*).

pluripara (plū-rip'ara): Multipara; a woman who has had two or more pregnancies resulting in viable offspring.

pluripotent (plū-rip'o-tent): Having the potential for affecting more than one organ or tissue. P. CELLS immature cells in the bone marrow that have the potential for developing into any of several types of tissue cells.

plutomania (plū'tō-mā'ni-a): The obsessional delusion that one possesses great wealth.

plutonium (plū-tō'ni-um): A radioactive metallic element (chemical symbol Pu), similar to uranium; used in nuclear weapons and as nuclear fuel. ^{238}Pu has been used as an energy source in pacemakers.

pneum-, pneumo-: Combining forms denoting: 1. Lungs. 2. Air or gas. 3. Respiration.

pneumat-, pneumato-: Combining forms denoting: 1. Air or gas. 2. Breathing.

pneumathaemia (nū-ma-thē'mi-a): Air embolus (*q.v.*), the presence of bubbles of air or gas in the blood.

pneumatic (nū-mat′ik): Relating to air or gas. P. BOOT or SLEEVE a boot or sleeve of varying lengths which is applied to a limb and rhythmically compressed by inflation with air; used to decrease swelling and to prevent post-operative thrombophlebitis; P. TOURNIQUET a narrow rubber band that is wrapped around a limb and then inflated with air to provide pressure on the limb.

pneumatocele (nū′mat-ō-sēl): 1. A thin-walled cavity that forms within the lung. 2. A hernial protuberance of lung tissue. 3. A tumour that contains gas, especially one occurring in the scrotum.

pneumatograph (nū-mat′-ō-graf): An instrument for recording the movements of the chest wall during breathing. Also called *pneumograph.*

pneumatosis (nū-ma-tō′sis): The presence of air or gas in an abnormal place in the body. P. CESTOIDES INTESTINALIS the presence of subserosal or submucosal gas-containing cysts in the wall of the intestine.

pneumatotherapy (nū′-mat-ō-ther′a-pi): Treatment with rarefied or condensed air. CEREBRAL P. treatment of certain psychoses by introducing oxygen into the subarachnoid space.

pneumaturia (nū-ma-tū′ri-a): The passage of flatus during or after urination; usually the result of a bladder-bowel fistula but may also be due to decomposition of bladder urine. *Pneumatinuria.*

pneumobacillus (nū-mō-ba-sil′us): See *Klebsiella pneumoniae.*

pneumocele (nū′mo-sēl): Pneumatocele (*q.v.*).

pneumocentesis (nū′mō-sen-tē′sis): Surgical puncture of a lung to allow drainage of accumulated fluid or pus, to evacuate a cavity, or to obtain material for diagnostic study.

pneumocephalus (nū-mō-kef′a-lus,-sef-): The presence of air or gas within the cerebral ventricles.

pneumococcus (nū-mō-kok′us): *Diplococcus pneumoniae.* A Gram-positive, encapsulated coccal bacterium, characteristically arranged in pairs; the common cause of lobar pneumonia; also causal agent for otitis media, mastoiditis, and leptomeningitis as well as many other infections. — pneumococcal, adj.

Pneumocystis (nū′mō-sis′tis): A genus of microorganisms considered to be protozoa. P. *carinii*, causative agent of a type of pneumonia in patients receiving immunosuppressive therapy for cancer or who have had an organ transplant, in premature infants, and in persons with acquired immunodeficiency syndrome.

May be called *interstitial cell pneumonia* or *pneumocystosis.*

pneumocyte (nū′mō-sīt): Any of the epithelial cells of the alveoli of the lungs. Also called *pneumonocyte.*

pneumoderma (nū-mō-der′ma): Subcutaneous emphysema; the presence of air or gas under the skin.

pneumodynamics (nū′mō-dī-nam′iks): The study of the mechanism and forces involved in breathing.

pneumoencephalogram (nū′-mō-en-kef′a-lō-gram,-sef′-): X-ray picture of the brain after replacement of the cerebrospinal fluid with gas or air.

pneumoencephalography (nū′mō-en-kef-a-log′ra-fi,-sef-): The making of an x-ray film of the brain after replacing the cerebrospinal fluid of the subarachnoid space with a gas, accomplished through spinal puncture; will reveal any distortion that may be caused by the presence of a tumour or a degenerative disease; may be done under local or general anaesthesia.

pneumogastric (nū-mō-gas′trik): Relating to the lungs and stomach. See VAGUS.

pneumography (nū-mog′ra-fi): 1. Roentgenology of the lungs. 2. The x-ray recording of the respiratory movements in breathing. 3. Roentgenology of a body organ or part after injection of a gas.

pneumohydrothorax (nū′mō-hī-drō-thaw′raks): The presence of either gas or air and fluid in the pleural cavity.

pneumolysis (nū-mol′i-sis): Separation of the two pleural layers, or the outer pleural layer, from the chest wall to collapse the lung. Also called *pneumonolysis.*

pneumomediastinogram (nū′mō-mē′-di-astī′no-gram): X-ray photograph of the mediastinum after rendering it opaque with air.

pneumomediastinum (nū′mō-mē-di-a-stī′num): The presence of gas or air in the mediastinal tissues; may result from emphysema or other pulmonary pathology such as respiratory distress syndrome in infants, cystic fibrosis, or asthma, or be introduced during certain diagnostic procedures.

pneumomelanosis (nū′mō-mel-a-nō′sis): A condition in which lung tissue becomes discoloured or black due to inhalation of such substances as coal dust.

pneumomycosis (nū′-mō-mī-kō′sis): Fungus infection of the lung such as aspergillosis, actinomycosis, moniliasis. — pneumomycotic, adj.

pneumon-, pneumono-: Combining forms denoting lung(s).

pneumonectomy (nū-mo-nek′to-mi): Excision of a lung or of lung tissue.

pneumonia (nū-mō′ni-a): Inflammation of the lung with the production of alveolar exudate, which consolidates, resulting in symptoms of fever, cough, lethargy, dyspnoea and/or apnoea, anorexia, and fine crackling rales. Traditionally, two main types were recognized on an anatomical or radiological basis, viz., lobar P. and broncho-P. The tendency now is to classify according to the specific bacterium or virus causing the infection (specific pneumonias) on the one hand, and the aspiration or secondary pneumonias on the other. ASPIRATION P., P. caused by inhalation by unconscious patients of foreign particles such as vomitus; ATYPICAL P. primary atypical P. caused by bacteria, most commonly diplococcus, staphylococcus, streptococcus, tuberculosis bacillus; ATYPICAL VIRAL P., P. caused by a virus; BRONCHAL P. an inflammation of the lungs that begins in the bronchioles; FRIEDLÄNDER'S P. acute P. characterized by massive exudation of mucoid material; caused by *Klebsiella pneumoniae*; HYPOSTATIC P. the result of stasis; occurs in debilitated patients from lack of movement in the dependent part of the lung; INFLUENZAL P. severe, often fatal P. caused by the influenza virus; characterized by high fever, prostration, sore throat, dyspnoea; may be complicated by bacterial pneumonia; INHALATION P. aspiration P.; LOBAR P. an acute febrile disease caused by the *Diplococcus pneumoniae*; characterized by inflammation and consolidation of one or more lobes of the lung, chills, dyspnoea, pain in the chest, cough, bloody expectoration; PNEUMOCOCCAL P. lobar P.; PRIMARY ATYPICAL P. an acute P. caused by *Mycoplasma pneumoniae* and various viruses; marked by fever, myalgia, sore throat, unproductive cough which later becomes productive; also called *VIRAL P.*; TERMINAL P., P. that develops during the course of another disease and often hastens death; VIRAL P., P. caused by a virus, most commonly adenoviruses, influenza virus, or varicella virus.

pneumonitis (nū-mō-nī′tis): Acute inflammation of lung tissue. ASPIRATION P. caused by inhalation of foreign matter into the lung; may be an extremely serious complication of anaesthesia; CHEMICAL P. caused by inhalation of an irritating chemical; GRANULOMATOUS P. farmer's lung; HYPERSENSITIVITY P. occurs in individuals whose occupations expose them to dusts containing animal or vegetable products or fungal spores, and who develop diseases such as farmer's lung or bagassosis.

pneumonoconiosis (nū′mō-nō-kō-ni-ō′sis): Dust disease. Fibrosis of the lung caused by long continued inhalation of dust in industrial occupations, such as coal mining, stone cutting, etc. The most important complication is the occasional superinfection with tuberculosis. Examples are silicosis, coal worker's P., asbestosis, siderosis, grinder's asthma and byssinosis, described elsewhere. — pneumonoconioses, pl.

pneumopericardium (nū′mōper-i-kar′di-um): The presence of air in the pericardial sac.

pneumoperitoneum (nū′mō-per-it-o-nē′um): Air or gas in the peritoneal cavity. May follow performated gastric ulcer, peritonitis, other pathological conditions, or may be introduced for diagnostic or therapeutic reasons.

pneumoradiography (nō′mō-rā-di-og′ra-fi): Radiographic examination of a region after injection of air, oxygen or other gas.

pneumoresection (nū′mō-rē-sek′shun): Surgical removal of part of a lung.

pneumorrhagia (nū-mō-rā′ji-a): Haemorrhage from the lungs.

pneumotachograph (nū-mō-tak′ō-graf): A device for measuring the flow of air going to and from the lungs. Some models also measure several other parameters of respiration, *e.g.*, tidal volume, inspired oxygen fraction, expired carbon dioxide.

pneumotaxic (nū-mō-tak′sik): Relating to pneumotaxis. P. CENTRE the centre in the pons that stimulates the expiratory centre in the medulla.

pneumotaxis (nū-mō-tak′sis): The control of the rate of respiration. — pneumotaxic, adj.

pneumothorax (nū-mō-thaw′raks): Air or gas in the pleural cavity; causes severe pain, dyspnoea, absence of breath sounds, abnormal distension of the chest. ARTIFICIAL P. induced in the treatment of pulmonary tuberculosis; OPEN P., P. caused by an injury to the chest wall that exposes the pleural cavity to the atmosphere; SPONTANEOUS P. occurs when an overdilated pulmonary air sac ruptures, permitting communication between the respiratory passages and pleural cavity; TENSION P. occurs when a valve-like wound allows air to enter the pleural cavity at each inspiration but not to escape on expiration, thus progressively increasing intrathoracic pressure.

pneumotoxin (nū-mō-tok′sin): An endotoxin produced by the pneumococcus and believed to be responsible for the systemic symptoms of lobar pneumonia.

pneumoventriculography (nū'mō-ven-trik'ū-log'ra-fi):): Examination of the cerebral ventricles by x-ray after removal of the fluid content and direct injection of air.

-pnoea: Combining form denoting (1) breath; (2) breathing.

pO₂: The symbol for the partial pressure of oxygen; in arterial blood normally about 100 mgHg; lower than 70 mmHg denotes a serious oxygen lack.

pock: A pustule, specifically the pustular lesion characteristic of chickenpox and, formerly, smallpox.

pockmark: The small, depressed mark, scar, or pit left after the pustular lesion of chickenpox heals.

pod-, podo-: Combining forms denoting foot or foot-like.

podagra (pō-dag'ra): Gout in the foot, especially that in the metatarsophalangeal joint of the big toe.

podalgia (pō-dal'ji-a): Pain in the foot or feet.

podalic (pōdal'ik): Pertains to accomplishment by means of the feet. P. VERSION see under VERSION.

podarthritis (pod-ar-thrī'tis): Arthritis of the joints of the feet.

podiatrist (po-dī'a-trist): One who specializes in the diagnosis and treatment of diseases and defects of the feet (primarily an American term). Syn., *chiropodist*. — podiatry, n.

podobromidrosis (pōd'ō-brō-mid-rō'sis): Offensive perspiration of the feet.

pododynia (pōd-ō-din'i-a): Pain in the foot or feet. Syn., *podalgia*.

podogeriatric (pōd-ō-jer-i-at'rik): Refers to foot care for the elderly.

podopompholyx (pōd-ō-pom'fo-liks): See CHEIROPOMPHOLYX.

-poiesis: Combining form denoting production or the formation of.

poikilocyte (poy'kil-ō-sīt): A large irregularly shaped red blood cell; frequently found in severe haemolytic anaemias.

poikilocytosis (poy'kil-ō-sīl tō'sis): 1. Variation in the shape of red blood corpuscles, *e.g.*, the pear-shaped cells found in the blood in pernicious anaemia. 2. The presence of poikilocytes in the circulating blood.

poikiloderma (poy'kil-o-der'ma): A skin disorder characterized by dryness, pigmentation, purpura, mottling, and atrophy. P. CONGENITALE a hereditary disorder characterized by erythema and pigmentation of the skin, telangiecstasia, skeletal defects, baldness, hypogonadism, and juvenile cataracts.

poison (poy'z'n): Any substance that is harmful or lethal when applied to or taken into the-body.

poison control centre: A facility equipped with personnel and reference works adequate to answer questions of the public about poisons and treatments for poisoning. Often associated with hospitals or medical schools, there are several in the United Kingdom.

poisoning (poy'z'ning): A state produced by the introduction of a poisonous substance into the body, or by exposure to such substance. ACID P. causes erosion of the tissues and skin; ALKALI P. corrosive P.; most often due to ingestion or contact with lye, or with sodium or potassium hydroxide; CARBON MONOXIDE P., P. due to inhalation of carbon monoxide gas which is contained in automobile exhaust, illuminating gas, sewer gas, and in mines.

poker back: Ankylosing spondylitis. See under SPONDYLITIS.

polarity (po-lar'i-ti): 1. In physics, the property of having two opposite poles, as in a magnet or storage battery. 2. The presence or manifestation of opposing or contrasting principles, tendencies or emotions, as love and hate, or femininity and masculinity.

polarization (pō'lar-ī-zā'shun): 1. The separation of the positive and negative charges in a molecule. 2. The production or acquisition of polarity. 3. A condition in which substances of opposite electrical charges are separated by a membrane, as in the cells of the body. — polarize, v.

poli-, polio-: Combining forms denoting relationship to the grey matter of the nervous system.

policy (pol'-i-si): 1. A course of action adopted and pursued by a government, party, ruler, or statesman. 2. Advantageous or expedient conduct.

policy-making: The decision process by which individuals, groups, or institutions establish a course of action pertaining to plans, programmes, or procedures.

polio: Colloquial term for poliomyelitis (*q.v.*).

polioencephalitis (pō'li-ō-en-kef-a-lī'tis,-sef-): Inflammation of the grey matter of the brain. Caused by poliomyelitis virus; marked by fever, headache, anxiety, confusion, trembling, twitching of facial muscles, insomnia, sometimes convulsions, lethargy; often fatal. — polioencephalitic, adj.

polioencephalomyelitis (pō'li-ō-en-kef'a-lō-mī'e-lī'tis,| sef'-): Inflammation of the grey matter of the brain and the spinal cord; caused by poliovirus.

poliomyelitis (pō'li-ō-mī'e-lī'tis): Inflammation of the grey matter of the spinal cord; an acute epidemic viral disease most commonly affecting children; marked by fever, headache, sore throat, stiff neck, gastrointestinal symptoms. May lead to paralysis and atrophy of one or more groups of skeletal muscles with resulting permanent deformity and disability. Many people who have had the disease have late effects, with symptoms that resemble those of the disease including pain in muscles along with weakness of muscles that had not been affected earlier, joint pain, fatigue, and general weakness; may require the use of braces and portable respirators; seldom fatal. ACUTE ANTERIOR P., P. in which the virus attacks the anterior horns of the grey matter of the spinal cord; ASCENDING P., P. that is first manifested in the legs and progresses upward; BULBAR P. a serious form of P. in which the virus attacks the medulla oblongata; there may be inability to swallow, paralysis, respiratory distress leading to respiratory failure; CEREBRAL P., P. that involves the brain stem and areas of the motor cortex; polioencephalitis; POSTINOCULATION P. symptoms of P. that appear, usually within three weeks, following some types of inoculation; SPINAL PARALYTIC P. the classic form of P. with flaccid paralysis of one or more limbs.

poliosis (pōl-i-ō'sis): Premature greying of the hair.

polio vaccine: Vaccine given for the purpose of conferring immunity to poliomyelitis.

poliovirus (pō'li-ōvī'rus): The causative agent of poliomyelitis. Three types are recognized serologically, of which Type One is the most frequent cause of paralytic poliomyelitis.

political parties: Groups within the established government system that hold particular beliefs/policies for conducting state affairs.

Politzer's bag: A soft, rubber, pear-shaped bag with a long tube and nozzle; used to inflate the inner ear via the nose and auditory tube. — politzerization, n.

pollex (pol'eks): The thumb. P. PEDIS the great toe. — pollices, pl.

pollinosis (pol-i-nō'sis): Allergic condition characterized by catarrh affecting the mucous membranes of eyes, nose, and respiratory tract; caused by sensitivity to pollen and recurs annually, usually in the spring or late summer. Hay fever and rose fever are examples of P. Also called *pollenosis*.

pollutant (po-lū'tant): Anything that acts to contaminate, befoul, dirty, or render impure the atmosphere or any other necessity for life; usually refers to agents that contaminate the human environment.

pollute (pol-lūt'): To render the environment or some substance impure, unclean, or unhealthful; to defile.

pollution (po-lū'shun): Defilement; uncleanness; impurity.

poly: Abbreviation and colloquial term often used to designate polymorphonuclear leukocyte.

poly-: Combining form denoting many several, diverse, excessive, multiple.

polyadenitis (pol'i-ad-e-nī'tis): Inflammation of several lymph nodes at the same time; refers especially to the cervical nodes.

polyaemia (pol-i-ē'mi-a): Excess amount of blood in the body.

polyandry (pol-i-an'-dri): A social setting in which a woman may be legally married to more than one man at the same time. — polyandrous, adj.

polyarteritis (pol-i-ar-te-rī'tis): Simultaneous inflammation of several arteries. P. NODOSA inflammation of the coats of the arteries in multiple circumscribed areas resulting in the formation of nodules; see PERIARTERITIS NODOSA.

polyarthritis (pol'i-ar-thrī'tis): Inflammation of several joints at the same time. See STILL'S DISEASE. Occasionally occurs in epidemic form, thought to be due to a virus; characterized by slight fever, rash, pain in joints of hands and feet.

polyarticular (pol-i-ar-tik'ū-lar): Relating to or affecting several joints simultaneously.

polyavitaminosis (pol'i-a'-vi-ta-min-ō'sis): A pathological condition in which there is a deficiency of more than one vitamin in the diet.

polyblennia (pol-i-blen'i-a): Excess production of mucus.

polycholia (pol-i-kō'li-a): Excessive secretion of bile.

polychondritis (pol-i-kon-drī'tis): Inflammation of cartilage in several parts of the body. RELAPSING P. an idiopathic condition in which recurring bouts of P. are accompanied by fever and malaise and may eventually result in deformities; affects chiefly the ears, nose, larynx, trachea, bronchi.

polychromasia (pol'i-krō-mā'zi-a): In physiology, variation in the amount of haemoglobin in the red blood cells.

polychromia (pol-i-krō'mi-a): Increased pigmentation or coloration in any part of the body.

polyclinic (pol-i-klin'ik): A clinic or hospital that cares for several types of diseases and injuries.

polycrotic (pol-i-krot'ik): Descriptive of a pulse that has several secondary waves following each pulse beat.

polycyesis (pol-i-sī-ē'sis): Multiple pregnancy.

polycystic (pol-i-sis'tik): Containing or composed of many cysts. P. KIDNEY DISEASE may be (1) congenital and slowly fatal, or (2) familial, with cysts forming in the medulla of the kidney, and usually seen in children. P. OVARY SYNDROME seen most often in women aged 15 to 30; characterized by large polycystic ovaries with small follicles that do not mature enough to ovulate but become cystic.

polycystoma (pol-i-sis-tō'ma): A condition in which a part of the body has many cysts; said especially of the breast.

polycythemia: A condition in which there is a net increase in the total circulatingerythrocyte mass of the body. Primary polycythemia (called polycythemia vera) occurs when excess erythrocytes are produced as a result of tumorous abnormalities of the tissues that produce blood cells. Secondary polycythemia is caused by increases in the production of erythropoietin that result in an increased production of erythrocytes.

polycytosis (pol'i-sī-tō'sis): An increase in the red and white cells of the blood with a reduction in blood volume.

polydactyly (pol-i-dak'ti-li): A congenital anomaly consisting of the presence of more than the normal number of fingers or toes. Also called *polydactilia* and *polydactylism.*

polydipsia (pol-i-dip'si-a): Frequent drinking because of excessive thirst, a characteristic of diabetes; may also be of psychogenic origin, due to a personality disorder.

polygalactia (pol'i-ga-lak'shi-a): Excessive secretion of milk.

polygene (pol'i-jēn): Any of a group of genes which, acting together, tend to influence the same character traits in the same way, resulting in a cumulative effect in the individual.

polyglandular (pol-i-glan'dū-lar): Relating to or affecting several glands and/or their secretions.

polygraph (pol'i-graf): An instrument that records several impulses or pulsations simultaneously; *e.g.*, pulse beat, blood pressure, and respiratory movements, any or all of which may be affected by emotional reactions, and thus useful in detecting lying or deception. Commonly called a *lie detector.*

polyhidrosis (pol'i-hīd-rō'sis): Excessive secretion of sweat; hyperhydrosis.

polyhydramnios (pol'i-hī-dram'ni-ōs): The presence of more than the normal amount of amniotic fluid in the uterus at term; appears to be associated with a high percentage of congenital anomalies, especially anencephaly and oesophageal atresia.

polyhydruria (pol-i-hī-drū'ri-a): The presence of an abnormally large fluid content of the urine.

polyhypermenorrhoea (pol'i hī'per-men-ō-rē'a): Frequent profuse menstruation.

polyhypomenorrhoea (pol'i-hī'pō-men-ō-rē'a): Frequent scanty menstruation.

polyinfection (pol-i-in-fek-shun): Mixed infection; infection with two or more organisms at the same time.

polyleptic (pol-i-lep'tik): Descriptive of diseases that have many remissions and exacerbations, *e.g.*, malaria.

polymastia (pol-i-mas'ti-a): The condition of having more than two breasts.

polymenorrhagia (pol'i-men-ō-rāj'i-a): Menstrual periods that are both too heavy and too frequent.

polymenorrhoea (pol'i-men-ō-rē'a): Menstrual periods that are normal in amount but occur too frequently.

polymer (pol'i-mer): A natural or synthetic chemical compound that results when two or more molecules of the same substance are combined to form a larger molecule.

polymerization (pol'i-mer-ī-zā'shun): The building up of large molecules, usually of high molecular weight, by combining identical smaller ones.

polymicrogyria (pol'i-mī-krō-jī'ri-a): A condition of the cerebral cortex, characterized by many small convolutions, caused by faulty brain development.

polymorphic (pol-i-mor'-fik): Multiform; existing or occurring in several forms.

polymorphonuclear (pol'i-mor-fō-nū'kli-ar): Having a many-shaped or lobulated nucleus; usually applied to the neutrophil leukocytes which constitute about 75% of the total white blood cell count and which function as phagocytes. See BASOPHIL; EOSINOPHIL.

polymorphous (pol-i-mor'fus): Occurring in many different morphologic forms; polymorphic.

polymyalgia (pol'i-mī-al'ji-a): Myalgia affecting several muscles at the same time. P. RHEUMATICA a syndrome affecting older people; marked by pain and stiffness in the proximal muscles and joints in the neck, and in the shoulder and pelvic girdles, accompanied by a high sedimentation rate; responds to corticosteroid therapy.

polymyositis (pol-i-mī-ō-sī′tis): Inflammation of several muscles at the same time. Often refers to a group of disorders characterized by slowly developing muscle pain and weakness, especially of the shoulder and pelvic girdles, dysphagia, arthralgia, fever, erythematous rash and purplish discoloration of the skin of the face, neck, chest, hands and elbows; seen most often in females. In older people often associated with malignancy.

polyneuritis (pol-i-nū-rī′tis): Inflammation of many peripheral nerves at the same time. Some of the causes are alcoholism; poisoning, particularly from metals; vitamin deficiency, especially of thiamine. ACUTE IDIOPATHIC P. may follow a febrile illness; characterized by sensory disturbances, muscular weakness, impaired reflexes; see also GUILLAIN-BARRÉ SYNDROME and LANDRY'S DISEASE.

polyneuropathy (pol′i-nū-rop′a-thi): Disease involving several nerves simultaneously, usually peripheral and/or cranial nerves; characterized by aching, burning, numbing, and tingling of the lower legs and feet; symptoms may extend to the arm; may be associated with such systemic disorders as diabetes, uraemia, carcinoma, alcoholism, poisonings.

polyopia (pol′i-ō′pi-a): Seeing many images of a single object simultaneously; multiple vision.

polyorchidism (pol-i-or′ki-dizm): The condition of having more than two testes.

polyp or polypus (pol′ip-us): A small, smooth, finger-like growth arising from the skin or a mucous surface (in the cervix, uterus, nose, rectum), usually attached by a stem. Most often benign but may become malignant. — polypi, pl.; polypous, adj.

polypectomy (pol-i-pek′to-mi): Surgical removal of a polyp.

polypeptides (pol-i-pep′tīdz): Proteins with long chains of amino acids linked together by peptide bonds.

polyphagia (pol-i-fā′ji-a): Pathological overeating; excessive appetite. See BULIMIA.

polypharmacy (pol-i-far′-ma-si): The concurrent use of many different medications, or drugs, in the treatment of a single patient.

polyphobia (pol-i-fō′bi-a): Morbid fear of many things.

polyphrasia (pol-i-frā′zi-a): Excessive or insane talkativeness. Syn, *verbigeration*.

polyplegia (pol-i-plē′ji-a): Paralysis of several muscles at the same time.

polypnoea (pol-ip-nē′a): Very rapid breathing; panting.

polypoid (pol′i-poyd): Resembling a polyp.

polyposis (pol′i-pō′sis): A condition in which there are numerous polypi in an organ. P. COLI a hereditary condition in which polypi occur throughout the large intestine, starting in childhood and increasing progressively with symptoms of colitis; it almost always leads to carcinoma of the colon when untreated. Also called *familial intestinal P*.

polysaccharide (pol-i-sak′a-rid): Any one of a class of carbohydrates containing a large number of monosaccharide groups $(C_6H_{12}O_6)_x$. Starch, inulin, glycogen, and cellulose are examples.

polysinusitis (pol′i-sīn-ūsī′tis): Inflammation of several sinuses at the same time.

polysomnography (pol′-i-sōm-nog′ra-fi): The continuous recording of such physical parameters as eye movements, heart rate, brain waves, muscle tonus, etc.; used in diagnosing sleep disorders.

polythelia (pol-i-thē′li-a): The condition of having supernumerary nipples; may be on the breast or elsewhere on the body.

polytrichia (pol-i-trik′i-a): Excessive hairiness.

polyunsaturated (pol′i-un-sat′ū-rā-ted): A chemical term referring to fatty acids that have two or more unsaturated bonds; they tend to be liquid at room temperature; found in soybeans; fish oil; corn; sunflower, safflower, and cottonseed oils. These oils, and foods made from them, are less likely to form plaque than saturated fats.

polyuria (pol-i-ū′ri-a): Excretion of excessive amounts of urine; may be due to intake of excess solute that has to be excreted, failure of the kidney to concentrate the urine, inadequate secretion of antidiuretic hormone, or renal pathology including atherosclerosis of renal arteries, congestive heart failure, hypertension, diabetes insipidus. — polyuric, adj.

polyvalent (pol′i-vā-lent, po-liv′-a′-lent): Usually refers to a serum or vaccine that is effective against several strains of a particular organism.

Pompe's disease: Glycogen storage disease, Type II; a hereditary condition characterized by excessive storage of glycogen in the heart, liver, and skeletal muscles; severe weakness and enlarged heart. Prognosis for life is poor.

pompholyx (pom′fol-iks): Vesicular skin eruption on the palms of the hands or soles of the feet. See CHEIROPOMPHOLYX.

pomphus (pom′fus): A blister or weal on the skin. — pomphoid, adj.

pons: A bridge; a process of tissue joining two sections of an organ. — pontine, adj. PONS

VAROLII the white convex mass of nerve tissue at the base of the brain which serves to connect the cerebrum, cerebellum and medulla oblongata.

pontine (pon'tēn): Relating to the pons varolii.

popliteal (pop-li-tē'al): Relating to the posterior surface of the knee. P. CYST see BAKER'S CYST; P. SPACE the diamond-shaped depression at the back of the knee joint, bounded by the muscles and containing the popliteal nerve and vessels.

popliteus (pop-li-tē'us): A muscle at the back part of the knee joint; it assists in flexing the leg at the knee and in rotating the leg.

Popper, Karl: A twentieth-century philosopher; a self-professed 'critical-rationalist', a dedicated opponent of all forms of scepticism, conventionalism, and relativism in science and in human affairs generally, a committed advocate and staunch defender of the 'open society', and an implacable critic of totalitarianism in all of its forms.

poradenitis (por'ad-e-nī'tis): A condition characterized by the formation of small abscesses in the iliac glands; occurs in lymphogranuloma venereum (q.v.).

pore: A small opening. One of the minute openings of the ducts that lead from the sweat glands to the surface of the skin; they are controlled by fine papillary muscles that contract in the cold, and dilate in the presence of heat.

porencephalia, porencephaly (por'en-ke-fā'li-a, kef'a-li,-sef'-): A condition in which there are abnormal cysts or cavities in the brain substance; may be congenital or due to imperfect development, infection, or injury following birth.

pores of Kohn: Small holes in the walls of the alveoli that allow communication between parts of the lung lobules that are supplied by different bronchioles.

pornography (por-nog'ra-fi): 1. The depiction of erotic behaviour in books or other media with the objective of arousing sexual excitement. 2. Devices such as pictures and books intended to arouse sexual excitement through depiction of erotic behaviour.

porosis (pō-rō'sis): The formation of cavities or holes in the tissue, e.g., osteoporosis (q.v.).

porosity (pō-ros'i-ti): 1. A pore, as in the skin. 2. The condition of being porous.

porphobilinogen (por'fō-bī-lin'o-jen): A chromogen involved in the biosynthesis of haem and porphyrin; found in the urine of some patients with acute intermittent porphyria.

porphyria (por-fir'i-a): A pathological state due to an inborn error of metabolism of blood pigments, resulting in the production of excess porphyrins in the blood, faeces, and urine. Symptoms include abdominal pain, profound neuritis, weakness that may progress to total paralysis, pathological changes in nervous and muscular tissue, a variety of mental symptoms, and excessive amounts of porphyrin precursors in the urine. ACUTE INTERMITTENT P. a rare form of P. that may be precipitated by certain drugs, infection, or pregnancy; seen mostly in young and middle-aged persons characterized by extreme sensitivity to light along with other symptoms of P.; CONGENITAL ERYTHROPOIETIC P. a rare form of P. seen in infants and young children; due to a defect in the synthesis of haemoglobin; characterized by cutaneous photosensitivity that leads to formation of mutilating lesions, enlarged spleen, haemolytic anaemia, and the presence of porphyrins in the blood; often causes early death; P. CUNEA TARDA a form of P. marked by photosensitivity, skin lesions, liver disease, and the presence of porphyrins in the urine; may be caused by the ingestion of certain drugs or alcohol; P. HEPATICA includes several types of P. including those that occur following hepatitis or heavy metal poisoning.

porphyrin (por'fi-rin): Any one of a group of organic pigments that are widely distributed in nature and also exist in small amounts in the human body.

porphyrinuria (por'fi-rin-ū'ri-a): Excretion of porphyrins in the urine. Such pigments are produced as a result of an inborn error of metabolism. The urine becomes red or dark brown in colour. See PORPHYRIA.

porrigo (po-rī'gō): Any disease condition of the scalp in which there is scaling or loss of hair or a tendency to spread.

porta: The depression (hilum) of an organ at which the vessels and nerves enter and, in some organs, excretory ducts leave. — portal, adj. P. HEPATIS the transverse fissure through which the portal vein, hepatic artery and bile ducts pass on the under surface of the liver.

portacaval (por'ta-kā'val): Relating to the portal vein and inferior vena cava. P. ANASTOMOSIS or P. SHUNT a fistula made between the portal vein and the inferior vena cava with the object of reducing the pressure within the portal vein in cases of cirrhosis of the liver.

portahepatitis (por'ta-hep-a-tī'tis): Inflammation around the transverse fissure of the liver.

portal (por'tal): 1. Relating to any porta or hilum, especially to the porta hepatis (see under PORTA). 2. The point of entrance of a pathogenic organism into the body; the most common P.S OF ENTRY are (1) through the mouth and/or nose to the respiratory tract, by inhalation; (2) through the mouth to the alimentary tract, by ingestion; and (3) through the skin to the deeper tissues, by inoculation. P. VEIN that conveying blood into the liver; about 7.5 cm long, it is formed by the union of the superior mesenteric and splenic veins.

Porter–Silber test: A laboratory test for the amount of 17-corticosteroids excreted in the urine as a means of evaluating adrenocortical function.

portfolio (port-fō'-li-ō): 1. A receptacle or case for keeping loose sheets of paper, prints, drawings, maps, music, or the like. 2. A body of work. 3. A collection of investments. P. OF EVIDENCE a collection of evidence produced by a candidate to prove his/her competence, comprising such items as certificates, examples of work, testimonials, etc. linked directly to the performance criteria (*q.v.*); PROFESSIONAL P. see APPENDIX 8.

portogram (por'tō-gram): X-ray film of the portal vein after injection of radiopaque liquid.

portosystemic (por'tō-sis-tem'ik): Relating to the portal system. P. ENCEPHALOPATHY see HEPATIC ENCEPHALOPATHY under ENCEPHALOPATHY.

port-wine stain or mark: A purplish-red superficial haemangioma of the skin occurring as a birthmark; a naevus (*q.v.*).

position: Posture; attitude. An arrangement of the parts of the body considered desirable or necessary for some medical or surgical procedure or for an examination. In obstetrics, the situation of the fetus in the pelvis as determined by the relation of an arbitrary point (occiput, chin, sacrum) to the right or the left side of the mother. ANATOMICAL P. the person stands erect with the arms at the sides and palms facing forward; DORSAL P. the person lies flat on the back; DORSAL RECUMBENT P. the person lies flat on the back with the knees lightly flexed and rotated outward; FOWLER'S P. the person's head or the head of the bed is elevated to about 125 cm above bed level; the knees are flexed and supported by a pillow; variations are specified as high, low, and semi-Fowler's; FROG P. P. sometimes assumed by premature infants or those with central nervous system disorders; the child lies prone with the thighs held in external rotation at the hips and abducted to about 90°; GENUPECTORAL P. the person kneels on the table with the head and upper part of the chest also resting on the table;

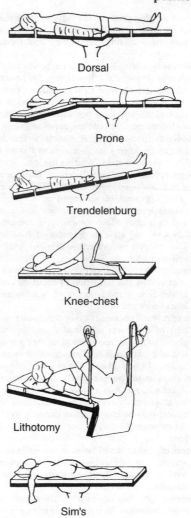

Dorsal

Prone

Trendelenburg

Knee-chest

Lithotomy

Sim's

Positions for various examinations.

the arms are raised and crossed over the head; GYNAECOLOGICAL P. the lithotomy P.; JACKNIFE P. the person lies on the back with the legs flexed and the thighs at right angles to the torso; KNEE–CHEST P. the genupectoral P.; LATERAL P. the person lies on the side with the knees slightly flexed; LITHOTOMY P. the person lies on the back with the thighs flexed and abducted; the feet may be supported by stirrups; PRONE P. the person lies flat and face

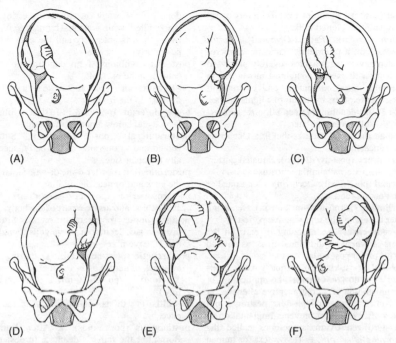

(A) (B) (C)

(D) (E) (F)

The pelvis brim showing the six fetal positions: (a) left occipitoanterior; (b) right occipitoanterior (c) left occipitolateral; (d) right occipitolateral; (e) left occipitoposterior; (f) right occipitoposterior.

downward; RECUMBENT P. the person lies on the back with knees slightly flexed and the arms crossed over the abdomen; SHOCK P. the patient is kept lying down in full Trendelenberg P. (q.v.), with the head of the bed lowered, or in a modified Trendelenberg P. in which only the legs are elevated; SIM'S P. the person lies on the left side, with the right knee and thigh drawn up well above the left, the left arm behind the person and hanging over the edge of the table, and the chest inclined forward so the person rests on it; SUPINE P. the dorsal P.; TRENDELENBERG P. the person lies on the back, with the body elevated at an angle of 45°, the head down.

positioning: Placing a patient in a bed or chair in a position that corrects postural faults, minimizes dangers of faulty posture, and helps correct impaired breathing.

positive: 1. Definite as opposed to negative. 2. Indicates that a substance, microorganism, or condition tested or examined for is present in the material or individual examined.

positive end expiratory pressure: The pressure in mechanical ventilation that is held at some preset level at the end of expiration, to keep the lungs partially inflated and to prevent collapse of the alveoli. Abbreviated **PEEP**.

positive pressure breathing: Inflation of the lungs with air (or oxygen) under pressure to produce inspiration. Exhaled air, hand bellows, or more sophisticated apparatus can be used. Elastic recoil of lungs produces expiration.

positivism (poz′-i-tiv-izm): 1. A system of philosophy that recognizes only positive facts and observable phenomena, with the objective relations of these and the laws that determine them, abandoning all enquiry into their ultimate origins. 2. A religious system founded upon this philosophy, in which humanity is the object of worship. 3. A general term referring to the view that every rationally justifiable assertion can be scientifically verified or is capable of logical or mathematical proof.

posology (pō-sol′o-ji): That branch of materia medica that is concerned with dosage.

posset (pos'set): In infant feeding, refers to regurgitation of clotted milk.

possum (pos'm): *P*atient-*O*perated *S*elector *M*echanism, a proprietary name for a microswitch device that enables severely paralysed patients with even the slightest movement to use telephones, computers, and to transmit messages to others by means of a lighted panel.

post-: Prefix denoting (1) behind, after, posterior; (2) subsequent to, later.

postanaesthetic (pōst'an-es-thet'ik): Occurring after anaesthesia.

postauditory (post-aw'di-tō-ri): Situated posterior to the external auditory meatus.

postcibal (pōst-sī'bal): Occurring after a meal or after taking food.

postclimacteric (pōst-klī-mak'ter-ik): Occurring after the end of the reproductive period.

post-code care: The rationing of care on the basis of where an individual lives, as defined by his or her post code.

postcoital (post-kō'i-tal): After sexual intercourse. P. CONTRACEPTION the application or administration of a contraceptive after the act of coitus; P. PILL a high-dose oestrogen pill taken after coitus; it prevents implantation of the fertilized ovum, sometimes called the *'morning after' pill*; P. TEST a test for human fertility, done as soon as possible after intercourse, one or two days before ovulation; involves microscopic examination of the cervical mucus for active and motile sperm. Also called *Huhner's test.*

postconcussional syndrome (pōst-kon-kush'onal sin'drōm): The headache, dizziness, and feeling of faintness that may follow a head injury and persist for a considerable length of time.

postdiphtheritic (pōst-dif'-ther-it'ik): Following an attack of diphtheria. Refers especially to paralysis of the limbs and palate.

postencephalitic (pōst-en-kef'-a-lit'ik,-sef'-): Following encephalitis lethargica. The adjective is commonly used to describe the syndrome of the parkinsonism which often results from an attack of this kind of encephalitis.

postepileptic (pōst-ep-i-lep'tik): Following or occurring as a consequence of an epileptic seizure. P. AUTOMATISM a fugue state following a fit, when the patient may undertake a course of action, even involving violence, without having any memory of this; see FUGUE.

posterior (pos-tēr'-i-or): 1. Situated towards the rear or behind a structure; opp. of anterior. 2. Situated or relating to the back of the body;

dorsal. P. CHAMBER OF THE EYE the ring-like space filled with aqueous human (*q.v.*) between the iris anteriorly and the ciliary body posteriorly.

postero-: Combining form denoting posterior, behind, at the back of.

posteroanterior (post'er-ō-an-tē'ri-or): From the back to the front.

posteroinferior (pos'ter-ō-in-fē'ri-or): Situated behind and below a part of the body.

posterolateral (pos-ter-ōlat'er-al): Situated behind and to one side of the body, specifically the outer side.

posteromedian (pos-ter-ō-mē'di-an): Situated at the back and/or near the midline.

posterosuperior (pos'-ter-ō-sū-pēr'i-or): Situated behind and above a part of the body.

postganglionic (pōst'gang-gli-on'ik): Situated distal to a collection of nerve cells (ganglion) as a P. nerve fibre.

postherpetic (po'st-her-pet'ik): Occurring after an attack of herpes or as a sequel.

posthetomy (pos-thet'o-mi): Circumcision (*q.v.*).

posthitis (pos-thī'tis): Inflammation of the prepuce.

posthumous (pos'tū-mus): 1. After death. 2. Born after the father's death. 3. In obstetrics, born by Caesarean section after the mother's death.

posthypnotic (post-hip-not'ik): After hypnosis. P. SUGGESTION one made while the person is under hypnosis but carried out after returning to a normal state, without the person being aware of the origin of the suggestion.

postictal (post-ik'tal): Following a sudden fall, attack, stroke, or seizure such as an epileptic seizure.

postmature (pōst-ma-tūr'): 1. Overly developed. 2. Past the expected date of delivery. A baby is postmature when labour is delayed beyond 40 weeks or 280 days. — postmaturity, n.

postmenopausal (pōst'-men-ō-paw'zal): Relating to or occurring in the period following menopause.

post-modernism: A complicated set of ideas that have emerged as an academic study in the past two decades. A concept that appears in a wide range of disciplines including art, architecture, music, film, literature, sociology, fashion, and technology.

postmortal (pōst-mor'tal): Occurring after death.

post-mortem (pōst-mor'tem): 1. Relating to the period after death. 2. Relating to an examination of the body after death. P. EXAMINATION

post-mortem 473 potassium

an examination of the dead body to determine the cause of death or the pathological changes produced by the disease; autopsy.

postmyocardial infarction syndrome (post'mī-ō-kar'di-al in-fark'shun sin'drōm): Pyrexia and chest pain associated with inflammation of the pleura, lung, or pericardium; due to sensitivity to products released from affected muscle. Also called *Dressler's syndrome*.

postnasal (pōst-nā'zal): Situated behind the nose and in the nasopharynx. — postnasally, adv. P. DRIP the continual dripping of nasal mucus down the back of the throat instead of out of the nostrils; often more annoying than significant. Causes include allergies, low-grade infections, cold or foggy climate, polluted air, excessive smoking.

postnatal (pōst-nā'tal): Occurring after birth. P. CARE includes the care of the mother for at least 6 weeks after delivery. P. PERIOD a period not less than 10 and not more than 28 days after the end of labour, during which the continued attendance of the midwife on the mother and baby is mandatory.

postocular (pōst-ok'ū-lar): Situated behind the eyeball.

postoperative (pōst-op'er-at-iv): Occurring or following soon after surgery. — postoperatively, adv.

postoral (pōst-o'ral): Situated behind or in the back part of the mouth.

postpartum (pōst-par'tum): Occurring soon after childbirth. P. DEPRESSION see under DEPRESSION; P. HAEMORRHAGE that occurring soon after childbirth and as a result of it; P. PSYCHOSIS a psychosis arising soon after childbirth, usually referring to one arising within three months of childbirth; often schizophrenic in nature; cause may be organic or emotional, or due to endocrine imbalance; symptoms include insomnia, instability of mood, hallucinations, withdrawal, restlessness, elation, suspiciousness.

postphlebitic syndrome (pōst-flē-bit'ik): A condition following thrombosis of a vein, especially a leg vein; the valves are destroyed and the thrombosed vein is obliterated resulting in chronic venous insufficiency.

postprandial (pōst-pran'di-al): Following a meal.

Post-Registration Education and Practice: See APPENDIX 8.

post-term (pōst-term): Refers to an infant born after more than 42 weeks of gestation.

post-tranfusion syndrome (pōst-trans-fū'zhun sin'drōm): A condition that may occur several weeks or months after blood transfusion or sometimes after heart surgery; symptoms resemble those of mononucleosis, including fever, hepatomegaly, splenomegaly, and the presence of atypical lymphocytes in the blood; thought to be caused by cytomegalovirus. Also called *postperfusion syndrome*.

post-traumatic stress disorder (traw-mat'-ik): A complex health condition that can develop as a response to a traumatic experience, see TRAUMA. Symptoms include anxiety, depression, sleep disturbance,frightening thoughts, nightmares, memories, flashbacks, and anger. Treatment options include cognitive-behavioural therapy, group therapy, and exposure therapy.

postulate (pos'tū-lat): A self-evident claim, demand, requirement, or basic principle, assumed without proof. KOCH'S P. a list of four experimental conditions that an organism must meet before it can be declared to be the cause of a disease.

postural (pos'tū-ral): Relating to or affected by posture. P. DRAINAGE usually infers drainage from the respiratory tract, by elevation of the foot of the bed, positioning the patient, or using a special frame; P. HYPOTENSION see ORTHOSTATIC HYPOTENSION under HYPOTENSION.

posture (pos-tūr): Active or passive arrangement of the whole body, or a part, in a definite manner.

postvaccinal (pōst-vak'sin-al): Following, or resulting from, vaccination.

pot: A street term for cannabis.

potassaemia (pot-a-sē'mi-a): The presence of more than the normal amount of potassium in the blood.

potassium (pō-tas'i-um): A soft, silvery-white alkaline, metallic element, occurring widely in nature but always in combination. Present in all animal cells and important for normal growth and development, in maintenance of acid–base balance, and in normal muscle activity, especially cardiac muscle. It is poorly conserved by the body but because it is present in many foods the daily requirement is easily met; symptoms of deficiency include changes in the electrocardiogram, weakness of muscles, thirst; see HYPOKALAEMIA. Its salts have long been used in medicine. P. ACETATE white powder or crystalline flakes; used as an alkaline diuretic, diaphoretic, and systemic and urinary alkalizer; P. BICARBONATE white crystals or powder; used as a diuretic, to acidify urine, and to correct electrolyte imbalance; P. CHLORIDE used to correct potassium deficiency; P. GLUCONATE used to correct hypo-kalaemia and as a replenisher of potassium; P. IODIDE white crystalline substance used in ex-pectorants; P. PERMANGANATE odourless purple crystals, used as an antiseptic and de-odorizer, and as an antidote in certain poison-ings.

pot-belly: A large, protruding belly, a fairly common condition in middle-aged males of sedentary occupations; due to a collection of fat in the omentum and weakening of the ab-dominal muscles. In children, often a symp-tom of disease conditions such as congenital megacolon, or the result of improper diet.

potency (pō-ten'si): 1. Inherent strength; force; or power. 2. The ability of a male to carry out sexual intercourse; often refers specifically to penile erection. See IMPOTENCE. 3. The strength of a drug.

potent (pō'tent): 1. Possessing inherent strength, force. 2. Describing a medicinal preparation that is highly effective. 3. Capable of produ-cing powerful mental or physical effects. 4. Of a male, able to engage in sexual intercourse.

potential (pō-ten'shal): Latent; existing as a possibility and having the power to eventually become an actuality. P. ENERGY energy that is stored in the body but not in actual use. See also ACTION POTENTIAL.

potentiation (pō-ten-shē-ā'shun): 1. The syner-gistic effect of a substance which, when added to another, increases the potency of that sub-stance. 2. The effect of combining two or more drugs which together produce an action greater than when the drugs are given separ-ately. — potentiate, v.

potion (pō'shun): A large draught of liquid medicine or other liquid mixture.

Pott: P.'S DISEASE spondylitis; occurs primarily in children and young adults. Usually of tu-berculous origin affecting one or more verte-brae; necrosis of the bone causes compression of the vertebrae and results in stiff spine, pain on motion, and kyphosis; P.'S FRACTURE a fracture at the lower end of the fibula and of the medial malleolus of the tibia with lateral and backward displacement of the foot; P.'S PUFFY TUMOUR osteomyelitis of the skull following injury without laceration; accom-panied by oedema. [Percival Pott, English physician, 1714–1788.]

Potter's syndrome: A rare congenital anomaly marked by skeletal and renal abnormalities; pulmonary hypoplasia; characteristic facies with widely spaced eyes, furrowed forehead, large low-set, floppy ears; and small jaw; clubbed feet. Often associated with oligohy-dramnios (*q.v.*). Affected infants are often stillborn or die soon after birth.

Potts' operation: A direct side-to-side anasto-mosis between the aorta and the pulmonary artery; used in cases of tetralogy of Fallot. [Willis J. Potts, American surgeon, 1895–1968.] — Also called *Pott–Smith–Gibson op-eration.*

pouch: A pocket, recess, or cul-de-sac. RECTOU-TERINE P. a cul-de-sac that lies between the posterior surface of the uterus and the anterior surface of the rectum; also called *Douglas' pouch*; RECTOVESICLE P. the fold of the peri-toneum that in the male extends downwards between the urinary bladder and the rectum; UTEROVESICLE P. the fold of the peritoneum that in the female lies between the anterior surface of the uterus and the urinary bladder.

poultice (pōl'tis): A soft, moist, pulpy mass spread between two layers of material and ap-plied, usually hot, to an external surface to relieve pain and congestion and improve circulation in the area, or to hasten suppur-ation. Materials used include bread, mustard, linseed.

Poupart's ligament: See INGUINAL LIGAMENT.

powder: 1. A mass of dry substance separated into minute particles; 2. A single dose of a drug in powdered form, usually contained in a paper. 3. To reduce a solid mass of a substance to fine particles.

power: 1. Ability to act so as to affect a person or thing. 2. A person, group, or body invested with authority or having influence. 3. A mental or bodily faculty or potential capacity. 4. Strength, force, energy, as actually exerted. 5. Influence, dominion, authority; legal authority or authorization. MATHEMATICAL P. (1) the product obtained by multiplication of a quan-tity or number by itself; (2) the index showing the number of times a factor is multiplied by itself.

powerlessness: Without power or ability; devoid of power; helpless.

pox: 1. Any disease characterized by an erup-tion, especially a pustular eruption. 2. An eruption. 3. Colloquial term for syphilis. See CHICKENPOX; SMALLPOX.

poxvirus (poks'vī'rus): Any of a group of rela-tively large viruses, including those that cause vaccinia and variola in humans.

PPD: Abbreviation for Purified Protein Deriva-tive (*q.v.*).

P–R interval: One of the segments of the elec-trocardiogram; it is a measure of the time between the beginning of the atrial depolarization and the beginning of the ventricular depolarization.

P–R segment: On the electrocardiogram, the interval between the end of the P wave and the beginning of the QRS complex.

practice development: A continuous process of improvement towards increased effectiveness of patient care.

practice nurse: A nurse employed within a general practice or health centre, providing a range of primary care services to patients in the community.

practicuum (prak-tik′-ū-um): A practice setting that simulates the real world, but which is relatively free of its distractions, risks, and pressures.

practitioner (prak-tish′un-er): A person engaged in practice in any profession. See NURSE, PRACTITIONER.

practitioner-based enquiry: A form of research in which practitioners explore their own practice using reflective and reflexive techniques.

practitioner-centred research: A process for converting personal learning from developments in professional practice, into shared knowledge available to all practitioners. It is concerned with increasing the stock of 'knowledge-of-practice', rather than increasing the stock of subject knowledge.

pragmatic (prag-mat′ik): Practical; matter-of-fact; concerned with practical aspects. P. EPISTEMIOLOGY relating to a belief that ideas are valuable only in terms of their consequences.

praxiology (prak′si-ol′o-ji): The science or study of behaviour.

praxis (prak′sis): A Greek term referring to the coming together of theory and practice as a single and indivisible whole. In nursing, a term employed to describe a model that integrates reflection on action (q.v.), reflection in action (q.v.), formal theory and informal theory, through hypothetico-deductive method (q.v.).

pre-: Prefix denoting (1) anterior, before, in front of; (2) preparatory, beforehand.

preanaesthesia (prē′an-es-thē′zi-a): Preliminary or light anaesthesia, usually produced by medication and induced prior to general anaesthesia.

preanaesthetic (prē′an-es-thet′ik): Relating to preanaesthesia, the period preceding anaesthesia, or to a drug given prior to general anaesthesia.

preauricular (prē′aw-rik′ū-lar): Situated in front of the auricle of the ear; used especially

with reference to the lymphatic nodes in this area.

precancer (prē′kan-ser): A condition that is expected eventually to become malignant.

precancerous (prē′kan′ser-us): 1. Occurring before cancer, with special reference to non-malignant pathological changes which are believed to lead on to, or to be followed by, cancer. 2. Tending to become malignant.

preceptor (prē′sep-tor): In nursing, a first-level professional nurse, with at least one year's experience in the relevant clinical field, who works on a one-to-one basis with a recently qualified nurse and who serves as a role model and clinical instructor, thus helping to reduce the reality shock often experienced by the new nurse on fully entering professional nursing practice. A preceptor may also be appointed to work with an experienced professional nurse during the orientation period when the nurse has moved into a new position or institution.

preceptorship (prē-sep′-ter-ship): A period of support for newly qualified nurses, midwives and health visitors or for those returning to nursing after a career break of five years or more. Preceptorship should be provided by the employer for a period of at least four months (UKCC 1993 recommendation).

precipitate (pre-sip′i-tāt): 1. To separate out or cause a substance in a solution or suspension to separate out. 2. A solid that is separated out from a solution or suspension. 3. Hasty or unduly rapid, as labour. — precipitation, n.

precipitin (pri-sip′i-tin): An antibody (q.v.) which forms a specific complex with precipitinogen (antigen); under certain physiochemical conditions this results in the formation of a precipitate.

preclinical (prē-klin′i-kal): Referring to the period before symptoms of a disease are recognizable.

precocious (pri-kō′shus): Exhibiting unusually early physical or mental development.

precomatose (prē-kō′ma-tōs): Relating to the state of consciousness which precedes the state of coma.

preconscious (prē-kon′shus): In psychoanalysis, thoughts that are submerged in the consciousness but which one can recall to mind when one wishes to do so.

precordial (prē-kor′di-al): Relating to the precordium. P. SHOCK a brief, high-voltage electric shock applied to the precordial area to convert abnormal arrhythmias to normal, or to correct ventricular fibrillation; P. THUMP a single sharp blow with the fist delivered over the midsternum from a distance of 20 to 25 cm above the sternum; an emergency measure that may be utilized by qualified personnel when a patient on a monitor develops ventricular fibrillation.

precordialgia (prē-kōr-di-al'ji-a): Pain in the precordium (q.v.).

precordium (prē-kōr' di-um): The area on the ventral surface of the body that lies immediately over the heart and stomach; comprises the epigastrium and lower, middle part of the thorax. — precordial, adj.

precursor (pre-kur'sor): Forerunner.

prediabetes (prē-dī-a-bē'tēz): Refers to potential predisposition to diabetes mellitus. Urine testing can detect the condition and it can sometimes be controlled by diet alone. — prediabetic, adj.; n.

prediction: 1. The action of foretelling future events. **2.** An instance of foresight, a prophecy.

predigestion (prē-di-jest'chun): Partial artificial digestion of foods before they are ingested.

predisposing (prē-dis-pōz'ing): Rendering one more vulnerable or susceptible to a disease condition.

predisposition (prē-dis-pō-zish'un): A latent or increased susceptibility to develop or contract certain diseases.

prednisolone (pred-nis'ō-lōn): A synthetic glucocorticoid having anti-inflammatory and anti-allergic effects.

pre-eclampsia (prē'ē-klamp'si-a): A condition characterized by albuminuria, proteinuria, oedema, azotaemia, hypertension, headache, confusion, irritability, and visual disturbances; arises usually after the 30th week of pregnancy, varies from mild to fatal; occurs most often in teenagers and women over 35; cause unknown. — preeclamptic, adj.

prefrontal (prē-fron'tal): Situated in the anterior portion of the frontal lobe of the cerebrum.

preganglionic (prē'gang-gli-on'ik): Preceding in front of a collection of nerve cells (ganglion) as a P. nerve fibre.

pregnancy (preg'nan-si): The state of having a developing embryo or fetus within the body; the state from conception to delivery of the fetus. The normal duration is 280 days (40 weeks or 9 months and 7 days) counted from the first day of the last menstrual period. ABDOMINAL P. development of the ovum in the peritoneal cavity; usually follows rupture of tubal P., primary abdominal implantation seldom occurs; EXTRAUTERINE P., P. developing outside the uterus; MULTIPLE P. more than one fetus in the uterus; PHANTOM P. see PSEU-

DOCYESIS; TOXAEMIA OF P., also known as *eclamphic toxaemia.*

pregnancy test: Any procedure used to diagnose pregnancy. See HUMAN CHORIONIC GONADOTROPHIN under GONADOTROPHIN.

pregnanediol (preg-nān-dī'ōl): A metabolite of progesterone found in the urine during pregnancy and during the progestational phase of the menstrual cycle; determinations during pregnancy indicate status of the placental function.

pregnant: Gravid; being with child; containing unborn young within the body.

prehensile (prē-hen'sīl): Equipped or adapted for grasping or seizing.

prehension (prē-hen'shun): The act of grasping or taking hold of.

prehypophysis (prē-hī-pof'i-sis): The anterior lobe of the pituitary body.

preictal (prē-ik'tal): Occurring before a stroke or a seizure, such as an epileptic seizure.

preinvasive (prē-in-vā'siv): Usually refers to malignant growths in which the cells are confined to their normal location and have not invaded surrounding tissues.

prejudice (prej'-u-dis): **1.** Preconceived opinion or judgement. **2.** Bias. **3.** Prepossession.

preload (prē'lōd): Refers to the volume of blood the heart has to pump out at each contraction, *i.e.*, the amount of blood that returns to the heart via the veins.

premature (prē-ma-tūr): Occurring before the usual or proper time. P. BABY one whose weight at birth is less than 5.5 pounds (2.5 kg); and therefore requires special treatment. Current synonyms are low birth weight, preterm or dysmature baby. Not all low birth weight babies are premature, but are included in the category 'small for dates'. See PLACENTAL INSUFFICIENCY; P. beat extrasystole (q.v.); P. LABOUR expulsion of the fetus before the 280th day of pregnancy.

premature ventricular contraction: A contraction that is out of regular sequence in the rhythm of the heartbeat; may or may not indicate the presence of heart disease.

premedication (prē-med-i-kā'shun): Drugs given before the administration of another drug, *e.g.*, those given before an anaesthetic for the purposes of allaying apprehension, producing sedation, inhibiting secretion of saliva and mucus from the upper respiratory tract, or to facilitate the administration of the anaesthetic.

premenarchal (prē-me-nar'kal): Relating to or occurring before menstruation has become established.

premenopausal (prē-men'ō-paw-zal): Before the menopause. P. AMENORRHOEA variation in the intermenstrual periods occurring before cessation of the menses.

premenstrual (prē-men'strōō'al): Preceding menstruation. P. SYNDROME or TENSION a cluster of symptoms that occur a few days prior to the appearance of the menses and subside with the onset of menstruation; most common in women over 30; exact cause unknown, but may be due to hormonal activity during the menstrual cycle. Symptoms include oedema of the hands and feet, breast tenderness, emotional instability, depression, anxiety, irritability. Mild analgesics are sometimes prescribed.

premolar (prē-mō'lar): One of 8 bicuspid teeth. There are two on each side of the jaw, between the canine and first molar.

premonitory (prē-mon'i-tōr-i): Relating to a warning experienced in advance of an event or a recognizable pathologic condition.

premunition (prē-mu-nish'un): A state of immunity that develops after an acute infection has become chronic and lasts as long as the causative organism remains in the body.

prenares (prē-nā'rēz): One of the anterior nares, nostril. — prenares, pl.

prenatal (prē-nā'tal): Occurring or existing before birth. Antenatal. — prenatally, adv.

pre-operative (prē-op'eī-at-iv): Before operation. — preoperatively, adv.

prep: Colloquial term meaning the preparation of an area (cleansing, shaving, etc.) for surgery, delivery, or other procedure.

preparalytic (prē-par-a-lit'ik): Before the onset of paralysis, often referring to the early stage of poliomyelitis.

prepartal (prē-par'tal): Before labour.

prepatellar (prē-pa-tel'ar): Situated in front of the kneecap. P. BURSITIS see under BURSITIS.

PREP: Abbreviation for Post-Registration Education and Practice; see APPENDIX 8.

preprandial (prē-pran'di-al): Before a meal.

prepuberty (prē-pū-ber-ti): The age preceding puberty. — prepubertal, adj.

prepuce (prē'pūs): The foreskin; the free fold of skin that covers the glans penis. In the female, a fold of tissue formed by the union of the labia minora anteriorly, the lower folds are attached under the surface of the clitoris.

preputium (prē-pū'shi-um): The prepuce (q.v.). — preputial, adj.

prerectal (prē-rek'tal): Situated in front of the rectum.

presacral (prē-sā'kral): Situated in front of the sacrum.

presacral air insufflation: Injection of air into retroperitoneal interstitial tissues, mainly used for x-ray demonstration of renal and adrenal outlines.

presby-, presbyo-: Combining forms denoting (1) old; (2) old age.

presbycardia (pres-bi-kar-di-a): Changes in the myocardium due to the ageing process along with pigmentation of the cardiac tissues; the heart reserve is decreased, but heart failure does not usually follow. Also called *senile heart disease*.

presbycusis (pres-bi-kū'sis): A sensorineural hearing loss which occurs typically in older persons; there is loss of sensitivity to sound, particularly those of high frequencies, and/or of the ability to distinguish words in speech; in addition to the ageing process, may be caused by long exposure to noise, certain drugs, or previous attacks of otitis media; usually bilateral and progressive. Also called *presbycusia, presbyacusia, presbyacusis*.

presbyope (pres'bi-ōp); A longsighted person.

presbyophrenia (pres-bi-ō-frē'ni-a): A mental disorder most often seen in the elderly, characterized by memory loss; disorientation, and confabulation. Often judgement remains relatively unimpaired. Also called *Wernicke's syndrome*.

presbyopia (pres-bi-ō'pi-a): Longsightedness due to loss of elasticity of the crystalline lens of the eye with consequent failure of accommodation; seen mostly in persons 45 and more years of age. — presbyopic, adj.; presbyope, n.

prescribe (prē-skrīb): To give directions orally or in writing for the administration of a remedy in the treatment of any disease condition.

prescription (pri-skrip'shun): A written formula, signed by a registered medical practitioner, directing the preparation and administration of a remedy. Also refers to instructions for grinding corrective lenses for eyeglasses. P. DRUG one that may be dispensed only on order of a registered medical practitioner.

Prescription Pricing Authority: A health organization that scrutinizes pricing and payment to contractors for the dispensing of NHS prescriptions, and management of the NHS low-income scheme. It also oversees the prevention of prescription and dispensing fraud within the NHS.

presenile dementia: See PRIMARY DEGENERATIVE DEMENTIA under DEMENTIA.

presenility (prē'sē-nil'i-ti): 1. Before senility is established. 2. Premature old age. — presenile, adj.

present 478 prickly heat

present (prē-sent'): **1.** To precede or appear first, as the part of the fetus that appears first at the os uteri. **2.** To come forward as a patient.

presentation (pre'zen-tā'shun): In obstetrics, the part of the fetus that is felt through the cervix at the start of labour and which first enters the brim of the pelvis. May be vertex, face, brow, shoulder or breech.

presenting symptoms: The symptoms or complaint for which a person seeks healthcare.

pressor (pres'or): **1.** A substance that tends to raise blood pressure. **2.** Involving or stimulating the vasomotor centre in the brain; P. DRUGS drugs that cause blood pressure to rise through increasing peripheral vasoconstriction.

pressoreceptor (pres'ō-rē-sep'tor): Baroreceptor (*q.v.*).

pressure: (presh'ur): **1.** A force or compression exerted against an area of the body. **2.** The sensation of touch aroused by compression against the skin. ARTERIAL P. the P. of blood within the arteries; BLOOD P. see BLOOD PRESSURE; CENTRAL VENOUS P., P. of the blood within the heart and great vessels of the thorax; can be measured accurately and automatically recorded; DIASTOLIC P. arterial blood pressure during the period of dilatation of the chambers of the heart; INTRACRANIAL P. the P. of the cerebrospinal fluid in the space between the brain and the skull; INTRAOCULAR P. see under INTRAOCULAR; MEAN ARTERIAL P. measured by means of an intra-arterial catheter; it is determined by averaging the systolic and diastolic pressure according to the formula:

$$\frac{\text{diastolic p.} + 2 + \text{systolic p.}}{-3}$$

NEGATIVE P., P. that is less than that of the atmosphere; P. AREAS bony prominences of the body, over which the flesh of bedridden patients is compressed between the bone and an external source of pressure; the latter is usually the bed, but may be a splint, plaster, upper bedclothes, etc. P. BANDAGE one applied so as to produce pressure; used to stop bleeding, prevent swelling, or to compress varicose veins; P. POINT a place at which an artery passes over a bone, against which it can be compressed, to stop bleeding; P. SORE decubitus ulcer; see under DECUBITUS; PULMONARY ARTERY P. pressure exerted on the pulmonary artery walls by blood being pumped out of the right ventricle; PULMONARY CAPILLARY WEDGE P. the blood pressure in the most distal peripheral capillaries of the pulmonary artery; measured by use of the Swan–Ganz catheter,

which is wedged into such a capillary; it is identical with left atrial pressure; PULSE P. the difference between the systolic and diastolic blood pressure; VENOUS P. may be either (1) peripheral, the constant pressure exerted by blood on venous walls, or (2) central, which is the venous blood pressure just before it enters the right atrium; read in centimetres of water and involving an invasive procedure utilizing either the cephalic or basilic vein; useful as a guide for treatment or for monitoring fluid replacement in patients with burns, shock, cardiac failure, or other critical condition.

pressure group: An association of people representing some special interest, who bring concerted pressure to bear on public policy.

presynaptic (pre'si-nap'tik): Located near or occurring before a synapse.

presystole (prē-sis'to-li): The interval just preceding the systole or contraction of the heart muscle. — presystolic, adj.

preterm: Refers to the birth of a child before the end of 37 weeks' gestation.

pretibial (prē-tib'i-al): In front of or on the front of the tibia.

prevalence (prev'-a-lens): In statistics, the total number of new cases of a specific disease at a particular point in time or during a specific period of time. P. RATE the number of cases present in a given geographical area or community at one time divided by the population of the area at the same time.

prevention: Rendering impossible an anticipated event or an intended act; see also PRIMARY PREVENTION.

preventive (prē-ven'tiv): Acting to prevent the occurrence of. P. MEDICINE that branch of medicine that deals with preventing the occurrence of disease in individuals or in the community at large.

prevesical (prē-ves'ik-al): Situated anteriorily to a bladder, especially the urinary bladder.

priapism (prī'a-pizm): [*Priapus*, the god of procreation.] Persistent and painful erection of the penis in the absence of sexual stimulation; usually due to disease; sometimes seen in sickle cell crisis and cord lesions.

priapitis (prī-a-pī'tis): Inflammation of the penis.

prickle cells: Cells of the stratum spinosum layer of the epidermis; so-called because of the rod-shaped processes that form intercellular bridges.

prickly heat: A non-contagious eruption that often occurs in hot humid weather; consists of small red pimples that itch, burn and tingle. See MILIARIA.

primary (prī'ma-ri): 1. First or most important in order of time and development. 2. First in rank or importance. PRIMARY COMPLEX Ghon's Focus; P. UNION healing by first intention, see under HEALING.

primary care: Initial point of contact for a client with the health service, ideally providing continuity and integration of healthcare. Its aims are to provide the patient with a broad spectrum of care, both preventive and curative, over a period of time and to co-ordinate all of the care the patient receives.

Primary Care Group: A group of primary healthcare professionals, including GPs, nurses and allied health professionals, working with a population of around 100,000. This group has been superseded by Primary Care Trusts (*q.v.*).

primary care nurse: See under NURSE.

Primary Care Trust: A self-governing body providing a range of services for primary care, where the health professional is the first point of contact with the patient. These health professionals include medical, dental, and ophthalmological practitioners, amongst others. The organization holds its own budget, and can provide services as it sees fit, appropriate to the local health need, without referral to the local health authority.

primary degenerative dementia, senile onset (before age 65 and at or after age 65): see SENILE PSYCHOSIS under PSYCHOSIS.

primary healthcare: Refers to either or both of two kinds of care: (1) care the person receives at his first point of contact with the health-care system usually within the community; (2) continued care of a health-care consumer by the same individual or team; it stresses holistic care and includes identification, management, and/or referral of health problems, integration of health-care services, restoration and maintenance of the consumer's health by preventive actions, which may be performed in the home, a health-care facility, or a community institution; the emphasis is on a close, long-term relationship between the consumer (the patient), his or her family, and the practitioner.

primary health-care system: Refers to the system or the context in which primary health-care is given, *e.g.*, occupational health unit, school health unit, public health service, clinic.

primary health-care team: Usually based in a health centre serving a defined geographical area. Consists of general practitioners, health visitors, domicillary midwives and district nurses supplemented as needed by paramedical staff, *e.g.*, a physiotherapist.

primary nurse: A nurse who is responsible and accountable for the assessment, planning, and implementation of the entire nursing care of a patient or group of patients for the duration of their stay in a hospital, hospice, care home, or community setting.

primary nursing: A model based on the therapeutic relationship between the nurse and the patient. A single nurse has primary responsibility for the planning, evaluation, and care of a patient throughout the course of illness, convalescence, and recovery.

primary prevention: 1. Stopping a disease or mental disorders form manifesting in susceptible individuals or populations, through promotion of health, including mental health, and specific protection, as in immunization, as distinguished from the prevention of complications or after-effects of existing disease. 2. Disease prevention at the earliest possible point.

primigravida (prim-i-grav'i-da): A woman who is pregnant for the first time. primigravidae, pl.

primigravidy (prī-mi-grav'i-di): The condition of being pregnant for the first time.

primipara (prī-mip'a-ra): A woman who has given birth to a viable child, whether alive or stillborn. — primiparous, adj.

primordial (prī-mor'di-al): Primitive, original; applied to the ovarian follicles present at birth.

primordium (prī-mor'di-um): The origin or earliest form of something, *e.g.*, the earliest recognizable part of an organ or part in an embryo.

principle (prin'si-p'l): 1. A fundamental truth, doctrine, or law. 2. A scientific law that explains the method of a natural action. 3. A rule of conduct, especially right conduct. 4. In pharmacology, the constituent of a drug or compound that is chiefly responsible for its action.

Prinzmetal's angina: See under ANGINA.

prison nursing: Nursing delivered in a custodial setting.

Private Finance Initiative (i-nish'-a-tiv): A government system enabling private capital to be employed in public sector projects.

privileged communication: Confidential information given by a patient to health-care personnel during physical examination or other procedures in connection with his diagnosis and treatment. See CONFIDENTIAL INFORMATION, CONFIDENTIALITY.

p.r.n.: Abbreviation for *pro re nata* [L.] (*q.v.*), meaning whenever necessary.

pro-: Prefix denoting (1) earlier than, prior to, before; (2) anterior to, located in front of; (3) projecting.

probability (prob-a-bil'-i-ti): The likelihood of being realized, which any statement or event bears in the light of present evidence. See also *p* value.

proband (prō'band): Propositus (*q.v.*).

probe (prōb): 1. A slender, somewhat flexible rod-like metal instrument with a blunt tip, used typically for exploring body cavities or wounds. 2. To use a probe for exploration purposes.

problem-based learning: An approach to learning which develops students' self-teaching skills. It aims to produce lifelong learning (*q.v.*) through encouraging students to consider specific clinical problems and discuss what they are learning in relation to their past and current experiences. It further challenges students to identify issues relating to the clinical situation that needs resolution. See EN-QUIRY-BASED LEARNING.

problem-oriented medical information system: A medical record system that records, manipulates, and retrieves, the entire health and health-care data on individual patients over time. It provides a framework for health-care professionals to analyse and improve health-care actions including nursing.

problem-oriented medical records: A system of record keeping in which an individual's health problems are listed in order of need for care at his entrance into the health-care system; all team members record care given and plan their care according to priorities implied by the list, which also becomes a checklist for the nursing audit. Consists of four logically sequenced parts: the database, the problem list, plans for care, and follow-up.

procedure (prō-sē'jur): In healthcare, a series of orderly steps followed in carrying out a treatment or operation.

procephalic (prō-ke-fal'ik,-se-): Related to or situated on or near the anterior part of the head.

process (pros'es): 1. A projection or outgrowth from the mass of an organism or part, especially from a bone. 2. A method system, or mode of action utilized in doing something. ACROMIAL P. the acromion; ALVEOLAR P. the parts of the mandible and maxilla that surround the teeth; ARTICULAR P. any of the four articulating processes of the vertebrae (two superior and two inferior); CAUDATE P. a P.

on the caudate lobe of the liver; DENDRITIC P. the branching processes of a nerve cell; a dendrite; ENSIFORM P. see under XIPHOID; ODONTOID P. the toothlike process extending upwards from the body of the axis; it articulates with the atlas; OLECRANON P. the olecranon (*q.v.*); TRANSVERSE P. a P. that projects laterally on either side of a vertebra. See also CORACOID, CILIARY, MASTOID, PALATINE, PTERYGOID, STYLOID, XIPHOID.

procidentia (prō-si-den'shi-a): Complete prolapse of an organ or part, especially the uterus so that it lies within the vaginal sac but outside the contour of the body.

proconvertin (prō-kon-vert'in): A blood factor required for the formation of a blood clot (Factor VII). Also called *stable factor*.

procreate (prō'krē-āt): To beget; produce offspring. Term applied usually to the male parent. — procreation, n.

proct-, procti-, procto-: Combining forms denoting anus or rectum, or both. See also words beginning RECT-, RECTO-.

proctalgia (prok-tal'ji-a): The occurrence of pain in the anal region or the rectum.

proctatresia (prok-ta-trē'zi-a): Imperforation of the anus. Anal atresia. See ATRESIA.

proctectomy (prok-tek'to-mi): Surgical removal of the rectum, usually because of the presence of a malignancy.

proctitis (prok-tī'tis): Inflammation of the mucous membrane of the rectum.

proctocele (prok'tō-sēl): Prolapse of the mucous coat of the rectum. Rectocele (*q.v.*).

proctocolectomy (prok'tō-kol-ek'to-mi): Surgical removal of the rectum and colon.

proctocolitis (prok'tō-ko-lī'tis): Inflammation of the rectum and colon; usually a type of ulcerative colitis.

proctology (prok-tol'o-ji): That branch of medicine that deals with the study of the anus, rectum and sigmoid and the treatment of their diseases.

proctoperineoplasty (prok'tō-per-i-ne'ō-plasti): An operation for the repair of the anus and perineum. Also called *proctoperineorrhaphy*.

proctopexy (prok'to-pek-si): Operation for surgical fixation of the rectum to some other part.

proctoplasty (prok'to-plas-ti): Plastic surgery of the anus and rectum.

proctoptosis (prok-top-tō'sis): Prolapse of the anus and rectum.

proctorrhagia (prok-to-rā'ji-a): Bleeding from the anus.

proctorrhaphy (prok-tor'a-fi): Suturing of a lacerated anus or rectum.

proctorrhoea (prok-to-rē′a): Discharge of mucus from the rectum.

proctoscope (prok′to-skōp): An instrument with a light at the distal end, used for dilating and visually examining the rectum. See ENDO-SCOPE. proctoscopic, adj.; proctoscopy, n.

proctoscopy (prok-tos′ko-pi): Examination of the rectum by means of a proctoscope (*q.v.*).

proctosigmoidectomy (prok′tō-sig-moi-dek′to-mi): Surgical removal of the anus, rectum, and sigmoid flexure.

proctosigmoiditis (prok′tō-sig-moy-dī′tis): Inflammation of the rectum and sigmoid colon.

proctosigmoidoscopy (prok′tō-sig-moy-dos′ko-pi): Direct inspection of the rectum and the sigmoid colon with a sigmoidoscope. — proctosigmoidoscopic, adj.

proctostasis (prok-tos′ta-sis): Constipation with retention of faeces in the colon due to the inability of the rectum to respond to the stimulus for defecation.

proctostenosis (prok′-tō-ste-nō′sis): Narrowing or stricture of the rectum or anus.

proctotomy (prok-to′to-mi): Incision of the rectum to relieve a stricture.

prodrome (prō′drōm): 1. An aura. 2. An early manifestation of a disease condition before signs and symptoms develop. Also called *prodroma*. — prodromata, pl.

proenzyme (prō-en′zīm): A precursor of an enzyme which requires some change to render it active, *e.g.*, pepsinogen. Zymogen.

profession (prō-fesh′un): 1. An avowed declaration of belief. 2. A calling or vocation requiring specialist knowledge and skills within a recognized system of learning authenticated by professional members. A profession functions autonomously and continuously strives to extend its body of knowledge whilst maintaining and regulating standards.

professional (pro-fesh′on-al): 1. Related to one's own profession or occupation. 2. A specialist in a particular occupation or speciality. ALLIED HEALTH P. a person with training who is supervised by a health-care professional with responsibilities for patient care; P. BODY an organization that represents the interests of a profession and contributes to the development of that profession; P. JUDGEMENT a complex skill, using cognition, intuition, a high level of professional education and experience to make a decision, often in emergency situations, without being conscious of using a logical process; P. ORGANIZATION an organization formed to deal with issues of concern to its members, who share professional status and common goals.

professionalisation (pro-fesh′-un-al-ī-zā′-shun): To render professional in character.

professionalism (pro-fesh′-un-al-izm): The qualities, character, method, or conduct expected of a particular profession.

profundus (prō-fun′dus): Deep; deep-seated; profound. Term usually applies to certain deep-seated muscles or nerves. Also called *profunda*.

progeria (prō-jer′i-a): Premature senility, particularly that occurring in childhood.

progestational (prō′jes-tā′shun-al): 1. Before pregnancy; favouring pregnancy. 2. Term applied to a phase of the menstrual cycle that immediately precedes menstruation. 3. Pertaining to a class of drugs that have similar effects to those of progesterone. P. AGENTS a group of hormones produced by the corpus luteum and placenta and in small amounts by the adrenal cortex, including progesterone, also produced synthetically, *e.g.*, progestin.

progesterone (prō-jes′te-rōn): A hormone produced by the corpus luteum, placenta, and adrenal cortex; plays an important part in regulation of the menstrual cycle and in pregnancy. Also prepared synthetically for use in certain gynaecological disorders.

progestin (prō-jes′tin): Name used for certain synthetic progestational agents. See PROGESTATIONAL, PROGESTERONE.

prognosis (prog-nō′sis): A forecast of the probable course, duration, and termination of a disease. — prognostic, adj.

progressive patient care: A system of caring for patients whereby the facilities are adapted to the needs of various types of patients. Acutely ill patients are cared for in an intensive care unit; those who are moderately ill are cared for in an intermediate care unit; those who need very little assistance with their physical care but who must remain in hospital, are cared for in a self-care unit. The objective is to allow patients to live as nearly normal lives as possible and to make the best use of the available nursing staff.

proinsulin (prō-in′sū-lin): A precursor of insulin, elaborated in the beta cells of the pancreas.

Project 2000: A system of pre-registration nurse education introduced in 1986. Nurses were educated to diploma level within higher education. The programme included a common foundation programme of 18 months and an 18-month branch programme for adult, child, mental health or learning disabilities nursing. The curriculum promoted a health-based rather than a sickness-based model, and focused on primary healthcare. See also MAKING A DIFFERENCE.

projectile vomiting: Sudden vomiting, usually without preceding nausea, so forcibly that the vomitus is projected for some distance.

projection (prō-jek'shun): 1. A prominence or extending process of a bone. 2. In psychology, a defence mechanism occurring in normal people unconsciously, and in an exaggerated form in mental illness, especially paranoia, whereby the person fails to recognize certain emotionally unacceptable motives, feelings, and behaviours in himself and attributes them to others, thus imparting his own faults to another.

prolactin (prō-lak'tin): A hormone produced by the anterior lobe of the pituitary gland; stimulates and sustains the production of milk by the mammary glands.

prolactinoma (prō-lak-tin-ō'ma): A large tumour of the pituitary gland which secretes prolactin, as does the gland itself.

prolapse (prō-laps'): 1. Descent; downwards displacement of an organ or body structure from its usual position. 2. A falling forward or down. P. OF THE CORD premature expulsion of the cord during labour; P. OF AN INVERTEBRAL DISC nucleus pulposis; see NUCLEUS; P. OF THE IRIS part of the iris bulges forward through a corneal wound; P. OF THE RECTUM the lower part of the intestinal tract extends downwards in varying degrees, sometimes protruding through the external anal sphincter; P. OF THE UTERUS the uterus descends into the vagina and may be visible at the vaginal orifice. See PROCIDENTIA.

proliferate (prō-lif'er-āt): To increase by cell division. — proliferation, n.; proliferative, adj.

proliferation (prō-lif-er-ā'shun): Rapid and increasing production, especially of cells and morbid growths.

prolific (prō-lif'ik): Fruitful, multiplying abundantly.

proline (prō'lēn): One of the amino acids.

prominence (prom'i-nens): A protrusion or projection. LARYNGEAL P., that in the front of the neck, formed by the thyroid cartilage of the larynx; Adam's apple.

PROMIS: Abbreviation for problem-oriented medical information system (q.v.).

promontory (prom'on-to-ri): A projection; a prominent part.

pronate (prō'nāt): To turn the ventral surface downward, e.g., to lie on the face; or to turn the palm of the hand downward. — pronation, n. Opp. of supinate.

pronation (prō-nā'shun): The position of the forearm and hand when the palm is turned down, or of the foot when the sole is turned downward.

pronator (prō-nā'tor): That which pronates, usually applied to a muscle. Opp. of supinator.

prone (prōn): Lying with the face downward. Opp. of supine.

pronormoblast (prō-nor'mō-blast): A precursor and the earliest recognizable form of the erythrocyte.

propagation (prop-a-gā'shun): 1. Growth. 2. Reproduction.

prophase (prō'fāz): The first stage in cell mitosis (q.v.) in which the chromosomes duplicate and the two parts move away from each other although still attached by a thread-like structure.

prophylactic (pro-fi-lak'tik): 1. Acting to defend against something, particularly infection or disease. 2. An agent that acts to protect or defend (as a condom) against infection or disease.

prophylaxis (pro-fi-lak'sis): Prevention. — prophylactic, adj.; prophylactically, adv.

propositus (prō-poz'i-tus): In studies in human genetics, the person whose particular mental or physical characteristics served as a stimulus for the study. Also called *proband*.

proprietary (prō-prī'e-ta-ri): Refers to any medicine that is protected from competition by secrecy as to its composition or manufacture, or by trademark, copyright, or patent.

proprioception (prō'pri-ō-sep'shun): The awareness of one's balance and position in space, and of the position of one's body parts without looking at them.

proprioceptive (prō'pri-ō-sep'tiv): Refers to neural stimuli arising from receptors in internal tissues.

proprioceptor (prō-pri-ō-sep'tor): One of the sensory nerve terminals of the afferent nerves in the deeper structures of the body, e.g., muscles, tendons, joints. They are responsible for the sensation of position of the body and its parts and of changes in position. — proprioception, n., proprioceptive, adj.

pro re nata: Whenever necessary; as the occasion arises. Sometimes used in prescription writing to indicate that the medicine is to be given according to the patient's need for it.

proso-: Combining form denoting forward or anterior.

prosopagnosia (pros'-ō-pag-nō'si-a): Inability to recognize faces, usually associated with other forms of agnosia (q.v.).

prosopo-: Combining form denoting (1) the face; (2) a person.

prosopoplegia (pros-ō-pō-plē'ji-a): Facial paralysis.

prospective medicine: Preventive medicine. Involves intervention before signs and symptoms of disease appear, and regulating life patterns to prevent disease through periodic appraisals of health hazards.

prostaglandins (pros-ta-glan'dins): A group of several hormone-like, physiologically active substances of similar chemical structure, formerly thought to be produced only in the prostate but now believed to be produced by most body tissues; found in high concentrations in seminal fluid, menstrual blood, amniotic fluid, and in maternal blood during labour. Apparently involved in normal body functioning and in certain pathological conditions. Six types have been recognized, some of which have been synthesized and may be administered by mouth, intravenously, or by nebulizer for use in certain endocrine, nervous system, and blood and blood vessel disorders, although the therapeutic usefulness of prostaglandins has not been fully established. Prostaglandin F₂ is used, usually with urea, in interruption of pregnancy when it is administered by intra-amniotic instillation.

prostate (pros'tāt): A small conical gland at the base of the male bladder and surrounding the first part of the urethra. It secretes a milky fluid that is discharged into the urethra and mixes with the semen at the time of emission. — prostatic, adj.

prostatectomy (pros-ta-tek'to-mi): Surgical removal of part or all of the prostate gland. RADICAL P. removal of the entire prostate gland and its capsule, the seminal vesicle and rim of the bladder neck; may be indicated in cancer; RETROPUBIC P. removal of a mass from the prostate via an incision into the prostatic bladder; SUPRAPUBIC P., P. through an abdominal incision into the urinary bladder; TRANSURETHRAL P., P. by means of an operating cystoscope.

prostatic (pros-tat'ik): Relating to the prostate gland. BENIGN P. HYPERTROPHY a common disorder of middle-aged men; the glandular and cellular tissue of the prostate enlarge putting pressure on the urethra and causing urinary problems; the usual treatment is surgical.

prostaticovesical (pros-tat'i-kō-ves'i-kal): Relating to both the prostate gland and the urinary bladder.

prostatism (pros'ta-tizm): The condition of chronic disorders of the prostate, particularly enlargement of the prostate gland, which obstructs the flow of urine.

prostatitis (pros-ta-tī'tis): Inflammation of the prostate gland.

prostatocystitis (pros'-ta-tō-sis-tī'tis): Inflammation of the prostatic urethra and the male urinary bladder.

prostatodynia (pros'ta-tō-din'i-a): Pain in the prostate.

prostatolithotomy (pros'tat-ō-li-thot'o-mi): Removal of a stone from the prostate gland.

prostatomegaly (pros'ta-tō-meg'a-li): Enlargement or hypertrophy of the prostate gland.

prostatorrhoea (pros'ta-tō-rē'a): A thin catarrhal discharge from the prostate gland; often occurs in prostatitis.

prostatoseminovesicular (pros'ta-tō-sem'i-nō-ve-sik'ū-lar): Relating to the prostate and seminal vesicles.

prostatoseminovesiculectomy (pros'ta-tō-sem'i-nō-ve-sik-ū-lek'tō-mi): Surgical removal of the prostate and the seminal vesicles.

prostatovesiculitis (pros'ta tō-ve sik'ū-lī'tis): Inflammation of the prostate and the seminal vesicles.

prosthesis (pros-thē' sis): An artificial substitute for a body part, e.g.., eye, tooth, heart valve, blood vessel, limb, breast. MYOELECTRIC P. a device that enables an amputee to carry out ordinary tasks such as picking up things. — prostheses, pl.; prosthetic, adj.

prosthetics (pros-thet'iks): The art and science of making and adjusting protheses.

prosthetist (pros'the-tist): One skilled in making and adjusting prostheses.

prosthodontics (pros'thō-don'tiks): The branch of dentistry that deals with the construction of prostheses to replace missing teeth, or other oral structures.

prosthodontist (pros'thō-don'tist): A dentist who specializes in prosthodontics.

prostitution (pros-ti-tū'shun): 1. The soliciting of or engaging in sexual intercourse for money. 2. The act of debasing oneself or one's abilities, especially when it is done for money.

prostration (pros-trā'shun): Complete exhaustion; extreme loss of strength. NERVOUS P. neurasthenia (q.v.). See HEAT EXHAUSTION.

prot-, proto-: Combining forms denoting; 1. First in time, formation, rank, status, or importance. 2. Giving rise to.

protanomaly (prō'ta-nom'a-li): A defect of vision in which the response of the retina to the colour red is diminished.

protanopia (prō'ta-nō'pi-a): Red–green colour blindness. Also called *protanopsia*.

protease (prō'tē-ās): Any protein-splitting enzyme. GASTRIC P. pepsin.

protein (prō'tēn): A highly complex, nitrogenous compound, found in all animal and vegetable tissues; the principal consitutent of cell protoplasm. Proteins are built up of amino acids and are essential for growth and repair of the body. Those from animal sources are of high biological value since they contain the essential amino acids. Those from vegetable sources contain some but not all of the essential amino acids. P. is hydrolysed in the body to produce amino acids which are then used to build up new body tissues. COMPLETE P., P. that contains all of the essential amino acids; INCOMPLETE P., P. that lacks one or more of the essential amino acids; SECOND CLASS P., P. that contains only slight amounts of some of the amino acids.

proteinaceous (prō-tin-ā'shus): Relating to protein or being protein in nature.

proteinaemia (prō-tin-ē'mi-a): More than the normal amount of protein in the blood.

proteinosis (prō-tin-ō'sis): Accumulation or increase of protein in the tissues; ALVEOLAR P. a chronic disorder of the lung characterized by the accumulation of eosinophilic proteinaceous material in the distal alveoli; symptoms include chest pain, dyspnoea, productive cough, haemoptysis, and weakness.

proteinuria (prō-tin-ū'ri-a): The presence of protein in the urine. May be an isolated finding or indicate some abnormality or pathology of the kidney. Syn., *albuminuria; nephrotic syndrome.* ORTHOSTATIC P., occurs when individuals with lumbar lordosis are in the upright position; usually no renal pathology is present.

proteolysis (prō-tē-ol'i-sis): The breaking down of proteins into simpler substances. — proteolytic, adj.

proteolytic (prō-tē-ō-lit'ik): Relating to or promoting proteolysis. P. ENZYME an enzyme that acts as a catalyst in the digestion of protein.

Proteus (prō'tē-us): A genus of Gram-negative, flagellated, motile, rod-shaped microorganisms; found in damp surroundings and putrefying material. May be pathogenic, especially in wound or urinary tract infections as a secondary invader; P. MIRABILIS usually saprophytic and found in putrefying materials; may be pathogenic and associated with prostatitis, cystitis, infections of the uterus, and wounds; P. MORGANI usually a normal inhabitant of the gastrointestinal tract and associated with summer diarrhoea of infants; P. VULGARIS

found in dirty wounds, particularly those soiled with animal dung or mud.

prothrombin (prō-throm'bin): A factor in the plasma of the blood; a precursor of thrombin. It is synthesized in the liver when the supply of vitamin K is adequate. In the presence of thromboplastin and calcium it is converted into thrombin. P. TIME is (1) a widely used one-stage test for clotting time (normal time is 12–18 seconds), or (2) the time it takes for clot formation after tissue prothrombin and calcium have been added to blood plasma; it is increased in certain haemorrhagic conditions.

prothymia (prō-thim'i-a): Mental alertness.

protocol (prō'-to-kolz): 1. The original draft of an official document or transaction, especially minutes or a rough draft of a diplomatic instrument or treaty, signed by the parties to a negotiation. 2. Customs and rules of etiquette governing any social or official occasion. 3. An official memorandum or account. 4. An annexe to a treaty which adds to its provisions or clarifies them.

protodiastolic (prō'tō-dī-a-stol'ik): Refers to the period immediately following the second heart sound; the initial one-third of the diastole.

protogyny (prō-toj'i-ni): A form of hermaphrodism in which the female gonad matures before the male gonad.

proton (prō'ton): One of the basic parts of the nucleus of the atom, around which the electrons revolve; it carries a positive charge.

protopathic (prō-tō-path'ik): Primary; primitive. P. SENSIBILITY, term applied to peripheral sensory fibres, of low sensibility, for degree and location of the sensations of pain and heat. Opp. to epicritic (q.v.).

protoplasm (prō'tō-plazm): The thick, viscid, complex chemical compound constituting the main part of tissue cells; it may be clear or granulated and is surrounded by membrane. P. is the physical basis of all living cells.

protoporphyria (prō'tō-por-fir'i-a): A condition in which there is an abnormal amount of protoporphyrin (q.v.) in the faeces. ERYTHROPOIETIC P. an inherited disorder characterized by increased faecal excretion of protoporphyrin, increased protoporphyrin in the red blood cells, and development of acute urticaria or eczema soon after exposure to sunlight.

protoporphyrin (prō-tō-por'fir-in): A porphyrin (q.v.) which is linked with iron to form the haem of haemoglobin.

protopsis (prō-top'sis): Protrusion of the eyeball; exophthalmos.

protosyphilis (prō-tō-sif'i-lis): Primary syphilis.

prototype (prō'tō-tīp): 1. The primitive or original member of a class or species on which subsequent members are modelled. 2. An individual or quality that exemplifies the standard for members of a particular class or species.

protozoa (prō-tō-zō'a): The smallest type of animal life; single-celled organisms, capable of asexual reproduction. Diseases produced by them include malaria, amoebic dysentery, leishmaniasis. — protozoon, sing.; protozoal, adj. See AMOEBA.

protozoiasis (prō'tō-zō-ī'a-sis): Any disease caused by protozoa.

protozoology (prō-tō-zō-ol' o-ji): The scientific study of protozoa.

protraction (prō-trak'shun): An extension forward or outward. FACIAL P. a facial anomaly in which some facial structure such as the jaw stands farther forward than usual. In dentistry, the extension of the teeth or other part of the upper and lower jaw to a position farther forward than usual.

protuberance (prō-tu'ber ans): A projecting part, outgrowth, swelling, knob.

proud flesh: Excessive growth of granulation tissue in a wound or ulcer with little tendency towards scar formation.

provitamin (prō-vi'ta-min): A principle in certain foods which the body is able to convert into a vitamin, e.g., carotene is converted into vitamin A.

proxemics (prok-sem'-miks): The study of the personal and cultural needs of people and of their interactions with various aspects of their environment, including urban overcrowding.

proximal (prok'si-mal): Nearest the head or source. In anatomy, the part of an extremity, nerve, vessel, etc. that is nearest the trunk or point of origin of the part. Cf. distal. — proximally, adv.

proximate (prok'si-māt): Nearest, immediate. P. CAUSE the particular cause, among several, which is the immediate cause of disease; P. PRINCIPLE the active part of a drug substance.

prudent (proo'-dent): Showing knowledge, judiciousness, and cautiousness in activities or behaviour.

prurigo (prū-rī'gō): A chronic skin disease marked by formation of papules that itch intensely, occurring most frequently in children. BESNIER'S P. a common skin condition usually called infantile eczema when it occurs in infants and atopic dermatitis when it occurs in adults; P. AESTIVALE, hydroa aestivale (q.v.); P. FEROX a severe form; P. MITIS a mild form; P.

NODULARIS a rare disease of the adult female in which intensely pruritic pea-sized nodules occur on the arms and legs.

pruritus (prū-rī'tus): An unpleasant sensation that produces itching and the desire to scratch; caused by drugs, bites, or disease, including allergy. P. ANI and P. VULVAE are considered to be psychosomatic conditions (neurodermatitis) except in a few cases where a local cause can be found, e.g., worm infestation, vaginitis. Generalized P. may be a symptom of systemic disease as in diabetes, icterus, Hodgkin's disease, carcinoma, etc. It may be psychogenic, e.g., widow's itch which occurs shortly after bereavement. P. ANI itching of the skin around the anus; P. AESTIVALIS occurs during the summer; associated with prickly heat; syn., summer itch; P. HIEMALIS occurs in cold weather; appears mostly on the legs; P. SENILIS common in the aged; probably due to lack of oil in the skin; worse in cold weather; may be associated with diabetes, gout, myxoedema, atherosclerosis, neurosis, liver disease; P. VULVAE irritative condition of the vulva with intolerable itching; causes are poor hygiene, vaginitis, allergies, carcinoma, skin disorders, jaundice, glycosuria, nutritional deficiencies, psychological factors, tissue changes following menopause.

prussic acid (prus'ik as'id): A 4% solution of hydrogen cyanide; hydrocyanic acid. Both the solution and its vapour are poisonous, with death occurring very rapidly from respiratory paralysis.

psammotherapy (sam-ō-ther'a-pi): Treatment by the use of sand baths.

psellism (sel'lizm): Stammering; stuttering; mispronunciation or substitution of letter sounds.

pseud-, pseudo-: Combining forms denoting: (1) false, counterfeit, faked, feigned, or illusory; (2) a deceptive resemblance; (3) abnormal, aberrant.

pseudaphia (sū-daf'i-a): A defect in the perception of touch.

pseudarthrosis (sū-dar-thrō'sis): A false joint, e.g., due to ununited fracture; also congenital. Occurs primarily in the long bones. Also called pseudoarthrosis. GIRDLESTONE P. the creation of a false joint by removing the head and neck of the femur and upper half of the wall of the acetabulum and suturing a mass of soft tissue in the gap to form a cushion between the bones.

pseudoaneurysm (sū'-dō-an'ū-riz-em): False aneurysm. May be a rupture of all of the arterial coats, with the blood being retained by the tissues surrounding the vessel, or it may be due to a haematoma that does not involve the walls but which presents the appearance of an aneurysm.

pseudoangina (sū-dō-an-jī′na): False angina. Sometimes referred to as left mammary pain, it occurs in anxious individuals. Usually there is no cardiac disease present. May be part of effort syndrome.

pseudoarthritis (sū′dō-ar-thrī′tis): A condition resembling or mimicking arthritis.

pseudoblepsis (sū-dō-blep′sis): A condition in which a person sees objects different from what they really are; visual hallucinations.

pseudobulbar palsy (sū-dō-bul′bar): See under PALSY.

pseudocide (sū′dō-sīd): Consciously acting to harm oneself in such a way as to attract attention or gain sympathy, without intending to take one's life.

pseudocrisis (sū-dō-krī′sis): A rapid reduction of body temperature resembling a crisis, followed by further fever.

pseudocroup (sū-dō-kroop′): Laryngismus stridulus (*q.v.*).

pseudocryptorchism (sū′dō-krip′tor-kizm): A fairly common condition in which both testes are in the inguinal canal but can be brought down into the scrotum without surgery.

pseudocyesis (sū-dō-sī-ē′sis): The existence of signs and symptoms simulating those of early pregnancy occurring in a childless person with an overwhelming desire to have a child and who believes she is pregnant when, in fact, this is not so.

pseudocyst (sū′dō-sist): A dilated space in an organ that resembles a cyst but which does not have the epithelial lining found in a true cyst. PANCREATIC P. the accumulation of pancreatic secretion in a space behind the peritoneum; occurs in chronic pancreatitis following the rupture of a pancreatic duct.

pseudodementia (sū′dō-dē-men′shi-a): Extreme apathy and indifference to environment and general behaviour that simulates dementia but without impairment of the mental faculties; usually reversible; often refers to the masked expression frequently seen in the elderly.

pseudodiabetes (sū′dō-dī-a-bē′tēz): Subclinical diabetes; a condition marked by abnormal glucose tolerance test findings but no other signs of diabetes.

pseudoexophthalmos (sū′dō-eks-of-thal′mos): Abnormal protrusion of the eyeball for any reason other than exophthalmos, *e.g.*, shallow orbits or extreme myopia.

pseudogout (sū′dō-gowt): A condition in which there is a deposit of calcium crystals rather than urate crystals in and around small joints but especially the cartilage of the knee; occurs mostly in older people; also called *pyrophosphate arthropathy*.

pseudogynaecomastia (sū′dō-gīn-ē-kō-mas′ti-a): Increase in the size of the male breast by deposit of adipose tissue rather than breast tissue.

pseudohaematuria (sū′-dō-hēm-a-tū′ri-a): False haematuria; reddish discoloration of the urine due to ingestion of certain drugs or foods, not to the presence of blood.

pseudohaemophilia (sū′dō-hē-mō-fil′i-a): A non-hereditary disease of both men and women in which the clotting time is normal but the bleeding time is prolonged. False haemophilia.

pseudohaemoptysis (sū′dō-hē-mop′ti-sis): The spitting of blood that does not come from the bronchial tubes or lungs.

pseudohallucination (sū′dō-ha-lū-si-nā′shun): The appearance to an individual of geometric forms and figures which the person recognizes as hallucinatory, not real.

pseudohermaphrodite (sū′dō-her-maf′rō-dīt): A person with the gonads of one sex but with external genitalia that resemble those of the opposite sex.

pseudohermaphroditism (sū′dō-her-maf′rō-dit-izm): A condition in which the gonads are definitely of one sex but there are morphologic contradictions in the individual's make-up. FEMALE P. pertaining to a genetic female with female gonads but with some masculine characteristics; MALE P. pertaining to a genetic male with male gonads but with some feminine characteristics.

pseudohypertrophic muscular dystrophy: A type of muscular dystrophy, occurring most often in young boys; probably hereditary. Marked by hypertrophy of the muscles, especially those of the calf and shoulder, difficulty in walking, and later dystrophy of the muscles.

pseudohypertrophy (sū′dō-hī-per′trō-fi): Increase in size, of some part of the body, that is not true enlargement, *e.g.*, in muscular P. in which the increase in size is due to infiltration of the muscle tissue by other tissues, not to enlargement of muscle fibres.

pseudohyponatraemia (sū′dō-hī-pō-na-trē′mi-a): Low serum concentration of sodium that is the result of hyperglycaemia or hyperlipaemia; it does not indicate a diminution in serum osmotic pressure.

pseudohypoparathyroidism (sū′dō-hī′pō-par-a-thī′royd-izm): A condition in which the symptoms are the same as in hypoparathyroidism, but which is due to the body's inability to respond to the parathyroid hormone rather than to lack of the hormone.

pseudologia (sū-dō-lō'ji-a): Pathological lying, manifested in either speech or writing. P. FANTASTICA a constitutional tendency to tell and defend fantastic lies plausibly; seen in some individuals with hysteria.

pseudolymphoma (sū'dō-lim-fō'ma): Lymphocytoma cutis; see under LYMPHOCYTOMA.

pseudomembrane (sū'dō-mem'brān): A false membrane such as that which forms on the mucous membrane of the throat in diphtheria.

pseudomembranous (sū'dō-mem'bra-nus): Relating to a pseudomembrane. P. ENTEROCOLITIS a serious, often fatal disease involving the mucosa of the small bowel thought to be caused by a staphlylococcus organism; a pseudomembrane forms over the mucosa causing the latter to become inflamed and necrotic; symptoms include vomiting and severe bloody diarrhoea; may occur in persons receiving antibiotics.

pseudomnesia (sū-dom-nē'zi-a): False memory. Memory of events that have never occurred.

Pseudomonas (sū-do-mōn'as): A bacterial genus. Gram-negative motile rods, found commonly in water, soil, and decomposing vegetable matter. Several species are recognized. Some are pathogenic to plants and animals and occasionally to humans *e.g., P. pyocyanea (Bacillus pyocyaneus)*, found commonly in intestinal infections, sinuses and suppurating wounds; a secondary invader in some urinary tract infections and wound infections; produces a blue or blue-green pigment which colours the exudate or pus; also called *P. aeruginosa*.

pseudonystagmus (sū'dō-nis-tag'mus): Rhythmic jerking movements of the eyeball occurring as a symptom in various diseases of the central nervous system.

pseudoparalysis (sū'dō-pa-ral'i-sis): See PSEUDOPLEGIA.

pseudopelade (sū'dō-pē'lahd): A form of alopecia characterized by small patches of folliculitis that are followed by a scarring type of alopecia.

pseudoplegia (sū'dō-plē'ji-a): Paralysis mimicking that of organic nervous disorders but usually hysterical in origin.

pseudopodia (sū'dō-pō'di-a): False legs. The temporary projection of protoplasmic processes of an amoeba or of amoebal cells (leukocytes) for the purposes of locomotion or for the ingestion of food or other particles. — pseudopodium, sing.

pseudopuberty (sū'dō-pū'ber-ti): A condition characterized by varying bodily and functional changes typical of puberty before the natural chronological age of puberty; may be due to the hormonal secretions of a tumour.

pseudosmia (sū-doz'mi-a): The subjective sensation of perceiving an odour that is not present.

pseudostrabismus (sū'dō-stra-biz'mus): The false appearance of convergent strabismus seen particularly in infants and Orientals in whom the nasal bridges are flat, the interpupillary distances are narrow, and there is less sclera showing at the nasal side of the eyes. See STRABISMUS.

pseudotumour (sū'dō-tū'mor): The appearance of signs and symptoms of tumour in the absence of a tumour; spontaneous recovery usually ensues. P. CEREBRI a condition marked by signs of an intracranial tumour in the absence of any neoplasm; sometimes seen in hypervitaminosis or prolonged use of steroids; recovery is usually spontaneous but the optic nerve may be affected and cause blindness unless treated.

PSI: Abbreviation for psycho-social intervention (*q.v.*).

psilosis (sī-lō'sis): 1. Sprue (*q.v.*). 2. Falling out of the hair.

psittacosis (sit-a-kō'sis): Viral disease of parrots, pigeons and budgerigars which is occasionally responsible for a form of pneumonia in humans.

psoas (sō'as): One of two muscles of the loins, the psoas major or the psoas minor.

psoriasis (so-rī'a-sis): A chronic skin condition characterized by bright red, slightly elevated, round or oval areas that are covered with dry adherent scales that leave bleeding points when removed; when scales are scraped they produce a shiny, silvery sheen that is diagnostic. Non-infectious; cause unknown. May occur on any part of the body but characteristic sites are extensor surfaces, especially over the knees and elbows; GUTTATE P. an acute form consisting of teardrop-shaped red, scaly patches 3 to 10 mm in diameter over the entire body; may accompany beta-streptococcal pharyngitis or other upper respiratory infection; unless adequate treatment is instituted, a more severe form of P. may develop. — psoriatic, adj.

psoriatic (sō-rī-at'ik): Relating to psoriasis, P. ARTHRITIS or ARTHROPATHY an arthritic condition associated with psoriasis, often involving the distal interphalangeal joints; may be a variant of rheumatic arthritis, or an unassociated condition.

psych-, psycho-: Combining forms denoting (1) the mind, mental processes; (2) spirit, soul.

psychalgia (sī-kal'ji-a): Mental pain or distress; sometimes caused by mental effort; seen especially in states of melancholia.

psychanopsia (sī-kan-op'si-a): Psychic blindness; the individual is able to see but does not recognize what he sees; usually due to a brain lesion.

psychasthenia (sī-kas-thē'ni-a): A form of psychoneurosis marked by mental fatigue, unreasonable fears, obsessions and compulsion, feelings of inadequacy, lack of self-control, a sensation of unreality of self and surroundings, preoccupation with minor details to the extent that nothing worthwhile is accomplished.

psyche (sī'ke): The mind; the intellect, including both conscious and unconscious mental processes. In psychoanalysis, includes the id, ego, superego, and all their conscious and unconscious processes.

psychedelic (sī-ke-del'ik): 1. Mind-manifesting or mind-expanding. 2. Relating to drugs that have the immediate action of producing highly creative and imaginative thought patterns, enlarging the vision, producing freedom from anxiety, and altering sensation or perception, *e.g.*, peyote and LSD. Also called *psychodelic*.

psychiatric (sī-ki-āt'rik): Relating to psychiatry. P. NURSE see under NURSE; P. SOCIAL WORKER a specially trained social worker who assists psychiatric patients with problems of employment, housing, family affairs, and other situational adjustments that need to be made following discharge from an institution, and who refers the patient to appropriate helping agencies.

psychiatrist (sī-kī'a'-trist): One who specializes in psychiatry (*q.v.*); specifically, a medical school graduate with postgraduate training in the treatment of mental disorders.

psychiatry (sī-kī'at-ri): That branch of medical science that is devoted to the origin, diagnosis, treatment and prevention of mental, emotional or behavioural disorders; by extension may include problems of personal adjustment. — psychiatric, adj.

psychic (sī'kik): 1. Relating to the psyche; of the mind; mental. 2. A person who is thought to have unusual sensitivity to non-physical forces; a spiritualistic medium. P. ENERGIZER popular term for a drug that elevates or stimu-

lates the mood of a depressed person; P. HEALING an ancient healing mode often called faith healing because the laying on of hands, which is one aspect of it, often has a religious connotation; the assumption is that a transfer of healing energy passes from the healer to the patient, which is the basis of the modern practice of 'therapeutic touch'.

psychoactive (sī-kō-ak'tiv): Usually pertains to psychopharmacologic agents that have the ability to alter mood, behaviour, and cognitive processes.

psychoanalysis (sī'kō-a-nal'i-sis): A specialized branch of psychiatry founded by Freud. Briefly, the method is based on recall and analysis of a person's past emotional experiences and dreams with the purpose of understanding the origin of the patient's symptoms and furnishing hints as to the kind of psychotherapy that may eventually alleviate the symptoms, which are seen as manifestations of unconscious conflicts. — psychoanalytical, adj.

psychoanalyst (sī-kō-an'al-ist): One who specializes in psychoanalysis (*q.v.*).

psychobiology (sī'kō-bī-ol'o-ji): A school of psychiatric thought that views the biological, psychological, and sociological experiences of an individual as an integrated unit, and believes that the interactions of body and mind have an important influence on the development of personality. Also called *biopsychology*.

psychochemotherapy (sī'kō-kē-mō-ther'a-pi): The use of drugs to improve or cure pathological changes in the emotional state. — psychochemotherapeutic, adj.; psychochemotherapeutically, adv.

psychodrama (sī'kō-dra'ma): Therapeutically controlled acting-out. A method of psychotherapy whereby patients act out their personal problems in spontaneous dramatic performances and receive instructive feedback about solving their stressful experiences.

psychodynamic (sī-kō-dī-nam'ik): Referring to mental or emotional processes or forces and their effects on behaviour and mental states.

psychodynamics (sī-kō-dī-nam'iks): The science of the mental processes, especially of the causative factors in mental activity.

psychoendocrinology (sī'kō-en'dō-kri-nol'o-ji): The study of inter-relationships between endocrine functions and mental states.

psychogenesis (sī-kō-jen'e-sis): The development of mental and emotional traits.

psychogenic (sī-kō-jen'ik): Arising from or originating in the psyche or mind as opposed to having a physical basis. P. BLADDER inability of the bladder to fill to any extent, resulting in incontinence or excessively frequent voiding; due to a number of nervous and/or emotional factors; P. SYMPTOM a neurotic symptom.

psychogeriatric (sī'-kō-jer-i-at'rik): Relating to the care and management of geriatric patients with psychological or psychiatric problems. P. CARE involves measures to relieve symptoms, treating conditions that are treatable, and providing long-term care when necessary.

psychogeriatrician (sī'-kō-jer-i-a-trish'un): A psychiatrist who specializes in the treatment of geriatric patients with emotional disturbances or mental illnesses. Also called *geropsychiatrist*.

psychogeriatrics (sī'-kō-jer-i-at'riks): 1. The branch of medical science dealing with geriatric patients who have psychological or psychiatric disorders. 2. Psychology applied to geriatrics.

psychokinesia (sī'kō-ki-nē'zi-a): Impulsive behaviour; a burst of violent behaviour, often maniacal, resulting from lack of inhibition.

psychokinesis (sī'kō-ki-nē'sis)· The production or alteration of movement by the direct influence of the mind without any somatic influence. — psychokinetic, adj.

psycholepsy (sī'kō-lep-si): A sudden temporary mood change involving mental inertia, feelings of helplessness, confusion, tachycardia; seen in hysterical persons. — psycholeptic, adj.

psychological (sī-kō-loj'i-kal): Relating to psychology. P. DEPENDENCE a craving or psychological need for an abused substance; P. STRESS stress relating to or affecting the mind; existing only in the mind; P. TESTING the use of diagnostic tools such as cognitive and projective tests by psychologists to aid in assessing and planning treatment for the patient.

psychologist (sī-kol'o-jist): One who specializes in the study of the mind, especially as it affects behaviour. CLINICAL P. generally one who holds a doctoral degree in psychology and who has had supervised experience in working with clients who have mental disorders or disturbances.

psychology (sī-kol'o-ji): The science that deals with emotions, mental processes, and behaviour of an organism in its environment. Medically, the study of human behaviour. ADLERIAN P. emphasizes man's social nature; emphasizes organic inferiority as a prominent cause of neuroses and the use of compensation and overcompensation to overcome feelings of inferiority and attain superiority; ANALYTICAL BEHAVIOURAL P. see BEHAVIOURISM; DEVELOP-

MENTAL P. deals with changes in human behaviour in relation to age; FREUDIAN P. based on the theory that abnormal behaviour can be modified or corrected by allowing patients to talk about their early experiences, memories, dreams, and so on to the therapist who remains objective and non-judgemental; GESTALT P. a German school of psychology that teaches that the whole is more than the sum of its parts; that the parts are not put together to make the whole but are derived from it and get their character from it; that humans respond to meaningful entities that cannot be broken down into component parts. From the German word *gestalt*, meaning the whole appearance or shape; HUMANISTIC P. a term invented by Kurt Goldstein to describe an existential approach to psychology, which holds that humans are unique in their subjectivity and their capacity for psychological growth; that humans are innately good and strive for such growth; and that humans control their destiny to a greater extent than was formerly believed possible; INDIVIDUAL P. Adlerian P., INDUSTRIAL P., P. that deals with the application of psychological principles to the activities and problems that arise in business and industrial situations; JUNGIAN P. utilizing the patient's imagination in the analytical process, often asking patients to paint or draw an image or to act out a fantasy; Jung also considered the libido the will to live rather than an expression of the sex instinct; PHYSIOLOGIC P. deals with the functions of the nervous system as they relate to behaviour; SOCIAL P. deals with the cultural, ecological, and social influences on mental life and mental disorders; TRANSPERSONAL P. an area of psychological study that investigates experiences that go beyond the ordinary limitations of time and space, including those involving psychic phenomena, biofeedback, meditation, and energy transformation. — psychological, adj.; psychologically, adv.

psychometric (sī-kō-met'rik): Related to or being a measurement of the duration and force of mental processes.

psychometrician (sī-kō-me-trish'un): A researcher in the field of geriatric health-care services who investigates the methods for assessing and measuring the health status of individuals in long-term care situations; may or may not be a physician.

psychometrics (sī-kō-met'riks): The measurement of mental potential, ability, and functioning by means of psychometric tests (often called *intelligence tests*).

psychometric testing: Assessment of psychological variables by the application of mathematical procedures.

psychometry (sī-kom'e-tri): The science of testing and measuring psychologic and mental ability and processes.

psychomotor (sī-kō-mō'tor): Relating to motor activities initiated by psychic or cerebral activity. P. EPILEPSY recurrent, periodic disturbances of behaviour in which the person carries out certain repetitive movements semiautomatically; P. RETARDATION general retardation in both physical and emotional development; P. TESTS usually measure such things as muscular coordination and behavioural activity.

psychoneuroimmunology (sī'-kōl-nū'-rō-im'-mū-nol'o-ji): A relatively new field of science which seeks to find precise connections between the body and mind. It is concerned with such issues as therapeutic touch in which its proponents believe there is a transfer of energy from the healer to the patient.

psychoneurosis (sī-kō-nū-rō'sis): A functional disorder of the mind, usually mild in character, based on psychogenic factors. Neurosis. — psychoneurotic, adj.

psychopath (sī'kō-path): An eccentric, unstable, or mentally ill person with a poorly balanced personality who engages in egocentric, impulsive, immoral, or anti-social behaviour, but who knows better and is not insane. See also SOCIOPATH and PSYCHOPATHIC PERSONALITY under PERSONALITY DISORDERS.

psychopathology (sī-kō-pa-thol'o-ji): The study of pathology of the mind, or of maladaptive psychological functioning, personality, and/or social adjustment. — psychopathologic, psychopathological, adj.

psychopathy (sī-kop'a-thi): Any disease or disorder of the mind, especially one that is associated with character or personality defect.

psychopharmaceuticals (sī'kō-far-ma-sū'ti-kals): Drugs used in the treatment of emotional disturbances.

psychopharmacology (sī'kō-far| ma-kol'o-ji): The study of the action of drugs on the emotional state and on behavioural activity. CLINICAL P. includes both the study of drugs and their effects in patients and their use in treatment of psychiatric conditions. — psychopharmologic, psychopharmacological, adj.

psychophysics (sī-kō-fiz'iks): A branch of experimental psychology dealing with the study of stimuli and the related psychological experiences. — psychophysical, adj.

psychophysiological (sī'kō-fiz-i-ō-loj'ik): 1. Relating to behaviour as it relates to physiologic body processes. 2. Denoting an illness that exhibits physical symptoms but has an emotional cause; often called *psychosomatic disorder*; see PSYCHOSOMATIC.

psychophysiology (sī'kō-fiz-i-ol'ō-ji): The physiology of the mental apparatus or structures. — psychophysiological, adj.

psychoprophylactic (sī'-kō-prō-fi-lak'tik): That which aims at preventing mental ill-health or distress; often referring specifically to education programmes in preparation for childbirth by the Lamaze method (*q.v.*). — psychoprophylaxis, n.

psychosensory (sī-ko-sen'-sor-i): Relating to one's conscious perception of sensation.

psychosexual (sī-kō-seks'ū-al): Relating to the emotional aspects of sexuality as contrasted to the physical aspects. P. DEVELOPMENT the characteristic changes that take place in the libido during the years from infancy to adulthood, including the phases described as anal, oedipal, oral, phallic, latent, and genital.

psychosis (sī-kō'sis): A major mental illness of an organic or emotional origin, arising in the mind itself, as opposed to a neurosis in which the mind is affected by factors in the environment. Marked by such abnormal mental function or behaviour as loss of contact with reality, distortions of perception, diminished control of elementary desires and impulses, delusions, hallucinations. The deterioration of personality may be so great as to be incompatible with self-sustained social adjustment. AFFECTIVE P., P. with the predominant disturbance being in the person's emotions and attitude; marked by mood changes ranging from elation to depression, and by disturbances in thinking and behaviour; includes (1) cyclothymic disorders which are marked by chronic mood disturbances lasting at least two years, and (2) dysthymic disorders, marked by loss of interest in all activities but not severe enough or sufficiently long lasting to be called depression; ALCOHOLIC P. that caused by excessive use of alcohol; see WERNICKE–KORSAKOFF SYNDROME; DEPRESSIVE P. that caused by depression; marked by self-doubt, melancholia, guilt feelings, physical symptoms, thoughts of death and/or suicide; DISINTEGRATIVE P., P. marked by normal development during the first few years, then loss of speech, social competence and mental acuity; cause sometimes unknown, but may follow measles, encephalitis, or other serious infection; DRUG P., P. induced by toxic effects of certain drugs; FUNCTIONAL P. schizophrenia, manic–depressive, and involutional P.; GESTATIONAL P., P. that develops during pregnancy; HYSTERICAL P., P. that is characterized by sudden onset, hallucinatory delusions, bizarre behaviour; occurs often in self-centred individuals with hysteric personalities; ICU P. intensive care syndrome; a transient state characterized by disorientation, confusion, hallucinations, and sometimes delusions; usually reversible when the patient leaves the ICU; INVOLUTIONAL P. a severe P. characterized by depression, insomnia, anxiety, delusions, somatic concerns; occurs in older persons; MANIC–DEPRESSIVE P. a mental disorder characterized by mood swings towards either excitement or depression; not all patients exhibit both phases, and many experience periods of complete recovery between the two phases. Also called *bipolar disorder*, ORGANIC P., P. resulting from brain disorder or injury; POSTPARTUM P. that occurring after delivery; may be organic or toxic in origin; SCHIZO-AFFECTIVE P. that seen in schizophrenic persons who exhibit manic–depressive features; SENILE P. mental deterioration in old age, often accompanied by eccentric behaviour and irritability; TOXIC P., that caused by drugs, chemicals, or the presence of toxins in the body.

psychosocial (sī-kō-sō′shul): Relating to a person's psychological development in relation to his social environment. P. INTERVENTION a therapeutic technique that uses cognitive, cognitive–behavioural (*q.v.*), behavioural, and supportive interventions to relieve pain. It includes patient education, relaxation techniques, psychotherapy and structured or peer support.

psychosomatic (sī′-kō-sō-mat′ik): Relating to the intimate relationship of mental and bodily functions and their effects upon each other. Most commonly used to describe symptoms of illnesses that are at least partly psychic or emotional in origin.

psychosomimetic (sī′kō-sō-mi-met′ik): 1. Relating to symptoms that resemble those of psychosis or to drugs that produce psychosis-like symptoms. 2. A hallucinogen. Also called *psychotomimetic*.

psychostimulant (sī-kō-stim′ū-lant): A substance that has psychoactive properties, *e.g.*, amphetamines, coffee, cocaine.

psychosurgery (sī-kō-ser′jer i): Treatment of severe psychiatric disorders by surgery on the brain, especially by prefrontal lobotomy; once widely used in treatment of schizophrenia (*q.v.*).

psychosynthesis (sī′-kō-sin′the-sis): A lay movement promoting the use of therapy aimed at restoring useful inhibitions; the opposite of psychoanalysis.

psychotherapist (sī′-kō-ther′a-pist): A health-care professional who is trained in psychotherapy; may be a psychiatrist, clinical psychologist, nurse, or psychiatric social worker.

psychotherapy (sī′-kō-ther′a-pi): A form of therapy that may be used either in the treatment of organic diseases or of neuroses and psychoses; it is based on psychological methods, *e.g.*, psychoanalysis, hypnosis, suggestion, or persuasion rather than medical, pharmaceutical, or surgical methods. see COGNITIVE BEHAVIOURAL THERAPY under COGNITIVE; DIALECTICAL BEHAVIOURAL THERAPY. GROUP P., see GROUP THERAPY under THERAPY. — psychotherapeutic, adj.

psychotic (sī-kot′ik): 1. Related to or characterized by psychosis (*q.v.*). 2. A person suffering from psychosis, usually out of touch with reality and incapable of reasonable behaviour.

psychotogenic (sī-kot′-ō-jen′ik): Producing a condition of psychosis; often refers to certain drugs. — psychotogenesis, n

psychotropic (sī-ko-trō′pik): That which exerts its specific influence upon the psyche or mind. Term often used to describe drugs that affect cognitive functioning, such as tranquillizers, antidepressants, and psychotomimetics such as LSD (*q.v.*).

psychro-: Combining form denoting cold, freezing.

psychrotherapy (sī-krō-ther′a-pi): Treatment of disease by the application of cold.

psyllium (sil′i-um): The seeds of an African plant. They contain mucilage, which swells on contact with water; useful as a bulk-forming laxative.

pterion (tē′ri-on): The point on the skull where the frontal, parietal, and temporal bones and the great wing of the sphenoid bone meet; is the thinnest portion of the skull, located about 3 cm behind the outer process of the bony orbit.

pterygium (te-rij′ē-um): 1. Web eye; a triangular patch of mucous membrane and blood vessels, usually seen on the nasal side of the eye with the apex pointing towards the pupil; a benign growth associated with exposure to wind and sun; encroachment on the cornea results in disturbance of vision. Treatment is surgical. 2. Any fold of skin that extends abnormally from one part of the body to another. P. COLLI a congenital condition in which a tight band of skin extends from the acromion to the mastoid; usually bilateral.

pterygoid (ter'i-goid): Resembling a wing. P. MUSCLES four muscles that originate on the pterygoid process and insert into the mandible; they open and close the jaw and move it forward and from side to side; P. PROCESS one of two processes that extend downwards from either side of the sphenoid bone at the junctions of the wings with the body of the sphenoid.

ptilosis (ti-lō'sis): Falling out of the eyelashes.

ptosis (tō'sis): A drooping, falling, or sinking down of an organ or part, particularly the drooping of an upper eyelid. May be an inherited condition or acquired, and may be unilateral, bilateral, or asymmetric. See VISCEROPTOSIS. SENILE P. usually refers to the ptosis of the upper eyelid; due to weakness of the elevator muscle and the presence of fat in the subcutaneous tissue. — ptotic, ptosed, adj.

-ptosis: Combining form denoting (1) sagging, falling; (2) prolapse of an organ or part.

PTSD: Abbreviation for post-traumatic stress disorder (q.v.).

ptyal-, ptyalo-: Combining forms denoting (1) saliva; (2) salivary gland(s).

ptyalagogue (tī-al'a-gog): An agent that increases the flow of saliva. Also called *ptyalogogue*. Syn., *sialagogue*.

ptyalism (tī'a-lizm): Excessive flow of saliva; salivation.

ptyalorrhoea (tīa-lō-rē'a): Abnormally heavy flow of saliva.

pubertas (pū'ber-tās): Puberty (q.v.). P. PRAE-COX premature (precocious) sexual development.

puberty (pū'ber-ti): The age at which the reproductive organs become functionally active and at which the person is potentially able to reproduce. It is accompanied by secondary sex characteristics. Occurs typically between 13 and 16 years of age in boys and 10 to 14 in girls. — pubertal, adj.

pubes (pū'bēz): 1. The hairy region covering the pubic bone. 2. Plural of pubis.

pubescent (pū-bes'ent): Approaching, or being at the age of, puberty. — pubescence, n.

pubic (pū'bik): Related to or concerning the os pubis. P. ANGLE that formed at the point where the right and left conjoined rami of the ischium and the pubic bones meet; P. ARCH, that formed by the union of the inferior rami of the two pubic bones at the symphysis; P. BONE the os pubis; the lower anterior part of the innominate bone; P. SYMPHYSIS the rather rigid joint at the centre of the front of the bony pelvis formed by the union of the two pubic bones by a thick pad of fibrocartilaginous tissue.

pubis (pū'bis): The pubic bone or os pubis; it is the centre bone of the front of the pelvis. — pubes, pl.; pubic, adj.

public health: Descriptive of all phases of health promotion and preventive medicine carried on in a community for the benefit of the public in general.

public health facilitator (fa-sil'-i-tā-tor): Someone who is based in the community and delivers public health to the local population and supports others involved in similar work, through inter-agency (q.v.) and collaborative ways of working. Responsible for leading a team of practitioners and support staff in public health roles.

Public Health Laboratory Service: A non-departmental body aimed at protecting the public from infection and preventing the spread of infectious diseases in England and Wales through a network of central and regional laboratories.

public involvement: The process of obtaining citizen's views in order that they can influence the design and access of services. See PATIENT ADVICE AND LIAISON SERVICES.

pubococcygeal (pū-bō-kok-sij'ē-al): Relating to the pubis and the coccyx or to the pubococcygeus muscle. P. MUSCLE the anterior part of the levator ani muscle; helps to support the pelvic viscera.

puddle sign: Observed in patients suffering from ascites. The patient is placed in knee–chest position and remains there for several minutes after which the examiner percusses the umbilical area; a dull sound is indicative of the presence of ascitic fluid.

pudendal (pū-den'dal): Of or relating to the pudendum. P. BLOCK rendering the pudendum insensitive by the injection of a local anaesthetic; used mostly for episiotomy and forceps delivery. See TRANSVAGINAL; P. CANAL a passageway through the obturator internus muscle providing for the transmission of the pudendal nerve and muscles; P. NERVE originates in the sacral plexus; branches are distributed to the pudendal and anal areas.

pudendum (pū-den'dum): The external genitalia. In the female, includes the labia majora and minor, mons pubis, clitoris, vestibule of the vagina, perineum, and the vestibular glands. In the male the P. includes the penis, testes, and scrotum.

puerilism (pū'er-il-izm): Childishness, particularly that seen in some older individuals; second childhood.

puerpera (pū-er'per-a): A woman who has just delivered a child.

puerperal (pū-er′pe-ral): Relating to the puerperium (*q.v.*). P. ECLAMPSIA convulsions that occur during the puerperium. See ECLAMPSIA; P. FEVER that which occurs after delivery and usually relates to P. infection; P. INFECTION, a general term for infection of the genital tract after delivery or abortion. Also called *childbed fever, lying-in fever, puerperal sepsis*; P. PSYCHOSIS a psychotic state that occurs during the puerperium.

puerperium (pū-er-pē′ri-um): The period immediately following childbirth to the time when involution is completed, usually 6 to 8 weeks. — puerperia, pl.

pulicosis (pō-li-kō′sis): Flea bites causing urticaria, sometimes haemorrhagic.

pulmo-: Combining form denoting lung(s).

pulmonary (pul′mo-ner-i): Relating to the lungs. P. ARTERY, leaves the right ventricle, divides into right and left branches that carry deoxygenated blood to the right and left lungs, respectively; P. CAPILLARY WEDGE PRESSURE see under PRESSURE; P. CIRCULATION see CIRCULATION; P. DISTRESS SYNDROME see RESPIRATORY DISTRESS SYNDROME; P. EMBOLISM the blocking or closing of the pulmonary artery by an embolus; a fairly common cause of death; P. OESINOPHILIA, refers to several conditions in which there are shadows on x-ray photographs of the lungs and a very high oesinophil count; P. FIBROSIS see under FIBROSIS; P. FUNCTION TEST any one of several tests to determine the functional ability of normal or diseased lungs, *e.g.*, one series of tests measures the ability of the lungs to move air in and out of the lungs; another series evaluates the ability of the alveoli to diffuse gas across the alveolar capillary membrane, and thus to adequately perfuse the blood with oxygen; P. HAEMOSIDEROSIS a rare condition caused by repeated haemorrhage of intra-alveolar capillaries; characterized by anaemia and sometimes haemoptysis which may be severe enough to cause death; occurs chiefly in children and young adults; P. INFARCTION a clot occluding a small blood vessel of the lung, causing death of the tissue supplied by the vessel; see INFARCTION; P. OEDEMA the extravascular accumulation of fluid in the air sacs and interstitial tissues of the lungs; P. PRESSURE the pressure in the pulmonary artery; P. SHUNT any condition that allows blood to move from the right side of the heart to the left side without circulating through the lungs. May be anatomical and occur as a congenital anomaly, or physiological, occurring most often in patients with atelectasis, bronchial obstruction, or pul-

monary disease, and resulting in anoxia; P. STENOSIS see under STENOSIS; P. TUBERCULOSIS see TUBERCULOSIS; P. VALVE the tricuspid valve at the junction of the pulmonary artery and the right ventricle; P. VEINS veins that leave each lung and carry oxygenated blood to the left ventricle of the heart. See also OBSTRUCTIVE PULMONARY DISEASE under OBSTRUCTIVE.

pulmonectomy (pul-mo-nek′to-mi): Pneumonectomy (*q.v.*).

pulmonic (pul-mon′ik): 1. Relating to or affecting the lungs. 2. A person suffering from a pulmonary disease. P. STENOSIS see under STENOSIS.

pulmonitis (pul′mo-nī′tis): Inflammation of the lung; pneumonia, pneumonitis.

pulmotor (pul′mō-tor): A portable apparatus for forcing oxygen or air or both, into the lungs and drawing out carbon dioxide; used to induce artificial respiration in emergencies such as drowning, asphyxiation by gas, smoke inhalation, etc. Most police and fire departments have at least one.

pulp: The soft, interior part of some organs and structures, DENTAL P. found in the P. cavity of teeth; carries blood, nerve and lymph vessels; DIGITAL P. the tissue pad at the finger tip. — pulpal, adj.

pulpitis (pul-pī′tis): Inflammation of the pulp of a tooth; usually caused by streptococcal or staphylococcal invasion. Odontitis.

pulsate (pul′sāt): To throb, move, or beat rhythmically; to vibrate.

pulsatile (pul′sa-tīl): Beating, throbbing.

pulsating mattress: Also called *alternating pressure mattress*. A mattress made of plastic and consisting of separate cells that are inflated alternately with air about every 3 minutes. Useful for patients who are long confined to bed, debilitated, or subject to decubitus ulcers.

pulsation (pul-sā′shun): 1. Beating or throbbing, as of the heart or arteries. 2. A single beat of the heart or pulse. 3. Rhythmic contraction, expansion, or vibration.

pulse (puls): The rhythmic impulse transmitted to arteries by contraction of the left ventricle and consequent expansion of an artery; customarily palpated by finger at the radial artery of the wrist. ABDOMINAL P. the P. over the abdominal aorta; ALTERNATING P. a regular P. with alternating beats of weak and strong amplitude; ARTERIAL P. the P. felt in an artery; BIGEMINAL P. coupled P.; a P. in which the beats occur in pairs, each pair being followed by a prolonged pause; BOUNDING P. one of large volume and force; CAROTID P. one felt in a

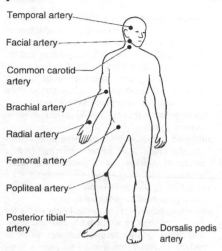

Temporal artery

Facial artery

Common carotid artery

Brachial artery

Radial artery

Femoral artery

Popliteal artery

Posterior tibial artery

Dorsalis pedis artery

The pulse can be felt in arteries lying close to the body surface.

carotid artery; DICROTIC P. one with a double beat, the second beat being weaker; ELASTIC P. one felt as full and elastic; FULL P. one that is easily felt and with good expansion of the blood vessel; HARD P. one of high tension; INTERMITTENT P. one characterized by intermittently dropped beats; PARADOXICAL P. one that is markedly lowered in amplitude during inspiration; QUADRIGEMINAL P. a P. in which there is a pause after every fourth beat; QUINCKE'S P. pulsations sometimes observable at the arterial end of skin capillaries as, for example, the alternate blanching and flushing of the nail bed, which can be elicited by putting pressure on the nail; so called *capillary*; THREADY P. a weak, usually rapid and scarcely perceptible P.

pulse deficit: The difference between the rate of the apical heartbeat, counted by stethoscope, and the pulse counted at the wrist; occurs when some of the ventricular contractions are too weak to open the aortic valve and hence produce a beat at the heart but not at the wrist.

pulse-echo technique: The use of ultrasonic energy directed into the body to obtain a graphic representation of any alterations in the structure of an organ or part.

pulse force or tension: Pulse strength estimated by the force needed to obliterate it by pressure of the finger.

pulseless disease: A group of disorders characterized by gradual occlusion of one or more arteries above their origin in the aortic arch,

resulting in loss of pulse in the neck and arms; other symptoms include headache, fever, dizziness, fainting, claudication, transient hemiplegia, atrophy of the retina, clouding or temporary loss of vision. Also called *aortic arch syndrome. Takayasu's disease, progressive obliterative arteritis,* and *brachiocephalic arteritis.*

pulse oximeter (ok-sim'-i-ter): A non-invasive monitor that measures the oxygen levels in haemoglobin.

pulse pressure: The difference between the systolic and diastolic pressures. See SYSTOLE; DIASTOLIC.

pulse rate: The same as the heartbeat; normally about 130 per minute in the newborn infant, 70 to 80 in the adult, and 60 to 80 in the elderly.

pulse rhythm: Refers to pulse regularity; can be regular or irregular.

pulse volume: Refers to the degree of expansion of the arterial wall during the passage of a pulse wave.

pulse-wave tracing: Produced by a painless diagnostic procedure which records low-frequency silent vibration from the jugular vein, carotid artery, or apex of the heart; helps to identify certain heart or circulatory disorders or abnormalities.

pulsimeter (pul-sim'i-ter): An instrument for measuring the rate, rhythm, and force of the pulse beat.

pulsus (pul'sus): Pulse. P. ALTERNANS a pulse beat that alternates between strong and weak.

pulvis (pul'vis): A powder.

pummelling (pum'mel-ling): A manoeuvre in massage; consists of mild pounding or thumping with the fist.

pump: An apparatus for forcing or drawing fluid or gas to or from a part. BREAST P. one for withdrawing milk from the breast; STOMACH P. one for withdrawing the contents of the stomach.

pump-oxygenator: An apparatus used during open heart surgery; it substitutes for both the heart and lungs in that it pumps the blood through the body and also oxygenates it.

punch biopsy: See under BIOPSY.

punch-drunk syndrome: A chronic neuropsychologic disorder, possibly due to repeated head injuries, especially when occurring in individuals who began a boxing career early in life; also occurs in alcoholics. Symptoms include mental, emotional, and motor dysfunction.

punctate (punk'tāt): Dotted or spotted, *e.g.*, punctate basophilia describes the immature red cells in which there are droplets of blue-staining material in the cytoplasm. P. ERYTHEMA a rash of very fine spots.

punctum (punk'tum): An extremely small point or spot. P. LACRIMALE the minute opening on either the upper or lower eyelid near the canthus through which excess tears enter the lacrimal duct and are carried to the nasal cavity. — puncta, pl.

puncture (punk'tūr): 1. A stab wound, hole, or other perforation made with a sharp pointed hollow instrument for the withdrawal or injection of fluid or other substance. 2. To make a stab wound or perforation. CISTERNAL P. insertion of a special hollow needle with stylet through the atlanto-occipital ligament between the occiput and atlas, into the cisterna magna. One method of obtaining cerebrospinal fluid; LUMBAR P. insertion of a special hollow needle with stylet either through the space between the third and fourth lumbar vertebrae or lower, or into the subarachnoid space, to obtain cerebrospinal fluid for examination, to remove excess fluid, or to inject a drug, e.g., an anaesthetic; P. WOUND see WOUND; STERNAL P. insertion of a special guarded hollow needle with stylet into the body of the sternum for aspiration of a bone marrow sample; VENTRICULAR P. a highly skilled method of puncturing a cerebral ventricle for a sample of cerebrospinal fluid.

pungent (pun'jent): Sharp, bitter, biting, acrid as to taste or odour.

PUO: Abbreviation for pyrexia of undetermined origin; see under PYREXIA.

pupil (pū'pil): The contractile circular opening in the centre of the iris that allows the passage of light rays to the retina. ADIE'S P. one characterized by slow accommodation, contracting or dilating only after prolonged stimulation; ARGYLL ROBERTSON P. one that responds to accommodation but not to light; PINHOLE or PINPOINT P. extremely contracted pupil, sometimes caused by miotics or certain brain disorders.

pupillary (pū'pi-ler-i): Relating to or concerning the pupil.

pupillotonia (pū'pil-ō-tō'ni-a): Tonic reaction of the pupil, as seen in Adie's syndrome (q.v.).

purgation (pur-gā'shun): Catharsis; vigorous evacuation of the bowels effected by a cathartic drug.

purgative (pur'ga-tive): 1. Causing copious evacuation of the bowels. 2. A drug that causes copious evacuation of the bowels. DRASTIC P. one which causes an unusually copious evacuation of watery faeces.

purge (purj): 1. To cause a thorough evacuation of the bowels. 2. A drug that causes such an evacuation.

Purified Protein Derivative: A purified protein derivative of tuberculin, used in intradermal test for tuberculosis. See MANTOUX TEST, TUBERCULIN.

purines (pū'rēnz): Constituents of nucleoproteins from which uric acid is derived. Gout is thought to be associated with the disturbed metabolism and excretion of uric acid; thus foods of high purine content are excluded in its treatment.

Purkinje: P. CELLS large flask-shaped cells with many branching dendrites, located in the middle layer of the cerebral cortex; they are important efferent neurons; P. FIBRES the terminal fibres of the right and left bundle branches (see BUNDLE OF HIS); they form a dense network in the walls of the chambers of the heart and make up the sinoatrial and atrioventricular nodes; are concerned with the electrical transmission of impulses through the heart. [Johannes E. von Purkinje, Bohemian anatomist, 1787–1869.]

purohepatitis (pū'-rō-hep-al ī'tis): Inflammation of the liver accompanied by suppuration.

puromucous (pū-rō-mū'kus): Containing both pus and mucous. Syn., mucopurulent.

purple (pur'p'l): A dark colour that is a blend of red and blue. VISUAL P. a photosensitive pigment in the rods and cones of the retina; rhodopsin.

purpura (pur'pū-ra): A physical sign rather than a disease entity, characterized by spontaneous extravasation of blood from the capillaries into the skin and manifest by either small red spots (petechiae) that darken to a purplish colour and gradually fade, or large plaques (ecchymoses), or by oozing into the mucous membranes. The condition may be idiopathic, or it can be due to impaired function of the capillary walls or to defective quality or quantity of blood platelets; it may also be associated with any of several infective, toxic, or allergic conditions. ALLERGIC P. non-thrombocytopenic P., due to ingestion of certain foods or drugs, or to insect bites; HENOCH–SCHÖNLEIN P. a type of idiopathic non-thrombocytopenic P. characterized by pain and tenderness in the abdomen, exanthema and purpuric skin lesions, mild fever, joint pains, vomiting of blood, bloody stools, nephritic symptoms; may be due to vasculitis; seen most commonly in male children. Also called *Henoch–Schönlein syndrome, acute vascular p.* HENOCH'S P. a variety of Henoch–Schönlein P.; IDIOPATHIC THROMBOCYTOPENIC P. an acute or chronic form of P., of unknown cause; characterized by red petechiae that are surrounded by blue-black areas occurring on the mucosa and skin of the face and neck, and upper and lower extremities; destruction of platelets; later symptoms include moon face, bleeding of gums, vomiting of blood, monorrhagia, stiff painful joints, prostration. Also called *autoimmune thrombocytopenia*. May be fatal; NON-THROMBOCYTOPENIC P., P. that is characterized by a normal platelet count and clotting time; P. HAEMORRHAGICA thrombocytopenic P., a common benign P., a P. characterized by greatly diminished platelet count and clotting time; P. SIMPLEX a type of non-thrombocytopenic P., a common benign recurring disorder not usually accompanied by systemic illness; characterized by bruising following trauma; seen most often on the arms, legs, and trunk; SENILE P. an ecchymotic eruption seen on the forearms and hands of elderly persons; SCHÖNLEIN–HENOCH P. see HENOCH-SCHÖNLEIN P.; THROMBOCYTOPENIC P., any of several forms of P. in which the platelet count is decreased; may be primary and idiopathic or secondary; THROMBOTIC THROMBOCYTOPENIC P. a disease of unknown origin characterized by thrombocytopenia, haemolytic anaemia, fever, neurological signs, intermittent nasal bleeding, purpura, and thrombosis occurring in terminal arterioles and capillaries; may be secondary to known disease or idiopathic, with prolonged bleeding time in either case; occurs chiefly in children and young adults. — Syn., *p. haemorrhagica*.

pursed lip breathing: Prolonged slow expiration with the lips pursed as in whistling.

purulence (pū'rū-lens): The state of being purulent, or of containing pus.

purulent (pū'rū-lent): Pertinent to, caused by, resembling, containing, or producing pus; suppurative (*q.v.*). Term is often combined with the part affected, *e.g.*, purulent meningitis.

pus: A thick, opaque fluid or semifluid substance; the product of inflammation; formed in certain infections, and composed of serum, leukocytes, tissue and dead cell debris, living and dead bacteria, fibrin, and various foreign elements; varying in colour, odour, and consistency with the particular causative organism.

pustulation (pus-tū-lā'shun): The formation of pustules.

pustule (pus'tūl): A small, circumscribed, superficial inflammatory elevation on the skin containing pus, *e.g.*, the lesions of acne, eczema, smallpox, chickenpox, impetigo. — pustular, adj. MALIGNANT P. cutaneous anthrax (*q.v.*).

putrefaction (pū'tri-fak'shun): The process of rotting; the destruction of organic material by bacteria. — putrefactive, adj.

putrescible (pu-tres'ib-l): Capable of undergoing putrefaction.

putrid ((pū'trid): Decayed, rotten.

Putti–Platt operation: An operation to shorten the subscapularis tendon in order to limit lateral rotation; done to correct recurrent anterior dislocation of the shoulder.

PV: Abbreviation for polycythaemia vera, see POLYCYTHAEMIA.

P value: The probability of the results of a test occurring by chance; the lower the value, the more significant the relationship between the test variables.

PVC: Abbreviation for premature ventricular contraction. (*q.v.*).

P wave: In the electrocardiogram it represents the contraction of the ventricles during the heartbeat.

py-, pyo-: Combining forms denoting (1) suppuration; (2) pus; (3) pus-producing infection.

pyaemia (pī-ē'mi-a): A grave form of general septicaemia (*q.v.*) in which blood-borne bacteria from an acute primary focus of infection lodge and grow in distant organs, *e.g.*, brain, kidneys, lungs, or heart, and form multiple abscesses. — pyaemic, adj.

pyarthrosis (pī-ar-thrō'sis): Pus or suppuration in a joint cavity.

pyel-, pyelo-: Combining forms denoting relationship to the pelvis of the kidney.

pyelitis (pī-e-lī'tis): Inflammation of the pelvis of the kidney. A mild form of pyelonephritis (*q.v.*) with pyuria but minimal involvement of renal tissue.

pyelocystitis (pī-e-lō-sis-tī'tis): Inflammation of the renal pelvis and the urinary bladder.

pyelogram (pī'e-lō-gram): An x-ray photograph of the renal pelvis and ureter. INTRAVENOUS P. a P. in which a radiopaque contrast material is given intravenously and excreted through the kidney, making possible radiographic visualization of the renal pelvis and ureter.

pyelography (pī-e-log'ra-fi): Radiographic visualization of the renal pelvis and ureter after injection of a radiopaque liquid. The liquid may be injected into the bloodstream whence it is excreted by the kidney (intravenous P.) or it may be injected directly into the renal pelvis or ureter by way of a fine catheter introduced through a cystoscope (retrograde P.). — Pyelogram, n.; pyelographic, adj.

pyelolithotomy (pī-e-lō-lith-ot'-ō-mi): The operation for the removal of a stone from the renal pelvis.

pyelonephritis (pī'e-lō-ne-frī'tis): An acute or chronic infection that spreads outwards from the pelvis to the cortex of the kidney. The origin of the infection is usually in or below the ureter, or in the bloodstream. EMPHYSEMATOUS P. a rare, usually fatal disease in which gas produced by bacteria accumulates in the kidney; occurs most often in older people who have diabetes. Nephrectomy is the usual treatment; XANTHOGRANULOMATOUS P. a rare chronic form of P., signs and symptoms include back pain, costovertebral tenderness, fever, weight loss, enlarged kidney with fibrosis of the parenchyma, enlarged histiocytes containing fat and cholesterol, staghorn calculi, diminished or absent kidney function.

pyelonephrosis (pī'e-lō-ne-frō'sis): A pathological condition of the kidney and its pelvis.

pyeloplasty (pī'e-lō-plas-ti): A plastic operation on the kidney pelvis.

pyeloscopy (pī-e-los'ko-pi): Fluoroscopic examination of the pelvis of the kidney after introduction of radiopaque material.

pyelostomy (pī e los'to mi): The operation of making an incision into the pelvis of the kidney and inserting a tube to divert the flow of urine from the ureter. The tube is connected with drainage apparatus in which the urine is collected.

pyelotomy (pī-e-lot'o-mi): An incision into the pelvis of the kidney, usually for the removal of a calculus.

pyemesis (pī-em'e-sis): The vomiting of material containing pus.

pyencephalus (pī-en-kef'a-lus,-sef'-): A purulent effusion or an abscess within the cranium. Also called *pyocephalus*.

pyesis (pī-ē'sis): The formation of pus; suppuration. — Syn., *pyosis*.

pygopagus (pi-gop'a-gus): A congenital anomaly in which conjoined twins are united at the sacral region and consequently are back to back.

pykn-, pykno-: Combining forms denoting (1) compact, dense, bulk; (2) frequent.

pyknic (pik'nik): A type of body structure; the P. individual has a large head and chest, broad shoulders, large body cavities, generally stocky body with considerable subcutaneous fat. Often associated with a personality that is an extrovert, happy and interested in others.

pyknocyte (pik'nō-sīt): A distorted erythrocyte, contracted and sometimes with spicules; small numbers are normally present in the blood of full-term infants; may also be seen in greater numbers in persons with haemolytic disorders.

pyknocytosis (pik'-nō-sī-tō'sis): Noticeable increases in the number of pyknocytes in the circulating blood. P. INFANTILE a transient haemolytic anaemia in the newborn; characterized by a high number of pyknocytes among the red cells; cause unknown; symptoms include jaundice, anaemia, splenomegaly; usually recovery is spontaneous in a few weeks.

pyl-, pyle-: Combining forms denoting the portal vein.

pylephlebitis (pī'-lē-flē-bī'tis): Inflammation of the veins of the portal system, usually secondary to intra-abdominal sepsis.

pylethrombosis (pī'-lē-throml bō'sis): Intravascular blood clot in the portal vein or any of its branches.

pylorectomy (pī'-lō-rek-tō-mi): Surgical removal of the pyloric end of the stomach.

pyloric (pī-lor'ik): Relating to the pylorus. P. ORIFICE the lower opening of the stomach into the duodenum; P. STENOSIS see under STENOSIS.

pyloroduodenal (pī lor'ol du-ō-dē'nal): Pertaining to the pyloric sphincter and the duodenum.

pyloromyotomy (pī-lor'-ō-mī-ot'ō-mi): Incision of the longitudinal and circular muscles of the pylorus to correct congenital stenosis.

pyloroplasty (pī-lor'ō-plas-ti): A plastic operation on the pylorus, designed to widen the passage.

pylorospasm (pī lor'ō spazm): Spasm of the pyloric sphincter muscle or of the pyloric portion of the stomach; usually due to the presence of a duodenal ulcer, but is also frequently of emotional origin.

pylorotomy (pī-lo-rot'o-mi): An operation on the pyloric muscle; usually done to relieve pyloric stenosis.

pylorus (pī-law'rus): The opening of the stomach into the duodenum, encircled by a sphincter muscle. — pyloric, adj.

pyochezia (pī-ō-kē'zi-a): The presence of pus in the faeces. Also called *pyofaecia*.

pyocolpocele (pī-ō-kol'pō-sēl): An accumulation of pus in the vagina or a vaginal tumour containing pus.

pyocolpos (pī-ō-kōl'pōs): Accumulation of pus in the vagina.

pyoderma (pī-ō-der'ma): Any inflammatory disease of the skin that is marked by formation of pus-containing lesions, *e.g.*, impetigo contagiosa, ecthyma. Also called *pyodermia*. P. GANGRENOSUM a form of P. occurring chiefly on the trunk and associated with ulcerative colitis and other wasting disease; STREPTOCOCCAL P. usually occurs in children of school age; spread primarily by person-to-person contact.

pyogen (pī'ō-jen): An agent that causes the formation of pus. — pyogenic, pyogenous, adj.; pyogenesis, n.

pyogenic (pī-ō-jen'ik): 1. Relating to or characterized by the formation of pus. 2. Pus-forming.

pyometra (pī-ō-mē'tra): Pus retained in the uterus and unable to escape through the cervix; may be due to malignancy or atresia. — pyometric, adj.

pyometritis (pī'ō-mē-trī'tis): Purulent inflammation of the musculature of the uterus.

pyonephritis (pī-ō-ne-frī'tis): Suppurative inflammation of the kidney.

pyonephrolithiasis (pī'ō-nef-rō-lith-ī'a-sis): A condition in which pus and stones are present in the kidney.

pyonephrosis (pī'ō-ne-frō'sis): Distension of the pelvis of the kidney with pus; there is suppurative destruction of the functional structures of the kidney with severe loss of renal function. — pyonephrotic, adj.

pyopericarditis (pī'ō-per-i-kar-dī'tis): Pericarditis with purulent effusion.

pyoperitonitis (pī'ō-per-i-to-nī'tis): Inflammation of the peritoneum, with suppuration.

pyopneumothorax (pī'ō-nūl mō-thaw'raks): Pus and gas or air within the pleural sac.

pyopoiesis (pī'ō-poy-ē'sis): Formation of pus.

pyoptysis (pī-op'ti-sis): The spitting of material containing pus.

pyorrhoea (pī-or-rē'a): A flow of pus. P. ALVEOLARIS an inflammatory condition involving the gums and the peridontal membrane, often with a discharge of pus from the alveoli; the breath has a foul odour and the teeth often become loose.

pyosalpingitis (pī'ō-sal-pinl jī'tis): Suppurative inflammation of a uterine tube.

pyosalpinx (pi-ō-sal'pinks): A uterine tube containing pus.

pyosis (pī-ō'sis): Pus formation. Also called *pyesis*.

pyothorax (pī'ō-thaw'raks): Pus in the pleural cavity; empyema (*q.v.*).

pyr-, pyro-: Combining forms denoting (1) fire, heat; (2) fever production.

pyramid (pir'a-mid): Descriptive of anatomical structures that are shaped like a wide-based, pointed cone. PETROUS P. the pyramid-like part of the temporal bone that contains the inner ear structures; RENAL P. one of the cone-shaped structures in the medulla of the kidney; contains the collecting tubules.

pyramidal (pi-ram'id-al): Applied to some conical-shaped eminences in the body. P. CELLS nerve cells in the pre-rolandic area of the cerebral cortex, from which originate impulses to voluntary muscles; P. TRACTS in the brain and spinal cord, transmit the fibres arising from the P. cells.

pyrectic (pī-rek'tik): 1. An agent that induces fever. 2. Pertaining to fever. 3. Feverish; febrile. Also called *pyretic*.

pyretherapy (pī're-ther'a-pi): Treatment of disease by artificially inducing fever; may involve the use of diathermy or the injection of malarial organisms. Also called *fever therapy*, *pyrotherapy*, *pyretotherapy*.

pyrexia (pī-rek'si-a): Fever; elevation of the body temperature above normal. P. OF UNDETERMINED ORIGIN a term often used in reference to a fever that occurs before the diagnosis of the condition causing it has been determined. Also often referred to as *fever of undetermined origin*; see under FEVER.

pyridoxine (pir-i-dok'sin): A water-soluble member of the vitamin B complex; may be connected with the utilization of unsaturated fatty acids and the conversion of tryptophan to niacin. Found in wheat germ, cereal grains, fish liver, meat (especially offal), molasses; an ordinary diet provides an adequate amount. Deficiency may result in symptoms of nervousness and convulsions (in infants), dermatitis, neuritis, anorexia, nausea, vomiting. Also called *vitamin B₆*.

pyrimidine (pī-rim'id-in): An organic compound that is the source of several nitrogen compounds found in nucleic acid and in some barbiturates.

pyrogen (pī'ro-jēn): A substance capable of producing pyrexia (*q.v.*). DISTILLED WATER P. a substance of unknown nature, found sometimes in distilled water; it causes a rise in the patient's temperature when used in solutions that are injected into the body. — pyrogenic, adj.

pyromania (pī-rō-mā'ni-a): Excessive preoccupation with fires; compulsive desire to set fires; in psychoanalysis, thought to be due to a desire to obtain erotic gratification. — pyromaniac, n.

pyrosis (pī-rō'sis): Heartburn; water-brash. The eructation of dilute acid content from the stomach into the pharynx or mouth, accompanied by bitter, burning sensation.

pyruvate (pi-rū'vāt): A salt or ester of pyruvic acid.

pyruvic acid (pī-rū'vik): An important intermediate compound produced during carbohydrate metabolism and dependent upon an adequate supply of thiamin(e) for its proper oxidation.

pyuria (pī-ū'ri-a): Pus in the urine (more than 3 leukocytes per high-power field). — pyuric, adj.

Q

QAA: Abbreviation for Quality Assessment Agency for Higher Education (*q.v.*).

QCA: Abbreviation for Qualifications and Curriculum Authority (*q.v.*).

Q fever: A mild rickettsial infection somewhat like Rocky Mountain spotted fever, characterized by fever, chills, muscle pain; transmitted by raw milk, contact with infected animals or dried particles, or by ticks which may serve as vectors.

Q law: The principle that as temperature decreases chemical activity also decreases; has been utilized in the form of treatment with cold to reduce acid secretion in patients with haemorrhaging gastric ulcer.

Q methodology (meth-o-dol'-o-ji): A method ology having the quality or function of describing; serving to describe; characterized by description. Invented in 1935 by Stephenson, it is often associated with quantitative research. However, it combines the strengths of both qualitative and quantitative research traditions through the process of analysis.

QRS complex: In the electrocardiogram, represents transmission of a group of waves created by the passage of the cardiac impulse through the ventricles, the R wave being the most prominent. Its width, along with the P–R interval, is important in interpreting cardiac rhythm. It represents depolarization of the ventricles.

q-sort: A personality assessment technique in which a person sorts cards carrying representations of certain objects according to the subject's interpretation of their meaning.

quack (kwak): One who fraudulently claims medical skill and knowledge; a medical charlatan; a fraud.

quackery (kwak'er-i): The pretensions and methods employed by a quack (*q.v.*). Charlatanism.

quadr-, quadri-, quadro-: Combining forms denoting four, fourth.

quadrant (kwo'drant): A quarter of a circle. In anatomy, an area that is roughly circular and may be divided into quadrants for descriptive purposes, *e.g.*, the surface of the abdomen.

quadrantanopsia (kwo'drant-an-op'si-a): Loss of vision in approximately one-fourth of the field of vision. Also called *quadrantanopia*.

quadrate (kwo'drat): Square; having four equal sides.

quadratus (kwo-drā'tus): Square. In anatomy, descriptive of skeletal muscles that are more or less four-sided, *e.g.*, the quadratus lumborum, which forms part of the posterior wall of the abdomen.

quadribasic (kwo'dri-bā'sik): Relating to an acid that has four replaceable hydrogen atoms.

quadriceps (kwo'dri-seps): Having four heads; denoting the great extensor muscle of the front of the thigh, which has four heads; the quadriceps femoris.

quadricuspid (kwo'dri-kus'pid): Having four cusps; said of (1) a tooth or (2) a semilunar valve (aortic or pulmonary) having four cusps.

quadridigitate (kwo'dri-dij'i-tāt): Having only four fingers or four toes on a hand or foot; tetradactyl.

quadrigeminum (kwo-dri-jem'-i-num): Quadruplet.

quadrilateral (kwo'dri-lat'er-al): **1.** Having four sides. **2.** A four-sided figure.

quadrilocular (kwo'dri-lok'-ū-lar): Having four chambers, cavities, or cells.

quadripara (kwo-drip'a-ra): A woman who has had four full-term pregnancies. — quadriparous, adj.

quadriparesis (kwo'dri-par'e-sis): Weakness of all four limbs.

quadripartite (kwo'dri-par'tīt): Divided into four parts or having four divisions.

quadriplegia (kwo'dri-plē-ji-a): Paralysis of both arms and both legs.

quadriplegic (kwo'dri-plē'jik): **1.** Relating to quadriplegia. **2.** A person with quadriplegia.

quadrisect (kwo'dri-sekt): To divide into four parts. Also called *quartisect*. — quadrisection, n.

quadritubercular (kwo'dri-tū-ber'kū-lar): Having four tubercles. In dentistry, refers to a molar with four cusps.

quadrivalent (kwo'dri-va'lent): Having a valence of 4.

quadruplet (kwo'drū-plet): One of four children born at a single birth.

quadruple vaccine: A vaccine to immunize against diphtheria, pertussis, poliomyelitis, and tetanus.

quale (kwā'lē): The quality of a thing, sensation in particular.

Qualifications and Curriculum Authority (kwol-i-fi-kā'-shunz, kur-rik'-ū-lum): Vocational accreditation body for England, Wales and Northern Ireland.

qualitative (kwo'li-tā'tiv): Relating to, connected or concerned with, quality or qualities. Now usually in implied or expressed opposition to quantitative (*q.v.*).

quality (kwo'li-ti): 1. A characteristic, distinguishing property or attribute. 2. A characteristic that denotes excellence, superiority, fineness.

quality-adjusted life years: A measure that assesses variations in the quality of life for the patient resulting from an intervention, in relation to cost and length of life. Used for measuring the clinical and cost effectiveness of interventions.

Quality Assessment Agency for Higher Education: An organization funded by the higher education institutions in the UK to monitor and ensure that the standard of their qualifications is maintained. See also APPENDIX 9.

quality assurance: In nursing, involves (1) setting standards for the achievement of excellent care; (2) taking steps for the achievement of excellent care; (3) utilizing peer review or audit to evaluate the quality of care given both in the past and currently; and (4) taking action to correct deficiencies in care as revealed by the evaluation.

quality circles: A participative philosophy woven around quality control and problem-solving techniques. It exemplifies the policy of people building, respect for human beings, and creates a participative management culture. This concept enables the grass-root level employees to play a meaningful and significant role in their organization. The responsibility for the attainment of quality depends on all the departments of an organization. Nurses and other health professionals in a clinical area are guided by a facilitator experienced in this process, to investigate a health-care intervention systematically and relate it to good standards of practice.

quality of care: The statutory duty of chief executives of NHS Trusts to ensure a level of quality in the provision of care.

quality of life: A term referring to the patient's level of comfort, enjoyment, and ability to pursue daily activities. Often used in discussions of treatment options. It takes into ac-

count the factors that allow an individual to cope with every aspect of his or her life.

quality management system: A set of processes that ensure a consistent approach to the management of an organization. ISO 9000 (*q.v.*) is the most commonly used international standard that provides a framework for an effective Q.M.S.

qualpacs (kwol'paks): A quality assurance tool used in the clinical situation by nurses to measure quality of nursing care. A predetermined scoring schedule is used and the process involves observation of randomly selected patients, reviewing care plans and listening to hand-over reports.

QUALYs: Abbreviation for quality adjusted life years (*q.v.*).

quantitative (kwon'ti-tā-tiv): 1. Something that is, or may be, considered with respect to the quantity or quantities involved. 2. Estimated or estimable by quantity. 3. Relating to, concerned with, quantity or its measurement.

Quant's sign: A T-shaped depression in the occipital bone; often seen in individuals with rickets.

quantum (kwan'tum): 1. A definite amount. 2. A unit of radiant energy.

quarantine (kwor'an-tēn): 1. To detain or isolate a person who has been exposed to a communicable disease for a period of time equal to the longest incubation period. 2. To restrict persons from an area or premises where a case of communicable disease exists. 3. To detain a ship coming from an infected port or carrying passengers who are suspected of having or having been exposed to a communicable disease, (originally for 40 days). 4. A place where persons under quarantine are kept, *e.g.*, an isolation hospital or ward. 5. To detain or isolate a carrier.

quartan (kwawr'tan): Recurring every fourth day, reckoning inclusively. Malaria in which the paroxysms occur every 72 hours.

quartipara (kwor-tip'a-ra): Quadripara (*q.v.*).

quasi (kwā'zī): Having some resemblance to a given thing; seemingly; in some sense or degree. Often joined by a hyphen to another word element naming the thing or condition that is resembled.

quassia (kwo'shi-a): A substance obtained from the bitterwood tree of Latin America; formerly much used as a bitter tonic and as an enema in the treatment for threadworms.

Queckenstedt's test: Normally, compression on the veins in the neck, on either or both sides, will result in a rapid rise in the pressure of the cerebrospinal fluid and the quick disappearance of the increase when the pressure is removed. When this manoeuvre produces little or no change in the pressure, the test is said to be positive for blockage in the spinal canal.

Queen Anne's sign: Loss of the outer portions of the eyebrows; often a sign of myxoedema in older persons.

Queensland: Q. COASTAL FEVER tsutsugamushi disease (*q.v.*). Q. TYPHUS FEVER a fever occurring in Queensland, Australia, where it is transmitted by marsupials and wild rodents; resembles Rocky Mountain spotted fever.

quellung (kwel'lung): Swelling. Q. REACTION swelling of the capsule of a bacterium when it comes into contact with its antigen.

querulent (kwer'ū-lent): Refers to an individual who is always suspicious, complaining, dissatisfied, and in opposition to suggestions of others; characteristic of the paranoid personality.

Quervain's disease (kair' vonz, kɛi'-vanz): Tenosynovitis due to inflammation of the tendons of the thumb muscles, characterized by swelling, tenderness, and pain.

questionnaire (kwes-chun-air', kɛs-chun-air'): A list of questions by which information is sought from a selected group.

Queyrat's erythroplasia (ka-rahz'-ē-rith-rō-plā'zi-a): A squamous-cell, precarcinomatous, circumscribed, erythematous lesion, velvety and papular in nature, occurring at the mucocutaneous junctions of the mouth, glans penis, or prepuce, and leading to ulceration and scaling.

quick: 1. Rapid. 2. Alive. 3. The stage of pregnancy when movements of the fetus can be felt. 4. The eponychium (*q.v.*).

quickening (kwik'en-ing): The first movements of the fetus that are perceptible to the mother at approximately the 18th to 20th week in a primigravid woman and at the 16th to 18th week in the multigravida.

quicklime (kwik'līm): Calcium oxide; unslaked lime. Formerly much used as a deodorant and mild disinfectant, particularly for excreta.

quicksilver (kwik'sil-ver): Mercury (*q.v.*).

quiescent (kwē-es'ent): Arrested; not active; causing no symptoms. Said especially of a skin disease which is settling under treatment.

quiet: Q. DELIRIUM delirium marked by quiet incoherent mumblings and the absence of uncontrolled psychomotor activity; Q. NECROSIS epiphysial aseptic necrosis; see under NECROSIS.

Quincke: Q.'S DISEASE angioneurotic oedema (*q.v.*); Q.'S MENINGITIS acute aseptic M., see ASEPTIC M. under MENINGITIS; Q.'S PULSE see under PULSE. [Heinrich Quincke, German physician, 1842–1922.]

quinidine (kwin'i-dēn): One of the alkaloids obtained from cinchona bark; an antimalarial; also used in treating arrhythmias.

quinine (kwi'-nēn): The chief alkaloid of cinchona, once the standard treatment for malaria. Now largely replaced by more modern drugs.

quininism (kwi-nē-nizm): A condition caused by an idiosyncratic reaction to, or long-continued use of, quinine or cinchona; symptoms include headache, noises in the ears and partial deafness, disturbed vision, and nausea.

quininoderma (kwin-i-nō-der'ma): Dermatitis following ingestion of quinine.

Quinlan's test: A spectroscopic test for the presence of bile.

quinquagenarian (kwin'kwa-jen-ar'i-an): An individual in his or her fifties.

quinquetubercular (kwin'-kwē-tū-ber'kū-lar): Having five tubercles or cusps.

quinquevalent (kwin'-kwē-vā'lent): Having a valence of 5; pentavalent.

quinsy (kwin'zi): Acute inflammation of the tonsil and surrounding loose tissue, with abscess formation. Peritonsillar abscess.

quint-, quinti-: Combining forms denoting five, fifth.

quintan (kwin'tan): Recurring every fifth day.

quintessence (kwin-tes'-ens): The highly concentrated essence of any substance.

quintipara (kwin-tip'a-ra): A woman who has had five full-term pregnancies. — quintiparous, adj.

quintiparity (kwin-ti-par'i-ti): The state of being a quintipara.

quintuplet (kwin'tup-let): One of five children born at a single birth.

quota (kwō'-ta): The part or share of a total which belongs, is given, or is due, to one.

quotidian (kwō-tid'i-an): Recurring daily. A form of malaria in which paroxysms recur daily. DOUBLE Q. recurring twice daily.

quotient (kwō'shent): A number obtained by division. ACHIEVEMENT Q. a percentage statement of the amount a child has learned in relation to his inherent intellectual ability; INTELLIGENCE Q. the estimate of intelligence; obtained by dividing the mental age, as determined by standard tests, by the chronological age, and multiplying the result by 100. Expressed as IQ; RESPIRATORY Q. the ratio between the CO_2 expired and the O_2 inspired during a specified time.

Q wave: The first deflection in the QRS complex; if it goes below the baseline it is considered a criterion for the diagnosis of myocardial infarction.

R

Ra: Chemical symbol for radium.

rabbeting (rab'et-ing): The fitting together of the jagged ends of a fractured bone.

rabic (rā'bik): Pertaining to rabies.

rabid (rab'id): 1. Relating to rabies. 2. Affected with rabies. 3. Extremely violent, furious.

rabies (rā'bēz): An acute, highly fatal, infectious disease of warm-blooded animals, especially the dog, cat, wolf, fox; caused by a filterable virus; attacks chiefly the nervous system; fatal if untreated. May be transmitted to humans through the infected saliva of a rabid animal, usually through a bite, primarily dog-bite. Characterized by the formation of Negri bodies (*q.v.*) in the brain, central nervous system excitement, wild madness, paralysis, and often, death. Syn., *hydrophobia.* — rabid, rabic, adj.

rabiform (rā'bi-form): Resembling rabies.

race: 1. A group within a species of animals or plants, connected by common descent or origin. 2. A tribe, nation, or people, regarded as of common stock.

rachi-, rachio-: Combining forms denoting relationship to the spine.

rachial (rā'ki-al): Relating to the vertebral column. Spinal.

rachialgia (rā-ki-al'ji-a): Pain in the spine.

rachianaesthesia (rā'ki-an-es-thē'zi-a): Spinal anaesthesia; see under ANAESTHESIA.

rachicele (rā'ki-sēl): Protrusion of the spinal canal contents to the exterior, as in spina bifida (*q.v.*).

rachicentesis (rā'ki-sen-tē'sis): Spinal puncture for the aspiration of fluid. Also called *rachiocentesis.*

rachidial (rā-kid'i-al): Spinal.

rachigraph (rā'ki-graf): An instrument for recording the curves of the spine.

rachiocampsis (rā-ki-ō-camp'sis): Curvature of the spine.

rachiochysis (rā-ki-ok'i-sis): The accumulation of fluid in the subarachnoid space of the spinal canal.

rachiodynia (rā'ki-ō-din'i-a): A painful condition of the spinal column.

rachiometer (rā-ki-om'i-ter): An apparatus for measuring curvatures in the spinal column.

rachiomyelitis (rā'ki-ō-mī-e-lī'tis): Inflammation of the spinal cord.

rachiopathy (rā-ki-op'a-thi): Any disease of the spine. Also called *Spondylopathy.*

rachioscoliosis (rā'ki-ō-skō-li-ō'sis): Lateral curvature of the spine.

rachiotomy (rā-ki-ot'o-mi): An incision into the spinal column or into a vertebra. See also LAMINECTOMY.

rachis (rā'kis): The spinal column.

rachischisis (ra-kis'ki-sis): A congenital fissure in the spinal column. Spina bifida (*q.v.*).

rachitic (ra-kit'ik): Relating to or affected with rickets. R. ROSARY or BEADS a row of bead-like nodules that form on the ribs at their junctions with the cartilage, sometimes seen in children with rickets.

rachitis (ra-kī'tis): 1. Rickets (*q.v.*). 2. An inflammatory condition of the spine.

rachitogenic (ra-kit-ō-jen'ik): Producing rickets.

racism (rā'-sizm): 1. The theory that distinctive human characteristics and abilities are determined by race. 2. Belief in the superiority of some races over others, and the resulting prejudice (*q.v.*).

rad: The standard unit of absorbed radiation dose; replaces the term roentgen as the unit of dosage; Gy (gray) is the SI unit. It is a measure of the x-ray energy absorbed per gram of tissue.

radectomy (rā-dek'to-mi): Surgical removal of all or part of the root of a tooth.

radiad (rā'di-ad): Towards the radius or the radial side.

radial (rā'di-al): In anatomy, relating to the radius. R. ARTERY the artery at the thumb side of the wrist; R. NERVE arises in the cervical plexus, runs around the back of the humerus and down the outer side of the forearm; supplies the extensor muscles of the elbow, wrist, and hand; R. PULSE the pulse felt by placing the fingers over the radial artery at the wrist.

radiant (rā'di-ant): Emitting rays or beams of light. R. ENERGY energy that is transmitted in the form of waves, including radiowaves, infrared and ultraviolet rays, visible light, x- and gamma rays.

radiate (rā'di-āt): 1. To spread from a common point or centre. 2. To emit radiation.
radiation (rā'di-ā'shun): 1. Divergence in all directions from a common centre. 2. In anatomy, a structure made up of divergent elements, particularly a group of nerve fibres which diverge from a common origin. 3. A general term for any form of radiant energy such as that emitted from a luminous body, x-ray tube or radioactive substance such as radium; R. RECALL a condition that occurs several weeks after the simultaneous administration of radiation and chemotherapy; presents as an erythema, with vesicle formation or desquamation and often followed by permanent pigmentation of the skin; R. SICKNESS that which follows the therapeutic use of radioactive substances or x-rays; symptoms include nausea, vomiting, anorexia, headache. The term is also used in reference to illness resulting from fallout of atomic bombs; R. THERAPY the therapeutic use of x-rays or radioactive elements.
radical (rad'i-kal): 1. In chemistry, a substance that, when dissolved in water, will dissociate into elements or groups of elements that will each carry a positive or negative charge. 2. A group of atoms which enters into and goes out of chemical combination without change, and which forms one of the fundamental constituents of a molecule. 3. Relating to or going to the root of a thing; in medicine, going to the root of a disease process. 4. The smallest branch of a vessel or nerve; a rootlet; FREE R. a radical, extremely reactive and having a very short half-life (10^{-5} seconds, less in an aqueous solution) which carries an impaired electron; R. OPERATION see RADICAL SURGERY under SURGERY.
radiculalgia (ra-dik'ū-lal'ji-a): Neuralgia of the sensory root, or roots of a spinal nerve or nerves; caused by irritation.
radiculectomy (ra-dik'ū-lek'to-mi): Excision of the root of a spinal nerve.
radiculitis (ra-dik-ū-lī'tis): Inflammation of the root of a nerve, particularly a spinal nerve.
radiculography (ra-dik'ū-log'ra-fi): Radiographic examination of the cauda equina and lumbar nerve roots of the spinal cord after injection of a water-soluble radiopaque medium.
radiculomeningomyelitis (ra-dik'ū-lō-menin'gō-mī-e-lī'tis): Inflammation of the spinal nerve roots, the meninges, and the spinal cord.
radiculomyelopathy (ra-dik'ū-lō-mī-e-lop'a-thi): Any disease of the nerve roots and the spinal cord.

radiculoneuropathy (ra-dik'ū-lō-nū-rop'a-thi): Any disease of the spinal nerve roots and spinal nerves.
radiculopathy (ra-dik-ū-lop'a-thi): Any disease of the spinal nerve roots.
radio-: Combining form denoting: 1. Radiation; radiant energy. 2. The radius. 3. Radium.
radioactive (rā'di-ō-ak'tiv): Relatings to a substance that gives off penetrating rays due to the spontaneous breaking up of its atoms. R. DECAY the decrease, over time, in the number of radioactive atoms in a radioactive substance; R. FALLOUT a mixture of debris and radioactive particles that fall to Earth following a nuclear explosion; R. GOLD see RADIOGOLD; R. IODINE see under RADIO-IODINE; R. ISOTOPES forms of an element that have an unstable nucleus; in becoming more stable they give off ionizing radiation; R. MERCURY used in investigation of brain lesions; R. TECHNETIUM used for investigation of visceral lesions; R. TRACER a labelled element that emits radiation and so can be traced throughout a chemical, biological, or physical process.
radioactivity (rā'di-ō-ak-tiv'i-ti): The quality or property of emitting radiant energy; possessed naturally by certain elements such as radium and uranium; certain other elements become radioactive after bombardment with neutrons or other particles.
radioautography (rā'di-ō-aw-tog'ra-fi): A form of photography that reveals the location and distribution of radioactive elements in a test material.
radiobicipital (rā'di-ō-bī-sip'i-tal): Relating to the radius and the biceps muscle of the arm.
radiobiology (rā'di-ō-bī-ol'ō-ji): The study of the effects of ionizing radiation on living tissue. — radiobiological, adj.; radiobiologically, adv.
radiocarcinogenesis (rā'di-ō-kar'si-nō-jen'e-sis): Cancer caused by exposure to radiation.
radiocarpal (rā'di-ō-kar'pal): Relating to the radius and the carpus.
radiochemistry (rā'di-ō-kem'is-tri): The branch of chemistry that deals with radioactive substances and their properties.
radiocurable (rā'di-ō-kūr'a-b'l): Refers to a condition that may be curable by radiation therapy.
radiode (rā'di-ōd): A metal container for a radioactive substance used in radiotherapy.
radiodermatitis (rā'di-ō-der-ma-tī'tis): Reddening and irritation of the skin due to overexposure to x-rays or radium.
radiodiagnosis (rā'di-ō-dī-ag-nō'sis): Diagnosis made by use of x-ray pictures.

radiodigital (rā'di-ō-dij'i-tal): Relating to the radius and the fingers on the radial side of the arm.

radioelectrocardiology (rā'di-ō-ē-lek'trō-kar-di-ol'ō-ji): A technique in electrocardiology whereby the heart impulses of a patient who is engaged in the normal activities of daily living are beamed by radio waves to a receiver placed at a distance from the patient.

radioencephalography (rā'di-ō-en-kef-a-log'ra-fi, -sef-): Recording of changes in the electrical potential of the brain by radio waves beamed from the patient directly to the recording apparatus.

radioepidermitis (rā'di-ō-ep'i-der-mī'tis): Destructive changes in the skin resulting from overexposure to radiation.

radioepithelitis (rā'di-ō-ep'i-thē-lī'tis): Disintegration and destruction of epithelium caused by overexposure to irradiation.

radiogenic (rā'di-ō-jen'ik): Produced by radiation.

radiogold (rā'di-ō-gōld'): A radioactive isotope of gold; has diagnostic and therapeutic uses.

radiogram (rā'di-ō-gram): An image produced on a radiosensitive surface by radiation, particularly by x-rays, or by photographing an image made by a radiopaque substance.

radiographer (rā-di-og'ra-fer): A professionally qualified healthcare worker who works within a diagnostic x-ray department or in a radiotherapy department.

radiography (rā-di-og'ra-fi): The making of a photograph or a record by the action of certain rays on a sensitized surface such as film; roentgenography. CONTRAST R. a technique involving injection of a radiopaque fluid into a cavity or tissue space before x-ray films are made; utilized in venography, arteriography, arthrography, and myelography; DIAGNOSTIC R. is concerned with obtaining roentgenographic information useful in making diagnoses; THERAPEUTIC R. treatment by radiation from x-rays, radium, or radioisotopes.

radiohumeral (rā'di-ō-hū'mer-al): Relating to the radius and the humerus.

radioimmunity (rā'di-ō-im-mū'ni-ti): Reduction of sensitivity to radiation which may be produced by repeated irradiation.

radioimmunoassay (rā'di-ō-im-mu-nō-as'ā): A sensitive investigative procedure utilizing a radioactive material and blood plasma to determine the presence and concentration of the particular hormone or other natural substance under study. Useful in diagnosis and treatment of diabetes, thyroid disease, sterility, growth disorders, certain types of hepatitis, and hormone-producing cancers.

radio-iodine (rā'di-ō-ī'ō-dēn): A radioactive isotope of iodine; ^{130}I and ^{131}I being most frequently used in medicine for diagnosis and treatment of disorders of the thyroid gland. R. UPTAKE TEST a test in which the person is given a small dose of radioactive iodine and the radioactivity of the thyroid gland is subsequently measured. If the gland is overactive, more than 45% of the iodine will be taken up by the gland within four hours. If the gland is underactive, less than 20% will be taken up after 48 hours.

radioisotope (rā'di-ō-ī'sō-tōp): A radioactive isotope (q.v.) of an element; an element that has the same atomic number as another but a different atomic weight, and exhibits the property of spontaneous decomposition. When fed or injected can be traced with a Geiger counter. R. SCAN pictorial representation of the distribution and amount of radioactive isotope present.

radiolesion (rā'di-ō-lē'zhun): A lesion produced by exposure to radiation.

radiologist (rā-di-ol'o-jist): One skilled in the use of x-rays and other forms of radiant energy for the diagnosis and treatment of disease.

radiology (rā-di-ol'ō-ji): The science that deals with radioactive substances, particularly that branch of medicine that is concerned with the use of the sources of radiant energy in the diagnosis and treatment of disease. — radiologic, radiological, adj.

radiolucent (rā-di-ō-lū'sent): Being entirely or partially permeable to x-rays or other forms of radiant energy. — radiolucency, n.

radiometer (rā-di-om'i-ter): An instrument used for detecting and measuring radiant energy, particularly small amounts of such energy.

radiomimetic (rā'di-ō-mi-met'ik): Producing effects similar to those of radiotherapy. See CYTOTOXIC.

radiomutation (rā'di-ō-mū-tā'shun): Changes in cells following exposure to radiation.

radionecrosis (rā'di-ō-ne-krō'sis): Ulceration or destruction of tissue caused by exposure to radiant energy.

radioneuritis (rā'di-ō-nū-rī'tis): Neuritis resulting from exposure to radiant energy.

radiopaque (rā-di-ō-pāk'): Referring to a substance that does not permit the passage of x-rays or other forms of radiation. Areas or organs treated with a R. substance prior to taking x-ray pictures appear light or white on the film. — radiopacity, n.

radioparent (rā-di-ō-par′ent): The characteristic of being penetrable by roentgen rays.

radiopathology (rā′di-ō-pa-thol′o-ji): The pathology of the effects of radioactive substances on cells and tissues.

radiopharmaceutical (rā′di-ō-far-ma-sū′ti-kal): Pertaining to (1) radiopharmacy, or (2) a radioactive chemical or substance used in diagnosis or treatment of disease.

radiopharmacy (rā′di-o-far′ma-si): The branch of pharmacy that deals with the preparation of radioactive substances used in therapy.

radioreceptor (rā′di-ō-ri-sep′tor): A receptor that is responsive to radiant energy such as heat or light.

radioresistance (rā′di-ō-ri-zis′tans): The resistance of cells or tissues to the effects of radiation, said especially of certain tumours.

radioscopy (rā-di-os′kō-pi): The examination of inner structures of the body by means of x-ray; fluoroscopy.

radiosensitivity (rā′di-ō-sen-si-tiv′i-ti): The condition of being sensitive to the effects of radiant energy; term often used to describe cells that can be destroyed by radiation. — radiosensitive, adj

radiotelemetry (rā′di-ō-tel-em′i-tri): Transmission of data, including biological data, by means of radio; a technique developed for monitoring vital signs of astronauts while in flight and now adapted for use by hospitals for monitoring patients at a distance.

radiotherapeutics (rā′di-ō-ther-a-pū′tiks): 1. Radiotherapy. 2. The body of knowledge concerning what is known about the therapeutic use of radiation therapy.

radiotherapist (rā′di-ō-ther′a-pist): One who specializes in radiotherapy (*q.v.*).

radiotherapy (rā′di-ō-ther′a-pi): Treatment of disease by x-rays, radium, radon seeds, cobalt, sunlight, or other forms of radioactive substances or radiant energy.

radiothermy (rā′di-ō-ther′mi): The use of radiant heat in therapy; short-wave diathermy.

radiotoxaemia (rā′di-ō-tok-sē′mi-a): Toxaemia produced by exposure to a radioactive substance.

radiotransparent (rā′di-ō-trans-par′ent): Refers to substances through which x-rays can pass without hindrance. — radiotransparency, n.

radiotropic (rā′di-ō-trōp;ik): Affected or influenced by radiation.

radioulnar (rā′di-ō-ul′nar): Relating to both bones of the forearm, the radius and ulna.

radium (rā′di-um): A rare radioactive element found in pitchblende and other uranium minerals; discovered in 1898 by Marie Curie, a Polish scientist in Paris. Used in radiotherapy, especially in the treatment of malignancies. R. IMPLANTATION the implanting of radium in a tumour for therapeutic treatment; R. NEEDLE a slender container containing R. that is inserted into tissue for treatment of malignant growths; R. THERAPY, treatment by radium or radon in cancer therapy.

radius (rā′di-us): 1. The bone on the outer side of the forearm. 2. A line radiating from the centre to the periphery of a circle or sphere. — radial, adj.

RAE: Abbreviation for Research Assessment Exercise (*q.v.*).

Raeder's syndrome: A rare condition characterized by trigeminal neuralgia followed by sensory loss on the affected side of the face, weakness of facial muscles, miosis, and ptosis of the upper eyelid; usually due to a lesion in the trigeminal ganglion.

rale (ral): An abnormal, non-continuous, bubbling, crackling, or gurgling sound associated with pneumonia, congestive heart failure, and long periods of recumbency; heard at the base of the lungs at inspiration when fluid is present in the small air passages and alveoli. Usually described as moist or dry, or as fine, medium, or coarse. Fine rales are high-pitched, crackling, or popping; they are indicative of fluid in the smallest airways. Medium rales are of lower pitch and have a wetter sound; they are indicative of fluid in the bronchioles. Coarse rales are low-pitched and loud; they indicate fluid in the bronchi and trachea.

ramify (ram′i-fī): To branch or diverge in different directions. — ramification, n.

Ramsay–Hunt syndrome: See HUNT'S SYNDROME.

Ramstedt's operation: An operation to relieve pyloric stenosis in infants by dividing the pyloric muscle, leaving the mucous lining intact.

ramulus (ram′ū-lus): A small ramus or branch.

ramus (rā′mus): 1. An elongated process of a bone. 2. A branch. Term used to describe the smaller structure formed when a larger one divides or forks; applied to bones, nerves, blood vessels. MANDIBULAR R. the upturned perpendicular part of the mandible on each side. — rami, pl.

random (ran′-dom): Relating to choices or occurrences without any perceivable pattern or logical connection.

randomization (ran′-dom-ī-zā′-shun): A process for the selection of subjects for a trial or study, which minimizes bias and other irrelevant factors, resulting in the production of statistically reliable data, using, for example, random-numbers tables or computer-generated random numbers. Using coin flips, odd–even numbers, patient social security numbers, days of the week, medical record numbers, or other such pseudo- or quasi-random processes, are not truly randomized.

randomized controlled trials (ran'-dom-īzd): Clinical trials that involve at least one test group and one control group (*q.v.*), concurrent enrolment and follow-up of the groups, and in which the treatments to be administered are selected by a random process, see RANDOMIZATION.

range: The difference between the upper and lower limits of a series of values.

range of motion (movement): Refers to the range through which a joint can move or be moved; measured in degrees of a circle. ROM EXERCISES exercises to restore motion in a joint or to keep joints functioning normally; may be active, *i.e.*, performed by the patient himself, or passive, *i.e.*, performed by a therapist who moves the body part through the possible range.

range statement: A description of the activities required to demonstrate competencies within the National Vocational Qualification/Scottish Vocational Qualification (*q.v.*) system.

ranine (rā'nīn): Relating to a ranula or to the lower surface of the tongue.

ranula (ran'ū-la): A retention cyst that forms underneath the tongue on either side of the frenum due to obstruction of the duct of a sublingual or mucous gland; contains stringy, mucoid material; surgery is usually needed. — ranular, adj.

Ranvier's nodes: Regularly spaced constrictions in myelinated nerve fibres; at these points the myelin sheath is absent.

rape (rāp): Unlawful sexual abuse or assault of one person by another, without consent, and obtained by force or deception; legally considered an act of violence.

rape trauma syndrome: A group of symptoms that sometimes develops in women (or men) who have been raped. Symptoms that develop immediately include fear, weeping, insomnia, terrifying dreams, nausea, loss of appetite, depression, suicidal behaviour; those that develop during the adjustment period include fears and phobias, nightmares, refusal to socialize, complete change in lifestyle.

raphe (rā'fē): A seam, suture, ridge, or crease marking the line of fusion of two similar parts, *e.g.*, the median furrow on the dorsal surface of the tongue.

rapid eye movements: Movements of the eye that occur in certain phases of the sleep cycle. REM SLEEP the period of deep normal sleep when one also has dreams which are thought to be the cause of rapid eye movements. See also NON-RAPID EYE MOVEMENTS.

rapport (ra-pawr'): A relation characterized by harmony and accord. In psychiatry, a conscious feeling of accord, trust, confidence, and responsiveness to another, particularly the therapist, with willingness to cooperate. Cf. TRANSFERENCE.

rapture of the deep: A psychotic experience of deep-sea divers, caused by sensory deprivation and disorientation.

raptus (rap'tus): 1. A sudden violent attack; may be physical, as a haemorrhage; or psychological, as an attack of intense nervousness. 2. Rape.

rarefaction (rar-e-fak'shun): Becoming less dense or thinning, but not being reduced in volume, as occurs in some bone diseases. — rarefy, v.

rash: A localized or general temporary skin eruption, often a characteristic of certain infectious diseases. NETTLE R. urticaria (*q.v.*); SERUM R. one following injection of a serum, *e.g.*, antitoxin; due to hypersensitivity.

raspberry mark: A congenital haemangioma (*q.v.*).

rating scale: A measure of the specific value of a property which is necessary for the optimal or standard use of a piece of equipment.

ratio (rā'shi-ō): The relationship in degree or number between two things. ALBUMINGLOBULIN R. the R. between the albumin and globulin in the blood serum which is normally 1.5 to 3; when lower than 1, some pathological condition is indicated.

rational (rash'un-al): 1. Of sound mind; not delirious. 2. Reasonable. 3. In medicine, treatment that is based on reason or general principles rather than empiricism.

rationale (rash-un-al'): The underlying reason or explanation for a practice, opinion, or phenomenon.

rational emotive therapy: A form of psychotherapy in which the patient is helped and encouraged to change his attitudes, his past ways of solving problems, and his general functioning in society in order to develop a more suitable and satisfying behaviour.

rationalization (rash'-un-al-ī-zā'shun): A mental process whereby a person explains an emotionally activated occurrence by substituting one that is more acceptable than the truth, both to himself and to others. The substitution must be plausible enough for self-deception and self-justification. In psychiatry, a defence mechanism used by the individual to justify a threat or event or make something unreasonable seem reasonable.

rattle: A rale or other sound heard on auscultation of the chest. DEATH R. a gurgling sound heard over the trachea in the dying; may also be heard as a respiratory sound.

rave (rāv): To speak incoherently, as in delirium; irrational speech.

raw: 1. Uncooked. **2.** Not pasteurized (*q.v.*), as applied to milk.

ray: 1. A beam of light or other radiant energy. **2.** A stream of particles from a radioactive substance. ALPHA R.S streams of fast-moving positively charged particles emitted from a disintegrating radioactive isotope; they are actually the nuclei of atoms; BETA R.S particles emitted from radioactive isotopes as streams of electrons; their penetrating power is greater than that of alpha rays; DIATHERMY R.S produced by an oscillating electric current; used to produce heat in the deeper body tissues; GAMMA R.S electromagnetic radiation similar to x-rays but of greater penetrating power; IN-FRARED R.S. long invisible rays beyond the red end of the visible spectrum; they emanate from a surface heated to 300–800°C, penetrate the skin and are felt as heat; hence used therapeutically to produce heat in the tissues; ROENTGEN R.S, see under X-RAY; ULTRAVIOLET R.S, the invisible rays beyond the violet rays of the spectrum; see ULTRAVIOLET.

Raynaud: R.'S DISEASE idiopathic phoneurosis, a common vasospastic disorder; characterized by bilateral paroxysmal spasm of the digital arteries producing severe hand-finger pain, numbness, tingling, and pallor of fingers or toes, or both, which become red as circulation returns; repeated attacks may result in osteoporosis of the fingers and toes, atrophy of the nails, and occasionally gangrene. Primarily a disease of young women who are under pressure; is brought on by emotion, any exposure to cold, even eating cold foods, or shock; R.'S PHENOMENON the occasional spasm of the digital arteries causing paleness and numbness of the fingers and toes. [Maurice Raynaud, French physician, 1834–1881.]

RCTs: Abbreviation for randomized controlled trials (*q.v.*).

re-: Prefix denoting: **1.** Again. **2.** Back, backward.

react (rē-akt'): **1.** To respond to a stimulus in a particular way. **2.** To undergo a chemical reaction. **3.** To tend to move towards a prior condition. **4.** To exert a counteracting or reciprocal influence.

reaction (rē-ak'shun): **1.** Response to stimulation. **2.** Result of a test to determine acidity or alkalinity of a solution; usually expressed as pH. **3.** The interaction of two or more different types of molecules with the production of a new type of molecule. ADVERSE R. an unpleasant or harmful physiological or psychological R. to a drug or treatment; ALLERGIC R. (see SEN-SITIZATION) is a hypersensitivity to certain proteins with which the patient is brought into contact through the medium of his skin, or his digestive tract or respiratory tract, resulting in eczema, urticaria, hay fever, etc. Inheritance and emotion contribute to the allergic tendency. The basis of the condition is probably a local antigen–antibody R.; ANAPHYLACTIC R., R. that occurs following the administration of a substance to which the individual has become sensitized; DELAYED R. a R. occurring after more than the usual reaction time; IDIOSYN-CRATIC R. an unexpected, unusual R.; in pharmacotherapy, the opposite R. from what was expected; IMMUNE R. a R. that indicates the presence of antibodies and probable high resistance to a specific infection; R. TIME the time interval between the application of a stimulus and the response to it; TRANSFUSION R., R. that occurs following transfusion of incompatible blood.

reactive (rē-ak'-tiv): **1.** Readily responsive to a stimulus. **2.** Occurring as a result of stress or emotional upset. R. DEPRESSION an emotional state characterized by a strong feeling of sadness and depression of spirit, usually occurring following an external incident or emotional situation, and is relieved when the incident or situation is removed or understood.

reactivity (rē-ak-tiv'i-ti): The property of reacting or the state of being reactive.

reactor (rē-ak'tor): In medicine, refers to a person who reacts positively to a foreign substance, particularly one who is sensitive to tuberculin (*q.v.*). In physics, an apparatus that houses a device that can initiate and control a nuclear fission chain reaction to generate heat or produce radiation.

Read coding system (rēd): A hierarchically arranged thesaurus, providing a numerical coding system for clinical conditions. It is being superseded by the Systemized Nomenclature of Medicine (*q.v.*) terms.

Read method: A method of preparing for childbirth introduced by Dr Grantly Dick-Read. The woman learns exercises that foster relaxation and conditioning of the muscles, and slow diaphragmatic breathing; the emphasis is on fearlessness.

reagent (rē-ā′jent): An agent capable of producing a chemical change; when added to a complex solution it may determine the presence or absence of certain substances.

reagin (rē-ā′jin): An antibody associated with allergic reactions; present in the serum of hypersensitive people. It is responsible for the liberation of histamines and other substances that cause symptoms of hay fever and asthma. — reaginic, adj.

reality (rē-al′-i-ti): The aggregate of all things that have an objective existence; not imaginary, fictitious, or pretended. R. ORIENTATION the performance of measures to increase one's awareness of time, place, and person; R. PRINCIPLE in psychoanalytical theory, awareness that the gratification of instinctual wishes is modified by the inescapable external demands of the physical environment in a way that meets these demands but also allows for gratification at a more appropriate time; R. TESTING a function of the ego in which certain actions are explored and their outcomes analysed so that when the stimulus to act in a given fashion occurs, the individual will know what outcome to expect.

reality orientation: A treatment approach for patients with Alzheimer's disease, based upon the belief that continual, repetitive reminders will keep the patient stimulated and lead to an increase in orientation. In order for this to be effective, reorienting techniques must be applied consistently by all of the people who come into contact with the patient, twenty-four hours a day.

rebore (rē-bor′): Boring out or recanalizing.

rebound phenomenon: The reaction that occurs when a limb that is being subjected to resistance moves in the intended direction and then, when the resistance is removed, rebounds in the opposite direction; spastic limbs respond with exaggerated rebound, whereas in patients with cerebellar disturbances, no rebound occurs.

rebreathing bag: A bag attached to a mask and which is used to pump air or an anaesthetic gas into the patient's lung when needed; it serves as an accessory source of anaesthetic gases during an operation.

recalcitrant (rē-kal′si-trant): Refractory. Describes medical conditions that are resistant to treatment.

recall (rē′kawl): The process of bringing a past mental image or event into consciousness; to remember. R. is one phase of memory, the other two being memorization and retention.

recanalization (rē′kan-a-lī-zā′shun): Re-establishment of patency of (1) a blood vessel, or (2) a bodily tube, e.g., the vas deferens.

recapitulation theory: The theory that an embryo goes through the same stages in its development that the species did in developing from lower to higher forms of life.

reception screening: A comprehensive mental and physical health screen of all new prisoners, undertaken by a health-care worker in a prison.

receptor (ri-sep′tor): Sensory afferent nerve ending capable of receiving and transmitting stimuli. ALPHA and BETA R.S are located on cell surfaces throughout the body; they react to stimulation by acetylcholine, noradrenaline, and adrenaline; ALPHA-1 R.S when stimulated, cause peripheral vasoconstriction. ALPHA-2 R.S respond to stimulation by inhibiting release of noradrenaline at the neuron terminal; ALPHA-ADRENERGIC R. any of the adrenergic parts of the receptor of a stimulus that react to certain chemical substances, adrenaline in particular, by causing constriction of peripheral vessels of the skin, mucosa, intestine, and kidney, and contraction of the pupil and pilomotor muscles; the opposite of BETA-ADRENERGIC R.; also called *alpha receptor*; BETA-1 R.S when stimulated, cause an increase in heart rate and heart contractility, and facilitate atrioventricular conduction; BETA-2 R.S when stimulated, cause relaxation of smooth muscle which results in peripheral and coronary vasodilatation.

recess (ri-ses′, rē′ses): A small empty space, depression, or cavity.

recession (ri-sesh′un): The gradual withdrawal of a part or a structure from its normal position.

recessive (ri-ses′iv): Receding; having a tendency to disappear. R. GENE one of a gene pair that determines the character trait in an individual only if the other member of the pair is also recessive; R. TRAIT an inherited characteristic that remains latent when paired with a dominant trait in selective mating. See MENDEL'S LAW. Opp. to dominant.

recidivation (ri-sid-i-vā′shun): Relapse of a disease or recurrence of a symptom; or the repetition of a crime or offence; or a tendency to relapse into a previous condition, or; more particularly, the recurrence of an undesirable behaviour pattern.

recidivist (ri-sid'i-vist): A person who is inclined towards recidivation.

recipe (res'i-pi): 1. A prescription. 2. A word at the head of a written prescription meaning *take*; usually represented by R$_x$.

recipient (ri-sip'i-ent): In medicine, one who receives; usually refers to the person who receives blood in a transfusion. UNIVERSAL R. one who can receive any type of blood in a transfusion without harmful effects.

Recommended Dietary Allowance: Refers to the recommended daily amounts of specific nutrients and/or vitamins and minerals required to maintain health.

recompression (rē-kom-presh'un): The gradual return to conditions of normal pressure after exposure to diminished atmospheric pressure, a procedure used in treating deep-sea divers or caisson workers to prevent decompression sickness after their return to the surface.

reconstructive surgery: Surgery to correct or repair a defect, congenital or acquired.

record keeping: Maintaining a collection of information about patients and clients. This is an integral component of professional practice, a mark of safe and skilled practitioners. Records should be written in terms that others can understand and be signed. Patients and clients have a right of access to records held about them. See DATA PROTECTION ACT 1998.

recovery room: A special room where patients are kept until they recover from anaesthesia. It is usually located near the operating suite so that if emergency care is needed it can be given quickly by the anaesthetist or surgeon. Specially trained nurses are present at all times to observe the patients and care for them.

recreation therapy: The use of such recreational activities as games, music, or theatre to provide relaxation for physically or mentally handicapped individuals, to improve their quality of life, and to help prepare them to re-enter the community following disease or injury.

recrement (rek're-ment): A secretion that performs its function and then is reabsorbed into the blood, *e.g.*, saliva, bile. — recrementitious, adj.

recrudescence (rē-kroo-des'ens): The return of symptoms, or of a pathological state, after a period of apparent improvement.

rectal (rek'tal): Pertaining to the rectum. R. ANAESTHESIA introduction of an anaesthetic into

the rectum to produce local anaesthesia, used particularly in labour. R. FEEDING introduction of fluid nutrients into the rectum. R. REFLEX the normal reflex that produces the desire to evacuate the rectum. R. TUBE a rubber tube used to introduce substances into the rectum or to assist in the expulsion of flatus.

rectalgia (rek-tal'ji-a): Proctalgia (*q.v.*).

rectectomy (rek-tek'to-mi): Excision of the rectum.

rectitis (rek-tī'tis): Inflammation of the rectum; proctitis.

rect-, recto-: Combining forms denoting: 1. Relationship to the rectum. 2. Straight. See also words beginning PROCT-, PROCTO-.

rectoabdominal (rek'tō-ab-dom'i-nal): Relating to the rectum and the abdomen, particularly to a rectal examination in which one hand of the examiner is placed firmly on the abdominal wall while one (or more) finger(s) of the other hand is inserted into the rectum.

rectoanal (rek'tō-ā'nal): Relating to the rectum and the anus.

rectocele (rek'tō-sēl): Hernial protrusion of anterior wall of the rectum through the vagina following injury to the posterior wall; may occur during childbirth or, in later life, by weakening of the muscles of the pelvic floor; usually repaired by posterior colporrhaphy. Proctocele.

rectoclysis (rek-tok'li-sis): Proctoclysis.

rectocolitis (rek'tō-ko-lī'tis): Inflammation of the rectum and colon. Proctocolitis.

rectoperineal (rek'tō-per-i-nē'al): Relating to the rectum and the perineum.

rectoperineorrhaphy (rek'tō-per-i-nē-or'a-fi): Repair of the rectal wall and the perineum.

rectopexy (rek'tō-pek-si): Surgical fixation of a prolapsed rectum.

rectoscope (rek'to-skōp): An instrument for examining the rectum. Proctoscope. See ENDOSCOPE. — rectoscopic, adj.

rectosigmoid (rek-tō-sig'moyd): The rectum and sigmoid portion of the colon. Also descriptive of the place where the rectum and the sigmoid join.

rectosigmoidectomy (rek'tō-sig-moy-dek'to-mi): Surgical removal of the rectum and sigmoid colon.

rectostenosis (rek'tō-ste-nō'sis): A narrowing or stricture of the rectum. Proctostenosis.

rectostomy (rek-tos'to-mi): The surgical creation of a permanent opening into the rectum to relieve stricture. Proctostomy.

rectourethral (rek-tō-ū-rē'thral): Relating to the rectum and the urethra. R. FISTULA a fistula between the rectum and the urethra.

rectouterine (rek-tō-ū'ter-in): Relating to the rectum and uterus.

rectovaginal (rek-tō-vaj-īn'al): Relating to rectum and vagina. R. FISTULA one between the rectum and vagina.

rectovasical (rek-tō-ves'i-kal): Relating to the rectum and urinary bladder. R. FISTULA one between the rectum and the bladder; R. POUCH the fold of peritoneum that extends between the urinary bladder and the rectum in the male.

rectovulvar (rek-tō-vul'var): Relating to the rectum and the vulva. R. FISTULA a fistula between the rectum and the vulva.

rectum (rek'tum): The lower part of the large intestine between the sigmoid colon and anal canal. — rectal, adj.; rectally, adv.

rectus (rek'tus): Straight; in anatomy, a straight muscle. R. ABDOMINIS MUSCLE one of a pair of straight muscles that extend from the pubis to the xiphoid process; they compress the abdomen and assist to flex the trunk; R. FEMORIS MUSCLE the large muscle on the front of the thigh; it flexes the thigh and extends the leg; R. MUSCLES OF THE EYE include the superior, inferior, lateral and medial; they control the movements of the eyeball.

recumbent (ri-kum'bent): Lying down or reclining. — recumbency, n.

recuperate (rē-kū'per-āt): To regain health or strength. — recuperation, n.

recurrent (ri-kur'ent): Occurring again at intervals after a period of quiescence or abatement, e.g., fever, haemorrhage.

recurvature (rē-kur'va-chur): A backward curvature or bending.

red: R. BLOOD CELL erythrocyte (q.v.); R. BONE MARROW see BONE MARROW; R. NUCLEUS a large distinctive oval nucleus in the upper part of the midbrain; it receives fibres from the cerebellum and projects fibres to the brain stem, spinal cord, and thalamus.

Red Cross: 1. Abbreviation for a local, national, or the International Red Cross Society. **2.** The insignia adopted by the various Red Cross Societies; consists of a red Geneva cross on a white ground. **3.** A sign of neutrality used for protection of the sick and wounded and those caring for them in time of war. See INTERNATIONAL RED CROSS.

reduce (ri-dūs'): **1.** To restore something to its normal place or position, as in hernia, fracture or dislocation. **2.** In chemistry, to remove oxygen from a chemical substance. **3.** To decrease in volume or size. — reduction, n.; reducible, adj.

reductase (ri-duk'tās): Any enzyme that has a reducing action on a chemical compound; a hydrogenase.

reduction (ri-duk'shun): In chemistry, the removal of oxygen or the addition of hydrogen to a compound. In medicine, the replacement of a part at its normal position in the body. CLOSED R. refers to reduction of a fracture by manipulation without making an incision; OPEN R. refers to reduction of a fracture after incision of the tissues over the site of the fracture.

reductionism (rē-duk'-shun-izm): The practice of describing a phenomenon (particularly one involving human thought and action) in terms of an apparently more 'basic' phenomenon, to which the first is then said to be equivalent; for example, the practice of describing organic processes in terms of the physico-chemical reactions that underlie them. It is supposed that reduction both explains, and also simplifies the phenomenon. However, reductionism is also used as a term of abuse for those theories that simplify too much, by reducing one phenomenon to another that is too basic to explain it.

Reed–Sternberg cell: An enlarged anaplastic reticuloendothelial cell with multiple hyperlobulated nuclei, characteristic of Hodgkin's disease but also seen in other conditions. Also called *Sternberg–Reed cell; Dorothy Reed's cell; Hodgkin's cell; giant cell.*

re-engineering: To design and construct a new an existing object or system.

re-epithelialization (rē'ep-i-thē'li-al-ī-zā'shun): **1.** The regrowth of epithelial tissue over an area that has been denuded of it. **2.** The surgical replacement of epithelial tissue over a denuded surface.

referred pain: Pain which is felt as occurring at a place distant from its origin, *e.g.*, the pain felt in the arm during an attack of angina pectoris.

reflection (ri-flek'shun): **1.** The turning back of a light ray from a surface that it does not penetrate. **2.** A turning or bending back. **3.** Deep continued thought on written or oral material, often a devotional act; meditation.

reflection in action: Contemplation that takes place whilst still engaged in the practice setting; the aim of such reflection is to immediately shape and modify practice through on-the-spot experimentation.

reflection on action: The retrospective contemplation of practice, usually away from the setting in which it took place, in order to identify best practice and areas for improvement.

reflective enquiry: Research that is predominantly concerned with the generation of informal theory and personal knowledge through the process of reflection on action.

reflective practice: The use of reflection in action (*q.v.*) or reflection on action (*q.v.*). The process has become increasingly important for practice-based professions; it is a valuable learning tool for the advancement of personal and professional knowledge and skills. See CRITICAL INCIDENT; CRITICAL INCIDENT ANALYSIS.

reflex (rē'fleks): In physiology, an unlearned, involuntary response to a stimulus. R. ACTION an involuntary response by the body or any of its parts to a stimulus; the testing of various reflexes provides information on the location and diagnosis of disorders involving the nervous system. ABDOMINAL R. contraction of the underlying muscles when the skin of the abdomen is stroked; ACCOMMODATION R. constriction of the pupils and convergence of the eyes for near vision; ACHILLES R. contraction of the calf muscles causing flexion of the foot when the Achilles tendon is stroked; BABINSKI'S R. movement of the great toe upwards (dorsiflexion) instead of downwards (plantar flexion) and fanning of other toes, on stroking the outer border of the sole of the foot. Occurs in young infants and in some cases of disease of the brain or spinal cord. Also called *Babinski's sign* and *Babinski's great toe sign.* [Joseph François Felix Babinski, French neurologist, 1857–1932.] BICEPS R. contraction of the biceps muscle when the biceps tendon is struck at the elbow; BLINK R. involuntary closing of both eyes when any stimulus is applied to the face; present in parkinsonism and in those with generalized brain disease, and sometimes in normal older persons; BRACHIORADIALIS R. contraction of the brachioradialis muscle when the lower end of the radius is tapped and the arm is held in supination at 45°; BRUDZINSKI'S R., see BRUDZINSKI'S SIGN; CALORIC R. see CALORIC TEST; CAROTID R. slowing of the heart rate and decreased blood pressure when pressure is applied to the carotid sinus; CHADDOCK R. extension of the great toe when a stimulus is applied to the area below the external malleolus; an indication of lesion in the pyramidal tract; CHEMICAL R., one initiated by hormones or other chemicals in the blood; CILIARY R. the normal pupillary constriction that occurs in accommodation; CILIOSPINAL R. ipsilateral dilatation of the pupil when a painful stimulus is applied to the skin of the neck; usually present in co-

matose patients when there is no lesion in the brain stem; CONDITIONED R. one that is not inborn but developed through training and repeated association with a definite stimulus; CONJUNCTIVAL R. involuntary closure of the eyelids when the conjunctiva is touched; CORNEAL R. the reaction of blinking when the cornea is touched lightly; COUGH R. clearing of the air passageways of foreign material; results from impulses carried to the medulla by the vagus nerve; CREMASTERIC R. reaction of the ipsilateral testis when the skin on the inner surface of the thigh is stimulated; DANCE or DANCING R. stepping R.; DEEP R. a R. elicited by irritating a deep structure; DOLL'S EYE R. the involuntary turning of the eyes upwards or downwards with flexion and extension of the head; GAG R. contraction of the constrictor muscle of the pharynx when the back of the pharynx is touched; GALANT'S R. seen in normal infants during the first months of life, running a finger parallel to the spine from the last rib to the iliac crest will cause the infant to flex its trunk towards the side that is stimulated; GASTROCOLIC R. an increase in intestinal and colic peristalsis following entrance of food into the empty stomach; GLUTEAL R. contraction of the muscles of the buttock when the skin over the area is stroked; GORDON R. extension of the thumb and index finger or all the fingers on pressure on the pisiform bone of the wrist; also called *finger phenomenon*; GRASP R. contraction of the flexor muscles and resistance to attempts to remove an object placed in the hand of a person with a prefrontal lesion; HERING–BREUER R. a nervous mechanism by which afferent vagal impulses inhibit the inspiratory centre in the brain; HIRSCHBERG'S R. adduction of the foot when the sole under the great toe is tickled; ILEOGASTRIC R. the inhibition of gastric motility when the ileum becomes distended; JAW JERK R. a quick closure of the jaws when the chin of a person whose mouth is open is tapped; implies damage to the cerebrum in the area that controls motor activity of the fifth cranial nerve (trigeminal); KNEE-JERK R. see PATELLAR R.; MONOSYNAPTIC R. any R. that involves only one synapse and no internuncial neurons, *e.g.*, the patellar R.; MORO R. the startle R., tested for in evaluating newborn's status; when a sudden noise is made the infant will throw out its arms and legs and bring them together as if to hold on. Also called the *Moro embrace* R.; NECK-RIGHTING R. when an infant's head is forcibly turned to one side the whole body tries to turn to that side; this R. disappears at about one year of age; OCULOCARDIAC R. slowing of the rhythm of the heartbeat following pressure on the eyes or on the carotid sinus; a slowing of 5 to 13 beats per minute is considered the normal range; OCULOCEPHALIC R. the doll's eye R.; OPPENHEIMER'S R. dorsiflexion of the great toe on downwards stroking of the medial surface of the tibia; PALMAR R. flexion of the fingers when the palm is tickled; PALMOMEN-TAL R. contraction of the mentalis muscle when a non-painful stimulus is applied to the palm; seen in patients with cerebral arterio-sclerosis; PATELLAR R. a forward jerk that occurs when the tendon immediately below the patella is struck; also called the *knee-jerk* R.; PLANTAR R. the involuntary movement of the toes when the sole of the foot is stroked; POSTURAL R. the ability to maintain body alignment against the effects of gravity; PU-PILLARY R. change in size of the pupil in response to a stimulus such as light; QUADRICEPS R. patellar R.; RIGHTING R. the ability to assume the optimal position when there has been a departure from it, either voluntary or involuntary; ROOTING R. occurs when a new-born's cheek is touched lightly; the infant turns its head towards the direction of the touch and purses its lips in preparation for sucking; STEPPING R. the stepping or dancing movement made by an infant when held up-right with its feet on a flat surface; SUCKING R. sucking movements of the lips, tongue, and jaw in response to contact of the lips with an object; normal in infants; SUPERFICIAL R. one that can be elicited by applying a stimulus such as stroking or scratching to the skin; SWALLOWING R. the act of swallowing when the palate, fauces, or posterior pharyngeal wall are touched; TENDON R. contraction of a stretched muscle when the skin over it is tapped lightly; includes the Achilles, biceps, patellar, and triceps reflexes; TONIC NECK R. a R. in the newborn when the infant, lying on its back with its head forcibly turned, extends the ipsilateral arm and sometimes the leg, in the direction the head is turned, while the contral-ateral limbs become flexed; this R. disappears after about four months; TRICEPS R. extension of the forearm when the triceps tendon is tapped at the elbow while the arm hangs loosely at right angles to the side; VOMITING R. contraction of the abdominal muscles, re-laxation of the cardiac sphincter of the stom-ach and of the throat muscles, elicited by a variety of stimuli, usually applied to the fauces.

reflex arc (rē′fleks ark): A sensory neuron, a connective neuron, and a motor neuron which, acting together, constitute the path that an im-pulse travels from a receptor to an effector organ or gland.

reflexive action research: Research that aims to bring about change in practice as part of the research itself, and which subsequently modi-fies the research process.

reflexivity (rē-fleks-iv′-i-ti): Critically examin-ing the research process, taking into consider-ation the subjectivity and experiences of the researcher in addition to social, political, and ethical contexts of the study.

reflexogenic (rē-flek-sō-jen′ik): Producing, in-creasing, or increasing the tendency to reflex action.

reflexograph (rē-flek′sō-graf): A device for recording a reflex action.

reflexology (rē-flek-sol′o-ji): A complementary therapy practising diagnostic foot massage, according to a theory that all the body's organs correspond to pressure points in the feet.

reflux (rē′fluks): Backward flow or return of a fluid; regurgitation. GASTROESOPHAGEAL R. often due to an incompetent gastroesophageal sphincter and associated with hiatus hernia; characterized by heartburn, regurgitation, an-terior chest pain; is aggravated by spicy foods, aspirin, chocolate; complications include oe-sophageal ulcer, haemorrhage, and perfor-ation; HEPATOJUGULAR R. distension of the jugular vein and elevation of blood pressure resulting from pressure on the liver; can be observed in the jugular vein and measured in the arm veins; VESICOURETERAL R. the passage of urine from the bladder back into the ureter. See also PEPTIC OESOPHAGITIS under OESOPHA-GITIS.

refraction (ri-frak′shun): 1. The bending of light rays as they pass through media of different densities. In normal vision, the light rays are so bent that they meet on the retina. 2. The process of measuring errors of refraction in the eyes and correcting them by eyeglass lenses. — refractive, adj.; refract, v.

refractometry (rē-frak-tom′e-tri): In ophthal-mology, the use of a refractometer to measure refractive errors in the eye.

refractory (ri-frak′tō-ri): 1. Stubborn, unman-ageable, rebellious; resistant to treatment. 2. Unable to accept a stimulus. ABSOLUTE R. PERIOD the time immediately after a nerve has been stimulated when the cells are depolarized and the nerve cannot respond to another stimulus, regardless of its strength; RELATIVE R. PERIOD the time period during which a neuron can respond to a stimulus if the stimulus is strong enough.

refracture (rē-frak'chur): The operation of rebreaking a bone that has united improperly after fracture.

refrigerant (ri-frij'er-ant): **1.** Allaying heat or fever. **2.** An agent that reduces fever and produces a feeling of coolness.

refrigeration (ri-frij-er-ā'shun): Cooling of the body or any part of it, to reduce basal metabolism or to render a part insensitive, as is needed for minor surgery. See HIBERNATION, HYPOTHERMIA.

refugee (ref-ū-jē'): A person who, for political, racial, or ideological reasons, or as a result of such crises as famine or disaster, has been forced to flee his or her home or home country.

refusion (re-fū'zhun): The return of blood to the circulation after it has been temporarily removed from the body or cut off from a part.

regeneration (rē-jen-er-ā'shun): The natural renewal or repair of tissue after injury. — regenerate, v.

regimen (rej'i-men): A systematic plan of diet, medication, and activities designed to restore or maintain a certain state of health or keep a certain condition under control.

region (rē'jun): In anatomy, a limited area of the surface of the body, e.g. the ABDOMINAL R. S include the epigastric, right and left hypochondriac, umbilical, right and left lumbar, hypogastric, right and left iliac.

registrar (re-jis'trar'): **1.** An experienced doctor working in a British hospital and training to be a specialist; **2.** An official recorder and keeper of records.

registration: In nursing, a process by which qualified individuals are listed on an official register maintained by the Nursing and Midwifery Council. R. OF BIRTHS AND DEATHS a legal requirement in the United Kingdom that all births and deaths are recorded with a Central Register Office. Births should be recorded within six weeks in England and Wales and within 21 days in Scotland. It is illegal to dispose of a dead person without a death certificate to indicate that the death has been officially registered.

regression (ri-gresh'un): **1.** A return to a former state or condition. **2.** The subsidence or abatement of symptoms or of a disease condition. **3.**

In psychiatry, a turning back to an earlier more comfortable stage of development in order to escape a frustrating or unbearable situation; occurs in dementia, especially senile dementia. — regressive, adj.; regress, v.

regulation (reg-ū-lā'-shun): The act of regulating, or the state of being regulated.

regurgitant (ri-gur'ji-tant): Flowing back or in the opposite direction from normal.

regurgitation (ri-gur-ji-tā'shun): Backward flow, as of stomach contents into or through the mouth, or of blood into the heart or between the chambers of the heart when the valves do not function properly, as in MITRAL R., in which blood flows back from the left ventricle into the left atrium, or in TRICUSPID R., in which blood flows back from the right ventricle into the right atrium. — regurgitation, adj.; regurgitate, v.

rehabilitation (rē-ha-bil-i-tā'shun): The restoration of an individual's ability to function as efficiently and normally as his condition will permit following injury, illness, or accident. It involves re-education and retraining of those who have become partially or wholly incapacitated by such conditions as blindness, deafness, heart disease, amputation, paralysis, etc. R. ENGINEERING the construction and use of a great number of devices used to restore or replace motor and sensory functions; R. MEDICINE all aspects of medicine involved in rehabilitative programmes. — rehabilitate, v.

rehabilitation programme: 1. The retraining of a person following imprisonment or illness. **2.** The restoration of industry, the economy, etc., after a war.

rehydration (re-hī-drā'shun): The restoration of water or fluid to a substance that has been dehydrated. — rehydrate, v.

Reichian therapy (rīk'-i-an): A type of psychotherapy characterized by emphasis on the necessity of full expression of the sexual libido as a cure for neurosis; introduced by Wilhelm Reich, German psychoanalyst [1897–1957].

Reil's island (rīls): See INSULA.

reimplantation (rē'im-plan-tā'shun): The replacement into its former position of a body part that has been removed.

reinfection (rē'in-fek'shun): A secondary infection, during convalescence or after recovery from a previous infection by the same or a very similar organism.

reinforcement (rē'in-fors'ment): Increasing the cumulative effect of something by strengthening it through repetition, addition, or similar action. In psychology, the strengthening of a response by offering a reward or by withholding punishment, an important process in operant conditioning. — reinforce, v.

reinfusion (rē'in-fū'zhun): The reinjection of blood serum, or cerebrospinal fluid.

reinnervation (rē'-in-er-vā'shun): The operation of restoring the nerve supply of an organ or muscle by grafting in a living nerve when the motor nerve supply has been lost.

reinoculation (rē'in-ok-ū-lā'shun): A second inoculation with the same virus or infection.

Reiter's syndrome: An arthritis-like syndrome with urethritis, conjunctivitis, and cutaneous lesions; of unknown origin; sometimes mistaken for acute gonorrhoeal arthritis. Likely to be chronic and to recur. Occurs most often in males. Also called *Reiter's disease.*

rejection (rē-jek'shun): 1. An immune reaction against a grafted tissue or organ. 2. In psychology, a denial; a refusal to accept, recognize, or grant.

relapse (rē-laps'): The return of a disease or of serious symptoms after the disease has apparently been overcome.

relapsing fever: Louse-borne or tick-borne infection caused by spirochaetes of genus *Borrelia.* Prevalent in many parts of the world. Characterized by a febrile period of a week or so, with apparent recovery, followed by a further bout of high fever.

relaxant (rē-lak'sant): 1. Causing relaxation. 2. An agent that produces relaxation or reduction of tension.

relaxin (rē-lak'sin): A factor secreted by certain pregnant animals and also prepared pharmaceutically for treatment of dysmenorrhoea and premature labour and to facilitate labour at term; it produces relaxation of the symphysis pubis and dilatation of the uterine cervix.

reliability (re-lī-a-bil'-i-ti): 1. The quality of being trustworthy and dependable. 2. In research, the likelihood of producing the same findings using the same research conditions over a period of time or with different researchers.

REM: Abbreviation for rapid eye movement (*q.v.*).

rem: The amount of ionizing radiation that will have the same effect as 1 rad or gray of x-ray radiation.

remedial (re-mē'di-al): Having curative properties.

remedy (rem'e-di): Any agent that prevents, cures, or alleviates a disease or its symptoms.

reminiscence (rem-i-nis'-ens): The act, process, or fact of remembering or recollecting; some-

times specifically the act of recovering knowledge by mental effort. R. THERAPY a treatment for older people or those with dementia, using objects from the past, such as photographs, food, and clothes, to trigger discussion and reflection.

remission (ri-mish'un): 1. Lessening or abatement of the symptoms of a disease. 2. A period of temporary abatement of the symptoms of a disease, *e.g.*, as in a fever.

remittent (ri-mit'ent): Characterized by periodic intervals of abatement of symptoms of a pathological condition.

ren-, reni-, reno-: Combining forms denoting the kidney.

renal (rē'nal): Relating to the kidney. R. ASTHMA hyperventilation of the lung occurring sometimes during uraemia, as a result of acidosis; R. CALCULUS a stone in the kidney; R. COLIC severe pain in the lower back, radiating down the groin and sometimes the leg; caused by a calculus in the kidney or ureter; R. DIALYSIS see HAEMODIALYSIS; R. DWARFISM dwarfism due to renal failure; R. FAILURE failure of the kidney to perform its functions; chronic failure is usually irreversible; R. FUNCTION TESTS various tests for measuring renal function, all requiring careful collection of urine specimens; some of those in common use are: para-aminohippuric acid clearance test for measuring renal blood flow; creatinine clearance test for measuring glomerular filtration rate; ammonium chloride test for measuring tubular ability to excrete hydrogen ions; urinary concentration and dilution tests for measuring tubular function; R. GLYCOSURIA that which occurs in patients with normal blood sugar and lowered renal threshold for sugar; R. HAEMANGIOPERICYTOMA a vascular neoplasm of the kidney in which the capillaries are often obscured by the growing tumour, which may be benign or malignant; R. HYPERTENSION systemic arterial hypertension resulting from kidney disease; R. INSUFFICIENCY inability of the kidney to perform its functions properly; R. MEDULLA the inner darker part of the kidney, composed of the renal pyramids; R. OSTEODYSTROPHY a chronic condition with onset in childhood, due to renal insufficiency, marked by increased resorption of bone with osteomalacia and osteoporosis; also called *renal rickets*; R. SHUTDOWN, R. failure; R. SYSTEM consists of the two kidneys, two ureters, bladder, urethra, renal arteries and veins; R. THRESHOLD the degree of concentration of a substance in the urine at which the kidney begins to excrete it;

R. TUBULAR ACIDOSIS a hereditary disorder characterized by inability to produce an acid urine; it occurs chiefly in males in whom it is the result of incomplete reabsorption of bicarbonate in the proximal tubule; R. URAEMIA uraemia that follows kidney disease in contrast to that caused by a circulatory disorder.

Rendu–Weber–Osler disease: Hereditary haemorrhagic telangiectasia; see under TELANGIECTASIA.

renin (rē′nin): A protein substance manufactured in the kidney that acts like an enzyme; when secreted into the bloodstream it acts as a powerful vasoconstrictor and raises the blood pressure; too high a level in the bloodstream will result in blood pressure that is higher than normal.

renin–angiotensin–aldosterone system: A system by which the kidneys control blood pressure. Renin, released by the kidney when blood pressure falls, combines with a plasma protein to form angiotensin I, then angiotensin II which is a potent vasoconstrictor that stimulates the production of aldosterone by the kidney cortex, which, in turn, promotes the reabsorption of sodium by the kidney tubules and results in the release of potassium and an increase in blood volume. Also called *renin–angiotensin* system.

renin–sodium profile test: Measures the sodium content in a 24-hour urine specimen during which time salt is restricted, and compares it with the renin content of the blood; useful in planning medical treatment of hypertension.

rennet (ren′et): An extract made of calf's stomach; contains rennin. Used in preparing certain foods and in cheese making.

rennin (ren′-in): Gastric enzyme that curdles milk.

renninogen (ren-in′ō-jen): The inactive precursor of rennin.

renogenic (rē-nō-jen′ik): Originating or arising in the kidney.

renogram (rē′nō-gram): The roentgenographic record showing the rate at which kidneys remove an intravenously injected dose of a radioactive substance from the blood, and aid in evaluating renal function.

renography (rē-nog′ra-fi): Radiography of the kidney.

renomegaly (rē′nō-meg′a-li): Abnormal enlargement of the kidney.

renopathy (rē-nop′a′-thi): Any disease of the kidney.

renorenal (rē-nō-rē′nal): Relating to or affecting both kidneys. R. REFLEX the mechanism by which pathology in one kidney will affect the functioning of the other kidney.

renotrophic (rē′nō-trōf′ik): Having the ability to cause an increase in the size of the kidney.

renovascular (rē′nō-vas′kū-lar): Relating to the blood vessels of the kidney. R. HYPERTENSION see under HYPERTENSION.

reorganization (rē-or′ga-nī-zā′shun): Healing by the formation of new tissue similar to that lost through some morbid process.

Reovirus (rē′ō-vi′rus): A genus of RNA viruses closely related to the echoviruses (*q.v.*) and the arboviruses (*q.v.*); have been found in the respiratory and intestinal tracts of both healthy and sick people, but not yet associated with any specific disease.

Rep.: See REPETATUR.

repellant (ri-pel′ent): 1. Capable of reducing a swelling. 2. An agent that is capable of reducing a swelling or oedema. 3. Capable of repelling insects or mosquitoes. 4. An agent that repels insects or mosquitoes.

repertory grid (rep′-er-to-ri): An index, list, catalogue, or calendar. Psychologist George Kelly developed the grid as a way of measuring an individual's dichotomous (bipolar) constructs. Also known as *ratings repertory grid.*

repetatur (re-pe-tā′tūr): Let it be renewed; a Latin term used in prescription writing.

replacement (rē-plās′ment): 1. The infusion of donor blood to replace lost blood. 2. The substitution of a prosthetic device to replace a missing part or one that has been lost by amputation or accident.

replantation (ri-plan-tā′shun): Usually refers to the replacement of teeth that have been extracted or otherwise removed. — replant, v.

repletion (rē-plē′shun): The state of having ingested food and drink sufficient to produce satiation. Fullness.

replication (rep-li-kā′-shun): The creation of one or multiple facsimilies of an object or information; for example, cellular mitosis (*q.v.*), genetic replication.

repolarization (rē′pō-lar-ī-zā′shun): The process by which a depolarized cell membrane becomes repolarized by the restoration of a positive charge on the outer surface of the cell and a negative charge on the inner surface. — repolarize, v.

reposition (rē′pō-zish′un): To replace an organ or part to its normal site.

repression (rē-presh′un): In psychiatry, a defence mechanism whereby an individual unconsciously refuses to recognize the existence of urges, thoughts, memories, or feelings that are unacceptable or painful, or in conflict with the person's accepted moral principles; these experiences may not be recalled at will, but may emerge as the source of anxiety neuroses.

reproduction (rē-prō-duk'shun): The process of producing offspring, usually by sexual means, *i.e.*, the union of male and female sex cells; may also occur asexually, *i.e.*, by some means other than the union of male and female sex cells.

reproductive (rē'prō-duk'tiv): Pertinent to or associated with reproduction. R. SYSTEM consists of the organs involved in reproduction. MALE R. SYSTEM includes the testes, efferent ducts, epididymis, ductus deferens, ejaculatory duct, urethra, prostate gland, penis. FEMALE R. SYSTEM includes ovaries, uterine tubes, uterus, vagina, vulva, and accessory glands.

repulsion (ri-pul'shun): The act of forcing or driving apart or away. Opp. of attraction.

research (re'serch): A search or investigation directed to the discovery of some fact by careful consideration or study of a subject; a course of critical or scientific enquiry.

Research Assessment Exercise: An investigative procedure, aimed at enabling the higher education funding bodies in the UK to distribute public funds for research selectively on the basis of quality. Institutions conducting the best research receive a larger proportion of the available grant, so that the infrastructure for the top level of research is protected and developed.

research ethics: The use and pursuit of new scientific knowledge with regard to widely held concepts of right and wrong.

research governance (guv' -er-nans): The enforcement of standards to ensure that research is carried out to a high quality and in a manner that the public can trust and support.

research methods: The techniques used to gather data in an investigation.

resect (rē-sekt'): To cut off or cut out part of a structure or organ.

resection (rē-sek'shun): Surgical removal of a section or segment of an organ or structure. SUB-MUCOUS R. a surgical procedure involving incision of the nasal mucosa, removal of deflected nasal septum, and replacement of mucosa; TRANSURETHRAL R. removal of the prostate utilizing an instrument passed through the urethra; WEDGE R. the removal of a small wedge-shaped portion of tissue from an organ or part.

resectoscope (rē-sek'tō-skōp): A tubular instrument for dividing or removing small structures from a body cavity under direct vision, without making an incision other than that used for passing the instrument; used particularly when removing the prostate gland through the urethra.

reserve (ri-serv'): In physiology, something that is held back or stored for future use. ALKALINE R. the amount of alkaline available in the body to act as buffer to maintain the normal pH of the blood; CARDIAC R. the amount of work the heart is able to perform in increasing its output to meet increased physiologic demands.

reservoir (rez'er-vwar): A place where anything is collected or stored. R. OF INFECTION anything that provides a place for infectious agents to live and multiply and from which such agents can transmit an infection to a susceptible host; may be a person, animal, plant, water, soil, or inanimate organic matter.

residential care: Accommodation, staffed 24 hours a day, providing board and general personal care to the residents. Such premises are provided for vulnerable persons (*e.g.*, children, the elderly, the physically disabled, those with dependence on alcohol/drugs and those with learning disabilities or who are mentally ill) who require ongoing care and supervision under circumstances where nursing care would normally be inappropriate.

residual (rē-zid'ū-al): Remaining. In physiology, refers to something remaining in a body cavity after normal expulsion has occurred. Also refers to a disability or deformity that remains after recovery from disease or operation, as a limp or a scar. R. AIR the air remaining in the lung after forced expiration; R. URINE urine remaining in the bladder after micturition; R. VOLUME the volume of air remaining in the lung after a maximal expiration.

residue (rez'i-dū): That which remains after removal of other substances. — residual, adj.

resilient (rē-zil'i-ent): Elastic. Having a tendency to return to previous shape, position, or condition. — resilience, n.

res ipsa loquitur (rās' -ip-sa-lok' -wi-toor): A legal term (Latin) that, literally, means 'the thing speaks for itself'. An important concept in malpractice lawsuits since it means specifically that the person or institution is being sued for an unfavourable or injurious injury or condition which could have been prevented if proper care had been used, *e.g.*, leaving a sponge in the patient's body after surgery.

resistance (ri-zis'tens): 1. Opposition to the passage of an electrical current. 2. Power of opposing an active force. 3. In psychology, the name given to the force that prevents repressed thoughts from reentering the consciousness. AIRWAY R. that usually offered to the airflow, mainly by the larynx, trachea, and bronchi; COGWHEEL R. stepwise jerking resistance felt by the examiner on passive stretching of muscle, as in passive flexion and extension of the elbow; occurs in patients with parkinsonism; PERIPHERAL R. that offered by the capillaries to the blood passing through them; R. TO INFECTION the power of the body to withstand infection; see IMMUNITY.

resolution (rez-ō-loo'shun): The subsidence or spontaneous arrest of an inflammatory process without suppuration; the breaking down and removal or absorption of the products of inflammation, as seen, e.g., in lobar pneumonia when the consolidation begins to liquefy.

resolve (rē-zolv'): To return to a normal state following a pathological condition, particularly when no suppuration has occurred.

resonance (rez'o-nans): The sound elicited when percussing a part that can vibrate freely, as for example, a hollow organ or a cavity containing air, VOCAL R. the reverberating note heard through the stethoscope on auscultation of the chest while the patient is speaking. — resonant, adj.

resorption (rē-sorp'shun): 1. The loss or disappearance of a body process or substance by absorption, lysis, or dissolution, e.g., callus following bone fracture, the root of a tooth, or blood from a haematoma. 2. The act of reabsorbing or assimilating an excretion, blood clot, pus, or exudative material.

respiration (res-pi-rā'shun): 1. The release of energy via chemical reactions within cells. The physical and chemical process by which the cells and tissues of an organism receive the oxygen needed for carrying on their physiological processes and are relieved of the carbon dioxide resulting from these activities. 2. The movement of gases across the alveolar–capillary membrane in the lungs. 3. The act or function of breathing. ABDOMINAL R. the use of the diaphragm and abdominal muscles in breathing; APNEUSTIC R. characterized by long inspirations and short expirations; ARTIFICIAL R. artificial methods to restore respiration such as mouth-to-mouth breathing, or by the use of a device that intermittently inflates the lungs by forcing either oxygen or air into them; BIOT'S R. jerky, rapid, irregular breathing that is inter-

rupted by apnoea after four or five breaths; seen in meningitis and other conditions resulting from increased intracranial pressure which depresses the respiratory centre; CAVERNOUS R., R. characterized by prolonged hollow resonance; usually indicates a cavity in the lung; CHEYNE–STOKES R. a type of breathing in which the respirations gradually increase in depth until they reach a maximum, then gradually decrease in depth, finally ceasing for a period of time after which the cycle is repeated; results from retarded blood flow to the cerebrum and is often seen in congestive heart failure; the prognosis is ominous; COGWHEEL R. jerky, interrupted breathing; DIAPHRAGMATIC R. abdominal R.; EXTERNAL R. the exchange between the oxygen in the air in the lungs and the carbon dioxide in the blood in the walls of the capillaries in the alveoli; INTERNAL R. the exchange of oxygen and carbon dioxide in the tissues; KUSSMAUL R. the deep, sighing or gasping respirations characteristic of diabetic acidosis; PARADOXICAL R. inward movement of the chest wall during inspiration and outward movement during expiration; occurs when the lung or part of it is deflated; STERTOROUS R. noisy, rattling R. due to breathing with the mouth open which causes vibration of the soft palate; often occurs in comatose patients; SONOROUS or STRIDENT R. in which a high-pitched crowing sound is heard; usually indicates a partial airway obstruction; THORACIC R., R. accomplished chiefly by the intercostal muscles.

respirator (res'pi-rā-tor): 1. An appliance worn over the nose and mouth and designed to filter out irritating or poisonous substances such as gases, fumes, smoke, or dust, or to warm the air before it enters the respiratory tract. 2. An apparatus that artificially and rhythmically inflates and deflates the lungs as in normal breathing, when for any reason the natural nervous or muscular control of respiration is impaired. The apparatus may work on either positive or negative pressure or on electrical stimulation. CURASS R. a R. in the shape of a shell; is worn over the front of the trunk; used for patients who have some ability to breathe on their own; DRINKER R. used when it is necessary to supply artificial respiration for a long period of time. Consists of a metal tank that encloses the entire body except the head; commonly called 'iron lung'.

respiratory (res-pi'ra-tō-ri): Relating to respiration. R. ACIDOSIS see under ACIDOSIS; R. ALKALOSIS see under ALKALOSIS; R. CENTRE the area in the medulla oblongata that regulates respiratory movements; it is stimulated by carbon dioxide in the blood and cerebrospinal fluid; R. FAILURE functional failure of the lungs and respiratory system to extract enough oxygen from the air to meet the body's needs; R. FUNCTION TESTS numerous available tests for vital capacity, forced vital capacity, forced expiratory volume, and maximal breathing capacity; R. SYSTEM consists of the nose, pharynx, larynx, trachea, bronchi, lungs, and pleura; accessory structures include the diaphragm, pleural sac, and muscles of the chest wall; R. TRACT the group of tubular and cavernous structures that, functioning together, accomplish the exchange of gases between the ambient air and the blood, the principal organs involved being the nose, larynx, trachea, bronchi, bronchioles, and lungs.

respiratory distress syndrome: 1. R.D.S. OF THE NEWBORN dyspnoea in the newly born; formerly called *hyaline membrane disease.* Occurs most often in preterm infants, and those born of diabetic mothers or by Caesarean section. A protein–lipid complex forms in the air spaces of the lungs on the first entry of air, causing reduced amounts of lung surfactant (*q.v.*); without adequate surfactant to decrease the surface tension of the fluids lining the alveoli, air cannot pass and there is partial or complete collapse of the lung (atelactasis); the chest wall retreats with every breath, cyanosis develops, the respiration rate increases and a characteristic grunt is heard on expiration. **2.** ADULT R.D.S. the name given to a severe obstructive lung disorder that results from the inflammatory response to such stresses as shock, chest injury, certain drug overdoses, or the effects of a viral, bacterial, chemical, or allergic agent; other causes include inhalation of smoke or corrosive chemicals, aspiration of stomach contents, or drowning. Symptoms are due to formation of a hyaline membrane in the alveoli which prevents formation of surfactant, causing suspension of oxygen–carbon dioxide exchange in the alveoli, which then become filled with exudate and fibrinous material. Symptoms include dyspnoea, hypoxia, interstitial oedema, and respiratory failure. Also called *acute respiratory distress syndrome, white lung, wet lung*, and *shock lung.*

respiratory sounds: May be (1) normal breath sounds heard on auscultation; often described as low-pitched, non-musical rustlings, or murmurs, or (2) adventitious sounds which are usually indicative of a pathological condition; may be popping or clicking, squeaking, wheezing, whistling.

respiratory syncytial virus (res-pi-ra-tō-ri sin-sish'-i-al vī'rus): A virus of the genus *Pneumovirus*; causes bronchitis and bronchopneumonia in children and minor upper respiratory infections in adults.

respiratory tract infection: Any infection affecting the respiratory tract; usually identified as (1) upper respiratory tract infections which include colds, tonsillitis, pharyngitis, sinusitis, rhinitis, and bronchial infections, and (2) lower respiratory tract infections which include those of the trachea and bronchi, and the various pneumonias.

respire (re-spīr'): To breathe.

respirometer (res-pi-rom'i-ter): An instrument used for studying and measuring the extent and character of the respiratory movements. Also called *Spirometer.*

respite care: Regular relief for the families of patients who are being cared for at home; may be provided on a daily or a weekly basis.

respondeat superior: The doctrine that an employer is responsible for wrongful or negligent acts of his employees in certain situations, and that both can be sued.

respondents: 1. One who answers or replies, *e.g.* to a questionnaire. **2.** One who defends a thesis against one or more opponents.

response (re-spons'): A reaction or movement following the application of a stimulus.

rest cure: Bed rest; usually combined with special diet, massage, physiotherapy, etc., to improve muscle tone and circulation and to promote relaxation; usually prescribed for individuals who are convalescing from debilitating illness or nervous system disorder.

restless legs syndrome: A condition characterized by weakness, coldness, and a disagreeable, prickly, creeping sensation in the muscles of the lower legs, and sometimes in the thighs, arms, and hands; begins after the person has gone to bed and can be relieved only by walking; the cause is unknown but thought to be a vascular condition; occurs most often in those suffering from a neurosis and in the elderly.

restoration (res-to-rā'shun): Repair or reconstruction of a part, or a return to a previous state of health; strength; or consciousness.

restorative (re-stor'a-tiv): **1.** An agent that serves to restore health, strength, or consciousness. **2.** Promoting or tending to restore health, strength, or consciousness.

rest pain: Pain that occurs mostly at night in patients with peripheral vascular disease; often severe and persistent; due to ischaemic neuritis. The peripheral pulses are absent and the toes may be red and tender; gangrene follows easily after injury.

restraint (r-strānt'): Forcible restriction of the movements of an excessively restless, irrational, or psychotic patient in order to prevent self-injury or injury to others.

restrictive pulmonary disease: Any disease or disorder that interferes with lung expansion, e.g., pulmonary fibrosis.

Resusci-Anne: A training manikin that responds to external cardiac massage and mouth-to-mouth resuscitation.

resuscitation (rē-sus-i-tā'shun): The restoration to life of someone who is in cardiac or respiratory failure or shock. CARDIOPULMONARY R. bringing an individual back to consciousness by keeping the airway open, and by mouth-to-mouth breathing or external cardiac massage; MOUTH-TO-MOUTH R. a method of giving artificial respiration in which the rescuer forces air from his own lungs into the mouth of the victim; also called *oral resuscitation*; OPEN-CHEST R. accomplished by massaging the heart in cases when the patient is in the operating room and the chest is already open, or when the patient is obese or barrel-chested, or in cases of tension pneumothorax or flail chest. — resuscitate, v.; resuscitative, adj.

resuscitator (ri-sus'i-tā-tor): An apparatus used to initiate breathing in persons whose respirations have ceased; consists of a mask that fits over the nose and mouth, a bag or reservoir for air, and a pump that may be electrically or hand-powered.

retardation (rē-tar-dā'shun): Delay; hindrance; slowing down; backwardness. MENTAL R. mental handicap (*q.v.*) lack of normal intellectual development, through impairment of learning, of social adjustment or of maturation. PSYCHOMOTOR R. abnormal slowness or lack of progress in both mental and physical development.

retch: To make a strong involuntary but ineffective effort to vomit.

retching: Straining at vomiting.

retention (ri-ten'shun): 1. Retaining information and facts in the mind; memory. 2. Accumulation of that which is normally excreted. 3. Keeping within the body that which normally belongs there, particularly food and liquid in the stomach. 4. Keeping in the body that which should normally be discharged. R. ENEMA one

given with the intent that it can be retained in order to provide nourishment, medication, or anaesthesia. R. OF URINE accumulation of urine within the bladder.

reticular (re-tik'ū-lar): 1. Resembling a net. 2. Relating to the reticuloendothelium (*q.v.*). R. ACTIVATING SYSTEM consists of the reticuloendothelium; maintains the person in the alert conscious state; lesions or chemical dysfunction of the system may produce lethargy, stupor, or coma.

reticulocyte (re-tik'ū-lō-sīt): A young circulating red blood cell, which still contains traces of the nucleus that was present in the cell when developing in the bone marrow. Increased numbers of reticulocytes in the blood are evidence of active blood regeneration. Reticulocytes normally constitute about 1% of the circulating red blood cells

reticulocytopenia (re-tik'-ū-lō-sī-tō-pē'ni-a): A decrease in the normal number of reticulocytes in the circulating blood.

reticulocytosis (re-tik'ū-lō-sī-tō'sis): A condition in which there is more than the normal number of reticulocytes in the peripheral blood, due either to irritation of the bone marrow or to excessive production; may occur after haemorrhage, in high altitude, and in treatment of some types of anaemia.

reticuloendothelioma (re-tik'ū-lō-en'dō-thē-li-ō'ma): A tumour that is derived from reticuloendothelial tissue.

reticuloendotheliosis (re-tik'ū-lō-en'dō-thē-li-ō'sis): A group of diseases affecting the reticuloendothelial system, including Hand–Schüller–Christian disease and Letterer–Siwe disease. Cause unknown; characterized by the proliferation of histiocytes; symptoms include otitis media, seborrhoeic rash, lymphoadenopathy, enlarged liver and spleen, anaemia.

reticuloendothelium (re-tik'ū-lō-en'dō-thē'li-um): A system of widely dispersed cells important in immunity because of their ability to remove bacteria, foreign particles, and cellular debris from the blood. Scattered throughout the body, these cells may be fixed or wandering, the fixed cells being found chiefly in connective tissue, thymus gland, lymph glands, bone marrow, liver, spleen, adrenals, hypophysis, and the microglia of the central nervous system, while the wandering cells are found in the blood. — reticuloendothelial, adj.

reticuloma (re-tik-ū-lō' ma): A tumour consisting chiefly of reticuloendothelial cells.

reticulosarcoma (re-tik'ū-lō-sar-ko'ma): Sarcoma composed of reticuloendothelial cells.

reticulosis (re-tik'ū-lō'-sis): Proliferative disease of the reticuloendothelial system. An ill-defined group of fatal conditions of unknown aetiology in which glandular and splenic enlargement are commonly found, and of which the three commonest members are Hodgkin's disease (lymphadenoma), lymphosarcoma, and reticulum cell sarcoma. See MYCOSIS. — reticuloses, pl.

reticulum (re-tik'ū-lum): A fine network of cells or of connective tissue fibres; the neuroglia.

retiform (ret'i-form): Resembling a net or network; reticular.

retina (ret'i-na): The delicate, light-sensitive, innermost of the three coats of the eyeball. The optic nerve enters the posterior of the eyeball and then expands to form the retina, which extends forward to the margin of the pupil. Thus it is composed of nerve tissue which receives stimuli from light and transmits them to the visual centre in the brain. It is soft in consistency, translucent, of a pinkish colour, and made up of layers, the outer one being pigmented and the seven inner ones being nerve tissue, the innermost of which contains the rods and cones, the receptors for light. In the centre of the posterior retina is the *macula lutea* or yellow spot, and in the centre of it is the *fovea centralis*, the area of most acute vision. DETACHED R. partial or complete separation of the retina from the choroid; may be due to trauma, or due to haemorrhage into the choroid. — retinae, pl.; retinal, adj.

retinaculum (ret-i-nak'ū-lum): 1. An instrument for holding tissues out of the way during surgery. 2. A band or structure that holds an organ or tissue in place. 3. A frenum (*q.v.*).

retinal (ret'i-nal): 1. Related to the retina. R. DETACHMENT see DETACHED R. under RETINA. 2. Part of a pigment extracted from the retina; the chief component of rhodopsin; can be converted into vitamin A by light and resynthesized into rhodopsin in the dark; allows for maximum vision in a dim light.

retinitis (ret-i-nī'-tis): Inflammation of the retina. R. CIRCINATA a condition of inadequate vascularity of the retina; characterized by the deposition of lipids in the pattern of a complete or incomplete ring in the deeper layers of the retina; seen most in the elderly; R. PIGMENTOSA a familial degenerative disease that leads to blindness following intraretinal pigmentation, narrowing of vision, and nyctalopia; often associated with other degenerative disorders; R. PROLIFERANS proliferation of the retinal vessels extending into the vitreous;

occurs in retrolental fibroplasia and diabetic retinopathy; usually seen in children and adolescents.

retinoblastoma (ret'i-nō-blas-tō'ma): A malignant tumour of the neuroglial element of the retina, occurring exclusively in children; usually bilateral. Often several in a family are affected.

retinomalacia (ret'i-nō-ma-lā'shi-a): Softening of the retina.

retinopapillitis (ret'i-nō-pap-i-lī'tis): Inflammation of the retina and the optic disc.

retinopathy (ret-i-nop'a-thi): Any non-inflammatory disease of the retina. DIABETIC R. that which occurs in diabetic patients; progressive disease of the retinal blood vessels with small punctate haemorrhages and dilation of the veins; severe haemorrhage into the vitreous may lead to visual disturbances or blindness; HIGH-ALTITUDE R. retinal changes associated with symptoms of hypoxia, including retinal haemorrhage; HYPERTENSIVE R. vascular R. associated with arteriosclerosis; characterized by 'cotton wool' exudate and linear haemorrhages.

retinopexy (ret'in-ō-pek'si): Fixation of a detached retina by surgery, freezing, laser beam, photocoagulation, or other methods.

retinoschisis (ret'i-nos'ki-sis): Splitting of the retina with the formation of an intra-retinal cyst; a benign and slowly progressive disorder.

retinoscope (ret'i-nō-skōp): Instrument for detection of refractive errors by illumination of the retina using a special mirror.

retinoscopy (ret'i-nos'ko-pi): A method of examining the eye and evaluating refractive errors by projecting a beam of light onto the retina and observing the refraction by the eye of the emergent rays.

retinosis (ret'i-nō'sis): A degenerative condition of the retina; retinomalacia.

retinotoxic (ret'i-nō-tok'sik): Having an injurious effect on the retina.

retract (ri-trakt'): To draw back, shorten, or contract.

retractile (ri-trak'tīl): 1. Capable of being drawn back. 2. The state of being drawn back.

retraction (ri-trak'shun): A drawing back or backward. R. OF NIPPLE frequently a sign of breast cancer.

retractor (ri-trak'tor): 1. An instrument for drawing apart the edges of a wound during surgery so as to expose the deeper structures or make them more accessible. 2. A muscle that draws a part backward.

retrad (rē'trad): Toward the back or posterior.

retro-: Combining form denoting: 1. Backward. 2. Located behind. 3. Contrary to a natural or ordinary course.

retroaction (ret'rō-ak'shun): Action in a direction that is the reverse of normal.

retroauricular (ret'rō-aw-rik'ū-lar): Behind the auricle of the external ear.

retrobuccal (ret'rō-buk'al): Pertinent to the back part of the mouth or cheek.

retrobulbar (ret'rō-bul'bar): 1. Behind the medulla oblongata. 2. Pertaining to or located at the back of the eyeball or behind it. R. NEURITIS inflammation of that portion of the optic nerve behind the eyeball.

retrocaecal (ret'rō-sē'kal): Behind the caecum, e.g., a retrocaecal appendix.

retrocalcaneobursitis (ret'rō-kal-kā'nē-ō-bur-sī'tis): Achillobursitis.

retrocele (ret'-rō-sēl)· Herniation of the rectum through the posterior vaginal wall.

retrocervical (ret'rō-ser-vī'kal): Behind the cervix of the uterus.

retrocession (ret-rō-sesh'un): 1. Going backward; a relapse. 2. A backward displacement, particularly of the uterus as a whole.

retrocolic (ret-rō-kol'ik): Behind the colon.

retrocollis (ret-rō-kol'is): Retrocollic spasm in which the head is drawn backward.

retrocrural (ret-rō-krū'ral): Relating to the back of the leg.

retrodeviation (ret'rō-dē-vi-ā'shun): A bending backward.

retrodisplacement (ret'rō-dis-plās'ment): Backward displacement of an organ or part.

retroflexed (ret'rō-flext): Bent backwards.

retroflexion (ret-rō-flek'shun): The state of being bent backwards, specifically the bending backwards of the body of the uterus at an acute angle, the cervix remaining in its normal position. Opp. to anteflexion. — retroflexed, adj.

retrograde (ret'rō-grād): Going backward. R. AMNESIA loss of memory for events that occurred just before trauma, illness, or emotional shock; R. CONDUCTION movement of impulses through the cardiac conduction system in a direction that is the reverse of the usual conduction pattern; R. PYELOGRAPHY see PYELOGRAPHY.

retrogression (ret-rō-gresh'un): 1. Reversal in a condition or development. 2. Degeneration; catabolism.

retroinfection (ret'rō-in-fek'shun): Infection of the mother by the fetus.

retrolental (ret-rō-len'tal): Behind the crystalline lens. R. FIBROPLASIA the presence of fibrous tissue in the vitreous, from the retina to the lens, causing blindness. Noticed shortly after birth, more commonly in premature babies who have had continuous oxygen therapy.

retrolingual (ret'rō-ling'gwal): Relating to the back of the tongue or the area behind it.

retro-orbital (ret'rō-or'bit-al): Behind the orbit of the eye.

retroperitoneal (ret'rō-per-i-to-nē'al): Behind the peritoneum. R. SPACE the space between the posterior peritoneum and the posterior abdominal wall; contains the kidneys and adrenal glands, the aorta, the vena cava, and the sympathetic nervous system.

retroperitoneum (ret'rō-per-i-to-nē'um): The space between the peritoneum and the posterior body wall.

retroperitonitis (ret'rō-per-i-to-nī'tis): Inflammation of tissues in the peritoneal space.

retropharyngeal (ret'rō-fa-rin'jē-al): Behind the pharynx. R. ABSCESS one between the pharynx and the spine.

retropharynx (ret'rō-far'inks): The posterior part of the pharynx.

retroplasia (ret'rō-plā'zi-a): Degeneration of a cell or tissue whereby lack of normal cellular activity results in reversion to an earlier more primitive form, or progresses to necrosis or death.

retroposed (ret'rō-pōzd): Displaced backwards but not bent.

retropubic (ret-rō-pū'bik): Behind the pubis. R. SPACE the space immediately above the pubis and between the peritoneum and the posterior side of the rectus abdominis muscle. Also called the *space of Retzius*.

retropulsion (ret-rō-pul'shun): 1. Forcing back of any part, e.g., the fetal head during labour. 2. The involuntary tendency to walk backwards as sometimes occurs in tabes dorsalis or Parkinson's disease.

retrospective (ret-rō-spek'-tiv): Referring to or pertaining to things in the past. R. CHART AUDIT an examination of patients' charts after care has been given; may take place while they are still in the hospital or after they have been discharged; the purpose is to evaluate the care in comparison to set standards. Nurses may conduct such an audit to evaluate effectiveness of the care that was given and alter their care plans for other patients accordingly.

retrosternal (ret-rō-ster'nal): Behind the breastbone.

retrosymphysial (ret-rō-sim-fiz'i-al): Behind the symphysis pubis.

retrotracheal (ret-rō-tra′ki-al): Behind the trachea.

retrouterine (ret-rō-ū′ter-īn): Behind the uterus.

retroversioflexion (ret′rō-ver-si-ō-flek′shun): Combined retroversion and retroflexion of the uterus.

retroversion (ret-rō-ver′zhun): Turning or tilting backward. Opp. of anteversion. R. OF THE UTERUS tilting of the whole of the uterus and the cervix backwards with the cervix pointing forwards may be developmental, acquired after childbirth, or due to some pelvic pathology such as the presence of a cyst, tumour, or adhesions.

retrovirus (ret-rō-vī′rus): Any of the Retroviridae family of complex viruses, some of which induce the development of certain tumours, *e.g.*, lymphoma and sarcoma.

revaccination (rē′vaks-in-ā′shun): Vaccination of an individual who has been successfully vaccinated previously.

revascularization (rē-vas′kū-lar-ī-zā′shun): 1. The regrowth of blood vessels in a tissue or organ after deprivation of the normal blood supply. 2. The re-establishment of the blood supply to a part by the operation of grafting a blood vessel.

reverse isolation: See under ISOLATION.

reversible brain syndrome: Also known as *acute brain syndrome* or *delirium*; caused by a variety of biological stressors and characterized by loss of cognition; recovery is possible.

reversion (rē-ver′zhun): 1. The appearance of an inherited characteristic in an individual after several generations in which it has not appeared. 2. A return to a previous state or condition.

Rh: Symbol of rhesus, rhesus blood groups in particular.

rhabdo-: Combining form denoting rod-shaped, or relationship to a rod.

rhabdocyte (rab′dō-sīt): A band cell; see under CELL.

rhabdomyoma (rab′dō-mī-ō′ma): A benign tumour of striated muscle.

rhabdomyosarcoma (rab′dō-mī-ō-sar-kō′ma): A rare malignant tumour, usually involving the striated muscle cells of the muscles of the extremities and the torso; grows rapidly and metastasizes early.

rhacoma (ra-kō′ma): Relaxation of the integument of the scrotum, causing it to become pendulant.

rhagades (rag′a-dēz): Cracks or fissures in the skin, especially around a body orifice, seen in vitamin deficiencies and syphilis. When they occur around the nares and mouth in cases of congenital syphilis, they leave superficial elongated scars that are pathognomonic for the disease.

-rhage, -rrhage, -rrhagia: Combining forms denoting haemorrhage, a bursting forth, or profuse flow.

-rhaphy, -rrhaphy: Combining forms denoting a joining together in a seam; suturing.

rhegma (reg′ma): A rupture, fracture, or tear.

rheo-: Combining form denoting flow, or relation to electricity.

rheocardiology (rē′ō-kar-di-ol′o-ji): The technique of measuring and recording the changes in electric conductivity of the body during the cardiac cycle.

rheocythaemia (rē′ō-sī-thē′mi-a): The presence of degenerated red blood cells in the peripheral circulation.

rheoencephalography (rē′ō-en-kef-a-log′ra-fi, -sef-): The measurement of blood flow through the brain.

rheometer (rē-om′i-ter): An instrument for measuring the flow of viscous substances, such as blood.

rheophore (rē′ō-for): A cord conducting an electric current, particularly as between a patient and an electrical apparatus; an electrode.

rheotometry (rē-ō-tom′e-tri): The measurement of blood flow.

rhesus (rē′sus): A genus of monkey from India much used in medical research and experimentation; *Macaca mulatta*. R. FACTOR usually called Rh factor, a substance with antigenic properties that is present in the red blood cells of most people. Blood that has this factor is designated as Rh-positive and that which does not is designated Rh-negative. If a person with Rh-negative blood is given Rh-positive blood in transfusion, antibodies develop in the recipient's blood and, in the event of a second transfusion, will cause agglutination of red cells and severe reaction in the patient. If a fetus with Rh-positive blood has a mother with Rh-negative blood, some of the Rh-positive blood enters the mother's bloodstream via the placenta; her blood builds up antibodies against this substance and they enter the fetus's circulation (again via the placenta) where they cause destruction of the red blood cells and the development of erythroblastosis fetalis (*q.v.*) in the infant.

rheum (room): A watery discharge from a mucous membrane, of the nose and eyes in particular.

rheumarthritis (roo-mar-thrī′tis): Rheumatism affecting chiefly the joints.

rheumatalgia (roo-ma-tal'ji-a): Rheumatic pain.

rheumatic (roo-mat'ik): Relating to or affected by rheumatism. R. FACTOR an antibody that reacts against human globulin; is diagnostic for rheumatic arthritis when it can be demonstrated in the blood serum; R. FEVER see ACUTE RHEUMATISM under RHEUMATISM; R. HEART DISEASE a serious form of rheumatic fever, consisting of inflammatory changes and damaged heart valves; may occur as an accompaniment to or sequela of that disease; usually involves the endocardium, including the mitral valve, the myocardium, and the pericardium. The heart may be seriously and permanently damaged. A frequent cause of death in children and young adults.

rheumatid (roo'ma-tid): A nodule or other skin eruption that may accompany rheumatism.

rheumatism (roo'ma-tizm): A non-specific term embracing a diverse group of diseases and syndromes that have, in common, disorder or disease of connective tissue and hence usually present with pain, or stiffness, or swelling of muscles and joints. The main groups are rheumatic fever, rheumatoid arthritis, ankylosing spondylitis, non-articular rheumatism, osteoarthritis and gout. ACUTE R. (rheumatic fever) a disorder tending to recur but initially commonest in childhood, classically presenting as fleeting polyarthritis of the larger joints, pyrexia and carditis within 3 weeks following a streptococcal throat infection. Atypically, but not infrequently, the symptoms are trivial and ignored, but carditis may be severe and result in permanent cardiac damage; the most common cause of mitral stenosis in later life because of scar tissue resulting from inflammation of the valve. GONORRHOEAL R. that which results from a systemic infection with the gonococcus; LUMBAR R. lumbago (q.v.); MUSCULAR R. term for a number of muscle conditions characterized by pain, tenderness and local spasm; includes myalgia, myositis, fibromyositis, torticollis; NON-ARTICULAR R. involves the soft tissues; includes fibrositis; (q.v.); OSSEOUS R. arthritis deformans, see under ARTHRITIS; PALINDROMIC R. a condition characterized by irregularly occurring attacks of afebrile arthritis and periarthritis of only one joint, which becomes red and swollen; the symptoms disappear within a short time without producing lasting deformity of the joints; TUBERCULOUS R. inflammation of the joints due to toxins of the tubercle bacillus.

rheumatoid (roo'ma-toyd): Resembling rheumatism. R. ARTHRITIS a chronic disease of unknown aetiology, characterized by polyarthritis affecting mainly the smaller peripheral joints, accompanied by general ill health and resulting eventually in varying degrees of ankylosis, crippling joint deformities, and associated muscle wasting; see STILL'S DISEASE; R. FACTOR a factor found in the serum of patients with rheumatoid arthritis; laboratory tests for its presence are useful in diagnosis.

rheumatologist (roo-ma-tol'o-jist): A physician who specializes in rheumatic conditions.

rheumatology (roo-ma-tol'o-ji): The study of rheumatic diseases.

rhexis (rek'sis): Rupture or bursting of an organ, blood vessel, or tissue.

Rh factor: Rhesus factor. See under RHESUS.

Rh haemolytic disease: Erythroblastosis fetalis. See ERYTHROBLASTOSIS.

rhigosis (ri-gō'sis): The perception of the sensation of cold.

rhin-, rhino-: Combining forms denoting the nose.

rhinal (ri'nal): Relating to the nose.

rhinalgia (ri-nal'-ji-a): Pain in the nose.

rhinallergosis (rin'al-er-gō'sis): Allergic rhinitis.

Rh incompatibility: see RHESUS FACTOR under RHESUS.

rhinelcos (ri-nel'kōs): An ulcer in the nose.

rhinencephalon (ri'nen-kef'a-lon, -sef'-): The part of the cerebral cortex concerned with the reception and interpretation of olfactory stimuli. — rhinencephalic, adj.

rhinenchysis (ri-nen'ki-sis): 1. The instillation of a medication into the nose. 2. The washing out of the nasal cavity, nasal douche.

rhiniatry (ri-ni'a-tri): The treatment of nasal defects and disorders of the nose.

rhinism (ri'nizm): A nasal quality of voice; rhinolalia.

rhinitis (ri-ni'tis): Inflammation of the nasal mucous membrane. ACUTE R. coryza; the common cold; ALLERGENIC R., R. caused by any effective allergen such as pollen; usually seasonal but may be perennial; R. MEDICAMENTOSA inflammation of the nasal mucosa resulting from overuse or improper use of topical medications; VASOMOTOR R. congestion of the nasal mucosa that is non-infectious and non-seasonal; catarrh.

rhinoantritis (ri'nō-an-tri'tis): Inflammation of the nose and either or both of the maxillary sinuses.

rhinobyon (ri-nō'bi-on): A nasal tampon or plug.

rhinocanthectomy (rī'nō-kan-thek'to-mi): Excision of the inner canthus of the eye.

rhinocheiloplasty (rī-nō-kī'lō-plas-ti): Plastic surgery on the nose and upper lip. Also called *rhinochiloplasty.*

rhinocleisis (rī-nō-klī'sis): Any obstruction in the nasal passageways.

rhinodacryolith (rī-nō-dak'ri-ō-lith): A lacrimal concretion formed in the nasal duct.

rhinodynia (rī-nō-din'i-a): Pain in the nose; rhinalgia.

rhinoedemá (rī'nē-dē'ma): Swelling of the nose or of the nasal mucosa.

rhinogenous (rī-noj'e-nus): Originating or arising in the nose.

rhinokyphectomy (rī'nō-kī-fek'to-mi): A plastic operation to removal an abnormal hump on the nose.

rhinokyphosis (rī'nō-kī-fō'sis): The presence of an excessively prominent hump on the bridge of the nose.

rhinolalia (rī'nō-lā'-li-a): Having a voice of nasal quality due to some defect of structure or pathology of the nose.

rhinolaryngitis (rī'nō-lar-in-jī'tis): Inflammation of the mucous membrane of the nose and of the larynx, occurring at the same time.

rhinomiosis (rī'-nō-mī-ō'sis): A plastic operation for reducing the size of the nose.

rhinomycosis (rī'nō-mī-kō'sis): A fungal infection of the mucous membrane of the nose.

rhinonecrosis (rī'nō-ne-krō'sis): Necrosis of the nasal bones.

rhinopathy (rī-nop'a-thi): Any disease of the nose or nasal structures.

rhinopharyngitis (rī'nō-far'in-jī'tis): Inflammation of the posterior nares and the upper part of the pharynx.

rhinopharyngocele (rī'nō-far-ing'gō-sēl): A tumour situated in the nasopharynx.

rhinopharyngolith (rī'nō-far-ing'gō-lith): A stone in the nasopharynx.

rhinopharynx (rī'nō-far'inks): The upper part of the pharynx which lies above the soft palate and communicates with the nasal cavity; the nasopharynx.

rhinophonia (rī'nō-fō'ni-a): Having a voice of nasal quality. Rhinolalia (*q.v.*).

rhinophycomycosis (rī'nō-fī-kō-mī-kō'sis): A fungal infection in which polyps form in the subcutaneous tissues of the nose and sinuses; may extend to paranasal sinuses, the cerebrum, and to the eye, causing blindness.

rhinoplasty (rī'nō-plas-ti): Plastic surgery to alter the shape or size of the nose or to repair a defect.

rhinopolypus (rī-nō-pol'i-pus): A polyp on the mucous membrane of the nose.

rhinorrhagia (rī-nō-rā'ji-a): Nosebleed.

rhinorrhoea (rī-nō-rē'a): 1. Free discharge of thin watery mucus from the nose. 2. The escape of cerebrospinal fluid through the nose.

rhinosalpingitis (rī'nō-sal-pin-jī'tis): Inflammation of the nasal mucosa and the auditory tube.

rhinoscleroma (rī'nō-sklē-rō'ma): A chronic infectious condition involving the nose, upper lip, and mouth; starts with the development of hard nodules in the nose and extends to the pharynx, larynx, trachea, and bronchi.

rhinoscopy (rī-nos'ko-pi): Examination of the nose by means of an instrument called a rhinoscope.

rhinostenosis (rī'nō-sten-ō'sis): Narrowing or constriction of the nasal passages.

rhinotomy (rī-not'o-mi): Any cutting operation on or in the nose.

rhinotracheitis (rī'nō-trak-ē-ī'tis): Inflammation of the nasal mucosa and the trachea.

rhinovaccination (rī'nō-vak-si-nā'shun): The application of an immunizing material to the mucous membrane of the nose.

rhinovirus (rī'nō-vī'rus): Any one of a large group of viruses considered to be the cause of common colds. More than 100 varieties have been identified.

rhitid-: For words beginning thus see those beginning RHYTID-.

rhizo-: Combining form denoting relationship to a root.

rhizoid (rī'zoyd): Resembling a root.

rhizomeningomyelitis (rī'zō-me-nin'gō-mī-e-lī'tis): Radiculomeningomyelitis (*q.v.*).

rhizotomy (rī-zot'o-mi): Surgical division of a root, especially that of a nerve. ANTERIOR R. sectioning of the anterior root of a spinal nerve for the relief of essential hypertension. POSTERIOR R. sectioning of the posterior root of a spinal nerve for the relief of intractable pain. CHEMICAL R. accomplished by injection of a chemical, often phenol.

Rh-negative: see RHESUS FACTOR under RHESUS.

rhombencephalon (rom-ben-kef' a-lon, -sef'): The hindbrain or after-brain; includes the pons, cerebellum, and medulla oblongata.

rhomboideus (rom-boy'dē-us): One of the two large muscles of the upper back; they lie under the trapezii and act to draw the scapula upwards and towards the median line and to rotate it.

rhoncus (ron'kus): 1. A whistling, turbulent, rattling, rumbling, or snorous sound heard on auscultation when there is exudate or fluid in the bronchi. **2.** A rattling in the throat. See SIBI-LUS. — rhonchi, pl.; rhoncial, rhoncal, adj.

Rh-positive: See RHESUS FACTOR under RHESUS.

Rh sensitivity: The state of being or becoming sensitized to the rhesus factor, *e.g.*, as happens when an Rh-negative woman is pregnant with an Rh-positive fetus. See BLOOD GROUPS.

-rhysis: A combining form denoting a flowing out.

rhythm (rith'em): The regular recurrence of a similar feature, action, or situation, *e.g.*, the heartbeat. ALPHA R., R. seen as uniform waves on the normal electroencephalogram when the subject's eyes are closed and the brain is at relative rest; average frequency is about 10 per second; BETA R., R. of smaller and faster waves, also seen on the EEG; the average frequency is about 25 per second; BIOLOGICAL R. cyclic variations in level of activity, physical and chemical functions of the body, and emotional states, CIRCADIAN R., R. having a cycle of 24 hours; CIRCAMENSUAL R., R. having a cycle of about 30 days. CIRCANNUAL R., R. having a cycle of about one year; CIRCASEPTAL R., R. having a cycle of about seven days; DIURNAL R., R. in which fluctuations are confined to the working day; GALLOP R. is of two types: (1) ventricular G.R., marked by a three-sound sequence in which two heartbeats occur close together followed by a third louder sound, the sound resembling that of a galloping horse; and (2) atrial G.R., R. in which a fourth sound is heard when the atrium contracts in resistance to ventricular filling; IDEOVENTRICULAR R. a slow ventricular rhythm controlled by an ectopic centre in the ventricle independently of the atrial rhythm; INFRADIAN R., R. having a cycle longer than 24 hours; may be weeks or months; NODAL R., R. initiated in the atrioventricular node and the main bundle of His; R. METHOD see under METHOD; SINUS R. normal heart rhythm as initiated by electrical impulses in the sinoatrial node; THETA R. the theta wave in the electroencephalogram; see under WAVE; ULTRADIAN R., R. having a cycle of less than 24 hours. — rhythmic, adj.

rhythmicity (rith-mis'i-ti): The property of rhythmic recurrence of an action or situation. In cardiology, the natural ability of the heart to beat rhythmically.

rhytidectomy (rit-i-dek'to-mi): The surgical removal of wrinkles. Face-lifting. Also called *rhytidoplasty*.

rhytidosis (rit-i-dō'sis): **1.** Wrinkling of the skin of the face. **2.** Wrinkling of the cornea. Also spelled *rhitidosis*.

rib: Any one of the paired bones, 12 on either side, which articulate with the twelve dorsal vertebrae posteriorly and form the walls of the thorax. The upper seven pairs are TRUE RIBS and are attached to the sternum anteriorly by costal cartilage. The remaining five pairs are the FALSE RIBS. The first three pairs of these do not have an attachment to the sternum but are bound to each other by costal cartilage. The lower two pairs are the FLOATING R.S which have no anterior articulation. CERVICAL R.S are formed by an extension of the transverse process of the seventh cervical vertebra in the form of bone or a fibrous tissue band; this causes an upward displacement of the subclavian artery; a congenital abnormality. R. CAGE the bony thorax; consists of the sternum, ribs, and thoracic vertebrae.

riboflavin (rī'bō-flā'vin): Vitamin B₆, a member of the vitamin B complex. Essential for growth and good vision; aids in digestion and carbohydrate metabolism. Found in liver, milk, eggs, kidney, lean meats, malt, yeast, green leafy vegetables, whole grain and enriched flour and cereals; also synthesized. Deficiency may result in lowered resistance and vitality, cracks at corners of the mouth and lesions on lips, glossitis, anaemia, retarded growth, photophobia, cataracts.

ribonuclease (rī'bō-nū'klē-ās): An enzyme present in various body tissues; is responsible for the breakdown of ribonucleic acid.

ribonucleic acid (rī'bō-nū-klē'ik as'id): A nucleic substance found in the nucleus and cytoplasm of all living cells and in many viruses; the medium by which genetic instructions from the chromosomes in the nucleus are transmitted to the rest of the cell and an important factor in the synthesis of protein within the cells. Differences in the molecular structure of the RNA particles determine the difference between messenger RNA, which is believed to transmit the genetic code, and transfer RNA, which carries amino acids to the ribosomes (*q.v.*) for protein synthesis.

ribonucleoprotein (rī'bō-nū'klē-ō-prō'te-in): Any of a large group of complex molecules which, on hydrolysis, yield ribonucleic acid and protein.

ribose (rī'bōs): A pentose sugar occurring in riboflavin and ribonucleic acids.

ribosome (rī'bō-sōm): One of the small complex particles within the cytoplasm of living cells that contain ribonucleic acid and various proteins and which synthesize protein within the cell.

ribosuria (rī-bō-sū'ri-a): The presence of ribose in the urine; occurs especially in patients with muscular dystrophy.

rice-water stool: The stool of cholera. The 'rice grains' are small pieces of desquamated epithelium from the intestine.

ricin (rī'sin): A poisonous substance found in the seeds of the castor-oil plant.

ricinism (ris'i-nizm): Poisoning by ricin or castor oil.

Ricinus (ris'i-nus): A genus of plants including the castor-oil plant, the seeds of which are the source of castor oil.

rickets (rik'ets): A disorder of calcium and phosphorus metabolism associated with a deficiency of vitamin D, and beginning most often between the ages of 6 months and 2 years. There is proliferation and deficient ossification of the growing epiphyses of bones, producing bossing, softening and bending of the long weight-bearing bones, muscular hypotonia, head sweating, delayed closure of the fontanelles, degeneration of the liver and spleen and, if the blood calcium falls sufficiently, tetany. FETAL R. see ACHONDROPLASIA; RENAL R. condition of decalcification of bones (osteoporosis) associated with chronic kidney disease and clinically simulating R. It occurs in later age groups than R., and is due to retention of phosphorus in the blood, which prevents absorption of calcium, and is characterized by excessive calcium loss in the urine.

Rickettsia (ri-ket'si-a): A group of small parasitic Gram-negative, non-filterable microorganisms that are like bacteria in some ways and like viruses in others. Their natural habitat is the gut of arthropods such as lice, mites, ticks, fleas. They are the vectors of many diseases, transmitting the organisms to humans through their bites. One clinical classification, based on groups of rickettsiae according to the diseases they cause, lists four groups: (1) typhus group, the causative agents in epidemic and endemic typhus; (2) spotted fever group, the causative agents in Rocky Mountain spotted fever, boutonneuse fever, and rickettsialpox; (3) tsutsugamushi group, the causative agents in tsutsugamushi disease and in both rural and scrub typhus; (4) miscellaneous group, the causative agents in trench fever and Q fever.

rickettsialpox (ri-ket'si-al-poks): An acute self-limited febrile disease resembling chickenpox; caused by the bite of a mite that infests house mice. Characterized by chills, fever, myalgia, headache, and a papulovesicular rash; a papule forms at the site of the bite, vesicates, and becomes escharotic. Usually non-fatal.

rickettsiosis (ri-ket-si-ō'sis): Infection with *Rickettsia*.

rickety (rik'i-ti): Suffering from rickets. R. ROSARY see RACHITIC ROSARY under RACHITIC.

Rift Valley fever: A highly infectious, virulent, viral disease, primarily of animals but transmissible to humans through many species of mosquitoes or the handling of infected animals; marked by headache, malaise, myalgia, pain in the bones, encephalitis, liver damage, retinitis that can lead to blindness. Seen particularly in certain parts of Africa and the Near East.

righting reflex: See under REFLEX.

rights: Legal or moral entitlements. The recognition in law that certain absolute freedoms should be respected. See HUMAN RIGHTS.

right to die: Refers to a debatable issue concerning employment by others of 'mercy killing' or 'involuntary euthanasia' when an individual cannot make that decision because of being in a condition such as irreversible coma, or of having suffered 'brain death', and cannot be expected to recover.

rigid (rij'id): Firm; hard; unyielding; inflexible.

rigidity (ri-jid'i-ti): Stiffness, inflexibility or rigor, particularly that which is abnormal or pathological. COGWHEEL R. muscle R. that progresses from rhythmic jerky movements to passive stretching; DECEREBRATE R. rigid contraction of the extensor and other muscles involved in maintaining the standing position; due to a lesion in the brain stem; HEMIPLEGIC R., R. of the paralysed limbs in paraplegia; LEAD-PIPE R. the muscular rigidity seen in persons with Parkinson's disease; POSTMORTEM R. see RIGOR MORTIS under RIGOR.

rigor (rig'or): 1. Stiffness, rigidity. 2. A sudden chill, accompanied by severe shivering. The body temperature rises rapidly and remains high until perspiration ensues and causes a gradual fall in temperature. R. MORTIS the stiffening of the body after death.

rigour: Severity in dealing with a person or persons; extreme strictness; harshness. The strict terms, application, or enforcement of some law, rule, etc.

rimose (rēm'os): Fissured; having many cracks going in all directions.

rimula (rēm'ū-la): A very small crack or fissure, particularly one in the brain or spinal cord.

ring: In chemistry, a closed chain of atoms in a cyclic compound, *e.g.*, the benzene R. In anatomy, a more or less circular structure that surrounds an opening or an area. EXTERNAL INGUINAL R. the opening in the fascia of the transversalis muscle through which the vas deferens or the round ligament passes into the inguinal canal; INTERNAL INGUINAL R. the opening in the aponeurosis of the external oblique muscle through which the spermatic cord or round ligament passes; WALDEYER'S R. the ring of lymphoid tissue in the throat; made up of the lingual, palatine, and pharyngeal tonsils.

Ringer's solution: A sterile isotonic solution containing a mixture of sodium chloride, potassium chloride, and calcium chloride in distilled water; used as a fluid and electrolyte replenisher. LACTATED R.S. contains sodium chloride, sodium lactate, potassium chloride, and calcium chloride in distilled water; it has the same uses as Ringer's solution. Also called *Hartmann's solution.*

ringworm: A broad general term used to describe a group of diseases of the skin and its appendages; caused by a fungus. So called because the common manifestations are circular, scaly patches. See TINEA and MYCOSIS.

Rinne test: Testing of air conduction and bone conduction hearing, by tuning fork. Discriminates between conduction and sensorineural deafness. [Heinrich Rinne, German otologist, 1819–1868.]

risk: A hazard; the possibility of harm. R. ASSESSMENT the qualitative or quantitative estimation of the likelihood of adverse effects that may result from exposure to specified health hazards or from the absence of beneficial influences, see CONTROL OF SUBSTANCES HAZARDOUS TO HEALTH; HEALTH AND SAFETY COMMISSION; R. FACTOR an element that increases the possibility or likelihood of harm or of a harmful occurrence; the systematic investigation and forecasting of risks in business and commerce; R. MANAGEMENT identifying, analysing, and controlling the risks from untowards occurrences in clinical and non-clinical areas; effective and timely incident reporting by all staff are essential components of effective practice.

Risser jacket: A specialized body cast used in correcting structural scoliosis; employs a spica jacket which usually incorporates the head and sometimes the arm; the cast is split on the side of the curve and a turnbuckle is incorporated into the two halves; as the two parts of the cast are opened out by the turnbuckle, correction takes place; when this is accomplished spinal fusion may be performed through a window in the jacket.

risus sardonicus (rī'sus sar-don'i-kus): An expression resembling a grin, caused by spasm of facial muscles; seen in tetanus (*q.v.*).

ritual (rich'ū-al): In psychiatry, any psychomotor activity that a person persists in performing when there is no need for it; a means of relieving anxiety. See OBSESSIONAL NEUROSIS under NEUROSIS.

RNA: Abbreviation for ribonucleic acid (*q.v.*).

Robert's Law of Progression: Describes a condition occurring in the elderly in whom early forgetfulness increases progressively until the individual cannot remember recent events whether or not they are important to his life and safety, but may remember earlier events clearly; the resulting development of hostility and resentment has a marked effect on the person's behaviour.

Robertson's pupil: See ARGYLL ROBERTSON PUPIL.

Rochelle salt: Potassium sodium tartrate, formerly much used as a saline cathartic.

Rocky Mountain spotted fever: An infectious rickettsial disease formerly thought to be confined to the Rocky Mountain area of the USA, but now known to occur in many other parts of the Western hemisphere. It is transmitted by the bite of an infected tick or by contamination of the broken skin with the crushed tissues or faeces of an infected tick. It is characterized by fever, headache, conjunctivitis, and a maculopapular rash. Also called *tick fever* and *spotted fever.*

rod: In anatomy, a slender mass of substance, specifically the rod-like bodies found in the retina. See also CONE; HARRINGTON ROD.

rodent (rō'dent): A gnawing animal. R. ULCER see BASAL-CELL CARCINOMA under CARCINOMA

rodonalgia (rō-dō-nal'ji-a): A condition characterized by cutaneous vasodilatation of the blood vessels of the feet and sometimes of the hand, causing redness, mottling, neuralgic pain, swelling, and increase in skin temperature of the extremities. Also called *erythromelalgia* and *acromelalgia.*

roentgenography (rent'gen-og'ra-fi): Examination of part of the body by means of a photograph made by exposure of the part to roentgen rays. See RADIOGRAPHY.

roentgenologist (rent'ge-nol'o-jist): One skilled in the use of roentgen rays for diagnostic and therapeutic purposes.

roentgenology (rent'ge-nol'o-ji): The study of roentgen rays and their diagnostic and therapeutic uses.

Rogers, Martha: The nursing academic who formulated the concept of unitary healthcare. She created the conceptual health-care system that became known as the Science of Unitary Human Beings.

rolandic (rō-lan'dik): Relating to structures first described by Rolando. R. AREA the area in the cortex of the cerebrum that is concerned with the control of motor activities; R. FISSURE the boundary between the frontal and parietal lobes of the cerebrum. [Luigi Rolando, Italian anatomist, 1773–1831.]

role: The kind of behaviour expected of a person because of his particular place in his or her social setting or situation, *e.g.*, the mother's role, nurse's role, the sick role, etc. Every person assumes or fulfils more than one role on occasion or as demanded by the situation, *e.g.*, the mother role and the nurse role may be enacted simultaneously.

rolfing: A technique, developed by Dr Ida Rolf, a chemist, based on the theory that the body is not a unit but an aggregate of large structures. It involves manipulating the muscles of the body with the purpose of helping the individual to establish relationships between deep structures that will result in symmetrical balanced functioning of the body when upright.

Romberg: R.'S DISEASE facial hemiatrophy, usually progressive and may involve most of the structures of the face. Symptoms may appear early in childhood along with epilepsy, trigeminal neuralgia, and alopecia; reconstructive surgery and orthodontia are often used successfully; R.'S SIGN a sign of ataxia (*q.v.*); inability to stand erect without swaying when the eyes are closed and the feet together; also called *rombergism, Romberg's phenomenon*, and *Romberg's test*. [Moritz Romberg, German neurologist, 1795–1873.]

rongeur (ron-zhur'): A type of forceps designed for cutting bone.

roof: A top covering membrane or structure. R. OF THE MOUTH the bony and muscular structure between the nasal and oral cavities; the palate.

rooming-in: The practice of keeping the neonate in a crib at the mother's bedside during the hospital stay; said to have psychological and physical advantages for both mother and infant and to facilitate 'on demand' feeding and bonding.

root: In anatomy, (1) the base, foundation, origin, beginning, or lowest part of a structure; (2) the embedded part of the structure; or (3) the proximal end of a nerve. R. OF THE LUNG the bronchus, pulmonary artery and veins, plexuses of pulmonary nerves, lymphatic vessels and lymph nodes, all of which are embedded in mediastinal tissue with the mass entering the lung at the hilus, thus forming the root.

rooting reflex: See under REFLEX.

Rorschach test (ror'shahk): A psychological test that also measures the elements of personality; consists of a series of ink blots, which the patient is told to look at and then simply tell what he sees. [Herman Rorschach, Swiss psychiatrist, 1884–1922.]

rosacea (rō-zā'shē-a): A chronic skin disease affecting the nose particularly; marked by flushing due to chronic dilatation of the capillaries, often complicated by the appearance of papules and acne-like pustules. Also called *acne rosacea, acne erythematosa, brandy face, rum nose, rum blossom*. Occurs most often in adult males.

rosaceiform (rō-zā'shē-i-form): Resembling acne rosacea; see under ACNE.

rosary: RACHITIC R. see under RACHITIC.

roseola (rō-zē-ō'la): A rose- or scarlet-coloured rash. EPIDEMIC R. rubella (*q.v.*); R. INFANTUM exanthem subitum; SYPHILITIC R. the rose-coloured eruption of early secondary syphilis; usually appears 6–12 weeks after the initial lesion of the disease; spreads over most of the body except for the skin of the hands and face. — roseolus, adj.

rose spots: The rose-coloured papular eruption that appears on the abdomen and loins during the first week of typhoid and paratyphoid fevers; the spots disappear on pressure.

Rose–Waaler test: A serological test formerly much used in the diagnosis of rheumatoid arthritis. The presence of rheumatoid factor is detected in the serum by the agglutination of sheep's red blood cells sensitized with rabbit gamma globulin.

rostrate (ros'trāt): Having a beak-like appendage or process.

rostrum (ros'trum): A beak-like or hook-like process. — rostral, adj.

rotary (rō'-ta-ri): 1. Relating to or causing rotation. 2. Resembling a body in rotation. R. NYSTAGMUS rotation of the eyeball around part of the visual axis.

rotate (rō'tāt): To turn about on an axis.

rotating tourniquet: See under TOURNIQUET.

rotation (rō-tā'shun): 1. The act of turning about on an axis that passes through the centre of the body, as R. of the head. 2. The turning of the fetus' head as it accommodates to the contours of the birth canal. EXTERNAL R. turning the anterior surfaces of a limb outwards; INTERNAL R. turning the anterior surface of a limb inwards or medially.

rotator (rō'tā-tor): A muscle having the action of turning a part.

rotator cuff: Name given to the tendinous cuff over the shoulder; consists of the upper half of the shoulder joint capsule and the insertion tendons of the supraspinatous, infraspinatous, teres minor, and scapularis muscles; it helps to stabilize the joint. R.C. INJURIES injuries that result from improper overhead or swing motion; occurs in those engaging in such sports as tennis, cricket, baseball, or volleyball; also called *rotator cuff impingement syndrome*.

rotavirus (rō-ta-vī'rus): A recently recognized virus resembling *Reovirus (q.v.)*; found worldwide; an important cause of infant diarrhoea, spread by oral–faecal route.

Rothmund–Thomson syndrome: See POIKILODERMA CONGENITALE.

rotula (rot'ū-la): 1 The patella or any similar disc-like bony structure. 2. A troche or lozenge. — rotular, adj.

roughage (ruf'ij): Coarse food such as unprocessed bran, fresh fruit, and vegetables, which contain much indigestible fibre composed of cellulose. It provides bulk in the diet and by this means helps to stimulate peristalsis and eliminate waste products. Lack of R. may cause atonic constipation. Too much R. may cause spastic constipation.

rouleau (roo'lō): A row of red blood cells, resembling a roll of coins. — rouleaux, pl.

round ligament: The ligament that passes from the anterior cornu of the uterus forward and downwards through the folds of the broad ligament and the inguinal canal and inserts into the subcutaneous fat of the labia; its function is to help hold the uterus in its proper position of anteversion and anteflexion.

rounds: The practice employed by health-care professionals of discussing and evaluating the status and care of patients for whom they are collectively responsible. Rounds may be conducted as 'sit-down' conferences or as 'teaching' or 'walking' rounds during which the patients are visited. Medical rounds are led by the physician in charge of the patients' care and are attended by junior medical staff, medical students; nurses and others who have some responsibility for the care of the patients involved may also attend medical rounds. Nursing rounds are attended by members of

the nursing staff and are usually conducted at the beginning of a shift; they may or may not include visits to patients' bedside. GRAND R.S formal conferences in which an expert gives a lecture or discussion regarding a clinical issue; slides, films, charts, etc. may be used, and the patient involved may or may not be presented.

roundworm: One of the more prevalent intestinal worms parasitic to humans, especially one of the class *Nematoda*; threadworm. See also *ASCARIS*.

route: In healthcare, the path of administration of a medication.

Roux (roo): ROUX-EN-Y DRAINAGE a surgically established system for draining the oesophagus, pancreas, and biliary tract directly into the jejunum, to prevent peristaltic reflux of intestinal content into these organs; ROUX-EN-Y JEJUNAL LOOP the segments of the jejunum as rearranged for establishing Roux-en-Y drainage. [Cesar Roux, Swiss surgeon, 1857–1926.]

Rovsing's sign: Pain in the right iliac fossa when pressure is applied in the left iliac fossa; a sign of acute appendicitis.

Royal College of Midwives: Established as the professional organization for midwives in 1881. Concerned with professional education: both statutory and postbasic, standards of professional practice and the negotiation of conditions of service and salaries. It is the only professional organization solely for midwives either as students or as qualified practitioners.

Royal College of Nursing: Founded in 1916 as the professional body for nurses and incorporated by Royal Charter in 1928. It is recognized as both an independent trade union and professional organization. Its main aim is to further both the art and science of nursing. The Royal College of Nursing also maintains the Institute of Advanced Nursing Education.

-rrhacis: Combining form denoting the spine.

-rrhage, -rrhagia: Combining forms denoting excessive flow.

-rrhaphy: Combining form denoting a joining together by sutures.

-rrhexis: Combining form denoting rupture or splitting.

-rrhoea: Combining form denoting discharge or flow.

rub: 1. Friction occurring when two surfaces are moved against one another. 2. The sound heard when two serous surfaces rub together. PERICARDIAL FRICTION R. a scraping or grating noise heard over the pericardium on auscultation when the pericardium is inflamed; PLEURAL

FRICTION R. the creaking or dry scuffing noise heard at the end of inspiration when the pleural membranes are roughened by inflammation, in the presence of a neoplasm, or in the absence or decrease of pleural fluid.

rubedo ((rū-bē′dō): Blushing or other temporary reddening of the skin.

rubefacient (rū-bē-fā′shent): 1. Producing redness of the skin. 2. An agent that acts as a counterirritant and produces a reddening when applied to the skin.

rubella (rū-bel′la): An acute, infectious, eruptive fever resembling both measles and scarlet fever, caused by the rubella virus and spread by droplet infection; symptoms include mild fever, coryza, conjunctivitis, a pink rash, possibly enlarged cervical glands, and arthralgia. The course is short and usually uneventful except when contracted in the first three months of pregnancy when it may produce fetal deformities. Also called *German measles* and *three-day measles*.

rubella syndrome: A congenital condition due to intrauterine rubella infection; characterized by deafness, cardiac anomalies, cataracts, thrombocytic purpura, hepatitis, retinitis, encephalitis, occasionally glaucoma.

rubeola (ru-bē-ō′la): See MEASLES.

rubeosis (rū-bē-ō′sis): Redness. R. IRIDIS the formation of numerous new blood vessels and connective tissue on the surface of the iris; usually bilateral; may occur in patients with diabetes and those with secondary glaucoma; R. RETINAE the formation of new blood vessels in front of the optic papilla in patients with retinitis; often occurs in diabetics as well as non-diabetics.

ruber (rū′ber): Red.

rubescent (ru-bes′ent): Reddish, or growing red.

rubiginous (rūbij′i-nus): Having a brownish or rusty colour; most often applies to sputum.

Rubin's test: A test for patency of the uterine tubes; carbon dioxide is insufflated into a tube and, if the tube is patent, the gas will pass out into the abdominal cavity where it can be visualized by x-ray. A manometer may be used to determine the pressure of the gas in the tube, which indicates the degree of patency.

rubor (rū′bor): Redness; one of the four classic signs of inflammation, the other three being pain, heat, and swelling.

rubricyte (rū′bri-sīt): An erythroblast (*q.v.*).

rubriuria (rū-bri-ū′ri-a): Red or reddish discoloration of the urine.

ructus (ruk′tus): Belching; eructation. R. HYSTERICUS a condition in which the individual belches air frequently and noisily. — ructation, n.

rudimentary (rū-di-men′ta-ri): Imperfectly or incompletely developed; elementary.

ruga (rū′ga): A wrinkle, corrugation, or fold; often of an impermanent nature and allowing for distension, *e.g.*, the wrinkles and folds seen on the inner surface of the stomach. — rugae, pl.; rugose, rugous, adj.

rugitus (rū′ji-tus): Rumbling sounds in the intestine caused by movement of flatus; borborygmus (*q.v.*).

rule of halves: The rule that states that half of the people in a specific group will take advantage of an available screening programme; half of those found to be at high risk will start a prevention programme; and half of those who start such a programme will reach their set goal.

rule of nines: See WALLACE'S RULE OF NINES, and LUND AND BROWDER'S CHART.

rumblossom: See ROSACEA.

rumination (rū-min-ā′shun): 1. The voluntary regurgitation of food, and the rechewing and reswallowing of it; most often seen in young children with emotional problems; also sometimes seen in the mentally handicapped and in psychiatric patients. 2. Chronic vomiting.

ruminative (rū′mi-na′tiv): 1. Having a tendency to be preoccupied with certain thoughts and ideas. 2. Having a tendency to regurgitate previously swallowed food; see REGURGITATION.

rump: The gluteal region; the buttocks.

Rumpel–Leede test: A test for capillary fragility. A tourniquet is applied to the upper arm for 5–10 minutes; if petechiae appear on the forearm, the test is said to be positive.

rupia (rū′pi-a): A skin eruption of vesicles and ulcers that appears especially in the tertiary stage of syphilis; the lesions are raised, dark yellow or brown, crusted and adherent, tending to develop into bullae. — rupial; rupoid, adj.

rupture (rup′chur): Tearing, splitting, bursting of a part. A popular name for hernia (*q.v.*).

rushes: Vigorous peristaltic movements producing sounds that are longer and higher pitched than normal bowel sounds.

Rush pin: A pin, rid, or nail used in surgical treatment of major long-bone fractures.

rutilism (rū′ti-lizm): Red-headedness.

R wave: In the ECG, an upwards deflection following the Q wave.

R_x: Symbol used at the head of a prescription; stands for the word 'recipe'. Dates back 5000 years to a picture of the eye of Horus, the Egyptian god of healing. See RECIPE.

Ryle's tube: A small-calibre rubber tube, with a weighted end, introduced via the nose into the stomach. It may be used for the withdrawal of gastric contents or for the administration of fluids.

S

Sabin's vaccine (sā'binz vak'sēn): A live, orally administered vaccine prepared from poliovirus and used to produce immunity to poliomyelitis; induces a poliovirus infection in the recipient, stimulating the production of antibodies and thus producing resistance to the disease. Also called *TOPV* (trivalent oral poliovaccine) and often used to immunize children. See also SALK VACCINE. [Albert Bruce Sabin, Russian-born virologist working in the USA.]

sabulous (sab'ū-lus): Sandy or gritty.

saburra (sab-bur'a): See SORDES.

sac (sak): A small pouch or bag-like cavity. AIR S. an air vesicle of the lung; an alveolus. AMNIOTIC S. the membrane that holds the fetus and amniotic fluid when *in utero*; CONJUNCTIVAL S. the potential space between the eyeball and the conjunctiva; HERNIAL S. the pouch of the peritoneum that contains a hernia; LACRIMAL S. the expanded portion of the upper part of the lacrimal duct; PERICARDIAL S. that formed by the pericardium. — saccular, sacculated, adj.

saccade (sa-kahd'): Rapid jerky movement of the eye as it moves from one fixation point to another, as occurs in reading. — saccadic, adj.

saccate (sak'āt): Shaped like a sac; pouched.

sacchar-, sacchari-, saccharo-: Combining forms denoting relationship to sugar.

saccharase (sak'a-rās): An enzyme that acts as a catalyst in the hydrolysis of sucrose to dextrose and levulose. — Syn., *invertase, invertin, sucrase*.

saccharic (sak'ar-ik): Relating to sugar.

saccharide (sak'a-rīd): 1. A simple sugar such as glucose. 2. A compound made up of sugar and another substance. 3. The carbohydrate grouping contained in each of the various types of carbohydrates which have been classified as monosacharides, disacharides, trisaccharides, polysaccharides, and heterosaccharides.

saccharify (sa-kar'i-fi): To make sweet or to convert into sugar.

saccharin ((sak'a-rin): A white crystalline compound several hundred times sweeter than sucrose; used as a non-calorific sweetening agent; but now proved to be carcinogenic in test animals.

saccharose (sak'ar-ōs): Cane sugar; sucrose.

saccharum (sak'ar-um): Sugar.

saccharuria (sak-a-rū'ri-a): The presence of glucose in the urine; glycosuria.

sacciform (sak'si-form): Resembling a sac or bag in shape.

saccular (sak'ū-lar): Sac-shaped.

sacculated (sak'ū-lā-ted): Containing or divided into small sacs. S. BLADDER a condition of the urinary bladder in which small pouches are formed by a pushing out of the mucous membrane lining between the muscular bundles; they contain urine that is not voided with a normal urination; may be caused by overdistension of the bladder or an obstruction in the bladder outlet.

sacculation (sak-ū-lā'shun): The formation of a saccule (*q.v.*).

saccule (sak'ūl): 1. A minute sac. 2. The lower portion of the vestibule of the inner ear. — saccular, sacculated, adj.

sacculus (sak'ū-lus): Saccule (*q.v.*).

sacr-, sacro-: Combining forms denoting sacrum.

sacrad (sā'krad): Towards the sacrum.

sacral (sā'kral): Involving, relating to, or in the area of the sacrum. S. BLOCK anaesthesia produced by injection of an anaesthetic into the sacral canal; S. NERVES the five pairs of nerves attached to the spinal cord at the sacral segment; they innervate the skin and muscles of the lower back and sacral region, pelvic viscera, the perineum, and the genitalia; S. VERTEBRAE the five lowest vertebrae which are fused into a single triangular bone, the sacrum.

sacralgia (sā-kral'ji-a): Pain in the sacral region.

sacrectomy (sā-krek'to-mi): Surgical removal of part of the sacrum.

sacroanterior (sā-krō-an-tē'ri-er): Describing a breech presentation in which the fetal sacrum is directed to one or the other acetabulum of the mother. — sacroanteriorally, adj.

sacrococcygeal (sā'-krō-kok-sij'ē-al): Relating to the sacrum and the coccyx.

sacrocoxalgia (sā'-krō-kok-sal'ji-a): Pain in the sacroiliac region or joint.

sacrocoxitis (sā'-krō-kok-sī'tis): Inflammation of the sacroiliac joint.

sacrodynia (sā-krō-din'i-a): Pain in the sacrum.

sacroiliac (sā-krō-il'i-ak): Relating to the sacrum and the ilium; or denoting the articulation between the two bones.

sacroiliitis (sā'krō-il-ē-ī'tis): Inflammation of the sacroiliac joint.

sacrolumbar (sā-krō-lum'bar): Relating to the sacrum and the loins.

sacroperineal (sā'krō-per-i-nē'al): Relating to the sacrum and the perineum.

sacroposterior (sā'krō-pos-tē'ri-or): Describing a breech presentation in which the fetal sacrum is directed to one or the other sacroiliac joint of the mother. — sacroposteriorly, adj.

sacropubic (sā-krō-pū'bik): Relating to the sacrum and the pubis.

sacrosciatic (sā'krō-sī-at'ik): Relating to both the sacrum and the ischium.

sacrospinalis (sā'krō-spī-nal'is): The long large muscle that passes up on either side of the vertebral column from the sacrum to the head. Extends the trunk, and bends the head and vertebral column to the side.

sacrouterine (sā'krō-ū'ter-in): Relating to the sacrum and the uterus. S. LIGAMENT a band of connective tissue that extends backwards from the cervix of the uterus, passes on either side of the rectum, and attaches to the posterior wall of the pelvis.

sacrovertebral (sā'krō-ver'te-bral): Relating to the sacrum and a vertebra or vertebrae above it.

sacrum (sā'krum): The triangular bone lying between the fifth lumbar vertebra and the coccyx; forms the back of the pelvis. It consists of five vertebrae fused together, and articulates on each side with the innominate bones of the pelvis, forming the sacroiliac joints. — sacral, adj.

SAD: Abbreviation for seasonal affective disorder (q.v.).

saddle: S. BLOCK anaesthesia produced by introducing an anaesthetic low in the dural sac to anaesthetize the buttocks, perineum, and inner aspects of the thighs; so called because these areas are in contact with the saddle in horseback riding, sometimes used for anaesthesia in childbirth and in surgical procedures on the rectum.

saddlenose: A nose with a flattened bridge; often a sign of congenital syphilis.

sadism (sā'dizm): The obtaining of pleasure from inflicting pain, violence or degradation on another person, or the sexual partner. Opp. to MASOCHISM.

sadist (sā'dist): An individual who practices sadism (q.v.).

sadistic (sad-is'tik): Relating to or marked by sadism.

sadomasochism (sād-ō-mas'o-kizm): The coexistence of sadism and masochism in a human relationship; the individual has a strong desire to inflict suffering and, at the same time, invites it.

'safe' period: A misleading term, used to describe the time in the menstrual cycle when conception is least likely to occur; the basis of a method of birth control used when mechanical or chemical means are not acceptable or obtainable; intercourse is avoided from the tenth to the twentieth day of the cycle inclusively.

safflower oil (saf'flow-er): Oil obtained from the safflower plant; used in diets of those in whom it is desirable to keep the blood cholesterol low.

sagittal (saj'it-al): 1. Shaped like an arrow; straight. 2. A lengthwise plane of the body, running from front to back; divides the body into right and left halves. S. SUTURE the immovable joint formed by the union of the two parietal bones.

sailor's skin· Pigmentation and keratosis of exposed areas of the skin due to excessive exposure to sunlight; may lead to squamous-cell carcinoma.

Sainsbury Centre for Mental Health (sānz'-be-ri): A registered charity, working to improve the quality of life for people with severe mental health problems. It aims to influence national policy and encourage good practice in mental health services. The Centre is affiliated to King's College, London.

Saint Anthony: SAINT ANTHONY'S DANCE Huntington's chorea; see under CHOREA; SAINT ANTHONY'S FIRE an old term for certain inflammatory or gangrenous conditions of the skin, including erysipelas. (q.v.).

Saint Vitus' dance: Chorea (q.v.). Named for a third-century child martyr who was invoked by sufferers of chorea.

sal: Salt or any substance resembling it.

salicylate (sa-lis'i-lāt): Any of a large group of salts of salicylic acid, commonly used in medicine for their analgesic effects in the treatment of such conditions as rheumatism, dysmenorrhoea, arthritis, and a variety of other aches and pains.

salicylic acid (sal-i-sil'ik as'id): A white crystalline substance; the basic component of aspirin.

salicylism (sal'i-sil-izm): A condition of toxicity resulting from large doses of salicylates; symptoms include nausea, vomiting, headache, dizziness, tinnitus, confusion.

saline (sā'lēn, sā'līn): **1.** Salty, containing salt, or resembling a salt. **2.** A solution containing salt. NORMAL or PHYSIOLOGICAL S. a 0.9% solution of sodium chloride in water that is of the same osmotic pressure as the blood; S. DEPLETION a condition existing when there is a deficiency of both water and sodium in the body; see HYPERTONIC, HYPOTONIC, ISOTONIC.

saliva (sa-lī'va): A secretion produced by the parotid, submaxillary, sublingual, and buccal glands; spittle. It contains water, mucus, and ptyalin. Its function is to keep the inside of the mouth moist, to moisten and dissolve foods, and to start the digestion of carbohydrates.

salivant (sal'i-vant): **1.** Stimulating the flow of saliva. **2.** An agent that stimulates the secretion of saliva.

salivary (sa-līve-ri, sal'i-ver-i): Relating to saliva. S. AMYLASE an enzyme which, in an alkaline medium, converts starch into dextrin and maltose; S. CALCULUS a stone formed in the salivary duct; S. DUCT one of several ducts that conduct the saliva; S. GLANDS those that secrete saliva, *e.g.*, parotid, submandibular, and sublingual; S. GLAND DISEASE cytomegalic inclusion disease (*q.v.*).

salivate (sal'i-vāt): To produce an excessive amount of saliva.

salivation (sal-i-vā'shun): An increased secretion of saliva. Ptyalism.

Salk vaccine: An inactivated poliovirus vaccine administered subcutaneously to infants, certain children, and unvaccinated adults to produce active artificial immunity to poliomyelitis; booster doses are required periodically. Introduced in 1955. See also SABIN'S VACCINE. [Jonas Salk, American immunologist.]

sallow (sal'low): Having a skin that is pale, yellowish, unhealthy looking.

Salmonella (sal'mo-nel'a): A genus of motile rod-shaped, Gram-negative bacteria of the family Enterobacteriaceae. Parasitic in many animals and humans in whom they are often pathogenic. Some species, such as *S. typhi*, are host-specific, infecting only humans. Others may infect a wide range of host species, usually through contaminated foods. Some species cause mild gastroenteritis, others a severe and sometimes fatal food poisoning.

salmonellosis (sal'mō-nel-lō'sis): Infection with a *Salmonella* organism.

salping-, salpingo-: Combining forms denoting: **1.** The uterine (formerly Fallopian) tube(s). **2.** Less often, the auditory (formerly Eustachian) tube(s).

salpingectomy (sal-pin-jek'to-mi): Excision of a uterine tube.

salpingian (sal-pin'ji-an): Of or relating to (1) the uterine tube; (2) the auditory tube.

salpingitis (sal-pin-ji'tis): Acute or chronic inflammation of one or both of the uterine tubes. The term is also sometimes applied to inflammation of the auditory tube. GONOCOCCAL S. infection of a uterine tube(s) with *Neisseria gonorrhoea*.

salpingocyesis (sal-ping'gō-sī-ē'sis): Tubal pregnancy. See ECTOPIC PREGNANCY under ECTOPIC.

salpingogram (sal-ping'gō-gram): Radiological examination of tubal patency after injecting an opaque substance into the uterus and along the tubes. — salpingography, n.; salpingographic, adj.; salpingographically, adv.

salpingography (sal-ping-gog'ra-fi): Radiographic demonstration of the uterine tube after it has been filled with a radiopaque medium.

salpingolithiasis (sal'ping-gō-li-thī'a-sis): The collection of calcareous material in the walls of the uterine tubes.

salpingolysis (sal-ping-gol'i-sis): The breaking up of adhesions involving the uterine tubes, a surgical procedure.

salpingo-oophorectomy (sal-ping'gō-ō'of-o-rek'to-mi): Excision of a uterine tube and ovary.

salpingo-oophoritis (sal-ping'ō-ō'of-o-rī'tis): Inflammation of both the uterine tubes and the ovaries.

salpingoperitonitis (sal-ping'gō-per'i-to-nī'tis): Inflammation of the uterine tube(s) and the peritoneum.

salpingopexy (sal-ping'gō-pek-si): Surgical fixation of one or both uterine tubes.

salpingoplasty (sal-ping'gō-plas-ti): Plastic repair of a uterine tube.

salpingoscope (sal-ping'gō-skōp): An instrument used for examining the nasopharynx and the auditory tube; nasopharyngoscope.

salpingostomy (sal-ping-gos'to-mi): An operation performed to restore tubal patency.

salpinx (sal'pinks): A tube, especially the uterine tube or the auditory tube.

salt: **1.** A chemical compound formed by the interaction of an acid and a base. **2.** Sodium chloride; common table salt. See also SALTS. IODIZED S. salt that has been treated with sodium iodide, usually 1 part to 10,000 parts of sodium chloride; used as a source of iodine in the diet to prevent the development of goitre.

salt-free diet: A diet low in sodium chloride; usually refers to a diet in which no salt is used in cooking, and none is added at the table.

saltpetre (salt-pe′ter): Potassium nitrate, often mistakenly claimed to be useful in decreasing sexual desire; its main effect is diuretic.

salt rheum (room): An old term for any of a variety of skin conditions resembling eczema.

salts: Usually refers to a saline cathartic such as magnesium sulphate (Epsom salts), Rochelle salt, or sodium sulphate.

salt-wasting disease: Chronic renal malfunctioning characterized by high excretion of sodium.

salubrious (sa-lū′bri-us): Wholesome; healthful. Usually refers to climate or environment.

saluresis (sal′ū-rē′sis): The excretion of sodium and chloride ions in the urine.

saluretic (sal′ū-rēt′ik): 1. Relating to or causing saluresis. 2. An agent that produces saluresis.

salutary (sal′ū-ta-ri): Heathful; remedial; curative.

salve (salv): An ointment.

sample: A relatively small quantity of material, or an individual object, from which the quality of the mass, group, species, etc. that it represents may be inferred.

sampling: The act of taking a part, example, or specimen to represent the whole.

sanative (san′a-tivc): Healing; curative.

sanatorium (san-a-taw-ri-um): An institution, usually private, for the treatment of patients with such chronic disorders as tuberculosis, and who are not extremely ill.

sand bath: See under BATH.

sandfly: A fly of the genus *Phlebotomus*; responsible for the 'sandfly' fever of the tropics, and for various types of leishmaniasis (*q.v.*).

sane: Of sound mind.

sangui-: Combining form denoting blood.

sanguifacient (sang′gwi-fā′shent): Forming blood.

sanguinary (sang′-gwin-er-i): Relating to, derived from, containing, or consisting of blood.

sanguine (sang′gwin): 1. Full-blooded, bloody, or resembling blood. 2. Hopeful, as of a cheerful temperament; optimistic.

sanguineous (sang-gwin′ē-us): Relating to or containing blood.

sanguinopurulent (sang′win-ō-pū′ru-lent): Relating to an exudate that contains both blood and pus.

sanguis (sang′gwis): Blood [L.]

sanies (sā′ni-ēz): A thin, greenish, fetid discharge from a wound or ulcer; consists of blood, pus, and serum.

sanitary (san′i-tāri): 1. Healthful; promoting health. 2. Characterized by cleanness, easily kept clean.

sanitation (san-i-tā′shun): The science of using measures that prevent diseases and that promote either individual or community health, or both.

sanitize (san′i-tīz): To clean or sterilize something so as to make it sanitary according to public health standards. — sanitization, n.

sanity (san′i-ti): Soundness of the mind.

San Joaquin Valley fever: Coccidioidomycosis.

saphenectomy (saf-ē-nek′to-mi): Excision of a saphenous vein.

saphenofemoral (sa-fē′nō-fem′o-ral): Pertinent to the saphenous and femoral veins.

saphenous (sa-fē′nus): Apparent; manifest. The name given to the two main superficial veins in the leg, the internal and the external, and to the nerves accompanying them.

saponin (sap′ō-nin): A group of glycosides obtained from certain plants growing widely in Europe; formerly used as a detergent and as an emulsifying agent, now largely replaced by synthetic products.

sapphism (saf′-izm): Lesbianism (*q.v.*).

sapr-, sapro-: Combining forms denoting (1) rotten, putrid, decayed; (2) dead or decaying organic matter.

sapraemia (sa-prē′mi-a): A pathological condition caused by the absorption into the bloodstream of toxins and breakdown products resulting from the action of saprophytic organisms on dead tissue. Septicaemia.

saprogen (sap′rō-jen): Any microorganism that causes putrefaction (*q.v.*).

saprogenic (sap-rō-jen′ik): Causing putrefaction or resulting from it.

saprophagous (sap-rof′a-gus): Denotes an organism that lives on decaying organic matter.

sarapus (sar′a-pus): A flat-footed individual.

sarc-, sarco-,-sarc: Combining forms denoting muscle tissue or resemblance to flesh.

sarcitis (sar-sī′tis): Inflammation of muscle tissue; old term for myositis.

sarcoblast (sar′kō-blast): An embryonic cell that becomes a muscle cell.

sarcocarcinoma (sar′kō-kar-si-nō′ma): Carcinosarcoma (*q.v.*).

sarcocele (sar′kō-sēl): A tumour of the testis.

sarcoid (sar′koyd): 1. Resembling flesh. 2. Sarcoidosis (*q.v.*).

sarcoidosis (sar-koy-dō′sis): A chronic granulomatous disease of unknown aetiology, characterized by the presence of tubercles that histologically resemble those of tuberculosis and range in size from that of a pinhead to that of a bean. May affect any organ of the body but most commonly presents as a condition of the skin, lymph nodes, lungs, liver, spleen, or the small bones of the hands and feet. See LUPUS.

sarcolemma (sar-kō-lem'ma): The delicate, outer elastic membranous covering of the striated muscle fibres.

sarcology (sar-kol'o-ji): Study of the soft tissues as distinguished from bone.

sarcoma (sar-kō'ma): A tumour of connective tissue, often highly malignant; tends to grow rapidly and to metastasize early to distant spots; may occur in any part of the body; seen most frequently in children and young adults. The tumour is usually soft, bulky, and highly vascular, and may give rise to ulceration and haemorrhage. The most common type is OSTEOSARCOMA, usually the tibia, femur, or humerus; also called *osteogenic s.* and *osteoid s.* CHONDROSARCOMA a S. containing much fibrous tissue; EPITHELOID S. a s. composed of a nest of epithelial cells that have sarcomatous properties; EWING'S S. malignant myeloma of bone, the long bones in particular; characteristic symptoms are pain, fever, swelling, and leukocytosis; KAPOSI'S S. a low-grade benign or malignant idiopathic neoplasm; occurs chiefly in the skin where it presents as purplish papules and nodules, particularly on the toes and feet, but may also affect lymph nodes and viscera where it is often haemorrhagic; MELANOTIC S. a very malignant type of s. containing melanin; NEUROGENIC S. neurofibroma (*q.v.*); OAT CELL s. a s. made up of cells that are long and blunted at the ends; OSTEOGENIC S. a malignant primary tumour of bone involving both the bone and cartilage; three subtypes are chondroblastic, fibroblastic, and osteoblastic; RETICULUM CELL s. a malignant tumour of lymphoid tissue in which the predominating cell is an anaplastic, sometimes multinucleated reticulum cell; ROUND CELL S. and GIANT CELL S. named for the type of cell that is predominant in the tumour; SYNOVIAL S. see SYNOVIOSARCOMA. — sarcomatous, adj.; sarcomata, pl.

sarcomatoid (sar-kō'ma-toyd): Resembling a sarcoma.

sarcomatosis (sar-kō'ma-tō'sis): A condition in which many sarcomata develop in the same individual.

sarcomatous (sar-kō'ma-tus): Resembling, or of the nature of, sarcoma.

sarcomphalocele (sar-kom-fal'ō-sēl): A fleshy tumour of the umbilicus.

sarcomyces (sar-kō-mī'sēz): A fleshy, tumorous growth that has a fungoid appearance.

Sarcoptes scabiei (sar-kop'tēz skā'bē-i): The itch mite that causes scabies (*q.v.*).

sarcosinaemia (sar'kō-si-nē'mi-a): An inborn error of metabolism marked by an increased amount of sarcosine (*q.v.*) in the plasma and urine; associated with mental and physical handicap.

sarcosine (sar'kō-sēn): An amino acid resulting from the hydrolysis of certain proteins.

sarcosis (sar-kō'sis): 1. The presence of multiple fleshy tumours. 2. Abnormal increase in body mass.

sarcous (sar'kus): Relating to muscle tissue or flesh.

sardonic grin (sar-don'ik): See RISUS SARDONICUS.

SARS: Abbreviation for severe acute respiratory syndrome (*q.v.*).

sartorius (sar-to'ri-us): A long muscle of the thigh; originates on the anterior superior spine of the ilium and inserts on the medical surface of the upper end of the tibia. It adducts the leg and enables one to sit with one leg crossed over the other; so called because tailors formerly sat in this cross-legged position while at their work.

satiety (sa-tī'e-ti): The condition of being satisfied or gratified in regard to appetite or thirst, with no desire to ingest more food or drink; limitation of intake is thought to result from stimulation of a satiety centre located in the ventromedial part of the hypothalamus.

saturated (satch'ū-rā-ted): Holding all of a substance that can be absorbed or taken up. S. FATS fats that are thought to encourage formation of plaque in blood vessels when taken in quantity; include animal fats, dairy products, and certain vegetable oils, *e.g.*, coconut oil and palm oils; S. SOLUTION a liquid that contains as much of a solute as it is capable of holding in solution.

saturnine (sat'ur-nīn): Relating to, resembling, or produced by the absorption of lead.

saturnism (sat'ur-nizm): Lead poisoning; plumbism. See LEAD.

satyriasis (sat-i-rī'a-sis): Excessive sexual craving in a male. Equivalent to nymphomania in a female.

sauna (saw'na): Steam bath followed by plunge in the snow; originated in Finland and adapted for use in other countries using a cold shower as a substitute for snow. Dry heat is also now used instead of steam.

Saunders, Cicely (sawn'-derz, sis'-e-li): An active missionary for the hospice movement, and founder, in 1967, of St Christopher's

Hospice, to provide total and active care for patients with incurable diseases.

sauriasis (saw-rī'a-sis): Ichthyosis (*q.v.*).

sausarism (saw'sa-rizm): 1. Dryness of the tongue. 2. Paralysis of the tongue.

Sayre's jacket: A cast applied for support and immobilization in the treatment of certain abnormalities of the spinal column.

scab: A dried crust forming over an open wound.

scabicide (skā'bi-sīd): Any agent that is destructive to *Sarcoptes scabiei*, the causative agent of scabies.

scabies (skā'bēz): A parasitic skin disease caused by the itch mite which bores beneath the skin; highly contagious. Characterized by intense itching and eczematous lesions caused by scratching. Sites most affected are the skin between the fingers and toes, axillae, genital region, around the breasts. NORWEGIAN S. a rare infectious form; marked by encrusted skin swarming with mites; may occur in epidemic form in small communities. Syn., *itch*.

scag: One of the street names for heroin.

scala (skā'la): Resembling stairs; refers particularly to the various passageways in the cochlea.

scald (skawld): 1. A burn caused by moist heat, either steam or a hot liquid. 2. To burn the skin with moist heat.

scale: 1. A small visible flake of skin that is cast off. 2. A system of marks at regular intervals on a strip of metal or glass that serves as a standard of measurement. 3. In dentistry, to remove tartar from the teeth.

scalene (skā'lēn): 1. Relates to a structure that has three unequal sides. 2. Part of a name given to any of several muscles with origins at the processes of cervical vertebrae and insertions at the two upper ribs; they act to flex and rotate the neck and assist in respiration by elevating the ribs. — scalenus, adj.

scalenectomy (skā'le-nek'to-mi): Surgical removal of a scalene muscle.

scalenotomy (skā'lē-not'o-mi): A surgical procedure in which the scalene muscles are severed close to their insertion into the ribs; the objective is to allow the apical part of the lung to rest; used in the treatment of pulmonary tuberculosis.

scalenus (skā-lē'nus): Descriptive of a structure that has three sides; refers particularly to the three muscles on each side of the neck, the anterior, medial, and posterior scalenus muscles; see SCALENE. S. ANTICUS SYNDROME pain over the shoulder radiating up the back or down the arm; caused by pressure on the nerves between the anticus (anterior scalenus) muscle and a cervical rib.

scaling (skā'ling): 1. Desquamation; the production of scales. 2. The removal of calculus material from the exposed part of a tooth.

scalp: Consists of the skin, subcutaneous tissue, muscles, and periosteum that cover the top of the cranium.

scalpel (skal'pel): A small, straight, pointed knife with a sharp edge, used in surgery.

scan: Usually used with another, designating word; *e.g.*, bone scan, brain scan, thyroid scan. See SCANNING.

scanner (skan'er): An apparatus consisting of a detector that scans a specific body region in a systematic manner to determine the distribution of a radiopaque substance, and a device for recording that distribution. GAMMA S. one in which the camera remains stationary; RECTILINEAR S. one in which the camera moves back and forth over the area being examined.

scanning (skan'ing): 1. Visually examining a small area or several isolated areas in great detail. In RADIOISOTOPE S. a two dimensional picture is made showing the gamma rays that are emitted by the isotope, which is concentrated in the particular tissue, *e.g.*, brain, thyroid. A useful technique for diagnosis and for detection of infections and lesions such as tumours. See also COMPUTERIZED AXIAL TOMOGRAPHY NUCLEAR MAGNETIC RESONANCE IMAGING. 2. The process of making a radioactive scan. S. SPEECH slow, hesitant speech with pronunciation of words a syllable at a time with a pause between each syllable; may be seen in individuals with multiple sclerosis.

scapegoating (skāp'gō-ting): Passing the blame for mistakes, misdemeanours, or problems to a person or persons other than the one(s) responsible.

scaphocephaly (skaf'-ō-kef'a-li, -sef-): A condition in which the skull is unusually long and narrow like the keel of a boat, with a ridge running from front to back; caused by premature closure of the sagittal suture; often association with mental handicap.

scaphoid (skaf'oyd): Boat-shaped, as the navicular bones of the tarsus and carpus. S. ABDOMEN refers to an abdomen in which the wall is thin, the contents small, and the contour concave rather than flat.

scaphoiditis (skaf-oy-dī'tis): Inflammation of the scaphoid bone.

scapholunate (skaf-ō-lū'nāt): Relating to the scaphoid and lunate bones of the wrist.

scapula (skap'ū-la): The shoulder blade — a large, flat, triangular bone; it articulates with the clavicle and the humerus.

scapulalgia (skap-ū-lal'ji-a): Pain in the scapular area.

scapular (skap'ū-lar): Relating to the scapula. s. LINE in anatomy, a vertical line drawn through the inferior angle of the scapula.

scapuloclavicular (skap'ū-lō-kla-vik'ū-lar): Relating to the scapula and the clavicle.

scapulocostal syndrome (skap'ū-lō-kos'tal): Pain in the shoulder girdle radiating to the neck and upper part of the triceps muscles, and numbness and tingling of the hands; caused by trauma, habitually poor posture, or friction between the scapula and the thoracic cage.

scapuloglenohumeral (skap'ū-lō-glen'ō-hū'mer -al): Relating to the scapula, glenoid cavity, and the humerus.

scapulohumeral (skap'ū-lō-hū'mer-al): Relating to the scapula and the humerus or the shoulder joint, or the muscles of the shoulder girdle.

scapulothoracic (skap'ū-lō-tho-ras'ik): Relating to the scapula and the thorax.

scar: The dense, avascular white fibrous tissue, formed as the end result of healing, especially in the skin. Cicatrix. See KELOID.

scarification (skar-i-fi-kā'shun): The making of a series of small superficial incisions or punctures in the skin. — scarify, v.

scarlatina (skar'la-tē'na): Scarlet fever. Acute infection by haemolytic streptococcus, producing a scarlet rash. Occurs mainly in children. Begins commonly with a throat infection, leading to pyrexia and the outbreak of a punctate erythematous eruption of the skin followed by desquamation. Characteristically, the area around the mouth escapes (circumoral pallor). — scarlatinal, adj.

scarlatinella (skar-lat-i-nel'a): Mild scarlet fever, with the rash but not the fever usually associated with scarlet fever. Also called *fourth disease* because it is the fourth member of a group of specific fevers including scarlet fever, morbilli, and rubella.

scarlet fever: See SCARLATINA.

scarlet red: A dye with some bacteriostatic action; in the past sometimes used to stimulate epithelial cell growth in treatment of burns, ulcers, and some other wounds, and as a covering for donor sites in skin grafting.

Scarpa's triangle: An anatomical area just below the groin. The base of the triangle is uppermost and is formed by the inguinal ligament. The vessels and nerves passing to and from the thigh are superficial here. [Antonio Scarpa, Italian anatomist and surgeon, 1747–1832.]

scat-, scato-: Combining forms denoting faeces, dung.

scatacratia (skat-a-krā'shi-a): Incontinence of faeces.

scataemia (ska-tē'mi-a): An autotoxic condition of the intestines, due to retained faeces.

scatology (ska-tol'o-ji): 1. The study and analysis of faeces. 2. Obsession with the obscene, particularly with the function of excretion and excreta.

scavenger cell: See MACROPHAGE; PHAGOCYTE.

SCBU: Abbreviation for special care baby unit (*q.v.*)

Schafer's method: A method of performing manual (prone pressure) artificial respiration. [Albert Edward Sharpey-Schafer, English physiologist, 1850–1935.]

schema (skē'ma): An outline or plan.

schematogram (skē-mat'ō-gram): An outline of the body or of some part of it that can be filled in following surgery or a physical examination.

Scheuermann's disease: Osteochondrosis of the vertebral bodies. Occurs chiefly in adolescents. [Holger Werfel Scheuermann, Danish orthopaedic surgeon, 1877–1960.]

Schick test: A test for susceptibility to the toxin of the organism that causes diphtheria, *Corynebacterium diphtheriae*. The toxin is injected into the skin of one arm and inactivated toxin is injected into the skin of the other arm. If the individual is susceptible, a red area will develop around the site of the toxin injection and persist for several days.

Schilder's disease: A chronic or subacute form of leukoencephalopathy (*q.v.*), characterized by destruction of white matter of the cerebral hemispheres resulting in progressive mental deterioration, varying degrees of bilateral spasticity, disorders of vision, deafness; occurs chiefly in children. Also called *encephalitis periaxialis diffusa*. [Paul Schilder, German-American psychiatrist, 1886–1940.]

Schiller's test: A test that involves painting an area, particularly the cervix, with iodine in order to determine from which sites a biopsy should be taken; normal cells stain brown, but abnormal cells do not.

Schilling test: A diagnostic test used to confirm the diagnosis of pernicious anaemia by detecting malabsorption or deficiency of vitamin B_{12}. Following the oral administration of a small dose of radioactive B_{12}, urine for the test is collected for 24 hours.

Schimmelbusch's disease: Cystic disease of the breast; see under CYSTIC.

Schiötz tonometer (shē'-erts): An instrument for measuring intraocular pressure.

Schirmer test: A test used for evaluating the secretion of the lacrimal glands.

schirro-: Combining form denoting hard.

-schisis: A combining form denoting fissure, split, cleft.

schistasis (shis'ta-sis): In anatomy, a split or splitting; usually refers to a congenital anomaly.

schisto-: Combining form denoting split, cleft.

schistocelia (shis-tō-sē'li-a): A congenital anomaly consisting of a fissure of the abdominal wall.

schistocephalus (shis-tō-kef'al-us, -sef'): A fetus with an unclosed cranium.

schistocyte (shis'tō-sīt): A fragment of a damaged red blood cell containing haemoglobin that appears as an irregularly shaped fragment on a stained glass smear; seen in patients with haemolytic anaemia.

schistocytosis (shis-tō-sī-tō'sis): The presence of many schistocytes in the circulating blood.

schistosome (shis'tō-sōm): Any of the species of the genus *Schistosoma*. s. DERMATITIS 'swimmers' itch' a dermatitis occurring after exposure to water in freshwater lakes, caused by penetration of the skin by a schistosome for which snails are the intermediate hosts.

schistosomicide (shis-tō-sō'mi-sīd): An agent that destroys schistosomes.

schiz-, schizo-: Combining forms denoting split or divided.

schizoaffective (skit'sō-af-fek'tiv): Relates to psychiatric disorders in which the individual exhibits a mixture of schizoid and major affective disorders.

schizogenesis (skit-sō-jen'e-sis): Reproduction by fission.

schizognathism (skit-sō-nath'izm): A congenital anomaly in which either the upper or lower jaw is fissured.

schizogony (skit-sog'o-ni): The asexual cycle of sporozoa, particularly the life cycle of the parasite that causes malaria.

schizoid (skit'-zoyd): Resembling schizophrenia. s. DISORDER OF CHILDHOOD or ADOLESCENCE a condition characterized by inability to make or keep friends, belligerence, irritability, seclusiveness, indecision; may be self-limited as the child matures; s. PERSONALITY DISORDER a disorder characterized by lack of ability to make and keep friends, coldness, aloofness, withdrawal, seclusiveness, eccentricity, detachment, and indifference to the feelings of others.

schizont (skīz'ont): A stage in the life cycle of the malarial parasite, *Plasmodium*.

schizonychia (skit-sō-nik'i-a): Splitting of the nails.

schizophrenia (skit-sō-frē'ni-a): A large group of mental illnesses characterized by disorganization of the personality, progressive withdrawal from reality, inappropriate responses, and often abnormal behaviour; may be a chronic lifelong illness with frequent hospitalizations. The onset, commonly in early life, may be sudden or insidious. Five main types are generally recognized: 1. DISORGANIZED type, in which the person exhibits silly purposeless behaviour, mannerisms, and speech; social withdrawal, fragmentary delusions or hallucinations; and incoherence, also referred to as *hebephrenic type*. 2. CATATONIC type, in which the person goes through stages of excitement alternating with stages of stupor, a peculiar sustained rigidity of the body, and mutism. 3. PARANOID type, a common chronic type characterized by delusions of persecution or of grandeur; anger, intense jealousy, argumentativeness, sometimes violence, and possibly doubts about one's gender identity. 4. RESIDUAL TYPE, in which the person has had one episode of schizophrenia in which the symptoms were not particularly prominent but signs of the illness still persist in the individual who may exhibit certain eccentric behaviours, social withdrawal, and illogical thinking; this type may be chronic or sub-chronic with remission and exacerbations. 5. UNDIFFERENTIATED TYPE in which the person may exhibit symptoms not noted under the other four types or which appear in more than one of them, *e.g.*, disorganized behaviour, incoherence, strong delusions, or hallucinations.

schizophrenic (skit-sō-fren'ik): Relating to schizophrenia. s. SYNDROME in childhood sometimes considered a truer diagnosis than autism or psychosis.

schizophreniform (skit-sō-fren'i-form): Having some of the characteristics of schizophrenia. s. DISORDER a condition in which the individual presents with some of the symptoms of schizophrenia, but the onset is acute and the condition responds to treatment within a few weeks or months.

schizophrenogenic (skit'sō-fren-ō-jen'ik): Having a tendency to result in schizophrenia.

schizotrichia (skit-sō-trik'i-a): Splitting of the hairs at the end.

schizotrypanosomiasis (skit′sō-tri-pa-nō-sō-mī′a-sis): Chagas' disease.

Schlatter's disease: Also called *Osgood–Schlatter's disease.* Osteochondritis of the tibial tuberosity. [Carl Schlatter, Swiss surgeon, 1864–1934. Robert Bayley Osgood, American orthopaedic surgeon, 1873–1956.]

Schneider nail: A nail used in surgical treatment of fractures of the femur.

Schölz's disease (sherlts): Genetically determined degenerative disease associated with mental handicap; the familial form of juvenile demyelinating encephalopathy.

school nurse: See under NURSE.

school nurse practitioner: A registered nurse who is qualified through satisfactory completion of a nurse practitioner (*q.v.*) programme to practise in a school.

school phobia: Term used to describe a child's irrational avoidance or fear of school, teachers, and classmates; thought to result from intense separation anxiety caused by dependency on the mother.

Schüffner's spots or dots: Small, round yellowish or pink granules that can be seen in stained red blood cells early in malaria.

Schultz–Charlton reaction: A skin test utilized in the diagnosis of scarlet fever; it is positive if the skin around the point of injection blanches when a person with a scarlatinaform rash is given an injection of human scarlet fever immune serum.

Schwabach's test: (shwā′-baks, shwā′-banks): A tuning fork test in which the bone conduction capability in a pathological ear is compared to the normal.

Schwann: S.'S CELLS the cells that make up the neurilemma (*q.v.*); S.'S SHEATH the neurilemma; S.'S TUMOUR a firm encapsulated neoplasm arising in the neurilemma of a nerve fibre, also called *schwannoma* and *neurilemmoma.* [Theodor Schwann, German anatomist, 1810–1882.]

sciatic (sī-at′ik): Relating to the ischium or the region of the hip. GREATER S. NOTCH a deep notch below the posterior spine of the ilium through which the sciatic nerve, other nerves, blood vessels, and the piriform muscle pass. LESSER S. NOTCH a notch between the spine and tuberosity of the ischium through which the tendon of the obturator muscle, nerves, and blood vessels pass; S. NERVE the largest nerve in the body; it extends from the hip down the back of the leg after passing under the buttock; at the level of the knee it divides into the tibial and common peroneal nerves.

sciatica (sī-at′i-ka): Pain along the line of distribution of the sciatic nerve (buttock, back of thigh, calf, and foot); may be caused by a herniated vertebral disc or an injury.

SCID: Abbreviation for severe combined immunodeficiency disease (*q.v.*).

science (sī′ens): Any branch of systematized knowledge that is a specific object of study or practice.

scillocephaly (sil-ō-kef′a-li, -sef′): A congenital anomaly in which the head is small and cone-shaped.

scintiphotography (sin′ti-fō-tog′ra-fi): Radioisotope scanning. PULMONARY S. scanning of the lungs after the patient has inhaled or been injected with radioactive particles.

scirrhous (skir′us): Pertaining to or of the nature of a hard tumour; indurated. Usually refers to a type of cancer. S. CARCINOMA chimneyweep's cancer; see SCROTAL EPITHELIOMA under EPITHELIOMA.

scirrhus (skir′us): A carcinoma which provokes a considerable growth of hard, connective tissue; a hard carcinoma of the breast. — scirrhoid, adj.

scissor gait: An abnormal gait in which the legs are abducted and the thighs cross each other alternately with the knees scraping together; seen in patients with bilateral hip joint disease or spastic diplegia or as a manifestation of Little's disease (*q.v.*). Also called *scissor leg.*

scissura (si-sū′ra): A splitting or a fissure; a cleft.

sclera (sklē′ra): The 'white' of the eye; the opaque bluish-white fibrous outer coat of the eyeball covering the posterior five sixths; it merges into the cornea at the front. — scleral, adj.; sclerae, pl.

sclera-, sclero-: Combining forms denoting: **1.** The sclera. **2.** Hard or dry.

scleradenitis (sklē′rad-e-nī′tis): An inflammatory induration or hardening of a gland.

sclerectasia (sklē-rek′-tā′zi-a): A bulging forward of the sclera.

sclerectoiridectomy (sklē-rek′tō-ir-i-dek′to-mi): A surgical procedure in which part of the sclera and part of the iris are removed; a treatment for glaucoma.

sclerectomy (sklē-rek′to-mi): **1.** Surgical removal of a portion of the sclera of the eye. **2.** Operation for the removal of sclerosed parts of the middle ear after otitis media.

sclerema (skle-rē′ma): Hardening and induration of the skin. S. OF THE NEWBORN a rare, often fatal, disease in the first few weeks of life, with a diffuse, rapidly spreading hardening of the

sclerema 541 sclerosis

subcutaneous tissues and associated limitation of movement.

scleriritomy (sklē-ri-rit′o-mi): Excision of the sclera and the iris.

scleritis (sklē-rī′tis): Inflammation of the sclera.

sclerochoroiditis (sklē′rō-kō-roy-dī′tis): Inflammation of the sclera and choroid.

scleroconjunctival (sklē′rō-kon-junk-tī′val): Relating to both the sclera and the conjunctiva.

scleroconjunctivitis (sklē′rō-kon-junk-ti-vī′tis): Inflammation of both the sclera and the conjunctiva.

sclerocorneal (sklē-rō-kor′nē-al): Relating to the sclera and the cornea, as the circular junction of these two structures.

sclerodactylla (sklē′rō dak-til′i-a). Thickening and hardening of the fingers, often associated with scleroderma.

scleroderma (skle-rō-der′ma): A progressive disease in which localized oedema of the skin is followed by hardening, atrophy, deformity, and ulceration. Occasionally it becomes generalized, producing immobility of the face, contraction of the fingers; diffuse fibrosis of the myocardium, kidneys, digestive tract and lungs. Cause unknown; occurs most often in women between 30 and 50 years of age; LINEAR s. *linea morphea*, a form of s. in which the lesions appear in a line or band, singly or as multiple ribbon-like lesions; LOCALIZED s., s. that is characterized by the formation of yellowish or whitish cutaneous patches that have a pinkish or purplish halo; occurs chiefly in women; also called *morphea*.

sclerodermatitis (sklē′rō-der-ma-tī′tis): Inflammation and hardening of the skin.

scleroedema (skle-re-dē′ma): A condition of oedema and induration of the skin; often follows an acute infection; more common in females than males. Frequently confused with scleroderma.

scleroid (skle′roid): Hard; firm; or of a firm nature.

scleroiritis (sklē′rō-ī-rī′tis): Inflammation of the sclera and iris.

sclerokeratitis (sklē′rō-ker-a-tī′tis): Inflammation of both the sclera and the cornea.

scleroma (skle′rō-ma): A circumscribed area or patch of hardened skin or mucous membrane.

scleromalacia (sklē′rō-ma-lā′shi-a): Softening or thinning of the sclera; sometimes seen in persons with rheumatoid arthritis.

scleronychia (skle-rō-nik′i-a): Thickening and drying of the nails.

sclerophthalmia (sklē′rof-thal′mi-a): Overgrowth of the cornea over the sclera so that only part of it remains clear.

scleroprotein (skle′-rō-prō′tē-in): A simple protein that is insoluble in water; of fibrous structure; serves a protective and structural function in the body. Also called *albuminoid* (*q.v.*).

sclerosant (skle-rō′sant): 1. An agent that hardens tissues. 2. A chemical agent that produces inflammation followed by fibrosis; sometimes used in treatment of varicose veins.

sclerose (skle-rōs′): To become hardened. — sclerosed, sclerotic, adj.

sclerosis (skle-rō′sis): Term used in pathology to describe abnormal hardening or fibrosis of tissue. AMYOTROPHIC LATERAL s. hardening of the motor tracts of the lateral columns of the spinal cord; results in progressive atrophy of the muscles; often fatal. Also called *Lou Gehrig disease*; DIFFUSE INFANTILE FAMILIAL S. a form of s. characterized by demyelinization of the cerebrum in infants; tends to affect several family members; also referred to as *globoid cell leukodystrophy* and *Krabbe's disease*; DISSEMINATED S. multiple S.; LATERAL S., s. of the pyramidal tracts in the spinal cord; results in slowly progressive weakness and disability of the legs; usually occurs after age 50; MULTIPLE S. a variably progressive chronic disease of the nervous system, most commonly first affecting adults between 20 and 40 years of age; may occur as a sequela to various viral infections including encephalitis, chickenpox, rubella, measles, or herpes; distribution is worldwide, with the highest incidence occurring in the colder regions and the lowest in the tropics. The disease begins with patchy degenerative changes occurring in the nerve sheaths in the brain, spinal cord, and optic nerves, followed by the formation of plaques and sclerosis. The disease may remain silent for years, and when the early signs appear they may be quite diverse, but usually include diplopia; nystagmus; numbness, weakness, and unsteadiness of a limb; ataxia; scanning speech; and loss of the sensations of pain and temperature; later signs include partial blindness, emotional lability, disturbances of micturition, and paralysis; remissions and exacerbations are characteristic with the intervals between them becoming progressively shorter; PROGRESSIVE SYSTEMIC S. characterized by thickening of tissues and skin of hands and face; fibrosis of tissues of lungs, oesophagus, and myocardium; osteoporosis of distal phalanges; dysphagia; dyspnoea.

sclerostenosis (skle-rō-ste-nō'sis): Hardening combined with contraction of tissues.

sclerostomy (sklē-ros'to-mi): A surgical procedure in which an opening is made into the sclera for the relief of glaucoma.

sclerotherapy (skle-rō-ther'-a-pi): A treatment for varicose veins or haemorrhoids; consists of the injection into the vein of a sclerosing fluid that damages the epithelium and causes an aseptic thrombosis, which progresses to fibrosis and obliteration of the vessel.

sclerothrix (skle-rō-thriks): Abnormal brittleness or dryness of the hair.

sclerotic (sklē-rot'ik): Relating to (1) the sclera of the eye; (2) sclerosis or the hardening of tissue.

sclerotitis (sklē-rō-tī'tis): Scleritis (q.v.).

sclerotomy (sklē-rot'o-mi): Incision of the sclera. ANTERIOR S. incision into the anterior chamber of the eye for the relief of acute glaucoma; POSTERIOR S. incision into the vitreous chamber of the eye for treatment of detached retina or removal of a foreign object.

sclerous (skle'rus): Indurated or hard.

SCM: Abbreviation for State Certified Midwife, see MIDWIFE.

scolio-: Combining form denoting twisted, crooked.

scoliokyphosis (skō'li-ō-kī-fō'sis): Combined lateral and posterior curvature of the spine.

scoliolordosis (skō'li-ō-lor-dō'sis): Combined scoliosis and lordosis.

scoliometer (skō'li-ō-mē'ter): An instrument for measuring the degree of curvature in scoliosis.

scoliorachitic (skō'li-ōra-kit'ik): Affected with both scoliosis and rickets.

scoliosis (skō-li-ō'sis): An appreciable lateral curve in the spine, causing a compensating deviation of the lumbar spine to the opposite side, and resulting in an S-shaped curve. May be functional and reversible, disappearing on flexion of the trunk, or structural and irreversible. Recognized types are lumbar, thoracolumbar, and thoracic. COXITIC S., S. in the lumbar area; caused by hip disease; HABIT S. caused by improper posture; IDIOPATHIC STRUCTURAL S. begins in childhood and increases progressively; cause unknown; often leads to development of marked deformity; OSTEOPATHIC S. caused by disease of the vertebrae; PARALYTIC S. caused by muscular paralysis; RACHITIC S. caused by rickets; SECONDARY STRUCTURAL S. the most common type; causes include congenital hemivertebra, neurofibromatosis, and poliomyelitis.

scoliotic (skol-i-ot'ik): Pertaining to or affected by scoliosis.

-scope: Combining form denoting an instrument for viewing or examining.

*Scope of Professional Practice***:** A guidance paper relating to the range of activities, knowledge and understanding, and competence of practitioners on the National Medical Council register.

scopophilia (skō'pō-fil'i-a): 1. An abnormal desire to be seen. 2. A sexual deviation in which the person derives sexual pleasure from viewing genitalia. 3. Voyeurism.

-scopy: Combining form denoting examination or inspection, usually referring to the use of an instrument for viewing.

scoracratia (skor-a-krā'shi-a): Incontinence of faeces.

scorbutic (skor-bū'tik): Relating to or affected by scurvy (formerly called scorbutus). S. BEADS a row of nodules at the costochondral junction; seen in patients with scurvy; they differ from rachitic 'rosary beads' in that they are sharper.

scorbutigenic (skor-bū'-ti-jen'ik): Causing scurvy.

scorbutus (skor-bū'tus): Scurvy (q.v.).

SCOTEC: Abbreviation for Scottish Technical Education Council (q.v.).

scoto-: Combining form denoting darkness.

scotochromogen (skō-tō-krō'mo-jen): Any microorganism whose pigmentation develops as well in the dark as in the light. — scotochromogenic, adj.

scotoma (skō-tō'ma): An area of darkness or blindness within the visual field; may be of varying size and shape; vision is normal in surrounding area. In psychiatry, refers to a 'blind spot' in a person's psychological awareness. ARCUATE S., S. marked by development of an arc-shaped defect in the field of vision; arises in the area near the blind spot and extends towards it. — scotomata, pl.

scotomization (skō'tō-mī-zā'shun): The development of blind spots or scotomata: In psychiatry, the development of blind spots for things the patient does not want to accept.

scotophilia (skō-tō-fil'i-a): Fondness for the night or for being in the dark. Nyctophilia.

scotopia (skō-tō'pi-a): Night vision.

scotopic vision: The ability to see well in poor light. Dark adaptation.

Scottish Qualifications Authority: A body responsible for developing, awarding and accrediting Scottish Vocational Qualifications (q.v.), although the accrediting and awarding functions are clearly separated.

Scottish Technical Education Council: Awarding body for the Scottish Technical Education Council.

Scottish Vocational Qualification: See NATIONAL VOCATIONAL QUALIFICATION/SCOTTISH VOCATIONAL QUALIFICATION.

scratch test: A test for allergy. The superficial layer of skin is scratched and the suspected allergen rubbed in. If a redness or weal appears at the site of the scratch the test is said to be positive. A safe test because so little of the allergen is used; as many as 30 may be done at one time.

screening: Mass examination of the population in a circumscribed area for the detection of such diseases as diabetes or tuberculosis. MULTIPHASIC S. the simultaneous use of several diagnostic tests with medical assessment at the end of the process; used for the detection of various diseases and pathological conditions such as anaemia, heart disease, tuberculosis; s. TEST (1) any test that separates those who are not, or who would not be, affected by a disease from those who are at risk for it and who will be given further tests, (?) a simple test for the purpose of uncovering a disease condition that is treatable.

scrivener's palsy (skriv'nerz pawl'zi): Writer's cramp (q.v.).

scrobiculus (skrō-bik'ū-lus): A small pit or cavity.

scromboid poisoning (skrom'boyd): Poisoning produced by a toxin elaborated by a marine bacterium that infests tuna, mackerel, and several other fishes; symptoms include headache, dizziness, flushing, nausea, vomiting, diarrhoea, urticaria.

scrotal (skrō'tal): Relating to the scrotum.

scrotectomy (skrō-tek'to-mi): Surgical removal of part of the scrotum.

scrotitis (skrō-tī'tis): Inflammation of the scrotum.

scrotocele (skrō'to-sēl): A hernia into the scrotum.

scrotum (skrō'tum): The pouch in the male which contains the testes and their accessory structures. — scrotal, adj.

scrub: S. NURSE an operating room nurse who has 'scrubbed' (see SCRUBBING), wears sterile mask, cap, gown, and gloves, and assists during an operation, e.g., by handing the surgeon instruments and other needed items during a surgical procedure; s. TYPHUS a rickettsial disease occurring mostly in Asia and Australia, characterized by a primary lesion at the site of attachment of an infected mite,

fever, headache, conjunctival infection, and maculopapular eruption. Seen mostly in adults who frequent scrub terrain. Mites and various rodents are reservoirs of infection. Syn., *tsutsugamushi disease*. See TYPHUS FEVER.

scrubbing: The thorough cleansing of the hands and nails with soap, water and a brush before carrying out or assisting with a surgical or other procedure requiring aseptic technique (q.v.).

scultetus binder (skul-tē'tus): A binder (or bandage) with many tails, which is applied with each tail overlapping the next.

scurf (skurf): A flaky desquamation of the epidermis, especially of the scalp; dandruff.

scurvy (skur'vi): A deficiency disease caused by lack of vitamin C (ascorbic acid). Clinical features include fatigue and haemorrhage. Latter may take the form of oozing at the gums or large ecchymoses. Tiny bleeding spots on the skin around the hair follicles are characteristic. In children painful subperiosteal haemorrhage (rather than other types of bleeding) is pathognomonic, INFANTILE S., S. caused by lack of vitamin C in infants whose feeding consists primarily of cow's milk; prevention involves supplementary administration of vitamin C. Also called *Barlow's disease*.

scutiform (skū'ti-form): Shield-shaped.

scybala (sib'a-la): Rounded, hardened masses of faecal matter in the intestine. — scybalum, sing.; scybalous, adj.

scyphoid (sī'foyd): Cup-shaped.

SD: Abbreviation for standard deviation.

SE: Abbreviation for standard error.

Seacole, Mary (sē'-kōl): Jamaican nurse, famous for overcoming racial prejudice to work in the Crimea among the troops.

sealant (sē'-lant): A liquid plastic substance brushed on the teeth, covering surface pits and fissures; reduces the number of cavities; used particularly in areas in which the water is not fluoridated.

seam: In anatomy, a line of union.

seamless care/services: Co-operation, collaboration, and co-ordination of activities between health and social services. Policy guidelines have stressed the need for this in order that the care for each individual passes seamlessly to different agencies at different stages of care. See INTER-AGENCY.

seasickness: See MOTION SICKNESS.

seasonal affective disorder: Winter depression, which can be particularly severe during December, January, and February in the UK. For some people, this is so disabling that they cannot function in winter without continuous treatment; others may experience a milder version, called *sub-syndromal SAD* or '*winter blues*'.

seatworm: Threadworm or pinworm; *Enterobius vermicularis* (*q.v.*).

sebaceous (sē-bā'shus): Relating to fat. S. CYST one due to the retention of sebaceous material in a sebaceous follicle; a wen; S. GLANDS the cutaneous glands which secrete an oily substance called sebum. The ducts of these glands are short and straight and open into the hair follicles.

seborrhoea (seb-ō-rē'a): A functional disturbance of the sebaceous glands, marked by overactivity and resulting in a greasy condition of the skin of the face, scalp, sternal region, and elsewhere, usually accompanied by itching and burning. The seborrhoeic type of skin is especially liable to conditions such as alopecia, seborrhoeic dermatitis, acne, etc. — seborrhoeal, seborrhoeic, adj.

seborrhoeic (seb-ō-rē'ik): Relating to or characterized by seborrhoea. S. DERMATITIS see under DERMATITIS; S. KERATOSIS see under KERATOSIS.

sebum (sē'bum): The normal secretion of the sebaceous glands; it contains fatty acids, cholesterol and dead cells.

secondary: Second or inferior in either time, place, or importance. S. ANAEMIA see under ANAEMIA; S. HEALING see HEALING, by SECOND INTENTION; S. INFECTION see INFECTION; S. SEX CHARACTERISTICS those that develop at puberty but are not directly associated with reproduction; S. SEX ORGANS those that are characteristic of one's sex but are not directly associated with reproduction, *e.g.*, the breasts in the female; S. SHOCK see under SHOCK; S. SYPHILIS the second stage of syphilis; usually occurs six weeks to three months after infection.

second intention: See HEALING.

secreta (si-krē'ta): The products of glandular secretion; secretions.

secretagogue (si-krēt'a-gog): A agent that stimulates secretion by a gland.

secrete (si-krēt'): 1. To produce or elaborate a new product from substances in the blood and either to pass it into the bloodstream or a body cavity, or transport it by a duct to the area where it is required or to the exterior of the body.

secretin (si-krē'tin): A polypeptide hormone secreted by the mucous lining of the duodenum and the jejunum; in the presence of chyme it stimulates the secretion of pancreatic juice and, to a lesser extent, bile and intestinal juice. S. TEST a test for pancreatic function; it involves the intravenous administration of secretin, measurement of the pancreatic secretion, and examining it for the level of lipase, trypsin, and chymotrypsin it contains.

secretinase (si-krē'tin-ās): A enzyme in the blood serum that inactivates secretin (*q.v.*).

secretion (si-krē'shun): 1. A fluid or substance, formed or concentrated in a gland, and passed into the alimentary tract, the blood or to the exterior. 2. The process of formulating such a substance.

secretory (si-crē'to-ri): Relating to a secretion or a gland that produces a secretion.

section: 1. The act of cutting. 2. A cut surface. 3. A thin slice that has been prepared for microscopic examination. 4. A segment or division of an organ or structure. ABDOMINAL S. laparotomy (*q.v.*); CAESAREAN S. incision through the abdominal and uterine walls for the delivery of a fetus; CORONAL S. a section of the skull that is parallel with the coronal suture; FROZEN S. a thin slice that has been cut from tissue that has been frozen; for microscopic study; SAGITTAL S. one that follows the sagittal suture that runs the entire length of the body, dividing it into right and left halves.

secundigravida (sē-kun'-di-grav'i-da): A woman pregnant for the second time.

secundines (sek'un-dins; sē'kun-dēns): The after-birth with its membranes which is expelled following delivery of an infant.

secundipara (sek-un-dip'a-ra): A woman who has borne two live children at different labours.

sedation (sē-dā'shun): The production of a state of lessened functional activity, especially when it is caused by a sedative drug. Also refers to a state of calmness.

sedative (sed'a-tiv): 1. Quieting; allaying physical activity and excitement. 2. Any agent that quiets, calms, or allays physical activity and excitement, and induces sleep; usually refers to a drug. S. BATH a prolonged warm bath.

sedentary (sed'en-tar-i): Usually refers to (1) an individual who is inclined to be physically inactive and who sits a great deal of the time, or (2) an occupation that requires the individual to work while seated most of the time.

sedimentation (sed-i-men-tā'shun): The settling of a solid substance in a fluid to the bottom of a container, or causing this to happen by the use of a centrifuge. ERYTHROCYTE S. RATE the rate at which red blood cells settle to the bottom of a tube of drawn blood; the rate differs in different diseases and in different stages of a disease; determination of the s. rate assists the doctor to follow the course of the disease.

seed: 1. The source or origin of anything. 2. Offspring or descendants. 3. Sperm or semen. 4. To plant with seed or to sow seed. 5. In radiotherapy, a small sealed container of radioactive material, often radon, that is inserted into the tissues to be treated. 6. In bacteriology, to inoculate a culture medium with a microorganism one wishes to grow and reproduce for purposes of study.

segment (seg'ment): A small section; a part of an organ or structure. — segmental, adj.; segmentation, n.

segregation (seg-ri-gā'shun): A setting apart, usually for a particular reason, e.g., to put those with the same or similar disease in a particular area.

Seidlitz powder: Consists of potassium sodium tartrate and sodium bicarbonate in one paper and tartaric acid in another paper; when the two are mixed in a solution just prior to taking, effervescence occurs; formerly much used as a cathartic.

Seiqol (se'kwol): Quality of life (q.v.) indicator.

seismotherapy. (sīz-mō-ther'a-pi): Treatment of disease by mechanical vibration or shaking.

seizure (sē'zhur): 1. A sudden attack or sudden occurrence of symptoms, e.g., convulsions. 2. An epileptic fit. ABSENCE S. occurs chiefly in children; there is no aura, but brief loss of consciousness with staring and twitching of the mouth and hands; AUDIOGENIC S. an epileptic seizure brought on by sound; CEREBRAL S. an epileptic s.; FOCAL S. one limited to a particular part of the body or to a single function and without loss of consciousness; often associated with such brain lesions as scars, inflammation, or tumour; may progress to generalized s.; GENERALIZED S. affects the entire body and all body functions; GRAND MAL S. see under EPILEPSY; JACK-KNIFE S. severe muscular contractions causing extreme flexion of the head, neck, and trunk, with extension of the extremities; occurs during the first months of life; JACKSONIAN S. see under EPILEPSY; LOCALIZED S. focal s.; PETIT MAL S. see under EPILEPSY; PHOTOGENIC S. an epileptic s. brought on by light; PSYCHOMOTOR S. psychomotor epileptic S., see under EPILEPSY.

selective action: 1. The tendency of disease-producing agents to attack certain parts of the body. 2. The ability to kill one group of microbes but not another.

selenium (se-lē'ni-um): A poisonous non-metallic element resembling sulphur; used in preparations for treating seborrhoea of the scalp. Selenium also occurs in the diet as an element.

self: 1. The total essence or being of a person; the individual. 2. Those affective, cognitive, and spiritual qualities that distinguish one person from another; individuality. 3. A person's awareness of his own being or identity; ego; consciousness.

self-actualization (self'-ak-tū-a-lī-zā'-shun): The perceived competence of an autonomous system to satisfy the basic needs for homeostasis, safety, protection, feedback and exploration.in due time.

self-analysis: In psychiatry, the practice of trying to gain insight into one's own psychic state and behaviour.

self-assessment: Assessment or evaluation of oneself, one's actions, or attitudes by oneself.

self-care: 1. The personal and medical care performed by the patient, usually in collaboration with and after instruction by a health-care professional. 2. The medical care by laypersons of their families, friends and themselves, to include identification and evaluation of symptoms, medication, and treatment. 3. Personal care accomplished without technical assistance, such as washing, eating, appearance, and hygiene. The goal of rehabilitative care is maximal personal self-care.

self-catherterization: Older children, male and female patients can be taught to pass a fine, non-retaining catheter into the urinary bladder to evacuate urine as required.

self-concept The mental self-image a person has, based on one's ideas and attitudes about oneself and one's personality.

self-efficacy (self-ef'-fi-ka-si): An individual's estimate or personal judgement of his or her own ability to succeed in reaching a specific goal.

self-esteem: Favourable appreciation or opinion of oneself.

self-examination: S.-E. OF THE BREASTS a procedure in which a woman examines her breasts at regular intervals to determine whether there are any changes that might indicate the presence of any structural change such as a lump or a tumour. S.-E. OF THE TESTICLES a procedure in which a man examines his testicles at regular intervals for evidence of change that could indicate malignant process.

self-harm: See DELIBERATE SELF-HARM.

self-help: The action or faculty of providing for oneself without assistance from others.

self-image: The total concept, idea, or mental image one has of oneself and of one's role in society: the person one believes oneself to be.

self-limited: Descriptive of a pathological condition that runs a definite course regardless of external factors or influences.

self-poisoning: A disorder resulting from absorption of the waste products of metabolism, decomposed matter from the intestine, or the products of dead and infected tissue as in gangrene.

self-regulation: Control or direction by or of oneself.

self-retaining catheter: A catheter which can be inserted into the urinary bladder to be retained by means of the inflation of a small balloon surrounding the tip. See BALLOON CATHETER, FOLEY CATHETER under CATHETER.

Sellick's manoeuvre: The procedure of placing pressure on the cricoid cartilage during endotracheal intubation in the anaesthetized person in order to prevent regurgitation.

semantic (sē-man'tik): Relating to the meaning of words. S. ALEXIA a form of alexia in which the person can read but does not comprehend the meaning of the words he or she reads; s. APHASIA inability to recognize broader significance of words and phrases although their individual meanings are understood.

semen (sē'men): The secretion from the testes and accessory male organs, *e.g.*, prostate. It contains the spermatozoa and is discharged during sexual intercourse.

semenuria (sē-me-nū'ri-a): The presence of semen in the urine. Also spelled *seminuria*.

semi-: Combining form denoting (1) half, in quantity or value; (2) partial, to some extent, incompletely.

semicircular canals (se-mi-sir'kū-lar ka-nalz): Three membranous semicircular tubes contained within the bony labyrinth of the internal ear. They are concerned with appreciation of the body's position in space.

semicoma (sem-i-kō'ma): A state of consciousness in which the individual will respond to painful stimuli by drawing away from the stimulus, but not make any spontaneous movements.

semicomatose (sem-i-kō'ma-tōs): Condition bordering on the unconscious. The person appears to be unconscious but can be aroused.

semiconscious (sem-i-kon'shus): Partly conscious.

semilunar (sem-i-lū'nar): Shaped like a crescent or half-moon. S. CARTILAGES the crescentic interarticular cartilages of the knee joint (me-

nisci); S. VALVES those guarding the opening between the right ventricle and the pulmonary artery and between the left ventricle and the aorta.

semimembranous (sem-i-mem'bra-nus): One of the three hamstring muscles of the inner and back part of the thigh.

seminal (sem'i-nal): Relating to semen. S. DUCTS ducts that convey the semen and spermatozoa; include the vas deferens and ejaculatory ducts; S. FLUID the fluid in which sperm are suspended; includes secretions from the seminal vesicles, prostate, and bulbourethral glands; is ejaculated during sexual excitement; s. VESICLES either of two sacculated glandular secretory structures lying between the male bladder and the rectum.

seminiferous (sem-i-nif'er-us): Carrying or producing semen. S. TUBULES convoluted channels in the testes in which the sperm develop and through which they leave the testes.

seminoma (sem-i-nō'ma): A malignant tumour of the testis; occurs most often in young male adults. — seminomata, pl.; seminomatous, adj.

semiography (sē-mi-og'ra-fi): A written description of the signs and symptoms of a disease or pathological condition.

semiological (sē-mi-o-loj'ik): Relating to the symptoms of a disease.

semiology (sē-mi-ol'o-ji): Symptomatology (*q.v.*).

semipermeable (sem-i-per'me-a-b'l): Relating to a membrane that allows the molecules of some substances to pass through, but not others.

semiplegia (sem-i-plē'ji-a): Hemiplegia (*q.v.*).

semispinalis (sem-i-spī-nal'is): One of the deeper longitudinal muscles on either side of the spine.

semi-structured interview: A somewhat flexible interview technique involving broad, open-ended questions to guide the respondent, but also giving him or her the opportunity to elaborate and expand on the subject at will.

semitendinous (sem-i-ten'di-nus): 1. Partially composed of tendon. 2. Referring to the semitendinosus, one of the three hamstring muscles of the posterior aspect of the thigh.

senescide (sen'e-sīd): The practice in some primitive groups of abandoning their elderly or neglecting to care for them as a way of disposing of them.

senescing (sen-es'-ing): The biological processes of ageing that accompany the passage of time as shown by the steady decrease of one's capacity for biologic repair; consists of the many changes that occur with ageing rather than a single predominant change.

Sengstaken–Blakemore tube: A tube with an attached inflatable balloon that is inserted into the oesophagus and retained there to cause pressure on bleeding oesophageal varices. [Robert Sengstaken, American neurosurgeon. Arthur H. Blakemore, American surgeon, 1897–1970.]

senile (sē'nīl): Relating to or characteristic of old age, particularly when associated with mental decline. S. CATARACT a cataract developing in old age due to the ageing process; S. DEMENTIA or S. PSYCHOSIS loss of intellectual power occurring in the elderly; characterized by loss of memory, irritability; and personality deterioration; S. LENTIGO see under LENTIGO; S. VAGINITIS see under VAGINITIS.

senile squalor syndrome: A condition occurring in an older person who withdraws from society, hoards rubbish, lives in filthy conditions; usually occurs in those living alone. Also called *Diogenes syndrome.*

senilism (sē'nil-izm): Premature ageing.

senility (se-nil'i-ti): 1. Feebleness or deterioration of mind and/or body when it occurs in the aged; progressive and irreversible. 2. Old age.

senior house officer: A doctor who supports the registrar and consultant.

senna (sen'a): The dried leaves of the plant *Cassia acutifolia*; has long been used as a cathartic.

senopia (sē-nō'pi-a): Improvement of vision in elderly people.

sensate (sen'sāt): Felt or perceived by the senses.

sensation (sen-sā'shun): The perception or mental image produced in the brain by a stimulus which has been carried there by a sensory nerve.

sense: 1. The property of perceiving. 2. Feeling or sensation. S. ORGAN a specialized structure for receiving certain stimuli, *e.g.*, the eye, ear; SPECIAL S. any one of the five senses of feeling, hearing, seeing, tasting, smelling.

sensibility (sen-si-bil'i-ti): Sensitivity; the capacity for feeling or perceiving.

sensible (sen'si-b'l): 1. Endowed with the sense of feeling. 2. Detectable by the senses. S. PERSPIRATION see PERSPIRATION.

sensitive (sen-si-tiv): 1. Capable of receiving and responding to a stimulus. 2. Responding to a stimulus. 3. Being unusually aware of

factors in interpersonal relations. 4. Being abnormally susceptible to a substance such as a drug or foreign protein.

sensitivity (sen-si-tiv'i-ti): 1. The capacity to feel and react to a stimulus. 2. The quality or state of being sensitive to certain agents such as a drug or antigen. S. GROUPS see ENCOUNTER GROUP THERAPY. S. TESTS tests for sensitization to various allergens; several methods are available: (1) cutaneous, as in the patch test (*q.v.*); (2) percutaneous, as in the scratch test (*q.v.*); (3) intradermal, in which a minute amount of dilute antigen is injected into the skin, usually of the inner arm; a weal develops at the site to a size that indicates the degree of sensitivity of the person. The percutaneous and intradermal methods may result in such symptoms as nausea, chills, flushing, and dyspnoea; S. TRAINING training to identify and deal with one's relationships; employed in group therapy during which groups meet for 8 to 10 hours a day for several days to develop self-assurance, self-awareness, sensitivity, and understanding that will enable the participants to have more satisfactory relationships; see ENCOUNTER GROUP THERAPY.

sensitization (sen-si-tī-zā'shun): Rendering sensitive. Persons may become sensitive to a variety of substances, such as certain foods (*e.g.*, shellfish), bacteria, plants, chemical substances, drugs, sera, etc. The sensitizing agent acts as an antigen leading to the development of antibodies in the blood. See ALLERGY; ANAPHYLAXIS.

sensor (sen'sor): 1. A sensory organ or structure. 2. A device that generates a measurable impulse in response to a specific stimulus.

sensorimotor (sen'so-ri-mō'tor): Both sensory and motor; descriptive of a nerve that has both afferent and efferent fibres.

sensorineural (sen'sor-i-nū'ral): Relating to a sensory nerve or nerves. S. HEARING LOSS deafness characterized by inability to discriminate sound; due to damage to the inner ear or to the sensory path from the inner ear to the brain.

sensoristasis (sen'sor-i-stā'sis): A mental state similar to the physical state of homeostasis; the individual receives sufficient sensory stimuli to allow for healthful adaptation to the environment and enjoys an optimum level of well-being.

sensorium (sen'saw'ri-um): A term that implies the presence of memory and orientation to time, place and person; roughly the same as consciousness. — sensorial, adj.

sensory (sen'so-ri): Relating to sensation. S. DE-PRIVATION being cut off from usual external stimuli by isolation, social withdrawal, loss of hearing or sight; S. NERVES those which convey impulses to the brain and spinal cord; S. PARALYSIS loss of sensation due to pathology of the nerves, their pathways, or centres in the nervous system.

sensual (sen'shū-al): Of or relating to the senses or to the sensory organs.

sensualism (sen'shū-al-izm): The condition of being unable to control one's emotions or the more primitive bodily appetites, or of being controlled by them.

sentient (sen'shi-ent): Capable of feeling; sensitive.

sentiment: An attitude or thought arising from an emotional experience, *e.g.*, love, hatred, contempt or self-regard, with reference to some particular situation, person or object.

separation anxiety: See under ANXIETY.

sepsis (sep'sis): The presence of pathogenic bacteria, especially pus-forming bacteria, and their toxins in the bloodstream or tissues. — septic, adj.

sept-, septi-: Combining forms denoting seven; seventh.

sept-, septo-: Combining forms denoting a septum.

septal (sep'tal): Of or relating to a septum. S. DEFECT usually refers to a defect in the septum between the right and left sides of the heart, allowing blood to flow from the right side to the left without having circulated through the lungs.

septectomy (sep-tek'to-mi): Excision of part or all of a septum; often refers to the nasal septum.

septic (sep'tik): Relating to or caused by the presence of pathogenic organisms or their poisonous products; infected. S. ABORTION see under ABORTION; S. SHOCK see under SHOCK; S. SORE THROAT streptococcal inflammation of the throat, usually accompanied by fever and prostration.

septic-: Combining form denoting poison; sepsis.

septicaemia (sep'ti-sē'mi-a): A systemic condition resulting from the invasion of the body by living pathogenic organisms and their persistence and multiplication in the bloodstream. — septicaemic, adj.

septigravida (sep'ti-grav'i-da): A woman pregnant for the seventh time.

septipara (sep-tip'a-ra): A woman who has had seven pregnancies resulting in viable infants.

septoplasty (sep'tō-plas-ti): Plastic surgery for reconstruction of the nasal septum.

septostomy (sep-tos'to-mi): The operation of creating an opening in a septum.

septotomy (sep-tot'o-mi): The operation of cutting a septum, the nasal septum in particular.

septum (sep'tum): A thin partition of bone or membrane that separates two cavities. ATRIO-VENTRICULAR S. the muscular wall that divides the heart into two sides; DEVIATED S. usually refers to a deviation of the nasal septum from the middle to one side or the other; may be a congenital anomaly, or be due to trauma or fracture; INTERATRIAL S. the partition that separates the two atria; INTERVENTRICULAR S. the partition that separates the two ventricles of the heart; NASAL S. the partition that divides the nasal cavity; is made up of bone, cartilage, and mucous membrane; RECTOVAGINAL S. the membranous partition between the rectum and the vagina; RECTOVESICAL S. the membranous partition separating the rectum from the prostate gland and the urinary bladder.

sequela (sē-kwel'a): Any morbid condition, lesion or affection that occurs following or consequent to a disease. — sequelae, pl.

sequestration crisis A situation that occurs in sickle cell anaemia, precipitated by decreased oxygen in the red blood cells causing the haemoglobin to crystallize and create obstructions in blood vessels to any of the organs; congestive heart failure or renal failure may ensue.

sequestrum (sē-kwes'trum): A piece of dead bone that has become entirely or partially detached from the sound bone and remains within a cavity, abscess, or wound.

sequoiosis (sē-kwoy-ō'sis): A type of penumonitis associated with inhalation of redwood sawdust that contains particles of fungus growth.

serine (ser'ēn): A naturally occurring amino acid, a component of many proteins.

sero-: Combining forms denoting: 1. A watery consistency. 2. The blood serum.

serocolitis (sēr-ō-ko-lī'tis): Inflammation of the external serous coat of the colon; pericolitis.

serodiagnosis (sē'rō-diag-nō'sis): Diagnosis that is based on the results of a test or tests on the serum of the blood or other serous fluids of the body.

seroenteritis (sē'rō-en-ter-ī'tis): Inflammation of the serous coat of the intestine.

serofibrinous (sē'rō-fi'bri-nus): Both serous and fibrinous in nature; often refers to an exudate.

serological (sē-rō-loj'ik): Relating to serology. S. TEST any test performed on serum.

serologist (sē-rol'o-jist): A person who specializes in serology (*q.v.*).

serology (sē-rol'oj-i): The branch of science dealing with the study of sera. — serologic, serological, adj.; serologically, adv.

serolysin (sē-rol'i-sin): A bactericidal substance normally present in the blood serum.

seroma (sē-rō'ma): An accumulation of serum, usually under the skin, which produces a swelling resembling a tumour.

seromembranous (sē'rō-mem'bra-nus): Relating to a serous membrane.

seromucous (sē'rō-mū'kus): Relating to a gland which produces a watery mixture that contains both serum and mucus.

seromuscular (sē'rō-mus'kū-lar): Relating to both the serous and muscular coats of the intestine.

seronegative (sē'rō-neg'a tiv): Having a negative reaction to a test for some condition; said especially of serological tests for syphilis.

seropositive (sē-rō-pos'i-tiv): Having a positive reaction to a test for some condition; said especially of serological tests for syphilis.

seropurulent (sē'rō-pū'roo lent): Relating to a discharge containing both serum and pus.

seropus (sē-rō'pus): Serum mixed with pus.

serosa (sē-rō'sa): A serous membrane covering a visceral structure, *e.g.*, the peritoneal covering of an abdominal organ. — serosal, adj.

serositis (se-rō-sī'tis): Inflammation of a serous membrane.

serosynovitis (sē'rō-sin-ō-vī'tis): Synovitis accompanied by copious serous effusion.

serotherapy (se-rō-ther'a-pi): Treatment by an injection of serum containing specific antibodies; may be either prophylactic or curative.

serotonin (sēr-ō-tō'nin): A potent vasoconstrictor found particularly in blood platelets, brain, and intestinal tissue; usually acts as a vasoconstrictor to large vessels and dilates arterioles and capillaries. During dissolution of blood platelets serotonin is liberated, along with histamine and, since both are vasoconstrictors, this may aid in the physiological control of blood loss.

serotoxin (sēr-ō-tok'sin): The presence of a toxin in the bloodstream.

serotype (sēr'-ō-tīp): The type of microorganism as identified by the kinds of antigens present in the cell. Used in taxonomy to classify certain sub-types of microorganisms.

serous (sēr'us): Relating to, containing, or producing serum. S. FLUID the normal lymph in a serous cavity; S. MEMBRANE one lining a cavity that has no communication with the external air and covering the organs that lie in those cavities.

serpiginous (ser-pij'i-nus): Snake-like; coiled; irregular; term often used to describe the margins of skin lesions, especially ulcers and ringworm which sometimes heal at one side while spreading from the other; also called *serpent ulcer*.

serpigo (ser-pī'go): Any creeping eruption of the skin. — serpiginous, adj.

serrated (ser'ā-ted): Having a sawtooth-like edge.

Serratia (ser-ā'shi-a): A genus of bacilli often found in water. S. MARCESCEN a Gram-negative, motile organism found in milk, water, soil, and human faeces; formerly thought to be a harmless saprophyte, now thought to be a cause of pulmonary diseases, septicaemia, and hospital infections.

serration (ser-ā'shun): A sawtooth-like notch. — serrated, adj.

serratus anterior (sēr-ā'tus un-tēr-i-or): A muscle that runs around the side of the thorax from the first nine ribs to the vertebral ridge of the scapula; it acts to stabilize, abduct, and rotate the scapula.

serum (sēr'um): **1.** Any thin, clear, watery fluid produced by serous membranes and which serves to keep serous surfaces moist. **2.** The fluid part of the blood that remains after the blood has clotted and thus removed the corpuscles. **3.** The fluid part of the blood of an animal that has been inoculated with a specific microorganism or its toxins and has become immunized against the disease; used to produce passive immunity in exposed or susceptible individuals. — sera, serums, pl. ANTITOXIC S. prepared from the blood of an animal that has been immunized by the requisite toxin; it contains a high concentration of antitoxin; CONVALESCENT S. that from a person who has recently recovered from a specific disease; given to exposed or susceptible individuals as a prophylactic measure or to modify the symptoms; used especially in measles, mumps, whooping cough, scarlatina, chickenpox, poliomyelitis; s. SICKNESS the symptoms arising as a reaction about 10 days after the administration of serum of a different species; symptoms include urticarial rash, pyrexia, joint pains.

serum albumin: The major protein in the blood plasma; present in amounts of 3.5 to 5.5 grams per 100 ml of plasma; important in maintaining the osmotic pressure and viscosity of the blood.

serum alkaline phosphatase: An enzyme that catalyses the cleavage of inorganic phosphate non-specifically from a wide variety of phosphate esters and having a high pH optimum (greater than 8). Found in bacteria, fungi and animals but not in higher plants.

serum gonadotrophin (sēr-um gō-nad-ō-trō′pin): An ovary-stimulating hormone obtained from the blood serum of pregnant mares. It is used in amenorrhoea (*q.v.*), often in association with oestrogens (*q.v.*).

sesqui-: Combining form denoting every half hour.

sessile (ses′il): Without a peduncle or stalk; having a broad base or attachment.

setaceous (sē-tā′shus): Like a bristle.

setting sun sign: A downwards drifting of the eyes when the patient's trunk is raised and then lowered quickly; occurs only if there is cerebral damage.

severe acute respiratory syndrome: A pneumonia-like disease having symptoms similar to those of influenza, including fever, headache, sore throat, and cough. There is no known vaccine, although treatment with a cocktail of antivirals and antibiotics may be of benefit. Attributed to the coronavirus (*q.v.*).

severe combined immunodeficiency disease: An inherited disorder consisting of a deficiency of T-cells, B-cells, and macrophages which results in lack of immunity that is dependent on these cells; the exact cause is unknown. Symptoms, which usually begin in early infancy, include a greatly increased susceptibility to infection, failure to thrive, diarrhoea, and respiratory problems. Usually fatal within the first year of life, if untreated. Complete immune function has been restored in some patients by bone marrow transplants from matched sibling donors.

Sever's disease: A harmless condition characterized by pain in the back of the heel; tenderness over the calcaneus; occurring usually in children between 8 and 13 years of age; symptoms subside gradually but spontaneously. *Calcaneus apophysitis.*

sex: 1. Either of two divisions of organisms that are distinguished as male and female. **2.** Coitus. S. CHROMOSOMES the X and Y chromosomes passed down in human reproduction and which determine the sex of the offspring; S. HORMONE one having an effect on growth and functions of the reproductive organs or on the development of secondary sex characteristics; S. LIMITED descriptive of conditions that affect one sex only; S. LINKED descriptive of characteristics that are transmitted by genes that are located on the sex chromosomes.

sexism: 1. The assumption that one sex is superior to the other and the resultant discrimination practised against members of the supposed inferior sex. **2.** Conformity with the traditional stereotyping of social roles on the basis of sex.

sexology (seks-ol′o-ji): The branch of science that deals with sex and relations between the sexes from a biological point of view.

sexopathy (seks-op′a-thi): Abnormality of sexual behaviour or expression.

sextipara (seks-tip′a-ra): A woman who has borne six viable infants.

sexual (sek′shū-al): Pertaining to sex. S. DEVIANCE abnormal or unacceptable expression of sexual drives such as sadism, pederasty, exhibitionism, nymphomania, or illegal acts such as rape; S. INTERCOURSE coitus.

sexual abuse: Performing a sexual act with a child or with an adult against the person's wishes. Victims tend to experience a traumatic feeling of loss of control of themselves.

sexuality (sek-shū-al′i-ti): The make-up of an individual in relation to sex drives, sexual activity, and other aspects of personality concerned with relationships.

sexually transmitted diseases and disorders: The veneral diseases and disorders, although some of those included in this category are also transmitted by means other than sexual contact. Included are acquired immunodeficiency syndrome; condyloma acuminata (genital warts); gonorrhoea; herpesvirus hominus (genital infection); non-gonococcal or non-specific urethritis; pediculosis pubis; scabies; syphilis; trichomonas vaginalis. Included within this category are the three legally defined venereal diseases of syphilis, gonorrhoea, non-specific urethritis.

Sézary syndrome: A condition involving the reticular lymphocytes; characterized by exfoliative erythroderma; associated with alopecia, skin disorders, and nail changes.

shaft: An elongated structure, *e.g.*, the long part of a bone between its wider ends or extremities.

shaking palsy: Paralysis agitans; PARKINSON'S DISEASE.

shamanism (sha′man-izm): A practice among certain cultures of the people throwing themselves into states of excitement for religious purposes; it developed into a form of ecstatic healing, with the practitioner achieving a heightened state of consciousness; the role of shaman is that of healer and seer and originally was assumed only by women.

shank: The shin or tibia.

sharps: Colloquial term for surgical instruments with a cutting edge.

shear (shēr): An applied force that causes a parallel sliding motion between the planes of an object or of a load, or the result of such application. Bone fractures may be brought about in this way and are referred to as *shearing fractures.*

sheath (shēth): A tubular or enveloping membrane covering a structure such as a muscle, nerve, or blood vessel. MYELIN S. the covering of many of the axons; composed of lipid and protein molecules; serves to increase the velocity of nerve impulses. S. OF SCHWANN the neurilemma (*q.v.*).

Sheehan's syndrome: Hypopituitarism due to necrosis or dysfunction of the anterior pituitary, occurring as a sequal to postpartum haemorrhage; the thyroid, adrenal, and gonadal glands are all affected. Also called *Sheehan's disease.*

sheep cell agglutination test: A test to determine whether T-lymphocytes are present in sufficient numbers in blood. Human blood cells are mixed with those of sheep and, if the T-lymphocytes are present, the sheep cells will be attracted to them in a characteristic rosette pattern; when this does not occur, or if only a few rosettes form, the reaction is considered diagnostic for certain diseases, *e.g.*, infectious mononucleosis. (*q.v.*).

sheepskin (shēp'skin): May be a real sheep's skin or synthetic; because it absorbs moisture and prevents friction, is used in prevention of decubitus ulcers.

shell shock: Term first used during World War I to designate a wide variety of psychotic or neurotic disturbances thought to be caused by the noise of bursting shells and other combat experiences. See SHOCK.

shiastic massage (shī-as'tik): Japanese massage, sometimes called acupressure (*q.v.*); pressure is exerted by hand, elbow, or knee along certain pathways, usually for 30 to 60 minutes; may cause discomfort but is not painful.

shiatsu (shi-at'-soo): A kind of massage, of Japanese origin, in which the practitioner applies pressure with his or her thumbs and palms to certain points on the client's body.

shield (shēld): A protecting tube or cover. BULLER'S S. a watch glass that is taped over one eye to protect it from infection in the other eye, *e.g.*, in gonorrhoeal ophthalmia; LEAD S.

a lead plate that is placed between the operator and an x-ray machine for protection from the x-rays; NIPPLE S. a device made of a glass dome and rubber teat that is placed over the nipple of a nursing mother when it is sore or not sufficiently protractile for the baby to suck.

Shiga's bacillus (*Shigella dynsenteriae*): One of the bacteria that produce dysentery. Most common in the Middle and Far East. Infection often serious. [Kiyoshi Shiga, Japanese bacteriologist, 1870–1957.]

Shigella (shi-gel'la): A genus of microorganisms, many of which are the causative agents of various forms of dysentery. The organism is found in the faeces of infected persons and carriers; it is also transmitted by infected food and flies; epidemic in underdeveloped areas of the world. S. FLEXNERI the most frequent cause of dysentery epidemics and often of infantile gastroenteritis; S. SONNEI a frequent cause of bacillary dysentery in temperate climates, and of summer diarrhoea in children.

shigellosis (shi-gel-ō'sis): Bacillary dysentery caused by one of the *Shigella* organisms; tends to be endemic in certain lower social and economic areas.

Shiley tube (shī'-li): A tube used in the management of a tracheostomy.

shin: The front of the leg below the knee. S. BONE the tibia; S. SPLINT pain, discomfort, and swelling along the shin bone caused by strain on the flexor digitoris longus muscle; an athletic injury, but may also be caused by running, jogging, or even walking. See ANTERIOR TIBIAL COMPARTMENT SYNDROME.

shingles: See HERPES ZOSTER under HERPES.

Shirodkar's suture: A purse-string suture placed around the cervix of a pregnant uterus and left in place until the 38th week of pregnancy after which it is separated, and labour soon begins; done to prevent abortion if the patient has had a previous abortion or has an incompetent cervix.

SHO: Abbreviation for senior house officer (*q.v.*).

shock: A grave, pathophysiological state in which the vital processes of the body are rapidly and profoundly depressed as a result of inadequate tissue perfusion due to a reduction in blood volume. Its features include a fall in blood pressure; weak, rapid, thready pulse; pallor, restlessness; cold, clammy skin; decreased respiratory depth, and decreased urinary output; ANAPHYLACTIC S. a violent attack of severe symptoms of shock produced when sensitized individuals receive a second injection of serum or foreign protein to which they have been previously exposed; an emergency situation that requires immediate attention. Symptoms include breathlessness; hypotension; pallor; weak, rapid, thready pulse; fever; vascular collapse; sometimes convulsions and unconsciousness; BACTERAEMIC S., s. caused by bacterial toxins liberated by bacterial organisms in the circulation; CARDIOGENIC S., s. due to inadequate cardiac output with inadequate peripheral circulation; caused by pump failure; often fatal; DRUG-INDUCED S. may occur following administration of drugs that are incompatible with each other or with some other substance in the blood; occurs chiefly with intravenous administration; ELECTRIC S. the sudden violent convulsive effect of an electric current passing through the body; ENDOTOXIC S. occurs in septicaemia as a result of pooling of blood caused by a decrease in effective circulating blood without actual blood loss; HAEMORRHAGIC S., s. due to excessive loss of blood; HYPOVOLAEMIC S. may be due to haemorrhage, trauma, burns, or diarrhoea, any of which may cause a slowly progressive reduction in the volume of circulating blood; INSULIN S. hypoglycaemia produced by (1) an overdose of insulin; or (2) a therapeutic measure used in certain psychoses; IRREVERSIBLE S. occurs when prolonged hypoxia causes damage to brain centres; NEUROGENIC S. results from interference with functions of the sympathetic nervous system; may be caused by drugs, anaesthesia, spinal injuries; OLIGAEMIC S. is associated with severe drop in blood volume; PRIMARY S. occurs immediately following an injury; SECONDARY S. occurs several hours, or even days, after trauma has occurred; often associated with life-threatening injury or illness and may or may not follow primary shock; symptoms include restlessness, weakness, progressive drop in blood pressure and body temperature, profuse sweating, reduced urinary output; SEPTIC S. a syndrome due to vasoconstriction; occurs in severe infections, particularly those caused by Gram-negative enteric bacteria; usually develops in persons already debilitated by an underlying disorder; characterized by chills, fever, hypotension, restlessness, irritability, tachypnoea, tachycardia, confusion, rapid pulse, gastrointestinal symptoms; may lead to respiratory insufficiency, heart failure, coma, and death; SHELL S. a type of psychoneurosis experienced by soldiers; a form of hysteria in which symptoms often indicate a functional disorder, e.g., blindness, deafness, paralysis; 'SPEED' S., s. caused by too rapid infusion of intravenous fluids; characterized by shock symptoms and syncope; may lead to cardiac arrest; SPINAL S. follows transection of the spinal cord; results in flaccid paralysis and loss of reflex activity in parts of the body below the lesion; the areflexia may be temporary or permanent; SURGICAL S. a condition in which there is serious impairment of circulation following surgery; may be caused by loss of blood, vasodilatation, prolonged anaesthesia, or inadequate cardiac output; VASOGENIC S., s. caused by marked vasodilatation; WARM S. occurs particularly in urological patients; characterized by warm, dry skin, fever, normal or excessive urine output; may occur after cystoscopy, urological surgery, or catheterization.

shock lung syndrome: Occurs after resuscitation following shock or serious insult to the body, when it appears that the patient is recovering. The first sign is rapid pulse followed by hypocapnia, pulmonary insufficiency, and anoxia in spite of the administration of high concentrations of oxygen. Also called *adult respiratory distress syndrome, stiff lung, wet lung, respiratory lung, hyaline membrane disease.*

shortsightedness: Myopia (*q.v.*).

shoulder: The part of the body on each side of the base of the neck where the arm joins the trunk and where the clavicle, scapula and humerus meet. FROZEN S. inability to abduct or rotate the arm due to inflammation of subacromial bursa; S. BLADE the scapula; S. GIRDLE formed by clavicle and scapula on either side.

shoulder–hand syndrome: Pain and limitation of motion of the shoulder and hand sometimes seen after injury to the neck or upper extremity, or after myocardial infarction.

show: A popular name for the bloodstained vaginal discharge at the commencement of labour.

shunt: 1. To turn to one side; divert from a normal path or course. 2. A naturally or surgically created passage between two natural channels to divert flow of blood or other body fluid, to allow for healing, or to bypass an obstruction. ARTERIOVENOUS S. passage of blood between an artery and vein, usually between a radial artery and a cephalic vein when repeated access to the arterial blood system is required for haemodialysis; CARDIOVASCULAR S. an abnormal flow of blood between the systemic and pulmonary circulation or between the two sides of the heart; LEFT-TO-RIGHT S. diversion of the blood from the left to the right side of the heart through a septal defect or patent ductus arteriosis; PORTACAVAL S. anastomosis of the portal vein with the inferior vena cava; RIGHT-TO-LEFT S. a diversion of the blood from the right to the left side of the heart through a patent ductus arteriosus, or in cases of pulmonary stenosis; SPLENORENAL S. an anastomosis of the splenic vein to the left renal vein, accompanied by removal of the spleen; done for the relief of portal hypertension; VENTRICULOPERITONEAL S. a surgically made communication between a lateral ventricle of the brain and the peritoneal cavity by means of a rubber tube, for relief of hydrocephalus; VENTRICULOATRIAL S., the surgical establishment of communication between the ventricles of the brain and a cardiac atrium to shunt cerebrospinal fluid to the heart; VENTRICULOURETERAL S. a surgically created shunt between a lateral ventricle of the brain and a ureter, a measure used in treatment of hydrocephalus.

Shy–Drager syndrome: A rare, progressive neurologic disorder characterized by orthostatic hypotension, rigidity, tremor, impotence, atonic bladder, anhidrosis in lower parts of the body, ophthalmoplegia, and fasiculations.

sial-, sialo-: Combining forms denoting (1) saliva; (2) salivary glands.

sialadenitis (sī′al-ad-e-nī′tis): Inflammation of a salivary gland. Also called *sialoadenitis*.

sialadenoncus (sī′al-ad-e-non′kus): A tumour of a salivary gland.

sialagogue (sī-al′a-gog): An agent that increases the flow of saliva.

sialic (sīal′ik): Relating to saliva.

sialism (sī′a-lizm): Excessive salivation; sialorrhoea.

sialoadenectomy (sī′al-ō-ad-e-nek′to-mi): Surgical removal of a salivary gland.

sialoaerophagy (sī′a-lō-ā-er-of′a-ji): The habitual swallowing of saliva and air.

sialoangiectasis (sī′a-lō-an-ji-ek′ -ta-sis): The dilatation of a salivary gland.

sialogenous (sī′a-loj′e-nus): Producing or resembling saliva.

sialogram (sī-al′ō-gram): Radiographic picture of the salivary glands and ducts, usually after injection of radiopaque medium. — sialography, n.; sialigraphic, adj.; sialographically, adv.

sialoma (sī-a-lō′ma): A tumour of the salivary gland.

sialorrhoea (sī′a-lō-rē′a): Excessive salivation. Syn., *sialism, ptyalism.*

sialostenosis (sī′a-lō-ste-nō′sis): Stenosis of a salivary duct.

Siamese twins: Twins that are joined together at birth, usually at the head, chest, or hip. When the union is slight it involves the skin, muscles and cartilage only; when it is extensive it may involve shared bones and organs. In some cases, surgical separation is possible.

sibilant (sib′i-lant): Having a dry, high-pitched, shrill, whistling, or hissing sound. S. RALE a whistling sound heard over the bronchi in cases of bronchial narrowing or spasm.

sibilus (sib′il-us): Rhonchus, or dry rale. Whistling sound heard on auscultation of the chest, *e.g.*, in cases of bronchitis, where the bronchi are narrowed by presence of oedema or exudate. — sibilant, adj

sibling (sib′ling): One of a family of children having the same parents. S. RIVALRY jealousy between brothers and sisters, often based on competition for parental affection.

siccant (sik′ant): 1. Drying. 2. A substance that speeds up drying.

siccative (sik′a-tiv): 1. Removing moisture, or drying. 2. An agent that causes drying.

sicchasia (si-kā′zi-a): Nausea, abhorrence of food.

siccus (sik′us): Dry.

sick: 1. Unwell. 2. Nauseated. S. HEADACHE see MIGRAINE.

sick bay: The infirmary or dispensary on a ship or in a boarding school.

sicklaemia (sik-lē′mi-a): The presence of sickle-shaped erythrocytes in the blood; see SICKLE CELL ANAEMIA under ANAEMIA.

sickle cell (sik′el): A red blood cell shaped like a crescent. S.C. ANAEMIA see under ANAEMIA; S.C. CRISIS recurring episodes of acute symptoms developing in patients with s.c. anaemia, usually occurring after infection, dehydration, or hypoxia; S.C. HAEMOGLOBINOPATHY the red blood cells contain an abnormal amount of haemoglobin and amino acid; results from inheritance of the sickle cell gene; symptoms include hypoaesthenia, priapism, pyelonephritis, pallor, weakness, and intermittent crises.

sickling disease: Sickle cell anaemia. See under ANAEMIA.

sickness: A disordered, weakened or unsound mental or physical condition; disease. AIR S. see MOTION SICKNESS; ALTITUDE S. condition characterized by giddiness, nausea, dyspnoea, thirst, prostration; caused by atmosphere that has less oxygen than one is accustomed to breathing; CAR S. see MOTION SICKNESS; DE-COMPRESSION S. see CAISSON DISEASE; FALLING S. epilepsy; RADIATION S., see RADIATION; SEA-SICKNESS see MOTION SICKNESS; SLEEPING S. see AFRICAN TRYPANOSOMIASIS.

sick role: Behaviour patterns consistent with those expected of an individual functioning in a state of ill health.

sideboards, siderails: Protective devices attached to the sides of the bed to prevent restless, delirious or aged persons from falling out of bed; bed rails.

side-chain theory: See EHRLICH'S SIDE-CHAIN THEORY under EHRLICH.

side effect: A result other than the one for which an agent or drug was administered; sometimes but not always an undesirable effect.

sider-, sidero-: Combining forms denoting iron.

sideroblast (sid'er-ō-blast): An immature red blood cell containing granules of iron.

siderocyte (sid'er-ō-sīt): A red blood cell containing granules of free iron.

siderocytosis (sid'er-ō-sī-tō'sis): The presence in the circulating blood of a considerable number of siderocytes.

siderofibrosis (sid'er-ō-fī-brō'sis): Fibrosis combined with multiple small deposits of iron.

sideropenia (sid'er-ō-pē'ni-a): A deficiency of iron in the circulating blood.

sideropenic dysphagia (sid'er-ō-pē'nik dis-fā'ji-a): See PLUMMER–VINSON SYNDROME.

siderophil (sid'er-ō-fil): A cell or tissue having an affinity for iron or that contains iron. — siderophilic, siderophilous, adj.

siderophilin (sid'er-ō-fil'in): Transferrin (*q.v.*).

siderosilicosis (sid'er-ō-sil-i-kō'sis): Pneumoconiosis caused by prolonged exposure to silica and iron dust.

siderosis (sid'er-ō'sis): **1.** Excess of iron in the blood or tissues. **2.** A form of pneumoconiosis caused by the inhalation of iron or other metallic particles.

SIDS: Abbreviation for sudden infant death syndrome (*q.v.*).

sigh (sī): A deep prolonged inspiration followed by a comparatively shorter expiration.

sight (sīt): **1.** The act of or the ability of seeing. **2.** The special sense involved in seeing.

sigmatism (sig'ma-tizm): **1.** A form of stammering in which the individual cannot properly articulate the letter S; lisping. **2.** The too frequent enunciation of the letter S.

sigmoid (sig'moyd): Shaped like the letter S, or the Greek sigma. S. COLON the part of the colon between the descending colon and the rectum; S. FLEXURE an S-shaped curve of

the intestine joining the descending colon above the rectum.

sigmoidectomy (sig-moy-dek'to-mi): Surgical removal of part of the sigmoid colon or all of it.

sigmoiditis (sig-moy-dī'tis): Inflammation of the sigmoid colon, especially the sigmoid flexure.

sigmoidopexy (sig-moy'dō-pek-si): An operation to correct prolapse of the rectum.

sigmoidoproctostomy (sig-moy'-dō-prok-tos'to-mi): The surgical creation of an anastomosis between the sigmoid colon and the rectum.

sigmoidorectostomy (sig-moy'dō-rek-tos'to-mi): The surgical creation of an artificial anus at the junction of the sigmoid colon and the rectum; a low colostomy.

sigmoidoscope (sig-moy'dō-skōp): An instrument for visualizing the rectum and sigmoid flexure of the colon. See ENDOSCOPE. — sigmoidoscopic, adj.; sigmoidoscopy, n.

sigmoidostomy (sig-moy-dos'to-mi): The surgical formation of a colostomy in the sigmoid colon.

sigmoidovesical (sig-moy-dō-ves'i-kal): Relating to the sigmoid colon and the urinary bladder. S. FISTULA a fistula between the sigmoid colon and the urinary bladder.

sign (sīn): Any objective of disease. VITAL S.S the signs of life, specifically the pulse, respirations, temperature, and blood pressure.

signature (sig'na-tūr): The part of a drug prescription that is placed on the label; it gives the directions for use to be followed by the patient.

sign language: A generic term given to the language of signs and gestures. BRITISH S.L. the indigenous language of the native deaf population of Great Britain. It is as distinct from English syntactically and grammatically as a foreign language. Also known as *fingerspelling, dactylology.* — signing, v.

silastic (sī-las'tik): A rubbery silicone material with various medical uses including drains, and for replacing tissues that have been removed, *e.g.*, breast tissue.

silent: **1.** A quiescent state of disease. **2.** Not showing the expected symptoms of a disease or disorder. **3.** Not responding to stimuli.

silica (sil'i-ka): A substance that occurs naturally and abundantly in the Earth in several forms; used in making glass and ceramic products and as an abrasive, adsorbent, and dehydrating agent.

silicon (sil'i-kon): An abundant natural element, found in soil, always found in combination;

combines with oxygen to form silica; used in manufacture of silicone, transistors, solar cells, ceramics.

silicone (sil'i-kōn): A plastic compound of silicon (*q.v.*) with many uses in medicine as a substitute for rubber, as in the manufacture of tubes and implants; also used in the manufacture of sealants, adhesives, and detergents.

silicosiderosis (sil'i-kō-sid-er-o'sis): A form of pneumonoconiosis caused by inhalation of dust containing particles of silica and iron.

silicosis (sil-i-kō'sis): A form of chronic pulmonary disease characterized by extensive nodular fibrosis of the lung; caused by inhalation of dust containing particles of silica; occurs in miners, metal grinders, stone workers, and those whose occupations bring them into contact with ceramics, sand, quartz, and other stones.

silicotuberculosis (sil'i-kō-tu-ber'-ku-lō'sis): Tuberculosis occurring in a person who already has silicosis.

silver (sil'ver): A soft, white, malleable metal; has several uses in medicine. S. NITRATE a compound of s. used as (1) a caustic; (2) in treatment of burns, in 1% solution, a disadvantage being that it stains linens an indelible black.

Simmond's disease: Hypopituitary cachexia. Results from destruction of anterior pituitary lobe with consequent absence of secretions which normally stimulate other endocrine glands, especially the gonads, thyroid, and the adrenal glands. The basal metabolic rate is very low, there is loss of pubic and axillary hair, loss of sexual desire, premature ageing, progressive emaciation.

Sims' position: See under POSITION.

Sims' test, Huhner test: A test to help determine the cause of infertility; involves examination of postcoital semen from the vaginal pool and endocervix soon after intercourse to ascertain the number and motility of the sperm.

simulation (sim-ū-lā'shun): 1. Malingering (*q.v.*). 2. The imitation of one disease or symptom by another.

sinciput (sin'si-put): The front part of the cranium just above and including the forehead, used in reference to the forehead. — sincipital, adj.

sinew (sin'ū): A ligament or tendon.

singer's node: A fibrous nodule that forms on the free margin of the vocal cords; occurs in singers, public speakers, and others who habitually strain their voices.

single blind: Descriptive of an experiment in which the researcher, but not the subject, knows which particular treatment is being used.

singultus (sing-gul'tus): A hiccup.

sinister (sin'is-ter): In anatomy, left, or on the left side.

sinistr-, sinistro-: Combining forms denoting the left; towards the left; on the left side.

sinistrad (sin'is-trad): Towards the left.

sinistral (sin'is-tral): Relating to the left side.

sinistrality (sin'is-tral'i-ti): The preferential use of the left member of any of the major paired organs or parts, *e.g.*, the eye, ear, hand, foot. Left-handedness.

sinistraural (sin'is-traw'ral): Hearing more acutely with the left ear.

sinistrocardia (sin'is-trō-kar'di-a): Displacement of the heart towards the left side of the body.

sinistromanual (sin'is-trō-man'ūal): Left-handed.

sino-, sinu-: Combining forms denoting sinus.

sinoatrial (sī'nō-ā'tri-al): Relating to the sinus venosus and the right atrium of the heart. S. NODE the heart's natural pacemaker; a collection of specialized conductive tissue at the junction of the superior vena cava and the right atrium; it emits regular impulses which control the rate of the heartbeat. S. BLOCK see under HEART BLOCK. Also called *sinoauricular* and *sinuatrial*.

sinobronchial syndrome (sī'nō-brong'ki-al sin'drom): Bronchitis associated with sinusitis; may be due to aspiration of purulent postnasal discharge; often caused by *Streptococcus pneumoniae* or *Haemophilus influenzae*.

sinobronchitis (sī'nō-bron-kī'tis): Inflammation of the paranasal sinuses and the bronchi.

sinogram (sī'nō-gram): Radiographic picture of a sinus after injection of radiopaque medium.

sinography (sī-nog'ra-fi): Roentgenography of any sinus following introduction of a radiopaque medium.

sinus (sī'nus): 1. A hollow or cavity, especially one in a cranial bone. 2. A channel containing blood, *e.g.*, the sinuses of the brain. 3. Any abnormal tract leading from a suppurating area; a fistula. CAROTID S. see under CAROTID; CAVERNOUS S. a channel for venous blood, on either side of the sphenoid bone; it drains blood from the lips, nose, and orbits; CORONARY S. the dilated portion of the great cardiac vein; it is about 2.5 cm in length and opens into the lower part of the right atrium; DERMAL S. a congenital fistula extending from the skin, between the vertebrae, to the spinal canal; ETHMOID S. one of a pair of paranasal sinuses; located in the ethmoid bone; FRONTAL S. one of a pair of paranasal sinuses, located in the frontal bone; INFERIOR SAGITTAL S. a small s. in the dura mater parallel to the superior sagittal s.; MAXILLARY S. (the antrum of Highmore) one of a pair of air cavities in the maxillae; PARANASAL S. one of the air spaces in the bones around the nose; they are lined with mucous membrane and communicate with the nasal passages; include the frontal, ethmoid, maxillary, and sphenoid sinuses; PILONIDIAL S. a s. containing hairs, usually occurring in the coccygeal region, especially in the cleft between the buttocks in hirsute people; RECTUS S. a s. of the dura mater; formed by the junction of the great cerebral vein and the inferior sagittal s.; also called *straight* s.; s. ARREST partial or complete obstruction of the heartbeat at its origin; s. BRADYCARDIA see under BRADYCARDIA; s. HEADACHE see under HEADACHE; s. NODE see under NODE; s. RHYTHM see under RHYTHM; s. TACHYCARDIA see under TACHYCARDIA. SPHENOID S. one of a pair of paranasal sinuses, located in the anterior part of the sphenoid bone; SUPERIOR SAGITTAL S. located in the sagittal suture of the dura mater; SINUSES OF VALSALVA three pouches between the wall of the aorta and each of the semilunar cusps of the aortic valve; VENOUS S. a large vein or canal for the circulation of venous blood.

sinusitis (si'nū-sī'tis): Inflammation of a sinus, particularly one or more of the paranasal sinuses. BACTERIAL S. may be caused by group A beta-haemolytic streptococci, *Haemophilus influenzae*, haemolytic *Staphylococcus aureus*, pneumococcus. NON-BACTERIAL S. may be due to a virus, vasomotor disturbances, obstruction.

sinusoid (sī' nū-soyd): 1. Resembling a sinus. 2. A dilated channel into which the arterioles open in some organs and which take the place of capillaries; found in such organs as the heart, spleen, liver, pancreas, and in the suprarenal, parathyroid, and carotid glands.

sinusotomy (sin-ū-sot'o-mi): An operation in which an opening is made into a sinus to remove pus; a drainage tube may be left in place for several days.

Sipple's syndrome: A condition characterized by phaeochromocytoma, cancer of the thyroid, and hyperparathyroidism.

sirenomelia (si're-nō-mē'li-a): A congenital anomaly in which the lower extremities are fused, and the feet are partially or completely fused; mermaid deformity.

-sis: Combining form denoting (1) a diseased state, or (2) a disease produced by the agent named in the stem, *e.g.*, amoebiasis. May appear as -aisis, -esis, -iasis, -osis.

sitieirgia (sit-ē-ir'ji-a): Morbid rejection of food; anorexia (*q.v.*).

sito-: Combining form denoting food; nutrition.

sitology (sī-tol'o-ji): The science of nutrition; dietetics.

sitomania (sī'tō-mā'ni-a): Abnormal craving for food; excessive hunger.

sitotherapy (sī'tō-ther'a-pi): Treatment of disease through diet; dietotherapy.

situs (sī'tus): Site or position.

SI units: The units of measurement generally accepted for all scientific and technical uses. Together they make up the International System of Units. The abbreviation SI, from the French *Système International d'Unites*, is used in all languages. There are seven base SI units, defined by specified physical measurements and two supplementary units. Units are derived for any other physical quantities by multiplication and division of the base and supplementary units. The base units and the prefixes used for multiples are shown in the tables in Appendix 1.

Sjögren–Larrson syndrome (syer' -gren-lah' - son): Genetically determined congenital ectodermosis. Associated with mental handicap and spasticity.

Sjögren's syndrome: A condition seen mostly in menopausal or postmenopausal women, characterized by deficient secretion from lacrimal, salivary and other glands; by keratoconjunctivitis, dry tongue, hoarse voice, tenderness of joints, muscular weakness, and anaemia. Thought to be due to an autoimmune process, possibly influenced by changes in the functioning of endocrine glands. [Henrik Samuel Conrad Sjögren, Swedish ophthalmologist.]

skelalgia (skē-lal'ji-a): Pain in the leg.

skeleton (skel'e-ton): The bony framework of the body supporting and protecting the soft tissues and organs. APPENDICULAR S. the shoulder girdle and upper extremities, and the pelvic girdle and lower extremities; AXIAL S. the skull, spine, ribs, and sternum, forming the bony structure of the trunk. — skeletal, adj.

Skene's ducts: Paraurethral ducts; see under PARAURETHRAL.

Skene's glands: Two small mucous glands at the entrance to the female urethra; the paraurethral glands. They empty into the vestibule via SKENE'S DUCTS located on either side of the urethra. [Alexander Johnson Chalmers Skene, American gynaecologist, 1838–1900.]

skenitis (skē-nī'tis): Inflammation of Skene's glands (*q.v.*).

skia-: Combining form denoting shadow, especially one produced by internal organs on x-ray film.

skiagram (skī'a-gram): An x-ray photograph.

skiagraphy (skī-ag'ra-fi): The making of x-ray pictures.

skiameter (skī-am'i-ter): An instrument for measuring (1) the intensity of x-rays, or (2) the refraction of the eye.

Skillern's fracture: A fracture in the lower one-third of the radius with a greenstick fracture of the ulna in the same region.

skill mix: The use of a variety of professionals, with varying qualities and expertise, to carry out roles traditionally performed by one health-care professional. Carried to its extreme, the theory is that all staff should be working to their maximum potential at all times, carrying out only those tasks which cannot be delegated to less highly trained professionals.

skin: The tissue that forms the outer covering of the body; it is an effective barrier against infection and trauma. Consists of the epidermis, or cuticle, the outermost coat which protects the cutis or true skin (cutis vera) which is extremely sensitive and vascular. The cutis contains nerve fibres that respond to pain, pressure, touch, and temperature. Appendages of the skin include hair, nails, sebaceous glands and sweat glands. S. GRAFT a procedure utilizing healthy skin from another part of the body to replace damaged or defective skin; see GRAFT; S. TEST an injection of a small amount of an antigen to test for immunity to a specific infection.

skin cancer: A fairly common disease among the elderly; may be caused by factors in the cells but is usually due to external factors such as exposure to ultraviolet rays in sunlight; light-skinned people are especially affected. Occurs more often in men; farmers and sailors seem to be especially susceptible. Ionizing radiation, including x-rays, gamma rays, and ultraviolet rays are common causes. The two most common types of skin cancer are basal cell carcinoma and squamous cell carcinoma; see under CARCINOMA.

skinfold (skin'fōld): The thickness of a fold of skin pinched between the thumb and forefin-

ger, usually the skin over the ribs; done to help in evaluating the patient's nutritional status. Calibrated calipers are used to measure the thickness of a fold of skin usually of the upper arm or over the lower ribs.

skin-popping: Term used by drug addicts for the subcutaneous injection of drugs; often produces characteristic abscess-like lesions at injection sites.

skin test: A frequently used method of determining induced sensitivity; involves applying an antigen to an abrasion in the skin or injecting it into the skin, and evaluating the inflammatory response this produces.

skull: The framework of the head. See CRANIUM.

slant: In microbiology, a test tube containing culture medium set at a slant to provide more area for growth of bacteria.

slapping. 1. A percussion movement in massage, consisting of an alternating series of sharp blows with the palm of the hand. 2. In walking, a gait in which the forefoot slaps the ground forcefully.

sleep: Recurring periods of rest for the body and mind, usually with the body in a lying-down, immobile position; the person is disengaged from the environment and voluntary acts are suspended. The physiological condition is readily reversible to one of wakefulness and response to external stimuli. Sleep patterns vary with age, state of health, and psychological state, and may be altered by medical regimens; however, scientists have described four stages of sleep as it occurs in the normal healthy adult: Stage 1, the time period immediately after falling asleep, during which the person is responsive to environmental stimuli and cerebral activity continues; lasts about 10 minutes. Stage 2, the time period during which the person is beginning to relax, cerebral activity slows down, with hearing being the last to go, and the individual falls asleep. Stage 3, the time period when the person becomes more relaxed, blood pressure, respirations and pulse decrease, metabolism slows down, and gastrointestinal activity increases. Stage 4, the time period beginning about 30 minutes after the person has fallen asleep; it is marked by deep sleep, very relaxed muscles, an increase in the release of growth hormones, and a very few rapid eye movements (REM). Within 10 to 30 minutes after Stage 4 begins, rapid eye movements become prominent; the person's pulse, respirations, and blood pressure rise, and vivid dreams occur which can often be recalled upon awakening. This REM sleep lasts about 20 minutes and the person then returns to Stage 2 and the cycle is repeated. TWILIGHT S. see TWILIGHT STATE.

sleeping sickness: 1. A disease endemic in Africa, characterized by increasing somnolence; caused by protozoal parasites transmitted by the tsetse fly. 2. Any one of the viral encephalitides that is characterized by somnolence, especially equine encephalitis.

sleepwalking Somnambulism (*q.v.*).

slide: A glass plate on which the object to be viewed through the microscope is placed.

sliding board: A board of appropriate length that is placed under the buttocks and thighs when transferring a paralysed individual; also useful for the emergency transfer of a spinal-cord-injured person.

sling: A bandage that supports any part of the body, particularly the arm. PELVIC S. see under PELVIC.

slipped disc: Herniated disc; see under HERNIATED.

slipped femoral epiphysis: See EPIPHYSIS.

slitlamp (slit'lamp): A special instrument for the microscopic viewing of the eye; it is fitted with a diaphragm with a narrow slit through which an intense beam of light is projected.

slough (sluf): 1. A mass of necrotic tissue that separates from the healthy tissue and is eventually washed away by exudated serum. 2. To separate or cast off necrotic tissue from the healthy tissue underneath.

sludge (sluj): To agglutinate or precipitate from a liquid, or the deposit formed by precipitation from a liquid.

small cell lung cancer: Accounts for over 80,000 deaths per annum in England and Wales. Cigarette smoking is a factor is most cases. Usually starts in the bronchi and disseminates rapidly; symptoms include cough, dyspnoea, hoarseness, dysphagia; metastasizes, often to the brain. See OAT CELL CARCINOMA.

small-for-dates: Term used to describe an infant who is smaller or lighter than expected for its gestational age. The definition may vary: some authorities include those below the 10th percentile and some below the 5th percentile.

small intestine: The part of the intestine between the stomach and the large intestine; consists of sections named duodenum, jejunum, and ileum; it is concerned chiefly with digestion and absorption of nutriments.

smallpox: Variola. Smallpox was eradicated from the world in 1977. Because of this, vaccination is no longer required for travellers to any part of the world where previously it had been endemic. It was an acute infectious disease, often fatal, caused by a virus linked with that of vaccinia (cowpox). Headache, vomiting, and high fever precede the eruption of a widespread rash which is papular, vesicular and finally pustular.

smear: A film of material spread on a glass slide and stained for microscopic examination. BUCCAL S. a s. containing scrapings from the mucous membrane of the mouth just above the line of the teeth; used in a cytological test for determining the somatic sex of an individual; 'PAP' S. see PAPANICOLAOU; VAGINAL S. a s. from the vagina plated for microscopic examination.

smegma (smeg'ma): An ill-smelling sebaceous secretion which accumulates under the male prepuce and in the folds of the vagina.

smell: 1. The sense that enables an individual to perceive and discriminate odours. 2. Odour. 3. To emit an odour.

smelling salts: A mixture of compounds usually containing some form of ammonia, which when inhaled acts as a stimulant or restorative, *e.g.*, to prevent or relieve fainting.

Smith-Petersen nail: See under NAIL.

smoker's cancer: Cancer of the lip, throat, or lung; seen in habitual smokers. C. of the lower lip is most often seen in pipe smokers.

snail fever: Term used for a type of schistosomiasis commonly occurring in the Middle East; a species of snail is the intermediate host.

snare (snār): A surgical instrument with a wire loop at the end; used for removal of polypi, tumours or any soft fleshy projection such as a tonsil.

Snellen's test type: A device employed for testing for acuity of distance vision; consists of block letters of varying sizes arranged on wall charts.

sniffing: Inhaling. In street language, the inhalation of such substances as carbon tetrachloride, gasoline, gluc, paint thinner, etc., or cocaine, to produce a state of euphoria; over time, indulgence may result in a pathological condition of liver, kidney, bone marrow or lung.

SNOMED: Abbreviation for Systemized Nomenclature of Medicine (*q.v.*).

snore: A rough sound produced during sleep; caused by vibration of the soft palate and the uvula.

snow: CARBON DIOXIDE S. solid carbon dioxide, dry ice. Used for local freezing of the tissues in minor surgery. s. BLINDNESS temporary blindness, with pain in the eyes and photophobia; caused by glare of the sun on snow. s. is also a street name for heroin.

snuffles (snuf'lz): A snorting inspiration due to congestion of nasal mucous membranes when the nasal discharge may be mucopurulent or bloody; seen in newborn infants. May be indicative of congenital syphilis.

soap: A cleansing agent formed by the action of an alkali on fatty acid. CASTILE s. hard soap made with olive oil; MEDICINAL SOFT s. made of vegetable oils; a soft soap used in treating certain skin conditions; also called *green soap* because of its colour.

social care: 1. The provision of resources necessary for the health and welfare of a person or group of people. 2. Any of various types of support or supervision provided by social workers and allied professionals.

social class: Classification of individuals in a population usually in terms of the householder's occupation or socioeconomic position. In the United Kingdom the Office of Population Censuses and Surveys recognises five classes based on occupations from (1) Professional to (5) Unskilled labouring.

social construction: A theory describing the influence of social processes on instinctive behaviours. See also CONSTRUCTIONISM.

social drift: The movement of individuals from one social category to another usually as a result of socioeconomic circumstances or as a result of morbid processes.

social exclusion: Alienation of an individual or group from human society; specifically exclusion or isolation from the health-care system and its rights and privileges, esp. as a result of poverty or membership of a particular social group. See SOCIAL INCLUSION.

social inclusion: An effort to incorporate individuals or groups into society. Promotes social justice and tackles disadvantage, by helping individuals, families and communities achieve economic independence and to access more and better opportunities. See SOCIAL EXCLUSION.

socialism: A theory or policy of social organization which advocates the ownership and control of the means of production, capital, land, and property by the community as a whole, and their administration or distribution in the interests of all.

socialization: The training or moulding of an individual through various relationships, educational agencies, and social controls, which enables him or her to become a member of a particular society.

socialized medicine: A type of medical care that is controlled, directed, and financed by the state or nation and which provides health-care for all the inhabitants.

social policy: A discipline within social science, relating to the support of well-being through social action. The focus is on the explanation or evaluation of policy. With the development of the Welfare State (*q.v.*) in the twentieth century, it has become the way that governments attempt to ensure that all citizens can lead a fulfilling and responsible lives through the provision of: education, health, employment, housing, and social security.

social sciences: The sciences that deal with social institutions, the functioning of human society, and the relationships between individuals in society.

social security: A system whereby the state provides financial assistance for those citizens whose income is inadequate or non-existent owing to disability, unemployment, and old age.

social services: Personal care services provided by local authorities for vulnerable people, including those with special needs because of old age or physical or mental disability, and children in need of care and protection.

social work: The deployment of professional skills to assist an individual in social adjustment within their community. Provided by a social worker who is employed by a local authority, hospital or other agency.

social worker: A professional trained in the recognition and treatment of individual social problems of patients, clients, and their families.

sociobiological (sō'shi-ō-bī'ō-loj'i-kal): Involving or relating to a combination of social and biological factors.

sociocultural (sō'-shi-ō-kul'chur-al): Relating to culture in its sociological setting.

sociodemographic (sō'shi-ō-dem-ō-graf'ik): Involving or relating to a combination of social and demographic factors.

socioecological (sō'shi-ō-ē'kō-log'ik): Involving or relating to a combination of social and ecological factors.

socioeconomic (sō'shi-ō-ē'kon-om'ik): Concerning or involving both social and economic factors.

sociogram (sō'shi-ō-gram): A diagram representing the pattern of relationships between individuals in a group.

sociology (sō-shi-ol′o-ji): The scientific study of interpersonal and intergroup social relationships. — sociological, adj.

sociomedical (sō′shi-ō-med′ik-al): Relating to the problems of medicine as they are related to society.

sociometry (sō-shi-om′e-tri): The branch of sociology that is concerned with the measurement of social relations and behaviour of humans. — sociometric, adj.

sociopath (sō′shi-ō-path): One who has an aggressively anti-social attitude and behaviour. Also called *psychopath*.

sociopathic (sō-shi-ō-path′ik): Relating to or characterized by asocial or anti-social behaviour. S. PERSONALITY see ANTI-SOCIAL PERSONALITY under PERSONALITY DISORDER.

socket (sok′et): 1. A hollow part or depression into which a part fits, as the eye socket. 2. The hollow part of a bone at a joint which receives part of another bone. DRY S. term given to a condition that occurs when a clot is lost following a tooth extraction and the bone is exposed to the air, causing considerable pain.

soda (sō′da): A term often loosely used in reference to the salts of sodium, *e.g.*, sodium carbonate (washing soda), sodium bicarbonate (baking soda).

sodium (sō′di-um): A soft, white metallic element, many of the salts of which are used in medicine. In the human body it occurs as a cation found chiefly in the extracellular fluid; its main function is to control the water balance in body tissues; its excretion by the kidneys is influenced by antidiuretic hormone and aldosterone. S. ACETATE colourless, odourless crystals with a saline taste, used as a diuretic and laxative; S. BICARBONATE an important constituent of blood; acts as a buffer substance helping to maintain the correct pH of the blood; S. CHLORIDE common salt, also an important constituent of blood and body tissues; an important factor in maintaining the water balance of the body; used for its diuretic effect, as a urinary acidifier, and to restore electrolyte balance; S. CITRATE a white powder, used as an anticoagulant in blood for transfusion; S. FLUORIDE a white crystalline powder, used as a dental prophylactic in drinking water; S. HYDROXIDE a compound of sodium that occurs in hard opaque flakes, pellets, or sticks; soluble in water; has a caustic effect; is used in preparation of certain chemicals and pharmaceuticals; not given internally; S. IODIDE a salt resembling potassium iodide, used as a source of iodine; S. IODOHIPPURATE a diagnostic agent used in urinary tract radiology; S. LACTATE a sodium salt of inactive lactic acid; may be administered parenterally to combat acidosis; S. NITROPRUSSIDE a reagent used in analysis to detect the presence of organic compounds; S. PHOSPHATE a form of phosphorus 32, used in treatment of polycythaemia vera and certain malignant conditions.

sodomist (sod′o-mist): A person who practises sodomy.

sodomy (sod′o-mi): Sexual relations including (1) anal intercourse between men; (2) copulation with an animal; (3) oral or anal copulation between members of the opposite sex.

soft chancre (shang′ker): Chancroid (*q.v.*).

soft palate: The soft, fleshy structure at the back of the upper part of the mouth; together with the hard palate in the front, it forms the 'roof' of the mouth.

soft sore: The primary ulcer of the genitalia occurring in the venereal disease chancroid (*q.v.*).

solar (sō′lar): Relating to, resembling, or derived from the sun. S. THERAPY treatment by exposure to the sun's rays; heliotherapy.

solarium (sō-lar′i-um): 1. A room or porch enclosed by glass; a sun room. 2. A room or place in a hospital where patients may expose their bodies to the sun for therapeutic purposes.

solar plexus: A large network of sympathetic nerve ganglia, situated behind the stomach and in front of the aorta, that sends nerve fibres to all of the abdominal organs; the pit of the stomach.

sole: The bottom of the foot.

soleus (sō′lē-us): Muscle at the back of the lower leg; lies over the gastrocnemius with which it unites at the lower end to form the tendon that attaches to the heel.

solipsism (sol′ip-sizm): The belief that the world exists only in one's mind and consists only of the individual and his or her life experiences.

soluble (sol′ū-b′l): Capable of being dissolved. — solubility, adj.

solute (sol′ūt): That which is dissolved in a fluid. S. LOAD refers to the concentration of soluble substances, especially electrolytes, delivered to the kidneys; is higher in artificially fed than breast-fed infants.

solution (so-lū′shun): A fluid that contains one or more dissolved substances that are evenly distributed throughout and chemically unchanged. The dissolving liquid is called the solvent and the dissolved substance is called the solute. NORMAL SALINE S. a solution of distilled water with sodium chloride dissolved in it in the same concentration as occurs in the blood; SATURATED S. one in which as much solid is dissolved as will be held in solution without precipitating or floating; SUPERSATURATED S. one that contains more of an ingredient than can be held in solution permanently, the excess being precipitated when the physical conditions are changed.

solvent (sol'vent): An agent, usually liquid, which is capable of dissolving other substances and holding them in solution.

soma (sō'ma): 1. The body as distinguished from the psyche or the mind. 2. The walls of the body as distinguished from the viscera. 3. The trunk of the body as distinguished from the appendages.

somaesthetic (sō-mas-thet'ik): Relating to the sensations of touch and proprioception (q.v.).

somasthenia (sō mas thē'ni-a): General chronic weakness of the body, Also called *somatasthenia*.

somat-, somato-: Combining forms denoting the body.

somataesthesia (sō'ma-tes-thē'zi-a): Being conscious of having a body; being sensitive to bodily sensation. Also called *somaesthesia*.

somatic (sō-mat'ik): 1. Relating to the body. 2. Pertaining to the trunk. 3. Relating to the wall of the body cavity rather than to the viscera. S. NERVES nerves controlling the activity of striated, skeletal muscle; S. NERVOUS SYSTEM see under NERVOUS SYSTEM; S. THERAPY in psychiatry, the biological treatment of mental disorders, as in electroconvulsive or psychopharmacological therapy.

somatization (sō'ma-tī-zā'shun): The conversion of anxiety into physical symptoms, *e.g.*, 'butterflies in the stomach', headache, diarrhoea, shortness of breath; an escape mechanism that often releases emotional tensions.

somatogenic (sō'ma-tō-jen'ik): Originating within the body, but resulting from the influence of external forces.

somatology (sō-ma-tol'o-ji): The study of the body, its structure, development, and functions.

somatomegaly (sō'ma-tō-meg'a-li): The condition of having an unusually large body; gigantism.

somatometry (sō'ma-tom'i-tri): Measurements of the entire body and the classification of individuals according to their form and size.

somatopathy (sō'ma-top'a-thi): Disorder of the body as distinguished from that of the mind.

somatoplasm (sōmat'-ō-plazm): The protoplasm of the cells of the body considered apart from the material constituting the germ cells.

somatopsychic (sō'mat-ō-sī'kik): Relating to states of depression or worry that occur as responses to physical disease states. Opp. of psychomatic (q.v.).

somatoscopy (sō'ma-tos'ko-pi): Physical examination of the body.

somatosensory (sō'ma-tō-sen'sō-ri): Relating to the bodily sensations.

somatostatin (so'ma-tō-stat'in): A tetrapeptide hormone produced in the hypothalamus that is capable of inhibiting the release of growth hormone from the anterior lobe of the pituitary gland, and of thyrotropin, as well as the enzymes, renin, pepsin, gastrin, and secretin; it also acts on the pancreas to suppress the secretion of both insulin and glucagon.

somatotonia (sō'ma-tō-tō'ni-a): A type of temperament manifested chiefly by enjoyment of activity and vigorous action.

somatotrophin (so'ma-tō-trō'pin). The growth-stimulating hormone secreted by the anterior lobe of the pituitary gland; it regulates body growth, stimulates healing of tissues, and lowers the cholesterol level in the body; secretion is increased during sleep. Also called *human growth hormone*.

somatotype (sō-mat'-ō-tīp): A particular type of body build as identified by certain physical characteristics; see *e.g.*, ECTOMORPH, ENDOMORPH, MESOMORPH.

somnambulism (som-nam'bū-lizm): Sleepwalking; a state of dissociated consciousness in which sleeping and waking states are combined; the individual performs purposeful and often complex acts but has no memory of them upon awakening. Occurs during the third and fourth stages of non-rapid eye movement sleep; see SLEEP. Considered normal in children but as an illness, having physical or psychological basis, in adults.

somnambulist (som-nam'bū-list): An individual who habitually sleepwalks.

somni-: A combining form denoting sleep.

somnia-: Combining form denoting a condition resembling sleep.

somnial (som'ni-al): Relating to dreams or sleep.

somniculous (som-nik'ū-lus): Sleepy.

somnifacient (som-ni-fā'shent): 1. Causing sleep; hypnotic, soporific. 2. An agent that causes sleep.

somniferous (som-nif'er-us): Producing sleep.

sommnific (som-nif'ik): Producing sleep.

somniloquism (som-nil'ō-kwism): Talking in one's sleep.

somnolence (som'nō-lens): Excessive or prolonged sleepiness or drowsiness. — somnolent, adj.

somnus (som'nus): Sleep.

Somogyi: s. EFFECT or PHENOMENON hypoglycaemia caused by overtreatment with insulin; followed by marked glycosuria and ketonuria resulting from increased production of glucose in the liver; occurs in diabetic patients; s. METHOD either of two methods developed by Somogyi for detecting amylase in the serum; s. UNIT a measure of diastase or amylase activity in the serum. [M. Somogyi, American biochemist, 1883–1971.]

sonicate (son'i-kāt): To treat with high-frequency sound waves. — sonication, n.

sonication (son-i-kā'shun): Exposure to high-frequency sound waves.

sonitus (son'i-tus): Tinnitus (q.v.).

Sonne dysentery (son'ne dis'en-ter-i): Bacillary dysentery caused by infection with *Shigella sonnei* [Carl Sonne, Danish bacteriologist, 1882–1948.]

sonochemistry (son'ō-kem-i-stri): The study of the chemical effects of high-frequency sound and ultrasonic waves.

sonogram (son'ō-gram): The recording of a diagnostic examination that utilizes ultrasound. See ULTRASONOGRAPHY.

sonography (son-og'ra-fi): Ultrasonography (q.v.).

sonometer (so-nom'i-ter): An instrument for testing hearing acuteness.

sonorous (so-no'-rus): Being resonant or having a loud sound. s. RALES rales that have a low-pitched or snoring sound; produced by the presence of mucous or viscid secretion in a bronchus.

sophomania (sof'ō-mā'ni-a): The deluded belief in one's own superior wisdom.

sopor (sō'por): Unnaturally deep or profound sleep; stupor.

soporific (so'por-if'ik): 1. An agent that induces profound sleep. 2. Producing sleep.

sorbefacient (sor-bi-fā'shent): 1. Causing absorption. 2. An agent that causes or promotes absorption.

sore: 1. Painful. 2. A general term for any ulcer or lesion on the skin or mucous membrane. BEDSORE or PRESSURE S. decubitus ulcer; CANKER S. an ulcer on the mucous membrane of the mouth; COLD S. herpes simplex, see under HERPES; SOFT S. chancroid (q.v.); VEN-

EREAL S. any lesion accompanying a venereal infection; usually refers to chancre (q.v.). See also ORIENTAL SORE.

souffle (soo'f'l): A murmur or soft blowing sound heard on auscultation of the heart. FUNIC S. a high-pitched sound heard on auscultation in pregnancy; it is synchronous with the fetal heartbeat and thought to be due to interference in the circulation of blood in the umbilical cord; UTERINE S. soft blowing murmur that can be auscultated over the uterus after the fourth month of pregnancy.

sound: 1. Vibrations that stimulate the receptors and organs of the sense of hearing and result in a mental image. 2. Normal or abnormal noise produced in an organ of the body and audible on auscultation, e.g., heart sound. 3. Sane or healthy. 4. A long, slender, cylindrical instrument to be inserted into a hollow organ for examination or exploration or to detect a foreign body, or into a duct to dilate it.

sovereignty (sov'-er-in-ti): 1. Supremacy or preeminence in respect of excellence or efficacy. 2. Supremacy in respect of power, domination, or rank. 3. Supreme dominion, authority, or rule.

soya bean: A highly nutritous legume that contains high-quality protein and little starch. Is useful in diabetic preparations. Also called *soybean.*

spa (spah): A place in which water, especially that from mineral springs, is used for therapeutic purposes; it is both drunk and used for bathing.

space: 1. A delimited area or region within the body. 2. The world outside or beyond the Earth's atmosphere. S. MEDICINE the branch of medicine that deals with the changes and effects on human physiology produced in those who are projected at high velocity through space and then returned to the Earth's atmosphere.

space-occupying lesions: Lesions such as abscesses, haematomata, or tumours which form in an area where there is little room for expansion and which therefore compress the normal structures in the area; frequently they occur in the skull.

spanaemia (spa-nē'mi-a): Thinness of the blood; anaemia.

Spanish fly: A species of beetle from which the powerful blistering agent, cantharadin, is derived. Formerly much used as a topical vesicant; not used in modern medicine.

Spansule (span-sūl): Trade name for a delayed-release form of capsule; it is prepared in such a way that some of the granules dissolve almost as soon as the capsule is administered, but the rest are coated with a substance that causes them to dissolve more slowly and further along in the gut.

spasm (spazm): Convulsive involuntary muscular contraction. CARPOPEDAL S., s. of the muscles of the hands, feet, thumbs, or great toe; seen in cases of rickets, tetany due to calcium deficiency, and laryngismus stridulus (q.v.); CLONIC S., s. in which fairly short periods of contraction alternate with periods of relaxation; HABIT S. an involuntary s. which recurs in a muscle that is ordinarily under voluntary control; a tic (q.v.); INFANTILE MASSIVE S. jackknife seizure; see SEIZURE; NODDING S. clonic s. of the sternocleidomastoid muscle causing bowing movements of the head; SALAAM S. nodding S.; TETANIC S. that which occurs in tetanus; TONIC S. that in which rigidity persists for some time; WINKING S. involuntary contraction of the muscles of the eyelid resulting in a wink; WRITER'S S. writer's cramp (q.v.).

spasmodic (spaz-mod'ik): 1. Recurring at intervals. 2. An agent that produces spasm. 3. Pertinent to or like a spasm.

spasmolygmus (spaz'mo-lig'mus): 1. Spasmodic sobbing. 2. Hiccup.

spasmolytic (spaz'mo-lit'ik): 1. Checking spasm(s). 2. An agent that checks spasm; an antispasmodic.

spasmophemia (spaz'mō-fē'mi-a): Stuttering.

spasmus (spaz'mus): Spasm. S. NUTANS headnodding spasm.

spastic (spas'tik): 1. Relating to spasm(s). 2. In a condition of muscular rigidity or spasm, e.g., spastic diplegia (Little's disease, q.v.). S. BLADDER see AUTONOMOUS BLADDER under BLADDER; S. GAIT see under GAIT; S. PARALYSIS see under PARALYSIS. — spasticity, n.

spasticity (spas-tis'it-i): A condition marked by sudden involuntary muscular spasm or rigidity.

spatula (spat'ū-la): A flat flexible knife with blunt edges for making poultices and spreading ointment. TONGUE S. a rigid, blade-shaped instrument for depressing the tongue.

special care baby unit: This is an intensive care unit for babies born prematurely.

special hospital: A hospital that provides conditions of high-security care for patients with mental health problems or learning disabilities. The majority of patients in special hospitals will have broken the law or present a severe danger to themselves or others.

specialist: In medicine, a doctor who limits his practice to certain diseases or disorders, or a certain type of therapy.

Special Olympics: A special recreation programme for any physically or mentally handicapped person. See PARALYMPICS.

speciality, specialty: A branch of nursing (or medicine) for which a health professional has qualified either through advanced study, experience, or having passed a qualifying examination.

species (spē'shēz): A subdivision of genus. A group of individuals having common characteristics and differing only in minor details.

specific (spe-sif'ik): 1. Special; characteristic; peculiar to. 2. Pertaining to a species. 3. A medication that has special curative properties for a particular disease, as quinine for malaria. S. DISEASE one that is always caused by a specified organism.

specific gravity: The weight of a substance, as compared with that of an equal volume of water. The specific gravity of urine is a measure of the relative proportion of the solvents in it.

specimen (spes'i-men): 1. A sample or small part of a substance or a thing taken for the purpose of determining the character of the whole, e.g., urine, sputum, blood, or a small portion of tissue. 2. A preparation of normal or abnormal tissue prepared for study or pathological examination.

spectroscopy: The use of a spectroscope in chemical analysis or in physics.

spectrum (spek'trum): 1. Range of activity; often refers to antibiotics, e.g., broad-spectrum antibiotics. 2. The components of a wave arranged in a particular order or sqence, such as wavelength or frequency, e.g., x-rays, or electric, ultraviolet, or infrared rays. — spectra, pl.; spectral, adj.

speculum (spek'ū-lum): An instrument used to hold the orifice or walls of a cavity apart, so that the interior of the cavity can be examined. — specula, pl.

speech: Oral communication of ideas by means of the utterance of vocal sounds. AUTONOMIC s. redundant speaking of words, as repeating the days of the week or months of the year; EXPLOSIVE s. loud, sudden speech, occurring in patients following nervous system injuries; INCOHERENT S., s. in which thoughts expressed are not related; MIRROR S. the practice of reversing the order of syllables in words; OESOPHAGEAL S. a technique learned following laryngectomy; the patient swallows air and then regurgitates it, producing vibrations in the column of air against the circopharyngeal sphincter; SCANNING S., s. in which the speaker pauses between syllables; s. DYS-FUNCTION any defect or abnormality in speech including sound production and enunciation, from whatever cause; s. PATHOLOGY the field of study that deals with the evaluation and treatment of communicative disorders such as occur in production of speech, use of language, and voice production; s. THERAPIST a person with special training in helping individuals to overcome their particular speech and language problems; STACATTO S., s. in which each syllable is uttered separately; occurs in persons with multiple sclerosis.

speed: Street term for amphetamine drugs.

sperm: Spermatozoon (*q.v.*).

sperm-, spermato-, spermo-: Combining forms denoting (1) spermatozoa; (2) semen.

spermatacrasia (sper′-ma-ta-krā′zi-a): A decrease or deficiency of spermatozoa in the semen.

spermatic (sper-mat′ik): Pertaining to or conveying semen. s. CORD suspends the testis in the scrotum and contains the s. artery and vein and the vas deferens.

spermatocele (sper-mat′ō-sēl): A localized enlargement of the spermatic cord; contains sperm; usually painless.

spermatocidal (sper-ma-tō-sī′dal): Destructive to spermatozoa.

spermatocide (sper-mat′-ō-sīd): Any agent that kills spermatozoa.

spermatocystitis (sper′ma-tō-sis-tī′tis): Inflammation of the seminal vesicles.

spermatogenesis (sper′mat-ō-jen′e-sis): The formation and development of sperm. — spermatogenetic, adj.

spermatorrhoea (sper′ma-tō-rē′a): Frequent involuntary discharge of semen without orgasm.

spermatozoon (sper′ma-tō-zō′on): A mature, male reproductive cell produced in the testes; consisting of a head or nucleus, neck, and tail; about 0.05 mm in length. — spermatozoa, pl.

spermaturia (sper′ma-tū′ri-a): The presence of spermatozoa or semen in the urine.

sperm bank: A facility where a male may deposit a quantity of semen, which is mixed with a protective fluid and stored at a very low temperature. At a later date the material may be thawed and used to induce pregnancy.

spermicide (sper′mi-sīd): An agent that kills spermatozoa. Also called *spermatocide*. — spermicidal, adj.

spermolith (sper′mō-lith): A concretion in the vas deferens or the seminal vesicle.

sphacelate (sfas′e-lāt): To slough or become gangrenous. — sphacelation, n.; sphacelous, adj.

sphagitis (sfā-jī′tis): 1. Sore throat. 2. Inflammation of a jugular vein.

sphen-, spheno-: Combining forms denoting (1) wedge-shaped; (2) the sphenoid bone.

sphenoid (sfē′noyd): 1. Wedge-shaped. 2. A wedge-shaped bone at the base of the skull, articulating with the occipital bone at the back, the ethmoid in front, and the parietal and temporal bones at the sides. s. SINUS see under SINUS.

sphenopalatine (sfē-nō-pal′a-tin): Relating to the sphenoid bone and the palatine bones.

spherocyte (sfē-rō-sīt): A red blood cell that is round instead of biconcave; characteristic of congenital haemolytic anaemia.

spherocytosis (sfē-rō-sī-tō′sis): The presence of spherocytes in the circulating blood. HEREDITARY S. a familial form of haemolytic anaemia in which the erythrocytes are abnormally fragile, spherocytes are present in the blood, the patient is jaundiced, and the spleen is enlarged.

sphincter (sfink′ter): A circular muscle, contraction of which serves to constrict a natural passage or to close a natural orifice. ANAL S. surrounds the anus; CARDIAC S. surrounds the oesophagus at its opening into the stomach; OCULAR S. surrounds the eye; ODDI′S S., an intricate muscular structure surrounding the bile and pancreatic ducts, where they join the duodenum; PUPILLARY S. surrounds the pupil; PYLORIC S. surrounds the junction of the stomach and the small intestine; S. OF BOYDFN surrounds the common bile duct just before its junction with the pancreatic duct.

sphincterectomy (sfink′ter-ek′tō-mi): The excision or resection of a sphincter (*q.v.*).

sphincteroplasty (sfink′ter-ō-plas-ti): Repair of or plastic surgery on a sphincter muscle.

sphingolipid (sfing′gō-lip′id): Any lipid that, on hydrolysis, yields sphingosine, a fatty acid attached to the nitrogen atom; found in membranes and particularly in brain and nerve tissue.

sphingolipidosis (sfing′gō-lip-i-dō′sis): A collective term for any of several inherited disorders of sphingolipid metabolism including Niemann–Pick disease, Gaucher's disease, and Tay–Sachs disease, which are characterized by the accumulation of certain glycolipids and phospholipids in some of the body tissues. CEREBRAL S. a condition characterized by progressive degeneration of the nervous system, with convulsions, ataxia, spasticity, weakness of extremities, lack of mental development, progressive blindness due to optic atrophy.

sphingomyelin (sfing'gō-mī'e-lin): One of a group of phospholipids found in brain, kidney, liver, and egg yolk; is composed of phosphoric acid, choline, a fatty acid, and sphingosine.

sphingosine (sfing'gō-sēn): A basic amino alcohol found as a constituent of sphingomyelin, cerebrosides, and several other phosphatides.

sphygmic (sfig'mik): Relating to the pulse.

sphygmo-: Combining form denoting pulse.

sphygmobolometer (sfig'mō-bō-lom'i-ter): An instrument for measuring and recording the energy of the pulse wave, which is an indirect means of measuring the strength of the systolic beat.

sphygmocardiograph (sfig'mō-kar'di-ō-graf): An apparatus for simultaneous graphic recording of the radial pulse and heartbeat. — sphygmocardiographic, adj.; sphygmocardiographically, adv.

sphygmograph (sfig'mō-graf): An instrument for recording the variations in blood pressure and in the pulse wave.

sphygmography (sfig-mog'ra-fi): The recording of the pulse wave, made with a sphygmograph.

sphygmomanometer (sfig'mo-ma-nom'i-ter): An instrument for measuring the force of the arterial blood pressure indirectly. Consists of an inflatable cuff usually applied to the upper arm and connected by a tube to a bulb used for inflating it; has a gauge that records the arterial pressure in millimetres on a graduated scale of a column of mercury.

sphyrectomy (sfi-rek'to-mi): Excision of the malleus of the ear.

spica (spī'ka): A bandage applied in a figure-of-eight pattern. S. CAST see under CAST.

spicule (spik'ūl): A small, spike-like fragment, especially of bone. — spicular, adj. Also called *spiculum*.

spider: S. ANGIOMA see under ANGIOMA. S. TELANGIECTASIA see TELANGIECTASIA.

spike: The pointed element in a graph or chart that is created by a rising and falling vertical line. The spikes on a fever chart represent the high temperatures that are recorded. The spike in an electroencephalogram represents a brief electrical discharge.

spiloma (spī-lō'ma): A naevus (q.v.).

spiloplania (spī-lō-plā'ni-a): Transient redness or erythema of the skin.

spiloplaxia (spī-lō-plak'si-a): A red spot that appears on the skin in leprosy and sometimes in pellagra.

spina bifida (spī'na bif'i-da): A congenital defect in which the vertebral neural arches fail to close properly, so exposing the contents of the vertebral canal posteriorly. The fissure usually occurs in the lumbosacral region. The contents of the canal may or may not protrude through the opening; paralysis, loss of sensation in the lower limbs, and bladder and bowel complications may occur; often occurs with other defects such as club feet, scoliosis, or sphincter incontinence. S.B. CYSTICA a protrusion of the meninges and/or the spinal cord through a defect in the spinal column; S.B. OCCULTA occurs when the contents of the spinal cord do not protrude through the fissure in the spinal column.

spinal (spī'nal): Relating to a spine or to the vertebral column. S. ANAESTHETIC a local anaesthetic solution, injected into the subarachnoid space so that it renders the area supplied by the selected s. nerves insensitive; S. BULB the medulla oblongata; S. CANAL the central hollow throughout the s. column; S. CARIES disease of the vertebral bones; S. CAVITY the s. canal; S. COLUMN a bony structure formed by 33 separate bones; the lower ones fuse together; the rest are separated by pads of cartilage; the backbone; S. CORD the continuation of the nervous tissue of the brain down the s. canal to the level of the first or second lumbar vertebra; S. CURVATURE an exaggerated curve in the s. column; see KYPHOSIS, LORDOSIS, SCOLIOSIS; S. FLUID cerebrospinal fluid (q.v.); S. FUSION an operation in which the articulations of vertebrae are destroyed, thus rendering a portion of the spine rigid (ankylosed); S. GANGLION a group of sensory nerve cells on the posterior root of a spinal nerve; S. NERVES 31 pairs leave the s. cord and pass out of the s. canal to supply the periphery; S. PUNCTURE or S. TAP lumbar puncture (q.v.).

spinalgia (spī-nal'ji-a): Pain in the spinal area.

spine (spīn): 1. A popular term for the bony spinal or vertebral column. 2. A sharp process of bone. ANTERIOR INFERIOR ILIAC S. a blunt projection of the lower part of the anterior edge of the ilium, just superior to the acetabulum; ANTERIOR SUPERIOR ILIAC S. a blunt projection at the anterior end of the crest of the ilium; S. OF THE SCAPULA a triangular plate of bone attached to the back of the scapula; extends from the vertebral edge of the scapula to the shoulder joint.

spinifugal (spī-nif′ū-gal): Conducting or moving in a direction away from the spinal cord, in particular, the efferent fibres of the spinal nerves.

spinipetal (spī-nip′e-tal): Conducting or moving in a direction towards the spinal cord, in particular, the afferent fibres of the spinal nerves.

spinnbarkeit (spin′bark-hīt): The clear, slippery, elastic consistency characteristic of cervical mucus during ovulation. It is a valuable sign of the peak fertile period in a woman's cycle as this usually coincides with the time at which the mucus can be drawn out on a glass slide to its maximum length.

spinobulbar (spī′nō-bul′bar): Relating to the spinal cord and the medulla oblongata.

spinocerebellar (spī′nō-ser-e-bel′lar): Relating to the spinal cord and cerebellum.

spinocortical (spī′nō-kor′ti-kal): Relating to the spinal cord and the cerebral cortex.

spinothalamic (spī′nō-thal′a-mik): Relating to (1) the spinal cord and the thalamus, or (2) the ascending pathways between the spinal cord and the thalamus. LATERAL S. TRACT is made up of nerve fibres that carry impulses for pain and temperature; VENTRAL S. TRACT is made up of fibres that carry impulses for touch and pressure.

spinous (spī′nus): Relating to or resembling a spine or a spine-like process. Also called *spinose*.

spirillicide (spī-ril′i-sīd): An agent that destroys spirilla. — spirillicidal, adj.

Spirillum (spī-ril′um): A bacterial genus; the organisms are corkscrew-shaped. Common in water and organic matter. S. MINUS found in rodents and may infect humans, in whom it causes one form of ratbite fever. — spirilla, pl.; spirillary, adj.

spirit: 1. An alcoholic solution. 2. A distilled solution.

spirochaete (spī′rō-kēt): Common term for any motile, slender, spiral-shaped, sometimes flagellated bacterium of the order Spirochaetales; among them are the causative organisms for syphilis, yaws, relapsing fever, and leptospirosis or Weil's disease.

spirochaetaemia (spī-′rō-kē-tē′mi-a): Spirochaetes in the bloodstream. This kind of bacteraemia occurs in the secondary stage of syphilis and in the syphilitic fetus. — spirochaetaemic, adj.

spirochaeticide (spī-rō-kē′ti-sīd): An agent that destroys spirochaetes. — spirochaeticidal, adj.

spirochaetosis (spī′-rō-kē-tō′sis): Infection with spirochaetes.

spirogram (spī′rō-gram): A recorded tracing of the chest movements and excursion of the chest during respiration. See SPIROGRAPH.

spirograph (spī′rō-graf): An apparatus which records the depth and rapidity of movement of the lungs. — spirographic, adj.; spirographically, adv.; spirography, n.

spirometer (spī-rom′i-ter): An instrument for measuring the air capacity of the lungs. See BRONCHOSPIROMETER. — spirometric, adj.; spirometry, n.

spirometry (spī-rom′i-tri): The measurement, with a spirometer, of the amount of air that can be moved in and out of the lungs.

spironolactone (spī′rō-nō-lak′tōn): A chemical compound in white crystalline form; used in medicine as a steroid diuretic because of its action in blocking the sodium-retaining action of aldosterone.

spissated (spis′āt-ed): Thickened.

spittle (spit′l): Sputum or saliva that is expectorated.

Spitz–Holter valve: A valve designed to drain cerebrospinal fluid from the cranium into the internal jugular vein and vena cava, thence into the right atrium, in cases of hydrocephalus.

splanchic (splank′nik): Relating to or supplying the viscera, especially the abdominal viscera. S. NERVES those of the sympathetic system that supply the abdominal viscera.

splanchnicectomy (splank-ni-sēk′to-mi): Surgical removal of the splanchic nerves, whereby the viscera are deprived of sympathetic impulses; occasionally performed in the treatment of essential hypertension or for the relief of certain kinds of visceral pain.

splanchnicotomy (splank-ni-kot′o-mi): The surgical division of a splanchnic nerve; may be done for the relief of hypertension.

splanchno-: Combining form denoting; 1. A viscus. 2. The splanchnic nerve.

splanchnology (splank-nol′o-ji): The study of the structure and function of the viscera.

splanchnomegaly (splank-nō-meg′a-li): Abnormal enlargement of one or more of the viscera.

splanchnopathy (splank-nop′a-thi): Any disease of the viscera.

splanchnoptosis (splank′nop-tō′sis): Visceroptosis (*q.v.*).

splayfoot (splā′foot): Flatfoot.

spleen (splēn): An elongated, oval, lymphoid, vascular organ lying in the upper left quadrant of the abdominal cavity, immediately below the diaphragm at the tail of the pancreas and behind the stomach. It is one of the blood-forming organs; stores blood, and acts as a blood filter. Apparently not essential to life as it can be removed without endangering the patient's life. — splenic, adj.

splen-:, spleno-: Combining forms denoting the spleen.

splenadenoma (splen-ad-e-nō'ma): Hyperplasia of the spleen.

splenectasia (sple-nek-tā'zi-a): Enlargement of the spleen.

splenectomy (sple-nek'to-mi): Surgical removal of the spleen.

splenic (splen'ik): Relating to the spleen. S. ANAEMIA Banti's disease; S. FLEXURE the bend in the colon just beneath the spleen where the transverse colon becomes the descending colon; S. VEIN the vein that transports blood from the spleen to the portal vein.

splenitis (splē-nī'tis): Inflammation of the spleen.

splenius (splē'nē-us): One of the flat muscles at the back of the neck and upper thoracic region.

splenocaval (splē nō kā'val): Relating to the spleen and inferior vena cava, usually referring to anastomosis of the splenic vein to the inferior vena cava.

splenocele (splē'nō-sēl): 1. Tumour of the spleen. 2. Hernia of the spleen.

splenocolic (splē'nō-kol'ik): Relating to the spleen and the colon; often refers to a fold of peritoneum that lies between the two organs.

splenodynia (splē'nō-din'i-a): Pain in the spleen.

splenogenous (splē-noj'e-nus): Arising in the spleen.

splenogram (splē'nō-gram): Radiographic picture of the spleen after injection of radiopaque medium. — splenograph, splenography, n.; sphenographical, adj.; splenographically, adv.

splenohepatomegaly (splē'nō-hep'a-tō-meg'a-li): Enlargement of the spleen and the liver.

splenoma (splē-nō'ma): An enlargement of the spleen; may or may not be due to the presence of a tumour.

splenomalacia (splē'nō-ma-lā'-shi-a): Abnormal softness of the spleen.

splenomegaly (splē'nō-meg'a-li): Enlargement of the spleen.

splenopancreatic (splē'nō-pan-krē-at'ik): Relating to the spleen and the pancreas.

splenopathy (splē-nop'a-thi): Any disease or disorder of the spleen.

splenophrenic (sple-nō-fren'ik): Relating to the spleen and the diaphragm; often refers to a fold of the peritoneum that lies between the two organs.

splenoportal (splē-nō-por'tal): Relating to the spleen and portal vein.

splenoportogram (splē'nō-port'ō-gram): Radiographic picture of the spleen and portal vein after injection of radiopaque medium. — splenoportograph, splenoportography, n.; splenoportographical, adj.; splenoportographically, adv.

splenorenal (splē'nō-rē'nal): Relating to the spleen and kidney, as an anastomosis of the splenic vein to the renal vein; a procedure carried out in some cases of portal hypertension. S. SHUNT see under SHUNT.

splenorrhagia (splē'nō-rā'ji-a): Haemorrhage from a spleen that has ruptured.

splint: An apparatus, usually rigid, used to support, protect, and immobilize an injured part temporarily, or to maintain an injured part in a specific position. AEROPLANE S. a plaster s. that holds the arm in elevation and abduction; the s. is supported by plaster which extends down the side of the thorax or around it; BANJO S. a device that exerts traction on the fingers; occasionally used to treat certain type of hand injuries; made of a metal rod shaped like a banjo; BARLOW'S S. holds the hips in extension; used for infants with congenital hip dysplasia, BRAUN S. a support that holds the leg in balanced traction, eliminating the need for traction equipment attached to the bed; COCKUP S. a s. used for treating injury to the wrist or hand or in cases of paralysis to support the wrist in a position of function, i.e., dorsiflexion; DOLL'S COLLAR S. a plaster collar used in treatment of fracture of cervical vertebrae; extends over the occiput, around the ears, over the chin, and down over the shoulders, sternum, and upper part of the back; DYNAMIC S. a s. that supplies support for an injured, operated on, or paralysed part, but allows for controlled motion to prevent stiffness and promote circulation; GUTTER S. a trough-like s. of wood or metal in which an injured arm or leg is placed to provide support and immobilization; HARE S. an adapatation of the half-ring Thomas s., has a ratchet mechanism to exert a stable amount of traction on the leg to establish its correct position in the splint; INFLATABLE S. a plastic, first-aid s. used to immobilize a fractured leg or arm; is inflated after application to conform to and support the limb; THOMAS S. a ring splint used for fixed traction in emergency care; the ring is placed in contact with the ischium, the leg supported on slings placed on the length of the splint, and the foot and ankle tied to the end of the s., providing traction. May also be used for balanced traction in combination with an attachment that allows for two lines of traction.

splinting: The application of a splint to provide fixation of a fracture or dislocation. Splinting an incision refers to the practice of pressing a pillow or similar object against the abdomen when the patient coughs, sneezes, or breathes deeply following abdominal surgery.

split: S. GRAFT split-thickness graft, see under GRAFT; S. PERSONALITY see under PERSONALITY DISORDER.

spondyl-, spondylo-: Combining forms denoting vertebra(e).

spondylalgia (spon'di-lal'ji-a): Pain in a vertebra.

spondylarthritis (spon-dil-ar-thrī'tis): Arthritis of the vertebrae. S. ANKYLOPOIETICA rheumatoid s.; see under SPONDYLITIS.

spondyle (spon'dil): A vertebra.

spondylitis (spon-di-lī'tis): Inflammation of one or more vertebrae involving the capsules and intervertebral ligaments; Pott's disease (q.v.). RHEUMATOID or ANKYLOSING S. a chronic inflammation of unknown aetiology, involving primarily the spine and girdle joints, the shoulder, neck, ribs, and jaw; characterized by pain, stiffness, ankylosis progressing upwards from the sacroiliac to the intervertebral and costocervical joints, and rigidity of the spine and thorax. Occurs mostly in men between 20 and 40 years of age; may be hereditary.

spondylodynia (spon'di-lō-din'ē-a): Pain in a vertebra.

spondylolysis (spon-di-lo-lī'-sis): The breaking down of the structure of a vertebra.

spondylopyosis (spon'di-lō-pī-ō'sis): Suppuration of a vertebra.

spondylosis (spon-di-lō'sis): Degeneration of the vertebral bodies or of the intervertebral discs, with an abnormal fusion or growing together of two or more vertebrae. Often called osteoarthritis of the spine. CERVICAL S. degenerative joint disease affecting the cervical vertebrae.

spondylosyndesis (spon'di-lō-sin-dē' -sis): Spinal fusion, surgical immobilization, or ankylosis of the vertebrae.

spondylus (spon'di-lus): A vertebra.

sponge: 1. The elastic, fibrous skeleton of a marine organism. 2. A folded piece of gauze or a piece of cotton used for mopping up fluids, for dressing, etc. S. BATH see under BATH.

spongiform (spun'ji-form): Resembling a sponge.

spongioblast (spun'ji-ō-blast): An embryonic cell, the processes of which develop into the neuroglia (q.v.).

spongiocytoma (spun'ji-ō-sī-tō'ma): Astrocytoma (q.v.).

spontaneous (spon-tān'ē-us): Occurring without apparent cause. S. ABORTION unexpected premature delivery of the contents of a pregnant uterus; S. FRACTURE one occurring without apparent injury; sometimes seen in certain diseases of the bone; S. GENERATION an obsolete theory in microbiology that microorganisms arise spontaneously.

spoonerism (spoon'er-izm): A speech or writing defect in which the person tends to transpose letters or syllables of words.

sporadic (spō-rad'ik): Scattered; occurring in isolated cases; not epidemic. — sporadically, adv.

spore (spawr): A phase in the life cycle of a limited number of bacterial genera where the vegetative cell becomes encapsulated and metabolism almost ceases. These spores are highly resistant to environmental conditions such as heat and dessication. The spores of important species such as *Clostridium tetani* and *Cl. botulinum* are ubiquitous and can survive for long periods of time without food or water; when water, a suitable food supply, and a suitable temperature become available, the spores grow, mature, and become pathogenic.

sporicidal (spor-i-sī'dal): Lethal to spores. — sporicide, n.

sporogenesis (spo-rō-jen'e-sis): The formation or reproduction of spores. — sporogenic, adj.

sporogony (spo-rog'o-ni): The sexual cycle of sporozoa; usually refers to the life cycle of the malarial parasite in the stomach and body of the mosquito.

sporonticide (spo-ron'ti-sīd): A drug that inhibits the growth of oocysts in the stomach wall of the mosquito and thus prevents the development of sporozoites (q.v.), making transmission of malaria by the mosquito impossible.

Sporozoa (spo-rō-zō'a): A class of Protozoa, some of which are parasitic to humans. — sporozoan, adj.

sporozoite (spo-rō-zō'īt): A spore that is formed after fertilization. In malaria, sporozoites are the forms of the causative organism that are liberated in the oocysts in the mosquito host and transferred to humans when the mosquito bites.

sport: An organism that varies entirely or partly from others of the same type and which may transmit this variation to its offspring; a mutation.

sporulation (spor-ū-lā'shun): The formation of spores. — sporulate, v.

spot: In medicine, a circumscribed area that differs from the surrounding area in colour, texture, elevation, or other characteristics; a macule. See KOPLIK'S SPOTS, LIVER SPOTS, ROSE SPOTS.

spotted fever: 1. A name given to several eruptive fevers that are characterized by the appearance of distinctive spots, including typhus and Rocky Mountain spotted fever. 2. Endemic cerebrospinal fever, caused by meningococcus.

spotting: The loss of a slight amount of blood between menstrual periods.

sprain: Injury to the soft tissues surrounding a joint, caused by forcible wrenching or hyperextension of the joint; sometimes ligaments or tendons are ruptured but the bone is not fractured or dislocated; accompanied by pain, swelling, and discoloration. Classified as first, second, and third degree, according to severity and extent of the injury.

SPSS: Abbreviation for Statistical Package for Social Sciences (*q.v.*).

spur: A calcar (*q.v.*). CALCANEAN S. occurs on the lower surface of the calcaneus; often follows injury and causes pain on walking; OCCIPITAL S. a small bony process on the occipital bone behind the posterior process of the atlas; OLECRANON S. an abnormal process of bone at the insertion of the triceps muscle on the olecranon.

sputum (spū'tum): Excess of secretion from the respiratory passages expectorated through the mouth; consists mainly of mucus and saliva, but may also contain blood, pus, microorganisms. PRUNE-JUICE S., S. with a dark reddish brown or bloody colour; seen in certain respiratory conditions including lobar pneumonia and cancer of the lung.

SQA: Abbreviation for Scottish Qualifications Authority (*q.v.*).

squama (skwā'ma): 1. A mass of plate-like tissue, especially of bone, as the s. of the temporal bone. 2. A flake or scale of the skin. — squamous, adj.

squame (skwām): Squama (*q.v.*).

squamo-columnar (skwā'mō-kol-um'nar): Relating to squamous and columnar cells usually refers to the junction of these two types of cells in the epithelial lining of the uterine cervix.

squamosa (skwā-mō'sa): The squamous part of the frontal, occipital, and, particularly, of the temporal bone.

squamous (skwā'mus): 1. Thin and flat like a fish scale. 2. Consisting of thin flat cells, as in the epithelium. 3. Relating to the thin scale-like portion of certain bones, *e.g.*, the temporal bone.

squamous cell carcinoma: See under CARCINOMA.

squint (skwint): 1. Strabismus. Incoordinated action of the muscles of the eyeball, such that the visual axes of the two eyes fail to meet at the objective point. CONVERGENT S. occurs when the eyes turn towards the medial line. DIVERGENT S. occurs when the eyes turn outward. 2. To partially close the eyes, as in a very bright light.

stable: Steady, regular, not easily moved or broken down.

staccato speech (sta-ka'tō): A jerky manner of speaking with interruptions between words or syllables; scanning speech (*q.v.*).

stage (stāj): 1. The platform-like part of a microscope upon which a slide is placed for viewing. 2. A phase or period in the course of a disease, in the life of an organism, or in the progress of labour.

staging (stāj'ing): Term used to describe the classification of malignant tumours according to their cellular make-up, their potential for responding to therapy, and the prognosis for the patient.

stain: 1. To discolour. 2. A dye or other pigment or colouring matter used to colour microorganisms or tissue for microscopic examination. See ACID-FAST; COUNTERSTAIN; DIFFERENTIAL STAIN under DIFFERENTIAL.

stakeholders: People or organizations that have a vested interest in an activity.

stalk (stawk): In anatomy, a narrow connecting or supporting structure.

stamina (stam'i-na): Endurance, vigour, strength.

stammer (stam'er): A speech disorder characterized by halting, repeating, mispronouncing, or inability to pronounce certain sounds; most often seen in children; may be caused by excessive nervousness, agitation, being constantly scolded, emotional states such as fear, worry, insecurity.

stammering bladder: Relates to a condition in which the urinary stream is frequently interrupted; may be a pathologic or psychogenic condition.

standardization (stand'dard-ī-zā'shun): The bringing of any drug or other substance into conformity with a set standard of purity, concentration, etc.

standard of care: In the health sciences, a measure against which a professional person's conduct is compared; comprises a list of those acts that a prudent professional person would have performed (or not performed) in like circumstances.

standing orders: A written set of general orders or policies prepared for a specific ward, or care facility unit to be followed for all patients and clients. They usually relate to the use of telephone, radio, or television; transfer activities, and so on.

standstill: The stoppage or cessation of a normal activity, as may occur with the heart. CARDIAC S. asystole; may be due to cessation of normal activity of the atrium, the sinoatrial node, or the ventricle; marked by complete absence of waves on the electrocardiogram.

stapedectomy (stā-pe-dek'to-mi): Surgical removal of stapes in treatment of otosclerosis.

stapediolysis (stā'-pē-dī-ol'i-sis): An operation to mobilize the foot of the stapes in treatment for conduction deafness from otosclerosis.

stapes (stā'pēz): The stirrup-shaped innermost bone of the middle ear. S. MOBILIZATION release of a stapes rendered immobile by otosclerosis.

staphyl, staphylo-: Combining forms denoting: 1. The uvula. 2. A structure or arrangement that resembles a bunch of grapes.

staphyle (staf'i-lē): The uvula.

staphylectomy (staf-i-lek'to-mi): Amputation of the uvula. Uvulotomy.

staphyline (staf'i-līn): 1. Relating to the uvula. 2. Shaped like a bunch of grapes.

staphylitis (staf-i-lī'tis): Inflammation of the uvula.

staphylocide (staf'i-lō-sīd): Destructive to staphylococci.

staphylococcaemia (staf'i-lō-kok-sē'mi-a): The presence of staphylococci in the bloodstream.

staphylococcal (staf'i-lō-kok'al): Relating to or caused by staphylococci.

staphylococcosis (staf'i-lō-kok-ō'sis): Infection with staphylococci.

Staphylococcus (staf-i-lō-kok'us): A genus of bacteria. Gram-positive cocci occurring in clusters. May be saprophytic or parasitic. Common commensals in humans, in whom they are responsible for much minor pyogenic infection and a lesser amount of more serious infection. A common cause of hospital cross-infection. S. ALBUS a white form often found in sputum; occasionally the cause of staphylococcal pneumonia; S. AUREUS produces a golden yellow pigment on culture media; responsible for many diseases and infections in humans; S. EPIDERMIDIS a species of s. commonly found on the skin. — staphylococcal, adj.

staphyloedema (staf'il-ē-dē'ma): Oedema or any enlargement or swelling of the uvula.

staphylolysin (staf'i-lol'i-sin): A substance produced by staphylococci that causes haemolysis (*q.v.*).

staphyloma (staf'i-lō'ma): A bulging outward of the cornea or sclera of the eye, caused by an inflammatory reaction.

staphyloncus (staf-i-lon'kus): A tumour or other enlargement of the uvula.

staphylopharyngorrhaphy (staf'i-lō-far-in-gor'a-fi): A plastic operation on the palate and pharynx for repair of a cleft palate.

staphyloptosis (staf'i-lop-tō'sis): Elongation of the uvula.

staphylorrhaphy (staf'i-lor'a-fi): The operation for closing or uniting a cleft uvula or cleft palate.

staphylotomy (staf'i-lot'o-mi): Excision of the uvula or of a staphyloma.

starch: A complex carbohydrate, classed as a polysaccharide, found abundantly in nature in rice, corn and other cereals, in vegetables, and in unripe fruits. S. BATH a bath using starch for relief of pruritus.

star ratings: A measure of performance issued for acute NHS Trusts. Highest scoring hospitals are awarded three stars, and the lowest, no stars. The rating carries funding implications and affects the degree of autonomy a Trust has.

'start hesitation': A sudden feeling of one's feet being extremely heavy and of being unable to walk.

startle reflex: See MORO REFLEX under REFLEX.

stasis (stā'sis): Stagnation, cessation, retardation, or stoppage of flow of blood, urine or other body fluid, or of the motion of a part *e.g.*, the intestines. INTESTINAL S., atony or sluggish bowel contractions resulting in constipation, auto-intoxication, neurasthenia and other symptoms; S. ULCER see ULCER.

-stasis: Combining form denoting (1) stoppage; (2) maintenance of a constant level.

stat: Abbreviation for statim (*q.v.*).

static (stat'ik): Not dynamic; not moving; resting.

statim (sta'tim): Latin abbreviation previously used in prescriptions, at once.

station (stā'shun): 1. An individual's attitude or manner when standing, *e.g.*, the position of his body and its parts. 2. A specific location to which the sick or wounded are taken for care.

Stationery Office: Government agency in London that issues the reports, etc. published by the government. (Formerly Her Majesty's Stationery Office, HMSO.)

Statistical Package for the Social Sciences: Probably the most widely used program for applied statistics in the health professions; also used by market researchers, health researchers, survey companies, government, education researchers, and others.

statistical significance: A measurement or score that is unlikely to have occurred by chance alone and might, therefore, be accounted for by some specific factor, such as an experimental treatment.

statistics (sta-tis'tiks): The science dealing with collecting, tabulating, and interpreting numerical data on any subject. See APPENDIX 6, RESEARCH.

statocyst (stat'ō-sist): One of the sacs of the labyrinth of the ear; thought to be involved in the maintenance of static equilibrium.

statolith (stat'ō-lith): An otolith (*q.v.*).

stature (statch'ur): The height or tallness of a person when standing; measured from the soles of the feet to the top of the head.

status (stā'tus): A state or condition; in medicine, often used in the sense of implying severe or intractable; s. ANGIOSUS angina that occurs during rest and is resistant to treatment; see ANGINA PECTORIS; S. ASTHMATICUS a prolonged and refractory attack of asthma; an acute emergency condition requiring immediate medical treatment; s. EPILEPTICUS repeated epileptic attacks in rapid succession without recovery between them; an emergency condition; s. LYMPHATICUS a morbid condition found mostly in children, in which there is hypertrophy of lymphoid tissue, particularly of the thymus; sudden death is not unusual in these patients, especially when they are under the influence of an anaesthetic.

statutory body (stat'-ū-to-ri): Groups established by law to regulate their specific professions. Each body keeps a register of its qualified practitioners and sets standards relating to entry, maintenance on, and removal from its professional register.

staunch (stawnsh): To stop the flow of blood; usually refers to bleeding from a wound. Also spelled *stanch*.

STD: Abbreviation for sexually transmitted disease, see under SEXUALLY TRANSMITTED DISEASES AND DISORDERS.

stearate (stē'a-rāt): Any compound of stearic acid.

stearic acid (sti-ar'ik as'id): A saturated fatty acid derived from animal fat; used in pharmaceutical preparations.

stearo-: Combining form denoting relationship to fat.

steat-, steato-: Combining forms denoting fat.

steatitis (stē-a-tī'tis): Inflammation of fatty tissue.

steatolysis (stē-a-tol'i-sis): The process by which fats are emulsified in the intestine and prepared for absorption.

steatoma (stē-a-tō'ma): 1. A retention cyst of a sebaceous gland; a wen. 2. A lipoma. Also called *steatocystoma*.

steatomatosis (stē'a-tō-ma-tō'sis): The presence of numerous sebaceous cysts.

steatonecrosis (stē'a-tō-ne-krō'sis): Necrosis of fatty tissue.

steatopathy (stē-a-top'a-thi): Any disease or disorder of the sebaceous glands.

steatopygia (ste-at-ō-pij'i-a): Excessive deposit of fat on the buttocks; most often seen in women.

steatorrhoea (ste-a-tō-rē'a): 1. An increase in sebaceous gland secretion. 2. A syndrome of varied aetiology associated with multiple defects in digestion and absorption of fat from the gut; characterized by the passage of pale, bulky, greasy stools.

Steele–Richardson–Olszewski syndrome: Progressive supranuclear palsy; see under PALSY.

Steinmann pin: An alternative to the use of a Kirschner's wire (*q.v.*) for applying skeletal traction to a limb. [Fritz Steinmann, Swiss surgeon, 1872–1932.]

stellate (stel'āt): Star-shaped. s. GANGLION a large collection of nerve cells (ganglion) on the sympathetic chain in the root of the neck.

Stellwag's sign: Occurs in exophthalmic goitre (Graves' disease). Patient does not blink as often as normal, and the eyelids close only imperfectly when he or she does so; also the upper eyelid is retracted so that the palpebral opening is widened. [Carl Stellwag von Carion, Austrian ophthalmologist, 1823–1904.]

stem: 1. A supporting structure; a stalk. 2. To check, as blood flow. 3. To originate in. BRAIN s. all of the brain except the cerebrum and the cerebellum; S. CELL a simple cell that gives rise to a line of specialized cells as occurs in haematopoiesis.

sten-, steno-: Combining forms denoting narrow, constricted.

stenagmus (ste-nag'mus): Sighing.

stenocardia (sten-ō-kar'di-a): Angina pectoris (*q.v.*).

stenopeic (sten-ō-pē'ik): Having a very narrow slit or a tiny hole for admitting light.

stenosed (ste-nozd'): Narrowed, constricted.

stenosis (ste-nō'sis): Abnormal narrowing or stricture of any canal or orifice. AORTIC S.

narrowing of the orifice between the heart and the aorta; AQUEDUCTAL S. narrowing or malformation of the aqueduct of Sylvius, resulting in an enlarged cranium, and hydrocephalus; may be caused by trauma or meningoencephalitis; characterized by headache, visual disturbances, possibly seizures; CARDIAC S. narrowing of any of the heart cavities or orifices; MITRAL S. narrowing of the bicuspid opening between the left atrium and ventricle; PULMONARY or PULMONIC S. narrowing of the orifice between the right ventricle and the pulmonary artery; PYLORIC S. narrowing of the orifice between the stomach and the small intestine; SUBAORTIC S., S. that obstructs the flow of blood from the left ventricle; due to a lesion subjacent to the aortic valve; TRICUSPID S. narrowing of the orifice between the right atrium and ventricle. — stenotic, stenosed, adj.

stenothermia (sten'ō-ther'mi-a): The condition of being able to develop only within a narrow range of temperature; said of certain bacteria.

stenothorax (sten'ō-thaw'raks): An unusually narrow chest.

stenotic (ste-not'ik): Characterized by abnormal narrowing or constriction.

Stensen's duct: The duct leading from the parotid gland and opening into the cheek opposite the upper second molar tooth. [Niels Stensen or Steno, Danish anatomist, 1638–1686.]

stercobilin (ster'kō-bī'lin): The brown pigment of faeces; it is derived from the bile pigments.

stercobilinogen (ster'kō-bī-lin'ō-jen): Urobilinogen (q.v.).

stercolith (ster'kō-lith): A hard, dry mass of faecal matter in the intestine.

stercoroma (ster-kō-rō'ma): A hard faecal mass in the rectum.

stereo-: Combining form denoting; (1) special qualities; (2) three-dimensionality; (3) firm, hard, solid, or a solid medium.

stereoarthrolysis (ster'ē-ō-ar-throl'i-sis): Loosening or manipulation of stiff joints so as to make them movable, especially in ankylosis.

stereopsis (ster-ē-op'sis): Stereoptic vision. See STEREOSCOPE.

stereoroentgenography (ster'ē-ō-rent'gen-og'ra-fi): The making of a stereoscopic roentgenogram.

stereoscope (ste'rē-o-skōp): An instrument that projects two images of the same object that, when blended, give an impression of depth and solidity in a single picture of that object,

presenting to the eyes as a three-dimensional view. — stereoscopic, adj.

stereotypy (ster'ē-ō-tī'pi): The persistent repetition of meaningless words or acts, often observed in persons with schizophrenia and in those with some forms of mental handicap.

sterile (ster'il): 1. Free from living microorganisms and their products. 2. Being unable to conceive; barren. S. TECHNIQUE a method of functioning that aims to maintain the sterility of sterilized objects.

sterility (ster-il'i-ti): 1. Freedom from microorganisms. 2. Inability to conceive or bear offspring.

sterilization (ster'i-lī-zā'shun): 1. The process of completely ridding material or tissue of live microorganisms, leaving no viable forms, including spores. 2. Rendering an individual incapable of reproduction. CHEMICAL S. destruction of microorganisms by means of a chemical substance; DRY HEAT S., S. by subjection to very high temperatures for several hours; FRACTIONAL S. subjection of materials to free-flowing steam for several hours several days in succession to kill spores that might have developed between sterilizations; GAS S. exposure of materials to a gas that kills microorganisms; MECHANICAL S. removing microorganisms by passing a fluid substance containing them through a filter; RADIATION S. utilizes x-rays, ultraviolet rays, and isotopes to sterilize certain substances; STEAM S. the destruction of microorganisms by exposure to free-flowing steam; STEAM-UNDER-PRESSURE S. utilizes the autoclave (q.v.) for sterilizing many materials and articles; ULTRASONIC S. a method destroying bacteria by exposing articles or materials to be sterilized to a transmitter that emanates ultrasonic waves which shatter the bacteria; used in certain industries and laboratories.

sterilize (ster'i-līz): To render sterile.

sterilizer (ster'i-līz-er): A mechanism, chemical, or method used for making any material or object free of living microorganisms.

stern-, sterno-: Combining forms denoting relationship to the sternum or breast.

sternal (ster'nal): Relating to or relating to the sternum. S. ANGLE that formed on the anterior surface of the sternum where the body of the sternum and the manubrium meet. Also called the *angle of Louis*; an anatomical landmark; S. PUNCTURE aspiration of bone marrow from the sternum for diagnosis of certain diseases of the blood or bone marrow.

sternalgia (ster-nal'ji-a): Pain in the sternum.

sternoclavicular (ster'nō-kla-vik'ū-lar): Relating to the sternum and the clavicle. Also called *sternocleidal*.

sternocleidomastoid (ster'nō-klī'dō-mas'-toyd): Relating to the sternum, clavicle, and the mastoid process. S. MUSCLE a strap-like muscle arising from the sternum and clavicle, and inserting into the mastoid process of the temporal bone. It draws the head towards the shoulder and assists in flexing the head and neck. See TORTICOLLIS.

sternocostal (ster'nō-kos'tal): Relating to the sternum and ribs.

sternodymus (ster-nod'i-mus): Conjoined twins united at the sternum.

sternodynia (ster-nō-din'i-a): Pain in the sternum.

sternohyoid (ster-nō-hī'oyd): Relating to the sternum and the hyoid bone.

sternomastoid (ster'nō-mas'toyd): Relating to the sternum and the mastoid process of the temporal bone.

sternotomy (ster-not'o-mi): The surgical division of the sternum.

sternum (ster'num): The breastbone; a narrow, flat bone, shaped like a dagger, with a handle (manubrium), blade (body), and tip (xiphoid); the first seven costal cartilages are attached to it on either side, and it articulates with the clavicles above. — sternal, adj.

sternutation (ster'nū-tā'shun): Sneezing, or a sneeze.

steroid (stēr'oyd): A term embracing a naturally occurring group of chemical compounds related to cholesterol, and including sex hormones, adrenal cortical hormones, progesterone, sterols, bile acids; by custom now often implies the natural adrenal glucocorticoids, *i.e.*, hydrocortisone and cortisone, or such synthetic analogues as prednisolone and prednisone.

steroidogenesis (stē-roy'-dō-jen'e-sis): The production of steroids by living tissue.

sterol (stēr'ol): Any one of a class of solid alcohols widely distributed in nature; they are waxy materials found in plant and animal tissues; cholesterol is the best known of the group.

stertor (ster'tor): A snore. Noisy or laborious breathing as occurs in deep sleep or coma. — stertorous, adj.

stertorous (ster'tor-us): Relating to or characterized by stertor or snoring.

steth-, stetho-: Combining forms denoting relationship to the chest.

stethometer (steth-om'i-ter): An instrument for measuring the expansion of the chest during respiration.

stethoscope (steth'ō-skōp): An instrument used for listening to the various body sounds, especially those of the heart and lungs. — stethoscopic, adj.; stethoscopically, adv.

sthenia (sthē'ni-a): A condition of great strength and activity. Opp. to asthenia.

sthenic (sthen'ik): Refers to a body type that is well developed, with broad shoulders and athletic appearance.

STI: Abbreviation for sexually transmitted infection, see under SEXUALLY TRANSMITTED DISEASES AND DISORDERS.

'stiff' lung: A lung that has low compliance and resists inflation.

stiff man syndrome: Intermittent, progressive, fluctuating muscular rigidity; cause unknown.

stiff neck: Torticollis; wryneck. Rigidity of neck muscles due to spasm.

stigma (stig'ma): In medicine (1) a spot or mark on the skin; or (2) any physical or mental mark or characteristic that aids in diagnosis of a particular condition, *e.g.* the facies of congenital syphilis. — stigmata, stigmas, pl.; stigmatic, adj.

stigmatosis (stig-ma-tō'sis): A skin disease characterized by the appearance of multiple ulcerated spots.

stilette (stī-let'): 1. A thin wire or metal rod for maintaining patency of a hollow instrument or rigidity of a catheter. 2. A small, slender, sharp surgical probe. Also called *stylet*.

stillbirth (stil'berth): The birth of an infant (after the 28th week of pregnancy) which after birth showed no signs of life. Stillbirths must be registered and the cause of death established before a certificate of stillbirth can be issued and a burial take place.

stillborn (stil'born): Born dead.

Still's disease: A form of rheumatoid polyarthritis, of unknown cause, characterized by high fever, skin rashes, abdominal discomfort, progressive pain and tenderness of joints, especially the larger joints; later by lymphadenectomy, splenomegaly, valvular heart disease, ankylosis, especially of the cervical spine, impaired growth and development. Occurs in young children. Also called *arthritis deformans juvenilis*. [George Frederic Still, English physician, 1868–1941.]

stimulant (stim'ū-lant): 1. Stimulating or promoting mental and physical activities or function. 2. An agent that excites or increases functional activity.

stimulate (stim'ū-lāt): 1. To excite to functional activity or growth. 2. To elicit a response in a special organ or system. — stimulation, n.

stimulus (stim'ū-lus): Anything that is capable of exciting functional activity or producing a response in an organ or part. ADEQUATE S. one that arouses a response in a particular receptor; INADEQUATE or SUBLIMINAL S. one that is too weak to arouse a response; THRESHOLD S. one that is just strong enough to arouse an appropriate response. — stimuli, pl.

stippling (stip'ling): A spotted appearance of a membrane or cell; often refers to blood cells. MALARIAL S. characteristic fine dots seen in the red blood cells in quartan malaria; also called *Ziemann's stippling.*

stirrup bone: The stapes (*q.v.*).

'stir-up' routine: The routine of turning, coughing, and deep breathing; a useful exercise to promote the removal of secretions from the respiratory tract.

stitch: 1. A sudden, sharp, darting pain. 2. A suture. 3. To fix an organ or part in a certain position or to bring the edges of a wound together with a needle and some suture material used as a thread. S. ABSCESS one that forms at the site of a stitch in a wound; due to non-sterile suture material or pus-forming bacteria on the skin.

stockinet, stockinette (stok-i-net'): A soft, circular-knit material, usually cotton, having elastic properties and used for bandages, under casts, etc.

stocking: See ELASTIC STOCKING.

stoic (stō'ik): A person who is indifferent to passion or feeling, or who does not allow pain to interfere with his or her plans and desires.

stoicism (stō'i-sizm): Indifference to pleasure or pain; an attitude of endurance and bravery.

Stokes–Adams syndrome: A fainting (syncopal) attack, commonly transient, which frequently accompanies heart block; characterized by slow and occasionally irregular pulse, vertigo, fainting, sometimes convulsions; Cheyne–Stokes respiration, and unconsciousness. Also called *Adams–Stokes* syndrome. [William Stokes, Irish physician, 1804–1878. Robert Adams, Irish physician, 1791–1875.]

stom-, stoma-, stomo-, stomata-: Combining forms denoting mouth or opening.

stoma (stō'ma): 1. Any minute pore, orifice or opening. 2. The mouth. 3. An artificial opening established surgically between an organ and the exterior or between two organs or parts. — stomal, adj.; stomata, pl.

stomach (stum'ak): The most dilated part of the digestive tube, situated between the oesopha-

gus (cardiac orifice) and the beginning of the small intestine (pyloric orifice); it lies just under the diaphragm in the epigastric, umbilical and left hypochondriac regions of the abdomen. The wall is composed of four coats; serous, muscular, submucous, and mucous. HOURGLASS S. one partially divided into two halves by an equatorial constriction following scar formation; S. PUMP a suction pump attached to a flexible tube that is passed into the stomach via the nose or mouth to remove stomach contents; S. TOOTH either of the canine teeth of the lower jaw in the first dentition; informal; S. TUBE a tube passed into the stomach through the mouth and used for feeding purposes or for lavage; UPSIDE-DOWN S. popular name for a THORACIC S. one that is in the thoracic cavity.

stomachalgia (stum'a-kal'ji-a): Pain in the stomach.

stomachic (stum-ak'ik): 1. Relating to the stomach. 2. An agent that increases the appetite and improves digestion, especially one of the bitters.

stomatic (stōm-at'ik): Relating to the mouth.

stomatitis (stō-ma-tī'tis): Inflammation of the mucous membrane of the mouth. ANGULAR S. fissuring in the corners of the mouth, usually due to riboflavin deficiency, pellagra, or sensitivity to dental materials; APHTHOUS S. recurring crops of small ulcers in the mouth; see APHTHAE; GANGRENOUS S. see CANCRUM ORIS; HERPETIC S. an acute infection of the oral mucosa with the formation of vesicles; caused by the herpes simplex virus; also called *vesicular s.*; S. NICOTINA inflammation of the mucous membrane of the palate, due to the irritating properties of tobacco, occurs chiefly in cigarette and cigar smokers; ULCERATIVE S., s. characterized by chronically recurring painful, shallow ulcers on cheeks, tongue, and lips; VINCENT'S S. see VINCENT'S ANGINA under ANGINA. See also THRUSH.

stomatocyte (stō'mat-ō-sīt): A red blood cell in which a slit or mouth-like area replaces the normal circle of pallor; may be observed in a rare form of haemolytic anaemia and in certain liver diseases.

stomatocytosis (stō'-ma-tō-sī-tō'sis): An uncommon form of congenital haemolytic anaemia characterized by the presence of stomatocytes in the peripheral blood.

stomatodynia (stō'ma-tō-din'i-a): Pain in the mouth.

stomatogastric (stō'ma-tō-gas'trik): Relating to the mouth and the stomach.

stomatomalacia (stō'ma-tō-ma-lā'shi-a): Softening of the tissues and structures of the mouth.

stomatomycosis (stō'ma-tō-mī-kō'sis): A fungal infection of the mouth.

stomatonecrosis (stō'ma-tō-ne-krō'sis): Gangrenous stomatitis. Also see STOMATONOMA. Noma.

stomatonoma (stō'ma-tō-nō'ma): Gangrene of the mouth.

stomatopathy (stō'ma-top'a-thi): Any disease or disorder of the mouth.

stomatoplasty (stō'ma-tō-plas-ti): Plastic surgery of the mouth.

stomatorrhagia (stō'ma-tō-rā'ji-a): Haemorrhage from the gums or other part of the oral cavity.

-stomy: Combining form denoting a surgical opening into a hollow organ or a new opening between two structures.

stone (stōn): Calculus; a hardened mass of mineral matter. 'INFECTION' STONES those that form in the urinary tract when the urine is highly alkaline and contains a high concentration of ammonia; commonly occur in patients with long-term indwelling catheters and those with recurrent infections; they damage tissue and encourage bacterial growth.

stool: Faeces discharged by the bowels. ALCOHOLIC S. a S. that is whitish in colour, due to lack of bile content; CURRANT-JELLY S. a S. that contains bloody mucus; FATTY S. one that contains fat; seen in malabsorption syndrome and diseases of the pancreas; MELANIN S. one that is dark coloured, often due to medications containing iron; PEA-SOUP S. the liquid s. seen in typhoid fever; RICE-WATER S. the watery s. that is characteristic of cholera; STEATORRHOEAL S. fatty s.; TARRY S. a s. that has the colour and consistency of tar; may be the result of taking medications containing bismuth, iron, or certain other substances, or of intestinal haemorrhage.

stopcock: A device to prevent fluid from flowing through tubing.

storage disease: A metabolic disorder in which some substances such as fats, proteins, and carbohydrates accumulate in certain body cells in abnormal amounts.

strabismus (stra-biz'mus): A condition in which the intraocular muscles do not balance, making it impossible for the eyes to function in unison. It is called CONVERGENT S. when the eye turns towards the nose (esotropia), and divergent when it turns outwards (exotropia). ACCOMMODATIVE S. overconvergence caused by excessive accommodation (*q.v.*); ALTERNATING S. a form of s. in which either eye may deviate; VERTICAL S. a form of s. in which one eye deviates either upwards or downwards.

strabotomy (stra-bot'o-mi): The cutting of an ocular tendon or muscle in treatment for strabismus.

straight back syndrome: A skeletal deformity marked by loss of the anterior concavity of the upper thoracic part of the spinal column which results in reduction of the anterior–posterior dimension of the upper part of the thorax and compression of the heart between the sternum and the vertebral column.

strain (strān): 1. To exert effort to the limit of one's ability. 2. Weakening or stretching of a muscle at the tendon area, resulting from overexercise, overuse, or improper use. 3. To overstretch some muscular part of the body. 4. To filter. 5. A group of microorganisms within a species whose common properties are maintained through successive generations.

strait (strāt): A constricted or narrow space or passage, as of the pelvic canal

straitjacket: Common name for a device formerly used to restrain irrational or restless patients; consists of a shirt with long sleeves which are fastened so as to restrict movement of the arms.

strangle (strang'-g'l): 1. To suffocate, choke, or cause one to be choked by compression or obstruction of the trachea sufficiently to prevent breathing. 2. To deny an organism or a body part of a vital substance such as blood, water, air.

strangulated (strang'gū-lat-ed): The condition of being compressed or constricted so as to cut off the supply of air, blood or other vital substance from a body part. S. HERNIA see HERNIA.

strangulation (strang-gū-lā'shun): 1. Choking caused by compression, constriction or obstruction of air passages, with consequent arrest of breathing. 2. Arrest of blood circulation to a part by compression or constriction of the blood vessels.

strangury (strang'gū-ri): Frequent desire to urinate with slow and painful micturition; due to spasm of the urethral muscles.

strapping: The application of strips of adhesive tape that overlap; used to cover, support, exert pressure on, or immobilize a part in such condition as strain, sprain, dislocation or fracture.

strategic health authority (stra-tē'-jik): Governing organization that manages the performance of the health-care system for an average population of around 1.5 million. It ensures the delivery of improvements in health and health services locally by Primary Care Trusts and NHS Trusts.

strategy (strat´-e-ji): In (theoretical) circumstances of competition or conflict, as in business administration, a plan for successful action based on the rationality and interdependence of the moves of the opposing participants.

stratified (strat´i-fid): Arranged in layers. S. EPITHELIUM epithelium in which the differently shaped cells are arranged in distinct strata or layers.

stratum (strah´tum): A lamina or layer, or a sheet-like mass of differentiated tissue, e.g., one of the layers of the skin. — strata, pl., stratified, adj.

strawberry mark: A congenital haemangioma; a bright red, soft, elevated, and often lobulated haemangioma present at birth; see HAEMANGIOMA.

streph-, strepho-, strepto-: Combining forms denoting twisted or a twisted chain.

strep throat: Lay term for an infection of the pharynx and tonsils caused by haemolytic *Streptococcus*; characterized by fever, chills, malaise, sore throat; spread by droplet infection; highly communicable.

strepticaemia (strep-ti-sē´mi-a): Streptococcaemia (*q.v.*).

streptococcaemia (strep´tō-kok-sē´mi-a): The presence of streptococcic organisms in the bloodstream.

streptococcal (strep´tō-kok´al): Relating to or caused by a streptococcus.

streptococci (strep´tō-kok´sī): Plural of streptococcus. BETA HAEMOLYTIC S. Lancefield's groups (*q.v.*).

Streptococcus (strep´tō-kok´us): A genus of more or less round, non-sporeforming, non-motile, Gram-positive bacteria that occur in chains of varying length; may be saprophytic or parasitic; some pathogenic species are capable of producing powerful exotoxins. S. FAECALIS an enterococcus normally present in the gastrointestinal tract; may on occasion be the cause of bacterial endocarditis; S. PNEUMONIAE organisms of this group produce lobar pneumonia and other acute pus-forming conditions, including middle ear infections and meningitis; S. PYOGENES organisms from this group produce haemolysis on blood agar medium; includes organisms that cause scarlet fever, septic sore throat, tonsillitis, erysipelas,

cellulitis, endocarditis, puerperal fever, rheumatic fever, acute glomerulonephritis, wound infections; S. SALIVARIUS a species normally present in the mouth, nose, and throat; may be associated with tooth abscesses and subacute bacterial endocarditis.

streptodornase (strep-tō-dor´nās): A enzyme used with streptokinase (*q.v.*) in liquefying pus and blood clots, thus promoting healing.

streptokinase (strep-tō-kī´nās): An enzyme derived from cultures of beta-haemolytic streptococci. Because it activates the formation of plasmin, a fibrinolytic enzyme that dissolves fibrin, it is often administered with streptodornase to liquefy and remove clotted blood, or fibrinous or purulent accumulations.

streptolysins (strep-tol´i-sinz): A group of filterable haemolysins (*q.v.*) produced by streptococci, *Streptocossus pyogenes* in particular. Antibody produced in the tissues against streptolysin may be measured and taken as an indicator of recent streptococcal infection. STREPTOLYSIN-O is antigenic and oxygenlabile. STREPTOLYSIN-S is not antigenic; is insensitive to oxygen but is destroyed by heat and acid.

streptosepticaemia (strep´tō-sep-ti-sē´mi-a): Septicaemia (*q.v.*) that is caused by a streptococcal organism.

stress: 1. Intense effort; emphasis; pressure; a constraining force or influence. **2.** A condition of strain caused by inability to adjust to factors in the environment, resulting in physiological tensions; may even contribute to the production of disease. **3.** The sum of physiological and psychological wear and tear caused by external influences that produce adverse reactions involving the entire body. S. INCONTINENCE see under INCONTINENCE; S. TEST Bruce treadmill test; a diagnostic test to determine the body's response to physical exertion; involves taking an ECG, taking blood pressure and pulse, and making observations while the patient is exercising by running in place, jogging, etc. S. ULCER see under ULCER.

stressor (stres´or): An agent or condition that serves as a stress-producing factor; may be biological, psychological, physical, or environmental in character.

stretcher (strech´er): A device for carrying and transporting the sick and injured.

stretch marks: See STRIA.

stria (strī´a): A streak; stripe; narrow band. STRIAE GRAVIDARUM lines which appear, especially on the abdomen, as a result of stretching of the skin in pregnancy; due to rupture of the lower layers of the dermis. They are red at first and then become silvery white. Striae may also result when the skin of the abdomen is stretched due to weight gained and then lost. — striae, pl.; striated, adj.

striated (strī'āt-ed): Striped. In anatomy, term usually applied to skeletal muscles in which the fibres are marked by cross striations.

stricture (strik'shur): An abnormal congenital or acquired narrowing of a tube, canal or passage; may be temporary or permanent; usually due to inflammation, infection, injury, scar formation, muscle spasm, or growth of abnormal tissue.

stridor (strī'dor): A harsh, high-pitched sound in breathing, caused by air passing through constricted air passages; often heard in acute constriction of the larynx. In absence of pathology may be due to poorly developed larynx, small glottis, or a large epiglottis.

stridulous (strid'ū-lus): Characterized by stridor (*q.v.*).

strip: 1. To force out the contents of a tube such as a blood vessel or the urethra by pressing a finger along the length of the tube. 2. To remove lengths of large veins or incompetent vessels by use of a stripper (*q.v.*); sometimes the treatment for varicose veins.

stripper: A surgical instrument consisting of a flexible metal tube with a cup or disc at the end; used in excising lengths of veins.

strobila (strō'bil-a): The segmented body of the adult tapeworm.

stroke (strōk): A sudden severe attack, particularly one resulting from the bursting or clogging of a blood vessel in the brain causing damage to nerve centres. APOPLECTIC S. one in which sudden unconsciousness occurs as a result of intracranial haemorrhage, thrombosis or embolism; HEAT S. one resulting from hyperpyrexia due to inhibition of the heat-regulating mechanism in conditions of high temperatures or high humidity or because sweating is interfered with; marked by dry skin, vertigo, headache, nausea, muscular cramps; PARALYTIC S. one in which injury to the brain or spinal cord causes paralysis of some part or parts of the body; S. VOLUME the amount of blood ejected by the left ventricle at each heartbeat.

stroke syndrome: Cerebrovascular accident (*q.v.*).

stroking (strōk'ing): A massage manoeuvre. See EFFLEURAGE.

stroma (strō'ma): The interstitial substance or supporting framework of a structure as distin-guished from its specific functional physiological element. — stromal, stromatic, adj.

stromal (strō'mal): Of or pertaining to the stroma of an organ or structure.

Strongyloides (stron'ji-loy'dez): A genus of widely distributed parasitic intestinal nematodes that infest animals, including certain animals and rodents as well as humans.

strongyloidiasis (stron'-ji-loy-dī'a-sis): Infestation with *Strongyloides stercoralis*, a roundworm widely distributed in tropical and subtropical areas. The larvae develop in the soil, penetrate the human skin and mucous membrane on contact, pass through the intestinal membrane, get into the bloodstream and are carried to all parts of the body including the lung where they may cause haemorrhage; other symptoms include abdominal pain, nausea, vomiting, and weight loss; severe cases may prove fatal. Occurs in persons with poor circulation who travel in tropical areas.

strontium (stron'ti-um): A metallic element, similar to calcium in its properties; its various salts are used therapeutically. The isotopes of strontium are used in radioisotope scanning; strontium 90 (⁹⁰Sr) is the longest-lived of the isotopes having a half-life of 28 years; it is the most dangerous component of atomic fallout. Chemical symbol, Sr.

structuralism (struk'-chur-a-lizm): The branch of psychology that is particularly interested in the basic structure or content of consciousness, including intellect and feeling as well as behaviour; the opposite of functionalism (*q.v.*).

struma (stroo'ma): 1. Goitre. 2. Any hardening of tissue. 3. Obsolete term for any enlargement. S. OVARII a rare teratomatous condition in which the ovary consists almost entirely of thyroid tissue. See HASHIMOTO'S DISEASE.

strumectomy (stroo-mek'to-mi): Thyroidectomy (*q.v.*).

strumitis (stroo-mī'tis): Thyroiditis (*q.v.*).

strumous (stroo'mus): 1. Relating to or having the characteristics of a struma. 2. Having goitre.

Strümpell–Marie disease: Rheumatoid spondylitis. See SPONDYLITIS.

strychnine (strik'nīn): An alkaloid obtained from the tree *Strychnos nux-vomica*; formerly much used as a central nervous system stimulant. It is poisonous.

Stryker wedge frame (strī'ker): An orthopaedic bed that allows the patient to be rotated as required to either the supine or prone position. The Stryker wedge frame is used in the immobilization of patients with unstable spines, management of severe burns and post-operative management of multilevel spinal fusions. Available in one size only, it caters for differing body builds by an adjustable crossbar on the anterior circle of the frame. When the crossbar is correctly adjusted, the patient is held firmly between the frames without the addition of pillows or extra padding.

S–T segment: The interval in the electrocardio-gram between the QRS complex and the be-ginning of the T wave.

Stuart–Power factor: See FACTOR X under FACTOR.

stump: The remaining distal end of a part that has been amputated.

stun: To render unconscious by a blow or other force; to daze.

stupefacient (stū-pē-fā′shent): 1. Inducing stupor. 2. An agent that causes stupor.

stupor (stū′por): A state of marked impairment of mental and physical activity but not com-plete loss of consciousness; may be due to cerebral vascular insufficiency or damage to brain tissue. The patient shows gross lack of responsiveness, usually reacts only to painful stimuli, and is disoriented as to person, time, and place, but the reflexes remain intact. In psychiatry, three main varieties are recog-nized — depressive, schizophrenic, and hys-terical. — stuporous, adj.

stutter (stu′ter): To speak with hesitation and spasmodic repetition of the initial consonant of a word or syllable; due to anxiety, nervous-ness, or an impediment.

sty, stye (stī): Inflammation of one of the seba-ceous glands at the edge of the eyelid. Syn., *hordeolum.*

styl-, styli-, stylo-: Combining forms denoting (1) a pillar, or pillar-like; (2) a projecting bony process.

styloglossus (stī′lō-glos′sus): A muscle that arises at the styloid process of the temporal bone and inserts into the tongue.

styloid (stī′loyd): Long and pointed, resembling a pen or stylus. Used especially in reference to a bony process, such as those at the distal end of the radius and of the ulna.

stylomastoid (stī-lō-mas′toyd): Relating to the styloid and mastoid processes of the temporal bone.

stylus (stī′lus): In pharmacology, a pencil-shaped stick of some substance containing a medicament such as a caustic.

sub-: Prefix denoting (1) under, below; (2) near, almost, moderately; (3) less than normal.

subabdominal (sub-ab-dom′i-nal): Below the abdomen.

subacromial (sub-a-krō′mi-al): Situated beneath the acromion.

subacute (sub-a-kūt): Moderately severe. Often the stage between the acute and chronic phases of a disease. S. BACTERIAL ENDOCARD-ITIS see ENDOCARDITIS.

subarachnoid (sub-a-rak′noyd): Beneath the arachnoid membrane. S. HAEMORRHAGE a haemorrhage into the subarachnoid space. S. SPACE the space between the arachnoid mem-brane and the pia mater; it contains cerebro-spinal fluid.

subaural (sub-aw′ral): Below the ear.

subception (sub-sep′shun): The reaction to a stimulus that one is not fully aware of having perceived.

subchondral (sub-kon′dral): Below or beneath a cartilage; usually refers to the cartilages of the ribs.

subclavian (sub-klā′vi-an): Beneath the clav-icle; usually refers to the subclavian artery or vein.

subclavian steal syndrome: A condition caused by the occlusion of one subclavian artery near the origin of the vertebral artery, causing, in turn, a reversal of blood flow through the ver-tebral artery; manifestations are visual symp-toms, lower blood pressure in the involved arm, pain in the occipital and mastoid regions, diminished or absent pulse on the affected side.

subclinical (sub-klin′i-kal): 1. The period in the course of a disease before the symptoms are severe enough to make the disease identifi-able. 2. A condition or infection not severe enough to cause the classic identifiable dis-ease.

subconjunctival (sub-con-jungk-tī′val): Under the conjunctiva. — subconjunctivally, adv.

subconscious (sub-kon′shus): 1. That portion of the mind outside the range of clear conscious-ness, but capable of affecting conscious mental or physical reactions. 2. Partially but not wholly conscious.

subcortical (sub-kor′ti-kal): 1. Beneath the cortex of an organ or structure. 2. Beneath the cerebral cortex.

subcostal (sub-kos′tal): Beneath a rib or ribs.

subcrepitant (sub-krep′i-tant): Only faintly crepitant; said of a rale.

subcutaneous (sub′kū-tā′nē-us): 1. Relating to the tissues beneath the skin. 2. Hypodermic.

subcuticular (sub-kū-tik′ū-lar): Beneath the cuticle or epidermis, as in a s. abscess.

subcutis (sub-kū'tis): The superficial fascia which lies immediately below the skin.

subdermal (sub-der'mal): Subcutaneous (*q.v.*).

subdiaphragmatic (sub'dī-a-frag-mat'ik): Below the diaphragm. — subphrenic, syn.

subdural (sub-dū'ral): Beneath the dura mater; between the dura and arachnoid membranes. S. HAEMATOMA see under HAEMATOMA; S. SPACE the space between the dura mater and the arachnoid.

subendocardial (sub-en-do-kar'di-al): Beneath the endocardium, that is, between the endocardium and the myocardium.

suberosis (sū-ber-ō'sis): Pneumonoconiosis (*q.v.*), which affects cork workers; characterized by bronchial asthma. Also called *cork workers' lung*.

subfertility (sub-fer-til'i-ti): A below normal capacity for reproduction.

subgaleal (sub-gal'ē-al): Beneath the galea aponeurotica.

subglenoid (sub-glē'noyd): Beneath the glenoid cavity.

subglossal (sub-glos'al): Sublingual; under the tongue.

subglossitis (sub-glos-sī'tis): Inflammation of the underside of the tongue and the tissues that lie beneath the tongue.

subglottic (sub-glot'ik): Beneath the glottis. S. STENOSIS GRANULOMATOUS a narrowing below the glottis, usually of cicatricial origin.

subhepatic (sub-hē-pat'ik): Below the liver.

subinvolution (sub-in-vō-lū'shun): The failure of an organ to return to its normal size and condition after enlargement; said especially of the uterus that fails to return to its normal size after childbirth. See INVOLUTION.

subjacent (sub-jā'sent): Lying below or under something.

subjective (sub-jek'tiv): Internal; personal; arising from the senses and not influenced by the environment or perceptible to others. Opp. of objective. S. EFFECTS mental and physical feelings a person reports while undergoing drug or other therapeutic regimen; S. SYMPTOMS those perceived only by the patient and not perceptible to the observer.

subjectivity (sub-jek-tiv'-i-ti): A personal view influenced by prior experience and education.

sublatio (sub-lā'shi-ō): The removal or detachment of a part; sublation (*q.v.*). S. RETINAE detachment of the retina.

sublation (sub-lā'shun): Detachment, removal, or elevation of an organ or part.

sublethal (sub-lē'thal): Almost fatal. S. DOSE one that contains not quite enough of a toxic substance to cause death.

sublimate (sub'li-māt): 1. A solid deposit resulting from the condensation of a vapour. 2. In psychiatry, to redirect an anti-social drive or primitive desire into some more socially acceptable channel, *e.g.*, a strong tendency to aggressiveness sublimated into athletic activity. — sublimation, n.

sublimation (sub-lim-ā'shun): 1. In psychiatry, an unconscious defence mechanism whereby unacceptable cravings, instinctive wishes, and repressed erotic data are channelled into socially acceptable behaviour. 2. In chemistry, the process whereby a solid is converted to a vapour without passing through a liquid state.

subliminal (sub-lim'in-al): Inadequate for perceptible response. Below the threshold of consciousness. See LIMINAL, STIMULUS.

sublingual (sub-ling'gwal): Beneath the tongue. S. ADMINISTRATION OF MEDICATION a method of administration in which the medication, in tablet form, is placed under the tongue and allowed to dissolve before swallowing; the substance is quickly absorbed by the oral mucosa; S. DUCT a duct leading from the sublingual gland to the oral cavity; S. GLAND a complex of small glands situated on each side of the floor of the mouth; their secretion forms part of the saliva.

sublinguitis (sub-ling-gwī'tis): Inflammation of the sublingual gland.

subluxation (sub-luk-sā'shun): Incomplete or partial dislocation of a joint. S. OF THE ELBOW the head of the radius is pulled backwards under the edge of a ligament, resulting in obstruction to rotation; often seen in young children. Characterized by sudden acute pain following a traction type force to the forearm, such as lifting a child by the arm; the elbow is held in a fixed position and the hand is pronated.

submandibular (sub-man-dib'ū-lar): Below the mandible.

submaxilla (sub-mak'sil-a): The lower jawbone; the mandible.

submaxillary (sub-mak'sil-a-ri): Beneath the lower jaw. S. DUCTS those that drain the submaxillary gland; they open on the floor of the mouth on either side of the frenum of the tongue; also called *Wharton's ducts*.

submucosa (sub-mū-kō'za): The layer of areolar connective tissue beneath a mucous membrane that attaches it to the underlying tissues. — submucous, submucosal, adj.

submucous (sub-mū′kus): Beneath a mucous membrane. S. RESECTION an operation for the correction of a deviated septum in the nose.

subnormal (sub-nor′mal): Having less of something than is normal; said especially of intelligence. Being inferior to an accepted standard.

subnormality: A state of arrested or incomplete development of mind, which includes s. of intelligence and is of a nature or degree that requires or is susceptible to medical treatment or other special care or training of the patient. Now an obsolete term.

suboccipital (sub-ok-sip′it-al): Beneath the occiput; in the nape of the neck.

suboccipitobregmatic diameter (sub-oks-sip′i-tō-breg-mat′ik): The measurement from the nape of the neck to the centre of the bregma; it is the presenting diameter in a vertex presentation of the fetus.

suborbital (sub-or′bi-tal): Beneath the orbit of the eye.

subpatellar (sub-pa-tel′ar): Beneath the patella.

subpericardial (sub-per-i-kar′di-al): Beneath the pericardium.

subperiosteal (sub-per-ios′ti-al): Beneath the periosteum of bone.

subperitoneal (sub-per-i-tō-nē′ al): Beneath the peritoneum.

subpharyngeal (sub-fa-rin′ji-al): Below the pharynx.

subphrenic (sub-fren′ik): Beneath the diaphragm. S. ABSCESS see under ABSCESS.

subpituitarism (sub-pi-tū′i-tar-izm): Hypopituitarism (*q.v.*).

subpleural (sub-ploo′ral): Beneath the pleura.

subpreputial (sub-prē-pū′shi-al): Beneath the prepuce.

subpubic (sub-pū′bik): 1. Situated below the pubic arch. 2. Pertaining to a surgical procedure that is performed below the pubic arch.

subpulmonary (sub-pul′mo-nar-i): Situated, or occurring, below the lungs. — subpulmonic, adj.

subscapular (sub-skap′ū-lar): Beneath the scapula.

subscription (sub-skrip′shun): The part of a prescription that gives directions to the pharmacist as to its preparation.

substance (sub′stans): The material of which something is made; in the body it refers to the materials that make up the organs and tissues to which they owe their characteristic qualities. Matter.

substance abuse: Usually refers to the use of a drug, alcohol, or tobacco to the extent that it

interferes with one's health and social functioning. See also SNIFFING, AEROSOL.

substandard (sub-stan′dard): Descriptive of something that falls short of the usual or accepted standard of quality.

substantia (sub-stan′shi-a): In anatomy, substance or tissue. S. COMPACTA the compact portion of bone; S. GELATINOSA a network of small nerve cells along the posterior horn of the grey matter of the spinal cord; they have the ability to interfere with incoming nerve impulses. S. NIGRA a broad thick layer of pigmented cells lying between the border of the pons and the hypothalamus; S. SPONGIOSA the cancellous portion of bone.

substernal (sub-ster′nal): Beneath the sternum. S. GOITRE one which lies partially beneath the sternum.

substitution (sub′sti-tū′shun): 1. In chemistry, the replacement of one substance in a compound by another substance. 2. Something that is used in place of another substance; may or may not be cheaper or inferior. 3. An artificial product used in place of a natural one; usually to correct a deficiency of the natural product, *e.g.*, a hormone. 4. In psychology and psychotherapy, the person who takes the place of or acts for another person in relation to the patient. 5. The unconscious acceptance of a suitable goal or emotion for one that is unacceptable or unattainable. S. THERAPY see under THERAPY.

substratum (sub-strā′tum): A lower stratum or layer; an underlying structure or part.

subtemporal (sub-tem′po-ral): Beneath the temporal area of the skull.

subtendinous (sub-ten′di-nus): Situated between a tendon, as a bursa.

subtotal (sub′tō-tal): Somewhat less than total or complete. S. HYSTERECTOMY see HYSTERECTOMY.

subungal (sub-ung′gwal): Beneath a finger or toe nail.

succorrhoea (suk-ō-rē′a): An abnormal increase in the flow of a secretion or a juice, *e.g.*, saliva, intestinal juice.

succus (suk′us): 1. A fluid secretion; usually refers to a secretion of a digestive fluid. 2. The fluid present in body tissues.

succussion (sū-kush′un): The shaking of a person to determine whether this produces a splashing sound in a body cavity, indicating the pressure of a fluid and gas or air; HIPPOCRATIC S. the splashing sound heard on shaking when fluid accompanies the presence of gas or air in the thorax or the stomach and intestine; S. SPLASH the sound heard when air or fluid moves about in a body cavity or hollow area.

sucking wound: A wound in the chest wall through which air is taken in and expelled.

suckle (suk′l): **1.** To suck or draw nourishment from the breast. **2.** To feed an infant at the breast.

sucrase (sū′krās): An intestinal enzyme that acts to split sucrose; invertase.

sucrosaemia (sū-krō-sē′mi-a): The presence of sucrose in the blood.

sucrose (sū′krōs): A sugar obtained from sugar cane, sugar beet, or sorghum; a disaccharide; is normally converted into glucose and fructose in the body.

sucrosuria (sū-krō-sū′ri-a): The presence of sucrose in the urine.

suction (suk′shun): The act or process of sucking up or aspirating. S. ABORTION abortion resulting from the use of a suction device inserted into the uterus; a technique utilized during the first trimester of pregnancy; S. LIPIDECTOMY a plastic operation for suctioning fat out of body tissue without leaving scars; a controversial procedure; WANGENSTEEN S. see under WANGENSTEEN.

sudarium (sū-dā′ri-um): A sweat bath.

sudation (sū-dā′shun): Sweating or excessive sweating.

sudden infant death syndrome: Unexplained cot death of an apparently healthy infant between 3 weeks to 5 months (approximately), occurs most often during sleep, with no warning cry; occurs chiefly during cold seasons and more often among children from low-income groups; most likely victims are premature or low birth weight infants. Cannot be predicted or prevented. It is now advised, based on research evidence, that babies should be put to sleep on their backs or sides, but not prone. Also called *crib* or *cot death.*

Sudek's atrophy: See under ATROPHY.

sudo-, sudor-: Combining forms denoting sweat, perspiration.

sudogram (sū′dō-gram): A graphic representation of the areas of the skin where sweat is produced.

sudor (sū′dor): Sweat. — sudoriferous, adj.

sudoresis (sū′dō-rē′sis): Profuse sweating; diaphoresis.

sudoriferous (sū′dō-rif′er-us): **1.** Conveying sweat. **2.** Producing sweat. S. DUCT, the duct leading from a sweat gland to the surface of the skin. S. GLAND, a gland in the skin that produces sweat (sudor); see under SWEAT.

sudorific (sū′dor-if′ik): **1.** Promoting the secretion of sweat. **2.** An agent that induces sweating; a diaphoretic.

sudorrhoea (sū′dō-rē′a): Excessive sweating; hyperhidrosis.

suffocation (suf-ō-kā′shun): Asphyxia (*q.v.*).

suffusion (su-fū′zhun): **1.** Extravasation or spreading of blood or other body fluid into surrounding parts. **2.** A sudden reddening of the surface of the skin as in blushing. **3.** The act of pouring a fluid over the body or wetting it.

sugar (shoo′gar): A generic name for any of a class of crystalline, sweet-tasting, water-soluble carbohydrates, mostly monosaccharides and disaccharides, of animal or vegetable origin; examples are glucose and lactose.

suggestibility (sug-jest′ti-bil′i-ti): Susceptibility to suggestion (*q.v.*); is heightened in hospital patients, due to the dependence on others that illness brings.

suggestion (sug-jest′shun): The implanting in a person's mind of an idea which is accepted by the individual without fully understanding the reason for acceptance. In psychiatric practice, s. is used as a therapeutic measure, sometimes under hypnosis or nacroanalysis (*q.v.*). See AUTOSUGGESTION.

suicide (sū′i-sīd): **1.** The act of killing oneself, now no longer a crime with the passing of the Suicide Act 1961. **2.** A person who has voluntarily and deliberately taken his or her own life.

suicide post-vention: A term denoting the study of the effects of suicide on survivors, families, and friends.

suicidology (sū′i-sī-dol′o-ji): The study of all aspects of suicide, its causes and prevention.

sulcus (sul′-kus): A furrow or groove, particularly one separating gyri or convolutions of the brain. CENTRAL S. the rolandic fissure, a groove on the lateral surface of the cerebrum; it separates the frontal from the parietal lobes of the brain; LATERAL S. the fissure of Sylvius, lies between the temporal lobe below and the frontal and parietal lobes above; PARIETO-OCCIPITAL S. marks off the boundaries of the occipital lobe.

Sulkowitch's test: A test for determining the presence and amount of calcium in the urine.

sulph-, sulpho-: Combining forms denoting the presence of sulphur in a compound.

sulpha: Abbreviation denoting the sulphonamides or sulphur drugs.

sulphanaemia (sul-fa-nē′mi-a): Anaemia caused by the use of sulphonamide drugs.

sulphanilamide (sul-fa-nil′a-mīd): The first sulphonamide (*q.v.*), and parent of the other sulpha drugs; derived from coal tar and effective especially against beta-haemolytic streptococci, meningococci, and gonococci; also against *Clostridium welchii* (*q.v.*) and *Escherichia coli* (*q.v.*); Not used as much as formerly because of its toxic reactions; symptoms of toxicity, include beta-haemolytic anaemia, agranulocytosis.

sulphatase (sul′fa-tās): An enzyme that acts as a catalyst in the hydrolysis of sulphuric acid esters into sulphuric acid and alcohol. A deficiency of sulphatase A is thought to be the cause of metachromatic leukodystrophy.

sulphate (sul′fāt): Any salt of sulphuric acid.

sulphide (sul′fīd): A compound of sulphur and another element or a base.

sulphite (sul′fit): Any salt of sulphurous acid.

sulphonamides (sul-fon′a-mīds): A group of synthetic drugs derived from sulphonic acid. Their action is bacteriostatic, thus, they prevent multiplication of bacteria and allow the body to build its defences against the organisms.

sulphones (sul′fōns): A group of synthetic drugs related to the sulphonamides, useful in treatment of leprosy; also sometimes used in tuberculosis.

sulphonic acid (sul-fon′ik as′id): Any of several acids containing the sulphonic group (— SO_3H).

sulphonylurea (sul′-fō-nil-ū-rē′a): Any one of several chemical agents that are related to the sulphanilamides and that act with the beta cells of the pancreas to stimulate the secretion of insulin; also used as oral antidiabetics.

sulphur (sul′fur): A pale yellow crystalline substance frequently used in various combinations in medicine.

sulphuric acid (sul-fū′rik): Heavy, colourless, odourless, oily liquid; extremely corrosive and caustic.

summer diarrhoea: Acute diarrhoea; occurs chiefly in children; caused by enteropathogenic bacteria and usually associated with poorly refrigerated food.

sump drain: A double-lumen drain of rubber or plastic with lateral openings and fish-tail end, used to remove accumulated fluids from the stomach, with or without suction; provides for continuous drainage, accurate measurement of drainage material, and prevents irritation to the skin from the gastric secretion.

sun: S. BATH exposure of the naked body to sunlight for therapeutic purposes; S. BLINDNESS caused by retinal damage from looking at the sun without proper eye protection; may be temporary or permanent.

sunburn: Reddening of the skin or dermatitis, caused by direct exposure to the rays of the sun. The reaction varies with the individual and the degree of exposure.

sundowning (sun-down′ing): A condition seen in some elderly individuals who become disoriented or confused towards the end of the day. These people have some loss of vision and/or hearing and of the sense of touch. With less light, they lose visual cues that help them to compensate for their sensory impairments. Also called *sundowner′s syndrome*.

sunstroke: A condition produced by overexposure to the direct rays of the sun; marked by convulsions, coma, and high temperature of the skin. See STROKE.

super-: Combining form denoting (1) situated above, over; (2) extra, in addition; (3) in excess; (4) higher in degree, quantity or quality.

superactivity (sū′per-ak-tiv′i-ti): Hyperactivity.

superacute (sū′per-a-kūt): Extremely acute.

superalimentation (sū′per-al-i-men-tā′shun): Overfeeding or overeating.

supercilium (sū′per-sil′i-um): The eyebrow. — supercilia, pl.; superciliary, adj.

superego (sū-per-ē′gō): That part of the personality that is concerned with moral standards and ideals, derived mainly from parents, teachers, and others in the environment. The theoretical part of the mind; popularly referred to as the conscience.

superfecundation (sū′per-fē-kun-dā′shun): The fertilization of more than one ovum during one intermenstrual period but at different acts of coitus; results in dizygotic twins.

superfetation (sū′per-fē-tā′shun): The presence of two fetuses of different ages in the uterus; they are not twins but the result of impregnation of two ova released at successive ovulations.

superficial (sū′per-fish′al): **1.** At or near the surface. **2.** Not serious or dangerous.

superficies (sū-per-fish′i-ēz): The outer surface.

supergenual (sū-per-jen′ū-al): Above the knee.

superinfection (sū-per-in-fek′shun): A second infection developing in a person who has not recovered from a different one; caused by a bacterium or fungus that is resistant to the drugs being used to treat the original infection; may occur at the site of the original infection or at a site remote from it.

superior (sū-pēr′i-or): Situated above. In anatomy, the upper of two parts. S. VENA CAVA the venous trunk that drains blood from the head, neck, upper extremities and chest and empties it into the right atrium.

superior vena cava syndrome: A condition characterized by engorgement of the vessels of the upper trunk, flushing of the face, neck, and upper arms; caused by pressure on the superior vena cava and its tributaries; most often seen in lung cancer.

superlactation (sū-per-lak-tā'shun): Excessive secretion of milk or excessive continuance of lactation.

superlethal (sū-per-lē'thal): Extremely lethal; refers to a dose of a drug that is larger than the dose that produces death.

supernumerary (sū-per-nū'mer-ar-i): In excess of the normal number; additional.

superscription (sū'per-skrip'shun): The R$_x$ sign at the beginning of a prescription; it stands for recipe.

supersensitive (sū'per-sen'si-tiv): Abnormally sensitive; usually referring to a foreign protein or other antigenic substance.

supinate (sū'pin-āt): 1. To turn the face upwards or to assume the supine position. 2. To turn the palm upwards or to turn the sole of the foot inward. Opp. of pronate.

supination (sū'pi-nā'shun): 1. The position of the forearm and hand when the palm is turned up or the foot when the sole is turned up and inward. 2. The position of lying on the back, face up. Opp. of pronation.

supinator (sū'pin-ā-tor): That which supinates (q.v.), usually applied to a muscle of the forearm. Opp. of pronator.

supine (sū-pīn'): Lying on the back with the face and palms of the hands turned upward. Having the palm of the hand turned upwards or outward. Opp. of prone.

supplemental air: That air that remains in the lung after an ordinary expiration but which can be exhaled when one makes a forcible effort to do so.

supportive (sū-por'tiv): Refers to any person, device, or measure that assists, supports, maintains, or, in any other way helps a patient. s. THERAPY any form of treatment that reinforces the patient's own defences or ability to overcome a physical or emotional disability.

suppository (su-poz'i-tō-ri): Medicament in a semisolid base that remains solid at room temperature but melts at body temperature, for insertion into a body orifice other than the mouth, e.g., rectum, vagina, urethra. Usually a cone or cylinder made of glycerinated gelatin, certain glycols, or cocoa butter.

suppressant (su-pres'ant): 1. Having a suppressing effect. 2. An agent that reduces or stops a secretion, excretion, or normal body discharge. In psychoanalysis, the conscious effort to ignore or control feelings, thoughts, or acts that are unacceptable.

suppression (su-presh'un): 1. Holding back; repressing; arresting; 2. Cessation or arrest of a secretion (e.g., urine) or a normal process (e.g., menstruation), as distinguished from retention (q.v.). In psychology, the conscious, intentional forcing out of the mind of unacceptable thoughts or feelings; may result in the precipitaton of a neurosis (q.v.); to be differentiated from repression (q.v.).

suppurant (sup'ū-rant): 1. Producing suppuration. 2. Any agent that promotes suppuration.

suppurate (sup'pū-rāt): To form or discharge pus.

suppuration (sup'ū-rā'shun): The formation or discharge of pus. — suppurative, adj,; suppurate, v.

supra-: Combining form denoting (1) a situation above, over, or higher; (2) beyond. Often used interchangeably with super-.

supracondylar (sū-pra-kon'di-lar): Situated above a condyle.

supradiaphragmatic (sū-pra-dī-a-frag-mat'ik): Situated above the diaphragm.

supraglottic (sū-pra-glot'ik): Situated above the glottis.

suprainfection (sū-pra-in-fek'shun): 1. An infection or disease occurring in a patient weakened by another disease. 2. An infection occurring after antibiotic treatment for another infection.

supraliminal (sū-pra-lim'i-nal): Above the threshold of consciousness; referring to a stimulus that is more than just strong enough to be perceived.

supraorbital (sū-pra-or'bit-al): Above the orbits. s. RIDGE the ridge formed by the prominence of the frontal bone; the eyebrows are situated over this ridge.

suprapatellar (sū-pra-pa-tel'ar): Situated above the patella. s. BURSA the bursa that lies between the tendon of the quadriceps muscle and the front of the lower end of the femur; s. REFLEX the sudden upwards movement of the patella when the quadriceps muscle contracts in response to a sharp blow on the examiner's finger, which rests on the upper border of the patella with the leg in extension.

suprapubic (sū-pra-pū'bic): Performed or situated above the pubic arch. s. CYSTOTOMY surgical opening of the bladder just above the pubis; S. PROSTATECTOMY see PROSTATECT-OMY.

suprarenal (sū-pra-rē'nal): **1.** Situated above the kidney. **2.** Tiny endocrine gland just above each kidney. Syn., *adrenal* (*q.v.*).

suprarenalectomy (sū'pra-rē-nal-ek'to-mi): Surgical removal of the adrenal gland(s).

suprascapular (sū-pra-scap'ū-lar): Situated above or in the upper part of the scapula.

supraspinal (sū-pra-spī'nal): Situated above a spine or the spinal column.

suprasternal (sū-pra-ster'nal): Situated above the sternum. S. NOTCH the U-shaped curve at the top of the manubrium of the sternum.

supraumbilical (sū-pra-um-bil'i-kal): Situated above the navel.

supraventricular (sū-pra-ven-trik'ū-lar): Located, occurring, or originating above a ventricle of the heart or above the branching of the bundle of His. S. RHYTHM any rhythm originating above the bifurcation of the bundle of His; S. TACHYCARDIA an arrhythmia characterized by atrial contractions at a very fast rate.

supravergence (sū-pra-ver'jens): The upwards movement of one eye while the other eye remains stationary.

sura (sū'rah): The calf of the leg. — sural, adj.

surdimutitas (sur-di-mū-tī-tas): Deafmutism.

surditas, surdity (sur'di-tas, sur'di-ti): Deafness.

Sure Start: A drive to eradicate child poverty in the UK. The programme aims to improve the health and well-being of families and children, before and from birth, so children have the opportunity to realize their full potential when they go to school.

surface: The exterior of any solid body. S. TENSION see under TENSION.

surfactant (sur-fak'tant): A lipoprotein substance that is manufactured in the alveoli of the lungs and lines them; it serves to decrease the surface tension of pulmonary fluids and permits the lungs to expand during inspiration and prevents them from collapsing during exhalation. In the newborn it reduces the adhesion between the unexpanded walls of the alveoli. See RESPIRATORY DISTRESS SYNDROME.

surfer's nodules: Traumatic nodules that form on the front of the legs and feet, due to repeated bumping from a surf board or other activity on which the leg is repeatedly hit.

surgeon (sur'jun): A medical practitioner who treats disease, disorders, or deformities by operative procedures.

surgery (sur'jer-i): The branch of medicine that treats diseases, deformities, and injuries, wholly or in part, by manual or operative procedures; usually involves making an opening in the body to remove, replace, or repair a part in order to cure or correct a pathological condition or damage caused by trauma, or to give the patient a period of remission from a disease. ASEPTIC S. that performed in a field kept free of pathogenic bacteria; CLOSED S. that done without making an incision, as in reducing a fracture; CLOSED-HEART S. that in which the myocardium is not invaded and normal cardiac circulation is maintained; can be utilized in performing valvulotomy; CONSERVATIVE S. that in which injured or diseased parts are repaired but removal is avoided if possible; ELECTIVE S. that which can be done at the patient's or surgeon's convenience when the delay would not endanger the health status or life of the patient; MAJOR S. important and serious operations that may involve risk to life; MINOR S. simpler, less serious operations that do not usually involve risk to life; OPEN-HEART s. involves opening the heart and establishing extral corporeal circulation; utilized in heart transplant operations, insertion of prosthetic heart valves, correction of congenital anomalies, or repair of ruptured aortic aneurysm; ORAL s. that done to treat disorders of the mouth and teeth; a branch of dentistry; ORTHOPAEDIC S. that which treats diseases or deformities of the skeletal system; PLASTIC S. that which repairs or reconstructs a tissue or part by such methods as skin grafting or transplanting of other tissue; RADICAL S. that which is extensive and thorough enough to be curative rather than palliative; often said of mastectomy that includes removal of the entire breast along with the pectoral muscles, axillary lymph nodes, and contiguous lymph tissue; TRANSSEXUAL S. that which alters the external appearance and characteristic of a person so as to make them resemble those of the opposite sex.

surgical (sur'ji-kal): Relating to or involving surgery.

surrogate (sur'ō-gāt): A substitute or replacement for something or someone.

survey: 1. The act of viewing, examining, or inspecting in detail, esp. for some specific purpose. **2.** A formal or official inspection of the particulars of something. **3.** A method used to gather data from a sample of the population. In studies of individuals the information is gathered using questionnaires, face-to-face or telephone interviews. Survey data are used to describe a population and used to establish trends. See CENSUS.

susceptibility (sus-sep-ti-bil'i-ti): The opposite of resistance. Usually refers to a disposition to infection.

suspension (sus-pen'shun): 1. Temporary cessation, as of a vital process. 2. A mixture in which finely divided particles are dispersed throughout a liquid and remain undissolved even after stirring or shaking vigorously. 3. A method of treatment whereby a part or the whole of a person's body is suspended in a desired position. 4. The fixation of an organ or part in correct position by suturing it to other tissues, *e.g.*, suspension of the uterus.

suspensory (sus-pen'so-ri): 1. Descriptive of a structure, often a ligament, that functions to hold an organ or part in correct position, *e.g.*, the suspensory ligament of the eye, which passes from the lens to the ciliary body and holds the lens in place. 2. A bandage or other material used to support a dependent part or organ, *e.g.*, the scrotum.

sustenance (sus'ten-ans): That which sustains life; nourishment; food.

sustentacular (sus'ten-tak'ūl lar): Supporting or sustaining; said of cells, fibres, tissues.

susurrus (su-sūr'us): A soft murmur.

sutura (sū-tū'ra): An immovable joint in which the bones are united by fibrous tissue that is continuous with the periosteum covering the bones, *e.g.*, the joints in the skull bones. Also called *suture*.

suture (sū'chur): 1. The fibrous joint where the opposed bony surfaces are very closely united by the connective tissue, permitting movement only in the neonate. 2. A stitch or series of stitches used to close a wound. 3. The act of stitching to close a wound. 4. The material used to close a wound by stitching; see LIGA-TURE; ABSORBABLE S. one made with a material that is liquefied in the body and absorbed; CONTINUOUS S. one of a series of sutures made with one length of material; INTERRUPTED S. one of a series of sutures, each one being made with a separate piece of material; MAT-TRESS S. strong non-absorbable suture that goes through the deeper tissues either vertically or parallel to the skin sutures; used to maintain strong repair in obese patients and those with weak musculature; NON-ABSORB-ABLE S. one that is not liquefied and absorbed by the body; made of cotton, silk, or nylon thread, or stainless stell; remains in the tissues when great strength is needed. Screws and plates used in bone repair are the equivalent of non-absorbable sutures in other tissues; PURSE-STRING S. a stitching around the edge of a circular opening that is then drawn up tightly to close the opening.

SVQ: Abbreviation for Scottish Vocational Qualification (*q.v.*).

SVT: Abbreviation for supraventricular tachycardia, see under SUPRAVENTRICULAR.

swab (swob): 1. To use a small tuft of cotton or similar material to cleanse an area or a cavity, absorb an exudate, or apply a medication. 2. A small piece of cotton or similar material wound firmly around one or both ends of a shaft of wire or wood; used to cleanse a cavity, apply a medication, or collect a specimen for laboratory examination; in the latter case it is sterilized and within a protective tube.

swallow: To pass food or any other material through the mouth, pharynx, and oesophagus into the stomach. BARIUM S. see under BARIUM.

Swan–Ganz catheter: See under CATHETER.

swan neck deformity: 1. A finger deformity in which the distal interphalangeal joint is flexed while the proximal joint is extended, giving the finger the appearance of a swan's neck. 2. An abnormality of the convoluted part of the kidney tubules which is distorted into the shape of a swan's neck; associated with rickets.

swathe (swāth): To envelop, cover, wrap or bind tightly as with a bandage.

S wave: The sharp downwards deflection in the electrocardiogram that follows the peak of the R wave to the beginning of the upwards curve of the T wave.

swayback: Increased lumbar lordosis accompanied by compensatory kypnosis.

sweat: 1. Sudor; a clear fluid secreted by the sweat glands in the skin; consists of water, salt, and waste products from the blood; is eliminated through channels that end in pores in the skin. 2. To perspire or sweat. S. TEST a diagnostic procedure used in cystic fibrosis of the pancreas; it is a measurement of the sodium and chloride in the sweat; see CYSTIC FIBROSIS; NIGHT S. profuse sweating while asleep; often a symptom of pulmonary tuberculosis and of AIDS. See PERSPIRATION.

swelling (swel'ling): A transient, abnormal elevation or enlargement of a body part or area, usually on the surface, that is not caused by new growth or proliferation of cells; may be due to injury, inflammation, or oedema.

swimmer's ear: Otitis media caused by an infection contracted in water, often that in swimming pools.

'swimmer's' shoulder: A syndrome sometimes seen in long-distance swimmers; the rotator cuff impinges over the shoulder and catches on the undersurface of the coracoacromial ligament.

'swimming pool' conjunctivitis: See under CONJUNCTIVITIS.

swineherd's disease: A disease caused by the *Leptospira pomona*, an organism that is harboured in swine; may be transmitted to humans, causing a form of leptospirosis characterized by aseptic meningitis.

swoon: A faint. See SYNCOPE.

SWOT analysis: A useful tool for industry, to gauge the strengths and weaknesses of a programme and to survey threats and opportunities.

sycoma (sī-kō'ma): A large soft wart-like growth.

Sydenham's chorea: See under CHOREA.

syllepsis (si-lep'sis): Pregnancy.

sylvatic (sil-vat'ik): Relating to or found in the woods. S. PLAGUE an endemic disease of wild rodents caused by *Yersinia pestis* and transmissible to humans by the bite of an infected flea. It is found on every continent except Australia.

Sylvius (sil'vi-us): FISSURE OF S. a deep fissure at the side of each cerebral hemisphere; the temporal lobe lies below. — sylvian, adj. [Franciscus de la Boë Sylvius, Dutch physician, 1614–1672.]

sym-: Combining forms denoting: **1.** Together; union of; association; similar to. **2.** At the same time.

symbiosis (sim-bi-ō'sis): In biology, close relationship between two similar organisms, or between organisms of different species, when this is necessary for the survival of both. In the family, s. usually refers to the relationship between mother and child. In psychiatry, s. refers to a close relationship between two disturbed individuals who are emotionally dependent on each other.

symblepharon (sim-blef'a-ron): Adhesion of one or both of the lids to the eyeball.

symbol (sim'bol): A letter, mark, or sign that represents an idea or word(s) or, in chemistry, an atom or group of atoms of an element.

symbolia (sim-bō'li-a): The ability to recognize objects through the sense of touch.

symbolic interaction: An approach to studying human behaviour that emphasizes the sharing and use of common symbols in human communication. Developed by the sociologist George Mead as an alternative to functionalism.

symbolization (sim'bol-ī-zā'shun): In psychiatry, the unconscious substitution of a symbol

to express thoughts or ideas that the individual had previously been unable or unwilling to accept or express.

symmetrical (sim-et'rik-al): Even; balanced; the same on both sides; in anatomy, refers to parts of the body.

symmetry (sim'e-tri): Correspondence or equality of size, shape, location, and general characteristics of things, or, in anatomy, of two parts of the body. — symmetric, symmetrical, adj.

sympathectomy (sim-pa-thek'to-mi): Surgical excision of a sympathetic nerve or surgical interruption of sympathetic nerve pathways which results in dilatation of blood vessels and increased blood flow to a part. — sympathectomize, v.

sympathetic (sim-pa-thet'ik): **1.** Exhibiting sympathy. **2.** Influenced by or produced by disease in another part of the body. S. NERVOUS SYSTEM see under NERVOUS SYSTEM.

sympatholytic (sim-path-ō-lit'ik): **1.** An adrenergic blocking agent (*q.v.*). **2.** Having an antagonistic effect on activity produced by a stimulant to the sympathetic nervous system.

sympathomimetic (sim-path-ō-mi-met'ik): Capable of producing changes similar to those produced in stimulation of the sympathetic nerves. S. AMINES a group of specific drugs that act as vasoconstrictors, bronchodilators, and sympathetic nervous system stimulants.

symphysiotomy (sim-fiz'i-ot'o-mi): The surgical separation of the mother's pubic bone, at its symphysis, to facilitate the birth of a living child.

symphysis (sim'fi-sis): A very slightly movable joint in which there is a fibrocartilaginous union of bones, as occurs between the two parts of the pubic bone, the vertebrae, and the sacrum and ilium. — symphyses, pl.; symphysiac, symphyseal, symphysial, adj.

symptom (simp'ton): Any morbid phenomenon, condition, or other perceptible evidence of disease. CARDINAL S. a major s., especially one that pertains to temperature, pulse, or respiration; DEFICIENCY S. one that indicates reduction in or lack of secretion of an endocrine gland, or lack of a vital element in the patient's diet; OBJECTIVE S. one apparent to the observer; PRESENTING S. the s. or group of symptoms the patient complains of most; PRODROMAL S. one that precedes the diagnostic symptoms of a disease; SUBJECTIVE S. one that is apparent only to the patient; SYMPTOM COMPLEX a group of symptoms which, occurring together, typify a particular disease or syndrome; WITHDRAWAL S. any of the physiological or psychological symptoms that occur when a drug or chemical to which an individual has become habituated, is withdrawn; also called *abstinence syndrome*.

symptomatic (simp'tō-mat'ik): Relating to, constituting, or of the nature of a symptom or symptoms.

symptomatology (simp'tom-a-tol'ol ji): 1. The branch of medicine concerned with symptoms. 2. The combined symptoms typical of a particular disease.

symptothermal method (sim-tō-therm'al): Term used to describe a rhythm method of natural family planning based on the woman's ability to recognize and keep a record of changes in basal body temperature, and changes in the cervical mucus during the menstrual cycle.

syn-: Combining form denoting with, together, union of, or association with.

synaesthesia (sin-es-thē'zi-a): A secondary or concomitant sensation accompanying a sensory response, or one perceived by a sense organ other than the one stimulated as happens, *e.g.*, when a certain sound produces a sensation of colour.

synapse (sīn'aps): The point of communication between two neurons; it is where the axon of one neuron comes into close proximity to the dendrites or cell body of another neuron and an impulse is chemically transmitted; impulses travel only in one direction at the synapse. — synapses, pl.; synaptic, adj.

synapsis (sī-nap'sis): The pairing of homologous chromosomes during the early stage of meiosis (*q.v.*).

synarthrosis (sin'ar-thrō'sis): An immovable articulation of bones that are held tightly together by fibrous connective tissue; two types of S. are sutures, as occur between the flat bones of the skull, and syndesmoses, as occur between the distal ends of the tibia and fibula.

synchondrosis (sin'kon-drō'sis): A type of joint in which the bones are held together by cartilage which, in certain joints, is eventually replaced by bone, as occurs in the epiphyses of long bones; the cartilage that joins the ribs to the sternum is not replaced by bone and is a permanent synchondrosis. — synchondroses, pl.

synchronous (sin'kro-nus): Occurring at the same time or together; simultaneous.

syncope (sin'kō-pi): A faint or temporary loss of consciousness, caused by cerebral ischaemia. May be a symptom of disease or may result

from a sudden change to the upright position, or may be associated with an emotional experience such as fright when the peripheral blood vessels dilate and drain the blood from the brain. The loss of consciousness is usually temporary. — syncopal, adj.

syncretio (sin-krē'shi-ō): The growing together, or development of adhesions between two opposing inflamed serous surfaces.

syncytiotrophoblast (sin-sish'i-ō-trō'fō-blast): The outer layer of the trophoblast (*q.v.*), consisting of a syncytium (*q.v.*).

syncytium (sin-sish'i-um): A mass of protoplasm with multiple nuclei, produced by the merging of cells. — syncytial, adj.

syndactyly (sin-dak'ti-li): A congenital anomaly in which the fingers and/or toes are webbed. Also called *syndactylism, syndactylia*. — syndactylous, adj.

syndesis (sin-dē'sis): The condition of being bound or fused together; see ARTHRODESIS.

syndesmitis (sin-des-mī'tis): 1. Conjunctivitis. 2. Inflammation of a ligament.

syndesmosis (sin'des-mō'sis): A fixed joint (synarthrosis) in which the surfaces of the bones are joined to each other by fibrous connective tissue, with the opposing surfaces being relatively far apart as occurs, *e.g.*, in the joints at the distal ends of the tibia and fibula.

syndrome (sin'drōm): A group of symptoms and/or signs that, occurring together, produce a pattern or symptom complex that is typical of a particular disease, disturbance, disorder, or lesion. — syndromic, adj.

synechia (si-nek'i-a): Abnormal union of parts, especially adhesion of the iris to the cornea in front, or to the lens capsule behind. — synechiae, pl.

syneresis (si-ner'e-sis): The action of drawing together the dispersed particles of a substance, as occurs in clotting of blood. S. OF THE VITREOUS liquefaction of the vitreous of the eye.

synergism (sin'er-jizm): Synergy (*q.v.*).

synergist (sin'er-jist): One of the partners in a synergistic action, *i.e.*, a drug, substance, or organ that stimulates or augments the action of another drug, substance, or organ. See SYNERGY. — synergistic, adj.

synergy (sin'er-ji): 1. In pharmacology, the combined action of two agents which is usually greater or more effective than the sum of their individual actions. 2. In anatomy, the coordination of actions of muscles and organs by the central nervous system, to produce specific motions or functions. — synergic, adj.

synophthalmus (sin'of-thal'mus): Cyclops (*q.v.*).

synorchism (sin'-ōr-kizm): Congenital fusion of the testes into one mass, usually within the abdomen.

synostosis (sin'os-tō'sis): The fusion of adjacent bones that are normally separate; also called *synosteosis*.

synovectomy (sin'-ō-vek'to-mi): Excision of synovial membrane. Current early treatment for rheumatoid arthritis, especially of the hands and of the knees.

synovia (si-nō'vi-a): The transparent, alkaline, viscous fluid secreted by the membrane lining a joint cavity; its function is to lubricate and thus minimize friction during joint movement. Syn., *synovial fluid*.

synovial (sin-ō'vi-al): Relating to or containing synovia (*q.v.*). S. BURSA in anatomy, a small synovia-filled sac that lies between two parts that move upon each other; s. CAPSULE the fibrous sheet that encloses a synovial joint; s. CHONDROMATOSIS an uncommon condition in which folds of the s. membrane change to cartilaginous bodies that often become calcified and then separate, becoming freely movable; s. FLUID synovia; s. JOINT a freely movable joint, as the elbow or hip; s. MEMBRANE the fluid-secreting membrane that lines a joint capsule.

synovioma (sin-nō-vi-ō'ma): A tumour of synovial membrane origin. BENIGN S. a giant-cell tumour of a tendon sheath; MALIGNANT S. synoviosarcoma; arises in the synovial membrane of joints, and sometimes in the synovial cells of tendons and bursae.

synoviosarcoma (si-nō'vi-ō-sar-kō'ma): Malignant synovioma (*q.v.*).

synovitis (sin-ō' vī'tis): Inflammation of a synovial membrane.

synovium (si-nō'vi-um): A synovial membrane lining a joint cavity.

synthesis (sin'the-sis): The forming of a complex substance by combining chemical elements or simpler compounds. — synthetic, adj.; synthesize, v.

synthesize (sin'the-sīz): To make or form chemically by means of synthesis.

synthetic (sin-thet'ik): Produced by artificial means.

syntonic (sin-ton'ik): Refers to a stable personality that responds to the various elements in the environment in a normal manner, as contrasted with the schizoid type of personality.

syphilid (e) (sif'i-lid,-līd): General term for any syphilitic skin lesion.

syphilis (sif'il-is): [Syphilis, syphilitic shepherd in poem by Fracastorius (1530), in which the term first appears.] A severe contagious venereal disease, caused by the *Treponema pallidum*. Infection is acquired, commonly by sexual intercourse, or the fetus may acquire it from the mother while *in utero*. CONGENITAL s. present at birth; marked by coryza, skin eruptions, malformed teeth, wasting of the tissues, and craniotabes (*q.v.*); ACQUIRED S. manifests in (1) the primary stage; appears 4 to 5 weeks (or later) after infection when a primary chancre associated with swelling or local lymph glands appears; (2) the secondary stage in which the skin eruption appears; (3) the third (tertiary) stage occurs 15 to 30 years after initial infection; gummata appear, or neurosyphilis and cardiovascular s. intervene. The commonest types of nervous system involvement are general paresis and tabes dorsalis (locomotor ataxia). Cardiovascular involvement produces cerebrovascular disasters, aortic aneurism, or destruction of the aortic valve. LATENT S., s. for which there is serological or historical evidence but no other symptoms; MENINGOVASCULAR S., s. affecting the meninges, with narrowing of the cerebral arteries in the leptomeninges, which may lead to occlusion and infarcts in the brain and spinal cord. — syphilitic, adj.

syphilitic (sif-i-lit'ik): Of, relating to, affected with, or caused by, syphilis.

syphiloid (sif'i-loyd): 1. Resembling syphilis. 2. A condition resembling syphilis.

syphiloma (sif-i-lō'ma): A tumour of syphilitic origin; a gumma.

syrigmus (si-rig'mus): Ringing in the ears.

syringadenoma (sir'ing-ad-e-nō'ma): An adenoma of a sweat gland.

syringe (si-rinj'): An instrument for injecting or withdrawing liquids; of differing sizes and designs depending upon the specific purpose for which it is used.

syringitis (sir'in-jī'tis): Inflammation of the auditory tube(s).

syringobulbia (si-ring'gō-bul'bi-a): The presence of a fluid-filled cavity or cavities in the medulla oblongata.

syringomyelia (si-ring'gō-mī-ē'li-a): An uncommon progressive disease of the nervous system, of unknown cause that may be due to trauma or defective embryonic development, beginning mainly in early adult life. Cavitation and surrounding fibrous tissue reaction, in the upper spinal cord and brain stem, interfere with sensations of pain and temperature, and sometimes with the motor pathways. The characteristic symptom is painless injury, particularly of the exposed hands. Touch sensation is intact.

syringomyelocele (si-ring'gō-mī'e-lō-sēl): Most severe form of meningeal hernia (spina bifida). The central canal is dilated and the thinned-out posterior part of the spinal cord is in the hernia which protrudes through a defect in the dorsal aspect of the vertebral column.

syrinx (sir'inks): 1. A pathologic tube or pipe. 2. A fistula. 3. The cavity that forms in spinal cord or brainstem in syringomyelia.

syrup (si'rup): A concentrated solution of sugar and water usually containing a drug.

system (sis'-tem): 1. A network of things so connected as to form a whole. 2. An established way of doing something; a method. 3. In anatomy, (a) a group of organs that work together to perform a particular function, or (b) the entire (physical) body organism. — systemic, systematic, adj.

systematic review: A review of clinical literature in a particular field that has set explicit tests to determine whether research is valuable enough to be included in an overview of the area. This is often combined with a statistical meta-analysis of clinical trial results.

systemic (sis-tem'ik): 1. Related to a particular system of the body. 2. Related to the body as a whole. s. CIRCULATION circulation of the blood through all parts of the body except the lungs; SYSTEMIC LUPUS ERYTHEMATOSUS see under LUPUS.

Systemized Nomenclature of Medicine: A coding system for clinical conditions, devised by the American College of Pathologists; superseding the Read Coding system (q.v.).

systems theory: A method of scientific inquiry whereby a particular entity involving human relationships is considered on the basis of resources, input, and outcomes, with feedback at each level leading to progress to the next level and allowing for ongoing evaluation. In nursing, the use of systems theory can be helpful in providing direction for assessment of patients, as well as planning and implementing care.

systole (sis'to-le): The contraction phase of the cardiac cycle; the total ventricular process. Alternates with diastole (q v.). EXTRA-SYSTOLE a premature contraction of an atrium or ventricle, or both, which does not alter the fundamental rhythm of contractions. — systolic, adj.

systremma (sis-trem'a): A cramp in the muscles of the leg, the calf muscles in particular.

T

tabacosis (tab-a-kō'sis): A chronic form of tobacco poisoning; usually caused by inhalation of tobacco dust.

tabella (ta-bel'a): A medicated troche or tablet.

tabes (tā'bēz): Progressive emaciation; wasting away. Term usually used in connection with tabes dorsalis. T. DORSALIS (*locomotor ataxia*), a variety of neurosyphilis in which there is progressive sclerosis of the posterior (sensory) columns of the spinal cord, the sensory nerve root and the peripheral nerves. It is marked by muscular incoordination, ataxia (*q.v.*), anaesthesia, joint disorders, neuralgia, sometimes paralysis; usually occurs after middle life. T. MESENTERICA tuberculous enlargement of the peritoneal lymph nodes; seen in children.

tabescense (ta-bes'ens): The state of wasting away, or progressive emaciation; atrophy. — tabescent, adj.

tabetic (ta-bet'ik): 1. Relating to tabes. 2. Affected with tabes. T. ARTHROPATHY Charcot's joint (*q.v.*); T. GAIT the ataxic gait of tabes dorsalis.

tablature (tab'la-tūr): The division or separation of the main cranial bones into two tables or plates which are separated by a layer of cancellous bone.

table: 1. In anatomy, the external or internal layer of compact bone, separated by a layer of cancellous bony tissue (diploe), that make up the main bones of the cranium. 2. An orderly presentation of numerical data or steps in an experiment, arranged in rows or columns showing the essential facts, for quick reference and comparison.

tablet: In pharmacology, a small disc of varying size and thickness, containing a dose of a medication, in either pure or diluted form. BUCCAL T. a T. that is inserted into the buccal pouch where it dissolves quickly and the essential ingredients are absorbed directly by the buccal mucosa; ENTERIC-COATED T. a T. coated with a material that delays release of the essential ingredients until after the tablet has left the stomach; SUBLINGUAL T. a T. that is placed under the tongue and held there until it is dissolved.

taboo, tabu (ta-boo'): 1. Any behaviour regarded as unacceptable or harmful to the social wel-

fare. 2. A prohibition imposed by social usage or for the protection of the group. INCEST T. relating to sexual activity between persons so closely related that marriage is prohibited.

taboparesis (tā'bō-par-ē'sis): A condition in which the spinal cord shows the same lesions as in tabes dorsalis (*q.v.*) and there is general paresis. Also called *taboparalysis*.

TABS: A useful acronym in checking the newborn's adjustment to the environment; refers to *t*emperature, *a*irway, *b*reathing, *s*ugar (blood glucose level).

tabular (tab'ū-lar): 1. Laminated or table-like, or having a flat surface. 2. Arranged in the form of a table, or resembling a table.

tachogram (tak'ō-gram): The graphic record made by tachography.

tachography (ta-kog'ra-fi): The recording of movement and velocity of arterial blood flow. Also called *tachygraphy*.

tachometer (ta-kom'i-ter): An instrument for measuring the speed of a moving object or substance. Also called *tachymeter*.

tachy-: Combining form denoting rapid, swift, accelerated.

tachyarrhythmia (tak'i-a-rith'mi-a): A heartbeat of 100 or more per minute; may or may not be regular.

tachycardia (tak'i-kar'di-a): Very rapid heart action (over 100 beats per minute in adults) with resulting increase in pulse rate; some of the causes are heart diseases, hyperthyroidism, high fever, toxaemia. PAROXYSMAL ATRIAL T. regular heart rhythm with an atrial rate of 150–250 per minute; often associated with acute respiratory disorders and with most forms of heart disease; PAROXYSMAL T. sudden marked increase in the pulse rate, lasting for various lengths of time and then disappearing; sometimes accompanies failing heart muscle action, but in some people it is of nervous origin; SINUS T., T. that originates in the sinoatrial node; SUPRAVENTRICULAR T. rapid heartbeat caused by an ectopic pacemaker located above the ventricles; see ECTOPIC BEAT; VENTRICULAR T. rapid regular heartbeat due to an ectopic stimulus in the conduction system of the ventricle. — tachycardiac, adj.

tachycrotic (tak'i-krot'ik): Relating to, causing, or characterized by an increased pulse rate.

tachylalia (tak-i-lā'li-a): Rapidity of speech.

tachylogia (tak-i-lō'ji-a): Extremely rapid or voluble speech.

tachyphagia (tak-i-fā'ji-a): Abnormally rapid eating, bolting of food.

tachyphrasia (tak-i-frā'zi-a): Volubility; extremely rapid flow of speech; may be seen in certain nervous disorders. Also called *tachyphasia*.

tachyphrenia (tak-i-frē'ni-a): Hyperactivity of the mental processes.

tachyphylaxis (tak-i-fi-lak'sis): The progressive decrease in response to a drug or other substance that produces a physiological action, following repeated administration of small doses.

tachypnoea (tak-ip-nē'a): Abnormal frequency of respiration, *i.e.*, over 20 per minute, in response to low oxygen or high carbon dioxide content of the blood; often seen in hysteria, neurasthenia, high fevers, respiratory infection; sometimes but not always accompanied by dyspnoea (*q.v.*), — tachypnoeic, adj.

tachypsychia (tak-i-sī'ki-a): Rapidity of psychic or mental responses or processes.

tachyrhythmia (tak-i-rith'mi-a): See TACHYCARDIA.

tachysystole (tak-i-sis'tō-lē): Tachycardia (*q.v.*).

tachytrophism (tak-i-trō'fizm): Unusually rapid metabolism.

tacit knowledge (ta'-sit): A term used to describe personal practical knowledge that cannot easily be put into words or articulated to others. Knowledge that is shared but not openly articulated.

tactile (tak'til): 1. Relating to the sense of touch. 2. Perceptible through the sense of touch. 3. Real, tangible. T. AGNOSIA loss of the ability to recognize objects by touch due to a cerebral lesion; T. ANAESTHESIA loss of the ability to perceive touch; T. CORPUSCLES see MEISSNER'S CORPUSCLES; T. SENSATION a sensation produced through the sense of touch.

tactometer (tak-tom'i-ter): An instrument for measuring an individual's acuity for the sense of touch.

tactual (tak'tū-al): Relating to or caused by touch.

tactus (tak'tus): Touch; the sense of touch.

Taenia (tē'ni-a): A genus of flat, parasitic worms; cestodes or tapeworms. In T. *echinococcus*, the adult worm lives in the intestines of dogs (the definitive host) and humans (the intermediate host) are infested by swallowing food contaminated by eggs from the dog's ex-

crement. These become embryos in the human small intestine, pass via the bloodstream to organs, particularly the liver, and develop into hydatid cysts. T. *saginata* larvae are present in infested, undercooked beef. In the human intestinal lumen they develop into the adult tapeworm, which, by its four suckers attaches itself to the gut wall. It grows to 3.5–7.5 m in length. Consists of a head and numerous segments, each one being capable of independent existence; consequently, in any treatment, it is necessary for the head to be expelled. T. *solium* resembles T. *saginata*, but has hooklets as well as suckers, length 2–3.5 m. The larvae are ingested in infested, undercooked pork; humans can also be the intermediate host for this worm by ingesting eggs which, developing into larvae in the human stomach, pass via the bowel wall to reach organs, and there develop into cysts. In the brain these may give rise to epilepsy.

taenia (tē'ni-a): 1. An organism of the genus *Taenia* (*q.v.*) 2. A flat band or strip of soft tissue. T. COLI three flat bands running the length of the large intestine and consisting of longitudinal muscle fibres; they pucker the walls of the colon to form pouches (haustra).

taeniasis (tē-nī'a-sis): Infestation with *Taenia* (*q.v.*).

tag: 1. A label; tracer. 2. To incorporate into a compound a substance that is more readily visible. 3. A small appendage, polyp, or outgrowth of skin.

tail: 1. The caudal extremity of an animal. 2. Anything resembling a tail, such as an elongated part of an organ. T. OF SPENCE the tissue of the mammary gland that extends into the axillary region; may become enlarged premenstrually or during lactation.

tailor's ankle: An abnormal condition of the bursa over the lateral malleolus of the tibia; due to sitting on the floor in a crossed-leg position.

taint (tānt): 1. Putrefaction or infestation. 2. A local discoloration or blemish. 3. A hereditary disposition to some pathological condition or unattractive attribute.

take: In medicine, a successful vaccination or inoculation. In plastic surgery, a successful transplantation of tissue, as a skin graft.

talalgia (tā-lal'ji-a): Pain in the heel.

talar (tā'lar): Of or relating to the talus.

talc, talcum: A naturally occurring soft white powder consisting of magnesium silicate.

talcosis (tal-ko'sis): A pulmonary disorder resembling silicosis (*q.v.*); occurs as an occupational disease of people who work in the talc industry.

taliped, talipedic (tal'i-ped) (tal-i-pēd'ik): Clubfooted.

talipes (tal'i-pēz): Descriptive of several types of congenital foot deformities, especially clubfootedness, of which there are four main types; (1) T. CALCANEUS dorsal flexion of the foot that results in walking with only the heel touching the ground; (2) T. EQUINUS hyperflexion of the foot, which results in walking with only the toes touching the ground; (3) T. VALGUS eversion of the foot, which results in walking on the inner edge of the foot; and (4) T. VARUS inversion of the foot, which results in walking on the outer edge of the foot only (opp. of valgus). Other types include; (1) T. CALCANEOVALGUS a deformity in which the heel is turned outwards and the anterior part of the foot is held elevated; (2) T. CALCANEOVARUS a deformity in which the heel is held towards the midline of the body and the anterior part of the foot is held in elevation; (3) T. EQUINOVALGUS the heel is held elevated and turned outward from the midline; (4) T. EQUINOVARUS the foot is plantar flexed, with the sole turned inward towards the midline; the heel does not touch the ground when the person is walking; this is the most common type of clubfoot. See also PES.

talipomanus (tal-i-pom'a-nus): A congenital or acquired fixed deformity of the hand that is analagous to clubfoot, *i.e.*, the hand is fixed in a position of strong flexion and adduction; also called *clubhand*.

talo-: A combining form denoting the talus.

talocalcaneal (tā'-lō-kal-kā'nē-al): Relating to the talus and the calcaneus. Also called *talocalcanean*.

talocrural (tā'lō-kroo'ral): Relating to the talus and the leg bones. T. ARTICULATION the ankle joint.

talofibular (tā'lō-fib'ū-lar): Relating to the talus and the fibula.

talomalleolar (tā'lō-ma-lē'o-lar): Relating to the talus and the malleolus.

talonavicular (tā'lō-na-vik'ū-lar): Relating to the talus and the navicular bone.

talotibial (tā'lō-tib'i-al): Relating to the talus and the tibia.

talus (tā'lus): The astragalus; situated between the tibia proximally and the calcaneus distally, thus directly bearing the weight of the body. It is the second largest bone of the ankle.

tama (tā'ma): Swelling of the feet and legs.

tampon (tam'pon): 1. A ball of absorbent cotton, gauze, sponge or similar substance used to pack or plug a cavity or canal to restrain haemorrhage, absorb secretions, or apply medication. 2. A type of sanitary towel to be worn internally to absorb menstrual fluid.

tamponade (tam-po-nod'): 1. The surgical insertion of a tampon as a device for checking internal haemorrhage by compression of a viscus. 2. Pathological compression of an organ as in cardiac T.; BALLOON T. oesophagogastric T., utilizing a device consisting of a three-lumen tube and two inflatable balloons; CARDIAC T. the accumulation of fluid in the pericardial sac, impairing heart function and resulting in decreased heart output, hypertension, tachycardia; may result in heart failure; OESOPHAGOGASTRIC T. exertion of pressure against a bleeding oesophageal varix using a tube-shaped balloon; see also VARIX; PERICARDIAL T. compression of the cardiac muscle by fluid accumulated in the pericardial sac; cardiac T.

tandem gait: See under GAIT.

tangentiality (tan-jen'shi-al'i-ti): In conversational speech, a pattern characterized by divergence from the original topic, often leading to an entirely different chain of thought. Also called *loose association*.

Tangier disease: A familial condition in which the lipoprotein in the blood serum is greatly reduced and cholesterol esters are deposited in the reticuloendothelial system; marked by enlarged, yellowish-grey tonsils, lymphadenopathy, and splenomegaly. In adults, the vascular and neurological systems are also involved.

tank: A large receptacle for fluid substances. HUBBARD T. a T. used for underwater exercises, for treatment of certain skin conditions, and for burn therapy.

tanner's disease: Anthrax (*q.v.*).

tannic acid (tan'ik as'id): A substance derived from tannin, which is obtained from nutgalls that form on twigs of certain trees, including the oak; used in medicine as a styptic and astringent, and sometimes in the treatment of burns.

tantrum: An unreasoning fit of anger accompanied usually by violent physical gestures, seen in children and sometimes in mentally disturbed patients. TEMPER T. loud, annoying behaviour, usually seen in children; thought by behavioural psychologists to result from failure of less violent ways of obtaining attention of parents or other significant persons.

tap: 1. A quick blow used in massage or by the physician during examination. 2. Paracentesis (*q.v.*).

tapeworm: See *taenia*.

taphophilia: (taf′ō-fil′i-a): A morbid attraction to graves and burial places.

taphophobia (taf′ō-fō′bi-a): A morbid fear of being buried alive.

tapinocephaly (ta-pi-no-kef′a-li,-sef′): The condition of having a flattened or depressed skull. — tapinocephalic, adj.

tar: A dark-coloured viscous substance obtained from bituminous coal or the wood of certain trees. COAL T. used as a base for some ointments and solutions used in treating skin disorders; PINE T. has several uses in medicine because of its antibacterial and irritant properties.

tarassis (ta-ras′is): The name given to hysteria occurring in a male person.

tardive (tar′div): Late; tardy. T. DYSKINESIA see under DYSKINESIA.

target: To direct or aim on a course.

tarry (tah′ri): Having the consistency and appearance of tar. T. STOOLS usually due to intestinal haemorrhage, but also occur when the patient is receiving certain medications that contain iron or bismuth.

tars-, tarso-: Combining forms referring to: 1. The eyelid. 2. The tarsus of the foot.

tarsadenitis (tar′sad-en-nī′tis): Inflammation of the tarsal edges of the eyelid and of the meibomian glands.

tarsal (tar′sal): 1. Relating to the eyelid or the plates of cartilage in the eyelid. 2. Relating to the seven bones of the tarsus (*q.v.*). T. PLATE the firm framework of connective tissue of the upper and lower eyelids which gives them their shape.

tarsalgia (tar-sal′ji-a): Pain in the tarsus or ankle.

tarsal tunnel syndrome: Pain and sensory loss in the medial anterior part of the foot and great toe; may be due to pressure on the medial plantar nerve or pressure on, or damage to, the posterior tibial nerve.

tarsectomy (tar-sek′to-mi): 1. Excision of a segment of the cartilaginous plate of the eyelid. 2. Excision of one or more of the tarsal bones.

tarsitis (tar-sī′tis): 1. Inflammation of the tarsal edge of the eyelid; blepharitis. 2. Inflammation of the tarsus or ankle.

tarsochiloplasty (tar-sō-kī′lō-plas-ti): Plastic surgery of the eyelid, the borders in particular.

tarsoclasis (tar-sok′la-sis): Surgical fracture of the tarsus of the foot in an operation for correction of clubfoot.

tarsomalacia (tar′sō-ma-lā′shi-a): Softening of the cartilaginous part of the eyelid.

tarsometatarsal (tar-sō-met′a-tar-sal): Relating to the tarsal and metatarsal regions.

tarso-orbital (tar′sō-or′bit-al): Relating to the eyelid and the orbit of the eye.

tarsophalangeal (tar-sō-fa-lan′jē-al): Relating to the tarsus and the toes.

tarsophyma (tar-sō-fi′ma): Any tarsal neoplasm.

tarsoplasty (tar′sō-plas-ti): Any plastic operation on the eyelid.

tarsoptosia (tar-sop-tō′si-a): Flatfootedness; falling of the tarsus.

tarsorrhaphy (tar-sor′ra-fi): Suturing together of the eyelids, partially, or entirely to shorten the palpebral fissure or to protect the cornea temporarily when there is paralysis of the obicularis muscle or to allow healing in case of chronic ulcer. Also called *blepharorrhaphy*.

tarsotibial (tar-sō-tib′i-al): Relating to the tarsus and the tibia.

tarsus (tar′sus): 1. The part of the foot that is behind the metatarsals; made up of seven bones; the calcaneus or heel bone, the talus or ankle bone, and the cuboid, navicular, and first, second and third cuneiform bones. 2. The thin elongated plates of dense connective tissue found in each eyelid, contributing to its form and support. — tarsal, adj.

tartar: A hard yellowish deposit that forms on the teeth.

tartaric acid (tar-tar′ik): A clear, colourless, crystalline acid found in vegetables and certain fruits; also produced commercially as a soluble white powder from potassium bitartrate, found in grape juice; has several pharmacological uses.

tartrate (tar′tr-āt): Any salt of tartaric acid.

tasikinesia (tas-i-ki-nē′zi-a): An uncontrollable desire to get up and walk about; inability to remain seated quietly.

task allocation (al-lo-kā′ -shun): The breaking down of a problem or tasks into smaller subsections. This was the method of delegating work employed prior to the more holistic approach espoused in the nursing process. Essentially it split the patient's care into tasks, so six nurses could attend the patient for six different procedures, instead of one primary nurse ensuring continuity of care.

taste: 1. The power to perceive and distinguish flavours. 2. The sensation produced when the specialized nerve endings in the taste buds are stimulated. T. BUDS small clusters of specialized cells located in the epithelium of the tongue and the inside of the mouth, epiglottis, and parts of the pharynx; they connect with the surface by small pores through which substances in solution enter and stimulate the nerve endings contained in the buds, thus giving rise to the sensation of taste. They are classified according to the composition of the substance to which they are sensitive; sweet, acid, salty, bitter.

tattoo (ta-tōō'): The insertion of permanent colouring matter into the skin by puncture. ACCIDENTAL T. the accidental embedding of small particles of foreign material into the skin.

taurine (taw'rin): An acid found in human bile; small amounts are also found in tissues of the lungs and muscles.

taurocholaemia (taw-rō-ko-lē'mi-a): The presence of taurocholic acid in the blood.

taurocholic acid (taw-rō-ko'lik): A bile acid that, on hydrolysis, splits into taurine and cholic acid.

taut (tawt): Tightly drawn or tensely stretched; not loose or flabby.

tauto-: A combining form meaning the same.

tautology (taw-tol'o-ji): The needless repetition of a word, phrase, or idea.

tautomenial (taw-tō-mē'ni-al): Relating to the same menstrual period.

-taxia,-taxis, taxy: Combining forms denoting order, arrangement.

taxis (tak'sis): 1. The restoration of a displaced part to its normal position by manual manipulation; term often used in relation to the reduction of a hernia by manipulation. 2. The reflex movement that occurs in response to a stimulus; term is usually attached to a word that designates the kind of stimulus, *e.g.*, chemotaxis, thermotaxis.

taxonomy (taks-on'-o-mi): The scientific and orderly classification of plants and animals, or the principles and laws upon which such classification is made. — taxonomic, adj.

TB: Abbreviation for tuberculosis (*q.v.*)

T-bandage: Also called *T-binder*.

Tc: Chemical symbol for technetium.

T-cell: See under CELL.

tds: *ter die sumendus*, Latin abbreviation previously used in prescriptions, three times daily.

teaching hospital: A large hospital or group of hospitals where medical students, junior medical staff and student nurses receive clinical instruction and experience.

team: A group of people working together with a common aim. In healthcare, includes people with a variety of skills and professional background. T. NURSING a practice in which a team of several nurses with varying degrees of experience and qualifications work together for a group of patients in planning nursing interventions and implementing care plans.

tear (taīr): 1. Laceration; a break in the continuity of a substance. 2. To pull apart by force.

tearing (tēr'ing): Excessive production of more tears than are carried off by the lacrimal duct, resulting in 'watering' of the eyes.

tears (tērz): The clear, slightly alkaline secretion constantly being formed by the lacrimal gland, and spread by blinking; function is to keep the conjunctiva moist. Contains the enzyme lysosome, which acts as an antiseptic. See LACRIMAL.

tease: To draw or pull out or separate into fine threads or minute shreds; refers especially to preparation of tissue for microscopic examination.

teat (tēt): A nipple, particularly the artificial nipple on infant's feeding bottle.

technetium (tek-nē'shi-um): A radioactive metallic element. Its most stable isotope is technetium 99m (^{99m}Tc) used in diagnostic tests and in scanning; has a half-life of only 6 hours.

technical (tek'ni-kal): Relating to a technique, or requiring a special skill.

technician (tek'nish'un): One who has had training in and uses the techniques required for carrying out specific procedures of a particular profession. In the health sciences the title often indicates the particular area in which the individual works, *e.g.*, histology technician.

technique (tek-nēk'): The detailed systematic manner in which a specific procedure, such as a mechanical or surgical operation or a test, is performed. ISOLATION T. the methods used to prevent the spread of pathogenic organisms or infection from a patient to other individuals.

technologist (tek-nol'o-jist): An individual who works in a particular technology (*q.v.*); often used with the name of the technology involved, *e.g.*, radiotherapy technologist.

technology (tek-nol'o-ji): The practical application of the knowledge and techniques of a profession or science.

tectocephaly (tek-tō-kef'a-li,-sef'): A condition in which the skull is abnormally long and narrow as a result of premature closing of the sagittal suture; usually associated with mental handicap. — tectocephalic, adj.

tectonic (tek-ton'ik): Relating to the reconstruction of a part by plastic surgery or the restoration of a lost part by grafting.

tectorial (tek-tor'i-al): **1.** Forming a roof or covering. **2.** Of the nature of a roof or cover.

tectospinal (tek-tō-spī'nal): T. TRACT a tract of white nerve fibres that pass from the tectum of the midbrain through the medulla oblongata to the spinal cord.

tectum (tek'tum): A roof-like structure. T. MESOENCEPHALI the membranous roof of the midbrain.

TEDs: Abbreviation for thromboembolic deterrent (stockings), see ELASTIC STOCKING under ELASTIC.

teenage (tēn'āj): The years between childhood and adulthood; usually considered to begin at about the age of 13 and to last until about the age of 19.

teeth: See TOOTH.

teething (tēth'ing): Dentition: the eruption of teeth, usually the first or deciduous set.

Teflon (tef'lon): A tradename for a synthetic material used in the manufacture of many medical and surgical supplies and prostheses, ranging from adhesive plasters to grafting material for blood vessels.

tegmen (teg'men): A structure that covers or roofs over a part. — tegmina, pl.

tegmentum (teg-men'tum): **1.** A covering. **2.** That part of the brain stem that lies behind the peduncles that connect the cerebrum with the pons. — tegmental, adj.

tegument (teg'ū-ment): The skin or covering of the animal body; the integument. — tegumental, tegumentary, adj.

teichopsia (tī-kop'si-a): The sensation of seeing flashing or shimmering lights appearing suddenly before the eyes in a zigzag pattern; may be associated with migraine headache and stress.

tel-, tele-, telo-: Combining forms denoting far off; at a distance; over a distance.

tela (tē'la): In anatomy, any web-like structure; a thin, delicate tissue. — telae, pl.

telaesthesia (tel-es-thē'zi-a): Extrasensory perception (*q.v.*).

telalgia (tel-al'ji-a): Referred pain.

telangiectasia (tel-an'ji-ek-tā'zi-a): Abnormal dilatation of the terminal skin capillaries; seen in certain disorders of the circulation, polycythaemia, alcoholism, overexposure to sunlight; often in the shape of a spider or a Medusa's head; see CAPUT MEDUSAE. HEREDITARY HAEMORRHAGIC T. hereditary T. characterized by the presence of multiple areas of T. and a tendency to haemorrhage, especially from the nose; develops chiefly after puberty. Also called *Osler's disease, Osler–Welser–Rendu disease*, and *spider angioma*.

telangiectasis (tel-an'ji-ek'ta-sis): Discoloration of the skin where the capillaries have dilated in telangiectasia (*q.v.*).

telangiectoma (tel-an'ji-ek-tō'ma): An angioma formed from dilated capillaries or arterioles.

telangiitis (tel-an'ji-ī'tis): Inflammation of capillaries.

telangioma (tel-an'ji-ō'ma): An angioma made up of dilated terminal capillaries.

telangiosis (tel-an'ji-ō'sis): Any disease of capillaries.

tele-: Combining form denoting: **1.** At the end. **2.** At a distance; far away.

telecardiography (tel'e-kar-di-og'ra-fi): The recording of an electrocardiogram utilizing an apparatus for transmitting the impulses to a point some distance from the patient.

telecardiophone (tel-e-kar'di-ō-fōn): A specially constructed stethoscope for making heart sounds audible to a listener at some distance from the patient.

telediagnosis (tel'e-dī-ag-nō'sis): Diagnosis made at a distance from the patient by means of data transmitted from the patient's monitoring equipment to a central monitoring station or an intensive care unit.

telefluoroscopy (tel'e-floo-ō-ros'kŏ-pi): Transmission by television of images on a fluoroscopy screen for observation at a distant point.

telematics (tel-ē-mat'-iks): The science of the long-distance transmission of computerized information.

telemedicine (tel-ē-med'-i-sin): The use of communications systems (such as electronic networks and visual display units) to provide remote diagnosis, advice, treatment, and monitoring. These are used in both primary care and hospital settings.

telemetry (te-lem'i-tri): Making measurements of a property such as blood pressure or temperature and transmitting the findings by radio signal to a receiver at a distance for interpretation and recording.

telencephalon (tel-en-kef'a-lon,-sef'): The anterior part of the embryonic forebrain which develops into the cerebral cortex, corpus striatum, and olfactory lobes.

teleneuron (tel-e-nū'ron): A nerve ending.

teleology (tē-lē-ol'o-ji): The belief that all physical phenomena can be explained in terms of their purpose. — teleological, adj.

teleopsia (te-lē-op'si-a): A visual disorder in which close objects appear to be far away, or objects perceived in space appear much denser than they are.

teleorganic (tel-e-or-gan′ik): Necessary to organic life.

telepathy (te-lep′a-thi): Mental communication, without any obvious means, between people who are at a distance from each other. Thought transference. Also called *extrasensory perception*.

teleradium (tel-e-rā′di-um): Radium whose radiation is directed into the body from an external source; radium beam.

teletherapeutics (tel′e-ther-a-pū′tiks): The use of hypnotic suggestion as a mode of treatment.

teletherapy (tel-e-ther′a-pi): 1. The external administration of radiotherapy; the radiation is delivered by an isotope placed in a mould or other container and applied to the skin, or by an external beam machine. 2. By custom, often refers to treatment by teleradium.

telethermometer (tel′e-ther-mom′e-ter): A device for registering temperature at a distance from the patient under observation.

telo-: Combining form denoting end.

telogen (tel′ō-jen): The final, quiescent stage in the cycle of hair in the follicle, lasting from the time the hair ceases to grow until it is shed. See CATAGEN. T. EFFLUVIUM transient loss of hair following a febrile illness, general anaesthesia, childbirth, or chemotherapy.

telognosis (tel′og-nō′sis): Diagnosis by examination of radiographs transmitted by special telephonic means.

telomere shortering theory: One of the most recent theories of ageing discovered by scientists at the Geron Corporation. It is understood that the telomeres (the sequence of nucleic acids extending from the ends of chromosomes) shorten every time a cell divides. The shortening of telomeres is beleived to lead to cellular damage due to the inability of the cell to duplicate itself correctly.

telophase (tel′ō-fāz): The final stage in cell mitosis when the chromosomes have been grouped at the ends of the cell and the cell divides, forming two new cells.

temperament (tem′per-a-ment): The habitual mental and emotional attitude of an individual as distinct from mood, which is temporary.

temperature (tem′per-a-chur): The degree of heat or coldness of an object or substance as measured by a thermometer. ABNORMAL BODY T. see HYPERTHERMIA, HYPOTHERMIA; AXILLARY T. that registered on a thermometer placed in the axilla; BODY T. refers to the internal or core temperature of vital organs,

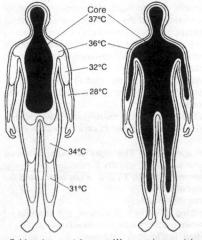

Core
37°C
36°C
32°C
28°C
34°C
31°C

Cold environmental temperature (20°-34°C)   Warm environmental temperature (35°C and above)

Body core and skin temperature

i.e., the heart, brain, lungs, abdominal viscera; remains constant in healthy individuals regardless of environmental temperature; INVERSE BODY T., T. that is lower in the evening than in the morning; MEAN T. the average T. of the atmosphere in an area over a period of time; NORMAL T. usually refers to that considered normal for the human body, 36.9°C; ORAL T. that registered on a thermometer placed in the mouth; RECTAL T. that registered on a thermometer placed in the rectum; ROOM T. the ordinary T. of the atmosphere in a room; SHELL T., the T. at or near the surface of the body; more variable than the core T., and more responsive to environmental influences; SUBNORMAL T. refers to body T. that is below the normal T. See also FEVER; PYREXIA.

temple: 1. The flattened area on either side of the head lying between the outer angle of the eye and the top of the ear flap. 2. One of the side supports for a pair of spectacles.

tempolabile (tem-pō-lā′bil): Having a tendency to change with the passage of time.

temporal (tem′por-al): 1. Limited in time or pertinent to time. 2. Relating to the temple (*q.v.*). T. ARTERITIS giant-cell arteritis, see under ARTERITIS; T. BONES one on either side of the head below the parietal bones; contain the middle ear; T. LOBE one of the five lobes of each hemisphere of the cerebrum; lies under the temporal bone and contains the auditory centre; T. LOBE EPILEPSY see under EPILEPSY.

temporofrontal (tem'po-rō-frun'tal): Pertaining to the temporal and frontal regions or bones.

temporomandibular (tem'po-rō-man-dib'ū-lar): Relating to the temporal region or bone and the lower jaw. T. JOINT SYNDROME often seen in the elderly who have ill-fitting dentures or degeneration of the soft tissue of the gums following tooth extraction; the pain may radiate to the ear, the mastoid area, or the mandible; sometimes causes trismus, tinnitus, and decreased hearing; also called *temporomandibular-pain dysfunction syndrome*.

temporomaxillary (tem'po-rō-mak'si-lar-i): Relating to the temporal and maxillary regions or bones.

temporo-occipital (tem'po-rō-ok-sip'i-tal): Relating to the temporal and occipital regions or bones.

temporoparietal (tem'po-rō-pa-rī'e-tal): Relating to the temporal and parietal regions or bones.

temporospatial (tem'po-rō-spā'shul): Relating to time and space.

temporosphenoidal (tem'po-rō-sfē-noy'dal): Relating to the temporal and sphenoid regions or bones.

tempostabile (tem'pō-sta'bǐ): Not subject to change over time.

tenacious (te-nā'shus): 1. Sticky, adhesive, holding fast. 2. Thick and viscid, usually said of sputum or other body fluid.

tenacity (te-nas'i-ti): The characteristic of being tough or resistant.

tenalgia (te-nal'ji-a): Pain in a tendon.

tenderness: Unusual sensitivity to touch or pressure. REBOUND T. a condition in which pain is felt when pressure over a part is released.

tendinitis (ten-din-ī'tis): Inflammation of tendons and of the tendon-muscle attachments. BICIPITAL T. swelling and enlargement of the biceps muscle sheath, causing discomfort in the upper anterior area of the tendon of the biceps muscle; caused by repetitive movements that put stress on the tendon. Also called *tendonitis; tenontitis*.

tendinoplasty (ten'di-nō-plas ti): Plastic surgery on a tendon. Also called *tendoplasty*.

tendinous (ten'din-us): Relating to, resembling, or composed of tendon.

tendon (ten'don): A band or cord of firm, white, inelastic, fibrous connective tissue that forms the termination of a muscle and attaches it to a bone or other structure. KANGAROO T., T. from

the tail of a kangaroo, used for sutures when delay of absorption of sutures is desired, as in orthopaedic surgery; T. OF ACHILLES the T. that attaches the gastrocnemius and the soleus muscles to the heel bone; see also ACHILLES; T. REFLEX, see under REFLEX. Syn., *sinew*. — tendinous, adj.

tendovaginitis (ten-dō-vaj-i-nī'tis): See TENOSYNOVITIS

tenectomy (te-nek'to-mi): Excision of part of a tendon. Also called *tenonectomy*.

tenesmus (te-nez'mus): Painful, ineffectual straining to empty the bowel or bladder. — tenesmic, adj.

tennis elbow: Pain and tenderness at the outer side of the elbow due to injury of the lateral epicondyle of the humerus and resulting from violent twisting of the hand as often occurs in playing tennis. Epicondylitis.

tennis leg: Severe burning pain in the popliteal area or calf; due to rupture or partial rupture of any of the muscles of the leg or popliteus; usually an athletic injury.

teno-: Combining form denoting tendon.

tenodesis (te-nod'e-sis): The fixation of a tendon, as to a bone, or the transferring of a tendon to a new point of attachment.

tenodynia (ten'ō-din'i-a): Pain in a tendon. Tenalgia.

tenomyoplasty (ten-ō-mī'ō-plas-ti): Plastic surgery on a tendon and a muscle.

tenonitis (ten-o-nī'tis): 1. Inflammation of Tenon's capsule (*q.v.*). 2. Inflammation of a tendon.

tenonometer (ten-ō-nom'i-ter): An instrument for measuring the amount of pressure exerted by the substances within the eyeball. Also called *tonometer*.

Tenon's capsule: The thin membrane that envelopes the eyeball from the optic nerve to the ciliary region and which forms a capsule or socket within which the eyeball moves. [Jacques R. Tenon, French anatomist and oculist, 1724–1816.]

tenoplasty (ten'ō-plas-ti): A plastic operation on a tendon. — tenoplastic, adj.

tenorrhaphy (te-nor'a-fi): Suturing together the cut or torn ends of a tendon.

tenositis (ten-ō-sī'tis): Inflammation of a tendon.

tenostosis (ten-os-tō'sis): Ossification of a tendon.

tenosuspension (ten'ō-sus-pen'shun): The surgical procedure of suturing, with tendon, the head of the humerus to the acromian for treatment of recurrent dislocation of the shoulder.

tenosynovectomy (ten′ō-sin-ō-vek′to-mi): The surgical removal of a tendon sheath.

tenosynovitis (ten′-ō-sin-ō-vī′tis): Inflammation of a tendon sheath; may be caused by irritation or by bacterial infection.

tenotomy (ten-ot′-oṁi): Division or cutting of a tendon; usually done to correct a deformity caused by a too-short muscle, *e.g.*, as occurs in strabismus.

tenovaginitis (ten′ō-vaj-i-nī′tis): Mild chronic inflammation or thickening of a tendon sheath; most often affects tendons of the finger, thumb, or wrist; cause unknown.

TENS: Abbreviation for transcutaneous electrical nerve stimulation (*q.v.*).

tense: Tight; strained.

tension (ten′shun): 1. The act of stretching. 2. The state of being stretched. 3. In psychology, a condition of inner unrest, striving or turmoil with a feeling of psychological stress, often manifested in increased muscular tone and other physiological signs of emotional imbalance. ARTERIAL T. that exerted by the blood on the arterial walls; INTRAOCULAR T. that exerted by the contents of the eyeball on the tunics of the eye; PREMENSTRUAL T. see PREMENSTRUAL SYNDROME; SURFACE T. the force that acts to preserve the integrity of a surface; it is based on differences in molecular attraction; T. PNEUMOTHORAX see under PNEUMOTHORAX.

tensor: Any muscle that stretches or causes tension in a part.

tent: 1. A conical cylinder of sponge, cotton, or similar material to be introduced into a canal or sinus to dilate it or keep it open. 2. A canopy of material arranged over a bed or part of a bed. CROUP T. a canopy arranged over the head of the bed in such a way as to maintain a high degree of moisture within it; used in treatment of croup; FACE or HOOD T. fits over the head, ties under the chin; used chiefly for providing high humidity for children on oxygen therapy; HUMIDITY T. a covering that may enclose the entire body or just the head; serves to prevent dispersal of mist created to assist in the delivery of oxygen to the terminal alveoli; ISOLATION T. a T. placed over a patient's bed as a means of achieving reverse isolation; see ISOLATION; OXYGEN T. a covering arranged over the bed or the head of it so as to maintain a high degree of oxygen when this is used in therapy.

tentacle (ten′ta-c′l): A slender process on an invertebrate, for prehension or locomotion; may also function as a sense organ.

tentiginous (ten-tij′i-nus): Lascivious; insanely lustful.

tentigo (ten-tī′gō): Lust.

tephromalacia (tef′rō-ma-lā′shi-a): Softening of the grey matter of either or both the brain and spinal cord.

tepid (tep′id): Lukewarm.

ter-: Combining form denoting three, threefold, three times.

teras (ter′as): A fetus with grossly malformed parts. — terata, pl.

terat-, terato-: Combining forms denoting a teras.

teratism (ter′a-tizm): The congenital anomaly of being a teras.

teratoblastoma (ter′a-tō-blas-tō′ma): See TERATOMA.

teratocarcinoma (ter′a-tō-kar-si-nō′ma): 1. A malignant tumour most often occurring in the testis. 2. A malignant epithelioma (*q.v.*) arising in a teratoma (*q.v.*).

teratogen (ter′a-tō-jen): Anything capable of disrupting normal fetal growth and producing malformation, *e.g.*, drugs, poisons, radiation, physical agents such as electroconvulsive shock, infections. — teratogenic, adj.; teratogenicity, teratogenesis, n.

teratogenesis (ter′a-tō-jen′e-sis): Embryonic development leading to gross physical abnormalities; may be the result of the mother's ingestion of chemical toxins, of radiation or of infection during pregnancy.

teratology (ter-a-tol′o-ji): The scientific study of malformations and other deviations from normal development. — teratologist, n.; tetralogical, adj.; teratologically, adv.

teratoma (ter-a-tō′ma): A tumour of embryonic origin, composed of various kinds of tissues, including epithelial and connective, none of which are native to the part where the tumour occurs; most commonly found in the ovaries where it is usually benign, and in the testes where it is usually malignant. — teratomata, pl., teratomatous, adj.

teratophobia (ter′a-tō-fō′bi-a): Abnormal fear of (1) deformed people, or (2) of giving birth to a deformed infant.

terebrachesis (ter′-e-brā-kē′sis): The surgical procedure of shortening the round ligament of the uterus.

teres (tē′rēz): Round, smooth and long; usually denotes certain muscles and ligaments.

tergal (ter′gal): Relating to the back.

tergum (ter′gum): The back.

term: In obstetrics, refers to an infant born any time between the thirty-eighth week and the end of the forty-first week of gestation. Also spoken of as full term. See POST-TERM; PRE-TERM.

terminad (ter'mi-nad): Toward a terminus.

terminal (ter'min-al): 1. Situated at or forming an end or extremity. 2. Related to the end, as the T. stage of a disease. T. CARE care given to the dying patient; T. DISINFECTION that which is done following a patient's illness, discharge from the hospital, or death; involves disinfecting any substance or object that has been used by the patient or been in contact with him; T. ILLNESS one from which the patient is not expected to recover; T. INFECTION infection with a pathogenic organism that occurs during the course of a chronic disease and causes death.

terminology (ter-mi-nol'o-ji): The particular words or expressions used in a special field of endeavour or science.

terror (ter'er): Excessive fear; fright. NIGHT T. that which occurs in sleep, especially in children; nightmare.

tertian (ter'shun): Occurring in three day cycles every second day. See MALARIA.

tertiary (ter'shi-ar-i): 1. Third in order. 2. Recurring every third day. 3. Pertinent to a third stage or order; often refers to the third stage of syphilis. T. HEALTHCARE includes services of specialists for serious long-term conditions and for treating complications of illnesses; often provided at regional medical centres; T. HEALTHCARE SYSTEM refers to the context in which care is given, usually large hospitals where critical, coronary, intensive, neonatal, and oncological care are given; the hospitals are often associated with universities and also engage in research and experimental work.

tertigravida (ter-ti-grav'ida): A woman who is pregant for the third time.

tertipara (ter-tip'a-ra): A woman who has had three pregnancies resulting in viable offspring. — tertiparous, adj.

test: 1. A means of examination. 2. A procedure done to determine the presence or absence of a substance. 3. To analyse a substance by the use of chemical reagents. 4. A trial. T. MEAL one given for later removal from the stomach for gastric analysis.

testalgia (tes-tal'ji-a): Pain in the testes.

testectomy (tes-tek'to-mi): Removal of a testis. Also *orchidectomy*.

testicle (tes'ti-k'l): Testis. — testicular, adj.

testis (tes'tis): One of the two glandular bodies contained in the scrotum of the male; they produce spermatozoa and also the male sex hormones. UNDESCENDED T. refers to the condition existing when a testis remains in the pelvis or inguinal canal; cryptorchism (*q.v.*). — testes, pl.; testicular, adj.

testitis (tes-tī'tis): Inflammation of the testes; orchitis.

testopathy (tes-top'a-thi): Any disease of the testes.

testosterone (tes-tos'te-rōn): 1. The hormone derived from the testes and responsible for the development of the secondary male characteristics. 2. A synthetic product prepared from cholesterol and used in treating carcinoma of the breast, to control uterine bleeding, and in male underdevelopment.

test tube: A slender tube of thin glass, closed at one end; has many uses in scientific laboratories. T.T. BABY one that results from impregnation of the mother by artificial insemination (*q.v.*).

test type: Letters of various sizes on cards used in testing visual acuity. SNELLEN'S T.T. square black letters on wallcharts; commonly used for testing distance vision.

tetanic (te-tan'ik): 1. Characterized by or relating to tetanus. 2. Producing tonic muscle spasm. 3. An agent that produces tonic muscle spasm.

tetaniform (te-tan'i-form): Resembling tetany or tetanus.

tetanigenous (tet'a-nij'e-nus): Tending to produce tetanus or tetanic spasms.

tetanize (tet'a-nīz): To produce tetany or tetanic muscle spasms.

tetanode (tet'a-nōd): The period of quiet between the tonic spasms of tetany.

tetanoid (tet'a-noyd): Resembling the muscle spasms of tetanus.

tetanospasmin (tet'a-nō-spaz'min): The potent exotoxin produced by the form of *Clostridium tetani* that causes tetanus and is responsible for the principle symptoms of that disease.

tetanus (tet'an-us): 1. Lockjaw. 2. An acute infectious disease induced by the toxin of *Clostridium tetani*, an anaerobic organism growing at the site of injury to body tissues; because the organism is present sometimes in road dust, manure, and cultivated soil, accidental wounds, particularly penetrating wounds, may become infected by it. T. is characterized by painful muscular contractions, chiefly of the face and neck, hence the appellation 'lockjaw'. Muscles of the back may become involved and result in opisthotonos (*q.v.*). 2. Sustained tonic spasm of a muscle or muscles, produced by repetition of stimuli so often that the muscle does not have a chance to relax between their application. CEPHALIC T. occurs following a head injury involving the facial, trigeminal, oculomotor, or hypoglossal nerve or all of them; spreads rapidly and seizures develop; DRUG T., T. that is produced by a drug such as strychnine; PUERPERAL or POST-PARTAL T., T. that develops from infection of the obstetrical wound.

tetanus antitoxin: Antibody to tetanus toxin, prepared from the serum of horses that have been hyperimmunized against the exotoxin of *Clostridium tetani*; produces passive immunity; used in prevention and treatment of wounds that may have become contaminated with the organism.

tetanus immune globulin: Used for short-term immunization when one may have been exposed to the causative organism of tetanus; prepared from the globulin of an immune person.

tetanus toxoid: Detoxified tetanus toxin; used to produce active immunity against tetanus in healthy individuals and those who may be at risk of developing tetanus following a dirty wound. Given by repeated subcutaneous doses.

tetany (tet'a-ni): 1. A condition of muscular hyperexcitability, due to abnormal calcium metabolism, in which mild stimuli produce cramps and spasms (carpopedal spasm). Seen in parathyroid deficiency, potassium deficiency, vitamin D deficiency, alkalosis, sprue. In infants it is associated with gastrointestinal upset and rickets. 2. Tetanus; see **definition 2** under TETANUS.

tetartanopia (tet'ar-ta-nō'pi-a): 1. Loss of vision in the corresponding quadrant in each field of vision. 2. A rare type of blue-yellow colour blindness.

tetr-, tetra-: Combining forms denoting four or having four parts.

tetra-amelia (tet'ra-a-mē'li-a): Absence of both upper and lower extremities.

tetrabrachius (tet'ra-brā'ki-us): A malformed fetus or individual with four arms.

tetrachirus (tet-ra-kī'-rus): A malformed fetus or individual having four hands.

tetrachloroethylene (tet'ra-klor-ō-eth'-i-lēn): A clear colourless liquid chemical used as an anthelmintic for hookworm.

tetrachromic (tet-ra-krō'mik): Relating to vision that is normal for four colours.

tetrad (tet'rad): A group of four.

tetradactyly (tet-ra-dak'ti-li): The condition of having only four digits on a hand or foot. — tetradactylous, adj.

tetrahydrocannabinol (tet'ra-hī'drō-ka-nab'i -nol): The active ingredient in cannabis sativa; has sedative and hallucinogenic effects.

tetralogy of Fallot: A form of congenital heart defect which includes four abnormalities — narrowing of the pulmonary artery, a septal defect between the ventricles, hypertrophy of the right ventricle, and displacement of the aorta to the right. The condition results in deficient oxygenation of the blood with cyanosis, dyspnoea, polycythaemia, clubbing of the fingers. [Etienne Louis Arthur Fallot, French physician, 1850–1911.]

tetramastia (tet-ra-mas'ti-a): The condition of having four breasts. — tetramastous, adj.

tetramelia (tet-ra-mē'li-a): Congenital absence of all four extremities.

tetrapeptide (tet-ra-pep'tid): A polypeptide composed of four amino acid groups.

tetraphocomelia (tet'ra-fō-kō-mē'li-a): Phocomelia affecting all four extremities.

tetraplegia (tet-ra-plē'ji-a): Paralysis of all four limbs. Quadriplegia.

tetrapus (tet'ra-pus): A fetus having four feet.

tetrascelus (tet-ras'e-lus): A fetus having four legs.

tetravaccine (tet-ra-vak'sēn): A vaccine containing dead cultures of the organisms causing typhoid, paratyphoid A, paratyphoid B and cholera.

tetravalent (tet-ra-vā'lent): Having a valence of four.

texiform (teks'i-form): Web-like; forming a mesh.

texis (tek'sis): Childbirth or childbearing.

textus (teks'tus): A tissue.

thalamectomy (thal-a-mek'tō-mi): Destruction of part of the thalamus by a chemical agent or by surgery.

thalamic (thal'a-mik): Relating to the thalamus. T. SYNDROME a condition characterized by mild hemiplegia and hemitaxia, pain with choreoathetoid movements of the affected side, and astereognosis, due to a lesion in the lateral part of the thalamus; is aggravated by fatigue, stress, and emotional disturbances.

thalamo-: Combining form denoting thalamus.

thalamotomy (thal-a-mot'o-mi): Usually operative (stereotaxic) destruction of a portion of the thalamus, sometimes done in treatment of psychotic disorders that have an emotional basis, or for relief of intractable pain.

thalamus (thal'a-mus): A collection of grey matter at the base of the cerebrum. Sensory impulses from the whole body (except olfactory) pass through on their way to the cerebral cortex. — thalami, pl.; thalamic, adj.

thalassaemia (thal-a-sē'mi-a): An ethnic, hereditary, genetically transmitted haemolytic anaemia in which there is interference with synthesis of haemoglobin; several types are recognized, according to the symptoms. There is no known cure; treatment consists of regular blood transfusions and bone marrow transplantation. Most victims are children of Greek or Italian descent; death usually occurs before the age of 25. The disease is marked by severe anaemia, headache, anorexia, darkened skin, enlargement of the liver, spleen, and bones. Also called *Cooley's anaemia, Mediterranean anaemia, familial erythroblastic anaemia.* BETA ZERO T. a type of T. characterized by defective structure of haemoglobin causing it to be fragile and break down easily, results in bone and heart problems and usually death in midlife; T. MINOR a heterozygous form of T., usually asymptomatic although there may be mild anaemia. [Name derived from the Greek word *thalassa*, meaning *sea*; the disease was first described in people in the Mediterranean Sea area.]

thalassophobia (thal'a-sō-fō'bi-a): Morbid fear of the sea.

thalassotherapy (thal'a-sō-ther'a-pi): The treatment of diseases by sea bathing or sea air.

thalidomide (tha-lid'o-mīd): A drug formerly used as a sleeping tablet and sedative; was the cause of several types of birth defects, primarily limb malformations, in infants born to mothers who took the drug during early pregnancy; it is no longer available in the UK but has a restricted use in some other countries.

thallitoxicosis (thal'i-toks-i-kō'sis): Poisoning by thallium (*q.v.*).

thallium (thal'i-um): A bluish-white lustrous metallic element, the salts of which are poisonous. T. SCAN, a scintillation scan. The radioisotope thallium-201 is administered intravenously and localizes in the myocardium. A scintillation camera produces an image of the distribution of the radioisotope, pinpointing occlusions of the coronary arteries; T. SULPHATE, is an ingredient of rat poisons. Chemical symbol, Tl.

thamuria (tha-mū'ri-a): Too-frequent urination.

thanat-, thanato-: Combining forms denoting death.

thanatologist (than'a-tol-o'jist): One who specializes in the study of the various aspects of death and dying.

thanatology (than'a-tol'o-ji): The study of the phenomenon of physical death.

thanatophoric (than'a-tō-for'ik): Lethal; causing death.

thanatopsia (than'a-top-si-a): Examination of the body after death; autopsy. Also called *thanatopsy.*

thanatos (than'a-tōs): In psychoanalysis, the death instinct.

thebesian (thē-bē'zi-an): T. VEINS the smallest of the coronary veins; they open into the cavities of the heart.

theca (thē'-ka): An enclosing or covering sac, capsule, membrane, or the sheath of a tendon. T. FOLLICULI the external connective tissue wall of an ovarian follicle; consisting of an external fibrous layer, the theca externa, and an internal vascular layer, the theca interna; it produces oestrogen and contributes to the formation of corpus luteum; T. VERTEBRALIS the dura mater of the spinal cord. — thecal, adj.

thecal (thē'kal): Relating to a capsule or sheath, often to a tendon sheath.

thecitis (thē-sī'tis): Inflammation of the sheath of a tendon.

thecoma (thē-kō'ma): A benign ovarian tumour. Also called *thelioma*

theine (thē'in): Caffeine.

thelalgia (thē-lal'ji-a): Pain in the nipple.

thelarche (thē-lar'ke): The beginning of breast development at puberty; may occur precociously in girls as young as eight years.

thele (thē'lē): The nipple.

theleplasty (thē'le-plas-ti): Plastic surgery on the nipple.

thelerethism (thē-ler'e-thizm): Erection of the nipple.

thelitis (thē-lī'tis): Inflammation of a nipple.

thelium (thē'li-um): 1. The nipple. 2. A papilla.

theloncus (thē-lonk'us): Tumour of a nipple.

thelorrhagia (thē-lō-rā'ji-a): Haemorrhage from a nipple.

thematic analysis: The identification of recurring issues that appear during the analysis of data.

thematic apperception test: A test used in psychiatry. The patient is asked to interpret a series of drawings that depict life scenes and situations and the interpretations given are thought to be indicative of the patient's moods and personality.

thenar (thē'nar): 1. Pertinent to the palm of the hand or the thumb. 2. The fleshy mound at the base of the thumb, also called the *thenar eminence.*

theobroma oil: A yellowish-white solid obtained from the roasted seeds of the *Theobroma cacao* tree; contains the glycerides of oleic, palmitic, stearic, and lauric acids; used in preparation of emollients, ointments, and suppositories. Syn., *cocoa butter*.

theobromin (thē-ō-brō′-min): An alkaloid derived from the seeds of the *Theobroma cacao* tree; has effects similar to those of caffeine; has been used in medicine as a vasodilator, heart stimulant, diuretic, and smooth muscle relaxant.

theomania (thē′ō-mā′ni-a): A type of religious insanity, especially one in which one imagines oneself to be God or to have divine attributes.

theory (thē′-ri): A reasoned proposed explanation of an occurrence, or of something that will occur or be produced, for which absolute proof is lacking; a theory is conjectural in nature but less speculative than a hypothesis.

theory–practice gap: The difference between what theory and research says should happen and what actually does happen in practice. This is particularly noticeable in nursing.

theotherapy (thē-ō-ther′a-pi): Treatment of disease by prayer or other religious expression.

therapeutic (ther-a-pū′tik): 1. Pertaining to the treatment of disease. 2. Curative. 3. Descriptive of an agent that has healing or curing properties. T. COMMUNITY a specially structured treatment and rehabilitative hospital milieu in which patients with severe behaviour problems are encouraged to assume responsibility for their own behaviour and to behave in a way that is socially acceptable. Peer group support increases self-awareness and motivation to change negative or damaging behaviours; T. DOSE the amount of a drug or other therapeutic agent prescribed; usually considered safe; T. INDEX the margin between the maximum tolerated dose of a drug and the minimal curative dose; based on kilograms of body weight; T. MILIEU T. community; T. RATIO the ratio of the minimal dose of a drug to its therapeutic dose; often used to estimate the safety of a drug. T. TOUCH a mode of treatment or a procedure based on an ancient practice, 'the laying-on of hands.' Modern health-care practitioners have added the concept that the body is an energy field that is constantly being influenced by forces outside itself and that body energies can be transferred from the hands of a person who has been trained to assume the role of healer to the body of a person who has some physical or mental disorder or condition that requires change. The procedure is not based on any religious tenet, nor is it performed in a religious context, but the psychological status of both healer and the person treated are considered fundamental to the outcome of the procedure.

therapeutic nursing: A philosophy that focuses on the therapeutic use of the nurse–patient relationship and is based on reflective presence. It attempts to capture the atmosphere of the nurse–patient relationship, exploring not only the interpersonal but also the intrapersonal

therapeutic relationship: Interactions between two people in the context of giving and receiving healthcare.

therapeutics (ther-a-pū′tiks): The branch of medical science dealing with the treatment of disease. — therapeutic, adj.; therapeutically, adv.

therapist (ther′a-pist): A person who is trained and skilled in the treatment of a disease or the effects of disease. The word is often used in combination with another that names the disorder being treated or the type of treatment employed, *e.g.*, speech T. physiotherapist.

therapy (ther′a-pi): The treatment of disease, or the means used in treating disease. AEROSOL T. see under AEROSOL; ART T. the therapeutic use of any art form to assist individuals who cannot express their feelings verbally; AVERSION T. sometimes used in treatment of alcoholism; a powerful emetic is administered, followed by alcohol; the effect often conditions the person against alcohol; COGNITIVE T., T. involving the correction of erroneous beliefs; COLLATERAL T., T. carried on with any two persons involved in a crisis, *e.g.*, mother and daughter; CONJOINT T., T. carried out with couples to help correct maladaptative relationships; CONVULSIVE T. electroconvulsive T. see ELECTROCONVULSIVE; CRISIS GROUP T., T. with a group of unrelated and unacquainted people who meet together, usually for about six sessions, and try to solve their individual problems; most of these groups are open-ended and people can enter or leave when they wish; DANCE T. the use of rhythmic body movement to disclose and express feelings and emotional conflicts, usually conducted in groups; ELECTROLYTE T., T. to correct electrolyte imbalance in the body; usually connected with intravenous T.; EMPIRIC T. that based on practical experience rather than scientific reasoning; ENDOCRINE T. treatment with hormones or glandular secretions; FAMILY T. group psychotherapy with a family or individual therapy applied to all family members simultaneously; FEVER T. treatment of disease by inducing high body temperatures; GOLD T. treatment of rheumatoid arthritis utilizing a solution containing gold given intramuscularly, in increasing doses, until symptoms abate; GROUP T., T. given to small groups of people who discuss their feelings and problems openly; HEAT T., T. utilizing some form of heat; IMPLOSIVE T. a counter-conditioning T. in which a great deal of anxiety is aroused and overcome; see FLOODING; INHALATION T. the administration of water vapour, gases, anaesthetics, and drugs by inhalation; INSULIN T. shock T.; consists of an injection of insulin in amounts sufficient to produce coma, followed by administration of glucose to restore consciousness; utilized in some psychoses; INTRAVENOUS T. the administration of medications and other substances by infusion into a vein; MILIEU T. psychiatric T. in a carefully constructed environment in which all elements enhance the medical T. and help the patient towards rehabilitation by developing needed social skills; MUSIC T. consists of participating in brass bands, opera groups, and choirs, as well as passive listening; used primarily in psychiatric patients; OCCUPATIONAL T. the teaching of specific skills, pursuits, crafts or hobbies that promote the rehabilitation of sick or handicapped people for independence in the activities of daily living; OXYGEN T. treatment that makes an increased amount of oxygen available to the patient; PARENTERAL T. refers to administration of therapeutic agents by injection or intravenously to maintain nutrition, or to replace water or other essential substances; PHYSIOTHERAPY the use of such physical agents as massage, exercise, etc. in treatment; PLAY T. a method of psychiatric treatment in which play is used as a medium of expression by the child thus enabling the psychiatrist to establish communication; REPLACEMENT T. used to replace loss of or deficient formation of body products; natural or synthetic substances are administered; ROENTGEN T. treatment by x-ray or other radioactive substances; SHOCK T. use of electric shock or a convulsant drug as a palliative or therapeutic measure in some psychoneurotic and psychotic disorders; SPECIFIC T. that which is directed towards the eradication of the specific cause of a disease; SPEECH T. the treatment of speech disorders. STEROID T., T. utilizing various steroid hormones especially those secreted by the adrenal cortex; patients on steroids must be closely monitored because of the many possible side effects; SUBSTITUTION T., T. that supplies a substance that is deficient or lacking in the body; SUPPORTIVE T. T. in which the therapist gives direct help and encouragement; SYMPTOMATIC T., T. directed towards relief of symptoms rather than their cause; WORK T. therapeutic use of work, either for or without compensation; ZONE T. treatment by stimulating a body area in the same longitudinal zone as the particular disorder.

therm-, thermo-: Combining forms denoting relationship to heat.

thermacogenesis (ther'ma-kō-jen'e-sis): The elevation of body temperature resulting from drug action.

thermacotherapy (ther'ma-kō-ther'a-pi): Treatment of disease by the application of heat, especially hot air.

thermal (ther'mal): Relating to heat. T. BURNS burns caused by hot liquid or flame; T. DISTURBANCES local or systemic reactions to the application or exposure to heat or cold in excessive amounts, as occurs in burns or frostbite.

thermalgesia (therm-al-jē'zi-a): Excessive sensitivity to heat, even heat of a fairly low degree. Also called *thermoalgesia*.

thermalgia (ther-mal'ji-a): Burning pain.

thermometer (ther'mel-om'i-ter): An electric thermometer.

thermistor (ther'mis-tor): A device for measuring small changes in temperature.

thermoaesthesia (ther'mō-es-thē'zi'a): The ability to recognize sensations of heat and cold and to distinguish between them. Also called *thermaesthesia*.

thermoanaesthesia (ther'mō-an-es-thē'zi-a): Loss or lack of the ability to recognize the sensations of heat and cold, or to distinguish between them; often due to spinal cord injury. Also called *thermanaesthesia*.

thermocauterectomy (ther'mō-kaw-ter-ek'tō-mi): The destruction of tissue by thermocautery.

thermocautery (ther'mō-kaw'ter-i): Cauterization by use of an instrument with a heated wire or point.

thermocoagulation (ther'mō-kō-ag'ū-lā-shun): Coagulation of tissue by electrocautery or by the passage of a high-frequency current.

thermodialysis (ther'mō-dī-al'i-sis): A technique utilized in producing hyperthermia therapeutically whereby the patient's blood is shunted through a controlled heat exchange and then returned to the body.

thermogenesis (ther'mō-jen'e-sis): The production of heat, specifically in the body. — thermogenetic, adj.

thermogenic (ther-mō-jen'ik): Relating to the production of heat. T. ACTION the action of certain foods and drugs that cause an increase in body temperature.

thermogram (ther'mō-gram): A regional surface map of the body or part of it obtained by an infrared sensing device.; it measures the radiant heat from the part and hence blood flow.

thermograph (ther'mō-graf): 1. The device or apparatus used in thermography (*q.v.*). 2. An instrument for recording variations in temperature.

thermography (ther-mog'ra-fi): A photographic technique that utilizes an infrared detector to measure variations in the surface temperature of the body; sometimes used in diagnosing underlying pathology such as tumours. Has also been used to differentiate pain of psychogenic origin from that of organic origin, since a painful disorder or injury may cause the temperature of the surrounding tissues to be lower than that in other parts of the body. — thermogram, n.

thermohyperaesthesia (ther'mō-hī-per-es-thē'zi-a): The condition of being extremely sensitive to variations in temperature.

thermolabile (ther-mō-lā' -bil): Subject to being easily altered or destroyed by heat.

thermolysis (ther-mol'i-sis): 1. The loss of body heat through evaporation, radiation, exhaled air, etc. 2. Chemical decomposition of a substance by use of heat. — thermolytic, adj.

thermomammography (ther'mō-mam-og'ra-fi): The use of thermography to examine for lesions of the breast.

thermomassage (ther'mō-mas-sazh'): A physical therapy technique utilizing a combination of heat and massage.

thermometer (ther-mom'i-ter): A device for determining temperature; consists of a substance such as mercury which expands and contracts with changes in temperature and which is enclosed in a sealed tube, usually glass, that is marked with a graduated scale. BATH T. one used for determining temperature of bath water; usually protected by a wooden case; CELSIUS or CENTIGRADE T. one marked with a 100-unit scale in which 0° is the freezing point and 100° the boiling point; the scale on the clinical Centigrade T. is from 34° or 36° to 42° with increments of 0.02°, CLINICAL T. one used for measuring the temperature of the body; FAHRENHEIT T. one marked with a 180-unit scale in which the freezing point is 32° and the boiling point is 212°. the scale on the clinical Fahrenheit T. is from 94° or 95° to 108° or 110°, with increments of 0.2°; FEVER T. a clinical T.; ORAL T. one used for taking temperature of the body by mouth; RECTAL T. one used fror taking temperature of the body by rectum; ROOM T. one used for determining the temperature of the air in a room.

thermoneurosis (ther' -mō-nū-rō'sis): Elevation of body temperature caused by vasomotor reactions to emotional influences.

thermonuclear (ther'mō-nū'klē-ar): Pertinent to or involving the nuclear fusion reaction that takes place between the molecules of a gas, hydrogen in particular, with the accompanying liberation of energy, when heated to temperatures of several million degrees.

thermophile (ther'mō-fil): A microorganism that thrives best at a relatively high temperature. — thermophilic, adj.

thermoplegia (ther'mō-plē'ji-a): Sunstroke; heat stroke.

thermopolypnoea (ther'mō-pol-ip-nē'a): Rapid respirations caused by exposure to excessive heat or fever.

thermoreceptor (ther'mō-rē-sep'tor): A nerve ending that is sensitive to heat.

thermoregulation (ther'mō-reg-ū-lā'shun): In physiology, the regulation of body temperature by an interrelated system consisting of the hypothalamus, the autonomic nervous system, and the cardiovascular system, which regulate the amount of heat produced or the amount lost, or both. — thermoregulatory, adj.

thermoresistant (ther'mō-rē-zis'tant): The quality of not being greatly affected by heat.

thermostable (ther'mō-stā'b'l): Remaining unaltered at a high temperature, which is usually specified. — thermostability, n.

thermostat (ther'mo-stat): A device that automatically regulates the temperature of a substance or area.

thermosterilization (ther'mō-ster-i-lī-zā'shun): Sterilization by the use of heat.

thermotaxis (ther-mō-tak'sis): 1. The normal regulation of the body temperature. 2. The reaction that occurs in an organism when stimulated by heat.

thermotherapy (ther'mō-ther'a-pi): Treatment of disease by the application of any form of heat including hot water, hot water bottle, hot wet pack, electric heating pad, infrared radiation, and diathermy. Body temperature may also be raised by artificial means such as induced fever, and decreased by induced hypothermia.

theta wave: See under WAVE.

thiamin(e) (thī'a-min,-mēn): Vitamin B_1 (aneurine hydrochloride), a member of the vitamin B complex; essential for metabolism of carbohydrates and fats, and for normal growth and healthy appetite; found in whole-grain cereals and flour, wheat germ, nuts, yeast, liver, lean pork, heart, kidney, milk, egg yolk, legumes, leafy vegetables, fruit; also produced synthetically; is slowly destroyed by heating. Deficiency may result in retardation of growth, loss of appetite, fatigue, mental apathy, impaired functioning of the nervous, digestive, muscular, circulatory, and endocrine systems, and, if severe and long-lasting, beriberi.

thiazides (thi'a-zids): A group of chemical compounds that promote the formation and excretion of urine; often used in treatment of hypertension and oedema; they tend to disturb the electrolyte balance in the body by increasing the excretion of sodium and potassium.

thigh (thi): The part of the leg between the hip and the knee. T. BONE the femur.

thigmaesthesia (thig'mes-the'zi-a): Having sensitivity to touch.

thio-: Combining form denoting the presence of sulphur. Usually refers to the replacement of the oxygen in a compound by sulphur.

thionin(e) (thi'o-nin,-nen): A dark green powder that gives a purple colour in solution; used as a stain in microscopic studies.

third: T. DEGREE BURN, see under BURN; T. DEGREE BLOCK, see under HEART BLOCK; T. HEART SOUND a sound heard at the end of rapid filling of the ventricles; also called *ventricular filling sound*; T. INTENTION, see under HEALING; T. NERVE PALSY palsy of the oculomotor nerve which affects certain extrinsic and intrinsic muscles of the eye.

thirst: A sensation of dryness in the mouth and throat, accompanied by a desire for drink.

Thomas: T. COLLAR, a stiff high collar usually made of metal and covered with leather, used as a support for the head in injuries of the neck and upper spine; T. SPLINT a metal splint used for emergency treatment or transporting a patient with a fractured leg or arm; it is shaped like a hairpin, the open end being equipped with a padded ring that is placed in the groin or axilla when the splint is applied; it is so constructed that traction can be applied to the limb. [H. O. Thomas, Scottish orthopaedic surgeon, 1834–1891.]

Thomsen's disease: Myotonia congenita (*q.v.*).

Thomson's sign: In scarlatina, the appearance of pinkish or red lines across the inner side of the bend of the elbow before the rash has erupted; they persist throughout the course of

the disease and, after desquamation, appear as pigmented lines. Also called *Pastia's lines*.

thorac-, thoraci-, thoraco-: Combining forms denoting chest or chest wall.

thoracectomy (tho-ra-sek'to-mi): Resection of all or part of a rib through an incision in the chest wall.

thoracentesis (tho'ra-sen-te'sis): Surgical puncture of the chest wall, usually with a large-bore needle, for the drainage of accumulated fluid; paracentesis. Also called *thoracocentesis*.

thoracic (tho-ras'ik): Relating to the thorax. T. BREATHING breathing in which the chest movements predominate; occurs in patients with certain gastric or abdominal conditions and those with paralysis; T. CAGE the bony framework that encloses the chest; T. CAVITY the space above the diaphragm; occupied by the thoracic artery and duct, the pulmonary veins and artery, vena cava, lungs, bronchi, mediastinum, heart, thymus gland, trachea, oesophagus; T. DUCT the duct that begins on the posterior abdominal wall in the cisterna chyli at the level of the second lumbar vertebra, and continues upwards along the bodies of the vertebrae to its termination at the junction of the left subclavian and left internal jugular veins; it drains lymph from the entire part of the body below the diaphragm and the upper left side of the structures above the diaphragm.

thoracicoabdominal (tho-ras'-i-ko-ab-dom'in-al): Relating to the thorax and abdomen. Also called *thoracoabdominal*.

thoracic outlet syndrome: A group of painful symptoms including weakness, coldness, and paraesthesia in the hand and arm, pain in the chest wall, and discomfort in the shoulder and neck muscles; may be caused by compression of a cervical disc or compression of a brachial plexus and subclavian artery by muscles of the clavicle and first rib.

thoracocyllosis (tho'rak-o-si-lo'sis): Deformity of the thorax.

thoracodorsal (tho'ra-ko-dor'sal): Relating to the thorax and the back.

thoracodynia (tho'-ra-ko-din'i-a): Pain in the chest.

thoracolaparotomy (tho'ra-ko-lap-a-rot'o-mi): A surgical procedure involving the opening of both the thorax and the abdomen.

thoracolumbar (tho-ra-ko-lum'bar): Relating to, arising in, or involving the thoracic and lumbar regions. Term often used in reference to the thoracic and lumbar spinal ganglia and their fibres that go to make up the sympathetic part of the autonomic nervous system.

thoracomyodynia (tho'ra-kō-mi-ō-din'i-a): Pain in the muscles of the chest.

thoracopagus (tho-ra-kop'a-gus): Conjoined twins united at the thoracic or epigastric region.

thoracopathy (tho-rā-kop'a-thi): Any disease of the organs of the thorax.

thoracoplasty (tho'ra-kō-plas-ti): 1. Plastic surgery on the chest. 2. An operation on the thorax in which the ribs are resected to allow the chest wall to collapse and the lung to rest; used in the treatment of pulmonary tuberculosis. Also called *thoracopneumoplasty*.

thoracoscope (tho-rak'o-skōp): A lighted instrument that can be inserted into the pleural cavity through a small incision in the chest wall to permit inspection of the pleural surface and treatment under visual control.

thoracostomy (tho-ra-kos'to-mi): The establishment of a surgical opening into the chest cavity to drain off accumulated fluid. T. TUBE one inserted through an opening in the chest wall; may be used in applying suction to the pleural cavity.

thoracotomy (tho-ra-kot'o-mi): Any surgical incision into the chest wall.

thorax (thaw'raks): The chest cavity; that part of the trunk situated below the neck and above the diaphragm, and within a bony framework formed by the sternum, ribs and thoracic vertebrae. Contains the trachea, bronchi, lungs, heart and oesophagus. — thoraces, pl.; thoracic, adj.

thorium (thaw'ri-um): A radioactive metallic element. Various compounds of T. are used in medicine. Chemical symbol, Th.

thought transference: Mental telepathy.

threadworm (thred'worm): *Enterobius (Oxyuris) vermicularis*, a nematode parasite in the colon of children. Pinworm.

thready (thred'i): Describes a pulse that can barely be felt.

three-day measles: See RUBELLA.

threonine (thrē'ō-nin,-nēn): A naturally occurring amino acid essential to human nutrition; found in most proteins.

threpsology (threp-sol'o-ji): The science of nutrition.

threshold (thresh'old): The lowest point at which a stimulus will evoke a response. PAIN T. the strength or amount of stimulus required to produce a sensation of pain or discomfort; RENAL T. the plasma level of a substance at which it begins to be excreted in the urine; T. DOSE the minimum dose that will produce a detectable response; T. STIMULUS see STIMULUS.

thrill: A fine vibration felt by the examiner on palpation over incompetent heart valves or an aneurysm.

thrix: Hair.

-thrix: Combining form denoting hair(s).

throat: The pharynx and fauces; the anterior part of the neck. SEPTIC SORE T. severe inflammation of the fauces and tonsils, usually caused by a streptococcal organism.

throb: 1. To beat or pulsate. 2. A beating or pulsation.

throe (thrō): A severe pain or pang, by custom referring to the pains of childbirth.

thromb-, thrombo-: Combining forms denoting (1) a blood clot; (2) the clotting of blood.

thrombasthenia (throm'bas-thē'ni-a): A rare hereditary platelet abnormality characterized by large platelets, prolonged bleeding time, defective clot formation, epistaxis, easy bruising, and excessive bleeding during or following surgery or other trauma. Also called *thromboasthenia* and *Glanzmann's disease*.

thrombectomy (throm-bek'to-mi): Surgical removal of a thrombus from within a blood vessel.

thrombin (throm'bin): An enzyme in shed blood that converts fibrinogen to fibrin; formed when prothrombin combines with calcium salts. Also called *thrombase*.

thrombinogen (throm-bin'ō-jen): Prothrombin (*q.v.*).

thromboangiitis (throm'bō-an-ji-ī'tis): Inflammation of the inner coat of a blood vessel with formation of a clot. T. OBLITERANS (syn., *Beurger's disease*) an uncommon disorder of unknown cause, occurring mainly in young adult males, characterized by patchy, inflammatory, obliterative vascular disease, principally in the limbs (sometimes in the cardiac or cerebral vessels), and presenting usually as calf pains, or more severely as early gangrene of the toes and following a chronic progressive course.

thromboarteritis (throm'bō-ar-ter-ī'tis): Inflammation of an artery with clot formation.

thromboblast (throm'bō-blast): A precursor of the thrombocyte; a giant megalocyte.

thromboclasis (throm-bok'la-sis): Thrombolysis (*q.v.*).

thrombocyte (throm'bō-sīt): Blood platelet; small non-nucleated disc-like body normally present in the blood in concentrations of approximately 300 000 per cu mm; its chief function is to assist in coagulation of the blood.

thrombocythaemia (throm'bō-sī-thē'mi-a): An increase in the normal number of circulating blood platelets; thrombocytosis.

thrombocytolysis (throm'bō-sī-tol'i-sis): Destruction of blood platelets.

thrombocytopathy (throm'bō-sī-top'a-thi): Refers to any disorder of the clotting mechanism that is caused by dysfunction of the blood platelets.

thrombocytopenia (throm'bō-sī-tō-pē'ni-a): A reduction in the number of platelets in the circulating blood. ACUTE T. may be caused by certain drugs, viruses, or bacteria; CHRONIC T. may be associated with such immune disorders as Hodgkin's disease or lupus erythematosus; ESSENTIAL T. idiopathic thrombocytopenic purpura; see under PURPURA.

thrombocytosis (throm'bō-sī-tō'sis): An increase in the number of blood platelets.

thromboembolectomy (throm'bō-em-bō-lek'to-mi): The surgical removal of an embolus of thrombic origin or of part of a thrombus.

thromboembolia (throm'bo-em-bō'li-a): Thromboembolism.

thromboembolism (throm'bō-em'bo-lizm): Obstruction of a blood vessel by a thrombus that has become detached from the site where it was formed and carried to another vessel which it blocks,—thromboemboli, pl., thromboembolic, adj.

thromboendarterectomy (throm'bō-end-ar-ter-ek'to-mi): Operation for the removal of a thrombus that is obstructing an artery.

thromboendarteritis (throm'bō-end-ar-ter-ī'tis): Inflammation of the inner lining of an artery with clot formation.

thrombogenesis (throm'bō-jen'e-sis): The formation of a blood clot.

thrombogenic (throm'bō-jen'ik): 1. Producing or capable of producing thrombi. 2. Capable of clotting blood. — thrombogenicity, n.; thrombogenetic, adj.; thrombogenetically, adv.

thromboid (throm'boyd): Relating to or resembling a thrombus.

thrombokinase (throm'bō-kī'nas): Thromboplastin (q.v.).

thrombolymphangitis (throm'-bō-lim-fan-jī'tis): Inflammation of a lymph vessel associated with the formation of a lymph clot.

thrombolysis (throm-bol'i-sis): The dissolving of a thrombus. — thrombolytic, adj.

thrombopathy (throm-bop'a-thi): Any disorder of the blood platelets that results in defective thromboplastin formation. Most often seen in kidney disease but also occurs in liver disease, and may be idiopathic.

thrombopenia (throm-bō-pē'ni-a): Thrombocytopenia (q.v.).

thrombophilia (throm-bō-fil'i-a): A tendency for thrombi to occur.

thrombophlebitis (throm'bō-flē-bī'tis): Inflammation of the wall of a vein with formation of a clot in the involved segment; sometimes caused by trauma to the vein as by an intravenous needle; may result in embolism. T. MIGRANS a form of recurring T. affecting principally the superficial veins; may occur at several sites at the same time or at intervals.

thromboplastin (throm'bō-plas'tin): A group of lipid and protein substances found in tissues, blood platelets and leukocytes, and which have an enzyme-like action in the conversion of prothrombin to thrombin in the clotting of blood.

thromboplastinogen (throm'bō-plas-tin'ō-jen): Factor VIII. See under FACTOR.

thromboplastinogenaemia (throm'bo-plas-tin-ō-jē-nē'mi-a): The presence of thromboplastinogen in the blood.

thromboplastinogenase (throm'bō-plas-tin-o-je-nās): An enzyme in the blood that acts as a catalyst in the conversion of inactive thromboplastinogen to thromboplastin.

thrombopoiesis (throm-bō-poy-ē'sis): The formation of thrombocytes.

thrombosed (throm'bōs'd): 1. Clotted. 2. Describing a blood vessel that contains a clot.

thrombosis (throm-bō'sis): The intravascular formation or presence of a clot, or other deposit that blocks an artery; CEREBRAL T., T. occurring in a cerebral vessel; may result in cerebral infarction; CORONARY T., T. occurring in a coronary artery and occluding it, thereby depriving the coronary muscle it serves of blood and usually leading to ischaemia and infarction of the myocardium; DEEP VEIN T. a serious condition where blood clots develop in the deep veins of the legs; MARASMIC T., T. that occurs usually in the longitudinal sinus of infants suffering a wasting disease; may also occur in the elderly; MESENTERIC T., T. occurring in a blood vessel of the mesentery; PUERPERAL T., T. occurring in a uterine vessel following childbirth; TRAUMATIC T., T. that occurs following injury to a part; VENOUS T., T. occurring in a vein. — thrombotic, adj.

thrombostasis (throm-bos'tā-sis): Stasis of blood in a vessel leading to, or resulting from, the formation of a thrombus.

thrombotic (throm-bot'ik): Relating to or affected by thrombosis. T. PHLEGMASIA see PHLEGMASIA ALBA DOLENS under PHLEGMASIA; T. THROMBOCYTOPENIC PURPURA see under PURPURA.

thrombotonin (throm-bō-tō'nin): Serotonin (*q.v.*).

thrombus (throm'bus): An intravascular clot composed of fibrin and solid blood elements that is formed by the coagulation of blood and that remains in the location in which it was formed; may more or less occlude a blood vessel or a heart cavity. — thrombi, pl.; thrombic, thrombotic, adj.

thrush: A disease associated with white spots on the mucous membranes of the mouth, which later become ulcerous; caused by *Candida albicans*. Occurs most often in malnourished and artificially fed infants and may involve the oesophagus and napkin area. Also sometimes seen in adults who have been weakened by infection, malnutrition or uncontrolled diabetes mellitus, or who have been treated with antibiotics for a long time. T. is also (colloquially) candidal vaginitis (*q.v.*) and occurs in pregnancy due to altered vaginal pH. See also CANDIDIASIS.

thrypsis (thrip'sis): A comminuted fracture; see under FRACTURE.

thumb: The first digit on the radial side of the hand; differs from the other digits in having only two phalanges and in having a freely movable metacarpal bone.

thym-, thymo-: Combining forms denoting: 1. The thymus gland. 2. The mind; emotions.

thymectomy (thī-mek'to-mi): Surgical excision of the thymus; usually done for removal of a tumour or in treatment of certain disease conditions such as myasthenia gravis.

thymelcosis (thī-mel-kō'sis): Ulceration or suppuration of the thymus gland.

-thymia: Combining form denoting mind or spirit.

thymic (thī'mik): Relating to the thymus gland. T. APLASIA a congenital disorder characterized by absence of the thymus and parathyroid glands, by cardiovascular deformities, susceptibility to fungal and viral infection, and tetany; often fatal; T. DYSPLASIA congenital lymphocytopenia characterized by early onset and susceptibility to viral and fungal infections; may be fatal.

thymitis (thī-mī'tis): Inflammation of the thymus.

thymocyte (thī'mō-sīt): A lymphocyte developed in the thymus; participates in the body's immune defences. Also called *T-lymphocyte* and *T-cell;* see under CELL.

thymol (thī'mol): A substance found in thyme oil and other volatile oils; also produced synthetically; used locally as a bactericide and fungicide.

thymoleptic (thī-mō-lep'tik): 1. Relating to agents that influence mood or spirit, particularly those that counteract depression. 2. A drug with mood-elevating action that counteracts depression.

thymoma (thī-mō'ma): A tumour arising in the thymus; usually benign; may be associated with myasthenia gravis.

thymopathy (thi-mop'a-thi): Any disease or disorder of the thymus gland.

thymosin (thī'-mō-sin): A hormone with immunologic properties, secreted by the thymus gland during childhood and decreasing as a person ages.

thymus (thī'mus): A gland-like structure lying behind the manubrium of the sternum and extending upwards as far as the thyroid gland. It is well developed in infancy and attains its greatest size towards the onset of puberty; then the lymphatic tissue slowly regresses and is replaced by fatty tissue. It has an immunological role in that it controls the production of T-cells (see under CELL), one of the body's defences against viruses, fungal infections, some bacterial infections, and cancer. See also LYMPHOKINES.

thyr-, thyro-: Combining forms denoting the thyroid gland.

thyroadenitis (thī-rō-ad-e-nī'tis): Inflammation of the thyroid gland.

thyroaplasia (thī'rō-a-plā'zi-a): Imperfect development and functioning of the thyroid gland.

thyrocalcitonin (thī'rō-kal-si-tō'nin): A polypeptide hormone containing 32 amino acids, secreted by the thyroid gland; acts to prevent resorption of bone; used therapeutically in treatment of Paget's disease. Formerly called *calcitonin*.

thyrocardiac (thī'-rō-kar'di-ak): 1. Relating to the thyroid gland and the heart. 2. Relating to disease of the thyroid gland in which cardiac symptoms predominate.

thyrocele (thī'rō-sēl): Enlargement of the thyroid gland; goitre.

thyrocervical (thī'rō-ser'vi-kal): Relating to the thyroid gland and the neck.

thyroepiglottic (thī'rō-ep-il glot'ik): Relating to the thyroid gland and the epiglottis.

thyrogenic (thī-rō-jen'ik): Originating in the thyroid gland.

thyroglobulin (thī-rō-glob'ū-lin): An iodine-containing glycoprotein secreted in the follicular cells of the thyroid and stored in the colloid substance of the gland; is concerned with the synthesis of thyroid hormones.

thyroglossal (thī-rō-glos′al): Relating to the thyroid gland and the tongue.

thyrohyoid (thī-rō-hī′oid): Relating to the thyroid cartilage and the hyoid (*q.v.*) bone.

thyroid (thī′roid): 1. Shaped like a shield. 2. The dried, powdered thyroid gland of the ox, sheep, or pig, used in the treatment of cretinism, myxoedema, and other conditions caused by thyroid dysfunction. 3. A highly vascular organ at the front of the neck, weighing approximately 30 g, consisting of bilateral lobes connected in the middle by a narrow isthmus. It secretes thyroxine directly into the blood and is part of the endocrine system of ductless glands. It is essential to normal body growth in infancy and childhood. LINGUAL T. a mass of thyroid tissue at or just beneath the base of the tongue; may or may not be associated with a normally situated thyroid gland; RETROSTERNAL T. a mass of thyroid tissue situated behind the sternum; T. CARTILAGE the large cartilage of the larynx, commonly called *Adam's apple*; T. CRISIS a serious condition resulting from the sudden increase in the basal metabolism rate due to hyperthyroidism; T. HORMONE see THYROXINE, LIOTHYRONINE, TRIIODOTHYRONINE, and THYROCALCITONIN; T. STORM a sudden increase in symptoms of thyrotoxicosis, particularly when it occurs following thyroidectomy; thyroid crisis.

thyroidectomy (thī-royd-ek′to-mi): Surgical removal of the thyroid gland. SUBTOTAL T. removal of only part of the thyroid gland.

thyroidism (thī′roy-dizm): Old term for a pathological condition caused either by overdoses of thyroid extract or by overactivity of the thyroid gland.

thyroiditis (thī-roy-dī′tis): Inflammation of the thyroid gland. HASHIMOTO'S T. see HASHIMOTO'S DISEASE; RIEDEL'S T. a chronic fibrosis of the thyroid gland; ligneous goitre; SUBACUTE T. usually occurs in association with viral diseases or upper respiratory infections; characterized by tenderness of the gland, malaise, fever, sore throat, pain that radiates to the ear and jaw; usually self-limited.

thyroidomania (thī′roy-dō-mā′ni-a): Mental disturbance due to hyperthyroidism.

thyroid-stimulating hormone: A substance secreted by the thyroid gland that stimulates the synthesis and release of thyroid hormone.

thyrolytic (thī′rō-lit′ik): Destructive to thyroid tissue.

thyromegaly (thī′rō-meg′a-li): Enlargement of the thyroid gland.

thyroncus (thī-ron′kus): Goitre; thyrocele.

thyroparathyroidectomy (thī′rō-par-a-thī′royddek′tō-mi): Surgical removal of the thyroid and parathyroid glands.

thyropathy (thī-rop′a-thi): Any disease of the thyroid gland.

thyropenia (thī′ -rō-pē′ni-a): Diminished activity of the thyroid gland.

thyroprival (thī′rō-prī′val): Relating to the effects of removal of the thyroid gland, or of loss of thyroid functioning.

thyroptosis (thī-rop-tō′sis): Downward displacement of the thyroid gland.

thyrosis (thī-rō′sis): Any disorder resulting from a malfunctioning thyroid gland.

thyrotherapy (thī-rō-ther′ a-pi): Treatment of thyroid disorders with preparations of the thyroid gland obtained from domesticated animals.

thyrotoxic (thī-rō-tok′sik): Relating to or affected by markedly increased thyroid gland activity. T. CRISIS see THYROID CRISIS under THYROID; T. HEART DISEASE a condition characterized by pericardial pain, weakness, sweating, weight loss; caused by hyperthyroidism which increases the work load of the heart and the amount of oxygen needed by the body.

thyrotoxicosis (thī′ -rō-tok-si-kō′sis): A condition due to excessive production of the thyroid gland hormone, thyroxine; signs and symptoms include increased metabolic rate, anxiety, nervousness, tachycardia, sweating, heat intolerance, emotional lability, increased appetite and loss of weight, a fine tremor of the hands when outstretched, and prominence of the eyes. In older patients, cardiac irregularities may be a prominent feature. Removal of the thyroid gland is usually necessary. APATHETIC T., occurs in a small percentage of cases in the elderly; characterized by severe apathy and inactivity; the classic symptoms of T. are often absent; cardiac and other organ pathology may be present; MASKED T. features of classic T. are absent but signs and symptoms of pathology affecting other organ systems may be evident.

thyrotrophic (thī′rō-trō′fik): 1. Directly affecting the secretory function of the thyroid gland. 2. A substance that stimulates the gland to activity, *e.g.*, the T. hormone secreted by the anterior pituitary gland.

thyrotrophin (thī-rot′rō-fin): A hormone originating in the anterior lobe of the pituitary gland; has the specific function of stimulating the thyroid gland. T. RELEASING FACTOR a hormone that originates in the hypothalamus of the brain; controls release of T. by the pituitary gland which, in turn, acts upon the thyroid gland causing it to release thyroid hormone; important in the diagnosis and treatment of disorders of the thyroid gland.

thyroxin(e) (thī-rok'sin,-sēn): An iodine-containing amino acid that is the chief active principle of the hormone secreted by the thyroid gland; essential for normal growth and metabolism. It is also prepared synthetically for use in disorders due to inadequate functioning of the thyroid gland.

TIA: Abbreviation for transient ischaemic attack (*q.v.*).

tibia (tib'i-a): The shinbone; the inner, thicker of the two bones of the leg below the knee; it articulates with the femur, fibula, and talus.

tibial (tib'i-al): Pertaining to the tibia. T. NERVE a branch of the sciatic nerve; supplies the muscles of the back of the leg.

tibialgia (tib-i-al'ji-a): Pain in the tibia or shin.

tibiocalcaneal (tib'i-ō-kal-kā'nē-al): Relating to the tibia and the calcaneus.

tibiofemoral (tib-i-ō-fem'o-ral): Relating to the tibia and the femur.

tibiofibular (tib-i-ō-fib'ū-lar): Relating to the tibia and the fibula.

tibionavicular (tib-i-ō-na-vik'ū-lar): Relating to the tibial and navicular bones.

tibiotalar (tib-i-ō-tā'lar): Relating to the tibia and the talus of the ankle, or to the articulation of these bones.

tibiotarsal (tib-i-ō-tar'sal): Relating to the tibia and the tarsal bones.

tic (tik): Minor, purposeless, repetitious, quick, involuntary gestures or muscular movements and twitchings, most often of the face, head, neck or shoulder, due to habit usually but also may be associated with a psychological factor. They disappear during sleep and are more common in boys and also in early life. T. DOU-LOUREUX trigeminal neuralgia; severe, brief but intense spasms of excruciating pain in an area supplied by one of the branches of the trigeminal nerve, especially the face or mouth.

tick (tik): A mite larger than others of the same class of bloodsucking arthropods. Some of them are transmitters of disease. See RELAPS-ING FEVER, Q FEVER, ROCKY MOUNTAIN SPOTTED FEVER, TULARAEMIA, TYPHUS.

tidal (tī'dal): T. AIR, see under AIR; T. DRAINAGE a method for continuous irrigation, most commonly used in treatment of a paralysed bladder; sometimes used for irrigating the chest after empyema; T. VOLUME the amount of air that flows in and out of the lungs with one breath at any level of activity.

Tietze's syndrome (tet'zēs): Low-grade costochondritis, characterized by pain in the costal cartilages that may radiate to the shoulder, neck, and arm, and resemble that of coronary heart disease; usually benign and self-limited. [Alexander Tietze, German surgeon, 1864–1927.]

tilt table: A table on which the patient lies prone and which can be rotated to a vertical position or various degress between horizontal and vertical; used in several examining and therapeutic procedures.

timbre (tim'b'r, tam-): The characteristic musical quality of sound.

time management: The planning and control of time resources to improve efficiency and effectiveness.

tincture (tink'-chur): An alcoholic pharmaceutical preparation made by extracting the useful principle from a vegetable material or a chemical substance; the amount of drug in the solution varies according to set standards for each drug.

tinea (tin'ē-a): A general term for several fungal infections of the skin; ringworm. T. BARBAE ringworm of the beard; barber's itch; T. CAPI-TIS ringworm of the scalp; T. CRICINATA or CORPORIS ringworm of the non-hairy surfaces of the body; T. CRURIS ringworm of the inner sides of thigh, perineal area or groin; more common in males; see DHOBIE ITCH; T. PEDIS chronic fungal infection of the feet, principally the areas between the toes; marked by intense itching, scaling, maceration and cracking of the skin; commonly called *athlete's foot*; T. UNGUIUM ringworm of the nails; see ONYCHOMYCOSIS; T. VERSICOLOR a common chronic disorder seen most often in tropical regions; usually symptomless and non-inflammatory; marked by the occurrence, usually on the trunk, of many macular patches of varying sizes and shapes which vary from white on darkly pigmented skin to fawn-coloured or brown on pale skin.

tine test: A skin test for tuberculosis. See HEAF MULTIPLE PUNCTURE TEST.

tingle: A slight, prickling, stinging, or throbbing sensation.

tinkles: Very high pitched bowel sounds that have a musical quality.

tinnitus (ti-nī'tus): Subjective noises such as buzzing, thumping, ringing, roaring, clucking, or humming that accompany certain types of hearing disorders. May also be a sign of impacted cerumen or of Ménière's disease (*q.v.*).

tissue (tish'ū): A collection of similar cells and the intercellular material surrounding them that form a structure, which, in turn, performs a particular function in the body. The five main classes of tissue are connective, epithelial, glandular, muscular, and nervous. ADIPOSE T. connective tissue containing masses of fat cells; AREOLAR T. loosely arranged, widely dispersed connective tissue; CANCELLOUS T. bony tissue that is spongy in appearance; COMPACT T. bony tissue that is dense and hard; CONNECTIVE T. made up of an interlacing mass of fibres; pervades, supports, and binds together tissues and organs; includes areolar, adipose, fibrous, elastic, and lymphoid tissues, cartilage and bone, blood and lymph; ENDOTHELIAL T. a single layer of flattened cells that lines serous cavities, blood vessels and lymphatics; EPITHELIAL T. one or more layers of flattened cells with little intercellular substance; lines tubes or cavities that connect with the exterior and covers the surface of the body; MUSCULAR T. made up of fibres that are capable of contracting and expanding; classified as skeletal, smooth or visceral, and cardiac. See MUSCLE; NERVOUS T. made up of highly differentiated cells that compose nerves and their fibres and the tissues that support them; PARENCHYMATOUS T. the specialized tissue of an organ that makes up its functioning part as differentiated from supporting tissues; SUBCUTANEOUS T. that found directly underneath the skin; it is a type of loosely organized connective T.

tissue culture: The culture of tissue cells in the laboratory.

tissular (tish'ū-lar): Relating to the tissues of the body.

titanium (tī-tā'ni-um): A dark grey hard metallic element. T. DIOXIDE an opaque white powder, used in creams and powders to protect the skin against irritation and solar rays. An alloy of the metal is used in making various orthopaedic prostheses.

titillation (tit-il-lā'shun): Tickling, or the sensation of tickling.

titrate (tī'trāt): To determine the strength of a solution, or the concentration of a substance in a solution, in terms of the amount of known concentration required to bring about a given effect in a reaction with a known volume of the test solution.

titration (tī-trā'shun): Determination of the quantity of a given constituent in a substance by observing the volume of a standard solution needed to change the constituent to a completely different form. — titrate, v.

titre (tī'tur): The strength of a solution or the quantity of a particular constituent of a solution as determined by titration (q.v.). A standard of strength or purity.

titubation (tit'ū-bā'shun): Incoordination, unsteadiness, and stumbling manifested when walking.

toco-: Combining form relating to obstetrics or childbirth.

tocodynamometer (tō'kō-dī-na-mom'i-ter): An instrument for measuring the frequency, strength, and duration of contractions of the uterus; used particularly during labour.

tocography (tō-kog'ra-fi): A process of recording uterine contractions graphically using a device called a tocograph or parturiometer.

tocologist (tō-kol'o-jist): An obstetrician.

tocology (tō-kol'o-ji): Obstetrics.

tocomania (tō-kō-mā'ni-a): Puerperal psychosis; see under PUERPERAL.

tocopherol (tok-of'er-ol): Any of a group of fat-soluble compounds containing vitamin E, of which alpha-tocopherol is the most physiologically active; is necessary for normal reproduction and believed to be necessary also for certain other physiological processes. Widely distributed in foods including wheat germ, some seeds, peanuts, cereal grains, rice, egg yolk, margarine, vegetable oils, milk, beef liver, fat and lean meats, all leafy green vegetables. Deficiency results in muscle degeneration, anaemia, infertility, liver and kidney damage.

tocophobia (tō-kō-fō'bi-a): Undue fear of childbirth.

Todd's paralysis: A transient paralysis that sometimes occurs in epileptics following a focal seizure; usually clears within 24 hours.

toe: Any of the digits of the feet. HAMMER T. claw-like deformity caused by the permanent flexion of the joint between the second and third phalanges; most often involves the second toe; may be congenital or caused by ill-fitting shoes; PIGEON T. deformity causing toeing in or walking with the toes turned towards the centre line of the body.

toeing in: Walking with the toes or the feet pointed towards the midline of the body.

togavirus (tō'ga-vī-rus'): Any of a subgroup of arboviruses (q.v.) including some that are transmitted by arthropods, especially ticks and mosquitoes; they cause haemorrhagic fever, yellow fever, dengue, and encephalitis; so-called because they are encapsulated in an envelope or toga.

toilet: 1. The cleansing of a wound area after surgery or delivery of an obstetric patient. **2.** A device for collecting and disposing of urine and faeces, or the room in which such a device is housed. **3.** The various activities involved in dressing and grooming. T. TRAINING teaching a child to control bowel and bladder function. Training methods used, parents' attitude about these, and the child's responses, are thought to influence the development of personality.

token economy: A means of shaping or changing the troublesome behaviour of the socially disabled, mentally ill, or mentally handicapped person. Acceptable or desired behaviour is rewarded by the giving of tokens on a defined and negotiated scale which can be exchanged for privileges or goods.

tolerance (tol'e-rans): **1.** The ability to endure the administration of unusually large amounts of a substance, usually a drug, without ill effects. **2.** Resistance to the effects of a medication administered over a period of time so that increasingly larger doses are required to get the effect of the original dose. CROSS T. the carrying over of tolerance for one drug to tolerance for another drug; PAIN T. the maximum amount of stimulation required to produce the sensation of pain or discomfort; REVERSE T. a condition in which response to a specific dose of a drug increases with repeated use so that smaller doses may be taken and still produce the effects that resulted from larger doses; SUGAR T. the amount of sugar a person can metabolize before it begins to appear in the urine.

tolerant (tol'er-ant): **1.** Possessing tolerance for the beliefs, opinions, and practices of others. **2.** The state of being resistant to the effects of continued or increasing use of a drug. **3.** The ability to survive and grow in a specific environment; said of bacteria particularly.

-tome: Combining form denoting cutting or sectioning, or a cutting instrument.

tomo-: Combining form denoting section or sectional.

tomogram (tom'o-gram): A radiographic study that provides segmental visualization of structures at selected levels by blurring structures in all other planes.

tomograph (to'mo-graf): A device for obtaining an x-ray image of an organ or tissue at a selected plane or layer in a specified region of the body while blurring images of structures in other planes. Can be a series of films taken at different depths. — tomography, n.; tomographic, adj.

tomomania (to'mo-mān'i-a): An abnormal desire to (1) perform surgery, or (2) to have surgery performed on one's self.

tomotocia (to'mo-to'si-a): Caesarean section.

-tomy: Combining form denoting incision; a cutting operation.

tone (ton): **1.** A particular quality or sound of voice. **2.** The normal firmness and strength of tissues. **3.** The normal healthy degree of tension in resting muscles.

tongs: In orthopaedics, a device with points that engages the skull and is attached to a traction apparatus; used for treatment of cervical fractures. Several types are available, the most common being Burton, Crutchfield, and Vincke.

tongue (tung): The mobile, muscular organ contained in the mouth; it is concerned with speech, mastication, swallowing, and taste. BIFID T. a T. in which the anterior part is divided by a longitudinal cleft; BLACK T. a T. with a black to brown fur-like patch at the back part where the papillae have become elongated, seen especially after the individual has been treated with antibiotics; COATED T. a T. covered with a layer of yellowish or whitish material consisting of bacteria, food debris, etc.; associated with high fever, and digestive disorders; ENCRUSTED T. a T. heavily coated with yellowish material; FURRED T. a T. coated with a surface that resembles white fur; due to extensive change in the papillae; GEOGRAPHIC T. a T. covered with migratory denuded patches that are surrounded by elevated thickened epithelium; HAIRY T. a T. in which the papillae have blackened and become elongated; may occur in individuals who have sucked on antibiotic lozenges; MAGENTA T. a purplish-red T., due to deficiency of riboflavin; RASPBERRY T. the T. is bright red, not coated; has elevated papillae; seen in scarlatina after the rash has been present for several days; SMOKER'S T. leukoplakia (q.v.) of the T.; STRAWBERRY T. a T. that has a whitish coat with reddened papillae; characteristic of scarlatina during the first 24 hours after the rash has appeared.

tongue-tie: Shortness of the frenum resulting in limited mobility of the tongue; may cause interference with sucking and articulation. — tongue-tied, adj.

-tonia: Combining form denoting degree or condition of tonus.

tonic (to'nik): **1.** A state of continuous or sustained contraction, said of muscles. **2.** Increasing or restoring physical or mental tone o strength. **3.** A drug that invigorates or restore strength. T. SPASM, refers to prolonged muscle spasm as differentiated from a clonic spasm; see CLONUS.

tonic: A combining form denoting: 1. The degree or quality of muscular contraction, *e.g.*, isotonic. 2. The concentration of a substance in solution, *e.g.*, hypertonic.

tonic–clonic: Relates to muscle spasms, especially those seen in generalized seizures in which there is both a tonic and clonic stage. See TONIC, CLONIC. Also called *tonicoclonic, tonoclonic.*

tonicity (tō-nis'i-ti): 1. The condition of possessing tone. 2. The state of normal tension or tone of a muscle or muscles. 3. The osmotic pressure or tension of a solution.

tono-: Combining form denoting: 1. Tone. 2. Tension. 3. Pressure.

tonography (tō-nog'ra-fi): Continuous recording of pressure using an electric tonometer (*q.v.*); used particularly for measuring intraocular pressure.

tonometer (tō-nom'i-ter): An instrument in measuring tension or pressure, especially intraocular pressure.

tonometry (tō-nom'e-tri): The measurement of pressure or tension, particularly the use of a tonometer to measure intraocular pressure.

tonsil (ton'sil): By custom referring to one of two small almond-shaped lymphoid bodies lying between the pillars of the fauces either side of the oropharynx and covered with mucous membrane; called palatine tonsils. CEREBELLAR T. one of a pair of rounded masses on the inferior surface of the cerebellum; LINGUAL T. an aggregation of lymph follicles at the root of the tongue; PHARYNGEAL T. an aggregation of lymphoid tissue situated in the roof and posterior wall of the nasopharynx. See WALDEYER'S RING. — tonsillar, tonsillary, adj.

tonsillectomy (ton'si-lek'to-mi): Usually refers to the surgical removal of one or both of the palatine tonsils.

tonsillitis (ton'si-lī'tis): Inflammation of the tonsils. FOLLICULAR T. inflammation of the tonsils involving the crypts, with development of projecting yellow or white spots.

tonsilloadenoidectomy (ton'sil-ō-ad' -e-noyd-ek'to-mi): Surgical removal of the palatine tonsils and the adenoids.

tonsillolith (ton-sil'ō-lith): Concretion arising in the body of a tonsil.

tonsillopharyngitis (tn'sil-ō-far-in-jī'tis): Inflammation of the palantine tonsils and the pharynx.

tonsillotome (ton-sil'ō-tōm): An instrument for excision of tonsils.

tonus (tō'nus): The normal condition of slight continuous contraction in body tissues, muscles in particular, when in a state of rest.

tooth: Any of the small bone-like structures that are set in the jaws and used for chewing; they also assist in articulation. Each tooth is made up of a pulp cavity which contains a soft pulpy substance that supports blood vessels and nerves, and a solid outer part consisting of dentin or ivory which is covered above the gum with enamel — the hardest substance in the body — and below the gum with cementum. The part outside the gum is called the crown and the part inside is the root. In humans, the deciduous, baby or milk teeth erupt between the 6th and 24th months of life and are shed by the age of approximately 7 years. The permanent set, 32 in number, is usually complete in the late teens and consists of 8 incisors, 4 canines (cuspids), 8 premolars (bicuspids), and 12 molars (tricuspids). CANINE or EYE T. a T. with sharp fang-like edge for tearing food; IMPACTED T. a T. so placed that it cannot erupt into its normal position; INCISOR T. a T. with a knife-like edge for biting food; PREMOLAR and MOLAR T., a T. that has a squarish termination for chewing and grinding food; STOMACH T. the lower canine T. one on each side; WISDOM T. the third and last molar, one at either side of each jaw.

toothache: An aching pain in a tooth or near a tooth; may be caused by trauma, infection, or caries. Odontalgia.

tooth grinding: See BRUXISM.

TOP: Abbreviation for termination of pregnancy.

top-, topo-: Combining forms denoting place; locality.

topaesthesia (tōp'es-thē'zi-a): The ability to localize a tactile sensation precisely.

topagnosis (top'ag-nō'sis): 1. Inability to locate the exact point at which some part of the body is touched. 2. Inability to find one's way about in a familiar location.

topalgia (tō-pal'ji-a: Localized pain.

topectomy (tō-pek'to-mi): Modified frontal lobotomy to treat a psychosis.

toper's nose: Rhinophyma.

tophaceous (tō-fā'shus): Gritty; sandy. T. GOUT see under GOUT.

topical (top'ik-al): 1. Relating to a definite spot; local. 2. Term often used to describe a substance that is to be applied to the surface of the body for its local effect as distinguished from one that is given internally for its systemic effect.

topognosis (top'og-nō'sis): The ability to localize a tactile sensation. Topaesthenia.

topography (to-pog'ra-fi): In anatomy, a description of the regions of the body. — topographical, adj.; topographically, adv.

topology (top-pol'o-ji): 1. Regional anatomy. 2. The description of the relation of the presenting part of a fetus to the pelvic canal.

toponarcosis (top'ō-nar-kō'sis): Loss of sensation or the development of anaesthesia in a localized area.

TOPV: Abbreviation for *t*rivalent *o*ral *p*olio-virus *v*accine, a live attenuated vaccine that includes all three strains of poliovirus; most recipients are protected after a single dose.

TORCH syndrome: The clinical manifestation of any of a certain kind of disease-producing agents, including T*oxoplasma gondii*, *o*ther, *r*ubella virus, *c*ytomegalovirus, and *h*erpes simplex virus in the fetus or newborn infant.

tormina (tor'mi-na): Gripping intestinal pains. — torminal, torminous, adj.

torpid (tor'pid): Sluggish; not reacting with normal vigour or ease.

torpor (taw'por): Sluggishness, inactivity, stupor, apathy, numbness; absence or slowness of reaction to ordinary stimuli.

torque (tork): The measurement of the force capable of producing rotation or torsion about an axis; a twisting force.

torsion (tor'shun): A twisting. T. OF THE OVARY a twisting of the ovary caused by the presence of an ovarian cyst or teratoma, resulting in severe pain, constipation, vomiting, and the presence of an adnexal mass; T. OF THE TESTICLE a twisting of the testicle on its mesentery, causing pain and interference with blood supply; T. OF THE UMBILICAL CORD more than the normal eight or ten twists of the cord; may follow death of the fetus. — torsive, adj.

torso (taw'sō): The trunk of the body without the head and extremities.

torticollis (tor'ti-kol'is): Wryneck; persistent involuntary contraction of the muscles on one side of the neck; the head is slightly flexed and drawn towards the contracted side, with the face rotated over the shoulder. CONGENITAL T. due to birth injury of the sternocleidomastoid muscle on one side only; INFANTILE T. arises during the first six months of life; due to a tight sternocleidomastoid muscle; the chin points to the opposite foot; MUSCULAR T. associated with fibrosis of the sternocleido-

mastoid muscle; MYOGENIC T. due to muscular contraction, particularly in rheumatism; NEUROGENIC T. due to irritation of the accessory nerve; STRUCTURAL T. due to congential hemivertebra. — torticollar, adj.

tortuous (tor'chū-us): Twisted, full of curves, turns or twists.

tortuosity (tor-chū-os'i-ti): 1. The quality of being bent, twisted, or winding. 2. Something twisted, winding, or curved.

torulus (tor'ū-lus): A minute projection or elevation; a papilla. — toruli, pl.

torus (to'rus): An elevation or prominence. T. PALATINUS the bony elevation along the midline of the hard palate. — tori, pl.; toric, adj.

total hip replacement: Reconstruction of both the head of the femur and the acetabulum and replacement of the head with a metal ball cemented into the shaft of the femur with methyl methacrylate.

total parenteral nutrition: Parenteral hyperalimentation. A way of supplying essential nutrients via intravenous infusion of a solution containing glucose, amino acids, vitamins, eletrolytes, and water, to meet the nutritional needs of the particular patient; used for patients with burns, severe infections, colitis, severe vomiting or diarrhoea, or for infants with congenital anomalies that interfere with normal feeding.

total patient care: 1. A planned therapeutic regime for a patient to which members of several different professional groups have contributed. 2. A term used to denote the inclusion of the physical, psychological, spiritual and social aspects of care for a person who requires nursing.

total quality management: The application of industrial management practice to systematically maintain and improve organization-wide performance. Effectiveness and success are determined and assessed by quantitative quality measures.

touch: 1. The special sense by which contact with objects makes one aware of their qualities. 2. To examine by touching with the finger or hand. THERAPEUTIC T. see under THERAPEUTIC.

Tourette syndrome: See GILLES DE LA TOURETTE SYNDROME.

tourniquet (toor'ni-ket,-kay): An apparatus for the temporary compression of the blood vessels of a limb. Designed for compression of a main artery to control bleeding. A T. is also often used to obstruct the venous return from a limb and so facilitate the withdrawal of blood from a vein. Tourniquets vary from a simple rubber band to a pneumatic cuff. RO-TATING T. a system of treatment in which tourniquets are applied to all four extremities in turn, as near the trunk as possible; every 10–15 minutes, the tourniquets are rotated so that a different arm or leg is free and three tourniquets are always in place.

tourniquet test: A test for capillary resistance. A blood pressure cuff on the patient's arm is inflated to a point midway between diastolic and systolic pressure and the pressure maintained for ten minutes; if petechiae appear on the forearm, the test is positive. Used in diagnosing diseases marked by capillary fragility, *e.g.*, scurvy, thrombocytopenic purpura, and purpura accompanying severe infections.

tox-, toxi-, toxo-: Combining forms denoting toxic, toxin, poison, poisonous.

toxaemia (tok-sē'mi-a): Generalized poisoning due to the accumulation of toxins in the bloodstream, usually as a result of bacterial action but may also be due to other causes. ALIMENTARY T., T. due to absorption of toxins generated in the gastrointestinal tract; ECLAMPTIC T., T. of pregnancy; HYDATID T., T. caused by the escape of fluid from a hydatid mole into the peritoneal cavity; *see* HYDATIDIFORM MOLE under MOLE, T. OF PREGNANCY a condition due to a disturbance of metabolism and characterized by hypertension, oedema, albuminuria, and sometimes eclampsia (*q.v.*). — toxaemic, adj.

toxanaemia (toks'a-nē'mi-a): Anaemia resulting from poisoning by a haemolytic agent.

toxic (toks'ik): 1. Poisonous. 2. Resulting from or caused by a poison. 3. Pertaining to a toxin. Syn., *poisonous*.

toxic-, toxico-: Combining forms denoting poison.

toxicant (toks'i-kant): A toxic or poisonous substance.

toxicity (tok-sis'i-ti): The quality or degree of the poisonousness of a substance.

Toxicodendron (toks'i-kō-den'dron): A plant species the sap of which causes dermatitis on contact with the skin; includes poison ivy and sumac.

toxicoderma (toks'i-kō-der'ma): Any skin disease caused by a toxin or poison.

toxicodermatitis (toks'i-kō-der-ma-tī' tis): Inflammation of the skin due to a poison.

toxicogenic (toks'ik-ō-jen'ik): 1. Caused by a poison. 2. Producing or capable of producing a poison.

toxicoid (toks'i-koyd): Resembling a poison, or having an action like that of a poison.

toxicologist (toks-i-kol'o-jist): A person who specializes in the study of poisons.

toxicology (toks-i-kol'o-ji): The science dealing with poisons and poisonings. — toxicological, adj.; toxicologically, adv.

toxicomania (toks'i-kō-mā'ni-a): A periodic or chronic state of intoxication, produced by repeated consumption of a drug harmful to the individual or society. Characteristics are: uncontrollable desire or necessity to continue using the drug and to try to get it by any means; tendency to increase the dose; and psychic and physical dependency as a result.

toxicopathy (toks-i kop'a-thi): Any disease or condition caused by a poison — toxicopathic, adj.

toxicopexis (toks' -i-kō-pek'sis): The neutralization of a poison in the body.

toxicosis (toks-i-kō'sis): The condition of systemic poisoning by a toxin or poison.

toxic shock syndrome: A rare, serious, potentially fatal condition characterized by high fever, headache, nausea, vomiting, diarrhoea, myalgia, erythematous rash, hypovolaemia, rapid drop in blood pressure, thrombocytopenia, resembles disorders caused by bacterial toxins. About 70% of cases have occurred in women using a tampon, but also it occurs in persons with infections of other origin. *Staphylococcus aureus* has been the usual causative organism.

toxic storm: A severe condition characterized by acute hypermetabolism. See THYROID CRISIS under THYROID.

toxiferous (tok-sif'er-us): Poisonous.

toxigenicity (toks'i-je-nis'i-ti): The degree of ability of an organism to produce toxic substances that may be injurious to human cells.

toxin (toks'in): Any poisonous substance produced by a plant or animal organism, usually referring to one produced by pathogenic organism.

toxinaemia (toks-in-ē'mi-a): Toxaemia (*q.v.*).

toxin–antitoxin: A mixture of diphtheria toxin and its antitoxin that was formerly used to produce immunity to diphtheria, now largely replaced by diphtheria toxoid.

toxinfection (toks-in-fek'shun): Infection caused by a toxin rather than a microorganism. Also called *toxoinfection*.

toxinic (tok-sin'ik): Relating to a toxin.

toxinosis (toks'in-ō'sis): Any pathological condition caused by the action of a toxin.

Toxocara (tok'sō-kar'a): A genus of nematode worms that are parasitic to humans, dogs (*T. canis*), and cats (*T. cati*).

toxocariasis (tol'sō-kar-ī'a-sis): A disease due to infection with the nematode worm of the genus *Toxocara*, which enters the circulation through the intestinal wall; characterized by inflammation, haemorrhage, and necrosis of the tissues of the organs to which the larvae of the worm migrate; may affect the brain, liver, heart, great vessels, or retina.

toxoid (tok'soyd): A bacterial toxin altered in such a way that it has lost its poisonous properties but retained its antigenic properties and thus is capable of producing active immunity. DIPHTHERIA T. that used to produce active immunity against diphtheria; it is prepared from products of the growth of *Corynebacterium diptheriae*; TETANUS T. used to produce active immunity against tetanus; prepared from the products of the growth of *Clostridium tetani*.

toxophore (tok'sō-for): The particular chemical group in the molecules of a poison that give it its toxic characteristics.

Toxoplasma (tok-sō-plaz'ma): A genus of protozoal parasites. *Toxoplasma gondii* causes toxoplasmosis (*q.v.*).

toxoplasmosis (tok'sō-plas-mō'sis): Infection by *Toxoplasma gondii*, a protozoan parasite, which commonly infects birds and mammals, including humans. Intrauterine fetal as well as infant infections are often severe, producing encephalitis, convulsions, hydrocephalus, and eye disease, resulting in death or, in those who recover, mental handicap and impaired sight. Infection in older children and adults may result in pneumonia, nephritis, or skin rashes. OCULAR T. posterior, granulomatous uveitis, characterized by chorioretinitis, pain, photophobia.

TPI test: *Treponema pallidum* immobilization test. A highly specific test for syphilis in which syphilitic serum immobilizes and kills spirochaetes grown in pure culture.

T piece: A T-shaped tube that may be used in conjunction with a tracheostomy tube to provide for delivery of humidity along with oxygen or air.

TPN: Abbreviation for total parenteral nutrition (*q.v.*).

TPR: Abbreviation for temperature, pulse, respiration.

TQM: Abbreviation for total quality management (*q.v.*).

trabecula (tra-bek'ū-la): In anatomy, one of the fibrous bands or septa of connective tissue that extend into the interior of an organ from its wall or the capsule that covers it, and that serve to hold the functioning cells of the organ in position. — trabculae, pl.; trabecular, adj.

trabeculation (tra-bek-ū-lā'shun): The formation or presence of trabeculae in a part of the body.

trabeculectomy (tra-bek'ū-lek'to-mi): A microsurgical procedure for the relief of glaucoma, involves the excision of a small rectangle of the sclera.

trace elements: Metals and other elements that are regularly present in very small amounts in the tissues and thought to be essential for normal metabolism (*e.g.* copper, cobalt, manganese, fluorine, iodine, zinc).

tracer (trā'ser): 1. An instrument used for dissecting blood vessels and nerves. 2. A substance or instrument used to gain information about the body and its functions. 3. A radioactive substance added in minute amounts to a given substance that is introduced into the body in certain x-ray examinations; useful in tracing the outline of organs or structures and determining the presence of tumours.

trach-, trachea-, tracheo-: Combining forms denoting the trachea.

trachea (tra'kē-a): The windpipe; the fibrocartilaginous tube lined with ciliated mucous membrane passing from the larynx to the bronchi. It is about 11.5 cm long and about 2.5 cm wide. — tracheal, adj.

tracheal (tra'kē-al): Relating to the trachea. T. BREATH SOUNDS bronchial breath sounds; see under BREATH SOUNDS; T. INTUBATION the insertion of a tube through the larynx into the trachea to maintain an airway; used especially in cardiopulmonary resuscitation and in patients having general anaesthesia.

trachealgia (tra-kē-al'ji-a): Pain in the trachea.

tracheitis (tra-kē-ī'tis): Inflammation of the mucous membrane lining the trachea. Also spelled *trachitis*.

trachel-, trachelo-: Combining forms denoting (1) the neck, or (2) a neck-like structure.

trachelagra (tra'ke-lag'ra): A gouty or rheumatic condition of the neck characterized by torticollis.

trachelectomy (tra'ke-lek'to-mi): Surgical removal of the neck of the uterus.

trachelismus (tra'ke-liz'mus): 1. Spasm of the neck muscles. 2. Bending backward of the neck, a sign that sometimes signals the imminence of an epileptic attack.

trachelitis (tra'ke-lī'tis): Inflammation of the cervix of the uterus.

trachelocystitis (tra'ke-lō-sis-tī'tis): Inflammation of the neck of the urinary bladder.

trachelokyphosis (tra'ke-lōkī-fō'sis): An abnormal anterior curvature of the cervical vertebrae; humpback.

trachelopexy (tra'ke-lō-pek'si): An operation for fixation of the neck of the uterus.

trachelophyma (tra'ke-lō-fī'ma): A swelling or tumour of the neck.

tracheloplasty (tra'ke-lō-plas-ti): Surgical repair of lacerations or other injuries to the neck of the uterus.

trachelorrhaphy (tra'ke-lor'a-fi): Operative repair of a lacerated uterine cervix.

trachelos (tra'ke-lōs): The neck.

tracheo-: Combining form denoting trachea.

tracheobronchial (tra'ke-ō-bron'ki-al): Relating to the trachea and the bronchi. T. TREE consists of the trachea, the bronchi, and their branching structures; a system of bifurcating tubes made up of muscular, cartilaginous, and elastic tissues.

tracheobronchitis (tra'ke-ō-bron-kī'tis): Inflammation of the trachea and bronchi.

tracheobronchomegaly (tra'ke-ō-bron'kō-meg'a li): A rare condition or syndrome of greatly enlarged lumen of the trachea and main bronchi, characterized by recurrent and chronic respiratory tract infections; thought to be congenital.

tracheobronchoscopy (tra'ke-ō-bron-kos'ko-pi): Inspection of the interior of the trachea and one or both of the bronchi by means of a bronchoscope.

tracheography (tra'ke-og'ra-fi): The process of making an x-ray picture of the trachea after instillation of a contrast medium.

tracheolaryngeal (tra' ke-ō-lar-in'je-al): Relating to the trachea and the larynx.

tracheomalacia (tra'ke-ō-ma-lā'shi-a): Softening and destruction of the walls of the trachea, especially of the cartilaginous rings.

tracheo-oesophageal (trak'ē-ō-ē-sof-a-je'al): Relating to the trachea and oesophagus. T. FISTULA an abnormal connection between the trachea and oesophagus, present at birth. The baby can swallow only with difficulty with coughing and choking as milk passes into the trachea, and there is a real risk of asphyxia. Early surgical correction is necessary.

tracheopharyngeal (tra'ke-ō-far-in'je-al): Relating to the trachea and the pharynx.

tracheophony (tra'ke-of'o-ni): The sound heard when auscultating over the trachea.

tracheoplasty (tra'ke-ō-plas-ti): Plastic surgery on the trachea.

tracheopyosis (tra'ke-ō-pī-ō'sis): Tracheitis with purulent effusion.

tracheorrhagia (tra'ke-ō-rāj'i-a): Haemorrhage from the trachea.

tracheorrhaphy (tra-ke-or'ra-fi): Suturing of the trachea.

tracheoscopy (tra'ke--os'ko-pi): Inspection of the interior of the trachea with a special instrument called a tracheoscope. — tracheoscopic, adj.

tracheostenosis (tra' -ke-ōste-nō'sis): Narrowing or constriction of the trachea.

tracheostoma (tra'ke-ō-stō'ma): An opening made into the trachea through the neck.

tracheostomy (tra-ke-os'to-mi): The surgical creation of a stoma or an opening into the trachea through the neck for the purpose of facilitating passage of air into the lungs or to remove secretions from the trachea; usually a tube is inserted to keep the opening patent and to facilitate passage of air or evacuation of secretions. T. TUBE a curved tube inserted into the trachea following a tracheostomy.

tracheotome (tra'ke-o-tōm): A tracheotomy knife, used for incising the trachea.

tracheotomize (tra'ke-ot'o-mīz): To perform a tracheotomy upon.

tracheotomy (tra-ke-ot'o-mi): The operation of making an incision into the trachea; may be done to remove a foreign body, secure a specimen for biopsy, or for exploratory purposes. — tracheotomize, v.

trachoma (tra-kō'ma): A chronic communicable disease of the cornea and conjunctiva, caused by the *Chlamydia trachomatis*; of worldwide distribution but occurs chiefly in the Middle East, Asia, and the Mediterranean area where it is the principal cause of blindness; of insidious or sudden onset and of long duration when untreated. Most often occurs in association with poverty, poor hygiene, crowded living conditions and exposure of the eyes to sun and sand in hot dry dusty regions; is transmitted by flies, fingers, and fomites. Symptoms include pain, tearing, photophobia, inflammation of the eyelids and conjunctiva with the formation of lesions and terminate in granulation and scar tissue, deformities of the eyelids, progressive visual disability, and, frequently, blindness.

trachyphonia (trak'i-fō'ni-a): Roughness or hoarseness of the voice.

tracing (trās'ing): A recording or pattern of lines made by a pointed instrument on paper or other surface to show movement or activity.

tract: In anatomy, (1) an area or region that is longer than it is wide, or (2) a path or track.

May consist of a number of separate organs arranged serially and engaged in performing a common function; or may consist of a bundle of nerve fibres that have the same origin, termination, and function. ASCENDING T. tracts that transmit afferent nerve impulses up the spinal cord to the brain; they include (1) the funiculus gracilis and funiculus cuneatus, which carry impulses of position movement, and touch–pressure, and terminate in the medulla oblongata; (2) the ventral spinothalamic T. which carries proprioceptive impulses and terminates in the thalamus; (3) the dorsal spinocerebellar T. which carries impulses of crude touch and pressure to the cerebellum; (4) the lateral spinothalamic T. which carries impulses of pain and temperature to the thalamus. DESCENDING TRACTS tracts that carry efferent impulses from the brain down the spinal cord; they include (1) the corticospinal T. which transmits impulses from the cerebral cortex to the muscles of the extremities, with some fibres going to the neck and trunk; (2) the vestibulospinal T. which transmits efferent impulses from the medulla oblongata that are concerned with the maintenance of muscle tone and equilibrium (also called *extrapyramidal tract*); (3) the reticulospinal T. which extends from the brainstem to the sympathetic ganglia and provides innervation for unconscious muscle coordination.

tractibility (trak-ta-bil′i-ti): The condition of being easily handled, managed, or controlled.

traction (trak′shun): 1. The process of pulling a part of the body along, through, or out of its socket or cavity, such as axis traction with obstetrics forceps in delivering an infant. 2. A steady drawing or pulling exerted manually or with a mechanical device to overcome muscle spasm, so that a fracture may be reduced, to keep the ends of fractured bones in position until healing can take place, to prevent deformities or contractures from fractures or other conditions, or to correct or lessen deformities such as scoliosis. Also refers to types of apparatus used to produce a steady pulling on a part, many of which involve the use of pulleys and weights. BUCK'S T. or EXTENSION an apparatus for obtaining extension of a fractured hip or femur; consists of a system of weights, ropes, and pulleys, and adhesive straps; also used in treatment of contractures and to realign the vertebrae in cases of scoliosis; CERVICAL T. continuous T. to immobilize the cervical spine in treatment of whiplash injuries or conditions due to arthritis; may consist of a head halter, sling, or tongs inserted into the skull; COTREL'S T. continuous opposing T. with a pelvic sling and a special head halter with a pulley system that allows the patient to increase the amount of T. by extending the legs which are placed in stirrups attached to the T. This T. plus exercises is used to stretch the muscles on the concave side of the scoliotic curve in preparation for casting or surgical treatment for scoliosis; FIXED T., T. exerted between two fixed points as, *e.g.*, on a Hare splint or T. between Steinmann pins that are incorporated in a cast; HALO-PELVIC T. applied to the spine by means of two metal hoops; one attached to the skull and one to the pelvis; joined by extension rods; used to correct deformity from scoliosis prior to fusion; HALO T. consists of a halo (circular band attached to the skull with surgical pins) which may be attached to direct T. or to a frame that is supported by the body; used to support the spine after injury or surgery; also used in post-operative treatment of scoliosis; HALTER T. a leather halter attached to a bar above the head and to a string that goes over a pulley to weights; the patient may be either sitting or lying down; used for treatment of cervical lesions; HAMILTON–RUSSELL T. a form of traction of the leg in which there is an upwards pull over a beam and the cord is continuous with a series of pulleys attached to the limb by skin traction horizontally; INTERMITTENT T., T. applied for certain periods each day; may be removed for performance of activities of daily living; used to relieve muscle spasm or to correct certain deformities; MANUAL T. a pull exerted by the hands; MECHANICAL T. skin or skeletal T. with weights to exert the necessary pull; SKELETAL T., T. exerted directly upon the skeleton with devices attached to pins or tongs inserted into the bone; used when long-term T. is necessary and when the amount of weight required is greater than the skin can tolerate, or when skin T. is contraindicated; SKIN T., T. attached to the skin and held in place with elastic bandage which compresses the soft tissue enough to exert indirect T. on the skeleton; SKULL T., used in dislocation or fracture–dislocation of the cervical spine; calipers are inserted into the temporal bones under anaesthesia, and a cord with a weight attached runs from the calipers over a pulley and then over the head of the bed, which is elevated.

tractotomy (trak-tot′o-mi): The operation of severing or making an incision into a nerve tract. Sometimes done for the relief of intractable pain.

trade name: Also called *proprietary name*. Usually refers to one registered by the Patent Office and is applied to a drug instead of the generic name. Sometimes there are several trade names for the same drug (*e.g.*, aspirin), since each pharmaceutical manufacturer may choose a different name for the same preparation.

trade union: An association of workers in a given trade or in allied trades for the protection and furtherance of their interests with regard to wages, hours, and conditions of labour, and for the provision, from their common funds, of pecuniary assistance to the members during strikes, sickness, unemployment, and old age.

tragacanth (trag′a-kanth): The dried gummy exudation of a shrub of the genus *Astralagus*; used in medicine as a demulcent and as an emulsifying, suspending, and thickening agent for medications. Gum tragacanth.

trait (trāt): A distinctive, enduring aspect of an individual's personality, reflecting his or her pattern of interpersonal relationships and adaptation to the environment, *e.g.*, friendliness, orderliness, punctuality. X-LINKED T. a genetically determined trait caused or controlled by a gene located on the X chromosome.

trance (trans): A state of profound unnatural stupor or sleep from which the patient cannot be aroused easily, or of partially suspended animation; may be induced by hysteria, catalepsy, hypnotism, or alcoholic indulgence; not due to organic disease; MYSTIC T., T. experienced by those practising intense meditation.

tranquillizer (trang′kwi-lī-zer): Any of a large group of drugs that act by alleviating agitation and anxiety without inducing hypnosis or narcosis, while calming the patient; they induce drowsiness, greatly exaggerate the effects of alcohol, and may result in drug dependency. MAJOR T. s drugs used in treatment of psychoses; MINOR T. s drugs used primarily in treatment of tension, mild anxiety, convulsive disorders, psychic distress, and, sometimes, in cases of alcohol withdrawal.

trans-: Prefix denoting (1) through, across; (2) to the other side.

transaminase (tranz-am′i-nās): An enzyme important in the catabolism of amino acids; found in large quantities in the cells of the heart, liver, kidney, pancreas, and muscles; becomes elevated when any disease of these organs exists. SERUM GLUTAMIC OXALOACETIC T. an enzyme normally present in blood serum and some body tissues, the heart and liver in particular; increases in certain liver diseases and when the heart muscle is damaged, as in infarction, severe arrhythmias, or angina, and following cardiac catheterization; may increase from 4 to 10 times the normal during the first 24 hours after infarction; SERUM GLUTAMIC PYRUVIC T. an enzyme normally present in the body, especially in the liver; the blood level increases markedly in hepatitis or following tissue injury of the liver.

transamination (tranz-am′-in-ā′shun): A reaction in which one or more amino groups transfer from one amino acid compound to another, or from one molecule to another in a substance.

transamniotic (tranz-am-ni-ot′ik): Through the amniotic fluid, as a T. transfusion to the fetus for haemolytic disease.

transanimation (tranz an′i-ma′shun): 1. Resuscitation. 2. Resuscitation by mouth-to-mouth breathing.

transcortical (trans-kor′ti-kal): Through or across the cortex of an organ; often refers to association tracts in the cortex of the brain.

transcultural nursing: Where the nurse is aware of the patient's cultural health beliefs and values and seeks to incorporate these into care planning.

transcutaneous (trans-kū-tā′nē-us): Relating to the passage of a substance through the unbroken skin, as occurs in inunction. Percutaneous.

transcutaneous electrical nerve stimulation: electrical stimulation of nerves and/or muscles to relieve pain. Electrodes may be placed along optimal trigger points that coincide with acupuncture analgesia points.

transdermal (trans-der′mal): Through the skin; usually refers to a medication applied to the skin either by inunction or by application of a gauze dressing that is impregnated with the medication which is released over time.

transdiaphragmatic (trans-dī′a-fra-mat′ik): Through or across the diaphragm.

transducer (trans-dū′ser): A device that converts one form of energy into another. In medicine, an electrode (attached to an individual) that converts the energy created by certain body functions into electrical impulses that can be transmitted to an oscilloscope and displayed as waves that can be measured by a monitoring device. DOPPLER ULTRASONIC T. a device that detects changes in the frequency of sounds along a blood vessel.

transect (tran-sekt'): To cut across or divide by cutting across.

transection (tran-sek'shun): A cutting made across the long axis of a structure. A cross section.

transfer: The moving of a patient from one surface to another, e.g., from bed to chair or from one unit/department to another. ACTIVE T., T. in which the patient assists with the moving; PASSIVE T., T. in which the patient is unable to assist and the moving is done entirely by another person(s) or by a lifting device; T. FACTOR see under FACTOR.

transferase (trans'fer-ās): Any of several kinds of enzymes that act as catalysts in the transfer of atoms or groups of atoms from one molecule to another.

transference (trans-fer'ens): 1. The conveying or shifting of something from one place to another. 2. The shifting of symptoms from one side of the body to the other; sometimes occurs in certain hysterical states. 3. The displacement by the patient of mental attitudes or emotions formerly directed to one object or person, often to the psychotherapist. THOUGHT T. the transfer of thoughts from one person to another; telepathy.

transferrin (trans-fer'in): A globulin of the blood serum concerned chiefly with the binding and the transportation of iron from the intestine to the bloodstream.

transfer RNA: Certain RNA molecules found in the majority of cells and which are essential for protein synthesis, where the amino acid arrangement is determined by the DNA in the chromosomes.

transfix (trans-fiks'): To pierce through completely, as with a sharp instrument.

transformation (trans'for-mā'shun): A decided change in structure, form, function, or behaviour. In cell biology, the conversion of a normal cell into one that is susceptible to carcinogenic influences.

transformer (trans-for'mer): An electrical apparatus that transfers electric energy from one or more alternating current circuits to one or more other circuits, with a change in voltage, current, phase, or other characteristic.

transfusion (trans-fū'zhun): The introduction of a fluid such as plasma, blood, saline or other solution directly into the bloodstream of the patient. BLOOD T. the transfer of blood, directly or indirectly, from one person into the vein of another person; DIRECT T., T. of blood from donor to recipient via a tube connecting two of their arteries; also called *arterial T.* and

immediate T.; EXCHANGE T. alternate withdrawal of part of the recipient's blood and replacement with donor blood until the greater part has been exchanged; used for Rhesus babies affected with erythroblastosis fetalis; INDIRECT T., T. of blood that has been previously collected and stored under suitable conditions; INTRAUTERINE T., T. of Rh-negative blood directly into the peritoneal cavity of the fetus in treatment of erythroblastosis fetalis; PERITONEAL T. the infusion of saline solution into the peritoneal cavity; PLATELET T., T. of platelets; used in treatment of individuals with severe thrombocytopenia (*q.v.*); TOTAL T. see exchange T. — transfuse, v.

transfusion reaction: The response of a recipient to the transfusion of blood that is in some way incompatible; may be due to erythrocyte incompatibility, an allergic condition, or some preservative substance in blood that has been stored. Symptoms begin early in the procedure and include headache, rapid thready pulse, dyspnoea, fever, cold clammy skin, and possibly, shock.

transient (tran'zi-ent): Passing quickly into and out of existence.

transient ischaemic attack: A sudden episode of ischaemia resulting in neurological signs that usually last from 5 minutes to several hours; incidence increase with age; recurrence is common. Symptoms include disturbance of vision, numbness of an extremity or of one side of the body, slurred speech, dizziness. May be associated with atherosclerosis or vertebrobasilar circulation.

transiliac (tranz-il'i-ak): Passing from one ilium to the other, or extending from one iliac spine to the other.

transillumination (tranz-i-lū-mi-nā'shun): The transmission of light through a cavity or sinus for diagnostic purposes.

transitional (tran-zish'un-al): Relating to or characterized by, change. T. CARE where neonatal nursing care is provided in the post-natal ward for the newborn infant alongside the mother; T. CELL CARCINOMA a malignant tumour containing anaplastic transitional cells.

transit time: Usually refers to the time it takes for ingested material to appear in the faeces.

translucent (tranz-lū'sent): Intermediate between opaque and transparent; describing a substance that allows the passage of light, but which diffuses the light so that objects are not clearly distinguishable through it.

transmigration (tranz-mī-grā'shun): A wandering across or through; usually refers to the passage of blood cells through a vessel wall; see DIAPEDESIS. OVULAR T. the passage of an ovum from an ovary to the uterine tube on the opposite side.

transmissible (tranz-mis'si-b'l): Capable of being transferred from one person to another; said of certain diseases.

transmission (tranz-mish'un): 1. The transfer of a disease from one person to another. 2. The passing on of an inheritable quality from parent to offspring. 3. The passage of a nerve impulse along a neural pathway or across a synapse.

transmural (tranz-mū'ral): Through the wall, *e.g.*, of a cyst, organ or vessel. — transmurally, adv.

transmutation (tranz-mū-tā'shun): A transformation or change in form, appearance, or nature. In physics, the conversion of one element into another by one or a series of nuclear reactions, or the changes of one nuclide into another.

transorbital (tranz-or'bit-al): Passing through the eye socket.

transpeptidase (trans-pep'ti-dās): An enzyme that acts as a catalyst in the transfer of an amino or a peptide group from one molecule to another.

transperitoneal (trans'per-i-to-nē'al): Through the abdominal wall or the abdomen.

transpiration (trans-pī-rā'shun): The giving off of vapour or moisture through the skin or a membrane, or of air through the lungs. — transpire, v.

transplacental (trans-pla-sen'tal): Through or across the placenta.

transplant (trans-plant', trans'plant): 1. To transfer living tissue from one part to another, or an organ from one person to another. 2. The tissue or organ that is transplanted from one part, or person, to another.

transplantar (trans-plan'tar): Denotes extension across the sole of the foot, particularly with reference to muscles and ligaments.

transplantation (trans-plan'tā'shun): Grafting, on to one part, tissue or an organ taken from another part or another body, *e.g.*, heart, kidney, tendon. — transplant, v.

transpleural (trans-ploo'ral): Through the pleura or across the pleural cavity.

transpose (trans-pōz'): To change from one location to another, may refer to a tissue or an organ.

transposition (trans-po-zish'un): 1. The location or displacement of an internal organ to the side of the body that is opposite its usual site. 2. An exchange of atoms within a molecule. 3. The attachment of a tissue flap to a new site without

separating it from the old one until it has united with the tissues at the new location. 4. In embryology, the shifting of genetic material from one chromosome to another, resulting in a congenital anomaly. T. OF THE GREAT VESSELS a congenital heart defect in which the aorta rises from the right rather than the left ventricle and the pulmonary artery arises from the left rather than the right ventricle.

transseptal (trans-sep'tal): Through or across the septum. T. CARDIAC CATHETERIZATION performed by puncturing the atrial septum in order to perform left heart studies.

transsexual (trans-seks'u-al): Term applied to persons who have the body and generative organs of one sex, but are convinced that they were meant to be a member of the other sex. Such persons distinguish themselves from homosexuals and transvestites and are often obsessed with the desire to be physically changed to the opposite sex; this is sometimes attempted through surgery and hormonal treatment.

transsynaptic (trans-si-nap'tik): Refers to the passage of a nerve impulse over a synapse.

transthoracic (tranz-tho-ras'ik): Across or through the chest wall or chest cavity.

transtracheal (trans-tra'kē-al): Refers to a surgical procedure performed by passage through the wall of the trachea.

transudate (trans'ū-dāt): A liquid substance that has passed over a membrane or through some other permeable substance. See TRANSUDE.

transude (trans-ūd'): To ooze or pass through a membrane or permeable substance, *e.g.*, the oozing of blood serum through intact vessel walls. — transudation, n.

transureteroureterostomy (tranz-ū-rē'ter-ō-ū-rē-ter-os'to-mi): The surgical procedure of transposing a ureter across the midline and suturing it to the opposite ureter in order to bypass an obstruction.

transurethral (tranz-ū-rē'thral): By way of the urethra. T. RESECTION prostatectomy or removal of part of the lower urinary tract by means of an instrument passed through the urethra; see PROSTATECTOMY.

transvaginal (tranz-vaj-īn-al): Through or across the vagina; surgery performed through the vagina. — transvaginally, adv.

transventricular (tranz-ven-trik'ū-lar): Through a ventricle. Term used mainly in connection with surgery on cardiac valves. — transventricularly, adv.

transverse (trans-vers'): Crosswise or situated at right angles to the long axis of the body or of a part. T. COLON the section of the large intestine that crosses the abdomen from the right to the left; T. FRACTURE a fracture in which the line of fracture is at right angles to the long axis of the bone; T. LIE or PRESENTATION, a crosswise position of the fetus in the uterus that must be altered before the child can be born normally.

transversectomy (trans-ver-sek'tōl mi): The surgical removal of a transverse process of a vertebra to relieve pressure on a nerve root.

transversus abdominis (trans-ver'sus abl dom'i-nis): A muscle that forms part of the muscular wall of the side of the abdomen.

transvesical (trans-ves'i-kal): Through the bladder, by custom referring to the urinary bladder. — transvesically, adv.

transvestite (tranz-ves'tīt): One who practises transvestitism (*q.v.*).

transvestitism (tranz-ves-ti-tism): A sexual deviation in which one has the desire to wear the clothes of, and in other ways masquerade as, a member of the opposite sex.

trapeze (tra-pēz'): A triangular device hung from the ceiling or from a bar over the bed which can be adjusted to the patient's reach; assists the person to change his position in bed or to sit up.

trapezium (tra-pē'zi-um): 1. An irregular four-sided figure. 2. The first bone on the thumb side of the second row of carpal bones. Also called the *greater multangular bone.* — trapezial, trapeziform, adj.

trapezius (tra-pē'zi-us): The large flat, triangular superficial muscle on either side of the posterior part of the neck and upper thorax; it draws the head backward, raises, depresses and rotates the scapula and draws it backward towards the spine.

trapezoid (trap'e-zoyd): 1. Resembling a trapezium (*q.v.*). 2. The second bone in the second row of carpal bones. Also called the *lesser multangular bone.*

trauma (traw'ma): A wound or injury caused by external force or violence. BIRTH T. injury to an infant during its delivery or, in psychology, the injury to the infant's psyche from the process of being born; PSYCHOLOGICAL T. an emotional shock or an experience that has a more or less permanent effect upon the mind, especially the subconscious mind. — traumatic, adj.

traumasthenia (traw-mas-thē'ni-a): Nervous exhaustion or neurosis following injury or violence.

traumatic (traw-mat'ik): Related to or caused by an injury or wound.

traumatize (traw'ma-tīz): To produce injury or trauma through accident or by carelessness.

traumatogenic (traw'ma-tō-jen'ik): Capable of causing a wound or injury.

traumatology (traw-ma-tol'o-ji): The branch of surgery that deals with wounds or accident surgery.

traumatopathy (traw-ma-top'a-thi): Any pathological condition resulting from injury or violence.

traumatophilia (traw'ma-tō-fil'i-a): The unconscious tendency to become injured, or the craving for injury.

traumatophobia (traw' -ma-tō-fō'bi-a): Morbid fear of being injured.

traumatosepsis (traw'ma-tō-sep'sis): Infection of or following a wound.

travail (tra-vāl'): The labour of childbirth.

travel sickness: See MOTION SICKNESS.

Treacher Collins syndrome: Mandibulofacial dysostosis; see under MANDIBULOFACIAL.

treadmill (tred'mil): A walkway that moves while the subject 'walks' on it while remaining in place. T. TEST Bruce treadmill test (*q.v.*).

treat: To give aid to a person suffering from a pathological, traumatic, or psychiatric condition by means of medical, surgical, nutritional, corrective, curative, or rehabilitative measures.

treatment: Medical, surgical or psychological care of a person, aimed at relieving symptoms of a disease or injury or curing the condition. CONSERVATIVE T. that in which surgery or other drastic measures are withheld if, and as long as, possible; CURATIVE T. that aimed at curing a disease; EMPIRIC T. that based on measures that experience has shown to be effective in the particular condition; KENNY T., see KENNY METHOD; MEDICAL T., T. by drugs, hygienic and other methods, that are distinguished from surgical methods; PALLIATIVE T., that which aims to relieve pain and distress but does not attempt to cure the causative disease; PROPHYLACTIC T. that which aims to prevent a person from being attacked by a specific disease; also called *preventive T.*; SHOCK T., consists of induction of coma or convulsions by injection of insulin or other drug or by passing an electric current through the brain; SPECIFIC T. that which is aimed at removing the specific cause of a disease; frequently refers to diseases caused by bacteriological invasion; SURGICAL T. includes T. by cutting operations and manual procedures such as reducing fractures without making an incision; SYMPTOMATIC T., T. of symptoms as they arise in the course of a disease rather than treating the cause. — treat, v.

trematodiasis (trem'a-tō-dī'a-sis): Infestation with a trematode.

tremens (trē'mens): Trembling; shaking. DELIRIUM T. a form of acute mental disturbance caused by excessive use of alcohol and marked by hallucinations, memory disturbances, sweating, restlessness, mental confusion, severe tremor.

tremograph (trem'ō-graf): A device for recording tremor.

tremolabile (trē'mō-lā'bil): Easily destroyed or inactivated by agitation or shaking.

tremor (trem'or): Involuntary, purposeless, rhythmic contraction of agonist and antagonist muscles causing trembling or quivering of a body part; may be due to disorders of the brain, e.g., Parkinson's disease, emotional disorders, effect of alcohol and other drugs on the nervous system, fear, or ageing. ANXIETY STATE T. a fine tremor, usually of the hands, which may be cold and clammy; COARSE T. violent T. in which the vibrations are not over six or seven per second; CONTINUOUS T. that which occurs constantly as seen in paralysis agitans. ESSENTIAL T. fine, isolated tremor, possibly familial; exaggerated by ingestion of alcohol, activity, and sedatives; disappears during rest; FINE T. slight trembling in which the vibrations may be 10 to 12 per second; seen in the outstretched hand of persons with thyrotoxicosis; the hands are usually warm; INTENTION T. occurs when voluntary movement is attempted; characteristic of disseminated sclerosis; PASSIVE T. occurs only when the person is at rest; disappears when active movement is undertaken; also called *resting T.*; SENILE T. a benign T. that occurs in older persons often without other symptoms; involves the head, jaw, and hands; at first seen only when the person uses the affected part; is increased by cold, fatigue, emotional states; TOXIC T. may be fine or coarse with no rigidity; seen in alcoholism and other drug intoxications. — tremulous, adj.

tremostable (trē'mō-stā'b'l): Not easily destroyed or inactivated by agitation or shaking.

tremulous (trem'ū-lus): Trembling; quivering; exhibiting tremor. — tremulousness, n.

trench: T. FEVER a rickettsial infection caused by the bite of an infected body louse; a major medical problem of World War I when the soldiers were in trenches for long periods of time with no opportunity to practise personal hygiene; T. FOOT a condition resembling frostbite; also a medical problem during World War I when men stood in trenches for long periods of time with wet, cold feet; T. MOUTH, see VINCENT'S ANGINA under ANGINA.

Trendelenburg: T. GAIT a gait that develops following paralysis of the gluteus medius muscle; the person leans the trunk towards the affected side with each step. Also called *gluteal gait*; T.'S OPERATION ligation of the long saphenous vein in the groin at its junction with the femoral vein. Used in treatment of varicose veins; T. POSITION in which the patient is supine on an inclined plane with the head lowered and the legs raised, thus causing the pelvic and abdominal organs to drop towards the thoracic cavity. T.'S SIGN seen in congenital dislocation of the hip, when the patient stands on the dislocated leg and flexes the hip and knee on the unaffected side, that side will sag, whereas in normal conditions it would rise; T.'S TEST test for competency of the veins of the leg; with the patient lying down, the leg is held upright until the veins are empty; then the leg is lowered and the patient quickly stands up; if the veins are normal they will fill from below, if not, they will fill from above. [Friedrich Trendelenburg, German surgeon, 1844–1924.]

trepanation (trep'a-nā'shun): The surgical procedure of trephining. Trephination.

trephination (tref'i-nā'shun): The operation of trephining; usually refers to opening the skull with a trephine. In dentistry, the surgical creation of an opening through the gum tissues to the root of a tooth.

trephine (trē-fin'): 1. An instrument with sawtooth-like edges used to remove a circular piece from a structure, e.g., cornea or skull. 2. To perform an operation with a trephine. Also called *trepan*.

trepidant (trep'i-dant): Exhibiting tremor; trembling.

Treponema (trep'ō-nē'ma): A genus of motile, slender, spiral-shaped bacteria, some of which are pathogenic to humans. T. PALLIDUM the causative organism of syphilis (q.v.) in humans. T. PERTENUE the causative organism of yaws (q.v.).

treponematosis (trep'ō-nē-mal tō'sis): Infection caused by a variety of *Treponema*. See YAWS.

treponemicidal (trep'ō-nē-mil sī'dal): Destructive to any organism of the genus *Treponema*.

trepopnoea (trē-pop'nē-a): An uncommon term that describes a situation in which breathing is comfortable in one position but not another;

usually occurs when the patient is turned to the left side.

-tresia: A combining form denoting perforation.

tresis (trē'sis): Perforation.

tri-: Combining form denoting three, three times.

triad (trī'ad): A group of three related objects or elements.

triage (trē'ahzh): The prompt sorting out and classification of injured or seriously ill persons in war, disaster, or emergency situation, whether in hospital or in the field, to determine who should be cared for, in what order, and where. In war, this along with giving first aid, is done at the front before evacuating casualties to the rear. Casualties are classified as (1) those who need immediate treatment in order to survive, (2) those who will survive without immediate treatment, and (3) those who cannot be expected to survive under any circumstances.

trial-and-error learning: The apparently random, haphazard activity that may precede acquisition of knowledge; may be overt and observable or covert and mental in character. Sometimes known as *learning from experience*.

triamelia (trī'a-mē'li-a): The congenital anomaly characterized by the absence of three limbs.

triangle (trī'ang-g'l): A geometric figure having three sides and three angles. In anatomy, a three-sided area the sides of which may be determined by natural structures or represented by arbitrarily drawn lines.

triangular (trī-ang'ū-lar): Resembling or having the shape of a triangle. T. BANDAGE see under BANDAGE.

triangulation (trī-ang-ū-lā'-shun): The process of combining different methods of research, data collection approaches, investigators, or theoretical perspectives in the study of one phenomenon.

TRIC: Actonym for agents that cause trachoma and inclusion conjuctivitis which is widespread in tropical areas, where trachoma is a common cause of blindness associated with poor living conditions and lack of hygiene. In temperate climates these agents cause conjunctivitis as well as urethritis and cervicitis.

tricephalus (trī-kef'a-lus,-sef'): A fetus having three heads.

triceps (trī'seps): Three-headed; specifically the three-headed muscle on the back of the upper arm that extends the forearm, and the triceps surae on the back of the lower leg (the gastrocnemius and soleus muscles considered as

one), that flexes the leg and extends the foot. T. SKINFOLD the skinfold measurement at midarm, used to determine the amount of stored fat; T. TENDON REFLEX see under REFLEX.

trich-, thricho-: Combining forms denoting: 1. Hair. 2. Filament.

trichatrophia (trik-a-trō'fi-a): A brittle dry state of the hair due to atrophy of the hair bulbs.

trichauxis (trik-awk'sis): Excessive growth of the hair.

-trichia: A combining form denoting hairiness, or the condition of the hair.

trichiasis (tri-kī'a-sis): Inversion or ingrowing of an eyelash causing irritation from friction on the eyeball.

Trichinella (trik'i-nel'la): A genus of nematode worms that infest both humans and animals. T. *SPIRALIS* the nematode that causes trichinosis in humans.

trichinosis (trik'i-nō'sis): A disease that results from eating raw or undercooked meat, pork in particular, that is infested with a parasitic worm, the *Trichinella spiralis*. The female worms live in the small intestine and produce larvae which invade the body and, in particular, form cysts in skeletal muscles; the usual symptoms are abdominal pain, diarrhoea, nausea, fever, facial oedema, fatigue, muscular pains, and stiffness. Also called *trichiniasis* and *trichenelliasis*.

trichitis (tri-kī'tis): Inflammation of the hair bulbs.

trichloroacetic acid (trī'klor-ō-a-sē'tik): An astringent and caustic escharotic used chiefly to remove warts.

trichloromethane (trī'klor-ō-meth'ān): Chloroform.

trichoaesthesia (trik'ō-es-thē'zi-a): 1. The sensation one feels when a hair is touched. 2. A form of paraesthesia in which one has a sensation as of hair being on the conjunctiva, the skin, or the mucous membrane of the mouth.

trichobezoar (trik'ō-bē'zor): A hairball; a concretion found in the stomach or intestine and containing hairs.

trichoclasia (trik'ō-klā'zi-a): Brittleness and breaking off of the hair.

trichocryptomania (trik'ō-krip-tō-mā'ni-a): An abnormal desire to pull out one's hair, usually that of the scalp.

trichocryptosis (trik'ō-krip-tō'sis): Any disease of the hair follicles.

trichoepithelioma (trik'ō-ep-i-thē-li-ō'ma): A small benign nodule, usually multiple, occurring on the skin, particularly that of the face, that has its origin in a hair follicle.

trichogen (trik'ō-jen): An agent that promotes growth of hair. — trichogenous, adj.

trichoglossia (trik'ō-glos'i-a): Hairy tongue; see under TONGUE.

trichologia (trik-ō-lō'ji-a): Constant pulling at the hair.

trichoma (tri-kō'ma): 1. Trichiasis (*q.v.*). 2. Trichomatosis (*q.v.*).

trichomatosis (tri-kō'ma-tō'sis): A matted, filthy condition of the hair, due to neglect, lack of hygiene, and infestation by parasites.

Trichomonas (tri-kom'ō-nas): A genus of flagellated protozoa, certain of which are parasitic in the intestinal tract, mouth, vagina, or urethra of humans. *T. VAGINALIS* the causative agent of a common, chronic disease of the genitourinary tract, trichomoniasis (*q.v.*).

trichomoniasis (trik'ō-mō-nī'a-sis): Infection of the genitourinary tract caused by the protozoan *Trichomonas vaginalis*. Characterized in women by vaginitis and profuse, foamy, yellowish discharge with a foul odour; in men the agent lives in the urethra, prostate, and seminal vesicles, and is usually asymptomatic. Transmitted through sexual intercourse.

trichomycosis (trik'ō mī-kō-sis): Formerly applied to any disease of the hair that is caused by a fungus; now known to be caused by a *Nocardia* (*q.v.*).

trichonosis (trik'ō-nō'sis): Any disease of the hair.

trichophagy (tri-kof'a-ji): The nervous habit of biting or eating hair.

Trichophyton (tri-kof' i-ton): A genus of fungi found on the skin, hair, and nails; often a cause of allergy; a causative agent in ringworm or tinea. *T. RUBRUM* causes chronic superficial infections of the skin and nails; *T. TONSURANS* a species of ringworm fungus that causes tinea capitis; see under TINEA.

trichophytosis (trik'ō-fī-tō'sis): Infection with a *Trichophyton* fungus, *e.g.*, ringworm of the hair or skin.

trichorrhoea (trik'o-rē'a): Rapid or excessive falling out of the hair.

trichosiderin (trik-ō-sid'er-in): An iron-containing pigment found in red human hair.

trichosis (tri-kō'sis): Any disease or abnormal condition of the hair.

Trichosporon (tri-kos'po-ron): A genus of fungi that grow on the hair shaft.

trichotillomania (trik'ō-til-lō-mā'ni-a): An uncontrollable compulsion to pull out one's own hair.

trichotomy (trī-kot' -o-mi): Being divided into three parts.

trichromatopsia (tri-krō' -ma-top'si-a): Normal colour vision.

trichromic (trī-krō'mik): 1. Having three colours. 2. Being able to perceive three colours; red, green, and blue.

trichuriasis (trik-ū-rī'a-sis): Infestation with *Trichuris trichiura*, a whipworm; a syndrome occurring most frequently in the tropics and often causing no symptoms although in some cases there is diarrhoea, vomiting, nervous disorders, and loss of weight.

Trichuris (trik-ū'ris): A genus of roundworms of the class Nematoda that infest humans. *T. TRICHIURA*, a whipworm with a coiled head that is parasitic in the large intestine of mammals including humans.

tricipital (trī-sip'i-tal): 1. Relating to a triceps muscle. 2. Having three heads.

tricrotic (trī-krot'ik): Pertinent to a pulse in which three waves are palpated during each heartbeat.

tricuspid (trī-kus'pid): Having three cusps or points. *T. TOOTH* a tooth having three cusps on the crown, as may occur on the second or third upper molar; *T. VALVE* that between the right atrium and ventricle of the heart; it allows blood to flow freely from the right atrium into the right ventricle and prevents backflow of blood from the ventricle into the atrium during ventricular contraction.

trifacial (trī-fā'shi-al): Denoting the 5th pair of cranial nerves. See TRIGEMINAL.

trifid (trī'fid): Split into three or having three corresponding parts.

trifocal (trī'fō-kal): Refers to eyeglasses that have three refractive powers in the same lens; to correct vision for distant, intermediate, and close objects.

trifurcation (trī'fur-kā'shun): A division into three prongs or branches — trifurcate, adj.

trigastric (trī-gas'trik): Having three bellies; usually said of a certain muscle.

trigeminal (trī-jem'in-al): Triple; separating into three sections, *e.g.*, the *T. NERVES* the 5th pair of cranial nerves, which have three branches and supply the skin of the face, tongue and teeth. *T. NEURALGIA* see TIC DOULOUREUX; *T. PULSE* pulsus trigeminus.

trigeminy (trī-jem'i-ni): 1. Occurring in threes. 2. A type of heartbeat in which the beats occur in groups of three.

trigger (trig'er): 1. An act or impulse that initiates an action. 2. To initiate an action. *T. FINGER* a condition in which the finger can be bent but cannot be straightened without help; usually due to a thickening on the tendon which prevents free gliding; T. THUMB tenderness at the base of the thumb and sometimes snapping or triggering movements; due to tenosynovitis of the pollicis longus muscle, often an occupational injury; T. POINT an area of hyperexcitability where the application of a stimulus will provoke pain or other phenomenon to a greater degree than in the surrounding area; T. ZONE an area of hypersensitivity where a stimulus will elicit a specific response.

triglyceride (trī-glis'er-īd): Any of a group of naturally occurring esters, composed of glycerol and three fatty acids (stearic, oleic, palmitic); found in most animal and vegetable fats; the chief constituent of adipose tissue and the major form in which fat is stored in the body.

trigone (trī'gōn): A triangular area, especially applied to the bladder base abounded by the ureteral openings at the back, and the urethral opening at the front. — trigonal, adj.

trigonitis (trī' gō-nī'tis): Inflammation of the trigone of the urinary bladder; characterized by frequency, urgency, and dysuria.

triiodothyronine (trī'ī-ō-dō-thī'rō-nēn): Either of two hormones present in the thyroid. See LIOTHYRONINE and THYROXINE.

trilateral (trī-lat'er-al): Having three sides.

trilobate (trī-lō'bāt): Having three lobes.

trilocular (trī-lok'ū-lar): Having three cells or chambers.

trilogy of Fallot: A congenital anomaly consisting of an atrial defect, pulmonic stenosis, and right ventricular hypertrophy. See TETRALOGY OF FALLOT.

trimensual (trī-men'sū-al): Occurring at intervals of three months.

trimester (trī-mes'ter): A period of 3 months. Usually refers to one-third of the length of a pregnancy.

triorchid (trī-or'kid): 1. Having three testes. 2. An individual who has three testes.

trip: In drug culture, an hallucinogenic drug experience. BAD T. temporary or chronic psychosis or a panic reaction following use of a hallucinogen (q.v.).

tripanopia (trip-a-nō'pi-a): Colour blindness for the colour blue, the third of the primary colours.

tripara (trip'a-ra): A woman who has had three pregnancies resulting in three live offspring. Also written *Para III*.

tripeptide (trī-pep'tīd): A peptide that yields three peptides in hydrolysis.

triplegia (trī-plē'ji-a): 1. Hemiplegia with one limb on the opposite side also affected. 2. Paralysis of the face and an upper and a lower extremity.

triplet (trip'let): One of three children born at the same birth.

triploidy (trip'loy-di): The state or condition of having three complete sets of chromosomes.

triplopia (trip-lō'pi-a): A defect of vision in which one sees three images of a single object.

tripsis (trip'sis): 1. Trituration (q.v.). 2. Massage.

-tripsy: A combining form denoting a crushing.

trisaccharide (trī-sak'a-rīd): A carbohydrate that yields three monosaccharide molecules on hydrolysis.

trismus (triz'mus): Spasm in the muscles of mastication caused by motor disturbance of the trigeminal nerve; an early sign of lockjaw. — trismic, adj.

trisomy (trī'sō-mi): A chromosomal anomaly; a state in which one of the chromosomes is present in triplicate rather than in a pair, *i.e.*, in human trisomy, the total number of chromosomes is 47 instead of the normal 46. Three main types are recognized (1) TRISOMY 13 or TRISOMY D, is relatively rare; the extra chromosome is from the 13–15 group, usually 13; in this condition there is cleft lip and palate, microcephaly, abnormalities of forehead, nose and eyes; polydactyly, mental handicap, failure to thrive; and a poor prognosis for life, with death occurring usually during the first year; also called *Patau's syndrome*. (2) TRISOMY 18 or TRISOMY E, usually occurs in children of parents over 30; characterized by low birth weight, abnormal facies with low-set malformed ears, micrognathia, heart defects, hypertonicity, severe mental handicap, and poor prognosis for life. Occurs most often in female children; also called *Edwards' syndrome* (3) TRISOMY 21 Down's syndrome (q.v.).

tristimania (tris-ti-mā'ni-a): Melancholia.

tritium (trit'i-um): A radioactive isotope of hydrogen; used as a tracer in metabolic studies.

triturate (trit'ū-rāt): To make into a fine powder.

trituration (trit'ū-rā'shun): The process of reducing a substance to a fine powder.

trivalent (tri-vā'lent): Having a valence of 3. T. ORAL POLIOVACCINE see SABIN'S VACCINE.

trocar (trō'kar): A sharp, pointed rod that fits inside a tube. It is used to pierce the skin and the wall of a cavity or canal in the body to aspirate fluids, to instill a medication or solution, or to guide the placement of a soft catheter.

trochanter (trō-kan'ter): One of two bony prominences on the upper end of the femur. The MAJOR or GREATER T. is on the outer side of the femur; the MINOR or LESSER T. is on the inner side of the femur between the shaft and the neck; they serve for the attachment of muscles. T. ROLL a large towel or other material rolled and placed under the greater trochanter of the patient in supine position; used to prevent external rotation of the lower limb. — trochanteric, adj.

troche (trō'ke): A medicated disc, tablet, or lozenge in a flavoured sweetened mucilaginous substance that is held under the tongue or in the cheek until it is dissolved.

trochlea (trok'lē-a): An anatomical term used to describe a part or structure that is like a pulley in function or appearance; usually a tendon or projection on a bone. — trochlear, adj.

trochlear (trok'lō ar): 1. Relating to a trochlea. 2. Name given to the 4th pair of cranial nerves; important in coordination and control of movements of the eyeball.

trochoides (trō-koy' dēz): A joint in which the only movement is pivotal, e.g., rotation around the longitudinal axis of the bone; an example is the rotation of the first cervical vertebra around the odontoid process of the second cervical vertebra.

troilism (troy'lizm): Sexual practices involving three people.

troph-, tropho-: Combining forms denoting nutrition or food.

trophic (trō'fik): Relating to nutrition.

-trophic: A combining form denoting (1) nutrition, or (2) a specific type of nutrition.

trophoblast (trof'ō-blast): A layer of ectodermal tissue that serves to attach the ovum to the wall of the uterus and supply nourishment to the embryo. — trophoblastic, adj.

trophoblastoma (trof-ō-blas-tō'ma): Choriocarcinoma (q.v.).

trophoneurosis (trof'ō-nū-rō'sis): Any trophic disorder such as atrophy or hypertrophy, caused by failure of nutrition resulting from disease or injury to the nerves of a part. See RAYNAUD'S DISEASE. — trophoneurotic, adj.

trophopathy (trō-fop'a-thi): Any disease or disorder of nutrition.

trophotherapy (trof-ō-ther'a-pi): Diet therapy.

trophotropism (trō-fot'rō-pizm): Repulsion or attraction to various nutritive substances, a characteristic of certain cells.

trophozoite (trof-ō-zō'īt): The active feeding stage of a protozoan as contrasted with the non-motile encapsulated stage.

tropia (trō'pi-a): An abnormal turning or deviation of the eye; strabismus (q.v.).

-tropia: Combining form denoting deviation in the visual axis.

-tropic: Combining form denoting: 1. Turning; changing. 2. Attraction to a specific tissue, organ, or system.

tropical: Relating to or common to tropic areas. T. DISEASE one which occurs in greater frequency and/or severity in tropical parts of the world; T. MEDICINE the branch of medicine that deals with diseases that most commonly occur in tropical or subtropical areas of the world.

tropism (trō'pizm): An innate tendency to react in a definite manner to specific stimuli.

tropomyosin (trō-pō-mī'ō-sin): A muscle protein that acts to inhibit muscle contraction.

troponin (trō' -pō-nin): A protein found in skeletal muscle; it assists in controlling heart muscle contraction.

Trousseau's sign: Carpopedal spasm [Armand Trousseau, French physician, 1801–1867.]

truncal (trun'kal): Relating to the trunk of the body or of a nerve, artery, etc.

truncate (trun'kāt): To cut off; amputate. To cut off at right angles to the long axis of the part. — truncated, adj.

truncus arteriosus (trun'kus ar-ter-i-o' -sis): An arterial trunk arising from the fetal heart; it develops into the pulmonary artery and the aorta and normally does not persist after birth.

trunk: 1. The torso or main part of the body to which the head and extremities are attached. 2. The main, undivided part of a nerve, blood vessel or duct. NERVE T. a collection of nerve fibres closely bound together and enclosed within a sheath of epineurium.

truss: An appliance consisting usually of a belt and a pressure pad, worn over a hernia to keep it in place after it has been reduced.

truth serum: Common name for a drug that acts to inhibit the nervous system and which is given to a person from whom it is desirable to obtain information not otherwise revealed.

trypanocide (tri-pan'ō-sīd): An agent that destroys trypanosomes; see *TRYPANOSOMA*.

Trypanosoma (tri-pan'ō-sō'ma): A genus of parasitic protozoa; a limited number of species are pathogenic to humans. The species that is the vector of trypanosomiasis (q.v.) in Africa lives part of its life cycle in the tsetse fly (q.v.) and is tranferred to new hosts, including humans, in the salivary juices when the fly bites.

trypanosome (trī-pan'ō-sōm): One of any of the species *Trypanosoma*; the protozoa are flagellated and live in the tissues and blood of the host.

trypanosomiasis (trī-pan′ō-sō-mi′a-sis): Disease produced by infection with *Trypanosoma*. In humans this may be *T. rhodesiense* in East Africa or *T. gambiense* in West Africa; both are transmitted by the tsetse fly and produce the illness known as African sleeping sickness, a severe, often fatal, disease marked by fever, intense headache, lymph node enlargement, anaemia, wasting, and somnolence. SOUTH AMERICAN T. Chagas' disease, caused by *T. cruzi* that is transmitted by bites of bloodsucking insects, is found in certain parts of South America.

trypsin (trip′sin): A proteolytic enzyme formed in the intestine when the trypsinogen from the pancreatic juice is acted upon by the enterokinase of the intestinal juice; it is the chief protein-digesting enzyme in the human.

trypsinogen (trip-sin′o-jen): The precursor of trypsin (*q.v.*), secreted by the pancreas; it is converted into trypsin when it comes into contact with enterokinase in the small intestine.

tryptophan (trip′tō-fān): One of the essential amino acids; necessary for optimal growth and for tissue repair; found in varying amounts in many proteins.

tryptophanuria (trip′tō-fan-ū′ri-a): The presence of tryptophan in the urine.

tsetse fly (tset′sē): A blood-sucking fly found in Africa; the vector of *Trypanosoma* (*q.v.*). Also called *tzetze*.

TSH: Abbreviation for thyroid-stimulating hormone (*q.v.*).

tsutsugamushi disease (tsoo-tsū-ga-moosh′ē): Scrub typhus that occurs in Japan and elsewhere; transmitted by mites.

T tube: A self-retaining drainage tube made in the shape of the letter T. T-TUBE CHOLANGIOGRAPHY see CHOLANGIOGRAPHY.

tubal (tu′bal): Pertaining to a tube. T. ABORTION, one in which an extrauterine pregnancy is terminated by rupture of the uterine tube; T. FEEDING see under FEEDING; T. INSUFFLATION insufflation of the uterine tubes to test for patency; see RUBIN'S TEST; T. LIGATION sterilization of a woman by closing off the uterine tubes with a ligature; may also involve crushing or severing the tubes; T. PREGNANCY see ECTOPIC PREGNANCY under ECTOPIC.

tube: An elongated, cylindrical structure or apparatus. For particular tubes, see ABBOT-MILLER, ALIMENTARY, AUDITORY, BRONCHIAL, DRAINAGE, ENDOTRACHEAL, EUSTACHIAN, FALLOPIAN, FEEDING, GASTRIC, INTUBATION, NASOGAS-

TRIC, NEPHROSTOMY, NEURAL, OESOPHAGEAL, RECTAL, RYLE'S SENGSTAKEN–BLAKEMORE, STOMACH, T. TEST, THORACOSTOMY, TRACHEOSTOMY, WANGENSTEEN.

tubectomy (tū-bek′to-mi): Plastic repair or excision of a tube, a uterine tube in particular; salpingectomy.

tube feeding: Usually refers to feeding an unconscious patient or one who has a throat problem by introducing pureed or liquidized food directly into the stomach via a tube that is inserted through either the nose or the oesophagus. May also refer to hyperalimentation (*q.v.*).

tuber: A localized swelling, knob, protuberance.

tubercle (tū′ber-k′l): 1. A small solid elevation or nodule on the skin, mucous membrane, or surface of an organ. 2. A small rounded eminence on a bone. 3. The specific lesion produced by the *Mycobacterium tuberculosis*. — tubercular, adj.

tuberculation (tū-ber′ -kū-lā′shun): The development of tubercles.

tuberculides (tū-ber′kū-līds): A group of erythematous, papular, or other skin manifestations thought to be due to the presence of tuberculosis elsewhere in the body.

tuberculin (tūber′kū-lin): A sterile extract of either crude (old T.) or refined (Purified Protein Derivative; PPD) complex protein constituents of the tubercle bacillus. Its most common use is in determining whether a person has or has not previously been infected with the tubercle bacillus, by injecting a small amount into the skin and reading the reaction, if any, in 48 to 72 hours; may be done by the Mantoux method, jet injection, or multiple injections (see MANTOUX TEST and HEAF MULTIPLE PUNCTURE TEST): negative reactors are those who have escaped previous infection. OLD T. a concentrated filtrate made from a 6-week-old culture of the tubercle bacillus; it does not contain the microorganisms, only the soluble products of bacterial growth.

tuberculitis (tū-ber′kū-lī′tis): Inflammation of a tubercle.

tuberculization (tū-ber′kū-lī-zā′shun): The formation of tubercles.

tuberculocele (tū-ber′kū-lō-sēl): Tuberculosis of a testis.

tuberculocidal (tū-ber′kū-lō-sī′dal): Having the ability to kill *Mycobacterium tuberculosis* (*q.v.*).

tuberculoid (tū-ber′kū-loid): Resembling tuberculosis or a tubercle.

tuberculoma (tū-ber'kū-lō'ma): 1. A large caseous tubercle, its size suggesting a tumour. 2. A tuberculous abscess. 3. Any new growth or nodule of tuberculous origin.

tuberculosis (tū-ber'kū-lō'sis): A specific, chronic, infectious disease caused by *Mycobacterium tuberculosis*, characterized by the formation of tubercles in the tissues. Often asymptomatic at first; later the local symptoms depend upon the part affected, and general symptoms are those of sepsis, *i.e.*, fever, sweats, emaciation. In humans the disease most commonly affects the lungs but may also affect the meninges, joints, bones, lymph nodes, kidney, intestine, larynx, or skin. AVIAN T. endemic in birds and rarely seen in humans; BOVINE T. endemic in cattle and transmitted to humans via cow's milk, causing T. of glands but rarely of the lungs; less common than formerly; MILIARY T. a generalized acute form of T. in which, as a result of bloodstream dissemination, minute, multiple tuberculous foci are scattered throughout many organs of the body; it is often rapidly fatal; PRIMARY T. infection with *Mycobacterium tuberculosis* for the first time; characterized by the formation, usually in the lung, of a local lesion that is most often benign, self-limited, and heals spontaneously; also called childhood T.; PULMONARY T., T. of the lung; the most common site of the disease in humans; also called *consumption, phthisis*; SECONDARY T. the adult type as distinguished from the primary or childhood type. — tuberculous, adj.

tuberculostatic (tū-ber'kū-lō-stat'ik): Inhibiting the growth of *Mycobacterium tuberculosis* which is the causative agent of tuberculosis, or an agent that inhibits such growth. — tuberculostat, n.

tuberculous (tū-ber'kū-lus): Relating to or affected by tuberculosis, or caused by the *Mycobacterium tuberculosis*. T. MENINGITIS see under MENINGITIS.

tuberculum (tū-ber'kū-lum): The anatomical term for a small eminence, nodule, knot or tubercle. — tubercula, pl.; tubercular, adj.

tuberosity (tū-be-ros'i-ti): A small rounded elevation or protuberance, particularly one from the surface of a bone.

tuberous (tū'ber-us): Knotting, knobby, covered with tubers.

tubo-: Combining form denoting a tube, or relationship to a tubal structure.

tuboabdominal (tū'bō-ab-dom'i-nal): Relating to the uterine tube and the abdomen. T. PREGNANCY the development of a fertilized ovum in the ampulla of a uterine tube and extending into the peritoneal cavity.

tubo-ovarian (tū'bō-ō-vai'ri-an): Relating to or involving both a uterine tube and an ovary, *e.g.*, a tubo-ovarian abscess.

tubo-ovariectomy (tū'bō-ō-vai-ri-ek'to-mi): Excision of the uterine tubes and ovaries. Salpingo-oophorectomy.

tubo-ovariotomy (tū'bō-ō-vai-ri-ot'o-mi): Surgical removal of a uterine tube and an ovary; usually refers to both right and left tube and ovary.

tubo-ovaritis (tū'bō-ōv-a-rī'tis): Inflammation of the uterine tubes and the ovaries.

tuboperitoneal (tū'bō-per-i-tō-nē'al): Relating to the uterine tubes and the peritoneum.

tuboplasty (tū'bō-plas-ti): Plastic surgery for repair of a uterine tube.

tuborrhoea (tū bō re'a). A discharge from the auditory tube.

tubotympanic (tū'bō-tim-pan'ik): Relating to the auditory tube and the tympanic cavity.

tubouterine (tū'bō-ū'ter-īn): Relating to the uterine tubes and the uterus.

tubovaginal (tū'bō-vag-īn'al): Relating to the uterine tubes and the vagina.

tubular (tū-bū-lar): In the form of or resembling a tube.

tubule (tū'būl): A small tube. COLLECTING T. straight tube in the kidney medulla conveying urine to the kidney pelvis; CONVOLUTED T. coiled tube in the kidney cortex; SEMINIFEROUS T. coiled tube in the testis; URINIFEROUS T. nephron (*q.v.*).

tubulocyst (tū'bū-lō-sist): A cyst-like dilatation in an occluded duct or tube.

tubulointerstitial nephritis (tū'bū-lō-in-ter-stish'al nef-rī'tis): An inflammatory disease of the kidney characterized by destruction of the tubules.

tubulus (tū'bū-lus): A small tube.

tuftsin (tuft'sin): A tetrapeptide that coats white blood cells; it promotes phagocytosis of particulate matter, bacteria, and aged cells.

tularaemia (tū'la-rē'mi-a): An endemic disease of rodents, caused by *Pasteurella tularensis*; transmitted by biting insects and acquired by humans in either handling infected animal carcasses, by the bite of an infected insect, or the bite of an infected animal. Suppuration at the inoculation site is followed by inflammation and suppuration of draining lymph glands and severe constitutional upset which may involve the spleen, liver, gastrointestinal organs, or lungs; symptoms include prolonged remittent fever, nausea, vomiting, lassitude, headache, myalgia; complications include pericarditis, bronchopneumonia, meningitis. Also called *rabbit fever, deer fly fever, tick fever*, and *O'Hara's disease*.

tulle gras (tūl'grah): A kind of dressing. Consists of mesh material impregnated with olive oil, paraffin, and balsam of Peru. Does not stick to the skin; useful in treatment of burns.

tumefy (tū'me-fī): To swell or cause to swell.

tumentia (tū-men'shi-a): A swelling.

tumid (tū'mid): Swollen.

tumoricidal (tū'mor-i-sī'dal): 1. Destructive to tumours. 2. An agent that is destructive to tumours.

tumorigenic (tū'mor-i-jen'ik): Initiating or promoting the growth of tumours. — tumorigenesis, n.

tumorous (tū'mor-us): Resembling a tumour.

tumour (tū'mor): 1. A swelling or enlargement occurring in inflammatory conditions. 2. A new growth of tissue characterized by progressive, uncontrolled proliferation of cells. Many types are described, often being named for the tissues from which they originate. BENIGN T. a simple, innocent, encapsulated T. that does not infiltrate adjacent tissue or cause metastases and is unlikely to recur if removed; MALIGNANT T. one that is not encapsulated, is likely to infiltrate adjoining tissue and to cause metastases, to progress, and ultimately to destroy life. See CANCER. — tumorous, adj.

tumour markers: Substances in the body that may indicate the presence of cancer. These are usually specific to certain types of cancer and are commonly found in the blood. Examples are alpha-fetoprotein (*q.v.*) and human chorionic gonadotrophin (see under GONADOTROPHIN). They may be indicators of tumour stage and grade, as well as being useful for monitoring responses to treatment and predicting recurrence, and in genetic screening to assess degree of risk.

tumultus (tū-mul'tus): Overaction; agitation; commotion.

Tunga penetrans: A sand flea found in Africa and in America; a chigger; it attacks between the toes causing a lesion that develops into a painful ulcer.

tungiasis (tung-gī'a-sis): A pustular skin disorder caused by the bite of the sand flea, *Tunga penetrans*.

tunic (tū'nik): A covering, coat, or lining, particularly of a hollow or tube-like structure. See TUNICA.

tunica (tū'nik-a): Anatomical term for a lining membrane or a coat, especially of a tubular

structure; usually named for the structure of which it is a part or for its location in that structure; also called *tunic*. The three tunica of the blood vessels are the T. ADVENTITIA or EXTERNA the outer supportive coat of blood vessels which is thicker in arteries than veins; the T. INTIMA the smooth inner lining of elastic endothelial tissue which also forms the valves in veins; and the T. MEDIA the middle coat, made up of muscular and elastic tissue which contains nerve fibres concerned with the regulation of the calibre of the vessels. T. DARTOS a layer of cutaneous tissue in the scrotum; helps form the septum of the scrotum; T. VAGINALIS TESTIS the serous membrane covering the testis and epididymus, and lining the cavity of the scrotum.

tuning fork: A small, two-pronged, fork-like instrument, usually of steel, that gives off a musical note when struck. Used in some hearing tests.

tunnel (tun'el): A closed passageway through a solid structure; of varying length; open at the ends for entrance and exit. See CARPAL TUNNEL SYNDROME.

turbid (tur'bid): Cloudy, unclear.

turbidity (tur-bid'i-ti): Cloudiness; usually refers to a solution in which the solid solutes have been disturbed.

turbinate (tur'bin-āt): Shaped like a top or inverted cone. T. BONES situated on either side of the nose, forming the lateral nasal walls. Syn., *concha nasalis*.

turbinated: Scroll-shaped, as the three bony prominences that project from the lateral nasal walls.

turbinectomy (tur'bi-nek'to-mi): Removal of a turbinate bone.

turgescence (tur-jes'ens): Swelling; distension; inflation. — turgescent, adj.

turgid (tur'jid): Swollen; firmly distended, as with blood by congestion. — turgescence, n.; turgidity, n.

turgor (tur'gor): Fullness, tension, resiliency. Usually refers to the skin and is exhibited when the skin springs back after being pinched.

turnbuckle cast or jacket: See under CAST.

Turner's syndrome: A chromosomal anomaly characterized by the absence of one X chromosome, congenital ovarian failure, genital hypoplasia, cardiovascular anomalies, short metacarpals, retarded growth, exostosis of tibia, and underdeveloped breasts, vagina and uterus. [Henry H. Turner, American endocrinologist, 1892–1970.]

turning frame: See STRYKER WEDGE FRAME.

TURP: Abbreviation for transurethral resection of tumour, see TRANSURETHRAL.

turpentine (tur'pen-tīn): A thin volatile oil obtained from the distillation of wood from certain pine trees; has several uses in medicine, e.g., in stimulating liniments and ointments, and as a vermifuge, counterirritant, diuretic, and expectorant.

tussiculation (tus-sik'-ū-lā'shun): A hacking cough.

tussis (tus'sis): A cough.

tussive (tus'iv): Relating to or due to a cough. T. SYNCOPE, occurs when prolonged coughing causes increased intrathoracic pressure resulting in inadequate return of blood to the heart; cardiac output falls and cerebral blood flow is diminished, causing syncope.

TV: Abbreviation for tidal volume, see under TIDAL.

T wave: In electrocardiology, the deflection that represents ventricular depolarization during which time the ventricles are in a relatively refractory period, it follows the QRS complex.

twilight state: A condition of indistinct or distorted consciousness and amnesia induced by the injection of morphine and scopolamine, in which awareness to pain is dulled and memory of it is dimmed or effaced, without total loss of consciousness.

twin: One of two children produced in the same pregnancy resulting from the fertilization of either one ovum or two ova at the same time.

twinge (twinj): A sudden sharp fleeting pain.

twinning (twin'ing): The simultaneous production of (1) two identical structures, by division, or (2) two embryos.

twitch: A brief spasmodic contraction of a muscle or muscle fibres. Resembles a tic but usually involves a larger muscle and is more noticeable.

tylectomy (tī-lek'to-mi): Surgical removal of a local lesion only, usually referring to a partial mastectomy in which only a carcinomatous lesion is removed.

tyloma (tī'lō'ma): Localized keratosis, as a callus.

tylosis (tī-lō'sis): See KERATOSIS PALMARIS ET PLANTARIS under KERATOSIS.

tympanectomy (tim'pa-nek'to-mi): Surgical removal of the tympanic membrane.

tympania (tim-pan'i-a): Tympanitis (q.v.).

tympanic (tim-pan'ik): Relating to the tympanum. T. MEMBRANE (membrana tympani) a thin semitransparent membrane in the middle

ear that transmits sound vibrations to the internal ear by means of the auditory ossicles. Also called *eardrum*.

tympanites (tim'pa-ni'tēz): Abdominal distension due to accumulation of gas in the intestine. Also called *tympanism*.

tympanitis (tim-pa-nī'tis): Inflammation of the tympanum and/or the tympanic membrane. Otitis media. Myringitis.

tympanocentesis (tim'pa-nō-sen-tē'sis): Surgical puncture of the tympanic membrane.

tympanoeustachian (tim'pa-nō-ū-stā'shi-an): Pertaining to both the tympanic cavity and the auditory tube.

tympanomandibular (tim'pa-nō-man-dib'ū-lar): Pertaining to the tympanum and the mandible.

tympanomastoiditis (tim'pa-nō-mas-toy-di'tis): Infection of the middle ear and the mastoid cells.

tympanoplasty (tim'pa-nō-plas-ti): A plastic operation involving the hearing mechanism of the middle ear.

tympanosclerosis (tim'pa nō-skle-rō'sis): The collection of masses of calcified connective tissue around the ossicles of the middle ear; may lead to deafness.

tympanotomy (tim-pa-not'o-mi): Incision of the tympanic membrane. Myringotomy.

tympanous (tim'pa-nus): Distended with gas, usually referring to the abdomen.

tympanum (tim'pa-num): The cavity of the middle ear.

tympany (tim'pa-ni): The drum-like resonant sound heard when a cavity containing air is percussed, e.g., an abdomen distended with gas; may be diagnostic. — tympanitic, adj.

Type 1 diabetes: See DIABETES.

Type 2 diabetes: See DIABETES.

type I error: In statistics, the erroneous rejection of a null hypothesis (q.v.). Also known as *alpha error*.

type II errors: In statistics, failure to reject an incorrect null hypothesis (q.v.). Also known as *beta error*.

typhaemia (tī-fē-mi-a): The presence of typhoid bacilli in the blood.

typhi-, typhlo-: Combining forms denoting: 1. The caecum. 2. Blindness.

typhinia (tī-fin'i-a): Relapsing fever (q.v.).

typhlectasis (tif-lek'ta-sis): Dilatation of the caecum.

typhlectomy (tif-lek'to-mi): Excision of the caecum.

typhlitis (tif-lī'tis): Inflammation of the caecum; caecitis. Term formerly used for appendicitis.

typhlodicliditis (tif′lō-dik-li-dī′tis): Inflammation of the ileocaecal valve.

typhloempyema (tif′lō-em-pī-ē′ma): The presence of an abscess in the caecum; may be associated with appendicitis or a sequela of caecitis.

typhloenteritis (tif-lō-en-ter-ī′tis): Inflammation of the caecum.

typhlolexia (tif-lō-lek′si-a): Word blindness; inability to recognize or comprehend words in written material.

typhlolithiasis (tif′lō-li-thī′a-sis): The presence of faecal concretions in the caecum.

typhology (tif-lol′o-ji): The study of blindness.

typhlomegaly (tif′lō-meg′a-li): Enlargement of the caecum.

typhlon (tif′lon): The caecum.

typhlopexy (tif′lō-pek′si): The surgical fixation of the caecum to the abdominal wall.

typhloptosis (tif′lō-tō′sis): Downward displacement of the caecum.

typhlosis (tif-lō′sis): Blindness.

typhlostenosis (tif′lō-ste-nō′sis): Stricture or narrowing of the caecum.

typhlostomy (tif-los′tō-mi): A colostomy into the caecum; a caecostomy.

typhloureterostomy (tif′lō-ū-rē′ter-os′to-mi): An anastomosis between the ureter and the caecum.

typhoid fever (tī′foid): A worldwide, often epidemic, systemic infectious disease caused by *Salmonella typhi*, which is transmitted by direct or indirect contact with a patient or carrier. Usual vehicles for spread of the disease are contaminated water or food, milk, milk products, or shellfish; flies are sometimes vectors. Average incubation period is 10–14 days. A progressive febrile illness marks the onset of the disease; there is anorexia, malaise, slow pulse, and rose spots (*q.v.*) on the abdomen and back. As the organism invades the lymphoid tissue, ulceration of Peyer's patches (*q.v.*) and enlargement of the spleen occur. Constipation is more often a symptom than diarrhoea, but when the latter occurs it is profuse with 'pea soup' stools which may become frankly haemorrhagic. Recovery usually begins at about the end of the third week. Protection is secured through scrupulous personal hygiene when in contact with patients or carriers and by inoculation with the appropriate vaccine. Community control is secured through public health measures concerning the disposal of sewage, purification of water supply, inspection and control of food handlers, and discovery of carriers. — typhoidal, adj.

typhous (tī′fus): Relating to typhus fever.

typhus (tī′fus): A group of acute, infectious, endemic diseases, many of which are named for the area in which they occur; caused by a rickettsial organism transmitted by arthropods; characterized by high fever, a skin eruption that may be macular or papular, severe headache, mental depression; lasts about two weeks. Spread by lice, fleas, and ticks; is a disease of war, famine, and catastrophe when large groups of people are concentrated in a small area and facilities for personal hygiene are lacking. Protection is secured by immunization with the appropriate vaccine. Community control during epidemics is secured through vigilant public health measures. MURINE T., T. transmitted to humans through the bite of the rat flea or rat louse; SCRUB T. seen mostly in Japan and the Orient; transmitted by a larval mite; marked by sudden onset and a rash that occurs several days after the first symptoms; tsutsugamushi disease (*q.v.*).

typing (tīp′ing): Classifying an individual microorganism, object, or substance in the category in which it belongs. BLOOD T. see BLOOD GROUPS.

tyremesis (tī-rem′e-sis): The vomiting of curd-like or cheese-like material by infants.

tyriasis (ti-rī′a-sis): **1.** Elephantiasis (*q.v.*). **2.** Alopecia (*q.v.*).

tyroma (tī-rō′ma): A tumour composed of caseous material.

tyromatosis (tī-rō-ma-tō′sis): Cheesy degeneration of tissue.

tyrosinaemia (tī-rō-si-nē′mi-a): A disorder of tyrosine metabolism in which there is an abnormally high level of tyrosine in the blood and urine; occurs in two forms (1) transient T. seen in the newborn and (2) hereditary T. which is associated with cirrhosis of the liver, glycosuria, and rickets.

tyrosine (tī-rō′sēn): An amino acid found in many proteins that is concerned with growth and is an essential element in any diet; may be present in the urine in some diseases, especially diseases of the liver. T. IODINASE an enzyme in the thyroid; important in the production of thyroxine.

tyrosinosis (ti′rō-si-nō′sis): A condition due to abnormal metabolism of tyrosine; *p*-hydroxyphenylpyruvic acid, an intermediate product of this metabolism is excreted in the urine. See PHENYLKETONURIA.

tyrosinuria (tī′rō-si-nū′ri-a): The presence of tyrosine in the urine.

U

U: 1. Chemical symbol for uranium. 2. Abbreviation for unit, units.

u: Symbol for micron, one millionth of a meter. Usually written μ.

uberus (ū'ber-us): Fruitful; plentiful; fertile.

UKCC: Abbreviation for United Kingdom Central Council for Nursing, Midwifery and Health Visiting (*q.v.*).

ul-, ule-, ulo-: Combining forms meaning: 1. Gingivae, or gums. 2. Scar.

ula (ū'la): The gums.

-ula,-ulum, -ulus: Suffixes denoting: 1. Abounding in. 2. Small one, *e.g.*, formula, capitulum, tubulus.

ulalgia (ū-lal'ji-a): Pain in the gums.

-ular: Suffix in adjectives denoting relationship to the thing named in the stem, *e.g.*, cellular.

ulatrophia (ū-la-trō'fi-a): Shrinkage of the gums.

ulcer (ul'ser): An open circumscribed lesion on the surface of the skin, or on serous or mucous membrane, due to destruction of tissue; characterized by necrosis, sometimes suppuration, and slow healing. BURROWING U. usually caused by microaerophilic streptococci and coexisting staphylococci; characterized by necrosis of large skin areas; may produce sinus tracts in underlying tissues; CORNEAL U. one occurring on the cornea of the eye; CURLING'S U. a peptic U. associated with extensive burns and scalds or severe bodily injury; CUSHING'S U. an acute U. of the stomach or duodenum; associated with central nervous disease; DECUBITUS U. see under DECUBITUS; DUODENAL U. one on the mucous membrane lining of the duodenum; peptic U.; GASTRIC U. one on the mucous membrane lining of the stomach; peptic U.; GRAVITATIONAL U. an U. of the leg that develops as a result of incompetency of the valves in varicosed veins; HARD U. chancre (*q.v.*); INDOLENT U. one with hard elevated edges and little or no granulation; occurs most frequently on the leg; very slow healing; MOOREN'S U. chronic, progressive, usually bilateral ulceration of the marginal cornea; seen in the elderly; cause unknown; PENETRATING U. a locally invasive U. may involve the wall of an organ, or may erode a blood vessel and result in haematemesis if the U. is in the stomach or duodenum; PEPTIC U. a U. that occurs in the mucous lining of the stomach or duodenum; caused by the action of the acidic gastric juice; PERFORATING U. one which erodes through the wall of an organ; RODENT U. one which grows slowly and is locally invasive of the skin, usually the face; see BASAL CELL CARCINOMA under CARCINOMA; SERPENT or SERPIGINOUS U. an U. that erodes at one margin while extending at another thus creating an undulating margin; STASIS U. a chronic ulcerative lesion, usually on the lower leg; due to venous stasis; a varicose U.; STRESS U. an U. that occurs in people who experience long periods of physiological or environmental stress; usually occurs in the stomach or duodenum and is usually multiple; SYPHILITIC U. chancre (*q.v.*); VARICOSE U. an indolent U. in which there is loss of skin surface in the area of a varicose vein; usually occurs on the lower third of the leg; also called *stasis* U. or *gravitational* U.; VENEREAL U. chancroid (*q.v.*).

ulcerate (ul'ser-āt): 1. To undergo ulceration. 2. To form an ulcer.

ulceration (ul-ser-ā'shun): 1. The process of forming and developing an ulcer. 2. An ulcer or ulcers.

ulcerative (ul'ser-a-tiv): Relating to, or of the nature of, an ulcer. U. BLEPHARITIS see under BLEPHARITIS; U. COLITIS see under COLITIS.

ulcerogenic (ul'ser-ō-jen'ik): Ulcer-producing or capable of producing an ulcer.

ulcerous (ul'ser-us): Affected with, resembling, or pertaining to an ulcer.

-ule: Suffix denoting little or diminutive, *e.g.*, capsule.

ulectomy (ū-lek'to-mi): 1. The surgical removal of diseased gingival (gum) tissue. 2. The surgical removal of scar tissue, as in iridectomy.

ulemorrhagia (ū'lem-ō-rā'ji-a): Bleeding from the gums.

-ulent: Suffix denoting abounding in, or full of, *e.g.*, flatulent, full of flatus.

uletic (ū-let'ik): Relating to the gums.

ulitis (ū-lī'tis): Inflammation of the gums; gingivitis.

ulna (ul'na): The bone on the inner side of the forearm extending from the elbow to the wrist parallel to the radius.

ulnar (ul'nar): Relating to the ulna. U. ARTERY, originates in the brachial artery; is distributed to the forearm, wrist, and hand; U. NERVE runs down the inner side and middle of the forearm; supplies the flexor muscles of the wrist and hand.

ulnocarpal (ul'nō-kar'p'l): Relating to the ulna and the ulnar side of the wrist.

ulnoradial (ul'nō-rā'di-al): Relating to the ulna and the radial side of the wrist.

ulo-: Combining form denoting the gums.

uloncus (ū-long'kus): A tumour or swelling on the gums.

ulorrhoea (ū-lō-rē'a): Bleeding from the gums.

ulotrichous (ū-lot'ri-kus): Having woolly hair or curly hair.

ulotripsis (ū-lō-trip'sis): Stimulation of the gums by massage.

ultra-: A prefix denoting (1) excess, excessive; (2) beyond in space, range, or limits; (3) beyond what is normal, ordinary, or natural.

ultrafiltration (ul'tra-fil-trā'shun): 1. The separation, by an ultrafilter, of all except the very smallest particles of a mixture. 2. The separation, by ultrafilters, of colloids or crystalloids from the medium in which they are dispersed or dissolved. See COLLOID; CRYSTALLOID.

ultramicroscope (ul-tra-mī'kro-skōp): A microscope for viewing objects too small to be seen with an ordinary microscope; it utilizes refracted instead of direct light. — ultramicroscopic, adj.; ultramicroscopy, n.

ultramicrotome (ul-tra-mī'kro-tōm): A cutting instrument for cutting sections of tissue extremely thin for examination under the electron microscope.

ultrasonic (ul'tra-son'ik): Relating to energy waves that are similar to sound waves but which have such a high frequency that they are inaudible to the human ear (above 20 000 cycles per second). U. STERILIZATION see under STERILIZATION.

ultrasonogram (ul-tra-son'ō-gram): The image obtained by ultrasonography. See also ECHOGRAM.

ultrasonography (ul'tra-so-nog'ra-fi): A diagnostic technique utilizing ultrasound; when ultrasound waves are passed over a body area the reflection or echo of the sound waves as they pass over the junction of tissues of differing intensities is converted into a visual pattern. Also called *sonography*. See also ECHOENCEPHALOGRAPHY.

ultrasound (ul'tra-sownd): Sound waves that are of such high frequency that they are inaudible to the human ear (over 20 000 vibrations per second); when they strike living tissue their energy is changed to heat which is reflected in differing degrees by various tissues. These reflections or echoes, which may be recorded pictorially, are used in making diagnoses since they detect heart abnormalities, delineate the deep body structures and determine the size and location of abnormal tissues or foreign bodies, *e.g.*, tumours, gallstones, foreign objects in the eye. Therapeutically, U. is utilized to destroy tissue, as in cancer treatment; in brain surgery; in physiotherapy for joint diseases; and in treatment of such conditions as Ménière's disease. U. is also useful in detecting multiple pregnancies and for determing fetal size, maturity, position, and abnormalities. See also ECHOENCEPHALOGRAPHY.

ultrastructure (ul-tra-struk'chur): 1. Very fine structure or particles seen with ultramicroscope. 2. The invisible ultimate structure of protoplasm.

ultraviolet (ul-tra-vī'ōlet): Denoting radiant energy waves that are beyond the violet end of the spectrum. U. RAYS invisible natural component of the sun's radiation; may also be produced artificially by a special lamp; important in the synthesis of vitamin D in the body, and for normal growth and development; also used in treatment of certain skin diseases and for their indirect effect in treatment of rickets and anaemia; their bacteriostatic effect has been utilized for de-germing inanimate objects and air in enclosed areas but is no longer widely used for this purpose.

ultravirus (ul-tra-vī'rus): A very small virus (*q.v.*).

ululation (ūl-ū-lā'shun): The loud, inarticulate wailing or crying of hysterical or emotionally disturbed persons.

umbilectomy (um-bil-ek'tō-mi): Excision of the umbilicus. Also called *omphalectomy*.

umbilical (um-bil'i-kal): Relating to the umbilicus. U. CORD the structure that connects the umbilicus of the fetus to the placenta in the gravid uterus; contains two U. arteries carrying deoxygenated blood and one umbilical vein carrying oxygenated blood, surrounded by Wharton's jelly and covered by amnion. It is usually 50–60 cm long, and has a spiral twist; U. HERNIA see under HERNIA.

umbilicated (um-bil'i-kāt-ed): Marked by depressed spots resembling the umbilicus.

umbilicus (um-bil′i-kus): The scar or pit in the centre of the abdominal wall left by the separation of the umbilical cord after birth; the navel. — Also called *navel* and *belly-button*.

umbo (um′bō): 1. A boss (*q.v.*). 2. Any central eminence on the surface of a structure. U. OF THE TYMPANIC MEMBRANE the elevated point in the tympanic membrane to which the manubrium of the malleus is attached.

un-: A prefix denoting (1) not, in-, non-; (2) contrary to, opposite of; (3) to remove, release, or free from.

unciform (un′si-form): Shaped like a hook. U. BONE the hamate bone, one of the eight bones of the carpus.

Uncinaria (un′si-nā′ri-a): A genus of the nematodes, including one of the causative agents of hookworm disease.

uncinariasis (un′-sin-a-rī′as-is): Hookworm disease (*q.v.*).

uncinate (un′sin-āt): 1. Being hooked or barbed; unsiform. 2. Pertaining to the uncinate gyrus in the cortex of the brain; see GYRUS. U. SEIZURE a psychomotor or temporal lobe seizure that is preceded by an aura involving an olfactory and gustatory hallucination of something unpleasant, often of something burning; occurs in epileptics and others suffering from a lesion in the region of the uncus or hippocampus. Also called *uncinate fit.*

unconditioned reflex: A reflex that is inborn, *e.g.*, salivation at the sight of food.

unconscious (un-kon′shus): 1. Insensible; not aware of, or perceiving, factors in the environment. 2. State of being unable to receive stimuli or to have subjective experiences. 3. A psychoanalytical term for that part of the mind that consists of personality factors and physiological drives of which one is unaware and that are not accessible to memory, although they may be studied by Psychoanalytical techniques. COLLECTIVE U. according to Jung, the accumulated memories and urges of the entire human race.

unconsciousness (un-kon′shus-nes): A physiological and psychological state of being unconsciousness (*q.v.*); lack of awareness and ability to perceive; insensibility. May result from shock, severe trauma, serious illness, alcoholism, overdose of certain drugs, sunstroke, toxaemia.

unction (unk′shun): 1. The application of a soothing ointment, salve or oil. 2. An ointment.

unctuous (unk′shu-us): Fatty; oily; greasy.

uncus (ung′kus): A hook-shaped structure or process, specifically the hooked process of the anterior end of the hippocampal gyrus.

undergraduate: A student in a university who has not yet taken a degree, and thus is still below the academic standing of a graduate.

underwater: U. SEAL DRAINAGE see under DRAINAGE; U. EXERCISE exercise performed under water in a pool or large tub; the buoyancy afforded by the water increases the effectiveness of the exercise.

undescended: Not descended; refers specifically to a testis that does not descend into the scrotum but remains within the abdomen.

undine (un′dīn): A small, thin glass flask used for irrigating the eyes.

undulant (un′dū-lant): Characterized by rising and falling, or wave-like motion. U. FEVER brucellosis (*q.v.*).

ung: Abbreviation for *unguent* (ointment).

ungual (ung′gwal): Relating to the fingernails or toenails.

unguent (ung′gwent): Ointment. Also *unguentum.*

unguis (ung′gwis): A fingernail or toenail. — ungues, pl.; ungual, adj.

uni-: Combining form denoting one; single.

uniarticular (ū′ni-ar-tik′ū-lar): Involving only one joint.

unicef: Abbreviation for United Nations International Children's Fund.

unicellular (ū-ni-sel′ū-lar): Consisting of only one cell.

unicornous (ū-ni-kor′nus): Having only one horn or cornu.

unigravida (ūn-i-grav′i-da): A woman who is pregnant for the first time.

unilateral (ū-ni-lat′er-al): Related to, or involving, only one side of a structure or of the body. — unilaterally, adv.

uniocular (ū-ni-ok′ū-lar): 1. Relating to, affecting, or involving only one eye. 2. Having only one eye.

union (ūn′yun): 1. The process of healing or growing together, as occurs between the edges of a wound or the ends of fractured bones. See INTENTION. DELAYED U. that in which the speed of callus formation following fracture is slower than usual.

uniovular (ū-ni-ov′ū-lar): Relating to, or arising from, one ovum; descriptive of certain twin pregnancies that result in identical twins. Cf. BINOVULAR.

unipara (ū-nip′a-ra): A woman who has borne only one child. — uniparous, adj.

Unison (ū'-ni-son): A trade union (*q.v.*) representing workers in the public sector.

unit: 1. A single person or thing, one part of a whole that is made up of identical or similar parts. **2.** A measurement of quantity, weight, or other quality that has been adopted as standard for that particular substance. U. DOSE a pharmacological preparation of a medication that contains the prescribed amount for a single dose.

United Kingdom Central Council for Nursing, Midwifery and Health Visiting: Established in 1979 as a result of the Nurses, Midwives and Health Visitors' Act. Together with the four national bodies representing England, Northern Ireland, Scotland and Wales, it was the statutory organization responsible for the education, training regulations and discipline of nurses, midwives and health visitors. See NURSING AND MIDWIFERY COUNCIL.

United Nations International Children's Fund: A fund established by the United Nations in 1946 to provide help for children in areas of the world that have suffered the devastation of war or other catastrophic event; provides food and clothing and acts to prevent such diseases as tuberculosis and diphtheria; children of over 50 nations have benefited from the Fund.

univalent (ū-ni-vā'lent): Having a valance (chemical combining power) of one.

universal: Without limit; including or covering every member of the class, genus, or group being considered. U. ANTIDOTE consists of a solution in warm water of 50% charcoal, 25% magnesium oxide, and 25% tannic acid; considered useful in many types of poisoning, including that from acids, alkaloids, certain heavy metals, and glycosides. U. DONOR an individual whose blood group is O and therefore compatible with most other blood types; U. RECIPIENT in transfusions, an individual whose blood group is AB and therefore compatible with A, B, and O types. See BLOOD GROUPS.

universal precautions: Prudent standard preventive measures to be taken by professional and other health personnel in contact with persons afflicted with a communicable disease, to avoid contracting the disease by contagion or infection. These include the wearing of gloves, gowns, and masks. Precautions are especially applicable in the diagnosis and care of patients with AIDS.

unmedullated (un-med'ū-lāt-ed): Descriptive of a nerve fibre that has no myelin sheath.

Unna's boot: A semirigid cast-like casing, using a paste made of glycerin, zinc oxide, and gelatin; applied to the entire leg or the lower leg and foot and covered with a spiral bandage, then more paste; this process is repeated until rigidity is obtained. Used in treating varicose veins and ulcers, oedema, and, sometimes, fractures of the ankle. [Paul Unna, German dermatologist, 1850–1929.]

unsaturated (un-sat'ū-rāt-ed): Descriptive of a solution that is capable of dissolving more of a solvent; not saturated.

unsex: To deprive an individual of the gonads, thus making reproduction impossible. To castrate.

unstriated (un-strī'ā-ted): Unstriped, referring usually to smooth muscle fibres.

untoward (un-to-ward'): Undesirable, adverse, unexpected, unfortunate; descriptive of effects of a drug or treatment.

upper GI series: The examination of the stomach and duodenum by x-ray, following the administration of a barium swallow.

upper motor neuron: A neuron that has its cell in the brain cortex and which conducts impulses to the nuclei of the cerebral nerves or the ventral grey columns of the spinal cord. See LOWER MOTOR NEURON.

upper respiratory tract: Composed of the nose and nasal cavity; the ethmoid, sphenoid, frontal, and maxillary sinuses; and the larynx and trachea; URT INFECTION infection confined to the structures of the upper respiratory tract.

ups or uppers: Slang for drugs that produce elated feelings, or 'highs'.

uptake: In medicine, a term used to describe the absorption of some substance by a tissue, *e.g.*, iodine by the thyroid gland.

ur-, uro-: Combining forms denoting: **1.** Urine; urination; urinary tract. **2.** Urea.

uracratia (ū-ra-krā'shi-a): The inability to retain urine in the bladder.

uraemia (ū-rē'mi-a): A clinical syndrome due to renal failure resulting from either disease of the kidneys themselves, or from disorder or disease elsewhere in the body, which induces kidney dysfunction and which results in gross biochemical disturbance in the body, including retention of urea and other nitrogenous substances in the blood. Depending on the cause it may or may not be reversible. The fully developed syndrome is characterized by nausea, vomiting, headache, hiccough, weakness, dimness of vision, convulsions, and coma. Also called *azotaemia*. — uraemic, adj.

uraemic (ū-rē'mik): Relating to or affected with uraemia. U. FROST whitish flakes that appear on the skin of some patients with advanced renal failure; due to inability of the kidneys to excrete urea compounds which are then excreted by the small capillaries in the skin where they collect on the surface.

uragogue (ū'-ra-gog): A diuretic (q.v.).

uran-, urano-: Combining forms denoting the palate or roof of the mouth.

uranicus (ū'ra-nis'kus): The palate.

uraniscoplasty (ū'ran-is'kō-plas-ti): Plastic surgery of a cleft palate. Also called *uranoplasty*.

uranium (ū-rā'ni-um): A hard, heavy, silvery-white, radioactive metallic element of the radium group; found chiefly in pitchblende; important in the work on atomic energy. Some of its isotopes have uses in medicine.

uranorrhaphy (ū-ran-or'-a-fi): An operation involving suturing of a cleft palate. Palatorrhaphy.

uranoschisis (ū-ran-os'ki-sis): Cleft palate; uraniscochasm.

urarthritis (ū'rar-thrī'tis): Inflammation of the joints, as occurs in gout.

urate (ū'rāt): Any of several salts of uric acid. Urates are present in blood and urine and are constituents of stones or concretions formed in the body.

uraturia (ū'ra-tū-ri'a): Excess of urates in the urine. — uraturic, adj.

urea (ū-rē'a): A white, crystalline substance, the major nitrogenous end waste product of protein metabolism; it is synthesized in the liver and carried to the kidney by the blood, thus is a normal constituent of blood, lymph and urine. The chief nitrogenous constituent of urine. Used in medicine as a diuretic. U. clearance, U. concentration, and U. range tests are all procedures for measuring the efficiency of kidney function. U. CYCLE a cyclic series of reactions involving several substances including arginine and ornithine, the end product being urea; this is the major route of removal from the body of the ammonia found in the liver and kidney during metabolism of amino acids.

Ureaplasma urealyticum (ū-rē'a-plaz'ma ū-rē'a-lit'i-kum): A small Gram-negative sexually transmitted microorganism found in both male and female genitourinary tracts and sometimes in the rectum and the pharynx; infections with the organism may be symptomless but may also be associated with non-gonorrhoeal urethritis in the male and with genitourinary tract infections, puerperal infec-

tions, and reproductive failure in the female, and with prematurity and neonatal death.

urease (ū'rē-ās): An enzyme elaborated by various microorganisms, it catalyses the change of urea into ammonia and carbon dioxide and is found in mucus and the urine of patients with inflammation of the bladder.

urecchysis (ū-rek'i-sis): Extravasation of urine into tissue, as may occur in rupture of the bladder caused by fracture of the pelvis.

uresis (ū-rē'sis): Urination.

ureter (ur're-ter, u-rē'ter): The tube that passes from each kidney to the bladder for the conveyance of urine; its average length is approximately 30 cm. — ureteric, ureteral, adj.

ureterectasia (ū-rē'ter-ek-tā'si-a): Dilation of a ureter.

ureterectomy (ū-rē-ter-ek'to-mi): Excision of a segment or all of a ureter.

ureteric (ū-rē-ter'ik): Relating to a ureter. U. CATHETER a fine-calibre catheter that can be passed up the ureter to the pelvis of the kidney in order to collect a specimen of urine. U. TRANSPLANTATION an operation in which the ureters are separated from the bladder and implanted in the ileus or colon; done to correct a congenital defect or because of a malignant growth.

ureteritis (ū-rē-ter-i'tis): Inflammation of a ureter.

uretero-: Combining form denoting ureter.

ureterocele (ū-rē'ter-ō-sēl): Prolapse and sacculation of the ureter at its junction with the bladder, resulting from stenosis of the meatus; may lead to hydronephrosis and kidney damage.

ureterocolic (ū-rē'ter-ō-kol'ik): Relating to the ureter and colon, especially to an anastomosis between the two structures when there is a pathological condition of the lower urinary system.

ureterocolostomy (ū-rē'ter-ō-ko-los'to-mi): Surgical transplantation of the ureters from the bladder to the colon so that urine is passed by the bowel.

ureteroenterostomy (ū-rē'te-ō-en-ter-os'to-mi): The formation of an anastomosis between the ureter and the intestine.

ureteroilcostomy (ū-rē'ter-ō-il-ē-os'to-mi): The formation of an anastomosis between a ureter and the ileum. Also called *ileoureterostomy*.

ureterolith (ū-rē'ter-ōlith): A stone in a ureter.

ureterolithotomy (ū-rē'ter-ō-li-thot'o-mi): Surgical removal of a stone from a ureter.

ureteroneocystostomy (ū-rē'ter-ō-nē'ō-sis-tos'to-mi): A surgical procedure in which the upper end of a divided ureter is implanted into the urinary bladder; most often performed during kidney transplant operation.

ureteronephrectomy (ū-rē'ter-ō-nef-rek'to-mi): Removal of a kidney and its ureter.

ureteropathy (ūrē'ter-op'a-thi) : Any disease or disorder of a ureter.

ureteropelvic (ū-rē'ter-ō-pel'vik): Relating to a ureter and the pelvis of the kidney to which it is attached.

ureteroplasty (ū-rē'ter-ō-plas-ti): Plastic surgery for repair of a ureter.

ureteroproctostomy (ū-rē'ter-ō-prok-tos'to-mi): The establishment of an anastomosis between a ureter and the rectum.

ureteropyelonephritis (ū-rē'ter-ō-pī 'e-lō-ne-frī' tis): Inflammation of a ureter, the pelvis of the kidney, and the kidney substance.

ureterosigmoidostomy (ū-rē'ter-ō-sig-moyd-os'to-mi): The surgical implantation of a ureter into the sigmoid colon.

ureterostenosis (ū-rē'ter-ō-ste-nō'sis): Stricture or narrowing of a ureter.

ureterostomy (ū-rē-ter-os'to-mi): The formation of a permanent fistula through which the ureter discharges urine. CUTANEOUS U. transplantation of the ureter to the skin in the iliac region.

ureterouterostomy (ū-rē'ter-ō-ū-rē'ter-os'to-mi): The establishment of an anastomosis between the two ureters.

ureterovaginal (ū-rē'ter-ō-vaj-īn'al): Relating to a ureter and the vagina. U. FISTULA one between the ureter and the vagina; may be congenital or the result of a pathological condition such as cancer of the cervix.

ureterovesical (ū-rē'ter-ō-ves'ik'l): Relating to a ureter and the urinary bladder.

urethr-, urethro-: Combining forms denoting urethra.

urethra (ū-rē'thra): The channel leading from the bladder through which urine is excreted; in the female it measures about 3.7 cm; in the male 20–22.5 cm. — urethral, adj.

urethralgia (ū-rē-thral'ji-a): Pain in the urethra.

urethrectomy (ū-rē-threk'to-mi): The surgical removal of all or part of the urethra.

urethremphraxis (ū'rē-threm-frak'sis): An obstruction preventing the free flow of urine through the urethra.

urethritis (ū-rē-thrī'tis): Inflammation of the urethra, characterized by pain on urination; often associated with an infection in the kidney or bladder. GONORRHOEAL U. caused by gonococcal infection; GOUTY U. that due to gout; NON-SPECIFIC U. that not due to a gonococcal or other specific organism.

urethrocele (ū-rē'thrō-sēl): In the female, (1) a prolapse of the urethra through the meatus urinarius, or (2) a pouch-like protrusion of the urethral walls into the vaginal canal.

urethrocystitis (ū-rē'thrō-sis-tī'tis): Inflammation of the urethra and urinary bladder.

urethrocystography (ū-rē'thrō-sist-og'ra-fi): X-ray of the urethra and bladder after the injection of a constrast medium. MICTURATING U., U. in which the bladder is filled with radiopaque fluid and several x-rays are taken with the bladder at rest, and during and after voiding; done to determine the efficiency of the internal sphincter of the bladder and the angle of the posterior junction of the urethra and the bladder. — urethrocystogram, n.

urethrogram (ū-rē'thrō-gram): An x-ray view of the urethra, usually following the introduction of a contrast medium. VOIDING U. a U. taken while the patient is voiding.

urethrography (ū-rē-throg'ra-fi): X-ray examination of the urethra. See UROGRAPHY.

urethroplasty (ū-rē'thrō-plas-ti): Any plastic operation on the urethra. — urethroplastic, adj.

urethrorectal (ū-rē'thrō-rek'tal): Relating to the urethra and the rectum.

urethrorrhoea (ū-rē'thrō-rē'a): Any abnormal discharge from the urethra.

urethroscope (ū-rē'thrō-skōp): An instrument designed to allow visualization of the interior of the urethra. — urethroscopic, adj.; urethroscopically, adv.; urethroscopy, n.

urethrostenosis (ū-rē'thrō-ste-nō'sis): Urethral stricture.

urethrostomy (ū-rē-thros'to-mi): The surgical creation of an artificial opening into the urethra in cases of severe stricture.

urethrotomy (ū-rē-throt'o-mi): Incision into the urethra; usually part of an operation for stricture.

urethrotrigonitis (ū-rē'thrō-trī-go-nī'tis): Inflammation of the urethra and the trigone of the urinary bladder; often due to damage to the urethra during sexual intercourse; marked by lower abdominal discomfort, frequent urination with pain and burning on voiding. See TRIGONE.

urethrovaginal (ū-rē'thrō-vaj-īn'al): Relating to the urethra and the vagina.

urethrovesical (ū-rē'thrō-ves'ik-al): Relating to the urethra and the urinary bladder.

-uretic: Combining form denoting urine.

urgency (ur'jen-si): Sudden strong desire to urinate.

urhidrosis (ūr-hī-drō'sis): The presence of urinous substances such as urea or uric acid in the sweat. The crystals of uric acid may be deposited on the skin as fine white particles.

-uria: Combining form denoting (1) urine; (2) some characteristic of urine.

uric acid (ū′rik as′id): An acid formed in the breakdown of nucleoproteins in the tissues, and excreted in the urine. It is relatively insoluble and liable to give rise to stones. Present in excess in the blood in gout.

uricaciduria (ū′rik-as-i dū′ri-a): The presence of more than the normal amount of uric acid in the urine. Uricaemia.

uricase (ū′ri-kās): An enzyme that acts as a catalyst in the decomposition of uric acid.

uricosuria (ū′rik-ō-sū′ri-a): Excessive excretion of uric acid in the urine.

uricosuric (ū′-rik-ō-sū′rik): An agent that enhances the excretion of uric acid in the urine; such substances are often used in treatment of chronic gout.

uridrosis (ū-ri drō′sis): Urhidrosis (q.v.).

urin-, urino-: Combining forms denoting urine.

urinal (ū-rīn′al, ū′rin-al): A vessel or container for receiving urine.

urinalysis (ū′ri-nal′i sis): A systematic examination and study of the physical, chemical, and microscopic properties of urine to obtain data that will be helpful in making diagnoses, serving as a guide for further tests, or checking on the progress of patients under treatment.

urinary (ū′ri-ner-i): Relating to urine. U. BLADDER the sac-like pelvic organ that serves as a reservoir for the collection of urine to be voided through the urethra; U. CALCULUS a concretion formed in the urinary tract; U. DIVERSION see ILEAL CONDUIT; U. FREQUENCY the urge to void more often than usual although the overall amount of urine voided is not increased; often associated with infection in the urinary bladder and accompanied by pain or a burning sensation; U. INCONTINENCE the involuntary voiding of urine; may be neurogenic or psychogenic in origin; U. OUTPUT the amount of urine secreted by the kidneys; U. RETENTION accumulation of urine in the bladder due to inability to void; U. STASIS the remaining still or pooling of urine as may occur in the kidney or bladder; U. SYSTEM or TRACT, consists of the kidneys, ureters, urinary bladder, and the urethra; U. TRACT INFECTION infection of any one of the structures in the urinary system; U. UNIDIVERSION an operation to re-establish continuity of the urinary tract following the creation of an ileal conduit.

urinate (ū′rin-āt): To discharge urine from the body.

urination (ū-ri-nā′shun): The discharge or passing of urine from the body; micturition.

urine (ū′rin): The amber-coloured fluid that is secreted by the kidneys, conveyed to the bladder by the two ureters, and stored there until it is discharged from the body. It has a normal pH of 4.5 to 8.0, and a specific gravity of 1.005 to 1.030, and consists of 96% water and 4% solids, the most important of which are urea and uric acid. Other solids found in urine include sodium chloride, potassium chloride, ammonia, hippuric acid, sulphuric acid, phosphoric acid, creatine. Solids that may be found in the urine of patients with various pathological conditions include bacteria, bile, blood, fat, glucose, ketone bodies, pus. The daily output varies, depending on various environmental factors, but the average is about 1.7 litres.

uriniferous (ū′ri-nif″er-us): Conveying urine; denoting particularly the tubules of the kidney.

urinogenital (ū′rin-ō-jen′it-al): See UROGENITAL.

urinoma (ū′ri-nō′ma): A cyst that contains urine.

urinometer (ū′rin-om′i-ter): An instrument for estimating the specific gravity of urine.

urinous (ū′rin-us): Having the characteristics of urine.

uro-, urono-: Combining forms denoting (1) urine; (2) urination; (3) urinary tract.

urobilin (ū′rō-bī′lin): A brownish pigment formed by the oxidation of urobilinogen and excreted in the urine and faeces.

urobilinogen (ū′ro-bī-lin′o-jen): A pigment formed from bilirubin in the intestine by the action of bacteria. It may be reabsorbed into the circulation and converted back to bilirubin in the liver. Small amounts are excreted in the urine and large amounts in the faeces.

urobilinuria (ū′rō-bī-lin-ū′ri-a): The presence of increased amounts of urobilin in the urine.

urocele (ū′rō-sēl): The escape of urine into the scrotal sac.

urochesia (ū-rō-kē′zi-a): The excretion of urine from the anus.

urochrome (ū′rō-krōm): The brownish or yellowish pigment that gives the urine its normal colour.

urodynamics (ū-rō-dī-nam′iks): The study of the forces involved in moving the urine along the urinary tract.

urodynia (ū-rō-din′i-a): Pain on urination; dysuria.

urogenital (ū-rō-jen′i-tal): Relating to the urinary and the genital organs.

urogenous (ū-roj′e-nus): Producing or excreting urine.

urogram (ū' rō-gram): The graphic recording of a radiograph of the urinary tract or any part of it, after injection of contrast medium.

urography (ū-rog'ra-fi): Radiological examination of any part of the urinary tract; usually involves use of a contrast medium. CYSTOSCOPIC U. with the contrast fluid being injected into the bladder; EXCRETORY U., U. with the contrast medium being taken by mouth; INTRAVENOUS U., U. with the contrast fluid being injected into a vein; RETROGRADE U. cystoscopic U.

urokinase (ū'rō-kī'nās): An enzyme normally found in the urine; important in the conversion of plasminogen to plasmin which acts as a fibrolytic enzyme.

urolagnia (ū-rō-lag'ni-a): Sexual stimulation produced by association with urine, *e.g.*, watching people urinate, or wishing to urinate on another person.

urolith (ū'rō-lith): A stone in the urinary tract, or one passed in the urine.

urolithiasis (ū-rō-li-thī'a-sis): A state in which there is marked tendency towards the formation of urinary stones.

urologist (ū-rol'o-jist): A physician who specializes in urology (*q.v.*).

urology (ū-rol'o-ji): That branch of medical science that deals with disorders of the female urinary tract and the male genitourinary tract.
— urologic, urological, adj.; urologically, adv.

uromelus (ū-rom'e-lus): A fetus with fused legs and a single foot.

uropathogen (ū'rō-path'o-jen): Any microorganism that causes disease of the urinary tract.

uropathy (ū-rop'a-thi): Any disease or disorder of the urinary tract or any part of it.

uropoiesis (ū'rō-poy-ē'sis): The formation or secretion of urine.

uroporphyria (ū'rō-por-fir'i-a): See PORPHYRIA.

uroporphyrin (ū'rō-por'fir-in): Any of the several porphyrins found in small amounts in normal urine and faeces; all contain four acetic acid groups and four proprionic acid groups.

uropsammus (ū-rō-sam'us): Calcerous sediment in the urine.

urorubin (ū'-rō-ru'bin): A red pigment in urine.

uroschesis (u-ros'ke-sis): 1. The retention of urine in the bladder. 2. The suppression of urine.

urosepsis (ū-rō-sep'sis): Septicaemia resulting from the retention and absorption by the tissues of substances normally excreted in the urine.

Urtica (ur'ti-ka): A herbaceous weed; nettle. Produces an intense stinging sensation on contact with the skin; has some uses in medicine.

urticaria (ur-ti-kā'ri-a): A skin eruption characterized by circumscribed, smooth, itchy, raised weals that are either redder or paler than the surrounding skin, developing very suddenly, usually lasting a few days, and leaving no visible trace. Common provocative agents in susceptible subjects are ingested foods such as shellfish, injected sera, and contact with, or injection of, antibiotics such as penicillin and streptomycin. Also called *nettle rash* or *hives*. ACUTE U., U. accompanied by mild constitutional symptoms; ALLERGIC U. weals due to sensitization and re-exposure to allergenic substances, usually from ingestion; CHOLINERGIC U. small weals produced by heat created by exercise or emotion; CHRONIC U., a form in which weals appear frequently or are persistent; COLD U., U. due to exposure to cold; GIANT U. angioneurotic oedema (*q.v.*); NEONATAL U. ill-defined white or yellow weals surrounded by blotches of bright erythema; SOLAR U., U. occurring in certain individuals on exposure to sunlight; U. MEDICAMENTOSA, U. due to ingestion of certain drugs; U. PIGMENTOSA a form of U. seen in mastocytosis (*q.v.*) in which the lesions have a brown or reddish colour when stroked.

urtication (ur-ti-kā'shun): 1. The development or production of urticaria (*q.v.*). 2. The sensation of having been stung by nettles.

urushiol (ū-roo'shē-ol): The irritating substance in certain plants, *e.g.*, poison ivy and related plants, that causes contact dermatitis and/or allergic reaction in susceptible individuals.

user involvement: A system in which there is greater equality between patients or users of services and professional practitioners. Users are seen to be involved at three levels: the policy-making process; disease management; and one-to-one relationships between users and their practitioners, where there is a dialogue and sharing of information. See PATIENT ADVICE AND LIAISON SERVICE.

uter-, utero-: Combining forms denoting uterus.

uteralgia (ū-ter-al'ji-a): Pain in the uterus.

uterectomy (ū-ter-ek'to-mi): Excision of the uterus; hysterectomy.

uterine (ū'ter-īn): Relating to the uterus. U. DYSFUNCTION inertia uteri (*q.v.*); U. PROLAPSE see PROLAPSE; U. TUBE formerly known as *fallopian tube* (*q.v.*). See also ANTEFLEXION, ANTEVERSION, RETROFLEXION, RETROVERSION.

uteritis (ū-ter-ī'tis): Inflammation of the uterus Also called metritis.

uterocervical (ū'ter-ō-ser'vi-kal): Relating to the uterine cervix, or to the uterus and the cervix.

uterofixation (ū'ter-ō-fik-ā'shun): Hysteropexy (*q.v.*).

uterography (ū-ter-og'ra-fi): X-ray examination of the uterus.

uterolith (ū'ter-ō-lith): A calculus in the uterus.

uteropexy (ū'ter-ō-pek'si): Hysteropexy (*q.v.*).

uteroplacental (ū'ter-ō-pla-sen'tal): Relating to the uterus and placenta. U. APOPLEXY see COUVELAIRE UTERUS and UTERUS.

uteroplasty (ū'ter-ō-plas-ti): Any plastic operation on the uterus.

uterorectal (ū'ter-ō-rek'tal): Relating to the uterus and the rectum.

uterosacral (ū'ter-ō-sā'kral): Relating to the uterus and sacrum. U. LIGAMENT the thickened pelvic fascia that curves along beside the lateral wall of the pelvis from the cervix to the front of the sacrum.

uterosalpingography (ū'ter-ō-sal-ping-gog'raf-i): X-ray examination of the uterus and uterine tubes after injection of a contrast medium.

uterotonic (ū'ter-ō-ton'ik): Giving tone to the muscles of the uterus, or an agent that gives tone to uterine muscles.

uterotubal (ū'ter-ō-tu'bal): Relating to the uterus and the uterine tubes. U. INSUFFLATION the blowing of air into the uterine tubes via the uterus; a test for tubal patency.

uterotubography (ū'ter-ō-tū-bog'ra-fi): Roentgenography of the uterus and uterine tubes after the injection of a radiopaque material.

uterovaginal (ū'ter-ō-vaj-īn'al): Relating to the uterus and the vagina.

uterovesical (ū'ter-ō-ves'ik-al): Relating to the uterus and the bladder.

uterus (ū'ter-us): The womb; a hollow, pearshaped muscular organ into which the ovum is received through the uterine tubes, where it is retained during development, and from which the fetus is expelled through the vagina. Situated in the pelvic cavity, between the bladder and the rectum, it is about 7.5 cm long and 5 cm wide at the widest part; is divided into 3 parts, the *fundus* or upper broad part, the cavity or *body*, and the neck or *cervix*; it opens into the vagina below and the uterine tubes above; it is maintained in position by ligaments, and lined with mucous membrane called endometrium. BICORNUATE U. a uterus with two horns; COUVELAIRE U. a serious condition involving separation of the placenta and infiltration of blood into the uterine musculature; may occur in association with abruptio placentae (*q.v.*); also called *uteroplacental apoplexy*. [Alexandre Couvelaire, French obstetrician, 1873–1948.]; GRAVID U. a pregnant uterus. — uteri, pl.; uterine, adj.

UTI: Abbreviation for urinary tract infection, see under URINARY.

utricle (ū'trik-l): 1. A little sac or pouch. 2. The small, delicate sac in the bony vestibule of the ear; the semicircular canals open into it.

UVA: Abbreviation for ultraviolet light A, see under ULTRAVIOLET.

UVB: Abbreviation for ultraviolet light B, see under ULTRAVIOLET.

uvea (ū've-a): The pigmented middle coat of the eye, including the iris, ciliary body and choroid. — uveal, adj.

uveitis (ū-vē-i'tis): Inflammation of the uvea or any part of it.

uveomeningitis (u've-ō-men-in-ji'tis): A condition marked by lesions of the uvea, accompanied by meningeal signs.

uveoparotid fever (ū've-ō-pa-rot'id): A form of sarcoidosis with symptoms of fever, uveitis, enlargement of the parotid gland, and sometimes temporary facial palsy. Also called *uveoparotitis*.

uvula (ū'vū-la): Any dependent fleshy mass; term usually refers to the central tag-like structure hanging down from the posterior of the soft palate. — uvular, adj.

uvulectomy (ū'vū-lek'to-mi): Excision of the uvula.

uvulitis (ū'vū-li'tis): Acute swelling and inflammation of the uvula; also called *staphylitis*.

uvuloptosis (ū'vū-lop'to-sis): A falling or relaxed condition of the palate.

uvulotomy (ū'vū-lot'o-mi): The operation of cutting off all or part of the uvula. Also called *staphylotomy*.

U wave: A deflection in the electrocardiogram that sometimes follows the T wave.

V

vaccinate (vak'sin-āt): To inoculate with a vaccine to produce immunity to the corresponding infectious disease.

vaccination (vak'sin-ā'shun): Originally, the process of inoculating persons with discharge from cowpox to protect them from smallpox. Now applied to the inoculation of any antigenic material for the purpose of producing active artificial immunity.

vaccine (vak-sēn'): A suspension or extract of the organisms that cause a disease, either killed or modified so as to reduce their power to cause the disease while retaining their power to cause the body to form antibodies against the disease. Used chiefly in prophylactic treatment of certain infections by producing active immunity; sometimes used for amelioration or treatment of certain infectious diseases. AUTOGENOUS V. one prepared from a culture of bacteria taken from the patient who is to receive the vaccine; MIXED V. one prepared from two species of bacteria; POLYVALENT V. one prepared from more than two species of bacteria; QUADRUPLE V. one that protects against diphtheria, tetanus, whooping cough, and poliomyelitis; TRIPLE V. one that protects against diphtheria, tetanus, and whooping cough. Vaccines are available for protection against many other diseases including cholera, influenza, measles, mumps, plague, rabies, typhoid and typhus fever, and yellow fever. See also BACILLUS CALMETTE–GUERIN (BCG); SABIN'S V.; SALK V.

vacuole (vak'ū-ōl): A very small space in the protoplasm of a cell, containing air or fluid. — vacuolar, vacuolated, adj.; vacuolation, n.

vacuolization (vak'-ū-ō-lī-zā'shun): The formation of vacuoles. Also called *vacuolation*.

vacuum (vak'ū-um): An empty enclosed space from which all air has been extracted. V. ASPIRATION the use of a vacuum extractor to assist in aborting the products of conception; done before the 14th week of pregnancy; V. EXTRACTION the employment of suction instead of obstetric forceps in the second stage of labour.

vagal (vā'gal): Relating to the vagus nerve (*q.v.*).

vagectomy (vā-jek'to-mi): Excision of a portion of the vagus nerve.

vagin-, vagini-, vagino-: Combining forms denoting the vagina.

vagina (va-jī'na): 1. A sheath or sheath-like structure. 2. The musculomembranous genital canal in the female lying between the urinary bladder and the rectum and extending from the cervix uteri to the vulva; measuring about 7.5 cm along the anterior wall and 10 cm along the posterior wall. — vaginal, adj.

vaginal (vaj-īn'al): 1. Like a sheath. 2. Relating to the vagina. V. HYSTERECTOMY surgical removal of the uterus by way of the vagina; V. SPECULUM an instrument used to open the vagina so as to facilitate inspection of it; V. SPERMICIDES contraceptives that are inserted into the vagina before coitus; they act by interfering with the viability of the sperm; available without prescription in the form of foams, jellies, and suppositories.

vaginate (vaj'in-āt): To ensheath, or to be enclosed in a sheath. See INVAGINATION.

vaginectomy (vaj-i-nek'to-mi): Colpectomy; excision of the vagina or part of it.

vaginismus (vaj-in-iz'mus): Painful spasm of the muscular wall of the vagina preventing satisfactory sexual intercourse.

vaginitis (vaj-i-nī'tis): A non-specific inflammation of the vagina. ATROPHIC V. characterized by a watery discharge, burning and itching of the vulva; usually occurs during and after menopause; may progress to kraurosis vulvae; often associated with leukoplakia; CANDIDAL V. caused by *Candida albicans*, a fungus; fairly common in pregnant women, diabetics, debilitated persons, and those taking oral contraceptives; characterized by a thick, curdlike discharge and severe pruritus; GONOCOCCAL V. caused by infection with *Neisseria gonorrhoea*; characterized by a thick yellow purulent discharge; HAEMOPHILUS V. caused by a Gram-negative organism, *Haemophilus vaginalis*; characterized by a scanty, malodorous, thin, creamy, grey discharge of frothy material; consistency and colour may vary; MONILIAL V. candidal v.; SENILE V. relatively common in older women; may be accompanied by profuse purulent or bloody discharge causing soreness; sometimes seen in cancer of the uterus; TRI-

642

vaginitis 643 valve

CHOMONAL V. Caused by *Trichomonas vaginalis*; characterized by frothy, greenish or yellowish copious discharge, intense itching and burning of vulva.

vaginocele (vaj'in-ō-sēl): Colpocele (*q.v.*).

vaginodynia (vaj'i-nō-din'i-a): Pain in the vagina; colpodynia.

vaginofixation (vaj'in-ō-fik-sā'shun): Surgical fixation of the vagina to the abdominal wall to correct vaginal relaxation or prolapse.

vaginohysterectomy (vaj'i-nō-his-ter-ek'to-mi): The surgical removal of the uterus through the vagina without any abdominal incision.

vaginolabial (vaj'i-nō-lā'bi-al): Relating to the vagina and the labia.

vaginomycosis (vaj'in-ō-mī'kō'sis): Infection of the vagina caused by a fungus.

vaginopathy (vaj-i-nop'a-thi): Any pathological condition of the vagina; colpopathy.

vaginoperineal (vaj'in-ō-per-in ō'al): Relating to both the vagina and perineum.

vaginoperineorrhaphy (vaj'in-ō-per-i-nē-or'a-fi): Surgical repair of a lacerated or ruptured vagina and perineum.

vaginoperineotomy (vaj'i-nō-per-i-ne-ot'o-mi): An incision at the outlet of the vagina and the adjoining perineum; done to facilitate childbirth.

vaginopexy (vaj-ī'nō-pek-si): Vaginofixation (*q.v.*).

vaginoplasty (vaj-īn-ō-plas-ti): Reparative plastic surgery on the vagina.

vaginovesical (vaj'i-nō-ves'i-kal): Relating to the vagina and the urinary bladder.

vagitis (va-jī'tis): Inflammation of the vagus nerve.

vagitus (va-jī'tus): The cry of an infant while being born or while still in the uterus.

vagolysis (vā-gol'i-sis): Surgical destruction of the vagus nerve.

vagolytic (vā-gō-lit'ik): 1. Relating to or causing vagolysis. 2. An agent that neutralizes the effect of a stimulated vagus nerve.

vagomimetic (vā'gō-mi-met'ik): Having an effect resembling that produced by vagal stimulation.

vagotomy (vā-got'o-mi): 1. Surgical division of the vagus nerve. 2. Interruption of the impulses carried by the vagus nerve.

vagotonia (vā-go-tō'ni-a): A condition of hyperexcitability of the vagus nerve; may result in vasomotor instability, sweating, bradycardia, constipation — vagotonic, adj.

vagus (vā'gus): The parasympathetic pneumogastric nerve; the tenth pair of cranial nerves, composed of both motor and sensory fibres, with a wide distribution in the neck, thorax, and abdomen, sending important branches to the heart, lungs, stomach, etc. — vagi, pl.; vagal, adj.

valence, valency (vā'lens): The degree of combining power of one atom of an element or a radical, using the combining power of one atom of hydrogen as the unit of comparison.

valgus (val'gus): Twisted or bent outward, denoting a displacement or angulation away from the midline of the body; term is used in connection with the noun it describes, *e.g.* hallux valgus. Opp. of varus. — valgoid, adj.

validity (val-id'-i-ti): The quality of being well founded on fact, or established on sound principles, and thoroughly applicable to a case or circumstances.

valine (val'ēn, vā'lēn): One of the essential amino acids; found in most protein foods; is synthesized in the body and considered essential for growth and development in infants and for maintaining nitrogen balance in adults.

vallate (val'āt): Cupped; describing a depression that is surrounded by an elevated rim. V. PAPILLAE the papillae that occcur in a V-shaped arrangement on the surface of the posterior part of the tongue.

Valsalva: V. MANOEUVRE forceful expiration of air against a closed glottis, which increases thoracic pressure, impedes venous return to the heart, and slows the heart rate; occurs normally in individuals when lifting heavy objects, straining at stool, or changing position when lying down; sometimes employed in treating paroxysmal tachycardia; V. SINUSES three small dilatations of the aorta behind the flaps of the valves at the opening of the aorta in the left ventricle; V. TEST a test for patency of the auditory tube; when the patient exhales forcefully while holding the nose and mouth tightly closed, air should pass into the middle air cavity and the person should hear a popping sound if the tube is patent. [Antonio Mario Valsalva, Italian anatomist, 1666–1723.]

value: 1. The material or monetary worth of a thing. 2. Tenet of morality.

Valuing People: A New Strategy for Learning Disability for the 21st Century: A White Paper (*q.v.*) published 20 March 2001, established the Learning Disability Taskforce (q.v.). It was the first White Paper on learning disability for thirty years and set out an ambitious and challenging programme of action for improving services.

valve (valv): In anatomy, a fold of membrane in a passage or tube, permitting the flow of contents in one direction only. AORTIC V. the V.

between the left ventricle and the ascending aorta; ATRIOVENTRICULAR V. either of the two valves between the atria and ventricles of the heart; BICUSPID V. one that has two cusps, *e.g.*, the v. between the left atrium and left ventricle; also called the *mitral* v.; HOUSTON'S V. three or four crescent-shaped membranous folds in the rectum; also called *Houston's folds* and *rectal valves*; ILEOCAECAL V. a v. consisting of membranous folds between the ileum and the large intestine; it prevents faecal matter from moving back into the ileum; MITRAL V. the bicuspid v. between the left atrium and left ventricle; PULMONARY V. the v. between the right ventricle and the pulmonary trunk; PROSTHETIC V. usually refers to a prosthetic heart valve used to replace a defective natural v.; PYLORIC V. a membranous fold at the junction of the stomach and the duodenum; SEMILUNAR V. a v. having three cusps, as the aortic and pulmonary valves; TRICUSPID V. a v. having three cusps, as the right atrioventricular v.; VENOUS V. any of the valves found in most veins except the venae cavae and the intestinal veins; they are semilunar pockets on the inner surface of the veins, with their free edges lying centrally in the direction of blood flow and preventing reversal of the direction of flow; most numerous in the lower extremities.

valvoplasty (val'vō-plas-ti): A plastic operation on a valve, usually reserved for the heart; includes valve replacement and valvulotomy (*q.v.*).

valvotomy (val-vot'o-mi): See VALVULOTOMY.

valvular (val'vū-lar): Relating to or resembling a valve. V. DISEASE OF THE HEART a condition resulting from deformity or constriction of one or more of the heart valves, making it impossible for them to reclose completely and allowing blood to regurgitate; may be congenital but more often a sequel of endocarditis resulting from rheumatic fever; V. PNEUMOTHORAX tension pneumothorax, a condition in which an open chest wound acts as a valve allowing inspired air to enter the pleural cavity but preventing its escape during exhalation.

valvulitis (val-vū-lī'tis): Inflammation of a valve, particularly one in the heart.

valvulotomy (val-vū-lot'o-mi): Surgical incision of a valve, by custom referring to a valve of the heart; specifically the operation of correcting a deformed or narrowed heart valve.

van den Bergh's test: A laboratory test for the presence of bilirubin in the blood serum.

vanillylmandelic acid (van'i-lil-man-del'ik): A metabolite of adrenaline and noradrenaline; its measurement in the urine is used as a test for phaeochromocytoma.

vaporizer (vā'por-ī-zer): An apparatus for converting a liquid, particularly a medicated liquid, into a vapour that can be inhaled; frequently used in treatment of bronchial conditions.

vapour (vā-por): The gaseous state of a liquid or solid, *e.g.*, steam, mist, gas, or an exhalation.

vapours (vā-pors): An obsolete term applied to hysterical nervousness, thought to be caused by bodily exhalations.

Vaquez's disease (va-kāz): Polycythaemia vera, an idiopathic condition in which the red cell count is very high. The white cell count platelets, volume and viscosity of the blood are also increased; and there is hyperaemia of all organs and enlargements of the spleen. [Louis Henri Vaquez, French physician 1860–1936.]

variable (va're-a-b'l): In research, any factor, characteristic, quality, or attribute under study. DEPENDENT V. the v. under investigation which the researcher wishes to observe so as to note the effect of an independent v. on it; INDEPENDENT V. the V. that the researcher manipulates or introduces into the situation.

variant Creutzfeldt−Jakob disease: A form of encephalopathy (*q.v.*), similar to, but presenting in younger patients than, Creutzfeldt−Jakob disease (*q.v.*) (average age of presentation 29 years, as opposed to 65 years). It has a relatively longer duration of illness, and is strongly linked to exposure to bovine spongiform encephalopathy (BSE) (*q.v.*).

varic-, varico-: Combining forms denoting varix (a twisted, tortuous vein, sometimes dilated).

varicella (var'i-sel'la): Chickenpox (*q.v.*). — varicelliform, adj.

varices (var'i-sēz): Pl. of varix (*q.v.*).

varicoblepharon (var'i-kō-blef'a-ron): A varicose swelling or tumour of the eyelid.

varicocele (var'i-kō-sēl): Varicosity of the veins of the spermatic cord.

varicography (var'i-kog'ra-fi): Roentgenology of a varicose vein.

varicophlebitis (var'i-kō-flē-bī'tis): Inflammation of a varicose vein.

varicose (var'i-kōs): 1. Unnaturally swollen or distended. 2. Related to or exhibiting varices (see VARIX). V. VEINS dilated veins that have lost their elasticity and in which the valves have become incompetent so that blood flow may be reversed or become static; may be due to trauma, thrombosis, inflammation, or heredity; usually seen in the lower legs, rectum (haemorrhoids) or lower oesophagus (oesophageal varices).

varicosity (var-i-kos′i-ti): 1. The state or condition of being varicose. 2. A varix (*q.v.*).

varicotomy (var-i-kot′o-mi): Excision of a varicose vein.

variola (va-rī′ō-la): Smallpox (*q.v.*). — variolar, variolic, variolous, adj.

varioloid (var′i-ō-loyd): Resembling smallpox.

varix (var′iks): A dilated, tortuous (or varicose) vein; less often an artery or lymphatic vessel. — varices, pl.

varus (vā′rus): Bent inward; denoting a displacement or angulation toward the midline of the body; term is used in connection with the noun it modifies, e.g., talipes varus (*q.v.*). Opp. of valgus.

vas: A vessel or canal for carrying a fluid. — vasa, pl. V. DEFERENS the excretory duct of the testes; it unites with the excretory duct of the seminal vesicle to form the ejaculatory duct. Also called *ductus deferens.*

vas-, vasi-, vaso-: Combining forms denoting a channel or vessel, especially a blood vessel.

vasa (vas′a, vā′za): V. PRAEVIA, (1) blood vessels that lie below the presenting part in labour; if they rupture there is danger of blood loss; (2) prolapsed umbilical cord; the cord precedes the infant in delivery; V. VASORUM the minute nutrient vessels in the outer and inner coats of the larger veins and arteries.

vascular (vas′kū-lar): Related to, supplied with, or containing vessels, referring especially to blood vessels. V. BED the total blood supply to an organ or body part, including arteries, veins, and capillaries; V. HEADACHE headache caused by painful dilatation of branches of the external carotid artery; see MIGRAINE; V. INSUFFICIENCY lack of adequate peripheral blood flow; may be due to damaged, blocked, or diseased vessels, causing cyanosis and swelling of an extremity, and intermittent claudication; V. SYSTEM the cardiovascular and lymphatic systems considered together.

vascularity (vas-kū-lar′i-ti): The condition of being supplied with blood vessels.

vascularization (vas′kū-lar-ī-zā′shun): The acquisition of a blood supply through the formation of new blood vessels in a part. The process of becoming vascular.

vasculature (vas′kū-la-chūr): The arrangement of the blood vessels in a structure or a part of the body.

vasculitis (vas′kū-lī′tis): Inflammation of a blood or lymph vessel. — vasculitides, pl.

vasectomy (vas-ek′to-mi): Resection of the vas deferens with ligation.

vasitis (vas-ī′tis): Inflammation of the vas deferens.

vasoactive (vas-ō-ak′tiv, vā′zō-): 1. Having an influence on the tone and calibre of the blood vessels. 2. A condition of blood vessels when they respond to various stimuli by changing their calibre.

vasoconstriction (vas-ō-kon-strik′shun, vā′zō): Narrowing of the lumen of the blood vessels, particularly the smaller ones, resulting in reduced blood flow to a part.

vasoconstrictor (vas-ō-kon-strik′tor, vā′zō-): Any agent that causes a narrowing of the lumen of blood vessels.

vasodepressor (vas-ō-dē-pres′or, va′zō-): Any agent that depresses circulation by lowering the blood pressure.

vasodilation (vas-ō-dī-la′shun, vā′zō-): Dilation of the blood vessels.

vasodilator (vas-ō-dī′lā-tor, vā′zō-): Any agent that causes a widening of the lumen of blood vessels.

vasoepididymostomy (vas′ō-ep-i-did-i-mos′to-mi, vā′zō-): An anastomosis between the vas deferens and the epididymus.

vasogenic (vas-ō-jen′ik, vā′zō-): Vascular in origin. V. SHOCK see under SHOCK.

vasography (vas-og′ra-fi, vā-sog′): Radiography of blood vessels.

vasoinhibitor (vas-ō-inhib′i-tor, vā′zō-): Any agent that interferes with or depresses the action of vasomotor nerves, thus causing dilation of the blood vessels. — vasoinhibitory, adj.

vasoligation (vas-ō-lī-gā′shun, vā-zō-): Ligation of a vessel, the vas deferens in particular.

vasomotor (vas-ō-mō′tor, v′a-zō-): Relating to or affecting the nerves and muscles that control the contraction and expansion of blood vessels.

vasopressin (vas-ō-pres′in, vā′zō-): The antidiuretic hormone formed in the hypothalamus and stored in the posterior lobe of the pituitary; also prepared synthetically. v. stimulates the muscular coat of the smaller blood vessels, thus raising the blood pressure, stimulates contraction of intestinal muscles, thus increasing peristalsis, has some effect on the muscles of the uterus, and has an antidiuretic effect. May be used in treatment of diabetes insipidus.

vasopressor (vas-ō-pres′sor, vā′zō-): Stimulating contraction of the musculature of the blood vessels, especially the smaller vessels, or an agent that has this effect.

vasoresection (vas-ō-rē-sek'shun, vā'zō-): Surgical division of the vas deferens.

vasospasm (vas'ō-spazm, vā'zō-): Constricting spasm of vessel walls, the smaller blood vessels in particular. Syn., *vasoconstriction*. — vasospastic, adj.

vasostomy (va-sos'to-mi, vā-zos'): The operation of making an opening into the vas deferens. Also called *vasotomy*.

vasotonia (vas-ō-tō'ni-a, vā'zō-): The tone of blood vessels, the smaller ones in particular. — vasotonic, adj.

vasotripsy (vas'ō-trip-si, vā'zo-): The arrest of haemorrhage by crushing an artery with a strong forceps. Angiotripsy.

vasovagal (vas-ō-vā'gal, vā-zō-): Referring to the vagus nerve and its action on the blood vessels. V. SYNDROME an autonomic nervous system response which may be caused by extreme fear; marked by faintness, pallor, sweating, anxiety, epigastric distress, feeling of impending death, respiratory difficulty, syncope. When part of the post-gastrectomy syndrome, it occurs a few minutes after a meal.

vasovasostomy (vas'-ō-va-sos'to-mi, vā'zō-): The surgical anastomosis of two cut ends of the vas deferens; usually done to restore fertility after a previous vasectomy.

vasovesiculectomy (vas'ō-ve-sik-ū-lek'to-mi, vā'zō-): Surgical removal of the vas deferens and the seminal vesicles.

vasovesiculitis (vas'ō-ve-sik-ū-lī'tis, vā'zō-): Inflammation of the vas deferens and the seminal vesicles.

vastus (vas'tus): Large or great. V. MUSCLES the large muscles of the thigh, named for their location: v. externus, v. intermedius, v. internus, v. lateralis, and v. medialis.

Vater: Ampulla of v., see under AMPULLA.

vault (vawlt): An anatomical part resembling an arched roof. PALATINE V. the roof of the mouth; VAGINAL V. the upper end of the vaginal canal into which the cervix inserts.

VC: Abbreviation for vital capacity, see under VITAL.

vCJD: Abbreviation for variant Creutzfeldt–Jakob disease (*q.v.*).

VDU: Abbreviation for visual display unit.

vection (vek'shun): The carrying of the organisms of a disease from an infected to an uninfected person; the transmission may be direct or through an intermediate host.

vector (vek'tor): **1.** A living carrier of disease that transmits the organisms causing a disease from one host to another, often an arthropod, *e.g.*, mosquito, fly, flea, louse. **2.** A quantity that expresses direction, magnitude, and polarity; may be represented by a straight line, and used to express velocity, force, or momentum.

vectorcardiogram (vek'tor-kar-di-ō-gram): A graphic record of the magnitude and direction of the heart's electric currents.

vectorcardiography (vek'tor-kar-di-og'ra-fi): Three-dimensional electrocardiography utilized for determining the direction and magnitude of the electrical forces of the heart.

vegan (vēg'an): An individual whose diet excludes all animal products.

vegetarian (vej-i-tā'ri-an): A person whose diet consists of foods of vegetable or plant origin, *i.e.*, vegetables, fruits, nuts, grains, and sometimes animal products such as milk or cheese.

vegetation (vej-e-tā'shun): A growth or accretion of any kind, especially a clot made up of fibrin and platelets occurring on the edge of the cardiac valves in endocarditis.

vegetative (vej'e-ta-tiv): **1.** Relating to growth or nutrition. **2.** Relating to the non-sporing stage of a bacterium. **3.** Functioning involuntarily or unconsciously. **4.** In psychiatry, describing a state of inactivity or sluggishness.

vehicle (vē'i-k'l): An inert or inactive substance, *e.g.*, water or syrup, used as a carrier for a drug that has a therapeutic action.

veil (vāl): **1.** In anatomy, any veil-like structure. **2.** A caul (*q.v.*).

vein (vān): A vessel carrying deoxygenated blood back to the heart (with the exception of the pulmonary veins). It has the same three coats as an artery, *i.e.*, inner, middle, and outer, but they are not as thick and they collapse when cut. Many veins have valves that prevent backflow of blood. All except the pulmonary veins carry dark, venous, deoxygenated blood.

velamentous (vel'a-men'tus): **1.** Being covered with a veil-like membrane. **2.** Veil-like or membranous. V. PLACENTA a P. with the umbilical cord arising from the outer border.

Velcro: A trade name for a textile used for closing a garment, appliance, or dressing; consists of two layers of material that adhere to each other.

vellication (vel-i-kā'shun): Spasmodic involuntary twitching of muscle fibrils.

vellus (vel'us): The fine downy hair that appears on all parts of the body except palms of the hands and soles of the feet. See also LANUGO.

velocity (ve-los'i-ti): Rapidity of motion; the rate of motion in a particular direction in relation to time.

velum (vē'lum): In anatomy, (1) any structure that resembles a veil or curtain; (2) the muscular portion of the roof of the mouth; it is elevated when one is speaking or swallowing, thus closing off the nasal passages.

ven-, veni-, veno-: Combining forms denoting (1) veins; (2) the vena cava.

vena (vē-na): Vein [L.] V. CAVA one of the two large veins which empty their contents into the right atrium of the heart; INFERIOR V.C. the vein which receives blood from the trunk of the body and lower extremities; it is formed by the union of the two common iliac veins; SUPERIOR V.C. the large vein which collects blood from the head, chest, and upper extremities; it is formed by the junction of the two innominate veins. — venae and venae cavae, pl.

venacavography (vē'na-kā-vog'ra-fi): Radiography of the vena cava; usually refers to the inferior vena cava.

venectasia (ven-ek-tā'si-a): Dilatation of a vein or veins.

venectomy (ven-ek'to-mi): The excision of part of a vein, a procedure sometimes used in treatment of varicose veins. Phlebectomy.

venenation (ven-e-nā'shun): Poisoning, or the condition of being poisoned.

veneniferous (ven-e-nif'er-us): Carrying or conveying poison.

venenific (ven-i-nif'ik): Poison producing.

venenous (ven'e-nus): Poisonous.

venepuncture (vē'ne-punk-tūr): The puncture of a vein, through the skin, usually with the needle of a syringe or a cannula to introduce a catheter for any purpose, most often to administer a medication or other fluid or to withdraw a blood sample. Also called *venipuncture*.

venereal (ve-nēr'-i-al): Relating to or transmitted by sexual contact. V. DISEASE contagious disease most often acquired by sexual contact, intercourse in particular; includes gonorrhoea, syphilis, chancroid, lymphogranuloma venereum, granuloma inguinale, balanitis gangrenosa, herpes simplex, Type 2; V. SORE see CHANCRE; V. WART see CONDYLOMA LATUM and WART.

venereologist (ve-nēr'i-ol'o-jist): A specialist in the study and treatment of venereal diseases.

venereology (ve-nēr-i-ol'o-ji): The study of venereal diseases.

venereophobia (ve-nēr-i-ō-fō'bi-a): Morbid fear of contracting a venereal disease.

venesection (vēn-e-sek'shun): Phlebotomy; opening the cubital vein with a scalpel for the purpose of letting blood; formerly a common clinical procedure. Also spelled *venisection*.

venin (ven'in): Any one of the various toxic substances in snake venom (*q.v.*).

venin–antivenin (ven-in-an'ti-ven-in): A mixture of venin and antivenin used as a vaccine in the treatment of bites by venomous snakes.

venoclysis (vē-nok'li-sis): The slow, continuous introduction of nutrient or medicinal fluids into a vein.

venogram (vē'nō-gram): A radiogram of veins after injection of a radiopaque substance.

venography (vē-nog'ra-fi): X-ray visualization of a vein or veins after injection with an opaque medium. — venographic, adj.; venographically, adv.

venom (ven'um): A poison, particularly the substance secreted by certain snakes, insects, and other arthropods, or animals, and that is transmitted to humans by a bite or sting.

venomous (ven'o-mus): Poisonous. Secreting or containing venom.

venoperitoneostomy (vē'nō-per-i-to-nē-os'to-mi): The surgical procedure of inserting a cut end of the saphenous vein into the peritoneum to drain ascitic fluid from the cavity into the vein.

venosclerosis (vē'nō-scler-ō'sis): Fibrous hardening of venous walls. Phlebosclerosis.

venostasis (vē-nō-stā'sis): 1. Slowing of the blood flow in the venous system. 2. A procedure for temporarily checking the return flow of blood by applying compression to the veins of the four extremities. See ROTATING TOURNIQUET under TOURNIQUET.

venotomy (vē-not'o-mi): Surgical incision into a vein. Phlebotomy.

venous (vē'nus): Relating to the veins or the circulation within them. V. HUM a continuous humming sound normally heard on auscultation in children and some healthy adults with high cardiac output; V. LAKES single or multiple bluish-black vascular lesions seen on exposed areas of the ears, face, and neck; V. PRESSURE the pressure of blood in the veins, often measured in the superior vena cava or right atrium and reported as central venous pressure; See CENTRAL VENOUS PRESSURE under PRESSURE; V. RETURN the blood that is returning to the heart through the great veins; V. STAR a small reddish-blue starlike spot often seen on the legs of elderly persons; V. STASIS the impairment or stoppage of blood flow in a vein or veins; V. THROMBOSIS the formation of a thrombus in a vein.

venovenostomy (vē-nō-vē-nos'to-mi): The surgical creation of an anastomosis between two veins.

venter (ven'ter): 1. Any belly-shaped part; a fleshy contractible part of a muscle. 2. The abdomen or stomach. 3. A hollowed part or cavity.

ventilate (ven'ti-lāt): 1. To remove stale air and supply fresh air to take its place; may be done artificially by mechanically propelling and extracting the air or naturally by opening windows, doors, etc. 2. To oxygenate the blood and remove the carbon dioxide from it; a function carried out by the capillaries and the alveoli in the lungs. 3. In psychiatry, to discuss problems and grievances. — ventilation, n; ventilatory, adj.

ventilation (ven'ti-lā'shun): 1. The process of bringing fresh air into the environment, *i.e.*, air with a higher oxygen content and lower carbon dioxide content than the air being replaced. 2. In physiology, the movement of air or a gas mixutre in or out of the lungs. 3. In psychiatry, the opportunity to express one's emotional problems verbally. ALVEOLAR V. see under ALVEOLAR. — ventilatory, adj.

ventilator (ven'til-ā-tor): Any of several available devices used in respiratory therapy to augment the respiratory exchange of gases in the lungs; a respirator (*q.v.*). Three main types are (1) VOLUME-CYCLED V. a v. that ends inspiration when a pre-set volume has been reached; (2) PRESSURED-CYCLED V. a v. that ends inspiration when a pre-set pressure has been reached, and (3) TIME-CYCLED V. a v. that ends respiration when a pre-set time interval has been reached. NON-INVASIVE PRESSURE SUPPORT V. can improve Oxygenation and CO_2 excretion without the complications associated with intubation, ventilation, and sedation.

ventilometer (ven-ti-lom'i-ter): A device for measuring the volume of air breathed in and out at various times during the respiratory cycle, and the capacity of the lungs under different environmental conditions.

ventr-, ventri-, ventro-: Combining forms denoting (1) the belly; (2) the anterior aspect of the body.

ventrad (ven'trad): Toward the ventral aspect of the body.

ventral (ven'tral): Relating to the abdomen or the anterior surface of the body. Opp., dorsal. — ventrally, adj.

ventricle (ven'trik-l): A small belly-like cavity. V.'S OF THE BRAIN four cavities filled with cerebrospinal fluid within the brain. V.'S OF THE HEART the two lower muscular chambers of the heart. — ventricular, adj.

ventricular (ven-trik'ū-lar): Relating to a ventricle. V. ANEURYSM see CARDIAC ANEURYSM under ANEURYSM; V. FIBRILLATION rapid, irregular, uncoordinated twitchings of muscle fibres that replace normal contractions of the muscular walls of the ventricles; V. GALLOP a sound heard over the right ventricle early in diastole; caused by early rapid filling of the ventricle with limited extensibility; the sound is likened to the word Ken-tuk'key; V. SEPTAL DEFECT a defect of the septum between the two ventricles, usually congenital; V. TACHYCARDIA see under TACHYCARDIA.

ventriculitis (ven-trik'ū-lī'tis): Inflammation of a ventricle, particularly one in the brain.

ventriculo-: Combining form denoting ventricle.

ventriculoatrial shunt (ven-trik'ū-lō-ā'tri-al): The surgical establishment of communication between a cerebral ventricle and the right atrium of the heart, to drain cerebrospinal fluid from the brain in cases of hydrocephalus. See SHUNT.

ventriculocisternostomy (ven-trik'ū-lō-sis-ter-nos'to-mi): The surgical establishment of communication between the lateral ventricle of the brain and the subarachnoid cisterns, usually the cisterna magna; used in the treatment of hydrocephalus. See SHUNT.

ventriculogram (ven-trik'ū-lō-gram): A radiograph of the brain after the injection of a gas or an opaque medium into the cerebral ventricles.

ventriculography (ven-trik-ū-log;'ra-fi): Radiography of the ventricles of the brain after injection of gas or an opaque medium into the ventricles to displace the cerebrospinal fluid normally present.

ventriculoperitoneal (ven-trik'ū-lō-per-i-tō-nē'al): Relating to a ventricle of the brain and the peritoneal cavity. V. SHUNT a shunt between the lateral ventricle of the brain and the peritoneal cavity; used in treatment of hydrocephalus. See SHUNT.

ventriculoscope (ven-trik'ū-lo-skōp): An instrument for viewing the inside of the ventricles of the brain.

ventriculostomy (ven-trik'ū-los'to-mi): An artificial opening into a ventricle. Usually refers to a drainage operation for hydrocephalus.

ventriculotomy (ven-trik-ū-lot'o-mi): Surgical incision into a ventricle, *e.g.*, into a ventricle of the heart for repair of a cardiac defect or into the third ventricle of the brain for the relief of hydrocephalus.

ventriculoureteral (ven-trik'ū-lō-ū-rē'ter-al): Relating to a ventricle of the brain and the ureter, particularly to a shunt between these two structures, used in treatment of hydrocephalus. See SHUNT. Also called *ventriculoureterostomy*.

ventrofixation (ven'trō-fik-sā'shun): Surgical fixation of a displaced organ to the abdominal wall.

ventrohysteropexy (ven'trō-his'ter-ō-peks-i): Surgical fixation of a displaced uterus to the abdominal wall.

ventrolateral (ven-trō-lat'er-al): Situated or occurring both ventrally and somewhat laterally.

ventrosuspension (ven'trō-sus-pen'shun): A surgical procedure in which the round ligaments are shortened to hold a retroplaced uterus forward. Also called *ventrofixation*.

Venturi effect: A principle stating that as the velocity of a fluid going through a constricted section of a tube increases, the pressure decreases; applies when measuring the flow of a fluid.

Venturi mask: A mask designed to mix room air with oxygen so that varying percentages of oxygen can be administered.

venule (ven'ūl): A minute vein; the smallest division or branch of a vein, continuous at one end with the vein and at the other end with a capillary. — venulae, pl.; venular, adj.

verbigeration (ver-bij-er-ā'shun): The constant uncontrollable repetition of meaningless words, phrases or sentences as seen in states of mental disorientation.

verbomania (ver-bō-mā'ni-a): A mania for words or talking.

vergence (ver'jens): A turning; usually said of one eye which turns vertically or horizontally as compared with the other eye.

vermicide (ver'mi-sī'd): An agent that kills intestinal worms. — vermicidal, adj.

vermiform (ver'mi-form): Worm-like in form. V. APPENDIX the vestigial, hollow, worm-like structure that is attached to the caecum, commonly called the *appendix*.

vermifuge (ver'mi-fūj): An agent that causes intestinal worms or parasites to be expelled. An anthelmintic.

vermin (ver'min): External parasites; usually refers to parasitic insects or worms. Broadly speaking, noxious small animals or insects that are hard to control, *e.g.*, rats, fleas, flies and depredating rodents.

vermis (ver'mis): 1. A worm. 2. The narrow middle part of the cerebellum; it lies between and connects the two hemispheres of the cerebellum.

vernix (ver'niks): A covering. V. CASEOSA the fatty substance covering the skin of the fetus.

It appears at about 30–32 weeks, is abundant at 36–37 weeks, and may remain until, or even past full term. It protects the fetal skin from the effects of the amniotic fluid.

verruca (ve-roo'ka): Wart. V. ACUMINATA a nonvenereal wart that appears on the external genitalia; V. NECROGENICA develops as a result

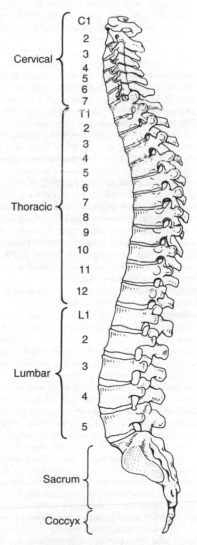

The vertebral column from the side.

of accidental inoculation with tuberculosis; V. PLANA JUVENILIS the common, multiple, flat, tiny warts often seen on childrens' hands and knees; V. PLANTARIS a flat wart on the sole of the foot; plantar wart; V. SEBORRHOEICA the brown, greasy wart commonly seen on the chest or back of seborrhoeic subjects; V. SENILIS superficial warty lesions that appear on the hands or face of older people, due to exposure to sunlight; may become malignant; V. VULGARIS the common wart of the hands, of brown colour and rough pitted surface. — verrucous, adj.; verrucae, pl.

version (ver'zhun): A change of direction; a tilting, or turning. In gynaecology, refers to a displacement or tilting of the uterus; varieties include anteversion, lateroversion, and retroversion. In ophthalmology, refers to the simultaneous rotation of both eyes in the same direction; may be upward, downward, or to the right or the left. In obstetrics, applies to the manoeuvre of altering the position of the fetus *in utero* from an abnormal to a normal or more favourable position; may occur spontaneously or by manual manipulation. Varieties of V. in obstetrics include: CEPHALIC V. turning the fetus so that the head presents; EXTERNAL V. turning the fetus by manipulation through the abdominal wall; INTERNAL V. turning the fetus with one of the obstetrician's hands in the uterus and the other on the mother's abdomen; PODALIC V. turning the fetus to a breech presentation.

vertebr-, vertebro-: Combining forms denoting (1) a vertebra, or (2) the vertebral column.

vertebra (ver'te-bra): One of the 33 small bones forming the vertebral (spinal) column. There are seven cervical, twelve thoracic, five lumbar, five sacral, and four coccygeal vertebrae. The sacral and coccygeal groups are fused in the adult. — vertebrae, pl.; vertebral; adj.

vertebral (ver'te-bral): Relating to the vertebrae. V. ARTERY either of two arteries, right and left, that arise in the subclavian artery and which supply the deep muscles of the neck, the spinal cord and its membranes, and the cerebellum; V. BODY the short column of bone in the vertebrae that forms the weight-bearing part of the spine; V. CANAL that formed by the foramina of the vertebrae; contains the spinal cord and its meninges; V. COLUMN the vertebrae from the cranium to the tip of the coccyx; the spine; V. CURVES seen when viewed from the side, the V. column curves slightly inward in the area of the cervical vertebrae, outward in the area of the thoracic vertebrae, and inward

at the area of the lumbar vertebrae; exaggeration of the thoracic (posterior) curve causes kyphosis (hunchback); of the lumbar curve (anterior) causes lordosis (swayback); normally there are no lateral curvatures, but when this does exist it is called scoliosis.

vertebrate (ver'te-brāt): Having a vertebral column or referring to an animal that has a vertebral column.

vertebrobasilar (ver'te-brō-bas'i-lar): Relating to the vertebral and basilar arteries. V. INSUFFICIENCY a syndrome caused by lack of sufficient blood to the hindbrain; may be progressive and episodic; symptoms include vertigo, nausea, ataxia, blindness, diplopia, hemiplegia due to transient cerebral ischaemia, drop attacks and signs of cerebellar dysfunction.

vertebrocostal (ver'te-brō-kos'tal): Relating to a vertebra and a rib.

vertex: A summit or top. In anatomy, refers usually to the top of the head. In obstetrics, an area of the fetal head bounded by the anterior and posterior fontanelles, and laterally by the parietal eminence.

vertiginous (ver-tij'i-nus): Relating to or affected with vertigo.

vertigo (ver'ti-gō): A sensation of whirling, either of oneself in space or of the world around one; may be a symptom of disease of the inner ear, eyes, stomach, heart, or brain, or of toxaemia. Also often a precursor to an epileptic seizure. Not the same as dizziness or faintness. BENIGN POSITIONAL V. occurs chiefly in the elderly, usually when walking, turning suddenly, or changing position of the head; may be due to peripheral neuropathy, cervical spine disease, or vestibular dysfunction; often associated with hearing loss and diminished vision.

vesic-, vesico-: Combining forms denoting: 1. A bladder. 2. A blister.

vesica (ves'i-ka): 1. A hollow organ or sac. 2. A bladder; a hollow organ with a musculomembranous structure that serves as a reservoir for a fluid, *e.g.*, the gallbladder or the urinary bladder.

vesical (ves'i-kal): Relating to a bladder, the urinary bladder in particular.

vesicant (ves'i-kant): 1. Causing blisters. 2. An agent that produces blisters.

vesication (ves-i-kā'shun): A blister or blisters, or the production of a blister or blisters.

vesicle (ves'ik-l): 1. A small bladder, cell, or hollow structure. 2. A small circumscribed superficial elevation on the skin containing clear or non-purulent serous fluid. SEMINAL V. one of two small sacs that stores the seminal fluid until it is ejaculated. — vesicular, adj.

vesicocele (ves'i-kō-sēl): Hernia of the bladder.

vesicocervical (ves-i-kō-ser-vī'kal): Relating to the urinary bladder and the cervix. V. FISTULA one between the bladder and the uterine cervix.

vesicocolonic (ves'i-kō-ko-lon'ik): Relating to the urinary bladder and the colon. V. FISTULA, one between the urinary bladder and the colon.

vesicoenteric (ves'i-kō-en-ter'ik): Vesicointestinal (q.v.).

vesicofixation (ves'i-kō-fiks-ā'shun): Surgical fixation of (1) the urinary bladder to the abdominal wall; (2) the uterus to the urinary bladder.

vesicointestinal (ves'i-kō-in-tes'tin-al): Relating to the urinary bladder and the intestine. V. FISTULA one between the urinary bladder and the intestine.

vesicopapular (ves'i-kō-pap' u lar): Relating to an eruption that consists of both vesicles and papules.

vesicoprostatic (ves'i-kō-pros-tat'ik): Relating to both the urinary bladder and the prostate gland.

vesicopustular (ves'i-kō-pus'tū-lar): Pertaining to an eruption that consists of both vesicles and pustules.

vesicorectal (ves-i-kō-rek'tal): Relating to the urinary bladder and the rectum. V. FISTULA one between the urinary bladder and the rectum.

vesicostomy (ves-i-kos'to-mi): Cystostomy (q.v.). CUTANEOUS V. a surgical procedure to divert drainage from the urinary bladder onto the anterior abdominal wall to which a collection bag is attached.

vesicotomy (ves-i-kot'o-mi): An incision into the urinary bladder.

vesicoureteral (ves'i-kō-ū-rē'ter-al): Relating to the urinary bladder and the ureters. V. REFLUX the backflow of urine from the bladder into the ureter.

vesicourethral (ves'i-kō-ū-rē'thral): Relating to the urinary bladder and the urethra.

vesicouterine (ves'i-kō-ū'ter-in): Pertinent to the urinary bladder and the uterus. V. POUCH the fold of the peritoneum that extends downward between the urinary bladder and the uterus.

vesicovaginal (ves-i-kō-vaj-īn'al): Relating to the urinary bladder and the vagina.

vesicular (ve-sik'ū-lar): Relating to or composed of vesicles. V. BREATH SOUNDS see BREATH SOUNDS.

vesiculation (ve-sik' -ū-lā'shun): 1. The presence of vesicles. 2. The formation of vesicles.

vesiculectomy (ve-sik'ū-lek'to-mi): Resection of all or part of both seminal vesicles; produces sterility.

vesiculitis (ve-sik'ū-lī'tis): Inflammation of a vesicle, particularly a seminal vesicle.

vesiculography (ve-sik'ū-log'ra-fi): X-ray of the seminal vesicles.

vesiculopapular (ve-sik'ū-lō-pap'ū-lar): Relating to or exhibiting both vesicles and papules.

vesiculoprostatitis (ve-sik'ū-lō-pros-ta-tī'tis): Inflammation of the urinary bladder and the prostate gland.

vesiculopustular (ve-sik'ū-lō-pus'tū-lar): Relating to or exhibiting both vesicles and pustules.

vessel (ves'el): A tube, duct or canal, holding or conveying fluid, especially blood and lymph.

vestibular (ves-tib'u-lar): 1. Relating to a vestibule. 2. Relating in particular to the vestibular part of the eighth cranial nerve that is concerned with equilibrium. V. GLANDS four small glands located in the vestibule of the vagina; two, called major or Bartholin's glands, are located on either side of the vaginal orifice; two, called minor V. glands are located in the mucous membrane around the urethral opening; V. NEURONITIS a disorder of the V. nerve that causes extreme vertigo but the hearing is not affected; V. SENSE the sense of balance, needed for maintaining posture, walking, and running; V. SYSTEM the structures in the vestibule of the inner ear that have to do with the maintenance of equilibrium.

vestibule (ves'ti-būl): 1. The middle part of the internal ear, lying between the semicircular canals and the cochlea. 2. The triangular area between the clitoris and the inner surfaces of the labia minora; it forms the entrance to the vagina. V. OF THE MOUTH the part between the teeth and alveolar ridges and the lips.

vestibulo-: Combining form denoting vestibule.

vestibulocochlear (ves-tib'ū-lō-kok'lē-ar): Relating to the vestibule and the cochlea of the inner ear. V. NERVE the acoustic nerve see under ACOUSTIC.

vestibulotomy (ves-tib'ū-lot'o-mi): Operation of making an opening into the vestibule of the inner ear.

vestibulourethral (ves-tib'ū-lō-ū-rē'thral): Relating to the vestibule of the vagina and the urethra.

vestigial (ves-tij'i-al): Rudimentary; indicating a remnant of something formerly present.

VF: Abbreviation for ventricular fibrillation, see under VENTRICULAR.

viability (vī-a-bil'i-ti): The state or quality of being viable.

viable (vī'a-b'l): Capable of independent life. A term applied to the fetus usually after 24 weeks of intrauterine life.

vial (vī'al): A small bottle for medicines or drugs; also spelled *phial*.

vibex (vī'beks): A linear mark or streak; a linear haemorrhage under the skin. — vibices, pl.

vibration (vī-brā'shun): 1. A rapid to-and-fro motion. 2. A manoeuvre in massage. 3. A therapeutic procedure in which the body is shaken rapidly.

vibrator (vī'brā-tor): A hand-held electric device that is set into vibration by an electric current; held over the thorax to assist in postural drainage or over a paralysed muscle to stimulate contraction.

Vibrio (vib-ri-ō): A genus of curved, motile microorganisms. *v. cholerae*, causes cholera. *v. parahaemolyticus*, an organism found worldwide that causes food poisoning from eating contaminated seafood, raw vegetables, or meat; characteristic symptoms are stomach pain, vomiting, diarrhoea, fever, chills.

vibrissae (vī-bris'ē): The hairs growing in the vestibule of the nose. — vibrissa, sing.

vicarious (vī-kair'i-us): 1. Acting as a substitute for something. 2. Occurring in an unexpected or abnormal situation. v. MENSTRUATION bleeding from the nose or other part of the body when menstruation is abnormally suppressed.

villous (vil'us): Relating to, resembling, or furnished with villi. v. ADENOMA a slow-growing neoplasm of the intestinal mucosa, usually occurring in the colon; potentially malignant; v. CARCINOMA carcinoma of the intestinal mucosa involving the villi.

villus (vil'us): A microscopic finger-like projection, such as is found in the mucous membrane of the small intestine, or on the outside of the chorion of the embryonic sac. — villi, pl.; villous, adj.

Vincent's angina: See ANGINA.

Vincke's tongs: See TONGS.

vinculum (ving'kū-lum): A band-like structure, ligament; or frenum (*q.v.*).

violaceous (vī'ō-lā'she-us): Refers to a violet discoloration, usually of the skin.

violence (vī'ō-lens): Unwarranted, extremely rough physical force or action exerted with the intent to injure or destroy oneself or another person. Rape is considered a form of violence.

viraemia (vī-rē'mi-a): The presence of virus in the bloodstream. — viraemic, adj.

viral (vī'ral): Relating to, caused by, or resembling a virus (*q.v.*). v. HEPATITIS see under HEPATITIS; v. INFECTION see under INFECTION; v. PNEUMONIA see under PNEUMONIA.

The thirteen generally acknowledged vitamins, their common synonyms and some biological functions.

Vitamins	Common synonyms	Some biological functions, mainly through co-enzymic action
A	Retinol	Vision, epithelial regeneration
B_1	Aneurine	Amino acid metabolism
	Thiamin	
B_2	Riboflavin	Fat metabolism; oxidation
B_5	Pantothenic acid	Carbohydrate and fat metabolism
B_6	Pyridoxine	Amino acid and protein metabolism
B_{12}	Cyanocobalamin	Replication of genes, red blood cell formation
C	Ascorbic acid	Collagen synthesis
D	Calciferol	Calcium metabolism and bone formation
	Cholecalciferol	
E	Alpha tocopherol	Neurological function, cell integrity; antioxidant
Folic acid	Folacin	Purine and pyrimidine synthesis for DNA
H	Biotin	Carbohydrate, amino acid metabolism
K	Menaphthone	Blood clotting mechanism
Niacin	Nicotinic acid	Oxidation and energy transfer

virgin (ver′jin): 1. A female who has never experienced sexual intercourse. 2. A person of either sex who has never experienced sexual intercourse. — virginity, n., virginal, adj.

viricidal (vi-ri-sī′dal): Virucidal (*q.v.*).

virile (vir′īl): 1. Energetic; vigorous; possessed of characteristics usually considered as belonging to men. 2. Specifically capable of functioning as a male in copulation.

virilism (vir′i-lizm): 1. Masculinity. 2. The appearance of secondary male characteristics in a woman.

virility (vi-ril′i-ti): The state of being a male and having the nature and characteristics of an adult male.

virilization (vir-il-ī-zā′shun): The acquisition of masculine characteristics by a female, *e.g.*, lowering of the voice pitch, loss of hair in the temporal area, amenorrhoea, hypertrophy of the clitoris. See ADRENOGENITAL SYNDROME. — virilizing, adj.

virion (vī′ri-on): A virus (*q.v.*) particle.

virologist (vī-rol′o-jist): One who studies viruses and viral diseases.

virology (vī-rol′o-ji): The study of viruses and the diseases caused by them. — virological, adj.

virucidal (vī-rū-sī′dal): Destructive or lethal to a virus. 2. Capable of destroying a virus.

virulence (vir′ū-lens): Infectiousness; the disease-producing power of a microorganism; the relative degree of the power of a microorganism to overcome host resistance and produce disease. — virulent, adj.

virulent (vir′ū-lent): 1. Extremely harmful or poisonous. 2. Having the power to overcome the hosts defences and produce disease.

virus (vī′rus): Any of a large group of disease-producing agents so small that they can be seen only under the electron microscope; are capable of passing through a filter that would hold back ordinary bacteria; can live and propagate only in the presence of living cells; and which produce a variety of pathological conditions. The virus particle, or virion, consists of a core of either deoxyribonucleic acid (*q.v.*) or ribonucleic acid (*q.v.*) that is enclosed in a protein sheath called a capsid; it varies greatly in size and shape. Viruses may gain entrance to the body through droplet infection from the respiratory tract; ingestion by the gastrointestinal system; blood transfusion; or a break in the skin, including bites by insect or animal carriers. Viruses have been classified according to several characteristics; the list according to anatomical area affected includes: (1) dermatropic (chickenpox, measles); (2) pneumotropic (common cold, influenza, atypical pneumonia); (3) neurotropic (rabies, poliomyelitis, herpes zoster, encephalitis); (4) viscerotropic (yellow fever, mumps).

viscera (vis′er-a): Plural of viscus (*q.v.*).

visceral (vis′er-al): Relating to a viscus or the viscera.

visceralgia (vis-er-al′ji-a): Pain in a viscus or the viscera.

viscero-: Combining form denoting viscera.

visceromegaly (vis′er-ō-meg′a-li): Abnormal enlargement of the viscera.

visceroperitoneal (vis′er-ō-per i tō-nē′al): Relating to the viscera and the peritoneum.

visceroptosis (vis′er op-tō′sis): Downward displacement or falling of the abdominal organs.

viscerotonic (vis′er-ō-ton′ik): Relating to the behaviour of a somatotype individual, characterized by love of food, sociability, friendliness, general relaxation. — viscerotonia, n.

viscid (vis′id): Glutinous or sticky.

viscidity (vi-sid′i ti): Adhesiveness; stickiness.

viscosity (vis-kos′i-ti): The quality of being glutinous, sticky, viscous. In physics, the tendency of a fluid to resist flow, due to the friction created by cohesion of its molecules.

viscous (vis′kus): Having a glutinous or ropy consistency and the quality of sticking or adhering.

viscus (vis′kus): Any one of the internal organs, especially those in the trunk of the body. — viscera, pl.

vision (vi′zhun): Sight; the special sense concerned with the perception of the particular qualities of an object, *e.g.*, colour, size, shape. ACHROMATIC V. colourblindness; BINOCULAR v. the normal perception of a single image when viewed with both eyes; DOUBLE V. diplopia (*q.v.*); NIGHT V. ability to see in dim light.

visual (vi′zū-al): Relating to vision. V. ACUITY acuteness of sight; V. CELLS usually refers to the rods and cones of the retina; V. FIELD the area within which objects can be seen; v. MEMORY see under MEMORY; V. PURPLE the light-sensitive purple substance contained in the rods of the retina; rhodopsin.

visuoauditory (vizh′ū-ō-aw′di-to-ri): Relating to both vision and hearing.

visuognosis (vizh′ū-og-nō′sis): The recognition and understanding of what is seen.

vital (vī′tal): Relating to or necessary to the maintenance of life. V. CAPACITY the maximal amount of air expelled from the lungs after a maximal inspiration; v. FUNCTIONS those necessary for the maintenance of life; v. SIGNS temperature, pulse, respiration, and blood pressure; V. STATISTICS records of births, deaths, marriages, and incidence of diseases in a specific area.

vitality (vī-tal′i-ti): 1. Vigour, liveliness, energy. 2. The power of surviving, living, and growing.

vitallium (vī-tal′i-um): An alloy that, in the form of nails, plates, tubes, prostheses, etc., can be left in the tissues. Often used to make knee and hip joint replacement.

vitals (vī′tals): Name sometimes given to the viscera.

vitamin (vi′ta-min, vī′): Any one of several complex chemical substances found in minute quantities in certain foodstuffs. As a group, vitamins are essential to life, growth, reproduction, good health, and resistan to infection. Sometimes classified as fat-soluble and water-soluble. Some can now be synthesized. Their absence or deficiency in the diet causes a variety of deficiency diseases. (See individual vitamin listings.)

vitamin A: A fat-soluble anti-infective vitamin that is necessary for growth, reproduction, the maintenance of healthy skin and mucous membranes, and for the formation of rhodopsin and prevention of night blindness. A carotene derivative, it is found in all animal fats, fish liver oils, egg yolk, liver, milk, butter, some leafy green vegetables, some yellow vegetables, carrots in particular, some fruits; also produced synthetically. Deficiency results in night blindness, xerophthalmia, keratinization of the skin and mucous membranes, predisposition to infections of the skin, bladder, and bronchi due to altered epithelial membranes in these organs, and retarded growth. Overdosage is possible, resulting in headache, anorexia, sparsity of hair, and certain bone changes as seen on x-ray. Also known as *anti-infective* vitamin. See also PROVITAMIN and CAROTENE.

vitamin B complex: An important group of water-soluble vitamins all of which are found in liver and yeast; various members of the group are also found in kidney, heart, pork, fish, egg yolk, nuts, soybeans, whole grain cereals, leafy green vegetables, dairy products, molasses. All are destroyed by heat or long cooking. Substances belonging to the complex, or that may be found associated with it include biotin, choline, folic acid, paraminobenzoic acid, riboflavin, thiamin.

vitamin B₁: See THIAMIN.

vitamin B₂: Old term for riboflavin (*q.v.*).

vitamin B₅: See PANTOTHENIC ACID.

vitamin B₆: See PYRIDOXINE.

vitamin B₁₂: See CYANOCOBALAMIN.

vitamin C: A water-soluble vitamin found in citrus and other fruits and fruit juices, the leafy green vegetables, tomatoes, sweet potatoes; also prepared artificially. Necessary for building strong teeth and bones; for strengthening small blood vessels, muscles, and connective tissue; for formation of intercellular cement; important in combating infections and preventing scurvy; facilitates absorption of iron. Deficiency results in sore bleeding gums, pyorrhoea, dental caries, sore joints, anaemia, tendency to bruise easily, scurvy. Also known as *ascorbic acid, antiascorbic vitamin,* and *cevitamic acid.* See ASCORBIC ACID.

vitamin D: A fat-soluble vitamin necessary for the absorption of calcium and phosphorus from the gut and for the proper development of bones and teeth. Found in fish liver oils, especially that of salmon, tuna, cod, and herring; milk and milk products, especially those which have been irradiated; oysters; and yeast. Deficiency results in rickets, osteoporosis, osteomalacia, and osteodystrophy. Overdosage is possible, producing anorexia, vomiting, diarrhoea, headache, drowsiness, high blood calcium, calcareous deposits in walls of blood vessels, heart and kidney tissues. Sometimes called the '*sunshine*' *vitamin* because it can be produced synthetically by irradiation of ergosterol as occurs when the skin is exposed to sunlight. VITAMIN D₂ calciferol (*q.v.*).

vitamin E: See TOCOPHEROL.

vitamin H: Name formerly designating biotin (*q.v.*).

vitamin K: Any of a group of fat-soluble vitamins that are essential for the formation of prothrombin and the clotting of blood and which are absorbed only in the presence of bile; found in fish liver and meal, animal liver, alfalfa, cabbage, spinach, tomatoes, all leafy vegetables, green vegetables, soybean oil, fats, pork, cheese, egg yolk; also produced synthetically. Also called *prothrombin factor* and *antihaemorrhagic factor.*

vitaminology (vi′ta-min-ol′o-ji): The scientific study of vitamins.

vitellin (vi-tel′in): The chief protein in egg yolk.

vitiate (vish′ē-āt): To contaminate or corrupt.

vitiation (vish-i-a′shun): 1. Contamination or injury. 2. Lessening of efficiency or impairment of usefulness.

vitiligo (vit-i-lī′gō): A skin disease characterized by formation of smooth, white, circumscribed irregular patches, with normal or increased pigmentation of the surrounding skin which darkens on exposure to sunlight. Occurs chiefly on the hands, most often in the elderly. Cause unknown. Most commonly seen in tropical zones.

vitrectomy (vi-trek'tō-mi): A microsurgical procedure for removing an opacity (usually consisting of old blood and protein) from the vitreous cavity of the eye.

vitreoretinal (vit-rē-ō-ret'i-nal): Relating to both the vitreous humour and the retina.

vitreous (vit'rē-us): **1.** Resembling glass. **2.** Resembling jelly. V. BODY the semifluid, transparent jelly-like substance filling the posterior cavity of the eye. Also called *vitreous humou.*

vivax malaria: Tertian malaria; see MALARIA.

vivi-: Combining form denoting alive; living.

viviparous (viv-ip'ar-us): Bringing forth or bearing the young alive.

vivisection (viv-i-sek'shun): The act of cutting or performing surgery on a living animal for purposes of research or experimentation; often extended to mean any form of animal experimentation.

vocal (vō'kal): Relating to the voice or the organ that produces voice. V. CORDS membranous folds enclosing ligaments that stretch anterioposteriorly across the larynx; usually referred to as TRUE and FALSE V. CORDS depending on their place of attachment to the thyroid and arytenoid cartilage. Sound is produced by their vibration as air from the lung passes between them. V. CORD NODULE see SINGERS' NODE; V. FREMITUS see FREMITUS. — vocalization, n.

vocalis (vō-kal'is): A muscle situated just beneath the true vocal cord; the musculus vocalis.

vocalization (vō'ka-lī-zā'shun): Use of the voice as in speaking or singing.

voice box: See LARYNX.

void: 1. To cast off or out, as waste matter from the body. **2.** To urinate.

vola (vō'la): The palm of the hand or the sole of the foot.

volar (vō'lar): Relating to the palm of the hand or the sole of the foot.

volatile (vol'a-til): **1.** Having a tendency to evaporate quickly. **2.** Having an explosive or violent nature or tending to change suddenly.

volition (vō-lish'un): The conscious act or power of adopting or refraining from a certain line of action. — volitional, adj.

volitional (vō-lish'un-al): Voluntary; describing an act of will.

Volkmann's contracture: See under CONTRACTURE.

volt (vōlt): The standard measure of electrical potential.

voltage (vōl'tej): Potential electromotive force measured in volts.

volubility (vol-ū-bil'i-ti): Garrulousness; loquaciousness; talkativeness.

volume (vol'yūm): Amount. **1.** The measure of a quantity of a substance. **2.** The space occupied by a substance, mass, bulk. BLOOD V. the total amount of blood circulating in the body; MINUTE V. the amount of air exhaled per minute; or the cardiac output per minute; RESIDUAL V. the amount of air that remains in the lungs after a maximum exhalation; STROKE V. the amount of blood the left ventricle ejects with each heartbeat; usual amount is about 75 ml per minute; TIDAL V. the amount of air that is breathed in and out in normal respiration.

voluntary (vol'un-ter-i): Under the control of the will; free and unrestricted; as opposed to reflex or involuntary; V. ORGANIZATION one that is organized and controlled by individuals who are not salaried but who may employ staff, and who may or may not be professional health care givers; may be supported by governmental or voluntary financing, *e.g.*, Action for Children Trust (ACT formerly NAWCH) or MIND (National Association for Mental Health). V. MUSCLES striated muscles that perform activities that are initiated and controlled by the individual.

Voluntary Service Overseas: An international development charity that works through volunteers.

volvulus (vol'vū-lus): A twisting of a section of bowel, so as to occlude the lumen. It causes obstruction of the bowel.

vomer (vō'mer): The thin ploughshare-shaped bone that forms the inferior and posterior part of the nasal septum.

vomit (vom'it): **1.** To forcibly eject the stomach contents through the mouth. **2.** Stomach contents ejected forcibly through the mouth.

vomiting (vom'i-ting): Forcible ejection of stomach contents through the mouth. CYCLIC V. recurrent spasms of vomiting; DRY V. retching and attempting to vomit without being able to do so; FAECAL V. vomiting of matter that contains faeces; PERNICIOUS V. uncontrollable v.; severe v. of pregnancy; PROJECTILE V. ejection of stomach contents with great force; PSYCHOGENIC V., v. without apparent physical cause; presumed to be of psychological origin;

STERCORACEOUS V. faecal V.; V. OF PREGNANCY see MORNING SICKNESS.

vomitus (vom'i-tus): Vomited matter. COFFEE-GROUND V. that which contains broken-down blood mixed with matter from the stomach; occurs in malignancy and some other diseases of the stomach where there has been bleeding in the stomach or upper respiratory tract and the blood has been acted upon by gastric enzymes.

von Gierke's disease (von-gēr'-kez): Glycogen storage disease, Type I; a hereditary condition characterized by hypoglycaemia, hepatomegaly, acidosis, and hyperuricaemia.

von Hippel–Lindau disease (von-hip'-p'l-lin'-dow): A hereditary condition involving the retina and cerebellum and sometimes the spinal cord; usually seen in association with lesions of the kidney, adrenal gland, pancreas, or other organ; characterized by seizures and lack of mental development.

von Pirquet disease (von-pēr'-kā): A skin test for tuberculosis. [Clemens Freiherr von Pirquet, Austrian paediatrician, 1874–1929.]

von Willebrand's disease: A hereditary disease in which the bleeding time is increased. There is a deficiency of Factor VIII and blood platelet abnormality. Symptoms include epistaxis, bleeding from the gastrointestinal tract, gums, uterus, and surgical incisions. Other names include von Willebrand's syndrome, *Willebrand–Jurgens syndrome, angiohaemophilia,* and *vascular haemophilia.*

voyeur (vwah'yer): One who derives sexual satisfaction from seeing the sexual organs of another or from watching sexual acts. A Peeping-Tom.

voyeurism (vwah'yer-izm): The characteristics, tendencies or acts of a voyeur (*q.v.*).

VSD: Abbreviation for ventricular septal defect, see under VENTRICULAR.

VSO: Abbreviation for Voluntary Service Overseas (*q.v.*).

VT: Abbreviation for ventricular tachycardia, see under TACHYCARDIA.

vulgaris (vul-gar'is): Ordinary.

vulnus (vul'nus): A wound or injury.

vulsellum (vul-sel'um): A forceps with claw-like hooks at the end of each blade.

vulva (vul'va): 1. The external genital organs in the female. 2. The pudendum (*q.v.*). — vulval, vulvar, adj.

vulvectomy (vul-vek'to-mi): Excision of the vulva. RADICAL V. excision of the vulva and of tissues from the anus to a few centimetres above the symphysis pubis, including the labia majora and minora, and the clitoris.

vulvismus (vul-viz'mus): Vaginismus (*q.v.*).

vulvitis (vul-vī'-tis): Inflammation of the vulva. DIABETIC V., V. occurring in women with diabetes; LEUKOPLAKIC V. kraurosis V., see under KRAUROSIS.

vulvo-: Combining form denoting (1) a covering, or (2) the vulva.

vulvopathy (vul-vop'a-thi): Any disorder of the vulva.

vulvorectal (vul-vō-rek'tal): Relating to the vulva and the rectum, as a v. fistula.

vulvovaginal (vul-vō-vaj-īn'al): Relating to the vulva and the vagina. V. GLANDS see BARTHOLIN'S GLANDS.

vulvovaginitis (vul'vō-vaj-in-ī'tis): Inflammation of the vulva and vagina or of the vulvovaginal glands.

W

waddle (wo'del): To walk with short steps and a swinging side-to-side movement of the upper part of the body, seen in certain neurological disorders.

wafer (wā'fer): A two-layered disc made of flour paste, with a dose of medicine between the layers; a cachet.

Wagner–Meissner corpuscles (vahg'-ner-mīs'-ner): Meissner's corpuscles (q. v.).

waist (wāst): The small part of the trunk of the body below the thorax and above the hips.

waiting list initiative: Prospective patient listings for appointments. Relates to the directive to reduce waiting lists for elective surgery through concentrated efforts.

Waldenström's disease (wald'-en-strōmz, val'-den-strermz): 1. Osteochondritis deformans juvenilis. See under OSTEOCHONDRITIS. 2. Macroglobulinaemia (q.v.).

Waldeyer's ring (vald'-i-erz, wald'ī-erz): A circle of lymphoid tissue that encircles the pharynx, the part above being called the pharyngeal tonsil, that on the sides the palatine tonsils, and that on the lower part the lingual tonsil. [Wilhelm von Waldeyer-Hartz, German anatomist, 1836–1921.]

walk-in centres: Clinics providing accessible services on a drop-in basis. They offer free consultations and treatment for minor injuries and illnesses, general health information, self-treatment advice and information about other health and care services. They are nurse-led services, although other professionals may be involved.

walking: SLEEP W. somnambulism (q.v.); w. CAST a cast so constructed as to allow the patient to be ambulatory; w. FRAME a freestanding metal frame for use as a walking aid by a person who holds or leans on the top; w. STICK a stick or short staff used as a walking aid; w. TYPHOID a mild case of typhoid fever in which the patient is not confined to bed.

wall: The structures that cover or surround an anatomical unit such as an organ, or that enclose a cavity, e.g., the chest cavity or the abdominal cavity.

Wallace's rule of nines: A rule for expressing the size of burns as a percentage of the body surface area involved; the head is estimated at 9% ($4\frac{1}{2}$% each for the anterior and posterior surface); the upper extremities at 9% ($4\frac{1}{2}$% each for anterior and posterior surfaces); the anterior and posterior trunk, 18% each; the lower extremities at 18% each (9% for each anterior and posterior surface). The perineum is estimated at 1%. See also LUND AND BROWDER'S CHART, APPENDIX.

wall climbing: An exercise sometimes prescribed for postmastectomy patients to prevent contraction of shoulder muscles and to restore full range of motion of the arm; the patient stands facing the wall, places her hands on the wall and moves them upwards until she reaches the point of pain, marks that place on the wall, and the next time she exercises tries to overreach it.

Wallenberg's syndrome: A condition characterized by occlusion of the posterior inferior cerebellar artery, which results in contralateral loss of temperature and pain sensation; occurs in fifth, ninth, and eleventh nerve palsies and in nystagmus, dysarthria, and dysphagia.

Wallerian degeneration: See under DEGENERATION.

walleye: 1. Opacity of the cornea. 2. A condition in which the iris is white or pale coloured. 3. A strabismus in which the eye turns outward.

wandering: 1. Moving about; not fixed in place. W. KIDNEY floating kidney; see under KIDNEY. 2. Disordered action of the mind due to illness or nervous exhaustion; rambling; delirium.

Wangensteen: W. SUCTION a method of continuous siphonage by suction, for the purpose of draining fluid from a body cavity, e.g., the stomach, employing a device that consists of a nasogastric catheter and a suction apparatus that operates on the principle of negative pressure. It is most commonly used for evacuating gas and fluids from the stomach and upper intestine; w. TUBE the catheter of the Wangensteen suction device. [Owen Wangensteen, American surgeon, 1898–1981.]

ward: A room in a hospital with beds for several patients.

ward clerk or secretary: An assistant to the ward or unit manager; assists with paper work,

657

answers the telephone, takes messages, orders supplies, etc.; is usually trained on the job.

ward or unit manager: A person on the management staff of a hospital who is responsible for the general management of a ward or unit; may or may not be assisted by a clerk or secretary.

warden: A custodian of a sheltered house.

warfarin (wor'fa-rin): A chemical substance that acts as an anticoagulant; in medicine, useful in prevention and treatment of such conditions as coronary thrombosis and pulmonary embolism. W. POISONING may occur as a result of overdosage of warfarin, or accidental ingestion of certain rodenticides that contain the chemical; marked by internal bleeding, epistaxis, haematuria; treatment is aimed at re-establishing coagulability of the blood.

wart: A benign horny projection on the skin caused by hypertrophy of the papillae of the corium. May also occur on mucous membrane. Believed to be caused by a virus; usually painless. Many varieties are described. See VERRUCA. GENITAL W. appears on the vulva especially during pregnancy; can be spread sexually; also called *venereal w.* and *condyloma acuminatum*; PERIUNGUAL W. a w. occurring commonly around or under a fingernail; may become fissured and painful; PLANTAR W. see under PLANTAR; SEBORRHOEIC W. seborrhoeic keratosis; see under KERATOSIS.

wash: A lotion for application to the skin or mucous membrane.

Wassermann test: The first serological test for syphilis; utilizes a complement-fixation technique; no longer in general use.

waste: In physiology, material that is of no use to the body and is cast off as refuse. W. THEORY the theory that ageing occurs as a result of the collection of chemical wastes in the body, which interferes with normal cell functioning.

wasting: Emaciation; pronounced loss of body weight, accompanied by decreased physical and mental activity.

water: A colourless, odourless, and almost tasteless liquid; makes up a large part of the body substance; boils at 100°C, 212°F and freezes at 0°C, 32°F; W. BALANCE the condition that exists when the intake of water equals the output; W. BRASH see PYROSIS; W. DEPLETION refers to loss of water alone as differentiated from dehydration, which may refer to loss of water and salt; is prevented by the sensation of thirst and drinking to relieve it; occurs chiefly in the person whose sensation of thirst is blunted or who is mentally or physically unable to respond to it; DISTILLED W., w. that has been heated to boiling, vaporized, and condensed into liquid form; the condensate has a pH of 7.0 and contains no minerals; HARD W., w. that contains calcium and magnesium ions which combine with fatty acids and prevent soap from making a lather in it; HEAVY W., w. in which most of the hydrogen atoms are heavy hydrogen (^{2}H), giving it properties that differ from those of ordinary w.; LIME W. calcium hydroxide; MINERAL W. contains certain mineral salts in sufficient quantity to be tasted and is considered to have some therapeutic properties; POLLUTED W., w. that is unfit for human consumption; POTABLE W., w. that is suitable for drinking; SODA W., w. that has been charged with carbon dioxide gas; SOFT W., w. that does not contain calcium and magnesium ions and in which soap will lather readily. VICHY W., w. from springs in Vichy, France; has a diuretic action; W. INTOXICATION a condition produced by the intake and retention of abnormal amounts of water and marked by subnormal temperatures, vomiting, depression, and possibly irreversible coma and death; W. MATTRESS a sealed rubber sack filled with water and used as a mattress for such purposes as preventing decubiti; W. OF HYDRATION W. in combination in a substance, but which may be expelled from it without any change in composition;

water-borne: Said of diseases that are spread largely by drinking-water, *e.g.*, cholera (*q.v.*), typhoid fever (*q.v.*).

water cure: Hydrotherapy.

water-hammer pulse: The full, bounding pulse felt in patients with aortic insufficiency. Also called *Corrigan's pulse.*

Waterhouse–Friderichsen syndrome: A fulminating meningococcal infection marked by headache, chills, fever, vomiting, diarrhoea, purpura, joint pain, shock, adrenal insufficiency, respiratory distress, convulsions; occurs mainly in children, especially those under ten years of age; an emergency condition.

Waterlow pressure sore prevention/treatment policy (waw'-ter-lō): A pressure ulcer risk scale developed by Judith Waterlow. It includes six criteria: build/weight for height; continence; skin type/visual risk areas; mobility; sex/age; appetite; plus additional special risks including: tissue malnutrition, neurological deficit, major surgery or trauma, and medication. See DECUBITUS ULCER, under DECUBITUS.

water on the knee: Lay term for synovitis (*q.v.*) of the knee joint; a sign of some underlying problem; not a diagnosis.

waters: Usually refers to the amniotic fluid (liquor amnii, (*q.v.*). BAG OF W. the closed sac that encloses the amniotic fluid.

water-seal drainage: A method of drainage in which the end of the tube is in water, thus allowing fluid and air to escape but preventing air from entering; used especially for draining and collecting fluid from the pleural space.

Waterston procedure: A surgical procedure performed on patients with tetralogy of Fallot; involves creating an anastomosis between the ascending aorta and the right pulmonary artery.

Watson–Crick helix: See HELIX.

watt (wot): The standard unit of electrical power.

wave: 1. A continuous, uniformly advancing, undulating rhythmic motion or series of movements that pass along a surface or through the air. **2.** BRAIN W. s the fluctuations in the electrical current set up in the cortex of the brain by brain action; they may be recorded during electroencephalography. ALPHA W. s in the EEG, occur chiefly in the occiput of the normal person, awake and at rest at a rate of about 8 to 13 per second; BETA W. s in the EEG, occur chiefly in the frontal and parietal areas during periods of intense nervous system activity, at a rate of about 18 to 30 per second; DELTA W. s in the EEG, occur during deep sleep and in serious brain disorders, at a rate of about 3 to 3.5 per second; F or FF W. s regular rapid atrial waves seen in the ECG; occur in cases of atrial flutter; J W. a positive deflection at the junction of the QRS and ST segments of the electrocardiogram of some patients with hypoglycaemia; P W. in the electrocardiogram, represents the depolarization of the atria; PULSE W. the beat felt with the finger over an artery or shown on a sphygmograph; Q W. in the ECG, the first downwards deflection in the QRS complex; represents the beginning of depolarization of the ventricles; R W. in the ECG, an upwards deflection, following the Q wave; S W. in the ECG, the negative deflection in the QRS complex, following the R wave; T W. in the ECG, is due to repolarization of the ventricles; THETA W.S in the EEG, occur chiefly in adults under stress and in children at a rate of about 4 to 7 per second; U W. in the ECG, a low amplitude upwards deflection following the T wave; not always present.

wavelength (wāv'length): In physics, the distance from a given point in the progression of a wave cycle to the corresponding point in the next wave cycle in a wave form having the same phase in two consecutive cycles.

wax: A solid fatty substance secreted by insects and obtained from plants; also made synthetically. BEESWAX a yellow wax secreted by bees; used as a base for ointments; EAR W. cerumen (*q.v.*); PARAFFIN W. a wax prepared from petroleum.

waxy flexibility: The condition of muscles that exists when a patient's limbs are held indefinitely in any position in which they are placed. See CATATONIA.

WBC: Abbreviation for white blood cell (*q.v.*)/count.

WDC: Abbreviation for Workforce Development Confederation (*q.v.*).

weal (wēl): The characteristic lesion of urticaria, but may follow insect bites or stings, or exposure to substances to which the person is allergic. Consists of an oedematous, circumscribed raised area of the skin, irregular in shape, redder or paler than the surrounding skin; usually accompanied by intense itching and usually transitory. Also spelled *wheal*.

wean (wēn): **1.** To discontinue feeding an infant at the breast or entirely on infant formula and substitute other methods of providing nutrition. **2.** To discontinue use of a respirator by gradually lessening the time the patient uses it; an important nursing responsibility to prevent the patient from becoming emotionally and physically dependent on artificial ventilation. **3.** To assist a person in withdrawing from something on which the person has become dependent.

wear and tear theory: A theory of ageing that poses the idea that the body is like a machine, and that various parts wear out, and that physiological functions deteriorate until, finally, they are unable to sustain life.

weaver's bottom: Inflammation of the bursa over the ischial tuberosity; occurs in sedentary people, especially those who sit cross-legged much of the time.

webbed: A congenital condition in which adjacent structures are connected by an abnormal band of tissue.

Weber–Christian syndrome: A disorder characterized by the formation of nodules and plaques in the subcutaneous fatty layer of the skin affecting chiefly the trunk and extremities, the thighs and legs in particular, and resulting in atrophy. Malaise, fever, hepatomegaly and splenomegaly may be present.

Weber's test: Tuning fork test for the diagnosis of conduction deafness. [Friedrich Eugen Weber, German otologist, 1832–1891.]

website: A document or a set of linked documents, usually associated with a particular person, organization, or topic, that is held on a computer system and can be accessed as part of the World Wide Web (*q.v.*).

Wechsler–Bellevue Intelligence Scale: Used in verbal and performance tests, for persons between 16 and 24 years of age, in converting test results into a conventional intelligence quotient. Comprises 11 subtests in various areas. Other scales developed by Wechsler are the WECHSLER INTELLIGENCE SCALE, WECHSLER INTELLIGENCE SCALE FOR CHILDREN, and WECHSLER PRESCHOOL AND PRIMARY SCALE OF INTELLIGENCE. [David Wechsler, American psychologist, 1896–1981.]

wedge pressure: See PULMONARY CAPILLARY WEDGE PRESSURE under PRESSURE.

weep: To exude, drop by drop, tears or other fluid such as serum.

weeping eczema (wē′ping ek′ze-ma): A type of eczema in which there is a vesicular eruption with the vesicles exuding serum.

Wegener's granulomatosis: Thought to be a variant of polyarteritis nodosa; a progressive disorder characterized by necrotizing lesions in the upper respiratory tract, the lungs, and arterioles; inflammation of all the organs of the body; and glomerulonephritis, which frequently results in renal failure and death.

Weigert's law (vī′ -gerts, wī′ -gerts): States that when a part of an organic structure is lost or destroyed, the repair and regeneration process is likely to result in overproduction of tissue.

Weight Watchers: A trade name for a behavioural self-management support group; the objective of members is to gain and retain control of their weight.

Weil–Felix reaction: Agglutination reaction useful in diagnosis of rickettsial diseases such as epidemic, marine, and scrub typhus; Rocky Mountain spotted fever; various other tick fevers. [Edmund Weil, German physician in Prague, 1880–1922. Arthur Felix, Prague bacteriologist, 1887–1956.]

Weil's disease (wīlz): A type of jaundice with fever and splenic enlargement caused by a small spirochaete voided in the urine of rats. A disease of miners, sewer workers, etc., who work in dirty water. Syn., *Spirochaetosis ictohaemorrhagica, leptospiral jaundice*. [Adolph Weil, German physician, 1848–1916.]

Welch's bacillus: *Clostridium perfringens*, the most common causative agent of gas gangrene.

Welfare State: A country in which the welfare of members of the community is underwritten by means of state-run social services for education, health, employment, housing, and social security.

well-baby clinic: A clinic devoted to the healthcare of well infants and children, usually through the first three to five years of life; provides guidance for parents regarding the child's nutrition, growth and development, immunizations, and general healthcare.

wellness: For the adult, a state of emotional, social, and spiritual health that permits clients, within the limits of their abilities and disabilities, to function effectively in their particular social group and to enjoy life. 'Wellness is a process of moving towards greater awareness of oneself and the environment, leading to ever increasing planned interactions with the dimensions of nutrition, fitness, stress, interpersonal relationships, and self-care.'

well-woman clinic: An establishment where women can have health checks. Health education and promotion advice aimed at women is also provided. See HEALTH EDUCATION; HEALTH PROMOTION.

welt: A raised ridge left on the skin by a slash or a blow, as of a whip. A weal.

wen: A retention cyst of a sebaceous gland of the skin. See CYST.

Wenckebach phenomenon: A second-degree atrioventricular heart block in which the P-R interval in the electrocardiogram becomes progressively longer until the P wave finally disappears and the sequence begins again; often a forerunner of complete heart block.

Werdnig–Hoffman syndrome or disease: A hereditary form of infantile muscular atrophy resulting from degeneration of the anterior horn cells of the spinal cord; characterized by wasting of the muscles, flaccid paralysis, and early death; usually occurs in siblings, rather than successive generations. Also called *infantile spinal muscular dystrophy* and *Werdnig–Hoffman paralysis*.

Werlhof's disease: Idiopathic thrombocytopenic purpura; see under PURPURA.

Wermer's syndrome: A rare hereditary condition characterized by hyperplasia of more than one endocrine tissue, involving most often the pituitary and parathyroid glands and the islets of Langerhans. Polyendocrine adenomatosis. Also called *multiple endocrine adenomatosis*.

Werner's syndrome: A condition involving many body systems, characterized by early senescence; cataracts; osteoporosis; scleroderma; and glandular dysfunction, particularly hypogonadism.

Wernicke–Korsakoff syndrome: Wernicke's encephalopathy (see under ENCEPHALOPATHY) and Korsakoff's syndrome (*q.v.*), which often occur together, particularly in alcoholics; due to nutritional deficiency, specifically of vitamin B_1.

Wernicke's syndrome: Wernicke's encephalopathy. See under ENCEPHALOPATHY.

Wertheim's hysterectomy (his-ter-ek'to-mi): An extensive operation for removal of carcinoma of the cervix, where the uterus, cervix, upper vagina, ovaries, and regional lymph glands are removed. [Ernest Wertheim, Austrian gynaecologist, 1864–1920.]

Westergren method: A laboratory test for determining the erythrocyte sedimentation rate; see SEDIMENTATION.

wet dreams: The discharge of semen during sleep, a natural occurrence during adolescence; may or may not be accompanied by a pleasurable dream.

wet lung syndrome: A condition of the lungs characterized by persistent cough and rales heard at the base of the lung; seen in those whose work exposes them to irritating dust, fumes, or vapour.

wet nurse: A woman who breast-feeds a child who is not her own offspring.

Wharton: W.'S DUCT that of the submaxillary salivary gland; W.'S JELLY a jelly-like substance contained in the umbilical cord. [Thomas Wharton, English physician, 1616–1673.]

wheelchair: A chair mounted on wheels for individuals who cannot walk; may be propelled by hand or be motor driven; some are collapsible for transportation by a vehicle.

wheeze (wēz): 1. To breathe noisily and with difficulty. 2. The hoarse whistling sound heard in conditions in which breathing is difficult; caused by partial obstruction of one or more of the air passages, may result from inflammation, trauma, presence of a foreign body, tumour.

whiplash injury (wip'lash in'jer-i): A popular term for injury of one or more cervical vertebrae, resulting from sudden jerking of the head. Symptoms are pain, swelling and limitation of motion.

Whipple's disease: A generalized disease involving the lymphatics and intestinal wall; marked by arthritis, steatorrhoea, emaciation, and lymphadenectomy. Syn., *intestinal lipodystrophy*.

Whipple's operation: See PANCREATODUODENECTOMY.

whipworm (wip'worm): See TRICHURIS TRICHIURA.

whirlpool bath: A bath in which the water is agitated and injected with air by a power device.

white blood cell: A blood cell that does not contain haemoglobin. A leukocyte (*q.v.*). The main types of white blood cells are polymorphonuclear, lymphocyte, and monocyte.

whitehead (wīt'hed): A small white papule, seen particularly on the face; probably caused by a blockage of a pilosebaceous follicle. See also MILIA.

whiteleg (wīt'leg): Phlegmasia alba dolens; see under PHLEGMASIA.

white matter: Nerve tissue that is whitish in colour as opposed to the grey matter. Consists of myelinated nerve fibres of the neurons and makes up the conducting matter of the brain and spinal cord.

White Paper: A government report containing statements of policy intentions.

whitlow (wit'lō): A felon (*q.v.*). MELANOTIC W., a malignant tumour that is characterized by changes about the border of the nail and in the nail bed. See PARONYCHIA.

WHO: Abbreviation for World Health Organization (*q.v.*).

whole time equivalent: Someone one works full time or equivalent hours.

whoop (hoop): The characteristic crowing intake of breath following a paroxysm of coughing in whooping cough. See PERTUSSIS.

whooping cough (hoo'ping kof): Pertussis (*q.v.*).

whorl (worl): A twist or spiral turn such as in the cochlea of the ear, in the muscle fibres at the apex of the heart, in the arrangement of the ridges in a fingerprint, or in an area in which the hairs grow in a radial manner.

Widal test or reaction: An agglutination test useful in diagnosing typhoid fever. Also called *Gruber–Widal reaction*.

will: The faculty of conscious and deliberate action; the power of choosing one's own actions.

Willis: See CIRCLE OF WILLIS.

willow fracture: Greenstick fracture; see under FRACTURE.

Wilms' tumour: A congenital, highly malignant tumour of the kidney, occurring chiefly in children; develops from abnormal epithelial tissue in the embryo; may start to grow before birth and may affect any part of the kidney; symptoms include hypertension, fever, anorexia, lethargy; metastasizes early to the lungs, liver, and long bones. [Max Wilms, German surgeon, 1867–1918.]

Wilson–Mikity syndrome: A condition of progressive pulmonary insufficiency seen in infants of low birth weight; characterized by dyspnoea, tachypnoea, cyanosis; often fatal.

Wilson's disease: Hepatolenticular degeneration (q.v.).

window: An opening in a structure or a wall, especially a window in the inner ear (oval window, round window).

windpipe (wind'pīp): The trachea.

wink: The involuntary opening and closing of the eyelids, a protective action by which the tears are spread over the front of the eyeball keeping the conjunctiva moist; can also be a voluntary act.

winter itch: Pruritus occurring in cold weather; affects chiefly the elderly and those with dry skin.

wiring: Fastening the ends of a fractured bone together with wire sutures. See KIRSCHNER'S WIRE.

Wirsung: w.'s DUCT the main excretory duct of the pancreas; runs the length of the pancreas and collects pancreatic secretions from many small ductules; usually joins the common bile duct before emptying into the duodenum. Also called *the canal of w.* and *hepatopancreatic duct.* [Johann Georg Wirsung, German physician, 1600–1643.]

wisdom tooth: The third molar on each side of the lower and upper jaws; wisdom teeth are the last to erupt, usually between the 17th and 21st years of age.

witch hazel: A shrub or small tree found in damp places in Asia and eastern and central North America. The dried leaves as well as an alcoholic solution have been used for treating minor wounds such as a bruise or contusion, inflammation, and headache, and for treatment of haemorrhoids. Also used as a skin toner.

withdrawal (with-draw'al): In medicine, the discontinuance of a medication or therapy. In psychiatry, the process by which a person retreats physically and/or psychologically to escape an emotionally disturbing situation. w. METHOD coitus interruptus; see under COITUS; W. SYNDROME the group of physical and psychological signs and symptoms exhibited by a drug addict upon withdrawal from an addictive drug; severity depends on the particular drug, the length of time of the addiction, and the size of the doses the person has been taking.

Wolff–Parkinson–White syndrome: An electrocardiographic pattern in which the PR interval is shortened and the QRS complex is lengthened; sometimes seen in paroxysmal tachycardia.

Wolman's disease: A rare inborn error of lipid metabolism characterized by large deposits of cholesterol, esters, and glycosides in the viscera, particularly the liver.

womb (woom): The uterus.

Women's Health Movement: Began in 1970 in the USA with the objectives of changing the attitude of physicians and others towards women's health problems and care, obtaining more participation by women in governing boards of hospitals and other community healthcare facilities, and providing literature and courses to inform women about their bodies and about healthcare services they may require.

Women's Royal Voluntary Service: One of the UK's largest voluntary services, dedicated to tackling social isolation or deprivation in communities throughout England, Scotland and Wales. It has over 95,000 volunteers, including 13,000 men.

Wood: w.'s GLASS a light filter that transmits only ultraviolet rays; useful in identifying fungi that are the causative agent in certain skin and scalp diseases; w.'s RAYS ultraviolet rays (q.v.).

wood alchohol: Methyl alcohol.

wood tick: Any one of several varieties of ticks that cling to bushes and fasten themselves to the body of an animal or person; the place of attachment often becomes an infected lesion. One variety is the vector for Rocky Mountain spotted fever.

woolsorter's disease: Pulmonary anthrax; an occupational disease that occurs in persons who handle the wool of animals that have had anthrax.

word blindness: A type of speech disturbance in which one is unable to perceive or understand certain sounds, syllables, or phrases. See also DYSLEXIA.

word salad: Term used to describe speech in which words and phrases are so combined that they have no logical coherence or comprehensive meaning; frequently seen in schizophrenic individuals.

workaholism (work'a-hol-izm): A state of exhaustion and a group of symptoms resulting from chronic compulsive overworking. — workaholic, adj.

work-based learning: The achievement of planned learning outcomes derived from the experience of performing a work role or function. Students are normally required to complement experiential learning with directed reading, research, or group work, to ensure that the learning is placed in the context of current theory or practice.

Workforce Development Confederation (kon-fed-er-ā′ -shun): Managment groups established to take on the central role in enabling the delivery of Strategic Health Authority franchise plans, through planning and development of the health-care workforce. They will work with Postgraduate Deaneries to commission education and training, and will manage the Department of Health's (England) annual investment in training of almost £3 billion.

work-up: Usually refers to the process of evaluating a patient's medical history; doing a complete physical examination, including any tests required; and gathering all possible data on the patient's present condition for the purpose of diagnosis and planning for his care.

World Health Organization: A 150-member agency of the United Nations, founded in 1948, the objective being the attainment, by all people of the world, of the highest possible level of health. Collects, analyses, and distributes data and statistics on health and environmental problems. It is a directing and coordinating authority on international health; supports and coordinates research in health problems and the control of communicable diseases; sets standards for the production of vaccines and bacteriological products; sets international sanitary regulations; supports the fight against pollution of air, water, and soil; provides technical assistance to member nations in the improvement of their health services. Headquarters are in Geneva, Switzerland.

world wide web: Sites (web pages) stored on computers, accessible through the Internet (q.v.), that provide information on virtually any subject. Sites can be set up by individuals or organizations.

wormian bones (wer′mi-an): Small, isolated, irregular bones found along the sutures of the skull.

worms: See *ASCARIS, TAENIA, TRICHURIS TRICHIURA.*

wound (woond): An injury to the body that involves a break in the continuity of tissues or of body structures; results from trauma or from a surgical procedure. CONTUSED W. one made with a blunt object and in which the skin is not broken; GUNSHOT W. one made by a bullet from a gun or small firearm; INCISED W. one made by a sharp cutting instrument; INFECTED W. one contaminated by microorganisms, or from debris, bits of clothing, etc.; LACERATED W. one in which the tissues are torn; OPEN W. one that opens to the surface; PENETRATING W. one that causes damage to subcutaneous tissues; has a W. of entrance but no W. of exit; PUNCTURE W. deep, narrow W. caused by penetration with a pointed object; SEPTIC W. one infected with pus-producing organisms; SUCKING W. a penetrating chest wound through which air is drawn in and out; W. HEALING see HEALING.

wrench (rench): 1. To twist something suddenly and forcibly. 2. A painful sudden violent twist, as of an ankle or wrist.

wrist (rist): The joint between the forearm and the hand; the carpus. Made up of eight carpal bones the scaphoid, lunate, triquetral, pisiform, trapezium, trapezoid, capitate, and hamate bones. W. DROP or WRISTDROP paralysis of the extensor muscles of the hand and fingers causing the hand to hang down at the wrist. Syn., *carpus.* — carpal, adj.

writer's cramp: Characterized by painful spasmodic cramps of the muscles of the fingers, hand or forearm whenever an attempt is made to write.

wryneck (wrī′nek): Torticollis (*q.v.*).

WTE: Abbreviation for whole time equivalent (*q.v.*).

Wuchereria (voo-ker-ē′ri-a): A genus of filarial worms that are parasitic in humans, inhabitating chiefly the lymphatic vessels; includes the causative parasite of tropical elephantiasis (*q.v.*).

wuchereriasis (voo-ker′ -e-rī′ -a-sis): Infestation with worms of the *Wuchereria* genus. *Filariasis.*

www: Abbreviation for world wide web (*q.v.*).

X

xanth-, xantho-: Combining forms denoting yellow or yellowish colour.

xanthine (zan'thīn): A yellow-white compound found in the liver, spleen, pancreas, muscle tissue, and in blood and the urine where it sometimes forms into a calculus; it is formed during metabolism of nucleoproteins and is a precursor of uric acid.

xanthinuria (zan-thin-ū'ri-a): The presence of abnormally large amounts of xanthine in the urine.

xanthism (zan'thizm): A congenital anomaly in black people characterized by reddish coloured skin and hair.

xanthochromatic (zan-thō-krō-mat'ik): Having a yellow or yellowish colour.

xanthochromia (zan-thō-krō'mi-a): 1. Yellow discoloration of the skin. 2. Yellow discoloration of the spinal fluid; due to haemolysis of blood in the subarachnoid space following subarachnoid haemorrhage.

xanthocyanopia (zan'thō-sī-an-ō'pi-a): A type of colour blindness in which the person cannot distinguish red and green but is able to discern yellow and blue. Also *xanthocyanopsia*.

xanthoderma (zan-thō-der'ma): Yellow-coloured skin.

xanthodontous (zan-thō-don'tus): Having yellowish-coloured teeth.

xanthogranuloma (zan'thō-gran-ū-lō'ma): A tumour that has characteristics of both granuloma (*q.v.*) and xanthoma (*q.v.*).

xanthogranulomatosis (zan'thō-gran'ū-lō-ma-tō'sis): A form of xanthomatosis (*q.v.*), in which the lipid deposits are granulomatous and are found chiefly in the skull bones. Also called *Hand–Schüller–Christian disease*.

xanthoma (zan-thō'ma): A condition characterized by a collection of histiocytes appearing as papules, nodules, or plaques under the skin around the orbital area, or around tendons and joints, and producing a yellow discoloration; several varieties are recognized; occurs chiefly in middle or later life and more often in women than men.

xanthomatosis (zan-thō-ma-tō'sis): A condition of faulty metabolism of cholesterol, characterized by yellowish or brownish discoloration of skin and other tissues and sometimes by formation of fatty tumours; may affect general health. See NIEMANN–PICK DISEASE.

xanthomatous (zan-thō'ma-tus): Relating to xanthoma.

xanthopia (zan-thō'pi-a): A condition in which all objects appear yellow or yellowish. Also called *xanthopsia*.

xanthoproteic (zan-thō-prō'tē-ik): x. TEST a laboratory test for (1) dextrose; (2) protein. *Mulder's test*.

xanthoprotein (zan-thō-prō'tēin): An orange pigment produced by treating protein with hot nitric acid.

xanthopsia (zan-thop'si-a): A condition in which all things are seen as yellow or yellowish; may occur in jaundice, digitalis poisoning, or picric acid poisoning.

xanthopsis (zan-thop'sis): Yellow pigmentation of the skin; seen especially in certain malignancies.

xanthosis (zan-thō'sis): Yellowish discoloration of the skin. Sometimes seen in degenerating tissues of malignant neoplasms. May also occur temporarily due to eating large quantities of foods containing carotene or from taking quinine over a long period of time.

xanthous (zan'thus): Of a yellow or yellowish colour.

xanthuria (zan-thū'ri-a): Xanthinuria (*q.v.*).

X chromosome: The female sex chromosome, present in all female gametes and only half male gametes. When union occurs two X-C.'s result in a female child (XX), one of each results in a male child (XY).

xeno-: Combining form denoting (1) strange; (2) foreign material.

xenogenesis (zen-ō-jen'e-sis): 1. The production of offspring unlike either parent. 2. Heterogenesis — xenogenic, adj.

xenogenous (ze-noj'e-nus): Caused by a foreign body or substance, or originating outside of the organism.

xenograft (zen'ō-graft): Transplantation of an organ or tissue from one species to another. Heterograft.

xenology (ze-nol'o-ji): The study of parasites that affect humans.

xenomenia (zen-ō-mē'ni-a): A condition in which (1) the physical changes that accompany menstruation occur, but there is no blood flow, or (2) menstrual blood is discharged from a part of the body other than the uterus.

xenon (zē'non): An inert gaseous element. Radioactive xenon is used in blood-flow clearance tests. Chemical symbol, Xe.

xenophobia (zen-ō-fō'bi-a): Morbid fear of strangers or foreigners.

xenophonia (zen-ō-fō'ni-a): An alteration in the voice, due to a speech defect.

xenophthalmia (zen-of-thal'mi-a): Conjunctivitis caused by a foreign body or trauma.

Xenopsylla cheopis (zen-op-sil'a che-op'is): The rat flea that transmits bubonic plague.

xer-, xero-: Combining forms denoting dry; dryness.

xeransis (zē-ran'sis): Gradual loss of moisture from the body tissues. — xerantic, adj.

xerasia (zē-rā'zi-a): Dryness and brittleness of the hair.

xerocheilia (zē-ro-kī'li-a): Dryness of the lips. Also *xerochilia*.

xeroderma (ze'rō-der-ma): Also called *xerodermia*. Dryness of the skin. See ICHTHYOSIS. X. PIGMENTOSUM, Kaposi's disease, a familial dermatosis thought to be caused by photosensitization. Pathological freckle formation (ephelides) may give rise to keratosis, neoplastic growth and a fatal termination. [Moritz Kaposi, Hungarian dermatologist, 1837–1902.]

xerodermatosis (zē'rō-der-ma-tō'sis): Sjögren's syndrome (*q.v.*).

xerography (zē-rog'ra-fi): A technique for obtaining an x-ray image utilizing a plate coated with selenium.

xeroma (zē-rō'ma): Abnormal dryness of the conjunctiva; xerophthalmia.

xeromammography (zē'rō-mam-og'ra-fi): Xeroradiography of the breast, a method that subjects the patient to less radiation than ordinary x-ray.

xeromenia (zē-rō-mē'ni-a): The presence of the usual physical disturbances that occur during menstruation but without the usual flow of blood.

xeronosus (zē-ron'o-sus): Dryness of the skin, mucous membranes, or conjunctiva.

xerophagia (ze-rō-fā'ji-a): Subsisting on dry foods only.

xerophthalmia (zē-rof-thal'mi-a): A serious disease of the eyeball, associated with vitamin A deficiency. The eyelids become inflamed, the conjunctiva dry and marked by appearance of yellow spots; the cornea becomes dry and ulcerated; night blindness develops and total blindness may develop in untreated cases.

xerosis (zē-rō'sis): Dryness.

xerostomia (zē'rō-stō'mi-a): Dryness of the mouth from lack of saliva.

xerotocia (zē'rō-tō'si-a): Dry labour.

xiph-, xipho-: Combining forms denoting the xiphoid process.

xiphisternum (zif-i-ster'num): The ensiform cartilage or process; the end section of the sternum. It is subject to much variety as to direction, shape and degree of ossification. — xiphosternal, adj.

xiphocostal (zif-ō-kos'tal): Relating to the xiphoid process and the ribs.

xiphodynia (zif-ō-din'i-a): Pain in the xiphoid process.

xiphoid (zif'oyd): Shaped like a sword. X. PROCESS the pointed process of cartilage at the lower end of the sternum; also called the *xiphisternum* and the *ensiform process.*

xiphoidalgia (zif-oy-dal'ji-a): A syndrome characterized by pain of a neuralgic character and tenderness over the xiphoid process.

xiphoiditis (zif-oy-dī'tis): Inflammation of the ensiform cartilage.

x-ray: 1. Roentgen ray; electromagnetic rays of short length and high frequency. X-rays produce a photographic effect and thus are useful in diagnosis; they also penetrate deeply, making them useful in therapy. So called because their nature was not known at the time of their discovery (1895). 2. An X-RAY PHOTOGRAPH, a radiographic image of organs or structures projected into a photographic plate.

xylene (zī'lēn): A clear inflammable liquid resembling benzene. Has been used as an ointment in pediculosis.

xylophobia (zī'lō-fō'bi-a): An abnormal fear of woods and trees.

xylose (zī'lōs): A pentose sugar found in woody materials; has a sweet taste; soluble in water and alcohol; used as a non-nutritive sweetener.

xylosuria (zī'lō-sū'ri-a): The presence of xylose in the urine.

Y

Y: Chemical symbol for yttrium.

yawning: The often involuntary act of opening the mouth widely, breathing in deeply, and then breathing out as the involved muscles relax; often due to suggestion or to sleepiness, but may also be a sign of vital depression following haemorrhage. — yawn, n.;v.

yaws: An infectious, non-venereal disease of the tropics, caused by the spirochaete *Treponema pertenue* and marked by fever, rheumatic pains and a characteristic lesion called a yaw. Lesions appear on hands, face, feet, external genitalia and are described as raspberry-like tubercles with a caseous crust; they may run together in fungus-like masses, form pustules and ulcerate. The organism enters through a break in the skin. Penicillin is the treatment of choice. Syn., *frambesia tropica, pian, bouba, parangi*. This and other diseases caused by the same organism closely resemble syphilis. The general name for this group of diseases is treponematosis.

Y chromosome (krō'mō-sōm): One of a pair of chromosomes (X and Y) carried in one-half of the male gametes and none of the female gametes; important in the determination of the sex of the offspring, since it is the differentiating chromosome for the male sex.

yeast (yēst): *Saccharomyces*. A unicellular fungus which reproduces by budding only. Used to produce alcoholic fermentation, leaven bread, and in some cases as a remedy. Some yeasts are pathogenic to humans, *e.g.*, the species causing thrush. BREWER'S Y. a by-product from the brewing of beer; a crude but adequate and complete source of vitamin B complex.

yellow bone marrow: See under BONE MARROW.

yellow fever: An acute, specific, infectious, febrile illness of the tropics, of short duration and varying intensity, caused by a virus. The urban type is transmitted from person to person by the bite of the *Aedes aegypti* mosquito; the sylvan type is transmitted from monkey to human by the bite of the forest mosquito. Characteristic features of a mild attack include headache, malaise, fever, bradycardia, jaundice, and proteinuria. More severe cases are characterized by icterus, haemorrhagic tendencies, liver necrosis, black vomit, anuria. Mortality rate is about 5% in victims who are native to areas of the world where the disease is endemic, but much higher for those from other areas. Vaccination with 17D strain of the virus produces immunity for several years. An attack of the disease results in lifetime immunity.

yellow spot: Macula lutea (*q.v.*).

yerba (yer'ba): A herb. Y. MATÉ the dried leaves of certain species of *Ilex*; grows in Paraguay and Brazil; contains caffeine and tannin and is used as a diaphoretic and diuretic, also as a beverage.

Yersinia: A genus of small bacilli, aerobic or anaerobic, that are pathological to animals and humans. Y. ENTEROCOLITICA a coccobacillary organism that causes enterocolitis and mesenteric lymphadenitis in humans; Y. PESTIS, a bacillary organism that causes plague in humans, Y. PSEUDOTUBERCULOSIS, the cause of lymphadenosis in humans.

yoga: A philosophy that emphasizes, among other concepts, the practice of a system of isometric exercises, breathing education, relaxation, and the assumption of certain positions, with the aim of achieving bodily, mental, and emotional well-being. The term is from the Sanskrit, meaning union, and refers to the union of the human spirit with the infinite.

yogurt, yoghurt (yog'ert, yōg'): A form of curdled milk produced by the action of *Lactobacillus bulgaricus*.

yolk sac: The embryonic membrane that connects to the midgut (*q.v.*).

youth: The period of life between childhood and maturity.

yttrium 90 (^{90}Y) (it'ri-um): A rare metallic substance emitting beta particles with a half-life of 64 hours; some of its radioactive isotopes are used in treatment of certain cancers.

Z

Zeis's glands (zīs'-iz): The sebaceous glands associated with the cilia at the edges of the eyelids.

Zenker's diverticulum: A diverticulum of the pharynx occurring at its junction with the oesophagus; also called *hypopharyngeal diverticulum* and *pharyngoesophageal diverticulum*.

zero (zē'rō): 1. Nothing; nought. 2. The numeral or symbol 0. 3. The point from which negative and positive quantities are measured on a graduated scale, as in a thermometer.

Ziehl–Neelsen procedure (zēl-nēl'-senz): A widely used laboratory method for detecting acid-fast bacteria, particularly the tubercle bacillus, *Mycobacterium tuberculosis*. [Franz Ziehl, German bacteriologist, 1857–1926. Friedrich Karl Adolf Neelsen, 1854–1894.]

Zieve's syndrome (zē'-vez): A condition associated with excessive intake of alcohol; characterized by enlargement of the liver and spleen, jaundice, cirrhosis, hyperlipaemia and hypercholesterolaemia, anaemia, lesions of the sclera, epigastric pain, and telangiectasia; the symptoms tend to disappear once the drinking stops.

ZIFT: Abbreviation for zygote intrafallopian transfer (*q.v.*).

zimmer (zim'a): Tradename for a light-weight metal walking aid or frame, used chiefly by the elderly.

zinc (zink): A bluish-white metallic element; many of its salts are used for their antiseptic and astringent action on skin and mucous membranes; made up in powder, solution and ointment form. Chemical symbol is Zn.

Zn: Symbol for zinc.

zo-, zoo-: Combining forms denoting (1) animal; (2) animal kingdom.

zoanthropy (zō-an'thro-pi): The delusion that one has become a dog or horse, or any other of the lower animals.

zoetic (zō-et'ik): Relating to life; vital.

Zollinger–Ellison syndrome: A familial condition characterized by tumour of the pancreatic islets of Langerhans, hypersecretion of gastric acid, fulminating ulceration of oesophagus, stomach, duodenum, and jejunum. Frequently accompanied by diarrhoea. [Robert M. Zollin-

ger, American surgeon, b.1903. E. H. Ellison, American physician, 1918–1970.]

zona (zō'na): 1. In anatomy, a delineated area in the body having characteristic structure or properties; a zone or girdle. 2. Herpes zoster (*q.v.*). Z. FACIALIS herpes zoster of the face; Z. OPHTHALMICA herpes zoster occurring along the distribution of the ophthalmic nerve; Z. ORBICULARIS COXAE a thickening of the fibres of the capsule of the hip joint that form a ring around the neck of the femur; Z. PELLUCIDA the thick transparent membrane surrounding the ovum.

zonaesthesia (zō-nes-thē'ze-a): A sensation of constriction about the body resembling that produced by a tight girdle or cord.

zone (zōn): A small belt or area. EROGENOUS, or EROTOGENIC Z. an area of the body that produces a sexual response when stimulated; GERMINATIVE Z. the deepest layer of the epidermis, lying just above the dermis; made up of the stratum spinosum and the stratum basale; Z. THERAPY see under THERAPY.

zonifugal (zō-nif'ū-gal): Passing outward from within a zone.

zonipetal (zō-nip'i-tal): Passing into a zone from without.

zonule (zon'ūl): A small zone or area. Z. OF ZINN the suspensory ligament that holds the crystalline lens in place.

zonulitis (zon-ū-lī'tis): Inflammation of the zonule of Zinn (*q.v.*).

zonulysin (zon-ū-lī'sin): A proteolytic enzyme used in surgery to dissolve the suspensory ligament of the crystalline lens.

zooblast (zō'ō-blast): An animal cell.

zoogenous (zō-oj'e-nus): Obtained or derived from animals.

zoograft (zō'ō-graft): A graft of tissue from a lower animal to a human.

zoolagnia (zō-ō-lag'ni-a): Sexual attraction of an individual to animals.

zoologist (zō-ol'ō-jist): A person who specializes in the science of zoology.

zoology (zō-ol'o-ji): The science that deals with the study of animals.

zoomania (zō'ō-mā'ni-a): Excessive love of animals.

zoonoses (zō-ō-nō′sēz): Diseases or infections of animals that may be transmitted to humans. — zoonosis, sing; zoonotic, adj.

zooparasite (zō-ō-par′a-sīt): An animal that exists as a parasite.

zoophagus (zō-of′a-gus): Carnivorous; living on animal foods only.

zoophilic (zō-ō-fil′ik): Preferring animals to humans.

zoophilism (zō-of′i-lizm): Abnormal fondness for animals. EROTIC Z. deriving sexual pleasure from handling animals.

zoophobia (zō-ō-fō′bi-a): Abnormal fear of animals.

zooplasty (zō′ō-plas-ti): Transplantation of skin or other tissue from one of the lower animals to man.

zoopsia (zō-op′si-a): A hallucination or delusion in which the individual thinks he or she sees animals.

zootoxin (zō′ō-tok′sin): A toxic substance produced by an animal, e.g., snake or spider venom.

zoster (zos′ter): Herpes zoster; see under HERPES.

zosteriform (zos-ter′i-form): 1. Resembling herpes zoster; see HERPES. 2. Referring to lesions that appear in bands following the course of a nerve.

Z-plasty (zed′plas-ti): A plastic operation for relieving the contraction of scar tissue in which a Z-shaped incision is made over the contracted scar.

Z-track: A method of intramuscular injection that prevents seeping of a medication into subcutaneous tissues or leakage from an injection site. The skin is pulled down and towards the median and held there while the injection is given; after 10 seconds the needle is removed and the skin returns to its normal position leaving a zigzag track from the point of insertion. Also called *zigzag method.*

zyg-; zygo-: Combining forms denoting joined or yoked.

zygodactyly (zī-gō-dak′ti-li): Syndactyly. The webbing or fusion of one or more fingers or toes.

zygoma (zī-gō′ma): The cheek bone. — zygomatic, adj.

zygomatic (zī′gō-mat′ik): Relating to the zygoma. Z. ARCH the bony arch formed by the zygomatic process of the temporal bone and the temporal process of the zygomatic bone that forms the prominence of the cheek; Z. PROCESSES projections on the frontal bone, maxilla, and temporal bone, all of which articulate with the zygoma.

zygote (zī′gōt): 1. The fertilized ovum before cleavage. 2. The organism produced by the union of two gametes (q.v.) See DIZYGOTIC, MONOZYGOTIC.

zygote intrafallopian transfer: In vitro fertilization (q.v.) with the transfer of a zygote into the Fallopian tube (q.v.). It is an assisted reproduction technique consisting of hormonal stimulation of the ovaries, laparoscopic follicular aspiration, in vitro fertilization and intrafallopian transfer of a zygote by abdominal cannulation.

zymogen (zī′mō-jen): The inactive granular precursor, with the secretory cell, of enzymes.

zymogenic (zī-mō-jen′ik): Causing fermentation.

zymologist (zī-mol′o-jist): One who specializes in the study of fermentation.

zymology (zī-mol′o-ji): The study of fermentation.

zymolysis (zī-mol′ī-sis): Digestion or fermentation brought about by an enzyme.

zymosis (zī-mō′sis): 1. Fermentation. 2. The process by which infectious diseases are thought to develop. 3. Any infectious disease.

zymotic (zī-mot′ik): 1. Relating to zymosis. 2. A general term sometimes used to designate endemic or epidemic infectious diseases that are caused by microorganisms.

APPENDICES

CONTENTS

Appendix 1:
NORMAL VALUES

1 Weights and measures

Linear measure

1	micrometre	(μm)	=	0.001	millimetres
1	millimetre	(mm)	=	0.001	metres
1	centimetre	(cm)	=	0.01	metres
10	centimetres		=	0.1	metres
100	centimetres		=	1.0	metre
1000	metres	(m)	=	1.0	kilometre (km)

Weight

1	microgram	(μg)	=	0.001	milligrams
1	milligram	(mg)	=	0.001	gram (g)
1000	milligrams		=	1.0	gram
1000	grams		=	1.0	kilogram (kg)

Volume

1	microlitre	(μl)	=	0.001	millilitres
1	millilitre	(ml)	=	0.001	litre (l)
1000	millilitres		=	1.0	litre

Conversion

Millimetres to inches	$\dfrac{mm \times 10}{254}$
Inches to millimetres	$\dfrac{in \times 254}{10}$
Kilograms to pounds	$\dfrac{kg \times 1000}{454}$
Pounds to kilograms	$\dfrac{lb \times 454}{1000}$

Grams to ounces	$\dfrac{g \times 20}{567}$
Ounces to grams	$\dfrac{oz \times 567}{20}$
Millilitres to fluid ounces	$\dfrac{ml}{30}$
Fluid ounces to millilitres	$fl\ oz \times 30$

Equivalent values

Metres	Centimetres	Millimetres	Feet	Inches
1.0	100.0	1000.0	3.2808	39.37
0.01	1.0	10.0	0.03281	0.3937
0.9144	91.44	914.40	3.0	36.0
0.3048	30.48	304.8	1.0	12.0
0.0254	2.54	25.4	0.0833	1.0

Grams	Kilograms	Ounces	Pounds
1.0	0.001	0.0353	0.0022
1000.0	1.0	35.3	2.2
28.35	0.02835	1.0	1/16
454.5	0.4545	16.0	1.0

Millimetres	Fluid ounces	Pints
1.0	0.333	0.0021
29.58	1.0	1/20
591.6	20	1.0

2   Temperature

'Celsius' and 'Centigrade' are equivalent. However, 'Celsius' is now the internationally recognized term.

Freezing Point: Fahrenheit 32   Celsius 0
Boiling Point: Fahrenheit 212   Celsius 100
Fahrenheit to Celsius $(F - 32) \times \frac{5}{9}$
Celsius to Fahrenheit $(C \times \frac{9}{5}) + 32$

Temperature conversion chart

F	C	C	F
92	33.33	33.00	91.4
93	33.89	33.5	92.3
94	34.44	34.0	93.2
95	35.0	34.5	94.1
96	35.56	35.0	95.0
97	36.11	35.5	95.9
98	36.67	36.0	96.8
99	37.22	36.5	97.7
100	37.78	37.0	98.6
101	38.33	37.5	99.5
102	38.89	38.0	100.4
103	39.44	38.5	101.3
104	40.0	39.0	102.0
105	40.56	39.5	103.1
106	41.11	40.0	104.0
107	41.67	40.5	104.9
108	42.22	41.0	105.8
109	42.78	41.5	106.7
110	43.33	42.0	107.6
		42.5	108.5
		43.0	109.4
		43.5	110.3

3   Laboratory values

Blood counts

Red cell count (RBC)
        Female $4.2 - 5.4 \times 10^{12}/l$
        Male $4.6 - 6.2 \times 10^{12}/l$

Haemoglobin (Hb)
        Female $12 - 15.5 \, g/dl$
        Male $14 - 18 \, g/dl$

Haemotocrit
        Female $0.3 - 0.45 (36 - 45\%)$
        Male $0.42 - 0.53 (42 - 53\%)$

Mean corpuscular volume (MCV) $77 - 97 \, fl$

Mean corpuscular haemoglobin (MCH) $27 - 33 \, pg/cell$

Mean corpuscular
  haemoglobin concentration (MCHC) $32 - 35 \, g/dl$

Reticulocytes $10 - 100 \times 10^9/l (0.2 - 2.0\%)$

Leukocytes   Female $3.9 - 11.1 \times 10^9/l$
                     Male $3.7 - 9.5 \times 10^9/l$

Differential count:

Neutrophils	$1.8-7.7 \times 10^9/\text{l}(40-75\%)$
Lymphocytes	$1.0-4.8 \times 10^9/\text{l}(20-45\%)$
Monocytes	$0-0.8 \times 10^9/\text{l}(2-10\%)$
Eosinophils	$0-0.45 \times 10^9/\text{l}(1-6\%)$
Basophils	$0-0.20 \times 10^9/\text{l}(<1\%)$
Platelets	$250 \times 10^9/\text{l}$

Blood constituents

As measured in whole blood (B), plasma (P) or serum (S)

Bilirubin (S)	$3-21\ \mu\text{mol/l}$
Calcium (S) (total)	$2.2-2.6\ \text{mmol/l}$
Cholesterol (P)	$3.2-8.5\ \text{mmol/l}$
Chloride (P)	$98-108\ \text{mmol/l}$
Creatinine (S)	$70-120\ \text{mmol/l}$
Folic acid (S)	$12-35\ \text{nmol/l}$
Glucose (P)	$4-7\ \text{mmol/l}$
Hb A_{1c}	$>7\%$
Iodine (protein bound) (S)	$0.28-0.63\ \mu\text{mol/l}$
Iron (S)	$14-31\ \mu\text{mol/l}$
	$11-29\ \mu\text{mol/l}$
Lactic acid (B)	$0.5-1.2\ \text{mmol/l}$
Nitrogen (non-protein) (S)	$10.7-25.0\ \text{mmol/l}$
Osmolality (P)	$278-295\ \text{mOsmol/kg}$
Phosphate (inorganic) (P)	$0.8-1.45\ \text{mmol/l}$
Potassium (S)	$3.4-5\ \text{mmol/l}$
pH (B)	$7.35-7.45$
PCO_2 (B)	$4.7-6.9\ \text{kPa}$
PO_2 (B)	$11.3-14.0\ \text{kPa}$
Protein (total) (S)	$62-83\ \text{g/l}$
albumin (S)	$35-50\ \text{g/l}$
globulin (S)	$20-40\ \text{g/l}$
fibrogen (P)	$1.8-4.2\ \text{g/l}$
Sodium (S)	$33-144\ \text{mmol/l}$
Urea (P)	$2.5-7.5\ \text{mmol/l}$

Cerebrospinal fluid

Calcium	$1.1-1.3\ \text{mmol/l}$
Chloride	$120-130\ \text{mmol/l}$
Potassium	$2.4-3.2\ \text{mmol/l}$
Sodium	$100-250\ \text{mmol/l}$
Glucose	$3-4.5\ \text{mmol/l}$
Protein	$20-30\ \text{mmol/l}$

Urine

Electrolytes	
calcium	2.5–7.5 mmol/24 h
chloride	50–250 mmol/24 h
potassium	40–120 mmol/24 h
sodium	100–250 mmol/24 h
17-Ketosteroids	
males	10–30 mg/24 h
females	5–15 mg/24 h
Reaction (pH)	4.5–7.5
Volume	0.5–3 l/24 h
Urea	250–300 mmol/24 h
Urea clearance	50–100 ml blood/min
Protein	< 150 mg/24 h

Faeces

Total fat	10–20% w/v
Free fatty acid	7.5–15% w/v
Neutral fat	2.5–5% w/v

Gastric secretion

Fasting volume	10–60 ml/h
pH	0.9–1.5
basal concentration	25 mmol/l
maximum pentagastrin stim.	50 mmol/h

4   Fractions and multiples

Fraction	Prefix	Symbol	Multiple	Prefix	Symbol
10^{-1}	deci	d	10	deca	da
10^{-2}	centi	c	10^2	hecto	H
10^{-3}	milli	m	10^3	kilo	K
10^{-6}	micro	μ	10^6	mega	M
10^{-9}	nano	n			
10^{-12}	pico	p			
10^{-15}	femto	f			

Conversion tables

Pressure			Energy		
mmHg	**kPa**		**kcal**	**kJ**	
1	0.13		1	0.0042	
10	1.33		100	0.42	
20	2.67		200	0.84	
30	4.00		300	1.26	
40	5.33		400	1.67	
50	6.67		500	2.09	
60	8.00		600	2.51	
70	9.33		700	2.93	
80	10.67		800	3.35	
90	12.00		900	3.77	
100	13.33		1000	4.19	
110	14.67		2000	8.37	
120	16.00		3000	12.56	
130	17.33				
140	18.67				
150	20.00				

5 Body mass index (BMI)

The optimum body weight for maximum longevity, based on life-insurance statistics, is arrived at using the body mass index (BMI), which is calculated as:

$$\frac{\text{Weight (kg)}}{\text{Height}^2 \text{ (m)}}$$

A BMI of 18–25 is considered to be the desirable range for both men and women. A BMI between 25 and 30 represents Grade I obesity; 30–40, Grade II; and upwards of 40, Grade III (Garrow JS (1981) *Treat obesity seriously: a clinical manual*, pp. 27–9, Churchill Livingstone, Edinburgh). BMI can also be expressed as percent body fat using a variety of simple prediction equations. For example:

Males: % fat = (1.281 BMI) − 10.13

Females: % fat = (1.480 BMI) − 7.0

Appendix 2:
USEFUL NURSING AND OTHER HEALTH-CARE ORGANIZATION ADDRESSES

American Nurses Association (ANA)
600 Maryland Avenue, SW, Suite 100 West, Washington DC 20024, USA
Web site: http.//www.nursingworld. org

British Medical Association (BMA)
BMA House, Tavistock Square, London WC1H 9JP, UK
Web site: http://www.bma.org.uk

British Red Cross
Information Services, 9 Grosvenor Crescent, London SW1X 7EJ, UK
Web site: http://www.redcross.org.uk

Chartered Society of Physiotherapy
14 Bedford Row, London WC1R 4ED, UK
Web site: http://www.csp.org.uk

College of Occupational Therapists
106–114 Borough High Street, Southwark, London SE1 1LB, UK
Web site: http://www.cot.org.uk

Commission for Health Improvement (CHI)
Finsbury Tower, 103-105 Bunhill Row, London EC1Y 8TG, UK
Web site: http://www.chi.nhs.uk

Commonwealth Nurses Federation
c/o Royal College of Nursing, 20 Cavendish Square, London W1M 0AB, UK
Web site: http://www the commonwealth.org

Community Practitioners' and Health Visitors' Association (CPHVA)
40 Bermondsey Street, London SE1 3UD, UK
Web site: http://www.msfcphva.org/

Department of Health
Richmond House, 79 Whitehall, London SW1A 2NL, UK
Web site: http://www.doh.gov.uk/

Department of Health, Social Services and Public Safety
Castle Buildings, Stormont, Belfast BT 4 3SJ, UK
Web site: http://www.dhsspsni.gov.uk/

Florence Nightingale Foundation
Suite 3, 38 Ebury Street, London SW1W 0LU, UK
Web site: http://www.florence-nightin-gale-foundation.org.uk/

Foundation of Nursing Studies
32 Buckingham Palace Road, London
SW1W 0RE, UK
Web site: http://www.fons.org/

General Medical Council
178 Great Portland Street, London
W1W 5JE, UK
Web site: http://www.gmc-uk.org/

Health Development Agency
Holborn Gate, 330 High Holborn,
London WC1V 7BA, UK
Web site: http://www.hda-online.org.uk

Health Service Ombudsman England
Millbank Tower, Millbank, London
SW1P 4QP, UK
Web site: http://www.parliament.
ombudsman.org.uk

International Council of Nurses
3, Place Jean Marteau, 1201 Geneva,
Switzerland
E-mail: icn@icn.ch
Web site: http://www.icn.ch

Irish College of Psychiatrists
123 St Stephen's Green, Dublin 2,
Ireland
Web site: http://www.irishpsychiatry.
com/

King's Fund
11–13 Cavendish Square, London W1G
0AN, UK
Web site: http://www.kingsfund.org.uk

Medical Research Council (MRC)
20 Park Crescent, London W1B 1AL,
UK
Web site: http://www.mrc.ac.uk

National Care Standards Commission
St Nicholas Building, St Nicholas
Street, Newcastle upon Tyne NE1 1NB,
UK
Web site: http://www.carestandards.org.
uk

National Institute for Clinical Excellence (NICE)
Web site: http://www.nice.org.uk/

NHS 24
Web site: http://www.nhs24.com/

NHS Direct
Web site: http://www.nhsdirect.nhs.uk/

NHS Direct Wales
Web site: http://www.nhsdirect.
wales.nhs.uk/

NHS Scotland
Web site: http://www.show.scot.nhs.uk/

NHS Wales
Web site: http://www.wales.nhs.uk/

Nursing and Midwifery Council (NMC)
23 Portland Place, London W1B 1PZ,
UK
Web site: http://www.nmc-uk.org

Office for National Statistics
1 Drummond Gate, London SW1V
2QQ, UK
Web site: http://www.statistics.gov.uk/

Royal College of General Practitioners
14 Princes Gate, Hyde Park, London SW7 1PU, UK
Web site: http://www.rcgp.org.uk/

Royal College of Midwives
15 Mansfield Street, London W1G 9NH, UK
Web site: http://www.rcm.org.uk

Royal College of Nursing
20 Cavendish Square, London W1G 0RN, UK
Web site: http://www.rcn.org.uk

Royal College of Obstetricians and Gynaecologists
27 Sussex Place, Regent's Park, London NW1 4RG, UK
Web site: http://www.rcog.org.uk/

Royal College of Pathologists
2 Carlton House Terrace, London SW1Y 5AF, UK
Web site: http://www.rcpath.org/

Royal College of Physicians
11 St Andrews Place, Regent's Park, London NW1 4LE, UK
Web site: http://www.rcplondon.ac.uk/

Royal College of Physicians and Surgeons of Glasgow
232–242 St Vincent Street, Glasgow G2 5RJ, Scotland, UK
Web site: http://www.rcpsglasg.ac.uk/

Royal College of Physicians of Edinburgh
9 Queen Street, Edinburgh EH2 1JQ, Scotland, UK
Web site: http://www.rcpe.ac.uk/

Royal College of Psychiatrists
17 Belgrave Square, London SW1X 8PG, UK
Web site: http://www.rcpsych.ac.uk/

Royal College of Psychiatrists Scottish Division
9 Queen Street, Edinburgh EH2 1JQ, Scotland, UK
Web site: http://www.rcpsych.ac.uk/college/division/scot.htm

Royal College of Surgeons in Ireland
123 St Stephen's Green, Dublin 2, Ireland
Web site: http://www.rcsi.ie/index.asp

Royal College of Surgeons of Edinburgh
Nicolson Street, Edinburgh EH8 9DW, Scotland, UK
Web site: http://www.rcsed.ac.uk/content/

Royal College of Surgeons of England
35–43 Lincoln's Inn Fields, London WC2A 3PE, UK
Web site: http://www.rcseng.ac.uk/

Royal Society for the Promotion of Health
38A St. George's Drive, London SW1V 4BH, UK
Web site: http://www.rsph.org/

Royal Society of Medicine
1 Wimpole Street, London W1G 0AE, UK
Web site: http://www.rsm.ac.uk/

Tavistock Institute
Tavistock House, 30 Tabernacle Street, London EC2A 4UE, UK
Web site: http://www.tavinstitute.org/index.php

UNISON
1 Mabledon Place, London WC1H 9AJ, UK
Web site: http://www.unison.org.uk

Welsh Division of Royal College of Psychiatrists
Postgraduate Centre, Whitchurch Hospital, Cardiff CF4 7XB, Wales, UK
Web site: http://www.rcpsych.ac.uk/college/division/welsh.htm#about

World Health Organization (WHO)
Avenue Appia 20, CH-1211 Geneva 27, Switzerland
Web site: http://www.who.int/en

Voluntary Organizations and Support Groups

There are numerous voluntary agencies in the field of health and social care and they can provide valuable information.

Contact addresses, e-mail and telephone numbers can be found by searching for them on the World Wide Web using a search engine such as Google (http://www.google.com) or Dogpile (http://www.dogpile.co.uk). Alternatively, you can seek information from local sources such as the telephone directory, Yellow Pages (http://www.yellow.co.uk), libraries, Social Services, or the Citizen's Advice Bureau.

Appendix 3:
NURSING AND OTHER JOURNALS

Each journal has the following information: the title, frequency of publication, publisher and web address.

1 General journals

Advances in Nursing Science
(Quarterly): Lippincott, Williams and Wilkins, USA
http://www.ans-info.net

American Journal of Nursing
(Monthly): Lippincott, Williams and Wilkins, USA
http://www.ajnonline.com

Annual Review of Nursing Research
(Yearly): Springer Publishing Co., USA
springerpub.com/store/ARNR.html

Applied Nursing Research
(Quarterly): WB Saunders, USA
www2.us.elsevierhealth.com

Australian Journal of Advanced Nursing
(Quarterly): Australian Nursing Federation, Australia
http://www.anf.org.au/pubs_ajan/pubs_ajan_guide.html

Australian Nurses Journal
(Monthly): Australian Nursing Federation, Australia
http://www.anf.org.au

British Journal of Nursing
(Fortnightly): Mark Allen Publishing, UK
http://www.britishjournalofnursing.com

Canadian Journal of Nursing Research
McGill University, Canada
http://www.cjnr.nursing.mcgill.ca

Canadian Nurse and Infirmière Canadienne
Canadian Nurses Association, Canada
http://www.infirmiere-canadienne.com

Evidence-Based Nursing
(Quarterly): RCN Publishing, UK
http://www.evidencebasednursing.com

International Journal of Nursing Studies
(Eight issues per year): Elsevier, UK
http://www.elsevier.com/locate/ijnurstu

International Nursing Review
(Quarterly): International Council of Nurses and Blackwell Science, UK
http://www.icn.ch

Journal of Advanced Nursing
(Twice monthly): Blackwell Publishing, UK
http://www.journalofadvancednursing.com

Nursing
(Monthly): Springhouse Corporation
and Nursing Center, USA
http://www.nursingcenter.com/library/
journals

Nursing Clinics Of North America
(Quarterly): WB Saunders, USA

Nursing Forum
(Quarterly): Nurscom Publications,
USA
http://www.nursecominc.com

Nursing Journal of India
(Monthly): Trained Nurses
Association, India

Nursing News
(Monthly): South African Nursing
Association, South Africa
http://www.sanc.co.za

Nursing Outlook
(Bi-monthly): Elsevier, USA
www2.us.elsevierhealth.com

Nurse Researcher
(Quarterly): RCN Publishing, UK
www.nurseresearcher.co.uk

Nursing Standard
(Weekly): Royal College of Nursing
Publishing, UK
http://www.nursing-standard.co.uk

Nursing Times
(Weekly): Macmillan, UK
http://www.nursingtimes.net

Professional Nurse
(Monthly): Mosby-Year Book Europe

RN: National Magazine for Nurses
(Monthly): Medical Economics, USA

http://www.rnweb.com/be_core/r/
index.jsp

*Research and Theory for Nursing
Practice*
(formerly *Scholarly Inquiry for
Nursing Practice*)
(Quarterly): Springer Publishing Co.,
USA http://www.springerpub.com/
journals/nursing/research_theory.html

World Of Irish Nursing
(Monthly): Irish Nurses Organization,
Eire
http://www.ino.ie

2   Specialist journals

Accident and Emergency Nursing
(Quarterly): Elsevier, UK
http://www.harcourt-
international.com/journals/aaen

*American Association of Nurse
Anaesthetics (AANA) Journal*
(Bi-monthly): American Association
of Nurse Anaesthetics, USA
http://www.aana.com

*American Association of Occupational
Health Nurses (AAOHN)*
(Monthly): AAOHN, USA
http://www.aaohn.org/practice/journal

British Journal of Community Nursing
(Monthly): Mark Allen Publishing, UK
http://www.britishjournalof
communitynursing.com

British Journal of Learning Disabilities
(Quarterly): Blackwell Publishing,UK
www.blackwell-synergy.com

British Journal of Midwifery
Mark Allen Publishing, UK
http://www.britishjournalofmidwifery.
com/

Cancer Nursing
(Bi-monthly): Lipincott, Williams and
Wilkins, USA
http://www.cancernursingonline.com

*Complementary Therapies in Nursing
and Midwifery*
(Quarterly): Elsevier, UK
http://www.harcourt-
international.com/journals/ctnm

European Journal of Cancer Care
(Quarterly): Blackwell Publishing,
UK
www.blackwell-synergy.com

*European Journal of Cardiovascular
Nursing*
Elsevier, UK
http://www.elsevier.com/locate/
jnlabr/ejcn

Geriatric Nursing
(Bi-monthly): Mosby, USA
www2.us.elsevierhealth.com

Health Expectations
Blackwell Publishing, UK
http://www.blackwell-synergy.com

*Health and Social Care in the
Community*
(Bi-monthly): Blackwell
Publishing, UK
http://www.blackwell-synergy.com

Intensive and Critical Care Nursing
(Bi-monthly): Elsevier, UK
http://www.harcourt-
international.com/journals/iccn/

*International Journal of Mental
Health Nursing*
Blackwell Publishing, Australia
www.blackwell-synergy.com

*International Journal of Nursing
Practice*
Blackwell Publishing, UK
www.blackwell-synergy.com

*International Journal of Trauma
Nursing*
(Quarterly): Mosby, USA
http://www2.us.elsevierhealth.com

Journal of Clinical Nursing
(Bi-monthly): Blackwell
Publishing, UK
http://www.blackwell-synergy.com

*Journal of Evaluation in Clinical
Practice*
(Quarterly): Blackwell Publishing,UK
http://www.blackwell-synergy.com

Journal of Nursing Management
(Bi-monthly): Blackwell
Publishing, UK
http://www.blackwell-synergy.com

Journal of Pediatric Nursing
(Bi-monthly): WB Saunders, USA
www2.pediatricnursing.org

Journal of Professional Nursing
(Bi-monthly): WB Saunders, USA
www2.professionalnursing.org

*Journal of Psychiatric and Mental
Health Nursing*
(Bi-monthly): Blackwell Publishing,
UK
http://www.blackwell-synergy.com

Journal of Vascular Nursing
(Quarterly): Elsevier, USA
www2.us.elsevierhealth.com

Learning in Health and Social Care
(Quarterly): Blackwell Publishing, UK
http://www.blackwell-synergy.com

Midwifery
(Quarterly): Elsevier, UK
http://www.harcourt-
international.com/journals/midw

NT Research
EMAP Publications, UK
http://www.NursingTimes.net

Nurse Education in Practice
(Quarterly): Elsevier, UK
http://www.harcourt-
international.com/journals/nepr

Nursing Education Perspectives
(Bi-monthly): National League of
Nursing, USA
http://www.nln.org/nlnjournal

Nurse Education Today
(Eight issues per year): Elsevier, UK
http://www.harcourt-
international.com/journals/net

Nurse Educator
(Bi-monthly): Lippincott, Williams
and Wilkins, USA
www.nurseeducatoronline.com

Nursing and Health Sciences
(Quarterly): Blackwell Publishing,
UK
http://www.blackwell-synergy.com

Nursing in Critical Care
Blackwell Publishing, UK
http://www.blackwell-synergy.com

Nursing Inquiry
(Quarterly): Blackwell Publishing,
Australia
http://www.blackwell-synergy.com

Nursing Older People
(Ten times a year): RCN Publishing,
UK
http://www.nursingolderpeople.co.uk

Nursing Philosophy
(2–3 times a year): Blackwell
Publishing, UK
http://www.blackwell-synergy.com

Nursing Research
(Bi-monthly): Lippincott, Williams
and Wilkins, USA
http://www.nursingresearchonline.com

Paediatric Nursing
(Ten times a year): RCN Publishing,
UK
http://www.paediatricnursing.co.uk

Public Health Nursing
(Bi-monthly): Blackwell Publishing,
UK
http://www.blackwell-synergy.com

*Scandinavian Journal of Caring
Sciences*
(Quarterly): Blackwell Publishing,
UK
http://www.blackwell-synergy.com

Sociology of Health and Illness
(Bi-monthly): Blackwell Publishing,
UK
http://www.blackwell-synergy.com

Appendix 4:
NURSING AND MIDWIFERY COUNCIL *CODE OF PROFESSIONAL CONDUCT*

Code of professional conduct

This *Code of professional conduct* was published by the Nursing and Midwifery Council in April 2002 and it came into effect on 1 June 2002.

As a registered nurse, midwife, or health visitor, you are personally accountable for your practice. In caring for patients and clients, you must:

- respect the patient or client as an individual
- obtain consent before you give any treatment or care
- protect confidential information
- co-operate with others in the team
- maintain your professional knowledge and competence
- be trustworthy
- act to identify and minimize risk to patients and clients.

These are the shared values of all the United Kingdom health-care regulatory bodies.

1 Introduction

1.1 The purpose of the *Code of professional conduct* is to:

- inform the professions of the standard of professional conduct required of them in the exercise of their professional accountability and practice
- inform the public, other professions, and employers of the standard of professional conduct that they can expect of a registered practitioner.

1.2 As a registered nurse, midwife, or health visitor, you must:

- protect and support the health of individual patients and clients
- protect and support the health of the wider community
- act in such a way that justifies the trust and confidence the public have in you
- uphold and enhance the good reputation of the professions.

1.3 You are personally accountable for your practice. This means that you are answerable for your actions and omissions, regardless of advice or directions from another professional.

1.4 You have a duty of care to your patients and clients, who are entitled to receive safe and competent care.

1.5 You must adhere to the laws of the country in which you are practising.

2 As a registered nurse, midwife, or health visitor, you must respect the patient or client as an individual

2.1 You must recognize and respect the role of patients and clients as partners in their care and the contribution they can make to it. This involves identifying their preferences regarding care and respecting these within the limits of professional practice, existing legislation, resources, and the goals of the therapeutic relationship.

2.2 You are personally accountable for ensuring that you promote and protect the interests and dignity of patients and clients, irrespective of gender, age, race, ability, sexuality, economic status, lifestyle, culture and religious or political beliefs.

2.3 You must, at all times, maintain appropriate professional boundaries in the relationships you have with patients and clients. You must ensure that all aspects of the relationship focus exclusively upon the needs of the patient or client.

2.4 You must promote the interests of patients and clients. This includes helping individuals and groups gain access to health and social care, information and support relevant to their needs.

2.5 You must report to a relevant person or authority, at the earliest possible time, any conscientious objection that may be relevant to your professional practice. You must continue to provide care to the best of your ability until alternative arrangements are implemented.

3 As a registered nurse, midwife, or health visitor, you must obtain consent before you give any treatment or care

3.1 All patients and clients have a right to receive information about their condition. You must be sensitive to their needs and respect the wishes of those who refuse or are unable to receive information about their condition. Information should be accurate, truthful, and presented in such a way as to make it easily understood. You may need to seek legal or professional advice, or guidance from your employer, in relation to the giving or withholding of consent.

3.2 You must respect patients' and clients' autonomy – their right to decide whether or not to undergo any health care intervention – even where a refusal may result in harm or death to themselves or a fetus, unless a court of law orders to the contrary. This right is protected in law, although in circumstances where the health of the fetus would be severely compromised by any refusal to give consent, it would be appropriate to discuss this matter fully within the team, and possibly to seek external advice and guidance (see clause 4).

3.3   When obtaining valid consent, you must be sure that it is:

- given by a legally competent person
- given voluntarily
- informed.

3.4   You should presume that every patient and client is legally competent unless otherwise assessed by a suitably qualified practitioner. A patient or client who is legally competent can understand and retain treatment information and can use it to make an informed choice.

3.5   Those who are legally competent may give consent in writing, orally or by co-operation. They may also refuse consent. You must ensure that all your discussions and associated decisions relating to obtaining consent are documented in the patient's or client's health-care records.

3.6   When patients or clients are no longer legally competent and thus have lost the capacity to consent to or refuse treatment and care, you should try to find out whether they have previously indicated preferences in an advance statement. You must respect any refusal of treatment or care given when they were legally competent, provided that the decision is clearly applicable to the present circumstances and that there is no reason to believe that they have changed their minds. When such a statement is not available, the patients' or clients' wishes, if known, should be taken into account. If these wishes are not known, the criteria for treatment must be that it is in their best interests.

3.7   The principles of obtaining consent apply equally to those people who have a mental illness. Whilst you should be involved in their assessment, it will also be necessary to involve relevant people close to them; this may include a psychiatrist. When patients and clients are detained under statutory powers (mental health acts), you must ensure that you know the circumstances and safeguards needed for providing treatment and care without consent.

3.8   In emergencies where treatment is necessary to preserve life, you may provide care without patients' or clients' consent, if they are unable to give it, provided you can demonstrate that you are acting in their best interests.

3.9   No-one has the right to give consent on behalf of another competent adult. In relation to obtaining consent for a child, the involvement of those with parental responsibility in the consent procedure is usually necessary, but will depend on the age and understanding of the child. If the child is under the age of 16 in England and Wales, 12 in Scotland and 17 in Northern Ireland, you must be aware of legislation and local protocols relating to consent.

3.10   Usually the individual performing a procedure should be the person to obtain the patient's or client's consent. In certain circumstances, you may seek consent on behalf of colleagues if you have been specially trained for that specific area of practice.

3.11 You must ensure that the use of complementary or alternative therapies is safe and in the interests of patients and clients. This must be discussed with the team as part of the therapeutic process and the patient or client must consent to their use.

4 As a registered nurse, midwife, or health visitor, you must co-operate with others in the team

4.1 The team includes the patient or client, the patient's or client's family, informal carers and health and social care professionals in the National Health Service, independent and voluntary sectors.

4.2 You are expected to work co-operatively within teams and to respect the skills, expertise and contributions of your colleagues. You must treat them fairly and without discrimination.

4.3 You must communicate effectively and share your knowledge, skill, and expertise with other members of the team as required for the benefit of patients and clients.

4.4 Health-care records are a tool of communication within the team. You must ensure that the health-care record for the patient or client is an accurate account of treatment, care planning, and delivery. It should be consecutive, written with the involvement of the patient or client wherever practicable and completed as soon as possible after an event has occurred. It should provide clear evidence of the care planned, the decisions made, the care delivered, and the information shared.

4.5 When working as a member of a team, you remain accountable for your professional conduct, any care you provide, and any omission on your part.

4.6 You may be expected to delegate care delivery to others who are not registered nurses or midwives. Such delegation must not compromise existing care but must be directed to meeting the needs and serving the interests of patients and clients. You remain accountable for the appropriateness of the delegation, for ensuring that the person who does the work is able to do it and that adequate supervision or support is provided.

4.7 You have a duty to co-operate with internal and external investigations.

5 As a registered nurse, midwife, or health visitor, you must protect confidential information

5.1 You must treat information about patients and clients as confidential and use it only for the purposes for which it was given. As it is impractical to obtain consent every time you need to share information with others, you should ensure that patients and clients understand that some information may be made available to other members of the team involved in the delivery of care. You must guard against breaches of confidentiality by protecting information from improper disclosure at all times.

5.2 You should seek patients' and clients' wishes regarding the sharing of information with their family and others. When a patient or client is considered incapable of giving permission, you should consult relevant colleagues.

5.3 If you are required to disclose information outside the team that will have personal consequences for patients or clients, you must obtain their consent. If the patient or client withholds consent, or if consent cannot be obtained for whatever reason, disclosures may be made only where:

- they can be justified in the public interest (usually where disclosure is essential to protect the patient or client or someone else from the risk of significant harm)
- they are required by law or by order of a court.

5.4 Where there is an issue of child protection, you must act at all times in accordance with national and local policies.

6 As a registered nurse, midwife, or health visitor, you must maintain your professional knowledge and competence

6.1 You must keep your knowledge and skills up-to-date throughout your working life. In particular, you should take part regularly in learning activities that develop your competence and performance.

6.2 To practise competently, you must possess the knowledge, skills, and abilities required for lawful, safe, and effective practice without direct supervision. You must acknowledge the limits of your professional competence and only undertake practice and accept responsibilities for those activities in which you are competent.

6.3 If an aspect of practice is beyond your level of competence or outside your area of registration, you must obtain help and supervision from a competent practitioner until you and your employer consider that you have acquired the requisite knowledge and skill.

6.4 You have a duty to facilitate students of nursing, midwifery, and health visiting and others to develop their competence.

6.5 You have a responsibility to deliver care based on current evidence, best practice and, where applicable, validated research when it is available.

7 As a registered nurse, midwife, or health visitor, you must be trustworthy

7.1 You must behave in a way that upholds the reputation of the professions. Behaviour that compromises this reputation may call your registration into question even if is not directly connected to your professional practice.

7.2   You must ensure that your registration status is not used in the promotion of commercial products or services, declare any financial or other interests in relevant organizations providing such goods or services, and ensure that your professional judgement is not influenced by any commercial considerations.

7.3   When providing advice regarding any product or service relating to your professional role or area of practice, you must be aware of the risk that, on account of your professional title or qualification, you could be perceived by the patient or client as endorsing the product. You should fully explain the advantages and disadvantages of alternative products so that the patient or client can make an informed choice. Where you recommend a specific product, you must ensure that your advice is based on evidence and is not for your own commercial gain.

7.4   You must refuse any gift, favour, or hospitality that might be interpreted, now or in the future, as an attempt to obtain preferential consideration.

7.5   You must neither ask for nor accept loans from patients, clients, or their relatives and friends.

8   As a registered nurse, midwife, or health visitor, you must act to identify and minimize the risk to patients and clients

8.1   You must work with other members of the team to promote health-care environments that are conducive to safe, therapeutic, and ethical practice.

8.2   You must act quickly to protect patients and clients from risk if you have good reason to believe that you or a colleague, from your own or another profession, may not be fit to practise for reasons of conduct, health, or competence. You should be aware of the terms of legislation that offer protection for people who raise concerns about health and safety issues.

8.3   Where you cannot remedy circumstances in the environment of care that could jeopardize standards of practice, you must report them to a senior person with sufficient authority to manage them and also, in the case of midwifery, to the supervisor of midwives. This must be supported by a written record.

8.4   When working as a manager, you have a duty toward patients and clients, colleagues, the wider community, and the organization in which you and your colleagues work. When facing professional dilemmas, your first consideration in all activities must be the interests and safety of patients and clients.

8.5   In an emergency, in or outside the work setting, you have a professional duty to provide care. The care provided would be judged against what could reasonably be expected from someone with your knowledge, skills, and abilities when placed in those particular circumstances.

Glossary

Accountable Responsible for something or to someone.
Care To provide help or comfort.

Competent Possessing the skills and abilities required for lawful, safe and effective professional practice without direct supervision.

Patient and client Any individual or group using a health service.

Reasonable The case of Bolam *v.* Friern Hospital Management Committee (1957) produced the following definition of what is reasonable.

The test is the standard of the ordinary skilled man exercising and professing to have that special skill. A man need not possess the highest expert skill at the risk of being found negligent ... it is sufficient if he exercises the skill of an ordinary man exercising that particular art.

This definition is supported and clarified by the case of Bolitho *v.* City and Hackney Health Authority (1997).

Further information

This *Code of professional conduct* is available on the Nursing and Midwifery Council's website at http://www.nmc-uk.org. Printed copies can be obtained by writing to the Publications Department, Nursing and Midwifery Council, 23 Portland Place, London W1B 1PZ, by fax on 020 7436 2924 or by e-mail at publications@nmc-uk.org. A wide range of NMC standards and guidance publications expand upon and develop many of the professional issues and themes identified in the *Code of professional conduct*. All are available on the NMC's website. A list of current NMC publications is available either on the website or on request from the Publications Department as above.

Enquiries about the issues addressed in the *Code of professional conduct* should be directed in the first instance to the NMC's professional advice service at the address above, by e-mail at advice@nmc-uk.org, by telephone on 020 7333 6541/6550/6553 or by fax on 020 7333 6538.

The Nursing and Midwifery Council will keep this *Code of professional conduct* under review and any comments, suggestions or requests for further clarification are welcome, both from practitioners and members of the public. These should be addressed to the Director of Policy and Standards, NMC, 23 Portland Place, London W1B 1PZ.

Summary

As a registered nurse, midwife or health visitor, you must

- respect the patient or client as an individual
- obtain consent before you give any treatment or care
- co-operate with others in the team
- protect confidential information
- maintain your professional knowledge and competence
- be trustworthy
- act to identify and minimize the risk to patients and clients.

Appendix 5:
EMERGENCY CARE

Nurses, by the very nature of their work, will at some time in their life need to provide emergency care to a patient or to a patient's relative. Emergency care goes beyond first aid and can be required in any setting (hospital, the community, or the GP's surgery). Nurses should take every opportunity to maintain their knowledge and update skills in this area of patient care.

In any emergency situation the nurse must follow some basic rules:

- Look after yourself; do not put yourself in danger.
- Obtain a history from the patient, relatives, or people at the scene.
- Use signs and symptoms to guide your assessment.
- Only do what you have to do to stabilize the patient's condition and prevent the situation becoming worse.
- Assess and intervene in a logical manner. Perform a rapid primary survey which includes assessment and life-saving intervention for airway, breathing and circulation. The secondary survey includes observation of vital signs (pulse, blood pressure, and respiration) and a head-to-toe assessment. Once the secondary survey is complete and problems identified, intervention can occur.

The unconscious patient

Many medical and traumatic conditions can cause a decrease in the patient's conscious level (see Disorders of consciousness). While not being able to prevent all patients from becoming unconscious, the nurse can, in some instances, prevent this situation from occurring (hypoglycaemia is a typical example). Unconsciousness is an abnormal state resulting from an interruption of the brain's normal activity. The patient does not respond to normal stimuli. An unconscious patient is at risk due to a loss of the body's reflexes.

Presentation
Patients with altered conscious levels will present in varying ways. Some may suddenly appear drowsy, confused, or disorientated. Others may fall to the ground and make no response to verbal or painful stimuli.

Assessment
The level of patient response should be assessed rapidly and life-saving intervention must occur immediately a problem is identified. Use of the 'AVPU' aide-memoir allows for quick assessment:

A   is the patient Alert?
V   does the patient only respond to Voice (speak loud and clear)?
P   does the patient only respond to Pain?
U   is the patient Unresponsive?

Also check for any spinal/neck injury/instability.
If there is no response from the patient, IMMEDIATELY go through the ABC formula:

- *Assess the airway.* Partial or total obstruction can be caused by the tongue, loose teeth, other foreign objects or fluid (blood/vomit). Total obstruction will cause a silent airway. Partial obstruction causes a noise as air passes by the obstruction (a noisy airway is an obstructed airway).
- *Assess breathing.* Look for chest movement. Listen for breath sounds. Feel for breath. If air is passing normally, when exhaled it will be felt on your hand or cheek.
- *Assess circulation.* Feel for the carotid pulse. Identify any major wounds.

Intervention

- *Airway.* Use of the jaw thrust will open a closed airway. Remove any foreign objects either manually or with the aid of a suction unit. (Portable suction units should be available for use in the GP's surgery or in the community.) Insertion of an oro-pharyngeal airway (Guedal) helps prevent the tongue obstructing the pharynx.
- *Breathing.* If breathing is absent, use positive-pressure ventilation. This is achieved by the mouth-to-mouth method, use of bag and mask, or the use of a double airway system (e.g. Brook's airway). If breathing is present, assess depth of breathing. If shallow, assist ventilation with the use of a bag and mask. If the patient is breathing normally, oxygen administration will be required.
- *Circulation.* If the carotid pulse is absent, it is essential that external cardiac compression be commenced immediately. Cover any major wounds with pressure dressings.

The unconscious patient who has a clear airway and is breathing should (unless injuries prevent) be placed on his or her side in the recovery position (see Fig. A1).

Cardiopulmonary resuscitation (CPR)

(Based on recommendations of the European Resuscitation Council http://www.er-c.edu/; for a full account, see the Resuscitation Council (UK) http://www.resus.org.uk. Other available sites (e.g. http://www.americanheart.org) may have subtle differences. Your country of residence predicts the site that should be accessed. See also http://omni.ac.uk/browse/mesh/c0007203L0007203.html./

Assessment criteria

- A patient suffering from cardiac arrest will suddenly collapse.
- There will be no response to verbal or pain stimuli.

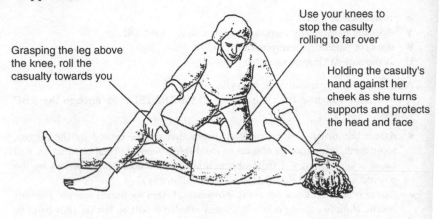

Grasping the leg above the knee, roll the casualty towards you

Use your knees to stop the casulty rolling to far over

Holding the casulty's hand against her cheek as she turns supports and protects the head and face

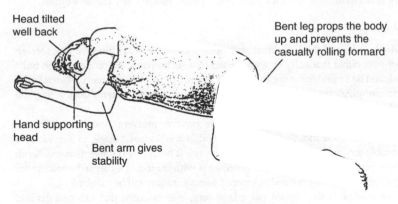

Head tilted well back

Bent leg props the body up and prevents the casualty rolling formard

Hand supporting head

Bent arm gives stability

The recovery position

- The skin will be pale or cyanosed.
- Breathing will be absent (in a witnessed arrest some respiratory effort may still be present).
- The major pulses (carotid or femoral) will be absent.

Performance criteria (Resuscitation Council Competencies in CPR 2000)

- Look for risks to self, the victim, and bystanders.
- Assess responsiveness.
- Position victim's head to ensure clear airway.
- Visible obstructions in the airway are sought and removed.
- Absence of normal breathing is established.
- Additional help is summoned as soon as possible.
- Victim is reassessed.

- Two rescuer breaths are given.
- Absence of circulation is established.
- Chest compressions are commenced with hands in the correct position on the sternum. 100 compressions per minute are recommended.
- CPR is continued with the correct ratio of compressions to rescuer breaths (15:2).

Intervention
If resuscitation is not commenced immediately, the brain will only survive for 2-4 minutes.

- Summon help (in hospital shout for help and direct respondent to use the emergency call system; in the community or GP surgery ask someone to call for an ambulance).
- Place the patient on a firm surface, establish a clear airway.
- Ventilate the patient's lungs twice (use mouth-to-mouth, bag and mask, or double airway, if it is available, always attach oxygen to bag and mask).

If you are alone:

- Commence cardiac massage, 15 compressions (place your middle finger on the xiphisternum and your index finger on the sternum; place the heel of your other hand on the sternum, just above your fingers; place the first hand on top of the hand on the sternum and leaning forward, with arms straight, compress the chest 4–5 cm).
- Ventilate the lungs twice (700–1000 ml per breath).
- Continue 15 to 2 ratio.
- Check carotid pulse; if this returns, continue with ventilation. Once breathing and circulation return, place the patient in the recovery position, administer oxygen and monitor progress.

If two persons are present:

- After the first two ventilations the second person should commence cardiac massage, 15 compressions.
- Ventilate the lungs once.
- Continue 15 to 2 ratio.

In the hospital setting, cardiac arrest equipment should be brought to the bedside, and in critical care areas, nurses should be taught to defibrillate.

Disorders of airway and breathing

Many problems of the airway or breathing can be dealt with by simple first aid intervention. For example, for *suffocation*, remove the physical barrier that is preventing air entering the system; for *smoke inhalation*, remove the patient from the scene and administer oxygen. Other disorders of the airway and breathing require more intervention. Two that can occur in any health-care setting are *choking* and an *acute asthmatic attack*.

Choking

In most cases this will be due to a foreign body becoming lodged in the air passages. In some instances the irritation from a foreign body (e.g. small fish bone) can cause muscular spasm and mucosal oedema.

Assessment

If the patient is coughing and is able to speak, the airway is not totally obstructed. If obstruction is present, the general signs are:

- difficulty with speaking and breathing
- reversed movement of the chest and abdomen: the chest wall will suck in and the abdomen will push out
- drawing in of the muscle of the chest wall, especially between ribs and the spaces above the clavicle and sterum
- cyanosis of lips, earlobes, and skin
- flaring of nostrils; this indicates severe asphyxia
- patient pointing to or grasping the throat.

Intervention

- If total obstruction has not occurred, reassure the patient. Help the patient bend forward. Using the flat of your hand, assist the coughing by applying five sharp blows between the patient's scapulae.
- If the problem is resolved, continue to monitor the patient and offer small sips of water.
- If there is total obstruction, give five sharp blows to the patient's back. If this fails to dislodge the foreign body use the abdominal thrust.
- Stand behind the patient, cradle the patient by interlocking your hands below the ribcage (epigastric area), pull sharply inwards and upwards. DO NOT COMPRESS THE RIBCAGE.
- If unsuccessful, try five times and rotate with five back blows.
- If the patient is or becomes unconscious, place the patient on the floor, kneel astride the patient and perform the abdominal thrust by placing the heel of one hand in the epigastric area and the other hand on top of the first. Press sharply inwards and upwards five times.

Asthma

Unfortunately, incorrect emergency care of a patient suffering an acute asthmatic episode is still a common occurrence.

Assessment

Respiratory distress is dependent on the degree of obstruction in the bronchioles. The patient will demonstrate:

- difficulty in breathing
- prolonged expiration
- respiratory wheeze

- distress and anxiety
- cyanosis.

Intervention

- Reassurance: a calm approach and the removal of other people will often help the individual become more relaxed.
- Help the patient sit upright; sitting upright allows for improved ventilation.
- If the patient has a relief inhaler, e.g. Ventolin, help the patient to use it. Preventative inhalers such as Intal will not be useful at this stage.

If relief does not occur:

- Administer oxygen (and nebulizer if available).
- In the community or surgery, send for an ambulance.
- DO NOT ASSUME THE PROBLEM WILL RESOLVE ITSELF.

Disorders of the circulation

Shock

The most common causes of shock in the pre-hospital situation are due to loss of body fluid (hypovolaemic shock) or cardiac disorders (cardiogenic shock). Nurses may, on rare occasions, witness anaphylactic shock and septicaemic shock. Emergency care of the patient in shock must relate to the cause. In hypovolaemic shock the aim must be to reduce the fluid loss and allow the circulating blood to return to the heart and then to the vital organs. In cardiogenic shock there is no fluid loss but the heart is unable to cope with the circulating volume. Restricting blood flow to the heart can often help. In anaphylactic shock the aim is to reduce the allergic reaction and systemic vasodilation.

Assessment of hypovolaemic and cardiogenic shock

- Pale skin is mainly seen in the hypovolaemic patient. Grey 'ashen' skin with cyanosis of lips and earlobes is more likely to indicate cardiogenic shock.
- The skin becomes cold and wet (clammy).
- Nausea and possibly vomiting may occur.
- The patient may complain of thirst.
- Weakness, giddiness, restlessness, and confusion are common signs.
- The breathing pattern changes and may become rapid with air hunger developing.
- The pulse will become rapid and weak in hypovolaemic shock but can become slow and irregular in cardiogenic shock.
- External signs (e.g. wounds, burns) may be present, or the patient may complain of pain, for example in the abdomen or chest.

Intervention

- Loosen tight clothing.
- Reassure the patient; explain to the patient that co-operation is essential.

- Administer high percentage oxygen if available.
- Protect the patient from the cold but do not overheat (overheating encourages peripheral vasodilation and reduces blood supply to the brain and other vital organs).
- Do not give fluids or food (due to reduced gastrointestinal activity, vomiting can occur).

Hypovolaemic shock

- Lie the patient down (improves venous return).
- Apply pressure dressings to any external wounds.
- Raise the legs to further improve venous return.
- Prepare for intravenous fluid replacement.

Cardiogenic shock

- Sit the patient in the semi-recumbent or upright position (this reduces venous return and aids breathing).
- If a coronary thrombosis is suspected (acute chest pain described as tight or vice-like and not related to movement or breathing) and there is no history of allergy to aspirin, bleeding disorder or peptic ulceration, give one aspirin tablet to the patient to chew. (Aspirin reduces the risk of myocardial infarction by assisting the breakdown of the coronorary thrombosis.)

Anaphylactic shock

This is due to an exaggerated allergic reaction. It can become life threatening.

Assessment

- A generalized skin itching and urticarial rash occurs.
- Respiratory wheeze, similar to the asthmatic attack, can be heard.
- Oedema, especially of the face and tongue, causes swelling and puts the airway at risk.
- A rapid pulse and low blood pressure causes general signs of shock.
- The patient can become unconscious and may suffer a cardiac arrest.

Intervention

- Summon help.
- If the patient is unconscious, but breathing, place the patient in the recovery position.
- Give adrenaline 1/1000 IM (local protocol should allow this without waiting for medical presence).
- Administer high percentage oxygen.

Fainting

Unlike shock this is simply a temporary reduction of blood flow to the brain.

Assessment

- The patient becomes giddy and complains of feeling light headed.
- Unconsciousness can occur within seconds.
- The patients skin becomes pale and often wet.
- The pulse rate is slow (radial pulse may be absent).

Intervention

- If the patient is feeling faint, either lay the patient flat or place the head between the knees. Do not attempt to walk the patient out to the fresh air.
- If the patient is unconscious, lay the patient flat, assess the airway. Recovery should occur within a few minutes. If unconsciousness persists, place the patient in the recovery position and summon further assistance (ambulance or the doctor).
- Do not use any inhalation stimulant. Do not sit the patient up until fully recovered.

Bleeding

Bleeding occurs either externally or internally.

Assessment

- Internal bleeding cannot be seen and therefore the history and signs of shock will be your only assessment tool.
- External bleeding can be seen, clothes should be removed or moved to allow assessment of the wound.
- Always look for any foreign body in the wound.
- Small puncture wounds (stab wounds, high velocity bullet wounds, etc.) may look innocent but extensive internal damage can occur.

Intervention
Internal bleeding:

- Treat the patient for hypovolaemic shock.

External bleeding:

- Apply pressure dressings to any wounds.
- If not fractured, arms and legs should be elevated.
- Foreign bodies should not be removed. Pad around the object. If necessary, treat the patient for hypovolaemic shock.
- Chest wounds should be covered with an airtight dressing, taped on three sides. One side should be left free in case of a developing tension pneumothorax. Monitor the patient's condition and support in the semi-recumbent position inclined towards the injured side.

- Abdominal wounds should be covered with a pressure dressing. If abdominal viscera are exposed, either cover with a polythene bag, cling film, or a warm saline dressing. If the wound is horizontal, raising and supporting the knees will help close the wound.
- Amputated limbs should be placed in a plastic bag and then surrounded with ice. The stump should have a dressing applied, using only sufficient pressure to prevent blood loss. (Pressure can damage nerve and vessel ends making replantation less successful.)
- Minor wounds should be cleaned and a suitable dressing applied.

Burning and scalds

Emergency care for burns and scalds is aimed at reducing the burning process, reducing pain, preventing infection, and, if severe, reducing the shock process. See http://www.prodigy.nhs.uk/guidance.asp?gt=burns%20and%20scalds#/

Assessment

- Assess the size of the burn/scald by using the 'rule of nines' calculation (see Fig. A2).
- If major burns have occurred, assess the airway, breathing, and circulation.
- Assess the depth of the burn. Redness without blistering. Partial skin loss, with or without blisters. Full thickness (black or white in colour and leathery in appearance).

Intervention

- Cool the burn or scald for 10 minutes or more using cold running water. Further irrigation will be required if a chemical is the cause of the burn.
- Remove rings, watches, etc. Only remove clothing if chemical contamination is suspected.
- Cover the burn or scald with cling film. Do not use cold soaks as this can lead to hypothermia.
- Do not apply any ointments or lotions. Do not burst blisters.
- Treat for shock.
- Minor burns/scalds can be cleaned and a non-adherent dressing applied.

Disorders of consciousness

As indicated at the beginning of this chapter, disorders of consciousness can be due to many causes. This section will deal with some of the more common causes. In the main, nursing assessment is restricted to determining the conscious level and intervention is aimed at airway maintenance.

General assessment

- If the patient is unconscious, assess the airway.

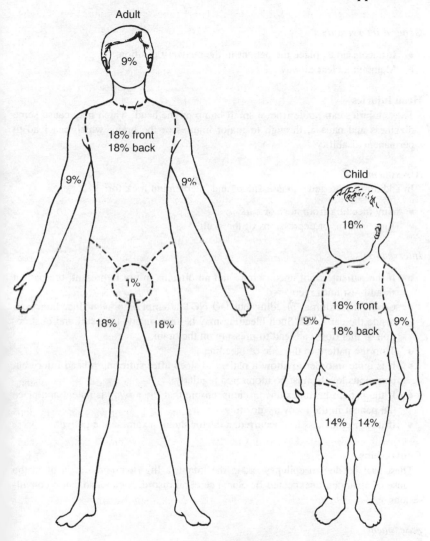

The rule of nines

- Obtain a history. Ensure you are not misled by things such as empty pill bottles. An empty pill bottle may indicate an overdose but it can also indicate that the patient has completed the course of medication.
- Assess the patient's level of consciousness.
- Look for any medic alert or other clues as to the problem.
- Examine the patient for any injuries.

General intervention

- If unconscious, place the patient in the recovery position.
- Maintain a clear airway.

Head injuries

These injuries can range from a small bump on the head, which may cause some dizziness and nausea, through to major injuries of the brain, which can lead to permanent disability.

Assessment

In addition to the general assessment and intervention look for:

- Any bleeding from nose or ears.
- Any bruising or depressions of the skull.

Intervention

- If the patient is not unconscious and no obvious injury is present, the patient should rest until recovered.
- Cover any external bleeding but DO NOT attempt to prevent bleeding from inside the ear canal. Such bleeding may be from inside the skull and obstruction of this flow can lead to pressure on the brain.
- Turn the patient to the side of bleeding.
- It is quite in order to allow a patient to sleep after suffering a head injury but conscious levels must be monitored regularly.
- If the patient becomes unconscious, ensure that the airway is patent and place the patient in the recovery position
- If unconsciousness has occurred, a doctor should examine the patient.

Convulsions

These can be due to epilepsy or, in the infant, a high temperature is often the cause of a sudden unexpected fit. Some cerebral disorders can also cause convulsions.

Assessment

- General assessment.
- Monitor the extent and duration of the fit.
- Identify whether any incontinence occurs.
- Monitor the airway.

Intervention

- The patient who is suffering a generalized convulsion should be protected from self-injury.

- Under no circumstances should limbs be held or objects used to lever the mouth open.
- Infantile convulsions should be treated with tepid sponging and, if the child is conscious, a dose of junior paracetamol may be given.
- Following the fit, if the patient is unconscious, place in the recovery position. Unless the patient is known to suffer from epilepsy an ambulance should be called or the patient seen by a doctor.

Cerebral vascular disorders

Cerebral thrombosis, while having a major effect on the patient's mobility, does not often cause unconsciousness. Cerebral haemorrhage is often the cause of unconsciousness and the patient is usually unresponsive even to painful stimuli.

Assessment

- General assessment
- The patient will become immobile. This immobility is usually unilateral.
- The patient will often lose the ability to speak.
- Unconsciousness can occur.

Intervention

- The patient's limbs should be supported.
- If conscious, the patient should be reassured in a sensible manner.
- There is no need to shout or talk slowly. The patient can often hear and understand, even though he or she may have lost the power of speech.
- If unconscious, the patient should be placed in the recovery position.

Hypoglycaemia

The most common occurrence of a hypoglycaemic episode is in a patient who is insulin dependent and has either missed a meal or over exercised. Either situation causes the blood sugar to drop below a level where normal cerebral activity can be maintained.

Assessment

- General assessment.
- The patient may present in a confused weak manner, become very agitated or aggressive and can often appear 'drunk'. Some patients will rapidly become unconscious.

Intervention

- If the patient is unconscious, maintain an open airway.
- If equipment is available, check the blood sugar level.
- If the patient is conscious, give an oral glucose if available, alternatively sugar, milk, chocolate, etc.

- If available, the unconscious patient can be given glucagon IM or glucose IV.
- See details on http://www.doh.gov.uk/nsf/diabetes/index.htm

Poisoning

Any poison can alter the conscious state. Most poisons are taken orally, though they can enter the body through inhalation, absorption, or injection.

Assessment

- General assessment.
- Is aimed at identifying the type of poison and the mode of entry.

Intervention

- DO NOT induce vomiting if a corrosive substance is involved or the patient is not in a clinical setting with medical presence (the patient may become unconscious and the airway compromised). To induce vomiting use Ipecac. For corrosive substances give the patient milk or water to drink.
- Patients who have inhaled poisons should be allowed fresh air and oxygen.
- Poisonous substances on the skin should be washed off with running water.
- Injected substances will be released more slowly if the limb is kept at rest.
- Antidotes may be required.
- DO NOT give oxygen if paraquat poisoning is suspected.

Injury to bone, muscle or joints

While the majority of injuries to bone, muscle, or joints are not life threatening, many of these injuries can cause permanent disability, especially if mishandled in the pre-hospital or hospital environment. Injury to some of the larger bones in the body, such as the femur or the pelvis, will cause major blood loss and lead to hypovolaemic shock.

Assessment

- History will often support the clinical findings. A history of direct or indirect trauma to the body, twisting of a limb, or over stretching of a limb can suggest injury to either bone, muscle, or joints. Compare with opposite limb to assess deformity.
- Pain at or near the site of injury. This pain may be described as a sudden sharp pain leading on to a very 'deep' intense pain.
- Inability to move the injured site or, in the lower limb, inability to weight bear indicates possible bone or joint damage.
- Swelling will occur at fracture sites or where muscle has been torn.
- Dislocated joints can often be seen to be out of place and the limb lies in an abnormal position.
- Nausea and vomiting often occur.

- Neurological abnormality, distal to the injury, indicates nerve damage at the site of injury. Absence of any abnormality does not in itself preclude a fracture. This is especially relevant in back injuries where a fracture of the vertebrae may be present but damage to the spinal cord has not occurred.
- Loss of a pulse and a degree of pallor distal to the injury indicate vascular involvement.

Intervention

- If a back injury is suspected, DO NOT MOVE the patient.
- Support the injured limb. This is best achieved by using simple items such as pillows, rolled blankets, etc. Only if you must move the patient should you consider splinting or tying limbs.
- If a compound fracture is present, the wound should be covered to prevent blood loss. If bone is exposed, padding should be placed around the bone and then the wound covered.
- Soft-tissue injuries such as sprains and strains should be treated with rest, ice packs, compression bandage, and elevation.

Conclusion

In the emergency care situation, it is essential that the nurse practises in a logical manner. Assessment and intervention of the *Airway, Breathing* and *Circulation* must always come first. Only after these three essential areas have been supported should further assessment and intervention be carried out.

Appendix 6:
UNDERSTANDING AND IMPLEMENTING CLINICAL NURSING RESEARCH

Introduction

The past century has seen dramatic changes in health care, with the rapid growth of care pathways, integrated care delivery systems, and changes in professional roles and boundaries, all of which require responsiveness from dynamic and critically reflective practitioners. In addition to local and national developments, globalization has led to widespread international progress in health-care education, practice, and research. This includes the drive towards evidence-based practice; the implementation of clinical and research governance frameworks in many countries; the changing roles of nurses; and the development of professional doctoral programmes for health-care practitioners. These and other initiatives converge to focus practitioners' attention on their unique role in establishing research-based practice.

It is almost three decades since Briggs (1972) and Chater (1975) argued that patient care should be based on defensible, research-based findings or, in other words, underpinned by scientific principles. However, as many writers have observed, this continues to be a challenge not only at a local level, but also nationally and internationally (Le May *et al.*, 1998; Tierney, 1998; Freshwater and Broughton, 2001; Freshwater and Rolfe, 2001).

Defining clinical research

There are numerous definitions of research to be found in the nursing and allied health-care literature, many of which centre around similar themes. An analysis of descriptions of research reveals that the generation of knowledge, using a variety of methodologies, is of high importance, although this is not always clearly related to potential outcomes. The difference that new knowledge might make to a practice-based discipline is not always evident, and it sometimes appears to be generated for its own sake.

The term 'clinical research' is commonly used in medical practice, but has not yet been accepted as normal within nursing. The main aim of clinical research in medicine is to identify best practice, with the purpose of adding to a general (generalizable) body of knowledge that can be shared with the larger scientific community as well as practitioners. Thus, clinical research in medicine has a tendency towards the quantitative end of the research methods continuum. However, not all research, or indeed practice, can be generalized. For this reason, nurse researchers have written at length about the importance of developing relevant and pragmatic approaches to research that reflect the real world of clinical nursing practice (see, for example, Rolfe, 1998; Freshwater and Rolfe, 2001; Holloway and Wheeler, 2002). This has had the effect of generating a long-running debate between two seemingly opposing approaches to research.

Nursing research is often perceived as an investigation into nurses, rather than the care they provide. In reality, nursing research may reach into any sphere relating to patient care and nursing interactions, professional roles and workforce issues and, just as importantly, the development of nursing knowledge. Changes in nursing care resulting from high patient turnover, new demands in the community, altered arrangements in service provision and, not least, major developments in technology and pharmacology, have changed what is expected of qualified practitioners. Areas to be researched need to reflect these dynamic changes. McKenna and Mason (1998) maintain that the goal of nursing research should be to carry out rigorous, systematic enquiry designed to make significant contributions to knowledge. They add that such knowledge should impact positively on the physical, mental, and social well being of the population. In addition, they argue that nurses have a series of key roles to play in health service research at strategic and operational levels, while retaining the flexibility to focus on issues and phenomena that are predominately the concern of the nursing profession.

Working collaboratively: international research

Nurses in different countries do not work in isolation and, as such, it is important for practitioners and researchers to locate themselves in the context of global developments. Established programmes of nursing research are now becoming more frequent, with the growth of graduate programmes in nursing in many countries. As our knowledge base increases, research evidence needs to be examined to assess whether it is applicable across international borders. In the scholarship of discovery, we must ask the question: Is this knowledge valid for use with persons in other countries? Evidence from replicated studies may provide some answers to this question. Also, as the pool of nurse researchers may be expanding unevenly in particular areas, collaboration is a means of bringing together nurses with similar research interests to share talents and resources in addressing common areas of concern. International research collaboration holds the promise of advancing nursing and health-care knowledge. The International Council of Nurses (ICN) concur with this and state that research-based practice is a hallmark of professional nursing (1999). They go on to add that nursing research is not just about generating new knowledge in practice, education, management, and research, but also about enhancing the awareness of the profession and its historical development (ICN, 1999). Nursing care is a global concern, and the movement of people across national boundaries makes it important to examine understanding of health and nursing care problems on an international basis.

Organization of nursing and health care is heavily influenced by a number of international agendas and agreements, often in negotiation with the World Health Organization (WHO) and members of the European Union. In the wider context, WHO sets the targets for health gain and health promotion, as in the Alma Ata Declaration (1978), which called for an acceptable level of health for all the people of the world by the year 2000. Complementing this strategy, one of the priorities of the International Council of Nurses (ICN) for the period between 1988 and 1993 was to work with national nurses' associations to encourage and facilitate the development of research in nursing and by nurses, and the dissemination of research findings (ICN, 1987). More recently, the ICN has identified research priorities in health, illness, and care-delivery services (ICN, 1997). Over a decade later, we can see that the international impact of nursing research is growing but it is still far from gaining the recognition and uptake that skilled and knowledgeable professionals deserve, and that the populations that they serve need. This provides all the more reasons to gather strong professional resolve and unite in our drive to improve health care.

In 1994, Oguisso wrote that reading nursing research reports and documents from all over the world convinced her that it was time for concrete actions, such as vigorous fostering of nursing research. She cites the ICN, an international federation with, at that time, 106 member associations, as having a facilitative role in networking and dissemination. However, it is the enthusiasm of the individual that empowers such organizations. Bishop commented on this nearly a decade ago, and it still holds true:

> The harnessing of the potential within the nursing profession to make a major impact on the quality of health care is indeed a challenge. It is a challenge that has triggered many initiatives both large and small, research based and practice driven. Nursing research is not the prerogative of an elite few; it belongs to the profession and must be bedded into practice . . . as we meet one challenge head on so another comes tumbling behind. What a blessing that we have such a large band of warriors, and how essential that we collaborate and strive together. (Bishop, 1994 p. 146)

Researching nursing practice

The nursing profession is charged with establishing its own credible research base. Some of the models of investigation used are less than satisfactory in the search for nursing outcomes, but are pursued because funding bodies deem them superior and thus essential. A great deal of debate has developed on the value of both qualitative and quantitative paradigms (Webb, 1996; Blaxter *et al.*, 2001; Rolfe *et al.*, 2001; Holloway and Wheeler, 2002) and anyone considering a career in research will find themselves, at some point, enmeshed in this argument. Much good work has been replicated using different approaches but, regrettably, despite the profession seeking to expand its body of knowledge through research into clinically effective practices, the knowledge gained has had little impact on health care. Implementation of research findings can be best described as patchy. While the reasons for this have been discussed widely, lack of career opportunities, pressure of time on practitioners, limited resources for practitioners, and shortsighted managers have, in many countries, conspired to make this a major issue that still needs to be addressed.

Stevens (1997) suggests that, while many clinical practitioners and academics are actively promoting the concept of clinical effectiveness through nursing research and development, we have failed, as a profession, to make it a part of everyday business. This is despite the raised awareness fostered in broader educational programmes. She goes on to suggest that a national strategic framework is needed to help nursing respond to the opportunities presented by evidence-based practice. At some level, this appears to conflict with what other authors term 'practitioner-based' approaches to research, but such a strategy may be necessary for the debate to be taken seriously (Jarvis, 2000; Freshwater and Rolfe, 2001).

Freshwater and Bishop (2003) contend that, while all practitioners need to be involved in practice-based enquiry, it is to be expected that practitioners will have different levels of involvement:

- First, a general level, at which nurses ensure that their practice is evidence-based, where good evidence exists, and are able to differentiate between good research and the not so good.
- Second, at a facilitative level, which ensures that those who have an aptitude for research are supported and encouraged, and are able to feed their work into the overall organization.
- Third, at a personal/professional development level, where research is undertaken.

Whatever the level of involvement, practitioners need to have an understanding of the most appropriate research methods for clinical research and the specific questions/problems involved in their work.

Methods for clinical research

Recent paradigm shifts in ways of understanding and explaining human experience mean that more fitting approaches to understanding and representing knowledge have come to be accepted within the scientific community. In what has been called the postmodern world, the certainties of a scientific truth that exists in codifiable and systematic form, have been subject to sharp scrutiny (Lyotard, 1984). In the realms of philosophy and social theory, postmodernism has encouraged the realization that, not only are there many ways of knowing and understanding the world, but also that the privileged position of particular forms of scientific discourse may be misplaced. As Polanyi (1962) has argued, this tacit knowledge can be explored, but not by the classic means of making explicit through reductive analysis.

Beliefs about the 'correct' way of researching the social world have led to numerous discussions and debates about the relative merits and limitations of quantitative and qualitative approaches to research. Indeed, as Blaxter *et al.*

(2001) note, the debate has at times resembled 'a veritable war zone' (p. 60). The quantitative and qualitative paradigms do offer a basic framework for dividing up knowledge into separate camps, yet even within these camps there are debates about what forms of knowledge and evidence are valid. While this debate continues, new approaches to research have been developed and are being refined; these include postmodern and poststructuralist approaches, interpretative and critical reflexivity, constructivist and narrative methods. For the new student, learning about research and evidence can be a minefield, let alone questioning and evaluating how specific research findings relate to professional practice.

One problem in qualitative research is that it has spent many years attempting to meet the standards of the traditional scientific forum, in terms of generalizability, reliability, and validity, which assume that the researcher must be kept outside the frame. Thus, attempts are made to eliminate any bias and to make the questioning process as neutral possible. This means that while the researcher is open to feedback in terms of the design of the question, he or she is attempting to eliminate his/her subjective response.

Objectivity and subjectivity

New ideas from Braud (1998), Rowan (1998), Freshwater and Rolfe (2001), Rolfe (2002) and Alvesson and Skoldberg (2000) on transformational research take a step beyond qualitative research in recognizing the impossibility of the neutrality of the questionnaire/researcher. Rather than trying to cancel out bias, they take this as an interesting element in the research process. Instead of simply acknowledging the impact of the researcher and trying, through intersubjective means, to minimize it, transformational research requires subjective reflexivity, necessary for exploring the subtle meaning of complex human experience. It requires a paradigm shift away from objectivity, not so much to intersubjectivity but to ideas of authenticity and inter-dependence. In nursing, for example, data do not arise solely from the patient but are gained through the collaboration of nurse and patient. In this new perspective, research is seen as an interdependent process that relies heavily on dynamic communication between researchers and practitioners. In transformational research, the researcher lives through the experience of the patient, rather than gaining knowledge about the patient experience.

Scientist-practitioner

Research based on the analysis of nursing outcomes (see Roth and Fonaghy, 1996; Hemmings, 1999; McLeod, 2001), is sometimes referred to as the 'scientist-practitioner' approach and arises out of practices and procedures in allied professions such as psychology and medicine. It is often the case that publicly funded and market-orientated therapy systems, such as public services, have to provide some evidence of efficacy using this methodology (Corney, 1999; Rose, 2000).

Producing evidence on therapeutic interventions (Hill and Corbet, 1993) involves detailed analysis of professional–patient interactions, with a view to identifying the therapeutic attitude and interventions, which are efficacious. This can be found in the work of Carl Rogers at Ohio State University in the 1940s and the University of Chicago in the 1950s. Rogers' work included the design of measures to evaluate the nature of the client response to practitioner attitudes and interventions. Again, this type of research falls foul of the social context within which it operates, often being undertaken by trained researchers rather than practitioners themselves, adopting similar practices to those of psychology.

Practitioner-researcher

Evidence based on the reflexive analysis of clinical experience, which is sometimes referred to as the 'practitioner-researcher' approach, addresses the research–practice gap. This is relevant to current public debates about health care, as some commentators have argued that problems have arisen because academically trained health professionals have been unable to integrate their knowledge with everyday practice. It arises out of the practice of nursing itself, is thus familiar to the vast majority of practitioners, and can only be undertaken by practitioners. Historically, it has given rise to the majority of documents produced by nurses and forms the central methodology on the majority of nursing courses.

It is worth noting that there are substantial differences in the way in which professional practice is viewed by the scientist-practitioner approach and practitioner- researcher approach. These can be summarized as:

- The scientist-practitioner looks for explanatory, predictive theories, whereas the objective of the practitioner-researcher is problem-solving.
- The scientist-practitioner attempts to arrive at general statements about a large area of reality, whereas the practitioner-researcher attempts to arrive at concrete statements about local and contingent situations.
- The scientist-practitioner tends to take the line of impersonal objectivity and minimizing bias, whereas the practitioner-researcher develops professional insights and findings based on a combination of knowledge, experience, and empathic understanding.

Motivation for research

The particular approach/perspective that individuals take when engaging in the research process will be dependent on their rationale for conducting the research. It is important that professionals spend sometime reflecting on their motivations, whatever paradigm they adopt. Indeed, it is crucial that the question and the motivation for research determine the methodological approach, rather than the method dictating the shape and nature of the question (Cormack, 2000).

Professionals need to reflect on the situations they are in and the actions they are taking, and to justify and verify their motives for certain choices. William Braud (1998) argues that there are three main motivations for conducting research:

- To learn as much as we can about others, the world and ourselves in order to predict and control.

- To understand the world in the service of curiosity and wonder.
- To learn to appreciate the world and delight in its bountiful nature.

The first motivation may be related to the scientist–researcher model. Braud (1998) argues that this particular motivation serves security and adaptation and also it brings in an important utilitarian dimension to research. Braud suggests that:

> The search for universal laws – a nomothetic approach – is quite consistent with these motivations; knowledge of principles of great generality increases the ability to predict and control (Braud, 1998, p. 53).

The methods that support this type of research are usually experimental and quasi-experimental.

The second two motivations have much in common with the practitioner-researcher model: 'There is an interest in discovering nature's themes and variations' (Braud, 1998, p. 54). The focus here is on the concept of discovery and the wonder that accompanies discovery, with unpredictable and unexpected aspects of professional practice being as valued as the predictable and the expected. Thus, a satisfying research outcome might be 'the presentation of a detailed map of some new territory or the revelation of some previously un-known trails and pathways in an old territory' (Braud, 1998, p. 54).

Whatever the motivation for the research, it is crucial that professionals begin with a question of great interest and importance to them, an area of enquiry that is driven by a heartfelt desire. This will affect not only the enthusiasm of the investigator and, thus, the successful completion of the project, but also the meaning and learning derived from the experience.

Literature may be given differing levels of importance across different meth-odological approaches, it is, nevertheless, of importance to all research at some point in the enquiry and is certainly crucial to the development of clinical nursing research.

Using literature to underpin clinical practice

A research study usually, although not always, starts off with a problem or question. Whatever the stimulus, the research question is not always immedi-ately suitable for focused research, as some exploration of its theoretical frame of reference may be required (Cormack, 2000).

Any nurse conducting a research project will almost invariably find them-selves involved in a significant amount of reading, although, as already men-tioned, the nature and timing of this reading will largely depend on the chosen research method. Blaxter *et al.* (2001), amongst others (see for example Hollo-way and Wheeler, 2002), argue strongly for the importance of reading when carrying out research, identifying ten reasons for doing so:

- To gain ideas.
- To ascertain what other researchers have done in a similar field.
- To expand perspectives and contextualize research questions.

- To enhance direct personal experience.
- To lend some weight to developing arguments.
- To help clarify one's own position and, perhaps, stimulate a change of opinion.
- To criticixe effectively what others have done.
- To have the opportunity to learn more about research methods and their application to practice.
- To identify gaps in research.
- Because writers need readers!

It is interesting to note that the motivation for reading embedded in this list appears to be mostly extrinsic; many practitioners and researchers read because they feel stimulated to do so by some intrinsic motivating factor. Indeed the motivation for research itself is usually based largely in intrinsic motivation, although this is almost always in the context of the individual's clinical practice. This is an important point, because the motivation for conducting a particular piece of research links directly to the amount of reading that is carried out, and indeed, what sort of reading is done.

Knoll Hoskins (1998) notes that the nature and purpose of the intended study directs the primary purpose of the literature review. She suggests that a study designed using quantitative methodologies will use the literature as an orientation to what is already known, to provide a conceptual or theoretical framework, and to gain an indication of the appropriate research design, instruments, and measurements. Although conducting a literature review prior to data collection is controversial in qualitative studies, a preliminary review of the literature may be carried out for a variety of reasons. It can open the researcher to the complex nature of phenomena under investigation, including contextual and cultural factors. It can also show how the study might contribute to existing knowledge (Knoll Hoskins, 1998).

Typically, research literature falls into two categories; primary sources, or those written by the investigators, and secondary sources, those prepared by someone other than the original researchers. Although it is important to read as many different sources or texts as possible, so as to encounter a range of views and forms of presentation, journal papers are often considered the prime source of information for keeping up to date.

As already indicated, research papers are just one form of literature to be explored. However, the verification of research findings as described by the scientist-practitioner community, usually takes place at the point of publication, with assessment for publication acting as the measure of the scientific quality of the research. In other words, peer review for publication in a scientific journal acts as one form of critical appraisal. Scientific journals make high demands on their authors and often do not publish papers when the methodology is not convincing or does not follow a traditional format. This obviously has implications for the publication of practitioner-researcher based research, which is often rejected by the more renowned international journals. It is important, therefore, to search the full range of literature sources to arrive at a fuller picture of the phenomena under consideration. In addition to exploring a full range of sources, including books, reports, letters and diaries, documents from meetings, reports in the popular media and computer-generated materials, it is also worth bearing in mind other distinguishing factors.

Critical appraisal can, and does of course, take place in other arenas. Conferences, seminars, and workshops can all support constructive criticism and enhance the quality of research. Academic institutions also act as critical verifiers of completed and ongoing research studies.

Developing critical appraisal skills and evaluating clinical research

It could be argued that a person needs to carry out research in order to be able to read research reports critically, and there is no doubt that the experience of conducting a study gives one more insight into the research process. However, as Stevens *et al.* (1993) argue, it is possible to evaluate research without having this type of practical experience.

There is no great mystery about the ability to read research critically. While it does require some knowledge, it is above all else a skill. As such, the more you practise it, the better you become, just as you would if you were learning to play a musical instrument or drive a car. Herein lies a concern, in that, as with any other learned skill, once the skills of critical appraisal are learnt, you can easily get into bad habits and start taking short cuts. From a research perspective, 'being critical' pertains to the justified and considered examination of what other authors or speakers have said about the subject under investigation. During this process, the researcher learns to entertain several contradictory ideas simultaneously, while concurrently comparing and contrasting these ideas with their own opinions. Developing the skills of critical reading feeds directly into the development of writing critically and analytically, and as such is fundamental to the evolution of a research portfolio based on publications, presentations and, of course, reflection on/in practice (Rolfe, 2001).

Critical reading of the literature, then, goes beyond a mere description of what has been read to inclusion of a personal response. Moreover, the personal response not only relates different writings to each other, but also offers alternative positions and vantage points. Critical appraisal of research is not just about identifying negative aspects of the literature under scrutiny. There are strengths and weaknesses in every paper, which need to be assessed and addressed in a balanced way. When reading a paper it is useful to divide your initial analysis into two components, the first focusing on the literary product itself (that is the wrapping), the second on the content (what is inside the wrapping). Learning to be critical of what you are reading helps you to assess the logic and rationale of arguments, and ask questions that go beyond the text and what it is saying (Peelo, 1994).

Research governance: conducting research in clinical practice

Research governance sets standards, and mechanisms to deliver and monitor them, thus improving research quality and safeguarding the public. This has been implemented largely as a result of high media exposure of unethical actions in medical practice and research. It is also a reflection of the realization that greater co-ordination and shared ethics are essential to prevent human exploitation, and to limit harm to patients, duplication of effort and misuse of limited resources. (For a contemporary view on limiting harm in research see Milligan and Robinson, 2003). Research governance defines the broad principles of 'good' research and is seen as key to ensuring that health and social care research is conducted to high scientific and ethical standards.

Any organization participating in research must now have a system in place to ensure that all ongoing studies are logged as having senior management and ethics committee approval. And as the ICN (1999) points out, a clear understanding of ethical guidelines is crucial for the delivery of nursing services. This does not just apply to research undertaken with patients and clients, but embraces research across the spectrum of health I care organizations. This includes projects by students, staff questionnaires, and other smaller studies that previously had sometimes been allowed to progress 'on the nod' and were never formally presented to research ethics committees. The reasoning behind this move to formalize all studies is sound. Not only will it prevent overtaxing specific populations (as occurred in the 1980s when HIV/AIDS patients were inundated with requests for information in the drive to tailor services to their needs), but it should ensure that data derived from small studies are, where possible, aggregated, thus adding to the overall development of a knowledge base.

The researcher has an ethical responsibility throughout the process of research to ensure that the work is carried out in accordance with the ethical proposal that has been approved, and that data are handled sensitively and, where necessary, in strict confidence. Once an ethics committee has approved a proposal, the lead researcher has an obligation to ensure that the protocol is adhered to, and that any proposed changes that arise once the study has begun (as is often the case), are formally approved. The degree of accountability and responsibility associated with this is not to be taken lightly and applies just as much to small projects as to grand scale research programmes.

Support for clinical research

Whether you are a novice researcher, a novice in your post or an accepted expert in your field, you need to keep abreast of changes to be able to assimilate and critique them and their relevance to clinical practice. One method of doing this is through critical reflection on practice, facilitated within an environment of either clinical supervision, research supervision, mentorship or journal clubs. This is lifelong learning, which is best done in good company! Find a peer group, or form one, network within your speciality, take the opportunity presented by attending conferences, and use e-mail and the web to dialogue with international colleagues.

Having found or developed a network for peer review you then need to pick a supervisor (either clinical, research, or both) who can challenge you without putting up hierarchical barriers or creating an uncomfortable power dynamic. Clinical supervision is gradually becoming a part of the nursing culture, changing it from one of didacticism to one of shared learning with a practice-based research philosophy (Bishop, 1998; Bishop and Scott, 2001).

Conclusion

Evaluating research is the business of every health professional, even those who do not consider themselves to be involved in research. Quality care hinges on the understanding, implementation, and development of research. The implementation of findings from sources other than your own area of practice must be undertaken with caution and only after critical appraisal. However, any practitioner interested and motivated to bring about change in their own practice should do so in a responsible and accountable manner, critically appraising their own findings and, of course, disseminating them to the wider audience for further critique.

References

Alvesson, M. and Skoldberg, K. (2000) *Reflexive Methodology*. London: Sage.

Bishop, V. (1994) Prevention and Primary Health Care Delivery Challenges. In Fitzpatrick, J.J., Stevenson J.S. and Polis N.S. (Eds) *Nursing Research and its Utilization*. New York: Springer Publishing Company.

Bishop, V. (Ed.) (1998) *Clinical Supervision in Practice*. London: Macmillan.

Bishop, V. and Scott, I. (2001) Introduction. In: Bishop, V. and Scott, I. (Eds) *Challenges in Clinical Practice. Professional Developments in Nursing*. Basingstoke: Palgrave.

Blaxter, L., Hughes, C. and Tight, M. (2001) *How to Research*, 2nd edn. Buckingham: Open University Press.

Braud, W. (1998) Integral Inquiry: Complementary ways of knowing, being, and expression. In: Braud, W. and Anderson, R. (Eds) *Transpersonal Research Methods for the Social Sciences*. London: Sage.

Briggs, A. (1972) *Committee on Nursing*. Cmnd.5115. London: HMSO.

Chater, S. (1975) *Understanding Research in Nursing*. Geneva: WHO.

Cormack, D. F. S. (2000) *The Research Process in Nursing*, 4th edn. Oxford: Blackwell Publishing.

Corney, R. (1999) Evaluating clinical counselling in primary care and the future. In: Lees, J. (Ed.) *Clinical Counselling in Primary Care*. London: Routledge.

Freshwater, D. and Bishop, V. (2003) *Nursing Research: Appreciation, Critique and Utilisation*. Basingstoke: Palgrave

Freshwater, D. and Broughton, R. (2001) Research and evidence based practice. In: Bishop, V. and Scott, I. (Eds) *Challenges in Clinical Practice. Professional Developments in Nursing*. Basingstoke: Palgrave, Ch 3.

Freshwater, D. and Rolfe, G. (2001) Critical Reflexivity: A politically and ethically engaged research method for nursing. *NTResearch* 6 (1), 526–537.

Hemmings, A. (1999) Assessment of psychological change and the future of practice in clinical counselling. In: Lees, J. (Ed.) *Clinical Counselling in Context*. London: Routledge.

Hills, C.E. and Corbett, M.M. (1993) A perspective on the history of process and outcome research in counselling psychology. *Journal of Counselling Psychology*. 40 (1), 3–24.

Holloway, I. and Wheeler, S. (2002) *Qualitative Research in Nursing*, 2nd edn. Oxford: Blackwell Publishing.

International Council of Nurses (1987) *Blueprint for ICN Programme 1988–1993 Toward More Effective Participation in Health Policy Making and Health Care Delivery* Auckland, New Zealand.

International Council of Nurses (1997) *Nursing Research: Building International Research Agenda*. Report of the Expert Committee on Nursing Research. Geneva: ICN.

International Council of Nurses (1999) Position statement on nursing research. www.icn.ch/psresearch99.htm

Jarvis, A. (2000) The practitioner-researcher in nursing. *Nurse Education Today* 20, 30–35.

Knoll Hoskins, C. (1998) *Developing Research in Nursing and Health*. New York: Springer.

Le May, A. Mulhall, A. and Alexander, C. (1998) Bridging the research-practice gap: exploring the research cultures of practitioners and managers. *Journal of Advanced Nursing* 28 (2), 428–437.

Lyotard, J. F. (1984) *The Postmodern Condition. A Report on Knowledge*. Manchester: Manchester University Press.

McKenna, H. and Mason, C. (1998) Nursing and the wider R & D agenda: Influence and contribution. *NTResearch* 3 (2), 108–115.

McLeod, J. (2001) *Practitioner Research in Counselling*. London: Sage.

Milligan, F. and Robinson, K. (Eds) (2003) *Limiting Harm in Health Care. A Nursing Perspective*. Oxford: Blackwell publishing

Peelo, M. (1994) *Helping Students with Study Problems*. Buckingham: Open University Press.

Polanyi, M. (1962) *Personal Knowledge: Towards a Post-critical Philosophy*. London: Routledge and Kegan Paul.

Rolfe, G. (1998) *Understanding and Researching your own Practice*. Oxford: Butterworth Heinemann.

Rolfe, G. (2002) Reflexive research and therapeutic use of self. In: Freshwater, D. (Ed.) *Therapeutic Nursing*. London: Sage, Ch. 10.

Rolfe, G., Freshwater, D. and Jasper, M. (2001) *Critical Reflection for Nurses and the Caring Professions: A users guide*. Basingstoke: Palgrave.

Rose, K. (2000) Counselling as a product or a process? *Psychodynamic Counselling* 3 (4), 387–400.

Roth, A. and Fonaghy, P. (1996) *What Works for Whom? A Critical Review of Psychotherapy Research*. London: The Guildford Press.

Rowan, J. (1998) Transformational Research In: Clarkson, P. (Ed.) *Counselling Psychology*. London: Routledge.

Stevens, J. (1997) Improving integration between research and practice as a means of developing evidence based health care. *NTResearch* 2 (1), 7–15.

Stevens, P.M.J., Schade, A.L., Chalk, B. and Slevin, O.D.A (1993) *Understanding Research*. Edinburgh: Campion Press.

Tierney, A. (1998) The politics of the NHS R and D agenda. *NTResearch* 3 (6), 419–420.

Clark, J. (2000) Action Research. In: Cormack, D. F. S. (Ed.) *The Research Process in Nursing*. Oxford: Blackwell Publishing, Ch 16.

Appendix 7:
INFORMATION TECHNOLOGY IN NURSING AND HEALTH CARE

Information technology (IT) has become an important part of our everyday lives, both at work and at home. Computers come in all shapes and sizes from a bank's cash dispenser, to a laptop or personal computer (PC). Although more and more nurses have access to, and an understanding of, computers and information technology, this appendix will give you an overview of how you can use it to your advantage.

The role of this technology is to help you with the storage, management, and retrieval of information. Increasingly there are more data and information available and without computers it would be difficult to access much of this.

Maslin-Prothero and Masterson (2003) were commissioned by the Nursing and Midwifery Council (NMC) to develop a policy paper on developments in information and communications technology (ICT). This involved reviewing key policy documents and related literature, and undertaking, analysing, and reporting on a series of telephone interviews undertaken with key stakeholders in relation to ICT and its likely impact on the education, regulation, and practice of nursing, midwifery, and health visiting in the UK. This is a summary of our findings.

The place of computers in health care

Since the 1982 computers have been incorporated into clinical practice, including: accessing laboratory results; planning and reporting patient/client care; and accessing evidence-based nursing. Information technology is there to make your working life easier. Significant moves are being made to bring modern clinical information systems into health and social service across the UK and to maximize the contribution of communications technologies in delivering telemedicine and telecare services [see, for example, Scottish Executive (SE) 2000; Department of Health (DoH) 2002a; Department of Health Social Services and Patient Safety (DHSSPS) 2002; Welsh Assembly (WA) 2001]. Initiatives have been launched over the past 5 years related to the development of electronic patient/health records; internet access to health information for patients, carers, and health professionals; electronic prescribing; and electronic booking of appointment systems, in order to provide a better service to patients. Key advantages identified in the policy documents reviewed include:

- improving the health-care experience;
- opportunities to re-engineer the processes through which health care is delivered;
- increasing accessibility to services for patients;
- reducing duplication in the collection of patient health-related information;
- enabling professionals to have immediate access to up-to-date clinical information, leading to improved outcomes and reduced risk;
- increasing patient and carer empowerment and participation in health care through provision of a range of information services in many languages;
- offering opportunities for more seamless care for patients through primary care, hospitals, and community services;
- promoting multi-professional care;
- giving health planners and managers the information they need to plan and deliver efficient and effective services;
- providing practitioners with on-line access to the latest local guidance and national evidence on treatment and the information they need to evaluate the effectiveness of their work and to support their professional development.

Specific initiatives under way involve the development of Electronic Health/ Patient Records that meet national standards; are integrated across all health and social care settings; designed around patients not institutions; and are able to support care pathways. Plans are in place to enable all NHS staff to have access to e-mail and basic Internet services. Electronic Patient Record (EPR) systems are seen as delivering information faster, but it is not believed that these will completely replace paper-based communications. Care pathways should ensure a smooth and fast journey for patients through the health system; however, in order for electronic care systems to be effective there must be reliable technical support, available for 24 hours, seven days a week. The following are priorities in relation to EPRs:

- anonymity of patient information
- appropriate use of the ICT system
- managing consent electronically.

There has been a growth in clinical decision support systems through the development of nurse-led services such as NHS Direct and Walk-in Centres, as well as significant developments in virtual monitoring of patients at home with a diverse range of conditions, and using video links from GP surgeries to hospital specialists for consultations, etc. Indeed, a recent Commons health select committee report recognized that telehealth had a key role to play as an alternative to hospital care (particularly for rural and island communities) and recommended that the Department of Health develop a strategy for this.

Important issues for nurses

Issues such as the impact on accountability, responsibility and delegation arrangements, and safeguards in relation to telemedicine, telehealth, and telecare, and the potential mis-match of current electronic patient record systems with uni-professional standards for record keeping, are rarely alluded to in policy documents. Yet there are frequent references to the need for standardization of clinical terms (although there are currently no nationally accepted nursing, midwifery, and health visiting specific coding systems) and auditing processes, all of which have implications for existing professional languages and accountability arrangements, etc. Issues that require our attention are:

- arrangements to ensure the accuracy of information available to practitioners
- sharing of information between systems and staff
- keeping information confidential and secure
- the slow speed of implementation of IT – key targets have already been re-scheduled several times
- agreed standards for information
- training and development of staff
- access to equipment in all settings and services

The way ahead

If practitioners are to take full advantage of the opportunities offered by ICT, then they need to be competent and confident in using the technology. Consequently there is a need to develop information- and knowledge-management skills in the nursing, midwifery, and health visiting professions from undergraduate level onwards. In England, Scotland, and Northern Ireland, the NHS has adopted the European Computer Driving Licence (ECDL) as the standard basic training for all staff, and it would seem reasonable to suggest that educational providers should be encouraged to integrate such learning outcomes into their pre- and post-registration programmes.

Allegations concerning poor record keeping were the second most common category of hearing brought before the UKCC in 2000–2001 (UKCC, 2001; NMC, 2002a) and the development of the Electronic Patient Record may, in time, improve the general standard of record keeping. However, current nursing, midwifery, and health visiting records are often in formats that most computer systems find it difficult to handle. Many practitioners still have no access to a computer, and still others have to keep paper records in addition to electronic records, which have implications for accuracy and the data entry time involved.

Systems must be extremely secure to ensure patient confidentiality. Patients want strict controls regarding who can access their health data and what they are allowed to see (NHSIA, 2002; NHSIA with the Consumers' Association and Health Which?, 2002). It is unclear how the tensions between the patients' desire for confidentiality and the need for shared information across professions, settings, and services are likely to be resolved satisfactorily in the short term. There is a draft code of practice for NHS professionals on the Web (NHSIA, 2002), which includes data protection, human rights, consent, and clinical governance. The NHSIA code is in keeping with the principles of the NMC Code of Conduct (2002b) but practitioners must understand how the NHSIA code impacts on their role and can be translated into practice in their setting and or service. There need to be:

- set levels of access
- password protection
- patient choice regarding information recorded electronically, and access.

Conclusion

As nurses, midwives, and health visitors need to be strategically and actively involved in planning and implementation of ICT at a national and local level, because informatics is fundamental to contemporary practice, and clinical skills are needed to apply ICT to practice; ICT has a contribution to make to the professions, for example through managing and co-ordinating care and accessing evidence via the Internet. There are cultural issues involved in ICT implementation, with increased patient access and the shift in balance of power from professionals to patients. Information systems must be fast, reliable, transferable, accurate, and easy to access if they are to improve and enhance practice.

This overview of information technology demonstrates the possibilities available to health-care professionals and their patients/clients. Nurses need to be open to developing their skills in using IT to aid their practice.

Bibliography

Department of Health (1998) *Information for Health*. London: DoH.

Department of Health (2000) *The NHS Plan: A Plan for Investment, a Plan for Reform*. London: DoH.

Department of Health (2001) *Building the Information Core: Implementing the NHS Plan*. London: DoH.

Department of Health (2002a) *Delivering 21st Century IT support for the NHS: Integrated Care Records Service* London: DoH.

Department of Health (2002b) *Making Information Count: A Human Resources Strategy for Health Informatics Professionals*. London: DoH.

Department of Health Social Services and Patient Safety (2001) *The Information and Technology Strategy Vision* http://www.dhsspsni.gov.uk/publications/archived/2001/vision.pdf

Department of Health Social Services and Patient Safety (2002) *Information and Communication Technology Strategy: for consultation*. Belfast, N. Ireland.

GB Parliament (1998) *Data Protection Act*. London: The Stationery Office.

GB Parliament (1999) *Modernising Government*. Cm. 4310. London: The Stationery Office.

GB Parliament (2000) *Human Rights Act*. London: The Stationery Office.

GB Parliament (2000) *egovernment: a framework for public services in the information age*. http://www.citu.gov.uk/iagc/strategy.htm

Maslin-Prothero, S. E. and Masterson, A. (2003) *Developments in Information and Communications Technology*. A report prepared for the Nursing and Midwifery Council. London: NMC.

NHSIA (NHS Information Authority) (2001) *Basic Information Technology Skills Standard for the NHS: Implementing the European Computer Driving License*. London: NHSIA. http://www.ecdl.co.uk/nhs/nurses.pdf

NHSIA (NHS Information Authority) (2002) *Confidentiality: A Code Of Practice For NHS Staff*. http://www.nhsia.nhs.uk/confidentiality

NHSIA (NHS Information Authority) in conjunction with the Consumers' Association and Health Which? (2002) *Share with Care! People's views on Consent and Confidentiality of Patient Information*. London: NHSIA

NHS Modernisation Board (2002) *The NHS Plan – A progress Report. The Modernisation Board's Annual Report 2000–2001*.

NMC (Nursing and Midwifery Council) (2002a) *Complaints about professional conduct*. London: NMC.

NMC (Nursing and Midwifery Council) (2002b) *Code of Professional Conduct*. London: NMC.

NMC (Nursing and Midwifery Council) (2002c) *Guidelines for Records and Record Keeping*. London: NMC.

Scottish Executive (2000) *Working Together to Build a Healthy, Caring Scotland*. Edinburgh: Scottish Executive.

Scottish Executive Health Dept (2002) *Facing the Future*. http://www.show. scot.nhs.uk/send/facingthefuture/

UKCC (United Kingdom Central Council for Nursing, Midwifery and Health Visiting) (2001) *Professional Conduct Annual Report 2000–2001*. London: UKCC.

Wanless, D. (2002) *Securing our Future Health: Taking a Long Term View*. London: HM Treasury.

Welsh Assembly (2001) *Improving Health in Wales: A Plan for the NHS and its Partners*. Cardiff: Wales.

Welsh Assembly (2001) *Better information, better health*. Cardiff: Wales.

Welsh Assembly (2002) *Informing Healthcare*. Cardiff: Wales.

Welsh Assembly (2002) *The National Assembly's Information Age Strategic Framework for Wales*. www.cymruarlein.wales.gov.uk

Appendix 8:
CONTINUING PROFESSIONAL DEVELOPMENT AND PREP

The Nursing and Midwifery Council (NMC) *Code of professional conduct* (2002) requires all nurses to maintain their professional knowledge and competence in order that they can retain their registration. 'Nurses are required to be up-to-date in their practice and to be aware of the limitations of their practice' (NMC, 2002). The Council expects that, wherever possible, all care provided should be evidence based, and that nurses have a duty to develop their competence throughout their working lives.

This approach to continuing development is not unique to nursing, continuous professional development (CPD) is an integral condition of many professions. Continuous professional development is not a body of theory, nor a collection of techniques; it is an approach to the management of learning. Continuous professional development means

- learning from real experiences at work
- learning throughout working life, not confined to useful but occasional injections of 'training'
- applying learning in your day-to-day work.

(Adapted from *The IPM Statement on Continuous Development: People and Work*, 1984.)

In nursing CPD has been inextricably linked to the United Kingdom Central Council for Nursing, Midwifery and Health Visiting (UKCC; now NMC) requirements for post-registration education and practice (PREP). In order to facilitate nurses' understanding of PREP, the UKCC prepared a number of briefing papers that outline ways for nurses to ensure they meet the requirements for continued registration. The following information is adapted from a number of UKCC and NMC papers.

In the Nursing and Midwifery Order (2001) it states that:

(1) The Council [NMC] may make rules requiring registrants to undertake such continuing professional development as it shall specify in standards.
(2) The rules may, in particular, make provision with respect to registrants who fail to comply with any requirements of the rules, including making provision for their registration to cease to have effect.
(3) The Council may by rules require persons who have not practised or who have not practised for or during a prescribed period, to undertake such education or training or to gain such experience as it shall specify in standards.

(4) If the Council makes rules under paragraph (1) or (3), it shall establish the standards to be met in relation to continuing professional development (CPD).

This legislation provided the Nursing and Midwifery Council with the authority to continue the work commenced by its predecessor, the UKCC, to encourage continuing professional development (CPD).

As part of the UKCC's PREP requirement, you are required by law to renew your registration every three years by providing a signed notification of practice form and payment of a registration fee. This form asks for details of your qualifications, specific area of practice, type of employer, and whether you work full or part-time. It also asks you to sign to declare that you have met your post-registration education and practice (PREP) requirements (see below). Your registration will only be renewed when the signed form with declarations, and your fee payment, have been received and processed by the UKCC.

If you do not comply with the PREP requirements, you will cause your registration to lapse. If you are not registered, you cannot practise as a registered nurse, midwife, or health visitor.

The Nursing and Midwifery Order 2001 also set out regulations for the Nursing and Midwifery Council (NMC); in this order it identified criteria for post-registration education and training which mirror the standards set by the UKCC.

The UKCC's PREP requirements

PREP requirements are professional standards for education and practice set by the UKCC. Your registration is affected by two separate PREP standards:

- The PREP continuing professional development standard
- The PREP practice standard.

The PREP (CPD) standard

This standard requires you to undertake and record your continuing professional development (CPD) over the three years prior to the renewal of your registration.

The PREP (CPD) standard means that you must have undertaken a minimum of 35 hours learning activity during the three year period leading up to your renewal of registration. Exactly how you meet this standard is entirely up to you. The important thing is that it helps you to do your job better. Whatever activity you choose, it needs to be recorded in your personal professional profile (PPP) and you must be able to explain how it has helped you develop your own practice. When you renew their registration, you must declare that you have met the standard on the Notification of Practice (NOP) form.

The PREP (practice) standard

The Nurses, Midwives and Health Visitors Act 1997 defines practising as ' ... working in some capacity by virtue of a qualification in nursing, midwifery or health visiting ... '.

Since 1995, the PREP (practice) standard has required you to have practised by virtue of your nursing, midwifery or health visiting registration for not less than 100 days (750 hours) during the five years prior to renewal of your registration. What this means to you since 1 April 2000 is set out below.

- If you are registered as a nurse or a health visitor, you need to have completed a minimum of 100 days (750 hours) of practice, irrespective of the number of your registrable nursing qualifications.
- If you are a practising midwife, Rule 37 of the midwives rules requires you to have practised for 12 weeks during the five years prior to your renewal of registration. From April 2001, this rule will be superseded by the PREP (practice) standard outlined above. You will, however, need to continue to submit your notification of intention to practise form annually.
- If you have both a nursing and a midwifery registration and you wish to continue to practise as both a nurse and a midwife, you will need to have practised for 100 days (750 hours) in respect of each of your nursing and midwifery registrations. This means that, if you wish to maintain both your nursing and midwifery registrations, you must have completed a minimum of 200 days (1500 hours) of practice, divided equally between nursing and midwifery.

From April 2000, the UKCC has required that you need to declare on your notification of practice form that you have met the practice standard when you renew your registration. If you do not meet this standard, you must undertake a return to practice course approved by a National Board before you can renew your registration. Contact details are set out on the back cover of this leaflet. These criteria have been reinforced by the NMC in the revised Code of Professional Conduct (UKCC/NMC, 2002) which states that 'You must maintain your professional knowledge and competence'.

As an accountable professional, you are responsible for ensuring that the 100 days (750 hours) of practice which you use to meet the PREP (practice) standard satisfies the definition of practice set out above.

Auditing PREP

From April 2001, the UKCC has been auditing compliance with the PREP (CPD) standard. Each month, up to 10% of those registrants who are due to renew their registrations will be selected for audit and issued with PREP (CPD) summary forms. These forms will be sent out between 14 and 90 days before the renewal date.

Registrants who are selected for audit will be asked to give a brief description of their learning activity, and the relevance of this learning to their work, on the forms provided. There is a copy of the PREP (CPD) summary form in the PREP handbook (page 24), but please note that only those who are chosen by UKCC to take part in the audit will have to fill in a form.

The completed form must show how the learning activity that you have undertaken has helped to improve care for your patients and clients. The key sentence

to be completed is: 'The way in which this learning has influenced my work is
...'.

All the information required by the UKCC is detailed on the form itself; no
further details, or evidence, will be asked for.

If you are required to fill in a PREP (CPD) summary form, the form must be
returned to the UKCC before your registration can be renewed. Failure to return the
forms will result in your registration lapsing until such time as you apply for re
entry.

Recording CPD: Personal Professional Profile

The UKCC PREP recommendations included the requirement that 'all practitioners must demonstrate that they have maintained and developed their professional
knowledge and competence; a personal professional profile should be completed
as a record of experience and achievements so that they develop their practice'.

Meeting the standard

In the year 2000, a pilot study of over 2300 practitioners, conducted by the
UKCC, found that more than 90% had completed the 35 hours minimum learning
activity requirement.

There are many ways for practitioners to meet the 35-hour target, for example:

• Attend team meetings to discuss ways of improving care.
• Study relevant articles in professional nursing journals.
• Take part in training days provided by your employer.
• Undertake more formal study activity relevant to your practice.

You also need to check that your PPP (personal professional portfolio) has been
kept up to date with details of how your learning activity has helped to improve
the care you provide for your patients and clients (the PREP handbook, developed by the UKCC provides some examples).

Professional development

The rapidly and constantly changing health-care environment in which practitioners work means that nurses, midwives, and health visitors have to develop their
knowledge and skills from the moment they first register until they retire. This
aspect of the PREP requirements is about keeping up to date in order to be safe
to practise in both today's and tomorrow's world.

As previously stated, the basic requirement is that you must undertake the equivalent of a minimum of five days (or at least 35 hours) of study activity for your
professional development every three years in order to renew and maintain your
registration. This does not mean five days of study leave or a five day course or even
a course at all. A wide range of possibilities is open to you. These include:

• conference or seminar attendance
• distance learning (including the education supplements in some professional
  journals)

- visits to other areas of practice to observe care delivery
- personal research, such as undertaking a literature search in a library or at home
- a course.

You may find it helpful to get together with a group of colleagues in order to undertake your PREP study activity collectively, through discussion, evaluation of your existing practice, and assessment of areas where the team needs to develop. *Neither the UKCC nor anybody else approves any study for PREP.* This is a deliberate decision as it is up to you to choose the most appropriate study for your personal professional development needs. It is your responsibility to keep yourself up to date. *It can be done without having to spend heavily on expensive courses and materials.* Indeed, there are many ways in which you can meet your PREP requirements without having to spend anything at all.

Please note that neither the Nursing Times or Royal College of Nursing's continuing education points systems, nor any other points systems, have anything to do with PREP and are not recognised by the UKCC. The study undertaken to acquire the points is, of course, acceptable in meeting your PREP requirements if that is your choice, but what you cannot do is simply collect points and then assume that this in itself means you have met the UKCC's requirements.

What are your personal professional development needs?

Study activity has to be relevant to your role and your registration. If you state on your notification of practice form that you are using more than one registerable qualification in your practice, you are only required to undertake five days of study activity – not five days per qualification. However, your learning activity must be relevant to all your areas of registration. If, in the three year period, you study for a specialist practice qualification or for any qualification relevant to your practice, you will have concurrently fulfilled the minimum study requirements.

To help you plan your studies, the UKCC has created five broad categories which indicate the range of activity and content you may choose. These are flexible to ensure that you meet your needs in the context of your practice. They are:

- patient, client and colleague support (supervision of clinical practice, counselling and leadership in professional practice)
- care enhancement (standard setting or new techniques and approaches to care)
- practice development (personal research/study or relevant visits to other practice settings)
- reducing risk (health promotion or screening)
- education development (personal research/study or exchange arrangements).

When planning your professional development, you may wish to work through the following stages:

1. Review your competence: What are your strengths, weaknesses and areas for further personal development?
2. Set your learning objectives: What do you want to achieve?
3. Develop an action plan: What learning activities will help you meet your needs? A literature search, course or visit?
4. Implement the action plan: Discuss your plan with your manager, clinical supervisor, supervisor of midwives, or tutor to ensure that it is feasible. Negotiate any study time or help with funding.
5. Evaluate what happened: Once the plan has been implemented, think what happened and what you learned. Did you meet your objectives? What was the value to patients and clients? How will you share your new knowledge?
6. Record your study time: Accurately record all your learning activities in and learning outcomes your personal professional profile. Keep these records for at least six years.

Common questions

If I choose to do distance learning, home study, library research or visiting another area of practice as my study for PREP, how do I prove it?
As an accountable practitioner, the UKCC expects that you will be honest when documenting study in your profile. You do not need others to confirm that you have undertaken study activity. All study, whether formal or informal, needs to be documented in your personal professional profile. This should show your objectives in undertaking the study, its content, duration, and relevance to your registration and role. You should also set out what you have gained from the study and how it has met the objectives that you set yourself. It is this documentation of how the study has contributed to your professional development, rather than simply collecting certificates of attendance, that will be regarded as evidence of study by the UKCC. Certificates of attendance prove nothing at all in terms of what you have learned and how it has helped you to improve your practice.

I'm practising abroad. Can I use study abroad to meet the PREP requirements?
Yes. Practitioners working abroad meet the PREP requirements in the same way as those in the United Kingdom.

I have three registerable qualifications (RGN, RMN, RSCN) which I am currently using in my practice. Does this mean I have to undertake five days of PREP study activity for each registerable qualification?
No. If you can identify a subject area which is relevant to all three registerable qualifications and is linked to your current professional role, then you need only meet the minimum requirement of five days of PREP study activity in a three-year period.

Bibliography

Institute of Personnel Management (1988) *The IPM Statement on Continuous Development*. London: IPM.

UKCC (1986) *Project 2000: A New Preparation for Practice*. London: UKCC

UKCC (1990) *The Report of the Post Registration Education and Practice Project* (discussion document). London: UKCC.

UKCC (1994) *The Future of Professional Practice – The Council's Standards for Education and Practice Following Registration. Position Statement 1*. London: UKCC.

UKCC (1995) *The Future of Professional Practice – The Council's Standards for Education and Practice Following Registration. Position Statement 2*. London: UKCC.

UKCC (1997) *PREP and You*. London: UKCC.

UKCC (2001) *The PREP Handbook*. London: UKCC.

UKCC/NMC(2002) *Code of Professional Conduct*. London: UKCC.

Appendix 9:
THE QUALITY ASSURANCE AGENCY FOR HIGHER EDUCATION: BENCHMARKING[1]

Subject benchmark statements provide a means of describing the nature and characteristics of programmes of study and training in health care. They also represent general expectations about standards for the award of qualifications at a given level and articulate the attributes and capabilities that those possessing such qualifications should be able to demonstrate.

Subject benchmark statements are used for a variety of purposes. Primarily, they are an important external source of reference when new programmes are being designed and developed. They provide general guidance for articulating the learning outcomes associated with the programme but are not a specification of a detailed curriculum. Benchmark statements provide for variety and flexibility in the design of programmes and encourage innovation within an agreed overall conceptual framework.

Subject benchmark statements also provide support in the pursuit of internal quality assurance. They enable the learning outcomes specified for a particular programme to be reviewed and evaluated against agreed general expectations about standards.

Finally, subject benchmark statements are one of a number of external sources of information that are drawn upon for the purposes of academic review[2] and for making judgements about threshold standards being met. Reviewers do not use subject benchmark statements as a crude checklist for these purposes, however. Rather, they are used in conjunction with the relevant programme specifications, the associated documentation of the relevant professional and statutory regulatory bodies, the institution's own self-evaluation documentation, together with primary data in order to enable reviewers to come to a rounded judgement based on a broad range of evidence.

The benchmarking of standards in health-care subjects is undertaken by groups of appropriate specialists drawn from higher education institutions, service providers, and the professional and statutory regulatory bodies. The statements represent the first attempt to make explicit in published form the general academic characteristics and standards of awards in these subjects in the UK. In due course, the statements will be revised to reflect developments in the subjects and the experiences of institutions, academic review, and others that are working with it.

Foreword

This benchmark statement describes the nature and standards of programmes of study in nursing, that lead to awards made by higher education institutions in the United Kingdom (UK) in the subject.

It has been developed in collaboration with a number of other health-care professions.[3] Although initial work was undertaken in subject specific groups, the analysis of these early drafts identified a number of features which all the subject groups shared. It was, therefore, agreed by each of the specialist benchmarking groups that their respective statements could be cast using a common structure. As work progressed it became increasingly apparent that there was considerable overlap within the details of the subject-specific statements and a common health professions framework was emerging. This emerging framework is, accordingly, displayed in each of the subject statements in order to illustrate, on the one hand, the shared context upon which the education and training of health-care professionals rests and, on the other, the uniquely profession-specific context within which programmes are organized. It is important to emphasize that benchmark statements are not cast in tablets of stone and will need to be revisited in the light of experience and further developments in health care. Moreover, we are confident that the emerging framework has the potential to embrace other health-related professions such as social work, dentistry, medicine, and other therapies. It is anticipated that further work in a second phase of the project could lead to an overarching health professions framework.

The initial section of this statement sets out the health professions framework under three main headings:

A   Expectations of the health professional in providing patient/client services;
B   The application of practice in securing, maintaining or improving health and well-being;
C   The knowledge, understanding, and skills that underpin the education and training of health-care professionals.

The main section of this statement, in addition to describing the nature and extent of programmes leading to awards in nursing, describes the profession-specific expectations and requirements under the same three categories.

The key feature in this statement, as in the associated statements, is the explicit articulation of the academic and practitioner standards associated with the award in nursing. This duality reflects the significance of the academic award as the route to registration for professional practice and formal recognition by the professional and statutory regulatory bodies. The threshold standards set out the expectations of health professionals entering their first post immediately on qualification.

The section on standards accords with the relevant level descriptor for awards in the qualifications frameworks published by the Quality Assurance Agency for Higher Education.

The section on teaching, learning, and assessment draws attention to the central role of practice in the design of learning opportunities for students and the importance of ensuring that professional competence developed through practice is adequately assessed and rewarded. It also notes how essential it is that the integration of theory and practice is a planned process within the overall arrangements made for teaching and learning.

The statement acknowledges the need to put the prospective client/patient at the centre of the student's learning experience and to promote within that experience the importance of team-working and cross-professional collaboration and communication. Implicit in the statement are the opportunities that exist for shared learning across professional boundaries, particularly in the latter stages of training when inter-professional matters can be addressed most productively. It is essential that the opportunities that exist for shared learning in practice are optimized, as well as best use being made of similar opportunities that prevail more obviously in classroom-based activities.

This statement and the associated statements will therefore allow higher education institutions, in partnership with service providers (where appropriate), to make informed curriculum choices about the construction of shared learning experiences. In this context shared learning is seen as one of a number of means of promoting improved collaborative practice and addressing a range of issues which span professional accountability and professional relationships.

Finally, the statement does not set a national curriculum for programmes leading to awards in nursing. It acknowledges that the requirements of the professional and statutory regulatory bodies need to be incorporated into the design of programmes. It seeks to encourage higher education institutions and service providers to work collaboratively in the design and delivery of their curricula. Its essential feature is the specification of threshold standards, incorporating academic and practitioner elements, against which higher education institutions are expected, as a minimum, to set their standards for the award.

n emerging health professions framework

The subject-specific statements for nursing have been set within the emerging health professions framework outlined below. As indicated in the foreword, this framework developed as a result of the benchmarking work undertaken collaboratively by 11 different health professional groups. Further evolution of the framework is anticipated through a second phase of the project which will address its goodness of fit with a range of other health and social care professions benchmark statements.

Expectations of the health professional in providing atient/client services

This section articulates the expectations of a registered professional within health and social care services. It describes what is regarded as a minimum range of expectations of a professional that will provide safe and competent practice for patients/clients in a variety of health and social care contexts.

A1 Professional autonomy and accountability

The award holder should be able to:

- maintain the standards and requirements of professional and statutory regulatory bodies;
- adhere to relevant codes of conduct;
- understand the legal and ethical responsibilities of professional practice;
- maintain the principles and practice of patient/client confidentiality;
- practise in accordance with current legislation applicable to health-care professionals;
- exercise a professional duty of care to patients/clients/carers;
- recognize the obligation to maintain fitness for practice and the need for continuing professional development;
- contribute to the development and dissemination of evidence-based practice within professional contexts;
- uphold the principles and practice of clinical governance.

A2 Professional relationships

The award holder should be able to:

- participate effectively in inter-professional and multi-agency approaches to health and social care where appropriate;
- recognize professional scope of practice and make referrals where appropriate;
- work, where appropriate, with other health and social care professionals and support staff and patients/clients/carers to maximize health outcomes;
- maintain relationships with patients/clients/carers that are culturally sensitive and respect their rights and special needs.

A3 Personal and professional skills

The award holder should be able to:

- demonstrate the ability to deliver quality patient/client-centred care;
- practise in an anti-discriminatory, anti-oppressive manner;
- draw upon appropriate knowledge and skills in order to make professional judgements, recognizing the limits of his/her practice;
- communicate effectively with patients/clients/carers and other relevant parties when providing care;
- assist other health-care professionals, support staff and patients/clients/carers in maximizing health outcomes;
- prioritize workload and manage time effectively;
- engage in self-directed learning that promotes professional development;
- practise with an appropriate degree of self-protection;
- contribute to the well-being and safety of all people in the work place.

A4 Profession and employer context
The award holder should be able to:

- show an understanding of his/her role within health- and social-care services;
- demonstrate an understanding of government policies for the provision of health and social care;
- take responsibility for his/her own professional development;
- recognize the value of research and other scholarly activity in relation to the development of the profession and of patient/client care.

B The application of practice in securing, maintaining, or improving health and well-being

All health-care professionals draw from the knowledge and understanding associated with their particular profession. This knowledge and understanding is acquired from theory and practice. It forms the basis for making professional decisions and judgements about the deployment in practice of a range of appropriate skills and behaviours, with the aim of meeting the health and social care needs both of individual clients/patients and of groups, communities, and populations. These decisions and judgements are made in the context of considerable variation in the presentation, the setting, and in the characteristics of the client/patient health and social care needs. They often take place against a backdrop of uncertainty and change in the structures and mechanisms of health- and social-care delivery.

Sound professional practice is essentially a process of problem solving. It is characterized by four major phases:

- the identification and analytical assessment of health- and social-care needs;
- the formulation of plans and strategies for meeting health- and social-care needs;
- the performance of appropriate, prioritized health promoting/health educating/caring/diagnostic/therapeutic activities;
- the critical evaluation of the impact of, or response to, these activities.

B1 Identification and assessment of health- and social-care needs
The award holder should be able to:

- gather relevant information from a wide range of sources, including electronic data;
- adopt systematic approaches to analysing and evaluating the information collected;
- communicate effectively with the client/patient, (and his/her relatives/carers), group/community/population, about their health- and social-care needs;
- use a range of assessment techniques appropriate to the situation and make provisional identification of relevant determinants of health and physical, psychological, social and cultural needs/problems;
- recognize the place and contribution of his/her assessment within the total health-care profile/package, through effective communication with other members of the health- and social-care team.

B2   Formulation of plans and strategies for meeting health- and social-care needs
The award holder should be able to:

- work with the client/patient, (and his/her relatives/carers), group/community/ population, to consider the range of activities that are appropriate/feasible/ acceptable, including the possibility of referral to other members of the health and social care team and agencies;
- plan care within the context of holistic health management and the contributions of others;
- use reasoning and problem-solving skills to make judgements/decisions in prioritizing actions;
- formulate specific management plans for meeting needs/problems, setting these within a timescale and taking account of finite resources;
- record professional judgements and decisions taken;
- synthesize theory and practice.

B3   Practice
The award holder should be able to:

- conduct appropriate activities skilfully and in accordance with best/evidence-based practice;
- contribute to the promotion of social inclusion;
- monitor and review the ongoing effectiveness of the planned activity;
- involve client/patient/members of group/community/population appropriately in ongoing effectiveness of plan;
- maintain records appropriately;
- educate others to enable them to influence the health behaviour of individuals and groups;
- motivate individuals or groups in order to improve awareness, learning and behaviour that contribute to healthy living;
- recognize opportunities to influence health and social policy and practices.

B4   Evaluation
The award holder should be able to:

- measure and evaluate critically the outcomes of professional activities;
- reflect on and review practice;
- participate in audit and other quality-assurance procedures;
- contribute to risk management activities.

C   Knowledge, understanding, and skills that underpin the education and training of health-care professionals

The education and training of health-care professionals draws from a range o well-established scientific disciplines that provide the underpinning knowledg and understanding for sound practice. Each health-care profession will draw fror these disciplines differently and to varying extents to meet the requirements of their specialty. It is this contextualization of knowledge, understanding, and skills that is characteristic of the learning in specific health-care programmes. Consequently, in this introductory section, the attributes and capabilities expected of the student are expressed at a generalized level.

C1 Knowledge and understanding
The award holder should be able to demonstrate:

- understanding of the key concepts of the disciplines that underpin the education and training of all health-care professionals, and detailed knowledge of some of these. The latter would include a broad understanding of:

− the structure and function of the human body, together with a knowledge of dysfunction and pathology;
− health- and social-care philosophy and policy, and its translation into ethical and evidence-based practice;
− the relevance of the social and psychological sciences to health and health care;
− the role of health care practitioners in the promotion of health and health education;
− the legislation and professional and statutory codes of conduct that affect health- and social-care practice.

C2 Skills
Information gathering
The award holder should be able to demonstrate:

- an ability to gather and evaluate evidence and information from a wide range of sources;
- an ability to use methods of enquiry to collect and interpret data in order to provide information that would inform or benefit practice.

Problem solving
The award holder should be able to demonstrate:

- logical and systematic thinking;
- an ability to draw reasoned conclusions and sustainable judgements.

Communication
The award holder should be able to demonstrate:

- effective skills in communicating information, advice, instruction, and professional opinion to colleagues, patients, clients, their relatives and carers; and, when necessary, to groups of colleagues or clients.

Numeracy
The award holder should be able to demonstrate:

• ability in understanding, manipulating, interpreting and presenting numerical data.

Information technology
The award holder should be able to demonstrate:

• an ability to engage with technology, particularly the effective and efficient use of information and communication technology.

Benchmark statement for nursing

Introduction

Nursing is an applied vocational and academic discipline that is often practised in a variety of complex situations across the health–illness continuum. There are a number of definitions of nursing but few, if any, that explicitly enable a benchmark nursing statement to be identified. The variety and diversity of nursing is articulated through the specialist branch structure that enables practitioners, upon successful completion of an approved programme, to register as either an adult, child, learning disability, or mental health nurse.

Nursing focuses on promoting health and helping individuals, families and groups to meet their health-care needs. Nursing work involves assisting people whose autonomy is impaired, who may present with a range of disabilities or health-related problems, to perform a range of activities, sometimes acting for, or on behalf of the patient. A defining feature of nursing is that it provides 24-hour care with a focus on meeting people's intimate needs.

Nurses work with patients, clients, families, and communities in primary care, acute and critical care, rehabilitation and tertiary care settings. The knowledge base for nursing is broad-based encompassing natural, human, and social sciences.

Nurses practise within a social, political and economic context. Through their *Code of professional conduct*, nurses embrace the concepts of inclusion, equal opportunities, individual rights, and empowerment of patients and client groups. Professional and patient/client autonomy is a key feature of the nurse's role.

Given the complex nature of nursing and diversity of health-care situations encountered, nurses must be skilled practitioners, knowledgeable in a range of subjects and able to appraise and adopt an enquiry-based approach to the delivery of care. Irrespective of the academic award, individuals undertaking programmes that lead to professional registration must demonstrate achievement of the nursing competencies required by the statutory regulatory body for entry to register.

The study of nursing encompasses the following principles:

• a commitment to provide high-quality patient-centred care;
• a commitment to the development of new roles that support the interface between health- and social-care practice;

- the application of current knowledge and research to nursing practice across the health and illness continuum;
- a commitment to working in partnership with other professionals;
- an evolution towards role transferability in support of patient-centred care;
- the development of educational programmes that enable nurses to demonstrate fitness for practice and a commitment to lifelong learning.

Nature and extent of programmes in nursing

Nursing is a large and complex profession and academic discipline. Approximately 100 UK universities provide programmes to enable over 11,000 nurses to enter the professional register each year, and to continuously update and develop additional and specialist knowledge and skills.

Pre-registration nursing education consists of a common foundation programme and four branch programmes to prepare nurses to work in either adult nursing, children's nursing, learning disabilities nursing, or mental health nursing.

Common foundation programme

The common foundation programme is the core element that underpins each branch and is shared by all nursing students. It introduces students to the four branches but also focuses on a range of subjects within and applied to nursing that are common to all branches.

Nursing programmes involve integrated study of the knowledge, skills and values from a range of subject disciplines applied to the practice of nursing. These are outlined in this benchmark statement. Core areas within these subjects are common to all of nursing, while other aspects within these disciplines are applied to specific branches. Regardless of the order that these subject areas appear in this benchmark statement, programmes within each of the four branches will place greater emphasis on certain subject areas.

Nursing competence requires the development of technical, cognitive and interpersonal skills and involves a variety of different ways of knowing and understanding. Technical skills are the most visible part of some branches of nursing, while for other branches interpersonal skills are the primary focus. Interpersonal and interactive skills are needed to enable nurses to form appropriate professional relationships, and for some branches the depth and breadth of interpersonal skills required is greater.

Through their educational preparation nurses become equipped to understand, contribute to, and work within the context of their profession and to analyse, adapt to, manage, and eventually lead the processes of change.

Adult nursing

Central to adult nursing is a commitment to patient-centred care that recognizes the need to assess physical, social, psychological, and spiritual needs to maximize potential for health and well-being. This is underpinned by a philosophy which embraces partnership working with patients, carers, and the multi-professional team. This approach enhances the development of values that promote independence, autonomy, and reciprocity in adult health care.

Adult nurses need to understand the differing health-care needs of adults within age groups that span adolescence, adulthood, and older people. Care is provided for adults in a wide variety of primary, acute, continuing, and rehabilitative care settings that include NHS trusts, the patient/client's own home, the workplace, the prison services and the independent and voluntary sector. Adult nurses acquire the knowledge, skills, and attitudes to meet the needs of adults in all care areas, support them through programmes of care and treatment, and maximize opportunities for health promotion.

A substantial part of adult nursing involves co-ordinating, integrating, and managing care, making referrals to other members of the care team and ensuring that effective communication channels are in place to support continuity of care. In order to fulfil this role, adult nurses need to be confident to make decisions and, where appropriate, challenge assumptions and practices.

Children's nursing

The developing needs of children from infancy to adolescence, in relation to physical and mental health and special needs, form the heart of children's nursing. Children's nursing is practised within a philosophy of child-focused and family-centred care in which, whenever possible, the child, parents, and carers are equal partners. This partnership enhances self-esteem, enables children to reach their full potential, and encourages the development of autonomy in care and decision making.

Ill children present with complex multi-dimensional problems, some being life limiting or life threatening, and many which persist through childhood into adult life. These problems impact upon the child's development, choices, and family life. This requires children's nurses to work collaboratively with other professionals in health and social care to promote health, minimize illness, and protect vulnerable children.

Children's nurses practise within the child's own home, hospital, school, community, and voluntary settings. The wide spectrum of health problems, care settings, and opportunities for health promotion require nurses to demonstrate confidence and competence in child-specific nursing. This involves the co-ordination of care and the use of refined interpersonal and communication skills with both children and adult carers, underpinned by knowledge of child development.

Children's nurses need to be politically aware, applying knowledge of health and social policy, law and ethics in order to champion the rights of children both as a group and as individuals receiving care.

Learning disabilities nursing

Programmes in the learning disabilities branch of nursing prepare nurses to work with people with a range of learning disabilities and with their families and significant others. Learning disability nurses' work is underpinned by the concepts of partnership, inclusion, and advocacy. The role of the learning disability nurse, specifically, is to assist and support people to become and remain healthy, to improve their competence and quality of life, and to fulfil their potential. Learning disability nurses work with people with a spectrum of needs and abilities in a wide variety of settings, often working collaboratively with professionals from a range of health- and social-care agencies. This support may take place in the National Health Service (NHS), voluntary or independent sector, or in the patient/client's own home.

Mental health nursing
Programmes in mental health nursing prepare nurses to work in a branch of nursing, the precepts of which acknowledge that nursing is essentially a human activity which has as its core the relationship between the nurse and his/her client(s) and carers. This relationship is premised on knowledge, attitudes, and skills that assist individuals with mental health problems to reach their maximum potential. The knowledge and practical skills required of the mental health nurse are those that facilitate the recognition and achievement of the interpersonal, emotional, behavioural, cognitive, and spiritual needs of clients. Mental health nurses approach these in a structured way through a systematic process that embraces the concepts of client-centredness, self-reflection, and self-awareness. This ensures that the nurse/client relationship is a dynamic one. The mental health nurse may be required to meet the health and/or nursing care needs of clients with acute, rehabilitative, or continuing care needs or health promotion requirements within community, residential, and hospital settings.

The statements in the rest of this document outline the knowledge, understanding and associated skills, and the application of these to nursing practice across all specialist nursing branches.

A   The nurse as a registered health-care practitioner; expectations held by the profession, employers and public

This section of the benchmark statement articulates the expectations of a registered nurse at the point of qualification. The core expectations that are common to all health-care professionals can be found in section A of the health professions framework within this benchmark statement. Listed below are those attributes and capabilities that are specific to nursing.

Pre-registration nursing programmes should ensure that students are able to demonstrate the following attributes and capabilities to be an award-holder.

A1   Professional identity and accountability
The award holder should be able to:

• maintain the standards and practices required of a registered practitioner by the nursing statutory regulatory body;
• adhere to the professional code of conduct for nurses, midwives, and health visitors;

- engage in clinical supervision and reflective practice;
- act autonomously, while acknowledging the boundaries of professional competence;
- apply ethical and legal knowledge to practice, ensuring the primacy of patients'/clients'/carers' interests.

A2   Professional relationships
The award holder should be able to:

- adopt partnership approaches with colleagues, patient/clients, families, and carers;
- demonstrate the principles of effective team-working;
- work with professional and support staff and delegate care appropriately;
- generate and maintain effective interactions with relevant external agencies.

A3   Personal and professional skills
The award holder should be able to:

- maintain therapeutic relationships through the use of appropriate communication and interpersonal skills;
- recognize moral/ethical dilemmas and issues in patient care;
- recognize own learning needs and draw up personal action plans to meet these;
- apply the principles of health promotion and health education;
- articulate and justify decision-making processes associated with managing practice.

A4   Professional and employer context
The award holder should be able to:

- initiate appropriate actions in emergency situations in accordance with employers' guidelines, policies and protocols;
- recognize the need for changes in practice from best available evidence;
- contribute to, and maintain, a safe working environment;
- maintain accurate records.

B   Principles and concepts: applications to nursing practice

Nursing draws upon nursing and health/social-related theories/models, frameworks and concepts as the basis for decision-making and judgements about the range of psychomotor, interpersonal, and other skills that are appropriate to meet the needs of individual patients/clients in different healthcare settings. Each branch within nursing requires a different emphasis in terms of the knowledge and skills required for best practice in that branch.

This section articulates these principles and concepts. Those that are held in common with other health-care professionals can be found in the Section B of the health professions framework of this benchmark statement.

B1 Identification and assessment of health-care need
In addition, core to all nursing programmes, regardless of branch, the award holder should be able to:
- undertake a comprehensive systematic assessment using the tools/frameworks appropriate to the patient/client taking into account relevant physical, social, psychological, and spiritual needs;
- discern relevant information from patients/clients/carers to determine and prioritize;
- apply relevant knowledge to the assessment of individuals, families, and communities;
- assess the potential for health promotion with patients, clients, and carers;
- assess priorities for clinical effectiveness including risk assessment.

B2 Formulation of plans and strategies for meeting health-care needs
The award holder should be able to:
- use evidence-based options to facilitate patient choice and inform nursing interventions;
- plan care delivery to meet identified needs;
- demonstrate initiative in planning and organizing care;
- formulate and document a plan of care in partnership with patient/client/family/carers and other health-care professionals.

B3 Nursing practice
The award holder should be able to:
- provide and document a rationale for nursing management of a patient/client that takes into account all the information gained from assessment;
- ensure that the primacy of the patient is upheld at all times;
- apply evidence-based knowledge to inform nursing care decisions;
- demonstrate standards of competence as laid down by the nursing statutory regulatory body;
- engage in appropriate therapeutic relationships using appropriate and sensitive communication and interpersonal skills;
- practise in a way that maintains human dignity, rights, and responsibilities;
- create and use opportunities to promote health and well-being of patient/clients;
- demonstrate sound clinical judgements across a range of nursing situations;
- recognize potential need and instigate care to prevent or minimize the risk of complications;
- interpret and present information in a clear and concise manner;
- demonstrate a commitment to safe practice for self and others through delegation and supervision of others;
- understand and interpret numerical data appropriately;
- prioritize one's own work;

- communicate effectively to promote partnerships in the planning and delivery of care;
- apply a knowledge-base to support and teach others;
- use information technology applied to the needs of the patient/client or client group;
- contribute to the development of protocols to guide quality provision of care.

B4   Evaluation

The award holder should be able to:

- use reflection on/in practice to appraise and evaluate the effectiveness of nursing care;
- interpret and respond to significant changes in health, medical, psychological, or social status;
- recognize situations in which quality of care might be compromised.

C   Knowledge, understanding, and associated skills that underpin the education and training of nurses

This section of the benchmark statement describes the subject knowledge, understanding, and associated skills that are essential to underpin the informed, safe and effective nursing practice of a registered nurse at the point of qualification.

The core knowledge, understanding and associated skills that are common to all health-care professionals can be found in section C of the health professions framework within this benchmark statement. Listed below is the knowledge, understanding, and associated skills that are specific to nursing and are additional to those identified in the health professions framework.

Nursing departments will put together different pathways or programmes that specifically represent the appropriate balance of knowledge applied to the different branches, as well as the different academic levels of these pathways/programmes. Therefore, the order in which each specific subject is presented below is arbitrary and does not indicate a degree of importance for specific pathways or programmes.

C1   Knowledge and understanding

The award holder should be able to demonstrate understanding of:

Nursing

- The nature of nursing;
- changing philosophical and historical perspectives in nursing and nursing theories appropriate to different client groups;
- the requirements of the statutory regulatory body associated with registration as a nurse;
- nursing, medical, and health-care language;
- nursing across the lifespan;

- professional nursing issues such as advocacy, accountability, informed consent, autonomy, partnerships, advocacy.

Natural and life sciences

- Pharmacology;
- immunology;
- microbiology;
- epidemiology;
- nutrition;
- genetics;
- anatomy;
- physiology;
- pathophysiology.

Application of these to nursing practice with specific client groups.

Social, health, and behavioural sciences

- Policy and politics;
- psychosocial determinants of health;
- health economics;
- sociology and health;
- psychology and health;
- models of health and illness;
- loss, change, and bereavement;
- anti-discriminatory practice including fairness, social inclusion, gender, sexuality, race and culture, and health promotion.

Application of these to nursing practice.

Ethics, law, and the humanities

- Ethico-legal frameworks within nursing and relevant legislation;
- issues related to spirituality;
- caring and the primacy of patient/client interest.

Application of these to nursing practice.

Management of self and others' reflective practice

- Teaching and learning;
- leadership;
- prioritizing care;
- principles of management within organizations;
- clinical governance and maintaining/monitoring standards.

Application of all of these to nursing care of clients and client groups.

C2   Associated skills

The statutory regulatory body for nursing has articulated the competency framework for nursing students in all branches relevant to expected achievements and upon completion of the relevant branch programme. Some of the core skills are common to health-care professionals and can be found in section C of the health professions framework. The additional core skills specific for all branches of nursing are identified below. However, each branch programme will place greater emphasis on certain of these skills.

Communication and interpersonal skills
The award holder should be able to demonstrate:

- counselling skills applied to specific client/patient situations;
- an ability to identify and manage challenging behaviours;
- an ability to recognize anxiety, stress and depression, give emotional support and identify when specialist counselling intervention is needed.

Information gathering
The award holder should be able to:

- use contemporary physical, and/or psychosocial assessment tools to gather clinical and other data;
- use audit tools;
- seek out research-based evidence related to specific client groups.

Care delivery
The award holder should be able to demonstrate:

- safe moving and handling of patients within specific client groups;
- cardiopulmonary resuscitation and other emergency first aid interventions;
- observational skills (physical, emotional, social);
- relevant physical, psychological, and social caring skills required of specific patients/clients or groups;
- pain management;
- risk management;
- delegate patients' care as appropriate.

Problem solving and data collection and interpretation
The award holder should be able to:

- assimilate and assess new concepts;
- think critically;
- analyse, interpret, and assess the value of evidence to inform problem-solving.

Information technology
The award holder should be able to:

- use word processing, e-mail, spreadsheets, and databases;
- access health care research and literature databases;
- use the Internet as an information source;
- use relevant electronic patient information systems.

Numeracy
The award holder should be able to:

- understand and carry out drug calculation and administration of drugs via appropriate routes;
- manage information relevant to the particular patient or client group;
- record patient data appropriate to the health-care setting;
- report changes in patient information/data appropriately.

Teaching, learning and assessment

Decisions about the strategies and methods for teaching, learning, and assessment are for institutions to determine, but should complement the learning outcomes associated with health profession programmes. It is not for benchmark statements to promulgate any one, or combination of, approaches over others. However, this benchmark statement promotes an integrative approach to the application of theory and practice. It underlines the significance attached to the design of learning opportunities that facilitate the acquisition of professional capabilities and to assessment regimes that ensure these are being both delivered and rewarded to an appropriate standard.

In developing the curriculum the relationship between theory and practice will require the use of practice in simulated and health- and social-care settings. Standards for preparing supervisors and assessors of practice should be explicit and conform to the recommendations of professional regulatory bodies.

Fundamental to the basis upon which pre-registration students are prepared for their professional career, is the provision of programmes of academic study and practice-based learning which lay the foundation for career-long professional development and lifelong learning to support best professional practice and the maintenance of professional standards.

The learning processes in nursing can be expressed in terms of four interrelated themes:

Cognitive and conceptual
Programmes should develop cognitive skills in students, e.g. the ability to reconstruct knowledge and apply it to individual situations. Such skills should be developed through a variety of teaching and learning methods in which students are encouraged to become actively and practically engaged with the process.

Clinical and technical
Nursing skills should be developed in both the university and the practice setting. These skills should be acquired through developmental learning experiences that are structured, supervised, and assessed. Students should receive formative and summative judgements and feedback on their performance throughout the programme.

Nursing social and personal context
The programme should enable students to develop an awareness of the cultural diversity, values, beliefs, and social factors that affect the context of nursing. This should be achieved from both theoretical and practice perspectives and by exposing students to clinical practice in a wide variety of settings.

Generic and enabling skills
Programmes should be designed to facilitate students' acquisition of effective communication skills, team working, problem solving, the use of IT, research methodology, and critical reasoning. The generic nature of these skills should enable them to be achieved through inter-professional education where their acquisition should be through activity based experiences.

The assessment strategy
Methods should match the teaching and learning strategy, meet learning outcomes and encompass a wide variety of tools. Academic assessment should be designed to develop and test cognitive skills, drawing on the context of practice and reflecting the learning and teaching methods employed. Methods should normally include case-study presentations and analyses, practice-focused assignments, essays, project reports, clinical assessments, and examinations of a written or practical nature. The assessment of competence to practise should be determined in partnership between nursing lecturers and placement staff. Professional registration is dependent upon meeting both statutory regulatory body assessment requirements and university requirements.

Academic and practitioner standards

The following standards are commensurate with the academic awards of the Diploma in Higher Education and the Honours Degree. They reflect the UKCC's competence requirements for pre-registration nursing programmes, UKCC Commission Report Fitness for Practice and the QAA national qualifications frameworks for higher education. The academic award standards for the Diploma in Higher Education together with the UKCC's competencies form the threshold standards for registration on the statutory body's professional register.

These standard statements are underpinned by the expectation of those who work as a professional in health care as identified in section A, the principles and concepts as applied to nursing as stated in section B and the subject knowledge and associated skills stated in section C. All of these apply to every branch within nursing.

A Working as a professional in health care: expectations

Diploma

- Manage oneself, one's practice, and that of others, in accordance with the *Code of professional conduct*, recognizing own abilities and limitations;
- transfer knowledge and skills to a variety of clinical settings and unexpected situations;
- work in partnership with patients, clients, and families, and recognize when this approach to patient care may be inappropriate;
- provide support to patients, clients, carers, families, and colleagues in changing and stressful situations;
- practise in accordance with the professional ethical and legal framework;
- demonstrate sound clinical judgement across a range of situations;
- contribute to public protection by creating and maintaining a safe environment of care;
- delegate care to others, as appropriate, ensuring effective supervision and monitoring;
- demonstrate understanding of the roles of others, by participating in multi-professional care.

Honours degree

- Manage oneself, one's practice and that of others in accordance with the *Code of professional conduct,* and critically evaluate own abilities and limitations;
- select and apply knowledge and skills to complex and unexpected situations;
- implement strategies to promote and evaluate partnership working;
- anticipate potential stressful situations and participate in minimizing risk;
- recognize the complexity of the professional ethical and legal framework and its impact on nursing care decision-making;
- demonstrate sound clinical judgement across a range of situations and critically evaluate the effectiveness of clinical judgement across a range of professional care contexts;
- participate in a range of quality assurance and risk management strategies to create and maintain a safe environment;
- provide appropriate levels of guidance, role-modelling, and support to others in the delivery of health care;
- critically analyse roles within the multi-professional team and propose ways to strengthen patient-centred care.

B Principles and concepts: application

Diploma

- Apply theories, concepts, and principles of nursing to deliver patient-centred care for individuals, families, and communities;

- recognize potential risk and intervene to prevent, where possible, complications occurring;
- analyse and interpret relevant health education/promotion information and use this knowledge to promote the health and well-being of patients, clients and groups;
- use appropriate research and other evidence to underpin nursing decisions that can be justified, even when made on the basis of limited information;
- undertake and document a comprehensive, systematic, and accurate nursing assessment of the physical, psychological, social, and spiritual needs of patients, clients, and communities;
- assess priorities in practice and deliver care competently to meet identified need;
- formulate and document a plan of nursing care in partnership with and the consent of patients, clients and where appropriate, their carers and families;
- demonstrate accountability for nursing care delivered, taking into account social, spiritual, cultural, legal, political, and economic factors;
- accurately document and evaluate the outcomes of nursing and other interventions;
- demonstrate knowledge and understanding of effective multi-professional/ multi-agency working practices and participate in team work that respects and uses the contributions of members of the health- and social-care team.

Honours degree
- Demonstrate critical understanding of research-based knowledge and the application to practice;
- contribute to the development of protocols to guide the provision of quality care and minimize risk;
- capitalize on the potential for health improvement for patients, clients, and groups through the development of health education/promotion strategies;
- articulate and justify decision-making and problem-solving processes associated with nursing practice;
- use relevant theoretical and research evidence to inform a comprehensive, systematic assessment of the physical, psychological, social, and spiritual needs of patients, clients, and communities;
- monitor and update priorities within a changing environment and communicate appropriately;
- critically evaluate research findings and suggest changes to planned care;
- demonstrate an ability to critically challenge the nursing care delivered taking into account the dynamic social, cultural, spiritual, legal, political, and economic factors;
- critically evaluate outcomes of nursing and other interventions, adjusting care accordingly;
- contribute with skill and confidence to effective multi-professional/multi-agency working.

C   Subject knowledge, understanding, and associated skills

Diploma

- Demonstrate knowledge and understanding of the subjects underpinning nursing (see section A) through application to a range of practice settings;
- discuss the political and social context within which the provision of health and social care takes place;
- understand and apply the values that underpin anti-discriminatory working practices;
- communicate effectively with patients, clients, carers, and other health-care professionals;
- demonstrate an understanding of research and other evidence and, where appropriate, apply findings to practice;
- engage in, and disengage from, therapeutic relationships through the use of effective interpersonal skills;
- provide safe and sensitive care through the use of practical skills and knowledge of current best practice;
- interpret and use data with the aid of technology to enhance the management of care.

Honours degree

- Use knowledge and understanding of the subjects underpinning nursing (see section A) to provide creative solutions to health-care situations;
- critically examine the impact of political and social contexts on the provision of health care;
- understand the differences in beliefs and cultural practices of individuals and groups and recognize and challenge discriminatory practice;
- confidently present information orally, in writing and, where appropriate through the use of technology, to provide coherent and logical arguments in the support of decision making;
- critically evaluate research findings, suggest changes to practice and contribute to health-care research to inform practice development;
- engage in, and disengage from, therapeutic relationships through the creative use of theories and skills, demonstrating ethical discernment and clinical judgement;
- use practical skills and knowledge with confidence and creativity to enhance the quality of care;
- critically analyse and interpret data and appraise the value for care delivery and management.

Notes

1. The Quality Assurance Agency for Higher Education (2003) *Subject benchmark sataements: Health care programmes – Nursing* http://www.qaa.ac.uk/

crntwork/benchmark/nhsbenchmark/newpdfs/nursing%5Ftextonly.htm#6 (accessed 05.09.03).

2. Academic review in this context refers to the Agency's arrangements for external assurance of quality and standards. Further information regarding these may be found in the *Handbook for academic review*, which can be found on the Agency's web site.

3. Dietetics, Health Visiting, Midwifery, Nursing, Occupational Therapy, Orthoptics, Physiotherapy, Podiatry (Chiropody), Prosthetics and Orthotics, Radiography, and Speech and Language Therapy.